# Supplements and New Media

## For Instructors

### Instructor's Resource Manual
ISBN: 0-13-143234-6

This manual contains a wealth of material to help faculty plan and manage the medical-surgical nursing course. It includes chapter overviews, detailed lecture suggestions and outlines, learning objectives, a complete test bank, answers to the textbook critical thinking exercises, teaching tips, and more for each chapter. The IRM also guides faculty on how to assign and use the text-specific Companion Website, www.prenhall.com/lemone, and the free student CD-ROM that accompany the textbook, as well as Prentice Hall's Research Navigator online.

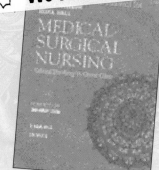

### Instructor's Resource CD-ROM
ISBN: 0-13-045581-4

This cross-platform CD-ROM provides discussion points and illustrations in PowerPoint from the new Third Edition of this textbook for use in classroom lectures. It also contains an electronic test bank, answers to the textbook critical thinking exercises, and animations from the Student CD-ROM. This supplement is available to faculty free upon adoption of the textbook.

### Companion Website Syllabus Manager
www.prenhall.com/lemone

Faculty adopting this textbook have free access to the online Syllabus Manager on the Companion Website, www.prenhall.com/lemone. Syllabus Manager offers a whole host of features that facilitate the students' use of the Companion Website, and allows faculty to post syllabi and course information online for their students. For more information or a demonstration of Syllabus Manager, please contact a Prentice Hall Sales Representative.

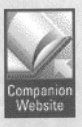

### Online Course Management Systems

Also available are online companions available for schools using course management systems. The online course management solutions feature interactive modules, electronic test bank, PowerPoint images, animations, assessment activities, and more. For more information about adopting an online course management system to accompany Medical-Surgical Nursing, please contact your Prentice Hall Health Sales Representative or go online to the appropriate website below and select "Courses," then "Nursing."

**WebCT:** http://cms.prenhall.com/webct/index.html/

**BlackBoard:** http://cms.prenhall.com/blackboard/index.html/

**CourseCompass:** http://cms.prenhall.com/coursecompass/

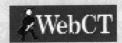
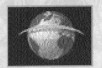

# Brief Contents

# MEDICAL-SURGICAL NURSING

## Critical Thinking in Client Care

**VOLUME TWO**
**THIRD EDITION**

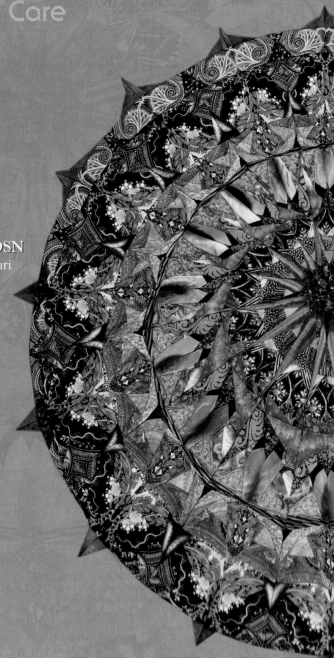

**PRISCILLA LEMONE,** RN, DSN
University of Missouri–Columbia, Columbia, Missouri

**KAREN BURKE,** RN, MS
Clatsop Community College, Astoria, Oregon

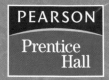

PEARSON

Prentice
Hall

Upper Saddle River, NJ 07458

## PART 3
## ELIMINATION PATTERNS 609

## Unit 6
## Responses to Altered Bowel Elimination 611

### Chapter 23
### Assessing Clients with Bowel Elimination Disorders 612

### Chapter 24
### Nursing Care of Clients with Bowel Disorders 617

## Unit 7
## Responses to Altered Urinary Elimination   693

**Chapter 25**
**Assessing Clients with Urinary System Disorders   694**

## Unit 11
## Responses to Altered Musculoskeletal Function   1177

### Chapter 37
### Assessing Clients with Musculoskeletal Disorders   1178

## PART 5
## COGNITIVE AND PERCEPTUAL PATTERNS 1287

### Unit 12
### Responses to Altered Neurologic Function 1289

## Chapter 49
## Nursing Care of Clients with Sexually Transmitted Infections   1598

At no other time in recent history has there been a greater need for nurses. In fact, the need for new nurses is projected to be at or greater than 1 million by 2010. Registered nurses are the largest group of health care professionals in the United States, numbering over 2.6 million. However, various forces are in effect that may decrease their numbers or challenge their ability to meet client needs. As our currently employed nurses age and retire, the population will also become older. As the population ages, more people will develop chronic illnesses and disabilities that require skilled nursing care. This means that your knowledge and skills will be in demand to meet health care needs well into the future.

Students are expected to build on a knowledge foundation of basic sciences, social sciences, and fundamentals of nursing to synthesize and critically analyze new knowledge necessary to provide holistic care that addresses the individualized human responses to potential or actual alterations in health. The third edition of *Medical-Surgical Nursing: Critical Thinking in Client Care* has been completely revised to provide you with that knowledge and the skills needed to care for clients to promote health, facilitate recovery from illness and injury, and provide support when coping with disability or grieving.

The kaleidoscope cover image is a strong reflection of health care today. The meditative aspect of focusing on the images in the kaleidoscope calms and helps to integrate the mind, spirit, and body. As with nursing care, healing benefits are discovered through various complementary and alternative therapy methods. Nursing care, like the kaleidoscope, is the integration of mind-body-spirit.

## GOALS FOR THIS TEXTBOOK

Although the information has been totally updated, we continue to believe that students learn best within a nursing model of care with consistent organization and understandable text. From the first edition, we have held fast to our vision that this textbook will:

- Provide the most current information possible about the art and science of nursing.

- Provide clear explanations of the pathophysiologic processes of human illnesses and injury, integrating that information as a vital component of treatment and nursing care.

- Emphasize the nurse's role as an essential member of the health care team.

- Prioritize nursing diagnoses and interventions specific to altered responses to illness.

- Provide case studies for each major illness or injury so students can envision the client as a person requiring care.

- Foster critical thinking and decision-making skills in clinical practice.

## NEW TO THIS EDITION

The third edition of this textbook includes new content on cultural diversity that is integrated throughout the narrative as well as incorporated into the following feature boxes: Focus on Diversity, Nursing Care of the Older Adult, Meeting Individualized Needs, Nursing Research, and Multisystem Effects. Additionally, new content covers health promotion, gerontology, complementary and alternative therapies, genetics, and diseases specific to bioterrorism. The new health-promotion heads can be found in the nursing care section in every disorder chapter. Complementary and alternative therapies are integrated throughout the textbook where appropriate. Genetics as a risk factor or that increases incidence of a disease is included with the disorders, such as Huntington's chorea, Von Willebrand's disease, sickle cell disease, and hemophilia. Diseases are included if more prevalent as the result of inheritance (such as diabetes). Genetic counseling is included in nursing care as appropriate. Information about infections that may be caused by bioterrorism is included in Chapter 8. Based on reviewer feedback, two new chapters have been added: Chapter 12 concerns care of clients with substance abuse and Chapter 39 deals with care of clients with musculoskeletal disorders (two separate chapters in the previous edition). This combined chapter is more consistent and easier for students to follow.

## ORGANIZATION

The book has six major parts, organized by functional health patterns. Each part opens with a concept map illustrating the relationship of each functional health pattern to possible nursing diagnoses. The parts are then divided into units based on alterations in human structure and function. Each unit with a focus on altered health states opens with an assessment chapter that provides a review of normal anatomy and physiology, questions for a health history, and assessment techniques with possible abnormal findings. Students will find a detailed health history questionnaire, using functional health patterns as a guide, on the Companion Website. Also on the CD, students will find a comprehensive review of anatomy and physiology complete with animations, three-dimensional structures, and exercises. This draws upon the student's prerequisite knowledge, and serves to reinforce basic principles of anatomy and physiology as applied to physical assessment.

Following the assessment chapter in each unit, information about major conditions and diseases follows a consistent chapter format. Key components of the clinical chapters include the following:

***PATHOPHYSIOLOGY.*** The discussion of each major illness or condition begins with an overview of pathophysiology, followed by manifestations and complications. In the new edition, we have increased coverage of pathophysiology and highlighted it as a section within the disease. A new feature, Focus on Diversity, is included with some disorders to demonstrate, for example, how race, age, and gender affect differences in incidence, prevalence, and mortality.

*COLLABORATIVE CARE.* Collaborative care considers the treatment of the illness or condition by the health care team. Information in this section includes, as appropriate, diagnostic tests, medications, surgery and treatments, fluid management, dietary management, and complementary therapies.

*NURSING CARE.* Because the prevention of illness is a critical factor in health care today, this section begins with health-promotion information. A brief section on assessment provides a focused health history interview and physical examination guides, as well as information about assessment of the older adult. Nursing care is discussed within a context of priority nursing diagnoses and interventions, with rationales provided for each intervention. As care is increasingly provided in the home, nursing care is followed by a list of topics and resources for teaching about home care. Lastly, for each major disorder or condition, a narrative Nursing Care Plan is provided. Each plan begins with a brief case study, followed by the steps of the nursing process in action. Critical thinking questions specific to the care plan conclude this part, with a section called Evaluate Your Response that provides additional guidance for critical thinking. Suggested guidelines are found in Appendix C.

*CHAPTER REVIEW.* This new section at the end of each chapter concludes with five multiple-choice review questions, to reinforce comprehension of the chapter content. The student will also find the section entitled EXPLORE MediaLink, which encourages students to use the CD-ROM and the Companion Website to apply what they have learned from the textbook in case studies, to practice NCLEX questions, and to use additional resources such as animation tutorials and more.

## HALLMARK FEATURES

Thoughtful attention was given to existing features that students and faculty liked in the previous edition. We give them more emphasis in the new edition.

- **Manifestations** boxes reinforce understanding of the effects of illness or injury, and guide assessments and interventions.
- **Pathophysiology Illustrated** and **Multisystem Effects** features provide visual illustrations of the causes and consequences of pathophysiology.
- **Nursing Implications** boxes provide students with nursing implications that they need to be aware of when their client is undergoing a particular diagnostic test. These boxes address nursing care and client/family teaching.
- **Meeting Individualized Needs** boxes contain information specific to altered health, age, gender, race, and culture.

- **Procedure** boxes describe common or important procedures in detail.
- **Nursing Care of the Client** boxes describe nursing care for various medical or surgical procedures.

## NEW FEATURES

In addition to the hallmark features that have made this textbook so popular with students and faculty, we provide new items that help students learn the concepts in this textbook, apply them in clinical settings, and hone their clinical judgment skills. These include the following:

- **MediaLink,** at the beginning of each chapter, lists specific content, animations, anatomy and physiology review, NCLEX review questions, tools, and other interactive exercises that appear on the accompanying student CD-ROM and the Companion Website. Special MediaLink tabs appear throughout the chapter in the margins, encouraging the students to use the media supplements for specific activities, applications, and resources. The purpose of the MediaLink feature is to further enhance the student experience, build on knowledge gained from the textbook, prepare students for NCLEX, and foster critical thinking.
- **Medication Administration** boxes provide examples of drugs commonly prescribed for specific illnesses, followed by nursing responsibilities and client/family teaching. The medication boxes reflect the role of nurses, who administer medications.
- **Focus on Diversity** boxes list incidence, prevalence, etiology, and more for a particular disorder as effected by race or ethnicity.
- **Nursing Care of the Older Adult** boxes are found throughout the text, as well as in the assessment sections for disorders. As the population continues to age, this is critical information for nursing care in any setting, and provides guidelines for assessing and teaching in home care for the elderly.
- **Nursing Care Plans** throughout the text help students approach care from a nursing process perspective. The care plan is followed by critical thinking questions for students to apply their knowledge to a plan of care for a specific client. Suggested responses to the critical thinking questions can be found in Appendix C. Additional care plan activities can be found on the Companion Website at www.prenhall.com/lemone. These activities provide students with client scenarios so they can write comprehensive care plans and email them to instructors as homework assignments.
- **NANDA, NIC, and NOC** charts illustrate the most up-to-date information on nursing language, and demonstrate how these items are related for specific disorders.
- **Nursing Research: Evidence-Based Practice** boxes are included to show how nursing research is used to provide rationales for nursing care.
- **Practice Alerts** are integrated into nursing care purposefully to help students consider all aspects of nursing even

though they may be focusing on only one aspect of client needs.

- **End of Chapter Review Section** provides students with an opportunity to evaluate their comprehension of the chapter. The student-friendly section includes:
- **Test Yourself**—Review questions at the end of every chapter.
- **EXPLORE MediaLink**—at the end of every chapter, encourages students to use the CD-ROM and Companion Website to apply their knowledge of the chapter through additional case studies, practice NCLEX questions, A&P review, animation tutorials, and additional resources.

## COMPREHENSIVE TEACHING-LEARNING PACKAGE

### Clinical Handbook ISBN: 0-13-048397-4

Serves as a portable, quick reference to medical-surgical nursing. Organized alphabetizing provides a succinct review of common disorders and conditions, including pathophysiology, nursing diagnoses, interventions, client teaching, and home care. This handbook will allow students to bring the information they learn from class into any clinical setting.

### Study Guide ISBN: 0-13-113666-6

Provides anatomy and physiology review, study tips, review exercises, case studies, care plan activities, NCLEX review, and more. MediaLinks refer students to activities on the CD-ROM and Companion Website.

### Student CD-ROM

Packaged *free* with the textbook, the student CD-ROM provides an interactive study program that allows students to practice answering NCLEX-style questions with rationales for right and wrong answers. It also contains an audio glossary, animations, anatomy and physiology review, and a link to the Companion Website (an Internet connection is required).

### Companion Website

A *free* online study guide is designed to help students apply the concepts presented in the book. Each chapter-specific module features objectives, audio glossary, chapter summary for lecture notes, NCLEX review questions, case studies, care plan activities, MediaLink applications, WebLinks, and nursing tools, such as functional health pattern concept maps, assessment guides, and more.

## SUPPLEMENTS AND NEW MEDIA FOR INSTRUCTORS

### Instructor's Resource Manual ISBN: 0-13-143234-6

This manual contains a wealth of material to help faculty plan and manage the medical-surgical nursing course. It includes chapter overviews, detailed lecture suggestions and outlines, learning objectives, a complete test bank, answers to the textbook critical thinking exercises, teaching tips, and more for each chapter. The IRM also guides faculty how to assign and use the text-specific Companion Website, www.prenhall.com/lemone, and the free student CD-ROM that accompany the textbook.

### Instructor's Resource CD-ROM ISBN: 0-13-045581-4

This cross-platform CD-ROM provides illustrations in PowerPoint from the new third edition of this textbook for use in classroom lectures. It also contains an electronic test bank, answers to the textbook critical thinking exercises, and animations from the student CD-ROM. This supplement is available to faculty free upon adoption of the textbook.

### Companion Website Syllabus Manager

www.prenhall.com/lemone

Faculty adopting this textbook has *free* access to the online Syllabus Manager on the Companion Website, www.prenhall.com/lemone. Syllabus Manager offers a whole host of features that facilitate the students' use of the Companion Website, and allows faculty to post syllabi and course information online for students. For more information or a demonstration of Syllabus Manager, please contact a Prentice Hall sales representative.

### Online Course Management Systems

Also available are online companions for schools using course management systems. The online course management solutions feature interactive modules, electronic test bank, PowerPoint images, animations, assessment activities, and more. For more information about adopting an online course management system to accompany *Medical-Surgical Nursing,* please contact your Prentice Hall Health sales representative or go online to one of the following websites and select "courses."

WebCT: http://cms.prenhall.com/webct/index.html/

Blackboard: http://cms.prenhall.com/blackboard/index.html/

CourseCompass: http://cms.prenhall.com/coursecompass/

# CONTRIBUTORS

## Text Contributors

**Jane Bostick, PhD, RN**
Sinclair School of Nursing
University of Missouri-Columbia
Columbia, MO

Chapter 12: Nursing Care of Clients
with Problems of Substance Abuse

**Roxanne W. McDaniel, PhD, RN**
Sinclair School of Nursing
University of Missouri-Columbia
Columbia, MO
Chapter 10: Nursing Care of Clients with
Cancer

**Elaine Mohn-Brown, RN, EdD**
Chemeketa Community College
Salem, OR

Chapter 8: Nursing Care of Clients with
Infection

Chapter 9: Nursing Care of Clients with
Altered Immunity

Chapter 45: Nursing Care of Clients with
Eye and Ear Disorders

**Margorie Whitman, RN, MSN, AOCN**
Sinclair School of Nursing
University of Missouri-Columbia
Columbia, MO

Chapter 7: Nursing Care of Clients Having
Surgery

## SUPPLEMENT AND MEDIA WRITERS
### Student CD-ROM

**Joseann DeWitt, RN, MSN, BC, CLNC**
Alcorn State University School of Nursing
Department of Baccalaureate Nursing
Natchez, MS

**Rebecca Gesler, RN, MSN**
Nursing Professor
Saint Catharine College
St. Catharine, KY

**Laurie Kaudewitz, RNC, BSN, MSN**
Assistant Professor
East Tennessee State University
Johnson City, TN

**Douglas Turner, PhD(C), RN, MSN, CNS, CRNA**
Lead Instructor
Forsyth Technical Community College
Winston-Salem, NC

**Linda White, PhD(C), MSN, CNS, RN**
Lead Instructor
Forsyth Technical Community College
Winston-Salem, NC

## Companion Website

**Joseann DeWitt, RN, MSN, BC, CLNC**
Alcorn State University School of Nursing
Department of Baccalaureate Nursing
Natches, MS

**Peggy Ellis, PhD, RNCS, ANP**
University of Missouri
Barnes College of Nursing
St. Louis, MO

**Lynne Bryant, PhD, RN, MSN**
Associate Professor, Nursing Technology
Broward Community College
Davie, FL

**Rebecca Gesler, RN, MSN**
Nursing Professor
Saint Catherine College
St. Catherine, KY

**Vincent Salyers, RN, EdD**
Associate Professor
Palomar College
San Marcos, CA
Adjunct Professor
University of Phoenix
San Diego, CA

## Study Guide

**Jacqueline B. Brinkman, RN, BSN, CPN**
College of the Redwoods
Eureka, CA

**Joseann DeWitt, RN, MSN, BC, CLNC**
Alcorn State University School of Nursing
Department of Baccalaureate Nursing
Natchez, MS

**Golden Tradewell, PhD, RN, MSN, MA**
Associate Professor
McNeese State University
College of Nursing
Lake Charles, LA

## Instructor's Resource Manual

**Joyce Hammer, RN, MSN**
Lourdes College
Sylvania, OH

**Edna Hull, RN, MSN, CPN**
Assistant Professor
Delgado Community College–Charity
School of Nursing
New Orleans, LA

# REVIEWERS

**Marianne Adam, MSN, RN, CRNP**
Assistant Professor
Moravian College—St. Luke's School of
    Nursing
Bethlehem, PA

**Ellise D. Adams, CNM, MSN, CD, ICCE**
Nursing Faculty
Calhoun Community College
Decatur, AL

**Martha Baker, PhD, RN, CS, CCRN**
Associate Professor
Missouri Southern State College
Joplin, MO

**Claudia P. Barone, EdD, RN, LNC, CPC**
Clinical Assistant Professor, Dean for the
    Master's Program,
Chairperson Department of Nursing Practice
University of Arkansas for Medical Sciences
Little Rock, AR

**Gail Bolling, MS, RN, CCRN**
Associate Professor
Montgomery College
Takoma Park, MD

**Joanne Bonesteel, MS, RN**
Nursing Faculty
Excelsior College
Albany, NY

**Tara Brenner, MS, RN, CS**
Assistant Professor
SUNY Brockport
Brockport, NY

**Polly Cameron Haigler, PhD, RN**
Clinical Assistant Professor
University of South Carolina
Columbia, SC

**Candice Cherrington, PhD, RN**
Assistant Professor
Wright State University
Dayton, OH

**Betty Christeson, BSNE, MN, EdD**
Adjunct Faculty
Greenville Technical College
Greenville, SC

**Patty Clark, RN, MSN**
Associate Professor
Abraham Baldwin College
Tifton, GA

**Janet M. Clifton, MS**
Instructor
Danville Area Community College
Danville, IL

**Maureen Cochran, RN, PhD**
Nursing Faculty
Suffolk University
Boston, MA

**Ruth F. Craven, EdD, RN, BC, FAAN**
Professor and Associate Dean
University of Washington
Seattle, WA

**Janice A. Cullen, EdD, RN**
Associate Professor
University of South Carolina-Aiken
Aiken, SC

**Cynthia L. Dakin, RN, PHD**
Clinical Specialist
Northeastern University
Boston, MA

**Ann Denney, RN, MSN**
Assistant Professor
Thomas More College
Crestview Hills, KY

**Nancy Dentlinger, AS, BS, MS**
Assistant Director
Redlands Community College
El Reno, OK

**Susan DeSanto-Madeya, RN, DNSc**
Assistant Professor
Moravian College—St. Luke's School of
    Nursing
Bethlehem, PA

**Susan Dipert-Scott, RN, MS**
Adjunct Faculty
Wright State University
Dayton, OH

**Mary Jo Distel, MS**
Assistant Professor
Midwestern State University
Wichita Falls, TX

**Jean Forsha, MSN, RN**
Nursing Faculty
Westchester University
Westchester, PA

**Rebecca Gesler, RN, MSN**
Director
Saint Catherine College
St. Catherine, KY

**Paula Gilbert, BS, RN, ANP**
Nursing Instructor
Arnot Ogden Medical Center
Elmira, NY

**LaVerne Grant, MS, RN**
Assistant Professor
University of Mississippi Medical Center
Jackson, MS

**Corinne Grimes, RN, MSN, DNSc,
AOCN**
Assistant Professor
Texas Women's University
Dallas, TX

**Barbara F. Harrah, RN, MSN**
Assistant Professor
Kent State University
East Liverpool, OH

**Anne Helm, RN, BSN, MSN**
Associate Professor
Owens Community College
Toledo, OH

**Mary Ann Helm, MSN, MRE, RN**
Assistant Professor
Nursing Faculty
Tennessee State University
Nashville, TN

**Beverly K. Hogan, MSN, RN, CS**
Nursing Faculty
University of Alabama-Birmingham
Birmingham, AL

**Susan P. Holmes, MSN, CRNP**
Nursing Faculty
Auburn University
Auburn, AL

**Karen C. Johnson-Brennam, EdD,
RN, MSN**
Professor and Associate Director
San Francisco State University
San Francisco, CA

**Paula R. Klemm, DNSc, RN, OCN**
Associate Professor
University of Delaware
Newark, DE

**Wilma La Cava, RNC, MSN**
Assistant Professor
Riverside Community College
Riverside, CA

**Kristine M. Lecuyer, RN, MSN**
Adjunct Assistant Professor
Saint Louis University
St. Louis, MO

**Camille Little, MS, RN, CS**
Assistant Professor
Illinois State University
Normal, IL

**Karen Martin, RN, MS**
Assistant Professor
Pikeville College
Paintsville, KY

**Arlene McGrory, DNSc, RN**
Associate Professor
University of Massachusetts-Lowell
Lowell, MA

**Shirley McIntosh, RNC, MSN, LNC**
Clinical Instructor
Kent State University
Kent, OH

## PRISCILLA LEMONE, RN, DSN, FAAN

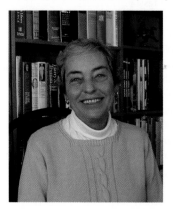

Priscilla LeMone has spent most of her career as a nurse educator, teaching medical-surgical nursing and pathophysiology at all levels from diploma to doctoral students. She has a diploma in nursing from Deaconess College of Nursing (St. Louis, Missouri), baccalaureate and master's degrees from Southeast Missouri State University, and a doctorate in nursing from the University of Alabama-Birmingham. She is currently an Associate Professor and Director of Undergraduate Studies, Sinclair School of Nursing, University of Missouri-Columbia.

Dr. LeMone has had numerous awards for scholarship and teaching during her over 30 years as a nurse educator. She is most honored for receiving the Kemper Fellowship for Teaching Excellence from the University of Missouri-Columbia, the Unique Contribution Award from the North American Nursing Diagnosis Association, and for being selected as a Fellow in the American Academy of Nursing.

She believes that her education gave her solid and everlasting roots in nursing. Her work with students has given her the wings that allow her love of nursing and teaching to continue through the years.

A widow, Dr. LeMone lives with her dog and shares time with her two children and her granddaughter. When she has time, she enjoys growing flowers and reading fiction.

## KAREN M. BURKE, RN, MS

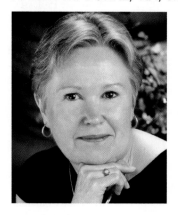

Karen Burke has practiced nursing in acute intensive and coronary care, in community-based settings, and in nursing education. As an educator, she has taught nursing skills, fundamentals, pathophysiology, and basic to advanced medical-surgical nursing. Ms. Burke has a diploma in nursing from Emanuel Hospital School of Nursing in Portland, Oregon, later completing baccalaureate studies at Oregon Health & Science University, and a master's degree at University of Portland.

Ms. Burke has been part of the nursing faculty at Clatsop Community College in Astoria, Oregon, since the inception of the Associate Degree Nursing program in 1983, most recently serving as Director of Health Occupations and Nursing. In this role, she is known as a leader and an innovator. She led the nursing faculty in developing an online program to deliver basic nursing education to a distant rural community. This program continues, serving as a model for other community college nursing programs to reach out to geographically isolated communities. Ms. Burke is actively involved in nursing education and developing strategies to address the nursing shortage in Oregon. She is a member of the Oregon Council of Associate Degree Nursing Programs (OCAP) and the Oregon Nursing Leadership Council (ONLC), currently serving as chair of the ONLC Education Committee. She is coauthor of several other texts: *Medical-Surgical Nursing Care,* with Priscilla LeMone and Elaine Mohn-Brown; *Fundamentals of Nursing: Concepts, Process, and Practice* (6th edition), with Barbara Kozier, Glenora Erb, and Audrey Berman; and a clinical handbook to accompany this text.

Ms. Burke sees herself as a nurse first, then a nurse educator and educational administrator. She strongly values the nursing profession and the importance of providing a solid education in the art and science of nursing for all students entering the profession.

When possible, Ms. Burke and her husband Steve spend time with their extended family and traveling. She enjoys a passion for quilting, and, when the weather allows, gardening.

# Guide to
# MEDICAL-SURGICAL NURSING

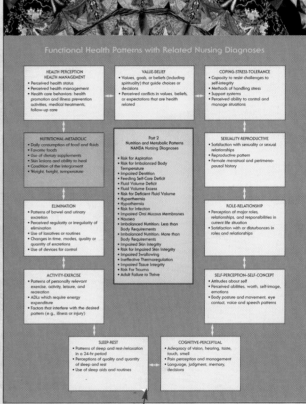

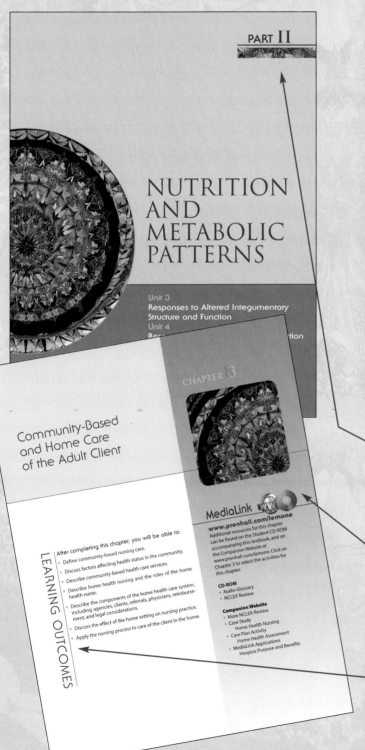

## PART II

## NUTRITION AND METABOLIC PATTERNS

Unit 3
**Responses to Altered Integumentary Structure and Function**

Unit 4
**Res...tion**

### Functional Health Patterns with Related Nursing Diagnoses

**HEALTH PERCEPTION HEALTH MANAGEMENT**
- Perceived health status
- Perceived health management
- Health care behaviors: health promotion and illness prevention activities, medical treatments, follow-up care

**VALUE-BELIEF**
- Values, goals, or beliefs (including spirituality) that guide choices or decisions
- Perceived conflicts in values, beliefs, or expectations that are health related

**COPING-STRESS-TOLERANCE**
- Capacity to resist challenges to self-integrity
- Methods of handling stress
- Support systems
- Perceived ability to control and manage situations

**NUTRITIONAL-METABOLIC**
- Daily consumption of food and fluids
- Favorite foods
- Use of dietary supplements
- Skin lesions and ability to heal
- Condition of the Integument
- Weight, height, temperature

**Part 2
Nutrition and Metabolic Patterns
NANDA Nursing Diagnoses**
- Risk for Aspiration
- Risk for Imbalanced Body Temperature
- Impaired Dentition
- Feeding Self-Care Deficit
- Fluid Volume Deficit
- Fluid Volume Excess
- Risk for Deficient Fluid Volume
- Hyperthermia
- Hypothermia
- Risk for Infection
- Impaired Oral Mucous Membranes
- Nausea
- Imbalanced Nutrition: Less than Body Requirements
- Imbalanced Nutrition: More than Body Requirements
- Impaired Skin Integrity
- Risk for Impaired Skin Integrity
- Impaired Swallowing
- Ineffective Thermoregulation
- Impaired Tissue Integrity
- Risk For Trauma
- Adult Failure to Thrive

**SEXUALITY-REPRODUCTIVE**
- Satisfaction with sexuality or sexual relationships
- Reproductive pattern
- Female menstrual and perimeno-pausal history

**ELIMINATION**
- Patterns of bowel and urinary excretion
- Perceived regularity or irregularity of elimination
- Use of laxatives or routines
- Changes in time, modes, quality or quantity of excretions
- Use of devices for control

**ROLE-RELATIONSHIP**
- Perception of major roles, relationships, and responsibilities in current life situation
- Satisfaction with or disturbances in roles and relationships

**ACTIVITY-EXERCISE**
- Patterns of personally relevant exercise, activity, leisure, and recreation
- ADLs which require energy expenditure
- Factors that interfere with the desired pattern (e.g., illness or injury)

**SELF-PERCEPTION–SELF-CONCEPT**
- Attitudes about self
- Perceived abilities, worth, self-image, emotions
- Body posture and movement, eye contact, voice and speech patterns

**SLEEP-REST**
- Patterns of sleep and rest-/relaxation in a 24-hr period
- Perceptions of quality and quantity of sleep and rest
- Use of sleep aids and routines

**COGNITIVE-PERCEPTUAL**
- Adequacy of vision, hearing, taste, touch, smell
- Pain perception and management
- Language, judgment, memory, decisions

## CHAPTER 3

### Community-Based and Home Care of the Adult Client

#### LEARNING OUTCOMES

After completing this chapter, you will be able to:

- Define community-based nursing care.
- Discuss factors affecting health status in the community.
- Discuss community-based health care services.
- Describe home health nursing and the roles of the home health nurse.
- Describe the components of the home health care system, including agencies, clients, referrals, physicians, reimbursement, and legal considerations.
- Discuss the effect of the home setting on nursing practice.
- Apply the nursing process to care of the client in the home.

### MediaLink

**www.prenhall.com/lemone**
Additional resources for this chapter can be found on the Student CD-ROM accompanying this textbook, and on the Companion Website at www.prenhall.com/lemone. Click on Chapter 3 to select the activities for this chapter.

**CD-ROM**
- Audio Glossary
- NCLEX Review

**Companion Website**
- More NCLEX Review
- Case Study
  Home Health Nursing
- Care Plan Activity
  Home Health Assessment
- MediaLink Applications
  Hospice:Purpose and Benefits

## Part Openers

Each Part Opener is followed by a Functional Health Pattern Concept Map. These concept maps relate nursing diagnoses to specific patterns covered in that part.

**MediaLink** introduces each chapter of the text and lists additional specific content, animations, NCLEX Review, tools, and other interactive exercises, which appear on the accompanying Student CD-ROM and the Companion Website.

**Learning Outcomes** appear at the start of each chapter, identifying important concepts students should know by the end of the chapter.

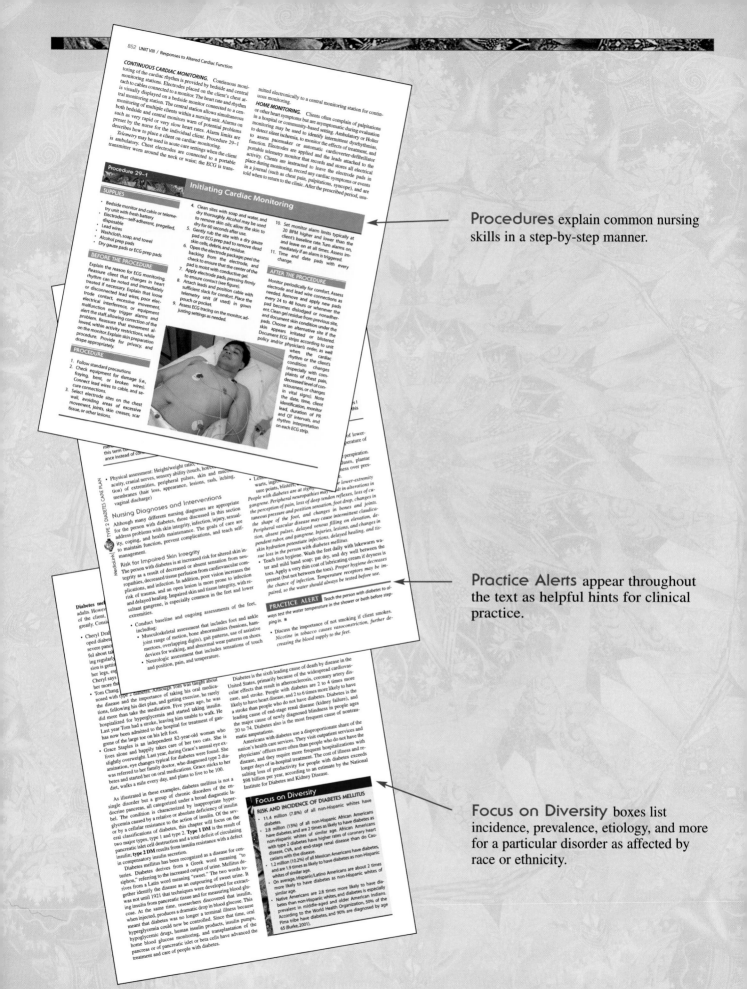

**Procedures** explain common nursing skills in a step-by-step manner.

**Practice Alerts** appear throughout the text as helpful hints for clinical practice.

**Focus on Diversity** boxes list incidence, prevalence, etiology, and more for a particular disorder as affected by race or ethnicity.

**Pathophysiology Illustrated** are three-dimensional illustrations that help students to visualize the pathophysiological process of a particular disorder. Additional animations can be found on the Student CD-ROM.

**Nursing Care Plan**

Throughout the text, nursing care plans help students approach care from a nursing process perspective. The care plan is followed by critical thinking questions for students to apply their knowledge to plan the care for a specific client. Suggested responses to the critical thinking questions can be found in Appendix C. Additional Care Plan activities can be found on the Companion Website.

**Multisystem Effects** are labeled illustrations that point out the effects a disorder has on various body systems.

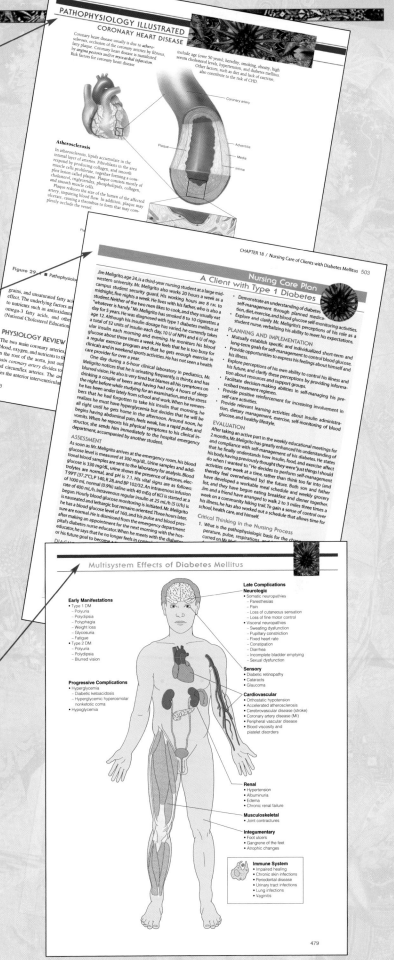

## Nursing Care of the Client

describes nursing care for various medical or surgical procedures.

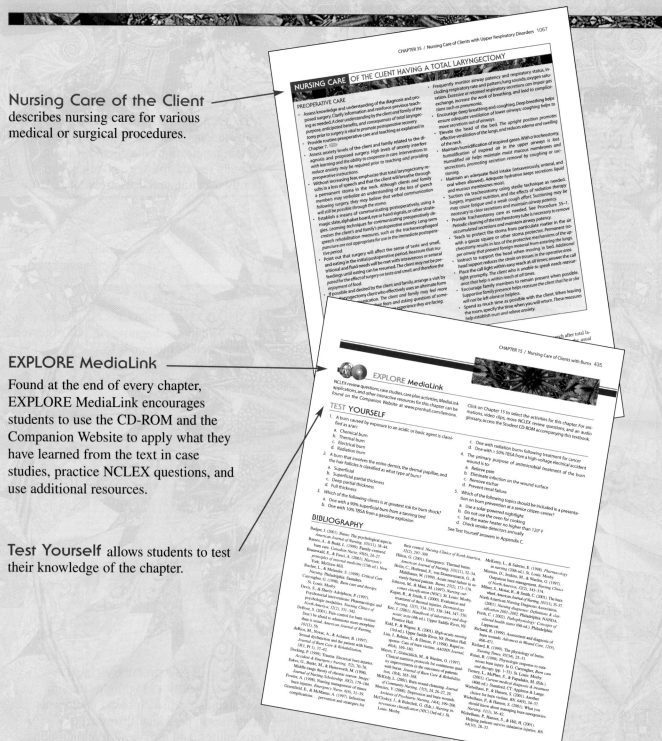

## EXPLORE MediaLink

Found at the end of every chapter, EXPLORE MediaLink encourages students to use the CD-ROM and the Companion Website to apply what they have learned from the text in case studies, practice NCLEX questions, and use additional resources.

**Test Yourself** allows students to test their knowledge of the chapter.

---

 **ADDITIONAL MEDIA RESOURCES:**

**Animation and Video Tutorials**—On the Student CD-ROM, the student will find animations illustrating difficult concepts or reinforcing content in the text.

**NCLEX Reviews**—Both the Student CD-ROM and the free Companion Website offer the student an abundance of NCLEX review questions for each chapter of the book. The questions provide comprehensive rationales, as well as identify how the questions correlate to the NCLEX test plan.

**Care Plan Activities**—Each clinical chapter on the Companion Website provides the student with a case scenario and asks the student to develop a care plan for the client. Students can e-mail these care plans to instructors as homework assignments.

**Case Studies**—For each clinical chapter on the Companion Website, the student can review a client scenario and answer critical thinking questions related to that client's care. Students can e-mail their responses to the case studies to instructors as homework assignments.

**MediaLink Applications**—Students are asked to go to websites to research the questions that are presented here.

# SPECIAL FEATURES

 Nursing Care Plans

 NANDA, NIC, and NOC Linkages

Procedures

 Multisystem Effects of ...

 Pathophysiology Illustrated

 Medication Administration

## Manifestations of ...

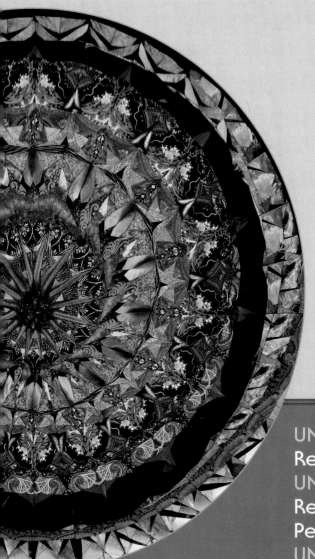

# ACTIVITY AND EXERCISE PATTERNS

# Functional Health Patterns with Related Nursing Diagnoses

### HEALTH PERCEPTION HEALTH MANAGEMENT
- Perceived health status
- Perceived health management
- Health care behaviors: health promotion and illness prevention activities, medical treatments, follow-up care

### VALUE-BELIEF
- Values, goals, or beliefs (including spirituality) that guide choices or decisions
- Perceived conflicts in values, beliefs, or expectations that are health related

### COPING-STRESS-TOLERANCE
- Capacity to resist challenges to self-integrity
- Methods of handling stress
- Support systems
- Perceived ability to control and manage situations

### NUTRITIONAL-METABOLIC
- Daily consumption of food and fluids
- Favorite foods
- Use of dietary supplements
- Skin lesions and ability to heal
- Condition of the integument
- Weight, height, temperature

### Part 4
Activity and Exercise Patterns
NANDA Nursing Diagnoses
- Activity Intolerance
- Risk for Activity Intolerance
- Bathing/Hygiene Self-Care Deficit
- Dressing/Grooming Self-Care Deficit
- Impaired Bed Mobility
- Risk for Disuse Syndrome
- Deficient Diversional Activity
- Fatigue
- Risk for Falls
- Impaired Home Maintenance
- Impaired Physical Mobility
- Impaired Wheelchair Mobility
- Impaired Transfer Ability
- Impaired Walking
- Delayed Surgical Recovery
- Decreased Cardiac Output
- Ineffective Breathing Pattern
- Ineffective Airway Clearance
- Impaired Gas Exchange
- Risk for Peripheral Neurovascular Dysfunction
- Impaired Tissue Perfusion
- Ineffective Tissue Perfusion
- Impaired Spontaneous Ventilation
- Dysfunctional Ventilatory Weaning Response

### SEXUALITY-REPRODUCTIVE
- Satisfaction with sexuality or sexual relationships
- Reproductive pattern
- Female menstrual and perimeno-pausal history

### ELIMINATION
- Patterns of bowel and urinary excretion
- Perceived regularity or irregularity of elimination
- Use of laxatives or routines
- Changes in time, modes, quality or quantity of excretions
- Use of devices for control

### ROLE-RELATIONSHIP
- Perception of major roles, relationships, and responsibilities in current life situation
- Satisfaction with or disturbances in roles and relationships

### ACTIVITY-EXERCISE
- Patterns of personally relevant exercise, activity, leisure, and recreation
- ADLs which require energy expenditure
- Factors that interfere with the desired pattern (e.g., illness or injury)

### SELF-PERCEPTION–SELF-CONCEPT
- Attitudes about self
- Perceived abilities, worth, self-image, emotions
- Body posture and movement, eye contact, voice and speech patterns

### SLEEP-REST
- Patterns of sleep and rest-/relaxation in a 24-hr period
- Perceptions of quality and quantity of sleep and rest
- Use of sleep aids and routines

### COGNITIVE-PERCEPTUAL
- Adequacy of vision, hearing, taste, touch, smell
- Pain perception and management
- Language, judgment, memory, decisions

*Reprinted from Nursing Diagnosis: Process and Application, 3rd ed., by M. Gordon, pp. 80–96, Copyright © 1994, with permission from Elsevier Science.*

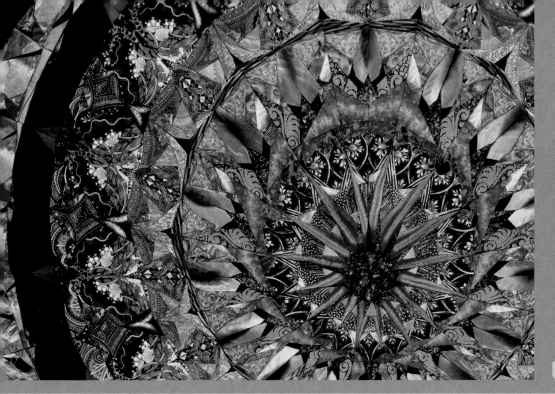

# RESPONSES TO ALTERED CARDIAC FUNCTION

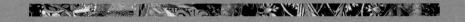

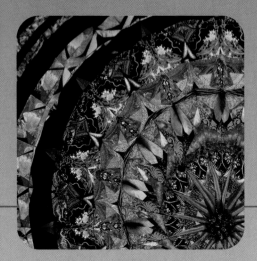

# Assessing Clients with Cardiac Disorders

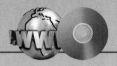

## MediaLink
### www.prenhall.com/lemone

Additional resources for this chapter can be found on the Student CD-ROM accompanying this textbook, and on the Companion Website at www.prenhall.com/lemone. Click on Chapter 28 to select the activities for this chapter.

**CD-ROM**
• Audio Glossary
• NCLEX Review

*Animations*
• Cardiac A&P
• Dysrhythmias

**Companion Website**
• More NCLEX Review
• Functional Health Pattern Assessment
• Case Study
  Chest Pain
• MediaLink Application
  Heart Sounds

## LEARNING OUTCOMES

After completing this chapter, you will be able to:

■ Review the anatomy and physiology of the heart.

■ Trace the circulation of blood through the heart and coronary vessels.

■ Identify the normal heart sounds and relate them to the corresponding events in the cardiac cycle.

■ Name and locate the elements of the heart's conduction system.

■ Define cardiac output and explain the influence of various factors in its regulation.

■ Identify specific topics for consideration during a health history interview of the client with health problems involving cardiac function.

■ Describe physical assessment techniques for cardiac function.

■ Identify abnormal findings that may indicate cardiac malfunction.

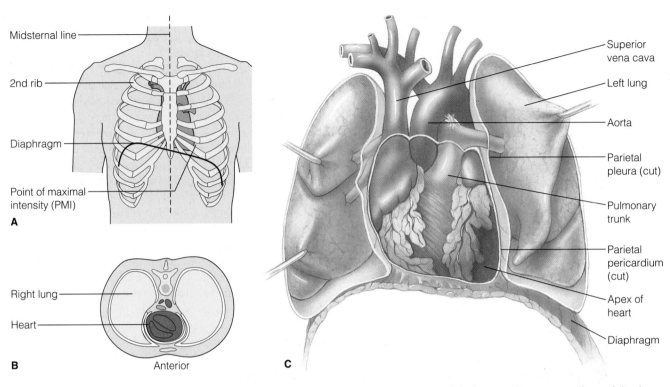

A

B        Anterior

C

**Figure 28–1** ■ Location of the heart in the mediastinum of the thorax. *A,* Relationship of the heart to the sternum, ribs, and diaphragm. *B,* Cross-sectional view showing relative position of the heart in the thorax. *C,* Relationship of the heart and great vessels to the lungs.

The heart, a muscular pump, beats an average of 70 times per minute, or once every 0.86 seconds, every minute of a person's life. This continuous pumping moves blood through the body, nourishing tissue cells and removing wastes. Deficits in the structure or function of the heart affect all body tissues. Changes in cardiac rate, rhythm, or output may limit almost all human functions, including self-care, mobility, and the ability to maintain fluid volume status, respirations, tissue perfusion, and comfort. Cardiac changes may also affect self-concept, sexuality, and role performance.

## REVIEW OF ANATOMY AND PHYSIOLOGY

The heart is a hollow, cone-shaped organ approximately the size of an adult's fist, weighing less than 1 lb. It is located in the mediastinum of the thoracic cavity, between the vertebral column and the sternum, and is flanked laterally by the lungs. Two-thirds of the heart mass lies to the left of the sternum; the upper base lies beneath the second rib, and the pointed apex is approximate with the fifth intercostal space, midpoint to the clavicle (Figure 28–1 ■).

## The Pericardium

The heart is covered by a double layer of fibroserous membrane, the pericardium (Figure 28–2 ■). The pericardium encases the heart and anchors it to surrounding structures, forming the pericardial sac. The snug fit of the pericardium prevents the heart from overfilling with blood. The *parietal pericardium* is the outermost layer. The *visceral pericardium* (or *epicardium*)

**Figure 28–2** ■ Coverings and layers of the heart.

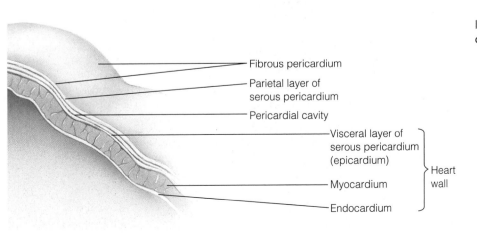

Fibrous pericardium

Parietal layer of serous pericardium

Pericardial cavity

Visceral layer of serous pericardium (epicardium)

Myocardium

Endocardium

Heart wall

MediaLink | CARDIAC ANATOMY & PHYSIOLOGY ANIMATIONS

adheres to the heart surface. The small space between the visceral and parietal layers of the pericardium is called the pericardial cavity. A serous lubricating fluid produced in this space cushions the heart as it beats.

## Layers of the Heart Wall

The heart wall consists of three layers of tissue: the epicardium, the myocardium, and the endocardium (see Figure 28–2). The outermost epicardium is the same structure as the visceral pericardium. The middle layer of the heart wall, the myocardium, consists of specialized cardiac muscle cells (myofibrils) that provide the bulk of contractile heart muscle. The innermost layer, the endocardium, is a sheath of endothelium that lines the inside of the heart's chambers and great vessels.

## Chambers and Valves of the Heart

The heart has four hollow chambers, two upper atria and two lower ventricles. They are separated longitudinally by the interventricular septum (Figure 28–3 ■).

The right atrium receives deoxygenated blood from the veins of the body: The superior vena cava returns blood from the body area above the diaphragm, the inferior vena cava returns blood from the body below the diaphragm, and the coronary sinus drains blood from the heart. The left atrium receives freshly oxygenated blood from the lungs through the pulmonary veins.

The right ventricle receives deoxygenated blood from the right atrium and pumps it through the pulmonary artery to the lungs for oxygenation. The left ventricle receives the freshly oxygenated blood from the left atrium and pumps it out the aorta to the arterial circulation.

Each of the heart's chambers is separated by a valve which allows unidirectional blood flow to the next chamber or great vessel (see Figure 28–3). The atria are separated from the ventricles by the two atrioventricular (AV) valves; the tricuspid valve is on the right side, and the bicuspid (or mitral) valve is on the left. The flaps of each of these valves are anchored to the papillary muscles of the ventricles by the *chordae tendineae*. These structures control the movement of the AV valves to prevent backflow of blood.

The ventricles are connected to their great vessels by the semilunar valves. On the right, the pulmonary valve joins the right ventricle with the pulmonary artery. On the left, the aortic valve joins the left ventricle to the aorta.

Closure of the AV valves at the onset of contraction produces the first heart sound, or $S_1$ (characterized by the syllable "lub"); closure of the semilunar valves at the onset of relaxation produces the second heart sound, or $S_2$ (characterized by the syllable "dub").

## Systemic and Coronary Circulation

Because each side of the heart both receives and ejects blood, the heart is often described as a double pump. Pulmonary circulation begins with the right heart. Deoxygenated blood from the venous system enters the right atrium through two large veins, the superior and inferior venae cavae, and is transported to the lungs via the pulmonary artery and its branches

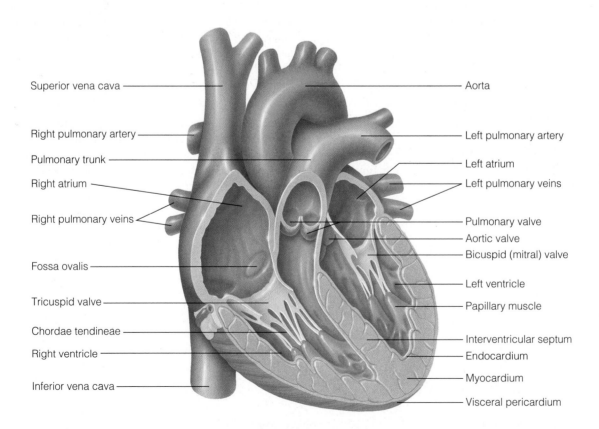

**Figure 28–3** ■ The internal anatomy of the heart, frontal section.

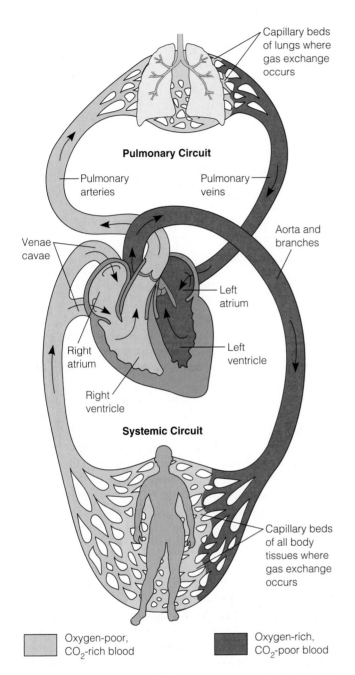

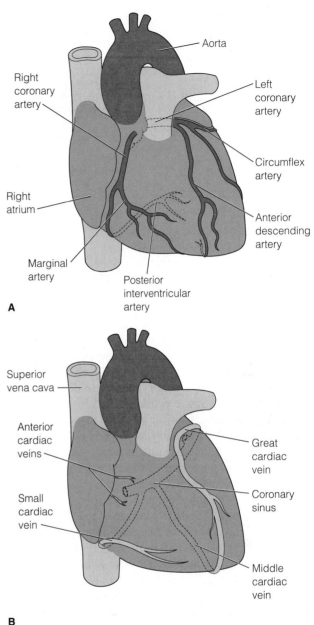

**Figure 28–5** ■ Coronary circulation. *A,* coronary arteries; *B,* coronary veins.

**Figure 28–4** ■ Pulmonary and systemic circulation. The left side of the heart pumps oxygenated blood into the arteries. Deoxygenated blood returns via the venous system into the right side of the heart.

(Figure 28–4 ■). After oxygen and carbon dioxide are exchanged in the capillaries of the lungs, oxygen-rich blood returns to the left atrium through several pulmonary veins. Blood is then pumped out of the left ventricle through the aorta and its major branches to supply all body tissues. This second circuit of blood flow is called the systemic circulation.

While this continuous circulation of blood through the heart meets the body's oxygen needs, the heart muscle itself is supplied by its own network of vessels through the coronary circulation. The left and right coronary arteries originate at the base of the aorta and branch out to encircle the myocardium

(Figure 28–5A■). While ventricular contraction delivers blood through the pulmonary and systemic circuits as described above, it is during ventricular relaxation that the coronary arteries fill with oxygen-rich blood. Then, after the blood perfuses the heart muscle, the cardiac veins drain the blood into the coronary sinus, which empties into the right atrium of the heart (Figure 28–5B).

## The Cardiac Cycle and Cardiac Output

The contraction and relaxation of the heart constitutes one heartbeat and is called the **cardiac cycle** (Figure 28–6 ■). Ventricular filling is followed by ventricular **systole,** a phase during which the ventricles contract and eject blood into the pulmonary and systemic circuits. Systole is followed by a

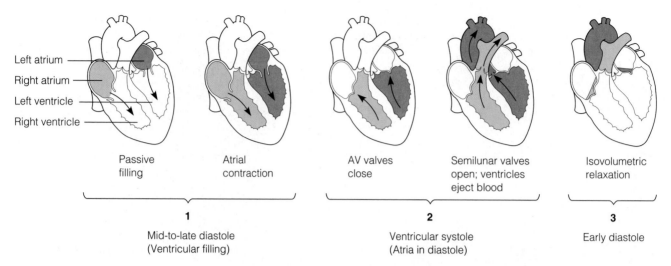

Left atrium

Right atrium

Left ventricle

Right ventricle

| Passive filling | Atrial contraction | AV valves close | Semilunar valves open; ventricles eject blood | Isovolumetric relaxation |

**1**

Mid-to-late diastole
(Ventricular filling)

**2**

Ventricular systole
(Atria in diastole)

**3**

Early diastole

**Figure 28–6** ■ The cardiac cycle has three events: (1) ventricular filling in mid-to-late diastole, (2) ventricular systole, and (3) isovolumetric relaxation in early diastole.

relaxation phase known as **diastole,** during which the ventricles refill, the atria contract, and the myocardium is perfused. Normally, the complete cardiac cycle occurs about 70 to 80 times per minute, measured as the heart rate (HR).

Each contraction ejects a certain volume of blood, called the **stroke volume (SV).** Stroke volume ranges from 60 to 100 mL/beat and averages about 70 mL/beat in an adult. The **cardiac output (CO)** is the amount of blood pumped by the ventricles into the pulmonary and systemic circulations in 1 minute. Multiplying the stroke volume by the heart rate determines the cardiac output: $CO \times HR = SV$.

The average adult cardiac output ranges from 4 to 8 L/min. **Ejection fraction (EF)** is the percentage of total blood in the ventricle at the end of the diastole ejected from the heart with each beat. The normal ejection fraction ranges from 50% to 70%. Cardiac output is an indicator of how well the heart is functioning as a pump: If the heart cannot pump effectively, cardiac output and tissue perfusion are decreased. Body tissues that do not receive enough blood and oxygen (carried in the blood on hemoglobin) become **ischemic** (deprived of oxygen). If the tissues do not receive enough blood flow to maintain the functions of the cells, the cells die.

Activity level, metabolic rate, physiologic and psychologic stress responses, age, and body size all influence cardiac output. In addition, cardiac output is determined by the interaction of four major factors: heart rate, preload, afterload, and contractility. Changes in each of these variables influence cardiac output intrinsically, and each also can be manipulated to affect cardiac output. The heart's ability to respond to the body's changing need for cardiac output is called **cardiac reserve.**

### Heart Rate

Heart rate is affected by both direct and indirect autonomic nervous system stimulation. Direct stimulation is accomplished through the innervation of the heart muscle by sympathetic and parasympathetic nerves. The sympathetic nervous system increases the heart rate, whereas the parasympathetic vagal tone slows the heart rate. Reflex regulation of heart rate

in response to systemic blood pressure also occurs through activation of sensory receptors known as baroreceptors or pressure receptors located in the carotid sinus, aortic arch, venae cavae, and pulmonary veins.

If heart rate increases, cardiac output increases (up to a point) even if there is no change in stroke volume. However, rapid heart rates decrease the amount of time available for ventricular filling during diastole. Cardiac output then falls because decreased filling time decreases stroke volume. Coronary artery perfusion also decreases because the coronary arteries fill primarily during diastole. Cardiac output decreases during bradycardia if stroke volume stays the same, because the number of cardiac cycles is decreased.

### Preload

**Preload** is the amount of cardiac muscle fiber tension, or stretch, that exists at the end of diastole, just before contraction of the ventricles. Preload is influenced by venous return and the compliance of the ventricles. It is related to the total volume of blood in the ventricles: The greater the volume, the greater the stretch of the cardiac muscle fibers, and the greater the force with which the fibers contract to accomplish emptying. This principle is called *Starling's law of the heart.*

This mechanism has a physiologic limit. Just as continuous overstretching of a rubber band causes the band to relax and lose its ability to recoil, overstretching of the cardiac muscle fibers eventually results in ineffective contraction. Disorders such as renal disease and congestive heart failure result in sodium and water retention and increased preload. Vasoconstriction also increases venous return and preload.

Too little circulating blood volume results in a decreased venous return and therefore a decreased preload. A decreased preload reduces stroke volume and thus cardiac output. Decreased preload may result from hemorrhage or maldistribution of blood volume, as occurs in third spacing (see Chapter 5). ⊙⊙

### Afterload

**Afterload** is the force the ventricles must overcome to eject their blood volume. It is the pressure in the arterial system ahead of the ventricles. The right ventricle must generate enough tension to open the pulmonary valve and eject its volume into the low-pressure pulmonary arteries. Right ventricle afterload is measured as pulmonary vascular resistance (PVR). The left ventricle, in contrast, ejects its load by overcoming the pressure behind the aortic valve. Afterload of the left ventricle is measured as systemic vascular resistance (SVR). Arterial pressures are much higher than pulmonary pressures; thus, the left ventricle has to work much harder than the right ventricle.

Alterations in vascular tone affect afterload and ventricular work. As the pulmonary or arterial blood pressure increases (e.g., through vasoconstriction), PVR and/or SVR increases, and the work of the ventricles increases. As workload increases, consumption of myocardial oxygen also increases. A compromised heart cannot effectively meet this increased oxygen demand, and a vicious cycle ensues. By contrast, a very low afterload decreases the forward flow of blood into the systemic circulation and the coronary arteries.

## Contractility

**Contractility** is the inherent capability of the cardiac muscle fibers to shorten. Poor contractility of the heart muscle reduces the forward flow of blood from the heart, increases the ventricular pressures from accumulation of blood volume, and reduces cardiac output. Increased contractility may overtax the heart.

## The Conduction System of the Heart

The cardiac cycle is perpetuated by a complex electrical circuit commonly known as the intrinsic conduction system of the heart. Cardiac muscle cells possess an inherent characteristic of self-excitation, which enables them to initiate and transmit impulses independent of a stimulus. However, specialized areas of myocardial cells typically exert a controlling influence in this electrical pathway.

One of these specialized areas is the sinoatrial (SA) node, located at the junction of the superior vena cava and right atrium (Figure 28–7 ■). The SA node acts as the normal "pacemaker" of the heart, usually generating an impulse 60 to 100 times per minute. This impulse travels across the atria via internodal pathways to the atrioventricular (AV) node, in the floor of the interatrial septum. The very small junctional fibers of the AV node slow the impulse, slightly delaying its transmission to the ventricles. It then passes through the bundle of His at the atrioventricular junction and continues down the interventricular septum through the right and left bundle branches and out to the Purkinje fibers in the ventricular muscle walls.

This path of electrical transmission produces a series of changes in ion concentration across the membrane of each cardiac muscle cell. The electrical stimulus increases the permeability of the cell membrane, creating an action potential (electrical potential). The result is an exchange of sodium, potassium, and calcium ions across the cell membrane, which changes the intracellular electrical charge to a positive state. This process of depolarization results in myocardial contraction. As the ion exchange reverses and the cell returns to its resting state of electronegativity, the cell is repolarized, and cardiac muscle relaxes. The cellular action potential serves as the basis for electrocardiography (ECG), the recording of the electrical impulses that immediately precede contraction of the heart muscle.

Cardiac conduction and electrocardiography are discussed in greater detail in Chapter 29. ⊖⊙

## Clinical Indicators of Cardiac Output

For many critically ill clients, invasive hemodynamic monitoring catheters are used to measure cardiac output in quantifiable numbers. However, advanced technology is not the only way to identify and assess compromised blood flow. Because cardiac output perfuses the body's tissues, clinical indicators of low

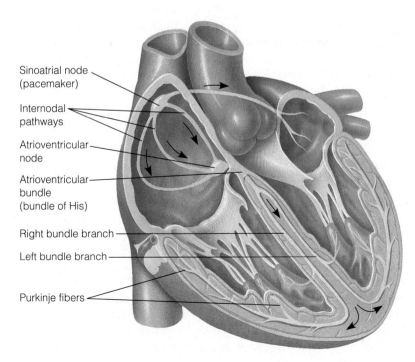

Sinoatrial node
(pacemaker)

Internodal
pathways

Atrioventricular
node

Atrioventricular
bundle
(bundle of His)

Right bundle branch

Left bundle branch

Purkinje fibers

**Figure 28–7** ■ The intrinsic conduction system of the heart.

cardiac output may be manifested by changes in organ function that result from compromised blood flow. For example, a decrease in blood flow to the brain presents as a change in level of consciousness. Other clinical manifestations of decreased cardiac output are discussed in Chapters 5 and 29. ⌘

*Cardiac index (CI)* is the cardiac output adjusted for the client's body size, also called the client's body surface area (BSA). Because it takes into account the client's BSA, the cardiac index provides more meaningful data about the heart's ability to perfuse the tissues and therefore is a more accurate indicator of the effectiveness of the circulation.

BSA is stated in square meters ($m^2$), and cardiac index is calculated as CO divided by BSA. Cardiac measurements are considered adequate when they fall within the range of 2.5 to 4.2 L/min/m². For example, two clients are determined to have a cardiac output of 4 L/min. This parameter is within normal limits. However, one client is 5 feet, 2 inches (157 cm) tall and weighs 120 lb (54.5 kg), with a BSA of 1.54 $m^2$. This client's cardiac index is $4 \div 1.54$, or 2.6 L/min/m². The second client is 6 feet, 2 inches (188 cm) tall and weighs 280 lb (81.7 kg), with a BSA of 2.52 $m^2$. This client's cardiac index is $4 \div 2.52$, or 1.6 L/min/m². The cardiac index results show that the same cardiac output of 4 L/min is adequate for the first client but grossly inadequate for the second client.

## ASSESSING CARDIAC FUNCTION

Conduct both a health assessment interview to collect subjective data and a physical assessment to collect objective data.

### The Health Assessment Interview

This section provides guidelines for collecting subjective data through a health assessment interview specific to cardiac function. A health assessment interview to determine problems with cardiac function may be conducted as part of a health screening or as part of a total health assessment, or it may focus on a chief complaint (such as chest pain). If the client has a problem with cardiac function, analyze its onset, characteristics, course, severity, precipitating and relieving factors, and any associated symptoms, noting the timing and circumstances. For example, ask the client:

- What is the location of the chest pain you experienced? Did it move up to your jaw or into your left arm?
- What type of activity brings on your chest pain?
- Have you noticed any changes in your energy level?
- Have you felt lightheaded during the times your heart is racing?

The interview begins by exploring the client's chief complaint (e.g., chest pain, palpitations, or shortness of breath). Describe the client's symptoms in terms of location, quality or character, timing, setting or precipitating factors, severity, aggravating and relieving factors, and associated symptoms (Table 28–1).

Explore the client's history for heart disorders such as angina, heart attack, congestive heart failure (CHF), hypertension (HTN), and valvular disease. Ask the client about previous heart surgery or illnesses, such as rheumatic fever, scarlet fever, or recurrent streptococcal throat infections. Also ask about presence and treatment of other chronic illnesses such as dia-

| TABLE 28–1 | Assessing Chest Pain |
|---|---|
| **Characteristic** | **Examples** |
| Location | Substernal, precordial, jaw, back Localized or diffuse Radiation to neck, jaw, shoulder, arm |
| Character/quality | Pressure; tightness; crushing, burning, or aching quality; heaviness; dullness; "heartburn" or indigestion |
| Timing: onset, duration, and frequency | Onset: Sudden or gradual? Duration: How many minutes does the pain last? Frequency: Is the pain continuous or periodic? |
| Setting/precipitating factors | Awake, at rest, sleep interrupted? With activity? With eating, exertion, exercise, elimination, emotional upset? |
| Intensity/severity | Can range from 0 (no pain) to 10 (worst pain ever felt) |
| Aggravating factors Relieving factors | Activity, breathing, temperature Medication (nitroglycerine, antacid), rest; there may be no relieving factors |
| Associated symptoms | Fatigue, shortness of breath, palpitations, nausea and vomiting, sweating, anxiety, lightheadedness or dizziness |

betes mellitus, bleeding disorders, or endocrine disorders. Review the client's family history for coronary artery disease (CAD), HTN, stroke, hyperlipidemia, diabetes, congenital heart disease, or sudden death.

Ask the client about past or present occurrence of various cardiac symptoms, such as chest pain, shortness of breath, difficulty breathing, cough, palpitations, fatigue, lightheadedness or dizziness, fainting, heart murmur, blood clots, or swelling. Because cardiac function affects all other body systems, a full history may need to explore other related systems, such as respiratory function and/or peripheral vascular function.

Review the client's personal habits and nutritional history, including body weight; eating patterns; dietary intake of fats, salt, fluids; dietary restrictions; hypersensitivities or intolerances to food or medication; and the use of caffeine and alcohol. If the client uses tobacco products, ask about type (cigarettes, pipe, cigars, snuff), duration, amount, and efforts to quit. If the client uses street drugs, ask about type, method of intake (e.g., inhaled or injected), duration of use, and efforts to quit. Include questions about the client's activity level and tolerance, recreational activities, and relaxation habits. Assess the client's sleep patterns for interruptions in sleep due to dyspnea, cough, discomfort, urination, or stress. Ask how many pillows the client uses when sleeping. Also consider psychosocial factors that may affect the client's stress level: What is the client's marital status, family composition, and role within the family? Have there been any changes? What is the client's occupation, level of education, and socioeconomic level? Are resources for support available? What is the client's emotional disposition and personality type? How does the client perceive his or her state of health or illness, and how able is the client to comply with treatment?

Further interview questions and leading statements, categorized by functional health patterns, can be found on the Companion Website.

## Physical Assessment

Physical assessment of cardiac function may be performed either as part of a total assessment or alone for clients with suspected or known problems with cardiac function. Assess the heart through inspection, palpation, and auscultation over the precordium (the area of the chest wall overlying the heart).

The equipment needed for an examination of the heart includes a stethoscope with a diaphragm and a bell, a good light source, and a ruler. Before the examination, collect all the equipment, and explain the examination to the client to decrease anxiety. A quiet environment is essential to hear and assess heart sounds accurately.

The client may sit or lie in the supine position. Movements over the precordium may be more easily seen with tangential lighting (in which the light is directed at a right angle to the area being observed, producing shadows). Assess the following types of movements.

- **Apical impulse** is a normal, visible pulsation (thrust) in the area of the midclavicular line in the left fifth intercostal space. It can be seen on inspection in about half of the adult population.
- **Retraction** is a pulling in of the tissue of the precordium; a slight retraction just medial to the midclavicular line at the area of the apical impulse is normal and is more likely to be visible in thin clients.
- **Lift** is a more sustained thrust than normal.
- **Heave** is an excessive thrust.

### Apical Impulse Assessment with Abnormal Findings (✓)

- First using palmar surface and then repeating with finger pads, palpate the precordium for symmetry of movement and the apical impulse for location, size, amplitude, and duration. The sequence for palpation is shown in Figure 28–8 ■. To locate the apical impulse, ask the client to assume a left lateral recumbent position. Simultaneous palpation of the carotid pulse may also be helpful. The apical impulse is not palpable in all clients.
  ✓ An enlarged or displaced heart is associated with an apical impulse lateral to the midclavicular line (MCL) or below the fifth left intercostal space (ICS).
  ✓ Increased size, amplitude, and duration of the point of maximal impulse (PMI) are associated with left ventricular volume overload (increased preload) in conditions such as HTN and aortic stenosis, and in pressure overload (increased afterload) in conditions such as aortic or mitral regurgitation.
  ✓ Increased amplitude alone may occur with hyperkinetic states, such as anxiety, hyperthyroidism, and anemia.
  ✓ Decreased amplitude is associated with a dilated heart in cardiomyopathy.

  ✓ Displacement alone may also occur with dextrocardia, diaphragmatic hernia, gastric distention, or chronic lung disease.
  ✓ A **thrill** (a palpable vibration over the precordium or an artery) may accompany severe valve stenosis.
  ✓ A marked increase in amplitude of the PMI at the right ventricular area occurs with right ventricular volume overload in atrial septal defect.
  ✓ An increase in amplitude and duration occurs with right ventricular pressure overload in pulmonic stenosis and pulmonary hypertension. A lift or heave may also be seen in these conditions (and in chronic lung disease).
  ✓ A palpable thrill in this area occurs with ventricular septal defect.
- Palpate the subxiphoid area with the index and middle finger.
  ✓ Right ventricular enlargement may produce a downward pulsation against the fingertips.
  ✓ An accentuated pulsation at the pulmonary area may be present in hyperkinetic states.
  ✓ A prominent pulsation reflects increased flow or dilation of the pulmonary artery.
  ✓ A thrill may be associated with aortic or pulmonary stenosis, aortic stenosis, pulmonary HTN, or atrial septal defect.
  ✓ Increased pulsation at the aortic area may suggest aortic aneurysm.
  ✓ A palpable second heart sound ($S_2$) may be noted with systemic HTN.

### Cardiac Rate and Rhythm Assessment with Abnormal Findings (✓)

- Auscultate heart rate.
  ✓ A heart rate exceeding 100 beats per minute (BPM) is **tachycardia.** A heart rate less than 60 BPM is **bradycardia.**
- Simultaneously palpate the radial pulse while listening to the apical pulse.
  ✓ If the radial pulse falls behind the apical rate, the client has a **pulse deficit,** indicating weak, ineffective contractions of the left ventricle.

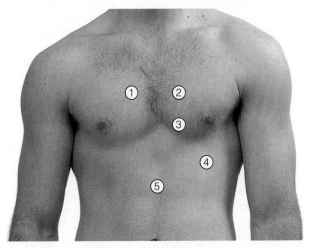

**Figure 28–8** ■ Areas for inspection and palpation of the precordium, indicating the sequence for palpation.

- Auscultate heart rhythm.
  - ✓ **Dysrhythmias** (abnormal heart rate or rhythm) may be regular or irregular in rhythm; their rates may be slow or fast. Irregular rhythms may occur in a pattern (e.g., an early beat every second beat, called *bigeminy*), sporadically, or with frequency and disorganization (e.g., atrial fibrillation). A pattern of gradual increase and decrease in heart rate that is within normal heart rate and that correlates with inspiration and expiration is called sinus arrhythmia.

## Heart Sounds Assessment with Abnormal Findings (✓)

See guidelines for cardiac auscultation in Box 28–1.

- Identify $S_1$ (first heart sound) and note its intensity. At each auscultatory area, listen for several cardiac cycles. See Figure 28–9 ■ for auscultation areas.
  - ✓ An accentuated $S_1$ occurs with tachycardia, states in which cardiac output is high (fever, anxiety, exercise, anemia, hyperthyroidism), complete heart block, and mitral stenosis.
  - ✓ A diminished $S_1$ occurs with first-degree heart block, mitral regurgitation, CHF, coronary artery disease, and pulmonary or systemic HTN. The intensity is also decreased with obesity, emphysema, and pericardial effusion. Varying intensity of $S_1$ occurs with complete heart block and grossly irregular rhythms.
- Listen for splitting of $S_1$.
  - ✓ Abnormal splitting of $S_1$ may be heard with right bundle branch block and premature ventricular contractions.
- Identify $S_2$ (second heart sound) and note its intensity.
  - ✓ An accentuated $S_2$ may be heard with HTN, exercise, excitement, and conditions of pulmonary HTN such as mitral stenosis, CHF, and cor pulmonale.

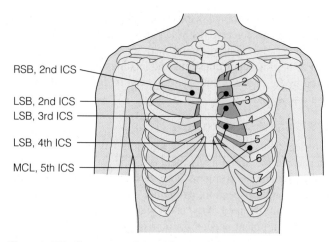

RSB, 2nd ICS
LSB, 2nd ICS
LSB, 3rd ICS
LSB, 4th ICS
MCL, 5th ICS

**Figure 28–9** ■ Areas for auscultation of the heart.

- ✓ A diminished $S_2$ occurs with aortic stenosis, a fall in systolic blood pressure (shock), pulmonary stenosis, and increased anterioposterior chest diameter.
- Listen for splitting of $S_2$.
  - ✓ Wide splitting of $S_2$ is associated with delayed emptying of the right ventricle resulting in delayed pulmonary valve closure (e.g., mitral regurgitation, pulmonary stenosis, and right bundle branch block).
  - ✓ Fixed splitting occurs when right ventricular output is greater than left ventricular output and pulmonary valve closure is delayed (e.g., with atrial septal defect and right ventricular failure).
  - ✓ Paradoxical splitting occurs when closure of the aortic valve is delayed (e.g., left bundle branch block).
- Identify extra heart sounds in systole.
  - ✓ Ejection sounds (or clicks) result from the opening of deformed semilunar valves (e.g., aortic and pulmonary stenosis).
  - ✓ A midsystolic click is heard with mitral valve prolapse (MVP).
- Identify the presence of extra heart sounds in diastole.
  - ✓ An opening snap results from the opening sound of a stenotic mitral valve.
  - ✓ A pathologic $S_3$ (a third heart sound that immediately follows $S_2$), or *ventricular gallop*, results from myocardial failure and ventricular volume overload (e.g., CHF, mitral or tricuspid regurgitation).
  - ✓ An $S_4$ (a fourth heart sound that immediately precedes $S_1$), or *atrial gallop*, results from increased resistance to ventricular filling after atrial contraction (e.g., HTN, CAD, aortic stenosis, and cardiomyopathy).
  - ✓ A less common right-sided $S_4$ occurs with pulmonary HTN and pulmonary stenosis.
  - ✓ A combined $S_3$ and $S_4$ is called a summation gallop and occurs with severe CHF.
- Identify extra heart sounds in both systole and diastole.
  - ✓ A pericardial friction rub results from inflammation of the pericardial sac, as with pericarditis.

## Murmur Assessment with Abnormal Findings (✓)

- Identify any **murmurs.** Note location, timing, presence during systole or diastole, and intensity. Use the following scale to grade murmurs:

---

**BOX 28–1** ■ **Guidelines for Cardiac Auscultation**

1. Locate the major auscultatory areas on the precordium (see Figure 28–9).
2. Choose a sequence of listening. Either begin from the apex and move upward along the sternal border to the base, or begin at the base and move downward to the apex. One suggested sequence is shown in Figure 28–9.
3. Listen first with the client in the sitting or supine position. Then ask the client to lie on the left side, and focus on the apex. Lastly, ask the client to sit up and lean forward. These position changes bring the heart closer to the chest wall and enhance auscultation. Carry out the following steps when the client assumes each of these positions:
   a. First, auscultate each area with the diaphragm of the stethoscope to listen for high-pitched sounds: $S_1$, $S_2$, murmurs, pericardial friction rubs.
   b. Next, auscultate each area with the bell of the stethoscope to listen for lower-pitched sounds: $S_3$, $S_4$, murmurs.
   c. Listen for the effect of respirations on each sound; while the client is sitting up and leaning forward, ask the client to exhale and hold the breath while you listen to heart sounds.

I = Barely heard
II = Quietly heard
III = Clearly heard
IV = Loud
V = Very loud
VI = Loudest; may be heard with stethoscope off the chest. A thrill may accompany murmurs of grade IV to grade VI.
- Note pitch (low, medium, high), and quality (harsh, blowing, or musical). Note pattern/shape, crescendo, decrescendo, and radiation/transmission (to axilla, neck).
  ✓ Midsystolic murmurs are heard with semilunar valve disease (e.g., aortic and pulmonary stenosis) and with hypertrophic cardiomyopathy.

✓ Pansystolic (holosystolic) murmurs are heard with AV valve disease (e.g., mitral and tricuspid regurgitation, ventricular septal defect).
✓ A late systolic murmur is heard with MVP.
✓ Early diastolic murmurs occur with regurgitant flow across incompetent semilunar valves (e.g., aortic regurgitation).
✓ Middiastolic and presystolic murmurs, such as with mitral stenosis, occur with turbulent flow across the AV valves.
✓ Continuous murmurs throughout systole and all or part of diastole occur with patent ductus arteriosus.

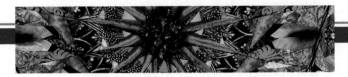

## EXPLORE MediaLink

NCLEX review questions, case studies, care plan activities, MediaLink applications, and other interactive resources for this chapter can be found on the Companion Website at www.prenhall.com/lemone.

Click on Chapter 28 to select the activities for this chapter. For animations, video clips, more NCLEX review questions, and an audio glossary, access the Student CD-ROM accompanying this textbook.

## TEST YOURSELF

1. Which circulatory process supplies the heart with blood?
   a. The systemic circulation
   b. The pulmonary circulation
   c. The coronary circulation
   d. The hepatic circulation

2. The amount of blood pumped by the ventricles in 1 minute is known as:
   a. Heart rate
   b. Ventricular contraction
   c. Stroke volume
   d. Cardiac output

3. The intensity of chest pain may be assessed by asking which question?
   a. "Did the pain move into your left arm?"
   b. "Was your pain relieved by resting?"

   c. "On a scale of 0 to 10, what number was your pain?"
   d. "Was the pain a pressure, a burning, or a tightness?"

4. At what anatomic location would you assess the apical impulse?
   a. Left midclavicular, 5th intercostal space
   b. Left substernal, 6th intercostal space
   c. Right midaxillary, 2nd intercostal space
   d. Right nipple line, any intercostal space

5. Your client's pulse rate is 50. You would document this as:
   a. Tachycardia
   b. Bradycardia
   c. Hypertension
   d. Hypotension

See Test Yourself answers in Appendix C.

## BIBLIOGRAPHY

Farla, S., & Flannery, J. (1999). Assessment of the patient in heart failure. *Home Care Provider, 4*(5), 184–188.

Kirton, C. (1996). Assessing normal heart sounds. *Nursing96, 26*(2), 56–57.

———. (1997a). Assessing a heart murmur. *Nursing97, 27*(9), 51.

———. (1997b). Assessing S₃ and S₄ heart sounds. *Nursing97, 27*(7), 52–53.

Ludwig, L. (1998). Cardiovascular assessment for home healthcare nurses: Part 1. *Home Healthcare Nurse, 16*(7), 450–456.

McAvoy, J. (2000). Cardiac pain: Discover the unexpected. *Nursing, 30*(3), 34–40.

McGrath, A., & Cox, C. (1998). Cardiac and circulatory assessment in intensive care units. *Intensive & Critical Care Nursing, 14*(6), 283–287.

Norrie, P. (1999). The parameters that cardiothoracic intensive care nurses use to assess the progress or deterioration of their patients. *Nursing in Critical Care, 4*(3), 133–137.

O'Hanlon-Nichols, T. (1997). Basic assessment series: The adult cardiovascular system. *American Journal of Nursing, 97*(12), 34–40.

Scrima, D. (1997). Foundations of arrhythmia interpretation. *MEDSURG Nursing, 6*(4), 193–202.

Weber, J., & Kelley, J. (2002). *Health assessment in nursing* (2nd ed.). Philadelphia: Lippincott.

Wilson, S., & Giddens, J. (2001). *Health assessment for nursing practice.* St. Louis: Mosby.

### CHAPTER 29

# Nursing Care of Clients with Coronary Heart Disease

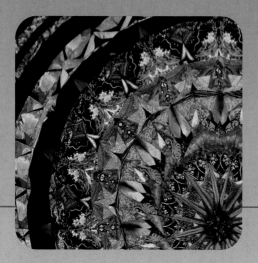

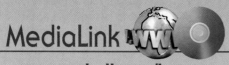

## www.prenhall.com/lemone

Additional resources for this chapter can be found on the Student CD-ROM accompanying this textbook, and on the Companion Website at www.prenhall.com/lemone. Click on Chapter 29 to select the activities for this chapter.

**CD-ROM**
- Audio Glossary
- NCLEX Review

*Animations*
- Coronary Heart Disease
- Nifedipine
- Propranolol

**Companion Website**
- More NCLEX Review
- Case Study
  Myocardial Infarction
- Care Plan Activity
  Perioperative Pacemaker Care
- MediaLink Application
  Women and Heart Attacks

## LEARNING OUTCOMES

After completing this chapter, you will be able to:

- Use knowledge of the normal anatomy and physiology of the heart in caring for clients with coronary heart disease.

- Discuss the coronary circulation and electrical properties of the heart.

- Compare and contrast the pathophysiology and manifestations of coronary heart disease and common cardiac dysrhythmias.

- Identify diagnostic tests and procedures used for clients with coronary heart disease and/or dysrhythmias.

- Discuss nursing implications for drugs used to prevent and treat coronary heart disease and dysrhythmias.

- Describe nursing care for the client undergoing diagnostic testing, an interventional procedure, or surgery for coronary heart disease or a dysrhythmia.

- Use the nursing process to plan and implement individualized nursing care and teaching for clients with coronary heart disease or dysrhythmias.

Changes in the conduction of electrical impulses through the heart, impaired blood flow to the myocardium, and structural changes in the heart itself affect the heart's ability to fulfill its major purpose: to pump enough blood to meet the body's demand for oxygen and nutrients. Disruptions in cardiac function affect other organ systems as well, potentially leading to organ system failure and death.

**Cardiovascular disease (CVD)** is a generic term for disorders of the heart and blood vessels. CVD is the leading cause of death and disability in the United States. Over 60 million people have some type of cardiovascular disease. The economic costs of CVD, both direct and indirect, to the nation are estimated at $329 billion annually (National Heart, Lung, and Blood Institute [NHLBI], 2002).

On an encouraging note, however, the incidence of new CVD cases per year is decreasing. Public education aimed at reducing fat intake, increasing exercise, and lowering cholesterol levels have made people more aware of risk factors associated with CVD. The mortality rate from heart disease peaked in 1963 and has shown a slow but steady decline since that time.

This chapter focuses on disorders of myocardial blood flow (coronary heart disease) and cardiac rhythm. Disorders of cardiac structure and function are discussed in Chapter 30. Review the normal anatomy and physiology and nursing assessment of the heart in Chapter 28 before proceeding with this chapter.

# DISORDERS OF MYOCARDIAL PERFUSION

## THE CLIENT WITH CORONARY HEART DISEASE

**Coronary heart disease (CHD),** or *coronary artery disease (CAD),* affects 12.6 million people in the United States and causes more than 500,000 deaths annually (NHLBI, 2002). CHD is caused by impaired blood flow to the myocardium (Porth, 2002). Accumulation of atherosclerotic plaque in the coronary arteries is the usual cause. Coronary heart disease may be asymptomatic, or may lead to angina pectoris, myocardial infarction (MI or heart attack), dysrhythmias, heart failure, and even sudden death.

Many risk factors for CHD can be controlled through lifestyle modification. In fact, with increased public awareness of risk factors related to CHD, mortality rates are declining by about 3.3% per year. Nevertheless, CHD remains a major public health problem. Heart disease is the leading cause of death for all U.S. ethnic groups except Asian females (NHBLI, 2002). Nurses are in a prime position to encourage and support positive lifestyle changes by teaching and promoting healthy living practices. Individual choices can and do affect health.

The highest incidence of CHD is in the Western world, mainly in white males age 45 and older. Both men and women are affected by coronary heart disease; in women, however, the onset is about 10 years later because of the heart-protective effects of estrogen. After menopause, women's risk is equal to that of men.

The causes of atherosclerosis are not known, but certain risk factors have been linked with the development of atherosclerotic plaques. The Framingham Heart Study provided vital research into the relationship between risk factors and the development of heart disease (Box 29–1). Research into CHD is ongoing, looking at causative factors, manifestations, and protective measures for many populations.

## RISK FACTORS

Risk factors for CHD are frequently classified as *nonmodifiable,* or factors that cannot be changed, and *modifiable,* those factors that can be changed (Table 29–1).

### Nonmodifiable

*Age* is a nonmodifiable risk factor. Over 50% of heart attack victims are 65 or older; 80% of deaths due to myocardial infarction occur in this age group. *Gender, race,* and *genetic factors* also are nonmodifiable risk factors for CHD. Men are affected by CHD at an earlier age than women. African Americans have a higher incidence of hypertension, which contributes to more rapid development of atherosclerosis.

### Modifiable

Modifiable risk factors include lifestyle factors and pathologic conditions that predispose the client to developing CHD. Pathologic conditions often can be controlled. Behavioral or lifestyle factors can be controlled or completely eliminated. Lifestyle changes require significant commitment by the client; ongoing support from the health care team is vital for success.

#### Pathologic Conditions

Disease conditions that contribute to CHD include hypertension, diabetes mellitus, and hyperlipidemia. Elevated homocystine levels and the metabolic syndrome are emerging risk factors. Although these conditions are not a matter of choice, they are modifiable risk factors that can often be controlled through medication, weight control, diet, and exercise.

*Hypertension* is consistent blood pressure readings greater than 140 mmHg systolic or 90 mmHg diastolic. Hypertension is common, affecting more than one-third of people over age 50 in the United States. Its prevalence is higher in African Americans than in Hispanics, and higher in Hispanics than in white Americans (NHLBI, 2002).

## BOX 29-1 ■ The Framingham Heart Study

The Framingham Heart Study (FHS) is an ongoing, significant clinical research study that has provided data about cardiovascular disease for over 50 years. The study was initiated in 1948 with an original study group of 5209 participants in the town of Framingham, Massachusetts. Every 2 years, this original group is evaluated for cardiovascular "events" via their medical history, physical findings, and diagnostic testing. Children of the original group have also been studied as part of the Framingham Offspring Study. It was in reports of the Framingham study that the term "risk factor" first appeared.

### IMPLICATIONS FOR NURSING

The data collected from both the Framingham Heart Study and the Framingham Offspring Study provide a rich database from which to develop evidence-based approaches for clients with heart disease. A major application of these research findings to practice is in primary preventive education, for example, through community cardiovascular health programs. As noted in the text, although research shows that increased public awareness of cardiovascular risk factors has lowered morbidity and mortality from heart disease, heart disease remains the number-one killer in the United States. Education about the effects of lifestyle on the cardiovascular system must begin in the early school years and be reinforced throughout the formative years. When healthy choices become habit, cardiac disease will be reduced.

A second application of these findings is in collaborative treatment. Nurses should keep up to date on the latest strategies for medical treatment so that they can provide accurate rationales to clients and formulate effective nursing treatment plans that complement medical management strategies. The result is better communication, a sense of collegiality and teamwork, and positive client outcomes.

### Critical Thinking in Client Care

1. What kinds of strategies can be used in elementary school settings to teach cardiovascular health in a fun, informative manner?
2. Which health care providers should be included in a multidisciplinary effort to encourage clients to modify their lifestyles?
3. What changes do you need to make in your lifestyle to role model heart healthy living?

### TABLE 29-1  Risk Factors for Coronary Heart Disease

| Nonmodifiable | Modifiable | |
| --- | --- | --- |
| | Pathophysiologic | Lifestyle |
| Age<br>Gender<br>Race/ethnic background<br>Heredity | Hypertension<br>Diabetes mellitus<br>Hyperlipidemia<br>Elevated homocystine levels<br>Metabolic syndrome<br>Women only: premature menopause | Cigarette smoking<br>Obesity<br>Physical inactivity<br>Diet<br><br>Women only: use of oral contraceptives, hormone replacement therapy |

### TABLE 29-2  Classification of Serum Cholesterol Values*

| | Total Cholesterol (mg/dL) | LDL Cholesterol (mg/dL) |
| --- | --- | --- |
| Optimal | | Less than 100 |
| Desirable | Under 200 | 100–129 |
| Borderline High | 200 to 239 | 130 to 159 |
| High | 240 or higher | 160 or higher |
| Very High | | >190 |

*As defined by the National Blood, Lung, and Heart Institute's National Cholesterol Education Program.

*Diabetes mellitus* contributes to CHD in several ways. Diabetes is associated with higher blood lipid levels, a higher incidence of hypertension, and obesity—all risk factors in their own right. In addition, diabetes affects blood vessels, contributing to the process of atherosclerosis. Hyperglycemia, altered platelet function, and elevated fibrinogen levels also are thought to play a role.

*Hyperlipidemia* is an abnormally high level of blood lipids and lipoproteins. Lipoproteins carry cholesterol in the blood. Low-density lipoproteins (LDLs) are the primary carriers of cholesterol. High levels of LDL (Memory cue: LDLs = less desirable lipoproteins) promote atherosclerosis because LDL deposits cholesterol on artery walls. Table 29–2 lists desirable and high-risk levels for total and LDL cholesterol. In contrast, high-density lipoproteins (HDLs = highly desirable lipoproteins) help clear cholesterol from the arteries, transporting it to the liver for excretion. HDL levels above 35 mg/dL appear to reduce the risk of CHD. Triglycerides, compounds of fatty acids bound to glycerol and used for fat storage by the body, are carried on very low-density lipoprotein (VLDL) molecules. Elevated triglyerides also contribute to the risk for CHD.

Recent research demonstrates a link between elevated serum *homocysteine levels* and CHD. Until menopause, women have lower homocysteine levels than men, which may partially explain their lower risk for CHD. Homocysteine levels are negatively correlated with serum folate and dietary folate intake; that is, increasing folate intake lowers homocysteine levels.

*Metabolic syndrome* is another emerging risk factor for CHD. Metabolic syndrome is a group of related risk factors occurring in the same individual: abdominal obesity, hyperlipidemia, hypertension, insulin resistance, and an increased tendency toward clotting and inflammation. The metabolic syndrome appears to significantly increase the risk for premature CHD.

## Nursing Research

### Evidence-Based Practice for Postmenopausal Women

The Women's Health Initiative (WHI) is studying the risks and benefits of strategies to reduce the incidence of heart disease, breast and colorectal cancer, and fractures in postmenopausal women (Writing Group, 2002). A group of 161,809 postmenopausal women between age 50 and 79 were originally enrolled in WHI trials. Of these women, a subgroup of 16,608 women with intact uteri became part of a randomized trial to assess the risks and benefits of HRT, using the most frequently prescribed combined hormone (estrogen and progestin [Prempro]) replacement in the United States.

After a mean of 5.2 years of follow-up, this study was stopped due to convincing evidence that the risk for invasive breast cancer exceeded the benefits of HRT. The study also demonstrated increased risks for coronary heart disease, stroke, deep vein thrombosis, and pulmonary embolism, although overall mortality was not affected. HRT reduced the risk for colorectal cancer and hip fracture in this study group. The risk for CHD appears to be independent of other CHD risk factors such as age, ethnicity, hypertension, diabetes, smoking, obesity, and other identified risk factors.

### IMPLICATIONS FOR NURSING

Nurses often are in position of advising women about menopause, its manifestations, and hormone replacement therapy. While HRT does reduce unpleasant menopausal effects such as night sweats and hot flashes, and it reduces the risk of osteoporosis and subsequent fractures, it carries associated risks. Advise each client about the risks and benefits of HRT, clearly presenting the evidence. Suggest alternative strategies to reduce menopausal symptoms, such as complementary medicines (see Chapter 48). Encourage measures such as weight-bearing exercise, calcium supplements, and a diet high in fiber and antioxidants to reduce the risks for osteoporosis, fracture, and colorectal cancer. Ultimately, each client will make her own decision about postmenopausal HRT.

### Critical Thinking in Client Care

1. What factors might you suggest that a client consider when deciding whether to use HRT for menopausal manifestations and risks?
2. In this study, the increased risk for CHD was not related to the duration of time taking HRT, whereas the increased risk for stroke and invasive breast cancer emerged more than 1 year after randomization (stroke in the second through fifth year of the study, breast cancer within several years following randomization). Will this data affect your advice to menopausal women inquiring about HRT? If so, how?

---

Risk factors unique to women include *premature menopause, oral contraceptive use,* and *hormone replacement therapy (HRT).* At menopause, serum HDL levels drop and LDL levels rise, increasing the risk of CHD. Early menopause (natural or surgically induced) increases the risk of CHD and MI. Women who have bilateral oophorectomy before age 35 without hormone replacement are 8 times more likely to have an MI than women experiencing natural menopause. Estrogen replacement therapy reduces the risk of CHD and MI in these women. Oral contraceptives, by contrast, increase the risk for myocardial infarction, particularly in women who also smoke. This increased risk is due to the tendency of oral contraceptives to promote clotting, and their effects on blood pressure, serum lipids, and glucose tolerance (Woods, Froclicher, & Motzer, 2000). The Women's Health Initiative randomized trial of HRT showed an increased risk for CHD in previously healthy women taking a commonly prescribed combination of estrogen and progestin (Writing Group, 2002). This well-controlled research study (see the box above) was terminated early when it showed a small but significant increase risk for CHD, stroke, pulmonary embolism, and invasive breast cancer in women taking HRT.

### Lifestyle Factors

*Cigarette smoking* is an independent risk factor for CHD, responsible for more deaths from CHD than from lung cancer or pulmonary disease (Woods et al., 2000). The male cigarette smoker has 2 to 3 times the risk of developing heart disease than the nonsmoker; the female who smokes has up to 4 times the risk. For both men and women who stop smoking, the risk of mortality from CHD is reduced by half. Second-hand (or environmental) tobacco smoke also increases the risk of death from CHD, by as much as 30% (Woods et al., 2000). Tobacco smoke promotes CHD in several ways. Carbon monoxide damages vascular endothelium, promoting cholesterol deposition. Nicotine stimulates catecholamine release, increasing blood pressure, heart rate, and myocardial oxygen use. Nicotine also constricts arteries, limiting tissue perfusion (blood flow and oxygen delivery). Further, nicotine reduces HDL levels and increases platelet aggregation, increasing the risk of thrombus formation.

*Obesity* (body weight greater than 30% over ideal body weight), increased body mass index (BMI), and fat distribution affect the risk for CHD. Obese people have higher rates of hypertension, diabetes, and hyperlipidemia. In the Framingham study, obese men over age 50 had twice the incidence of CHD and acute MI of those who were within 10% of their ideal weight. Central obesity, or intra-abdominal fat, is associated with an increased risk for CHD. The best indicator of central obesity is the waist circumference. A waist-to-hip ratio of greater than 0.8 (women) or 0.9 (men) increases the risk for CHD.

*Physical inactivity* is associated with higher risk of CHD. Research data indicate that people who maintain a regular program of physical activity are less prone to developing CHD than sedentary people. Cardiovascular benefits of exercise include increased availability of oxygen to the heart muscle, decreased oxygen demand and cardiac workload, and increased myocardial function and electrical stability. Other positive effects of regular physical activity include decreased blood pressure, blood lipids, insulin levels, platelet aggregation, and weight.

*Diet* may be a risk factor for CHD, independent of fat and cholesterol intake. Diets high in fruits, vegetables, whole

Coronary heart disease usually is due to *atherosclerosis*, occlusion of the coronary arteries by fibrous, fatty plaque. Coronary heart disease is manifested by *angina pectoris* and/or *myocardial infarction*. Risk factors for coronary heart disease include age (over 50 years), heredity, smoking, obesity, high serum cholesterol levels, hypertension, and diabetes mellitus. Other factors, such as diet and lack of exercise, also contribute to the risk of CHD.

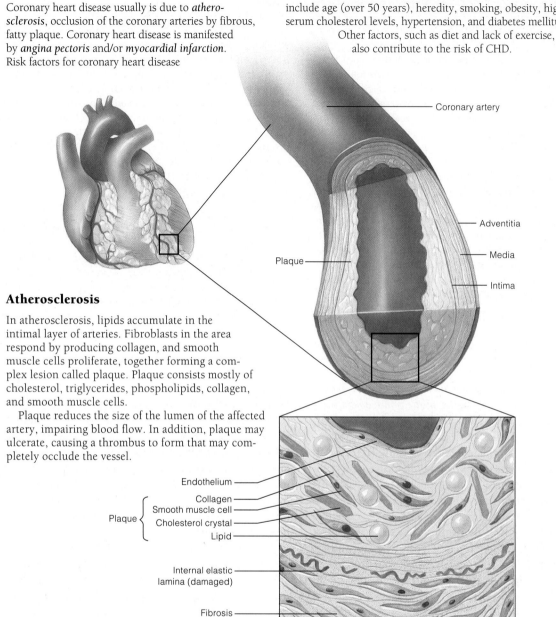

### Atherosclerosis

In atherosclerosis, lipids accumulate in the intimal layer of arteries. Fibroblasts in the area respond by producing collagen, and smooth muscle cells proliferate, together forming a complex lesion called plaque. Plaque consists mostly of cholesterol, triglycerides, phospholipids, collagen, and smooth muscle cells.

Plaque reduces the size of the lumen of the affected artery, impairing blood flow. In addition, plaque may ulcerate, causing a thrombus to form that may completely occlude the vessel.

grains, and unsaturated fatty acids appear to have a protective effect. The underlying factors are not clear, but probably relate to nutrients such as antioxidants, folic acid, other B vitamins, omega-3 fatty acids, and other unidentified micronutrients (National Cholesterol Education Program, 2001).

## PHYSIOLOGY REVIEW

The two main coronary arteries, the left and the right, supply blood, oxygen, and nutrients to the myocardium. They originate in the root of the aorta, just outside the aortic valve. The *left main coronary artery* divides to form the anterior descending and circumflex arteries. The *anterior descending* artery supplies the anterior interventricular septum and the left ventricle. The *circumflex* branch supplies the left lateral wall of the left ventricle. The *right coronary artery* supplies the right ventricle and forms the posterior descending artery. The *posterior descending* artery supplies the posterior portion of the heart (see Figure 28-4).

Blood flow through the coronary arteries is regulated by several factors. Aortic pressure is the primary factor. Other factors include the heart rate (most flow occurs during diastole, when the muscle is relaxed), metabolic activity of the heart, blood vessel tone (constriction), and collateral circulation. Although there are no connections between the large coronary arteries, small arteries are joined by **collateral channels.** If large vessels are gradually occluded, these channels enlarge, providing alternative routes for blood flow (Porth, 2002).

### Angina Pectoris

Angina is characterized by episodes of chest pain, usually precipitated by exercise and relieved by rest. When myocardial oxygen needs are greater than partially occluded vessels can supply, myocardial cells become ischemic and shift to anaerobic metabolism. Anaerobic metabolism produces lactic acid that stimulates nerve endings in the muscle, causing pain. The pain subsides when the oxygen supply again meets myocardial demand.

### Myocardial Infarction

Myocardial infarction occurs when complete obstruction of a coronary artery interrupts blood supply to an area of myocardium. Affected tissue becomes ischemic and eventually dies (infarcts) if the blood supply is not restored. The necrotic area is bordered by an area of injured or damaged tissue, which is in turn surrounded by an area of ischemic tissue.

As myocardial cells die, they lyse and release various cardiac isoenzymes into the circulation. Elevated serum levels of creatinine kinase (CK) and cardiac-specific troponins are specific indicators of myocardial infarction.

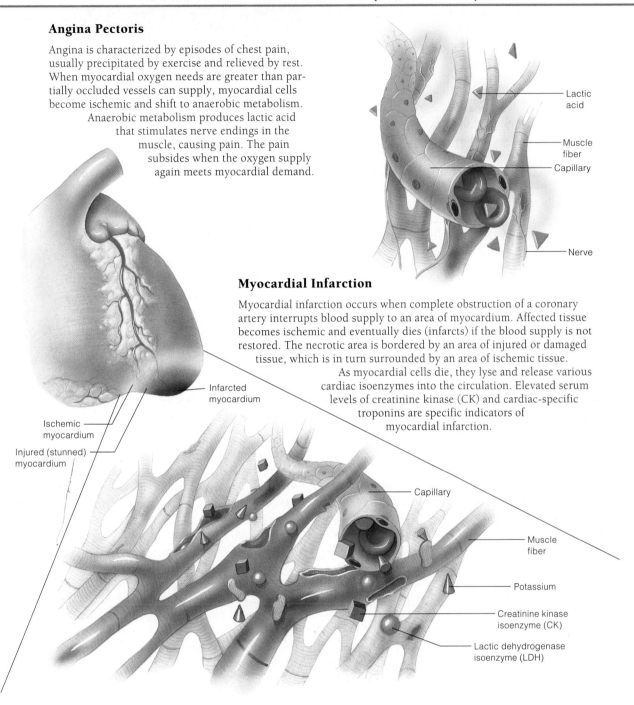

## PATHOPHYSIOLOGY

### Atherosclerosis

Coronary atherosclerosis is the most common cause of reduced coronary blood flow. **Atherosclerosis** is a progressive disease characterized by *atheroma* (plaque) formation, which affects the intimal and medial layers of large and midsize arteries. See *Pathophysiology Illustrated,* above.

Atherosclerosis is initiated by unknown precipitating factors that cause lipoproteins and fibrous tissue to accumulate in the arterial wall. Although the precise mechanisms are unknown, the most accepted theory is that atherosclerosis begins with an injury to or inflammation of endothelial cells lining the artery. Endothelial damage promotes platelet adhesion and aggregation, and attracts leukocytes to the area.

At the injury site, *atherogenic* (atherosclerosis-promoting) lipoproteins collect in the intimal lining of the artery. Macrophages migrate to the injured site as part of the inflammatory process. Contact with platelets, cholesterol, and other blood components stimulates smooth muscle cells and connective tissue within the vessel wall to proliferate abnormally. Although blood flow is not affected at this stage, this early lesion appears as a yellowish fatty streak on the inner lining of the artery. Fibrous plaque develops as smooth muscle cells enlarge, collagen fibers proliferate, and blood lipids accumulate. The lesion protrudes into the arterial lumen and is fixed to the inner wall of the intima. It may invade the muscular media layer of the vessel as well. The developing plaque not only gradually occludes the vessel lumen but also impairs the vessel's ability to dilate in response to increased oxygen demands. Fibrous plaque lesions often develop at arterial bifurcations or curves or in areas of narrowing. As the plaque expands, it can produce severe stenosis or total occlusion of the artery.

The final stage of the process is the development of *atheromas,* complex lesions consisting of lipids, fibrous tissue, collagen, calcium, cellular debris, and capillaries. These calcified lesions can ulcerate or rupture, stimulating thrombosis. The vessel lumen may be rapidly occluded by the thrombus, or it may embolize to occlude a distal vessel.

Plaque formation may be *eccentric,* located in a specific, asymmetric region of the vessel wall, or *concentric,* involving the entire vessel circumference. Manifestations of the process usually do not appear until about 75% of the arterial lumen has been occluded.

## Myocardial Ischemia

Myocardial cells become ischemic when the oxygen supply is inadequate to meet metabolic demands. The critical factors in meeting metabolic demands of cardiac cells are coronary perfusion and myocardial workload (Copstead & Banasik, 2000). The oxygen content of the blood is a contributing factor. Table 29–3 lists factors that may lead to myocardial ischemia.

Myocardial cells have limited supplies of adenosine triphosphate (ATP) for energy storage. When myocardial workload increases or the supply of blood and oxygen falls, cellular ATP stores are quickly depleted, affecting their contractility. Cellular metabolism switches from an efficient aerobic process to anaerobic metabolism. Lactic acid accumulates, and cells are damaged. If blood flow is restored within 20 minutes, aerobic metabolism and contractility are restored, and cellular repair begins (McCance & Huether, 2002). Continued ischemia results in cell necrosis and death (infarction).

Coronary heart disease is generally divided into two categories, chronic ischemic heart disease and acute coronary syndromes. *Chronic ischemic heart disease* includes stable and vasospastic angina, and silent myocardial ischemia. *Acute coronary syndromes* range from unstable angina to myocardial infarction (Porth, 2002). These disorders are discussed in the following sections of this chapter.

## COLLABORATIVE CARE

Care of clients with coronary heart disease focuses on aggressive risk factor management to slow the atherosclerotic process and maintain myocardial perfusion. Until manifestations of chronic or acute ischemia are experienced, the diagnosis often is presumptive, based on history and the presence of risk factors.

### Diagnostic Tests

Laboratory testing is used to assess for risk factors such as an abnormal blood lipid profile (elevated triglyceride and LDL levels and decreased HDL levels).

- *Total serum cholesterol* is elevated in hyperlipidemia. A *lipid profile* includes triglyceride, HDL, and LDL levels as well, and enables calculation of the ratio of HDL to total cholesterol. The ratio should be at least 1:5, with 1:3 being the ideal ratio. Elevated lipid levels are associated with an increased risk of atherosclerosis (see Table 29–2). For the most accurate results, dietary cholesterol intake should be consistent for 3 weeks prior to testing, and the client should fast for 10 to 12 hours before the sample is drawn. Alcohol intake and many medications can affect results.

Diagnostic tests to identify subclinical (asymptomatic) CHD may be indicated when multiple risk factors are present.

- *C-reactive protein* is a serum protein associated with inflammatory processes. Recent evidence suggests that elevated blood levels of this protein may be predictive of CHD.
- The *ankle-brachial blood pressure index (ABI)* is an inexpensive, noninvasive test for peripheral vascular disease that may be predictive of CHD. See Chapter 33 ⊙ for more information about this test.
- *Exercise ECG testing* may be performed. ECGs are used to assess the response to increased cardiac workload induced by exercise. The test is considered "positive" for CHD if myocardial ischemia is detected on the ECG (depression of the ST segment by greater than 3 mm; see Figure 29–1), the client develops chest pain, or the test is stopped due to excess fatigue, dysrhythmias, or other symptoms before the predicted maximal heart rate is achieved.
- *Electron beam computed tomography (EBCT)* creates a three-dimensional image of the heart and coronary arteries that can reveal plaque and other abnormalities. This noninvasive test requires no special preparation, and can identify clients at risk for developing myocardial ischemia.

### TABLE 29–3 Factors Contributing to Myocardial Ischemia

| Coronary Perfusion | Myocardial Workload | Blood Oxygen Content |
|---|---|---|
| • Atherosclerosis | • Rapid heart rate | • Reduced atmospheric oxygen pressure |
| • Thrombosis | • Increased preload, afterload, or contractility | • Impaired gas exchange |
| • Vasospasm | • Increased metabolic demands (e.g., hyperthyroidism) | • Low red blood cells and hemoglobin content |
| • Poor perfusion pressure | | |

• *Myocardial perfusion imaging* (see the section on angina that follows) may be used to evaluate myocardial blood flow and perfusion, both at rest and during stress testing (exercise or mental stress). These diagnostic tests are further explained in the section on angina. Perfusion imaging studies are costly, and therefore not recommended for routine CHD risk assessment.

## Risk Factor Management

Conservative management of CHD focuses on risk factor modification, including smoking, diet, exercise, and management of contributing conditions.

### Smoking

Smoking cessation rapidly reduces the risk for CHD and improves cardiovascular status. People who quit reduce their risk by 50%, regardless of how long they smoked before quitting. For women, the risk becomes equivalent to a non-smoker within 3 to 5 years of smoking cessation (Woods et al., 2000). In addition, stopping smoking improves HDL levels, lowers LDL levels, and reduces blood viscosity. All smokers are advised to quit. Health promotion activities focus on preventing children, teenagers, and adults from starting to smoke.

### Diet

Dietary recommendations by the National Cholesterol Education Program (2001) include reduced saturated fat and cholesterol intake, and strategies to lower LDL levels (Table 29–4). Most fats are a mixture of saturated and unsaturated fatty acids. The highest proportions of saturated fat are found in whole-milk products, red meats, and coconut oil. Nonfat dairy products, fish, and poultry as primary protein sources are recommended. Solidified vegetable fats (e.g., margarine, shortening) contain *trans* fatty acids, which behave more like saturated fats. Soft margarines and vegetable oil spreads contain low levels of trans fatty acids, and should be used instead of butter, stick margarine, and shortening. Monounsaturated fats, found in olive, canola, and peanut oils, actually lower LDL and cholesterol levels. Certain cold-water fish, such as tuna, salmon, and mackerel, contain high levels of omega-3 (or n-3) fatty acids, which help raise HDL levels, and decrease serum triglycerides, total serum cholesterol, and blood pressure.

In addition, increased intake of soluble fiber (found in oats, psyllium, pectin-rich fruit, and beans) and insoluble fiber (found in whole grains, vegetables, and fruit) is recommended. Folic acid and vitamins $B_6$ and $B_{12}$ affect homocystine metabolism, reducing serum levels. Leafy green vegetables (e.g., spinach and broccoli) and legumes (e.g., black-eyed peas, dried beans, and lentils) are rich sources of folate. Meat, fish, and poultry are rich in vitamins $B_6$ and $B_{12}$. Vitamin $B_6$ also is found in soy products; $B_{12}$ is in fortified cereals. Increased intake of antioxidant nutrients (vitamin E, in particular) and foods rich in antioxidants (fruits and vegetables) appears to increase HDL levels and have a protective effect on CHD.

In middle-aged and older adults, moderate alcohol intake may reduce the risk for CHD (National Cholesterol Education Program, 2001). Consumption of no more than two drinks per day for men or one drink per day for women is recommended. A drink is 5 ounces of wine, 12 ounces of beer, or 1 1/2 ounces of whiskey. People who do not drink alcohol, however, should not be encouraged to start consuming it as a heart-protective measure.

People who are overweight or obese are encouraged to lose weight through a combination of reduced calorie intake (maintaining a nutritionally sound diet) and increased exercise. High-protein, high-fat weight loss programs are not recommended for weight reduction.

### Exercise

Regular physical exercise reduces the risk for CHD in several ways. It lowers VLDL, LDL, and triglyceride levels, and raises HDL levels. Regular exercise reduces the blood pressure and insulin resistance. Unless contraindicated, all clients are encouraged to participate in at least 30 minutes of moderate-intensity physical activity 5 to 6 days each week.

### Hypertension

Although hypertension often cannot be prevented or cured, it can be controlled. Hypertension control (maintaining a blood pressure lower than 140/90 mmHg) is vital to reduce its atherosclerosis-promoting effects and to reduce the workload of the heart. Management strategies include reducing sodium intake, increasing calcium intake, regular exercise, stress management, and medications. Hypertension management is discussed in Chapter 33. ∞

### Diabetes

Diabetes increases the risk of CHD by accelerating the atherosclerotic process. Weight loss (if appropriate), reduced fat intake, and exercise are particularly important for the diabetic client. Because hyperglycemia apparently also contributes to atherosclerosis, consistent blood glucose management is vital.

| TABLE 29–4 Dietary Recommendations to Reduce Total Cholesterol, LDL Levels, and CHD Risk ||
| --- | --- |
| **Nutrient** | **Recommendation** |
| Total fat | 25%–35% of total calories |
| • Saturated fats | • <7% of total calories |
| • Polyunsaturated fat | • Up to 10% of total calories |
| • Monounsaturated fat | • Up to 20% of total calories |
| • Cholesterol | • <200 mg/day |
| Carbohydrate (primarily complex carbohydrates, such as whole grains, fruits, and vegetables) | 50%–60% of total calories |
| Dietary fiber | 20–30 g/day |
| Protein | About 15% of total calories |

*Note: Compiled from* Adult Treatment Panel III Report *by the National Cholesterol Education Program, 2001.*

## Medications

Drug therapy to lower total serum cholesterol and LDL levels and to raise HDL levels now is an integral part of CHD management. It is used in conjunction with diet and other lifestyle changes, and is based on the client's overall risk for CHD.

Drugs used to treat hyperlipidemia act specifically by lowering LDL levels. The goal of treatment is to achieve an LDL level of < 130 mg/dL. Medications to treat hyperlipidemia are not inexpensive; the cost–benefit ratio needs to be considered, as long-term treatment may be required. The four major classes of cholesterol-lowering drugs are statins, bile acid sequestrants, nicotinic acid, and fibrates. The nursing implications and client teaching for these drug classes are outlined in the Medication Administration box on the next page.

The statins, including lovastatin (Mevacor), pravastatin (Pravachol), simvastatin (Zocor), and others, are first-line drugs for treating hyperlipidemia. They effectively lower LDL levels and may also increase in HDL levels. The statins can cause myopathy; all clients are instructed to report muscle pain and weakness or brown urine. Liver function tests are monitored during therapy, as these drugs may increase liver enzyme levels.

The other cholesterol-lowering drugs, such as the bile acid sequestrants, nicotinic acid, and fibrates, are primarily used when combination therapy is required to effectively lower serum cholesterol levels. They also may be used for selected clients, such as younger adults, women who wish to become pregnant, or to specifically lower triglyceride levels.

Clients at high risk for MI are often started on prophylactic low-dose aspirin therapy. The dose ranges from 80 to 325 mg/day (Tierney et al., 2001). Aspirin is contraindicated, however, for clients who have a history of aspirin sensitivity, bleeding disorders, or active peptic ulcer disease. Angiotensin-converting enzyme (ACE) inhibitors also may be prescribed for high-risk clients, including diabetics with other CHD risk factors.

## Complementary Therapies

Diet and exercise programs that emphasize physical conditioning and a low-fat diet rich in antioxidants have been shown to be effective in managing CHD (Box 29–2). Supplements of vitamins C, E, $B_6$, $B_{12}$, and folic acid may be beneficial. Other potentially helpful complementary therapies include herbals such as ginkgo biloba, garlic, curcumin, and green tea; and consumption of red wine, foods containing bioflavonoids, and nuts. Behavioral therapies of benefit for clients with CHD include relaxation and stress management, guided imagery, treatment of depression, anger/hostility management, and meditation, tai chi, and yoga.

## NURSING CARE

### Health Promotion

Present information about healthy lifestyle habits to community and religious groups, school children (grades K through 12), and through the print media. In promoting healthy lifestyle habits, nurses can positively affect the incidence, morbidity, and mortality from CHD.

---

**BOX 29–2** ■ **Complementary Therapies: Diet for CHD**

Two diet programs have been shown to have a beneficial effect on CHD. The *Pritikin diet* is basically vegetarian, high in complex carbohydrates and fiber, low in cholesterol, and extremely low in fat (< 10% of daily calories). Egg whites and limited amounts of nonfat dairy or soy products are allowed. The Pritikin program requires 45 minutes of walking daily and recommends multivitamin supplements, including vitamins C and E and folate.

The *Ornish diet* also is vegetarian, although egg whites and a cup of nonfat milk or yogurt per day are allowed. No oil or fat is permitted, even for cooking. Two ounces of alcohol a day are permitted. The Ornish program also calls for stress reduction, emotional social support systems, daily stretching, and walking for 1 hour three times a week.

---

Strongly encourage all clients to avoid smoking in the first place, and to stop all forms of tobacco use. Discuss the adverse effects of smoking and the benefits of quitting. Provide information about dietary recommendations to maintain a healthy weight and optimal cholesterol levels. Discuss the benefits and importance of regular exercise. Finally, encourage clients with cardiovascular risk factors to undergo regular screening for hypertension, diabetes, and hyperlipidemia.

### Assessment

Nursing assessment for CHD focuses on identifying risk factors.

- Health history: current manifestations such as chest pain or heaviness, shortness of breath, weakness; current diet, exercise patterns, and medications; smoking history and pattern of alcohol intake; history of heart disease, hypertension, or diabetes; family history of CHD or other cardiac problems
- Physical examination: current weight and its appropriateness for height; body mass index; waist-to-hip ratio; blood pressure; strength and equality of peripheral pulses

### Nursing Diagnoses and Interventions

#### Imbalanced Nutrition: More than Body Requirements

This nursing diagnosis may be appropriate for clients who are obese, have a waist-to-hip ratio greater than 0.8 (female) or 0.9 (male), or whose diet history or serum cholesterol levels indicate a need to reduce fat and cholesterol intake. See Chapters 19 and 20 for more information about assessing obesity.

- Encourage assessment of food intake and eating patterns to help identify areas that can be improved. *Clients often are unaware of their fat and cholesterol intake, particularly when many meals are eaten away from home. Careful assessment increases awareness and allows the client to make conscious changes.*
- Discuss American Heart Association and therapeutic lifestyle change (TLC) dietary recommendations, emphasizing the role of diet in heart disease. Provide guidance regarding specific food choices with healthy alternatives. *Specific diet information and suggestions help the client make better food choices.*

# Medication Administration

## Cholesterol-Lowering Drugs

### STATINS

> Lovastatin (Mevacor)
> Pravastatin (Pravachol)
> Simvastatin (Zocor)
> Fluvastatin (Lescol)
> Atorvastatin (Lipitor)

Statins inhibit the enzyme HMG-CoA reductase in the liver, lowering LDL synthesis and serum levels. The statins are first-line treatment for elevated LDL, used in conjunction with diet and lifestyle changes. Although their side effects are minimal, they may cause increased serum liver enzyme levels and myopathy.

#### Nursing Responsibilities
- Monitor serum cholesterol and liver enzyme levels before and during therapy. Report elevated liver enzyme levels.
- Assess for muscle pain and tenderness. Monitor CPK level if present.
- If taking digoxin concurrently, monitor for and report digoxin toxicity.

#### Client and Family Teaching
- Promptly report muscle pain, tenderness, or weakness; skin rash or hives, or changes in skin color; abdominal pain, nausea, or vomiting.
- Do not use these drugs if you are pregnant or plan to become pregnant.
- Inform your doctor if you are taking any other medications concurrently.

### BILE ACID SEQUESTRANTS

> Cholestyramine (Questran)
> Colestipol (Colestid)
> Colesevelam (Welchol)

Bile acid sequestrants lower LDL levels by binding bile acids in the intestine, reducing its reabsorption and cholesterol production in the liver. They are used in combination therapy regimens and for women who are considering pregnancy. Their primary disadvantages are inconvenience of administration due to bulk and gastrointestinal side effects such as constipation.

#### Nursing Responsibilities
- Mix cholestyramine and colestipol powders with 4 to 6 oz of water or juice; administer once or twice a day as ordered with meals.
- Store in a tightly closed container.

#### Client and Family Teaching
- Promptly report constipation, severe gastric distress with nausea and vomiting, unexplained weight loss, black or bloody stools, or sudden back pain to your doctor.
- Drinking ample amounts of fluid while taking these drugs reduces problems of constipation and bloating.
- Do not omit doses as this may affect the absorption of other drugs you are taking.

### NICOTINIC ACID

> Niacin (Nicobid, Nicolar, Niaspan, others)

Nicotinic acid in both prescription and nonprescription forms lowers total and LDL cholesterol and triglyceride levels. The crystalline form and Niaspan, a prescription extended release tablet, also raise HDL levels. Because the doses required to achieve significant cholesterol-lowering effects are associated with multiple side effects, nicotinic acid generally is used in combination therapy, particularly with the statin drugs.

#### Nursing Responsibilities
- Give oral preparations with meals and accompanied by a cold beverage to minimize GI effects.
- Administer with caution to clients with active liver disease, peptic ulcer disease, gout, or type 2 diabetes.
- Monitor blood glucose, uric acid levels, and liver function tests during treatment.

#### Client and Family Teaching
- Flushing of face, neck, and ears may occur within 2 hours following dose; these effects generally subside as treatment continues. Alcohol use during nicotinic acid therapy may worsen this effect.
- Report weakness or dizziness with changes in posture (lying to sitting; sitting to standing) to your doctor. Change positions slowly to reduce the risk of injury.

### FIBRIC ACID DERIVATIVES

> Gemfibrozil (Lopid)
> Fenofibrate (Tricor)
> Clofibrate (Atromid-S)

The fibrates are used to lower serum triglyceride levels; they have only a slight to modest effect on LDL. They affect lipid regulation by blocking triglyceride synthesis. They are used to treat very high triglyceride levels, and may be used in combination with statins.

#### Nursing Responsibilities
- Monitor serum LDL and VLDL levels, electrolytes, glucose, liver enzymes, renal function tests, and CBC during therapy. Report abnormal values.
- Up to 2 months of treatment may be required to achieve a therapeutic effect; rebound, with decreasing benefit, may occur in the second or third month of treatment.

#### Client and Family Teaching
- Take with meals if the drug causes gastric distress.
- Promptly report flulike symptoms (fatigue, muscle aching, soreness, or weakness) to your doctor.
- Do not use this drug if you are pregnant or plan to become pregnant. Use reliable birth control measures while taking this drug.
- Contact your doctor before stopping this drug and before taking any over-the-counter preparations.

- Refer to clinical dietitian for diet planning and further teaching. Suggest cookbooks that offer low-fat recipes to encourage healthier eating, and provide American Heart Association and American Cancer Society recipe pamphlets and information on low-fat eating. *These resources provide tools for the client to use as eating patterns change.*
- Encourage gradual but progressive dietary changes. *Drastic changes in eating patterns may cause frustration and discourage the client from maintaining a healthy diet over the long term.*
- Discourage use of high-fat, low-carbohydrate, or other fad diets for weight loss. *These diets may adversely affect serum cholesterol and triglyceride levels, and often are too drastic to maintain over the long term.*
- Encourage reasonable goals for weight loss (e.g., 1.0 to 1.5 lb per week and a 10% weight loss over 6 months). Provide information about weight loss programs and support groups such as Weight Watchers and Take Off Pounds Sensibly (TOPS). *Gradual but steady weight loss is more likely to be sustained. Recognized programs that emphasize healthy eating provide support and incentive for making lifetime dietary changes.*

### Ineffective Health Maintenance

Clients with risk factors for CHD may be unable to identify or independently manage their risk factors.

- Discuss risk factors for CHD, stressing that changing or managing those factors that can be modified reduces the client's overall risk for the disease. *Clients with significant nonmodifiable risk factors may be discouraged, reducing their ability to eliminate or control modifiable risk factors.*
- Discuss the immediate benefits of smoking cessation. Provide resource materials from the American Heart Association, the American Lung Association, and the American Cancer Society. Refer to a structured smoking cessation program to increase the likelihood of success in quitting. *Long-time smokers may assume that the damage from smoking has already been done, and quitting would not be "worth the price."*
- Help the client identify specific sources of psychosocial and physical support for smoking cessation, dietary, and lifestyle changes. *Support persons, groups, and aids such as nicotine patches help the client achieve success and provide encouragement during difficult times (such as withdrawal symptoms).*
- Discuss the benefits of regular exercise for cardiovascular health and weight loss. Help identify favorite forms of exercise or physical activity. Encourage planning for 30 minutes of continuous aerobic activity (i.e., walking, running, bicycling, swimming) four to five times a week. Encourage identification of an "exercise buddy" to help maintain motivation. *Engaging in preferred activities with a partner maintains motivation and increases the likelihood of maintaining an exercise program. Encourage continuation of the plan, even when days are missed. Exercise is cumulative, so increasing the duration of exercise on subsequent days can "make up" for a lost day.*
- Provide information and teaching about prescribed medications such as cholesterol-lowering drugs. Discuss the relationship between hypertension, diabetes, and CHD. *Teaching is important to promote understanding of and compliance with the prescribed drug regimen.*

## Home Care

Encourage participation in some form of cardiac rehabilitation program. Formal programs provide comprehensive assessment of, interventions for, and teaching of clients with cardiac disease. Monitored exercise and information about risk factors help clients identify ways to lower their risk for CHD.

Because clients themselves are primarily responsible for maintaining the lifestyle changes necessary to reduce the risk of CHD, provide teaching and support as outlined in the previous section. Assist the client to make healthy choices and reinforce positive changes. Emphasize the importance of regular follow-up appointments to monitor progress.

## THE CLIENT WITH ANGINA PECTORIS

**Angina pectoris,** or *angina,* is chest pain resulting from reduced coronary blood flow, which causes a temporary imbalance between myocardial blood supply and demand. The imbalance may be due to coronary heart disease, atherosclerosis, or vessel constriction that impairs myocardial blood supply. Hypermetabolic conditions such as exercise, thyrotoxicosis, stimulant abuse (e.g., cocaine), hyperthyroidism, and emotional stress can increase myocardial oxygen demand, precipitating angina. Anemia, heart failure, or pulmonary diseases may affect blood and oxygen supplies as well, causing angina.

## PATHOPHYSIOLOGY

The imbalance between myocardial blood supply and demand causes temporary and reversible myocardial ischemia. **Ischemia,** deficient blood flow to tissue, may be caused by partial obstruction of a coronary artery, coronary artery spasm, or a thrombus. Obstruction of a coronary artery deprives cells in the region of the heart normally supplied by that vessel of oxygen and nutrients needed for metabolic processes. Cellular processes are compromised. Reduced oxygen causes cells to switch from aerobic metabolism to anaerobic metabolism. Anaerobic metabolism causes lactic acid to build up in the cells. It also affects cell membrane permeability, releasing substances such as histamine, kinins, and specific enzymes that stimulate terminal nerve fibers in the cardiac muscle and send pain impulses to the central nervous system. The pain radiates to the upper body because the heart shares the same dermatome as this region. Return of adequate circulation provides the nutrients needed by cells, and clears the waste products. More than 30 minutes of ischemia irreversibly damages myocardial cells (necrosis).

Three types of angina have been identified:

- *Stable angina* is the most common and predictable form of angina. It occurs with a predictable amount of activity or stress, and is a common manifestation of CHD. Stable angina usually occurs when the work of the heart is increased by physical exertion, exposure to cold, or by stress. Stable angina is relieved by rest and nitrates.

- *Prinzmetal's (variant) angina* is atypical angina that occurs unpredictably (unrelated to activity), and often at night. It is caused by coronary artery spasm with or without an atherosclerotic lesion. The exact mechanism of coronary artery spasm is unknown. It may result from hyperactive sympathetic nervous system responses, altered calcium flow in smooth muscle, or reduced prostaglandins to promote vasodilation.
- *Unstable angina* occurs with increasing frequency, severity, and duration. Pain is unpredictable and occurs with decreasing levels of activity or stress and may occur at rest. Clients with unstable angina are at risk for myocardial infarction.
- *Silent myocardial ischemia,* or asymptomatic ischemia, is thought to be common in people with CHD. Silent ischemia may occur with either activity or with mental stress. Mental stress increases the heart rate and blood pressure, increasing myocardial oxygen demand (McCance & Huether, 2002).

## MANIFESTATIONS

The cardinal manifestation of angina is chest pain. The pain typically is precipitated by an identifiable event, such as physical activity, strong emotion, stress, eating a heavy meal, or exposure to cold. The classic sequence of angina is activity–pain, rest–relief. The client may describe the pain as a tight, squeezing, heavy pressure, or constricting sensation. It characteristically begins beneath the sternum and may radiate to the jaw, neck, or arm. Less characteristically, the pain may be felt in the jaw, epigastric region, or back. Anginal pain usually lasts less than 15 minutes and is relieved by rest. Additional manifestations of angina include dyspnea, pallor, tachycardia, and great anxiety and fear. The manifestations of angina are summarized in the box below.

## COLLABORATIVE CARE

Acute angina care focuses on relieving pain and restoring coronary blood flow. Long-term management is directed at the causes of impaired myocardial blood supply. As for CHD, risk factor management is a vital component of care for the client with angina (see the preceding section of this chapter).

### Manifestations of Angina

- Chest pain: Substernal or precordial (across the chest wall); may radiate to neck, arms, shoulders, or jaw
- Quality: Tight, squeezing, constricting, or heavy sensation; may also be described as burning, aching, choking, dull, or constant
- Associated manifestations: Dyspnea, pallor, tachycardia, anxiety, and fear
- Precipitating factors: Exercise or activity, strong emotion, stress, cold, heavy meal
- Relieving factors: Rest, position change; nitroglycerine

## Diagnostic Tests

The diagnosis of angina is based on past medical history and family history, a comprehensive description of the chest pain, and physical assessment findings. Laboratory tests may confirm the presence of risk factors, such as an abnormal blood lipid profile and elevated blood glucose. Diagnostic tests provide information about overall cardiac function.

Common diagnostic tests to assess for coronary heart disease and angina include electrocardiography, stress testing, nuclear medicine studies, echocardiography (ultrasound), and coronary angiography.

### Electrocardiography

A resting ECG may be normal, may show nonspecific changes in the ST segment and T wave, or may show evidence of previous myocardial infarction. Characteristic ECG changes are seen during anginal episodes. During periods of ischemia, the ST segment is depressed or downsloping, and the T wave may flatten or invert (Figure 29–1 ■). These changes reverse when ischemia is relieved. For more details about the ECG, its waveforms, and its uses, see the section of this chapter about dysrhythmias.

### Stress Electrocardiography

Stress electrocardiography (exercise stress test) uses ECGs to monitor the cardiac response to an increased workload during progressive exercise. See the previous section on coronary heart disease for more information about exercise stress tests.

### Radionuclide Testing

Radionuclide testing is a safe, noninvasive technique to evaluate myocardial perfusion and left ventricular function. The

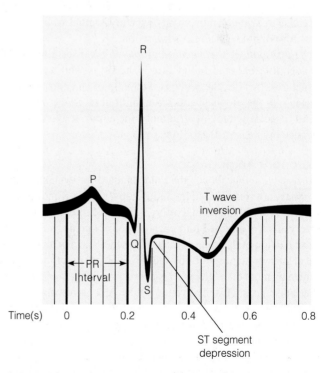

**Figure 29–1 ■** ECG changes during an episode of angina. Note characteristic T wave inversion and ST segment depression of myocardial ischemia.

amount of radioisotope injected is very small; no special radiation precautions are required during or after the scan. Thallium-201 or a technetium-based radiocompound is injected intravenously, and the heart is scanned with a radiation detector. Ischemic or infarcted cells of the myocardium do not take up the substance normally, appearing as a "cold spot" on the scan. If the ischemia is transient, these spots gradually fill in, indicating the reversibility of the process. With severe ischemia or a myocardial infarction, these areas may remain devoid of radioactivity.

Left ventricular function can also be evaluated. Whereas the ejection fraction, or portion of blood ejected from the left ventricle during systole, normally increases during exercise, it may actually decrease in coronary heart disease and stress-induced ischemia.

Radionuclide testing may be combined with pharmacologic stress testing for clients who are physically unable to exercise or to detect subclinical myocardial ischemia. A vasodilator is injected to induce the same ischemic changes that occur with exercise in the diseased heart. Coronary arteries unaffected by atherosclerosis dilate in response to the drugs, increasing blood flow to already well-perfused tissue. This reduces flow to ischemic muscle, called *myocardial steal syndrome.*

## Echocardiography

*Echocardiography* is a noninvasive test that uses ultrasound to evaluate cardiac structure and function. High-frequency sound waves emitted from a transducer are reflected off of heart structures back to the transducer as echoes. These echoes are displayed on a screen. Echocardiography is usually performed with the transducer held to the chest wall. It may be done at rest, during supine exercise, or immediately following upright exercise to evaluate movement of the myocardial wall and assess for possible ischemia or infarction.

*Transesophageal echocardiography (TEE)* uses ultrasound to identify abnormal blood flow patterns as well as cardiac structures. In TEE, the probe is on the tip of an endoscope inserted into the esophagus, positioning it close to the posterior heart (especially the left atrium and the aorta). It avoids interference by breasts, ribs, or lungs.

## Coronary Angiography

*Coronary angiography* is the gold standard for evaluating the coronary arteries. Guided by fluoroscopy, a catheter introduced into the femoral or brachial artery is threaded into the coronary artery. Dye is injected into each coronary opening, allowing visualization of the main coronary branches and any abnormalities, such as stenosis or obstruction. Narrowing of the vessel lumen by more than 50% is considered significant; most lesions that cause symptoms involve more than 70% narrowing. Vessel obstructions are noted on a coronary artery "map" that provides a guide for tracking disease progression and for elective treatment with angioplasty or cardiac surgery. During angiogram, the drug ergonovine maleate may be injected to induce coronary artery spasm and diagnose Prinzmetal's angina. Nursing care of the client undergoing a coronary angiogram is summarized in the box on the next page.

## Medications

Drugs may be used for both acute and long-term relief of angina. The goal of drug treatment is to reduce oxygen demand and increase oxygen supply to the myocardium. Three main classes of drugs are used to treat angina: nitrates, beta blockers, and calcium channel blockers.

### Nitrates

Nitrates, including nitroglycerin and longer-acting nitrate preparations, are used to treat acute anginal attacks and prevent angina.

Sublingual nitroglycerin is the drug of choice to treat acute angina. It acts within 1 to 2 minutes, decreasing myocardial work and oxygen demand through venous and arterial dilation, which in turn reduce preload and afterload. It may also improve myocardial oxygen supply by dilating collateral blood vessels and reducing stenosis. Rapid-acting nitroglycerin is also available as a buccal spray in a metered system. For some clients, this may be easier to handle than small nitroglycerin tablets.

Longer-acting nitroglycerin preparations (oral tablets, ointment, or transdermal patches) are used to prevent attacks of angina, not to treat an acute attack. The primary problem with long-term nitrate use is the development of *tolerance,* a decreasing effect from the same dose of medication. Tolerance can be limited by a dosing schedule that allows a nitrate-free period of at least 8 to 10 hours daily. This is usually scheduled at night, when angina is less likely to occur.

Headache is a common side effect of nitrates, and may limit their usefulness. Nausea, dizziness, and hypotension are also common effects of therapy.

### Beta Blockers

Beta blockers, including propranolol, metoprolol, nadolol, and atenolol, are considered first-line drugs to treat stable angina. They block the cardiac-stimulating effects of norepinephrine and epinephrine, preventing anginal attacks by reducing heart rate, myocardial contractility, and blood pressure, thus reducing myocardial oxygen demand. Beta blockers may be used alone or with other medications to prevent angina.

Beta blockers are contraindicated for clients with asthma or severe COPD (see Chapter 36 ) because they may cause severe bronchospasm. They are not used in clients with significant bradycardia, or AV conduction blocks, and are used cautiously in heart failure, Beta blockers are not used to treat Prinzmetal's angina because they may make it worse.

### Calcium Channel Blockers

Calcium channel blockers reduce myocardial oxygen demand and increase myocardial blood and oxygen supply. These drugs, which include verapamil, diltiazem, and nifedipine, lower blood pressure, reduce myocardial contractility, and, in some cases, lower the heart rate, decreasing myocardial oxygen demand. They are also potent coronary vasodilators, effectively increasing oxygen supply. Like beta blockers, calcium channel blockers act too slowly to effectively treat an acute attack of angina; they are used for long-term prophylaxis. Because they may actually increase ischemia and mortality in clients with heart failure or left ventricular dysfunction, these drugs are not usually prescribed in

# NURSING CARE OF THE CLIENT HAVING CORONARY ANGIOGRAPHY

## PREOPERATIVE CARE

- Assess the client's and family's knowledge and understanding of the procedure. Provide additional information as needed. Explain that the client will be awake during the procedure, which takes 1 to 2 hours to complete. A sensation of warmth (a "hot flash") and a metallic taste may occur as the dye is injected. A rapid pulse or a few "skipped beats," also are common and expected during the procedure. *A good understanding of the procedure and expected sensations reduces anxiety and improves cooperation during the procedure.*
- Provide routine preoperative care as ordered (see Chapter 7). ∞ *Although the client remains awake, sedation may be given. Signed consent is required, and preprocedure fasting may be ordered.*
- Administer ordered cardiac medications with a small sip of water unless contraindicated. *Regularly ordered medications are continued to prevent cardiac compromise or dysrhythmias during the procedure.*
- Assess for hypersensitivity to iodine, radiologic contrast media, or seafood. *An iodine-based radiologic contrast dye is typically used for an angiogram. Iodine or seafood allergy increases the risk for anaphylaxis and requires an alternative dye or special precautions.*
- Record baseline assessment data, including vital signs, height, and weight. Mark the locations of peripheral pulses; document their equality and amplitude. *The data provide a baseline for evaluating changes after the procedure.*
- Instruct to void prior to going to the cardiac catheterization laboratory, *to promote comfort.*

## POSTOPERATIVE CARE

- Assess vital signs, catheterization site for bleeding or hematoma, peripheral pulses, and neurovascular status every 15 minutes for first hour, every 30 minutes for the next hour, then hourly for 4 hours or until discharge. *The data provide vital information about the client's status and potential complications such as bleeding, hematoma, or thrombus formation.*
- Maintain bed rest as ordered, usually for 6 hours if the femoral artery is used, or 2 to 3 hours if the brachial site is used. The head of the bed may be raised to 30 degrees. *Bed rest reduces movement of and pressure in the affected artery, reducing the risk of bleeding or hematoma.*
- Keep a pressure dressing, sandbag, or ice pack in place over the arterial access site. Check frequently for bleeding (if the access site is in the groin, check for bleeding under the buttocks). *Arteries are high-pressure systems. The risk for significant bleeding after an invasive procedure is high.*
- Instruct to avoid flexing or hyperextending the affected extremity for 12 to 24 hours. *Minimizing movement of the affected joint allows the artery to effectively seal and promotes blood flow, reducing the risk of bleeding, hematoma, or thrombus formation.*
- Unless contraindicated, encourage liberal fluid intake. *An increased fluid intake promotes excretion of the contrast medium, reducing the risk of toxicity (particularly to the kidneys).*
- Promptly report diminished peripheral pulses, formation of a new hematoma or enlargement of an existing one, severe pain at the insertion site or in the affected extremity, chest pain, or dyspnea. *While the risk of complications is low, myocardial infarction or insertion site complications may occur. These necessitate prompt intervention.*
- Provide instructions about dressing changes, follow-up appointments, and potential complications prior to discharge.

the initial treatment of angina. They are used cautiously in clients with dysrhythmias, heart failure, or hypotension.

The nursing implications of antianginal medications are summarized in the Medication Administration box on page 818.

## Aspirin

The client with angina, particularly unstable angina, is at risk for myocardial infarction because of significant narrowing of the coronary arteries. Low-dose aspirin (80 to 325 mg/day) is often prescribed to reduce the risk of platelet aggregation and thrombus formation.

## Revascularization Procedures

Several procedures may be used to restore blood flow and oxygen to ischemic tissue. Nonsurgical techniques include transluminal coronary angioplasty, laser angioplasty, coronary atherectomy, and intracoronary stents. Coronary artery bypass grafting (CABG) is a surgical procedure that may be used.

### Percutaneous Coronary Revascularization

*Percutaneous coronary revascularization (PCR)* are procedures used to restore blood flow to the ischemic myocardium in clients with CHD. Approximately 600,000 PCR procedures are done annually in the United States. PCR is used to treat clients with:

- Moderately severe, chronic stable angina unrelieved by medical therapy.
- Mild angina but objective evidence of coronary ischemia.
- Unstable angina.
- Acute myocardial infarction (Braunwald et al., 2001).

PCR procedures are similar to the procedure used for coronary angiography. A catheter introduced into the arterial circulation is guided into the opening of the narrowed coronary artery. A flexible guidewire is inserted through the catheter lumen into the affected vessel. The guidewire is then used to thread an angioplasty balloon, arterial stent, or other therapeutic device into the narrowed segment of the artery. The procedure is performed

# Medication Administration

## Antianginal Medications

### ORGANIC NITRATES

Nitroglycerin (Nitropaste, Nitro-Dur, Nitro-Bid, Nitrol, Transderm-Nitro, Nitrogard, Nitrodisc, Tridil)

Isosorbide dinitrate (Isordil)

Isosorbide mononitrate (ISMO)

Amyl nitrite

Nitrates dilate both arterial and venous vessels, depending on the dose. Coronary artery vasodilation increases blood flow and myocardial oxygen supply. Venous dilation allows peripheral blood pooling, reducing venous return, preload, and cardiac work. Arterial dilation reduces vascular resistance and afterload, also reducing cardiac work. Sublingual nitroglycerin (NTG) tablets are used to treat and prevent acute anginal attacks (when taken prophylactically before activity). Nitrates are administered sublingually, by buccal spray, or intravenously for immediate effect; or orally or topically for sustained effect.

#### Nursing Responsibilities

- Dilute intravenous nitroglycerin before infusing; use only glass bottles for the mixture. Nitroglycerin adheres to PVC bags and tubing, affecting the amount of drug that is delivered. Use non-PVC infusion tubing.
- Wear gloves when applying nitroglycerin paste or ointment to prevent absorbing the drug through the skin. Measure dose carefully and spread evenly in a 2-by-3 inch area.
- Remove nitroglycerin patches or ointment at night to help prevent tolerance.

#### Client and Family Teaching

- Use only the sublingual, buccal, and spray forms of nitrates to treat acute angina.
- If the first nitrate dose does not relieve angina within 5 minutes, take a second dose. After 5 more minutes, you may take a third dose if needed. If the pain is unrelieved or lasts for 20 minutes or longer, seek medical assistance immediately.
- Carry a supply of nitroglycerin tablets with you. Dissolve sublingual nitroglycerin tablets under the tongue or between the upper lip and gum. Do not eat, drink, or smoke until the tablet is completely dissolved.
- Keep sublingual tablets in their original amber glass bottle to protect them from heat, light, and moisture. Replace your supply every 6 months.
- You may experience a burning or tingling sensation under the tongue and develop a transient headache when you take the drug. These are expected; the headache will diminish over time.
- Use caution when standing from a sitting position; nitroglycerine may make you lightheaded.
- Rotate ointment or transdermal patch application sites. Apply to a hairless area; spread ointment evenly without rubbing or massaging. Remove the patch or residual ointment at bedtime daily. Apply a fresh dose in the morning.
- If you are using a long-acting nitrate, keep a supply of immediate-acting nitrates to treat acute angina.

### BETA BLOCKERS

Atenolol (Tenormin)

Metoprolol (Lopressor)

Propranolol (Inderal)

Nadolol (Corgard)

Beta blockers decrease cardiac workload by blocking beta receptors on the heart muscle, decreasing heart rate, contractility, myocardial oxygen consumption, and blood pressure. Beta blockers also reduce *reflex tachycardia*, which may develop with other antianginal drugs. Beta blockers are frequently prescribed as antianginal and antihypertensive agents.

#### Nursing Responsibilities

- Document heart rate and blood pressure before administering the medication. Withhold drug if the heart rate is below 50 BPM or the blood pressure is below prescribed limits. Notify the physician.
- Assess for and report possible contraindications to therapy, including heart failure, bradycardia, AV block, asthma, or COPD.
- Do not abruptly discontinue these drugs after long-term therapy, as this can increase heart rate, contractility, and blood pressure, and cause fatal dysrhythmia, myocardial infarction, or stroke.

#### Client and Family Teaching

- Beta blockers help prevent angina but will not relieve an acute attack. Keep a supply of fast-acting nitrates on hand for acute anginal attacks.
- Do not suddenly stop taking this medication. Discuss discontinuing this medication with your doctor.
- Take your pulse daily. Do not take the drug, and contact your doctor if your heart rate is below 50 BPM. Check your blood pressure frequently.
- Report a slow or irregular pulse, swelling or weight gain, or difficulty breathing to your doctor.

### CALCIUM CHANNEL BLOCKERS

Nifedipine (Adalat, Procardia)

Diltiazem (Cardizem)

Verapamil (Isoptin, Calan)

Bepridil (Vascor)

Felodipine (Plendil)

Isradipine (DynaCirc)

Nicardipine (Cardene)

Nimodipine (Nimotop)

Calcium channel blockers are used to control angina, hypertension, and dysrhythmias. By blocking the entry of calcium into cells, these drugs reduce contractility, slow the heart rate and conduction, and cause vasodilation. Calcium channel blockers increase myocardial oxygen supply by dilating the coronary arteries; they decrease the workload of the heart by lowering vascular resistance and oxygen demand. Calcium channel blockers are often prescribed for clients with coronary artery spasm (Prinzmetal's angina).

#### Nursing Responsibilities

- Do not mix verapamil in any solution containing sodium bicarbonate. Administer IV push verapamil over 2 to 3 minutes.
- Document blood pressure and heart rate before administering the drug. Withhold the drug if the heart rate is below 50 BPM. Notify the physician.

## Medication Administration

### Antianginal Medications (continued)

- The nifedipine capsule may be punctured and administered by extracting the liquid with a syringe and squirting the dose under the client's tongue (discard the needle first!).
- Use caution when giving a calcium channel blocker with other cardiac depressants, such as beta blockers. Concomitant administration with nitrates may cause excessive vasodilation.
- Manifestations of toxicity include nausea, generalized weakness, signs of decreased cardiac output, hypotension, bradycardia, and AV block. Report these findings immediately. Maintain intravenous access, and slowly administer intravenous calcium chlo-

ride. Do not infuse large volumes of fluid to treat hypotension as heart failure may result.

#### Client and Family Teaching

- Take your pulse before taking the drug. Do not take the drug and notify physician if your heart rate drops below 50 BPM.
- Keep a fresh supply of immediate-acting nitrate available to treat acute anginal attacks. Calcium channel blockers will not work fast enough to relieve an acute attack.

---

in the cardiac catheterization laboratory using local anesthesia. The hospital stay is short (1 to 2 days), minimizing costs.

For *balloon angioplasty* (also called percutaneous transluminal coronary angioplasty or PTCA), a balloon-tipped catheter is threaded over the guidewire, with the balloon positioned across the area of narrowing (Figure 29–2 ■). The balloon is inflated in a step-by-step fashion for about 30 seconds to 2 minutes to compress the plaque against the arterial wall, with a goal of reducing the vessel obstruction to less than 50% of the arterial lumen. When used alone, balloon angioplasty is associated with a relatively high risk of abrupt vessel closure and restenosis. Its primary current use is in combination with stent placement or atherectomy.

*Intracoronary stents* are metallic scaffolds used to maintain an open arterial lumen. Stents reduce the rate of restenosis following angioplasty by about one-third, and are now used in 70% to 80% of all PCR procedures (Braunwald et al., 2001). The stent is placed over a balloon catheter, guided into position, and expanded as the balloon is inflated (Figure 29–3 ■). It then remains in the artery as a prop after the

balloon is removed. Endothelial cells will completely line the inner wall of the stent to produce a smooth inner lining. Antiplatelet medications (aspirin and ticlopidine) are given following stent insertion to reduce the risk of thrombus formation at the site.

In contrast to balloon and stent procedures which enlarge the artery by displacing plaque, *atherectomy* procedures remove plaque from the identified lesion. The directional atherectomy catheter shaves the plaque off vessel walls using a rotary cutting head, retaining the fragments in its housing and removing them from the vessel. Rotational atherectomy catheters pulverize plaque into particles small enough to pass through the coronary microcirculation. Laser atherectomy devices use laser energy to remove plaque.

Complications following PCR procedures include hematoma at the catheter insertion site, pseudoaneurysm, embolism, hypersensitivity to contrast dye, dysrhythmias, bleeding, vessel perforation, and restenosis, or reocclusion of the treated vessel.

Nursing care of the client undergoing PCR is outlined in the box on the next page.

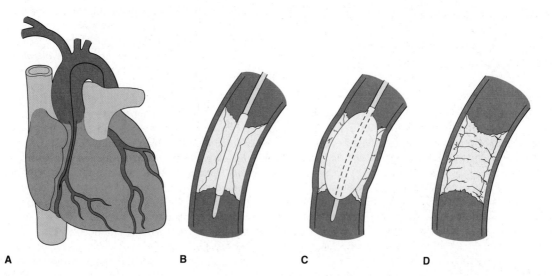

**Figure 29–2** ■ Balloon Angioplasty. *A,* The balloon catheter is threaded into the affected coronary artery. *B,* The balloon is positioned across the area of obstruction. *C,* The balloon is then inflated, flattening the plaque against the arterial wall, *D.*

**Figure 29–3** ■ Placement of the balloon expandable intracoronary stent. *A,* The stainless steel stent is fitted over a balloon-tipped catheter. *B,* The stent is positioned along the blockage and expanded. *C,* The balloon is deflated and removed, leaving the stent in place.

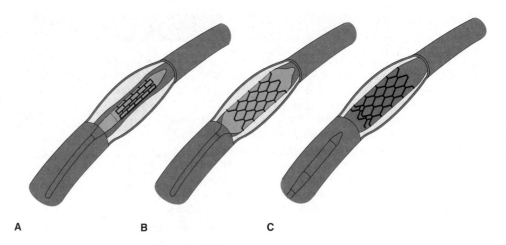

A　　　　B　　　　C

## Coronary Artery Bypass Grafting

Surgery for coronary heart disease involves using a section of a vein or an artery to create a connection (or bypass) between the aorta and the coronary artery beyond the obstruction (Figure 29–4 ■). This then allows blood to perfuse the ischemic portion of the heart. The internal mammary artery in the chest and the saphenous vein from the leg are the vessels most commonly used for coronary artery bypass grafting (CABG).

Bypass grafts are safe and effective. Angina is totally relieved or significantly reduced in 90% of clients who undergo

# NURSING CARE   OF THE CLIENT HAVING PCR

## BEFORE THE PROCEDURE

- Assess knowledge of the procedure and expectations of treatment. *This allows information to be tailored to the client's needs and provides an opportunity to clarify misconceptions.*
- Describe the cardiac catheterization laboratory and the planned PCR procedure, including:
  - Preoperative preparation (see Chapter 7). ⊖⊖
  - Planned anesthesia or sedation to be used.
  - Drugs that may be given during the procedure, such as anticoagulants to reduce the risk of thrombus formation, and intravenous nitroglycerine and a calcium channel blocker to dilate coronary arteries and prevent anginal pain.
- Discuss possible sensations during the procedure, including flushing or warmth and a metallic taste in the mouth as the contrast dye is injected, and a feeling of pressure or chest pain during balloon inflation. *Advanced preparation for expected sensations reduces anxiety and improves outcomes.*

## AFTER THE PROCEDURE

- Complete a head-to-toe assessment. Note any complaints of chest pain, or evidence of decreased cardiac output or myocardial infarction. *Assessment provides a baseline for subsequent assessments and allows early identification of possible complications.*
- Monitor vital signs and cardiac rhythm continuously. Treat dysrhythmias as ordered. Obtain a 12-lead ECG if signs of ischemia develop, and notify physician. *Vital signs reflect cardiac output. Dysrhythmias may develop with reperfusion of the ischemic myocardium. ECG changes may indicate infarction or restenosis of the affected vessel.*
- Maintain intravenous nitroglycerin infusion. Administer anticoagulant and antiplatelet medications, nitrates, and calcium channel blockers as ordered. *These drugs decrease oxygen de-*

*mand and increase oxygen supply by dilating the coronary arteries and systemic vasculature. They also reduce the risk of thrombus formation.*
- Monitor for and treat or report chest pain as indicated. *Chest pain may indicate ischemia and possible myocardial infarction.*
- Maintain bed rest as ordered with the head of the bed at 30 degrees or less. Prevent flexion of the leg on the affected side. Following sheath removal, follow protocol for pressure dressing or device or sandbag placement. *A large puncture wound occurs at the insertion site. Immobilization allows the wound to seal; a pressure dressing helps prevent bleeding.*
- Monitor distal pulses, color, movement, sensation, and temperature of the affected leg, and insertion site every 15 minutes for the first hour, every 30 minutes for the next hour, every hour for the next 8 hours, then every 4 hours. *A clot may form at the site, reducing perfusion of the affected leg. The site and dressing are monitored for excessive bleeding hematoma formation, or pseudoaneurysm. Pseudoaneurysm occurs as a result of inadequate hemostasis after catheter removal.*
- Monitor intake and output, serum electrolytes, blood urea nitrogen (BUN), creatinine, complete blood count (CBC), partial thromboplastin time (PTT), and cardiac enzymes. Report abnormal results to the physician. *Contrast dye causes osmotic diuresis and may cause renal damage or a hypersensitivity reaction. Electrolyte imbalances increase the risk of dysrhythmias. Cardiac enzymes are monitored for indications of possible myocardial damage during the procedure. The PTT monitors the effectiveness of heparin therapy.*
- Monitor for bradycardia, lightheadedness, hypotension, diaphoresis, and loss of consciousness during sheath removal. Keep atropine at bedside during sheath removal. *Bradycardia and signs of decreased cardiac output may occur during sheath removal because of a vasovagal reaction. Atropine decreases vagal tone and increases heart rate.*

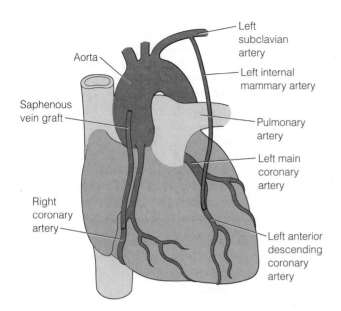

**Figure 29–4** ■ Coronary artery bypass grafting using the internal mammary artery and a saphenous vein graft.

complete revascularization. While anginal pain may recur within 3 years, it rarely is as severe as before surgery. Coronary artery bypass graft has a positive effect on mortality in many cases. It is recommended for clients who have multiple vessel disease and impaired left ventricular function or diabetes, and for clients who have significant obstruction of the left main coronary artery (Braunwald et al., 2001).

A median sternotomy is used to access the heart. The heart is usually stopped during surgery. The *cardiopulmonary bypass (CPB) pump* is used to maintain perfusion to the rest of the organs during open-heart surgery. Venous blood is removed from the body through a cannula placed in the right atrium or the superior and inferior venae cavae. Blood then circulates through the CPB pump, where it is oxygenated, its temperature regulated, and is filtered. Oxygenated blood is returned to the body through a cannula in the ascending aorta (Figure 29–5 ■). Cardiopulmonary bypass enables surgeons to operate on a quiet heart and a relatively bloodless field. Hypothermia can be maintained to reduce the metabolic rate and decrease oxygen demand during surgery.

When the saphenous vein is used, it is excised from its normal attachments in the leg, flushed with a cold heparinized saline solution, and then reversed so that its valves do not interfere with blood flow. It is *anastomosed* (grafted) to the aorta and the coronary artery, distal to the occlusion (see Figure 29–5). This provides a bridge or conduit for blood flow past the obstruction. If the internal mammary artery (IMA) is used, its distal end is excised and anatomosed to the coronary artery distal to the obstruction. The IMA often is used to revascularize the left coronary artery because of the greater oxygen demand of the left ventricle.

Once grafting is completed, cardiopulmonary bypass is discontinued and the client is rewarmed. Rewarming stimulates the heart to resume beating. Temporary pacing wires are sutured in place and passed through the chest wall in case temporary pacing is necessary. Chest tubes are placed in the pleural space

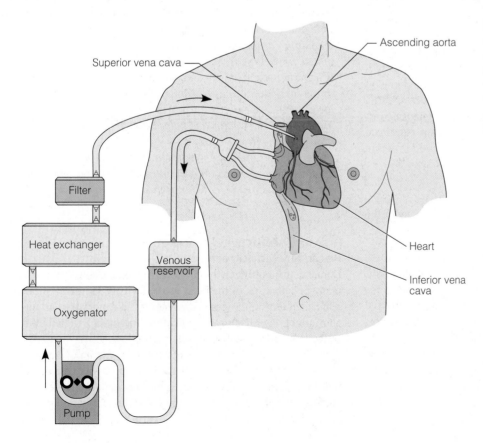

**Figure 29–5** ■ A diagrammatic representation of cardiopulmonary bypass. A cannula in the superior and inferior venae cavae removes venous blood, which is then pumped through an oxygenator and heat exchanger. After filtering, oxygenated blood is returned to the ascending aorta.

and mediastinum to drain blood and reestablish negative pressure in the thoracic cavity. The sternum is closed using heavy wires and bone wax, the skin is closed with sutures or staples, and sterile dressings are applied over sternal and leg incisions.

Pre- and postoperative nursing care and teaching for the client having a coronary artery bypass graft or other open-heart surgery are outlined on pages 823–825.

### Minimally Invasive Coronary Artery Surgery

*Minimally invasive coronary artery surgery* is a potential future alternative to CABG. Two approaches may be used: *port-access coronary artery bypass* uses several small holes, or "ports" in the chest wall to access vessels for connection to the CPB pump and the surgical site; CPB is avoided altogether using the *minimally invasive coronary artery bypass (MIDCAB)* approach. With MIDCAB, a small surgical incision and several chest wall ports are used to graft a chest wall artery to the affected coronary vessel while the heart continues to beat.

### Transmyocardial Laser Revascularization

A new development in myocardial revascularization techniques is called *transmyocardial laser revascularization (TMLR)*. In this procedure, a laser is used to drill tiny holes into the myocardial muscle itself to provide collateral blood flow to ischemic muscle. Clients whose coronary artery obstructions are too diffuse to bypass are candidates for this new surgical treatment.

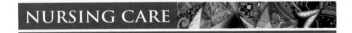

## NURSING CARE

## Health Promotion

In addition to health promotion measures identified for CHD, emphasize the importance of active CHD risk factor management to slow progression of the disease. Encourage clients to stop smoking. Discuss the use of cholesterol-lowering drug therapy with clients who have hypercholesterolemia. Encourage regular aerobic exercise and a diet based on American Heart Association or National Cholesterol Education Program guidelines.

## Assessment

Focused assessment data for the client with angina includes the following:

- Health history: chest pain, including type, intensity, duration, frequency, aggravating factors and relief measures; associated symptoms; history of other cardiovascular disorders, peripheral vascular disease, or stroke; current medications and treatment; usual diet, exercise, and alcohol intake patterns; smoking history; use of other recreational drugs
- Physical assessment: vital signs and heart sounds; strength and equality of peripheral pulses; skin color and temperature (central and peripheral); physical appearance during pain episode (e.g., shortness of breath, apparent anxiety, color, diaphoresis)

## Nursing Diagnoses and Interventions

The focus of nursing care for clients with angina is similar to the collaborative care focus: to reduce myocardial oxygen demand and improve the oxygen supply. Angina usually is treated in community settings; the primary nursing focus is education. High-priority nursing problems for clients with angina include ineffective cardiac tissue perfusion and management of the prescribed therapeutic regimen.

### Ineffective Tissue Perfusion: Cardiac

The pain of angina results from impaired blood flow and oxygen supply to the myocardium. Nursing interventions can both prevent ischemia and shorten the duration of pain.

- Keep prescribed nitroglycerin tablets at the client's side so one can be taken at the onset of pain. *Anginal pain indicates myocardial ischemia. Nitroglycerin reduces cardiac work and may improve myocardial blood flow, relieving ischemia and pain.*
- Start oxygen at 4 to 6 L/min per nasal cannula or as prescribed. *Supplemental oxygen reduces myocardial hypoxia.*
- Space activities to allow rest between them. *Activity increases cardiac work and may precipitate angina. Spacing of activities allows the heart to recover.*
- Teach about prescribed medications to maintain myocardial perfusion and reduce cardiac work. Emphasize that long-acting nitrates, beta blockers, and calcium channel blockers are used to *prevent* anginal attacks, not to *treat* an acute attack. *It is important for the client to understand the purpose and use of prescribed drugs to maintain optimal myocardial perfusion.*
- Instruct to take sublingual nitroglycerin before engaging in activities that precipitate angina (e.g., climbing stairs, sexual intercourse). *This prophylactic dose of nitroglycerin helps maintain cardiac perfusion when increased work is anticipated, preventing ischemia and chest pain.*
- Encourage to implement and maintain a progressive exercise program under the supervision of the primary care provider or a cardiac rehabilitation professional. *Exercise slows the atherosclerotic process and helps develop collateral circulation to the heart muscle.*
- Refer to a smoking cessation program as indicated. *Nicotine causes vasoconstriction and increases the heart rate, decreasing myocardial perfusion and increasing cardiac workload.*

### Risk for Ineffective Therapeutic Regimen Management

Denial may be strong in the client with angina pectoris. Because many people think of the heart as the locus of life itself, problems such as angina remind people of their mortality, an uncomfortable fact. Denial may lead to "forgetting" to take prescribed medications or to attempting activities that will precipitate angina. Some clients, by contrast, may become "cardiac cripples," afraid to engage in activities because of anticipated chest pain. Their inactivity may actually hasten the atherosclerotic process and inhibit collateral circulation development, worsening angina.

# NURSING CARE OF THE CLIENT HAVING A CORONARY ARTERY BYPASS GRAFT

## PREOPERATIVE CARE

- Provide routine preoperative care and teaching as outlined in Chapter 7. ⊖⊕
- Verify presence of laboratory and diagnostic test results in the chart, including CBC, coagulation profile, urinalysis, chest X-ray, and coronary angiogram. *These baseline data are important for comparison of postoperative results and values.*
- Type and crossmatch four or more units of blood as ordered. *Blood is made available for use during and after surgery as needed.*
- Provide specific client and family teaching related to procedure and postoperative care. Include the following topics.
  - Cardiac recovery unit; sensory stimuli, personnel; noise and alarms; visiting policies
  - Tubes, drains, and general appearance
  - Monitoring equipment, including cardiac and hemodynamic monitoring systems
  - Respiratory support: ventilator, endotracheal tube, suctioning; communication while intubated
  - Incisions and dressings
  - Pain management

  *Preoperative teaching reduces anxiety and prepares the client and family for the postoperative environment and expected sensations.*

## POSTOPERATIVE CARE

- Provide routine postoperative care as outlined in Chapter 7. In addition to the care needs of all clients having major surgery, the cardiac surgery client has specific care needs related to open-heart and thoracic surgery. These are outlined under the nursing diagnoses identified below.

### Decreased Cardiac Output

Cardiac output may be compromised postoperatively due to bleeding and fluid loss; depression of myocardial function by drugs, hypothermia, and surgical manipulation; dysrhythmias; increased vascular resistance; and a potential complication, *cardiac tamponade,* compression of the heart due to collected blood or fluid in the pericardium

- Monitor vital signs, oxygen saturation, and hemodynamic parameters every 15 minutes. Note trends and report significant changes to the physician. *Initial hypothermia and bradycardia are expected; the heart rate should return to the normal range with rewarming. The blood pressure may fall during rewarming as vasodilation occurs. Hypotension and tachycardia, however, may indicate low cardiac output. Pulmonary artery pressure (PAP), pulmonary artery wedge pressure (PAWP), cardiac output, and oxygen saturation are monitored to evaluate fluid volume, cardiac function, and gas exchange.* Hemodynamic monitoring is further discussed in Chapter 30.
- Auscultate heart and breath sounds on admission and at least every 4 hours. *A ventricular gallop, or $S_3$, is an early sign of heart failure; an $S_4$ may indicate decreased ventricular compliance. Muffled heart sounds may be an early indication of cardiac tamponade. Adventitious breath sounds (wheezes, crackles, or rales) may be a manifestation of heart failure or respiratory compromise.*

- Assess skin color and temperature, peripheral pulses, and level of consciousness with vital signs. *Pale, mottled, or cyanotic coloring, cool and clammy skin, and diminished pulse amplitude are indicators of decreased cardiac output.*
- Continuously monitor and document cardiac rhythm. *Dysrhythmias are common, and may interfere with cardiac filling and contractility, decreasing the cardiac output.*
- Measure intake and output hourly. Report urine output less than 30 mL/h for 2 consecutive hours. *Intake and output measurements help evaluate fluid volume status. A fall in urine output may be an early indicator of decreased cardiac output.*
- Record chest tube output hourly. *Chest tube drainage greater than 70 mL/hr or that is warm, red, and free flowing indicates hemorrhage and may necessitate a return to surgery. A sudden drop in chest tube output may indicate impending cardiac tamponade.*
- Monitor hemoglobin, hematocrit, and serum electrolytes. *A drop in hemoglobin and hematocrit may indicate hemorrhage that is not otherwise obvious. Electrolyte imbalances, potassium, calcium, and magnesium in particular, affect cardiac rhythm and contractility.*
- Administer intravenous fluids, fluid boluses, and blood transfusions as ordered. *Fluid and blood replacement helps ensure adequate blood volume and oxygen-carrying capacity.*
- Administer medications as ordered. *Medications ordered in the early postoperative period to maintain the cardiac output include inotropic drugs (e.g., dopamine, dobutamine) to increase the force of myocardial contractions; vasodilators (e.g., nitroprusside or nitroglycerin) to decrease vascular resistance and afterload; and antidysrhythmics to correct dysrhythmias that affect cardiac output.*
- Keep a temporary pacemaker at the bedside; initiate pacing as indicated. *Temporary pacing may be needed to maintain the cardiac output with bradydysrhythmias, such as high-level AV blocks.*

**PRACTICE ALERT** *Assess for signs of cardiac tamponade: increased heart rate, decreased BP, decreased urine output, increased central venous pressure, a sudden decrease in chest tube output, muffled/distant heart sounds, and diminished peripheral pulses. Notify physician immediately. Cardiac tamponade is a life-threatening complication that may develop postoperatively. Cardiac tamponade interferes with ventricular filling and contraction, decreasing cardiac output. Untreated, cardiac tamponade leads to cardiogenic shock and possible cardiac arrest.* ■

### Hypothermia

Hypothermia is maintained during cardiac surgery to reduce the metabolic rate and protect vital organs from ischemic damage. Although rewarming is instituted on completion of the surgery, the client often remains hypothermic on admission to cardiac recovery. Gradual rewarming is necessary to prevent peripheral vasodilation and hypotension.

*continued on page 824*

## NURSING CARE OF THE CLIENT HAVING A CORONARY ARTERY BYPASS GRAFT *(continued)*

- Monitor core body temperature (e.g., tympanic membrane, pulmonary artery, bladder) for the first 8 hours following surgery. *Oral and rectal temperature measurements are not reliable indicators of core body temperature during this period.*
- Institute rewarming measures (e.g., warmed intravenous solutions or blood transfusion, warm blankets, warm inspired gases, radiant heat lamps) as needed to maintain a temperature above 96.8 F (36° C). Administer thorazine, morphine, or diltiazem as ordered to relieve shivering. *Low body temperature may cause shivering, increasing oxygen demand and consumption. Hypothermia also increases the risk for hypoxia, metabolic acidosis, vasoconstriction and increased cardiac work, altered clotting, and dysrhythmias.*

### Acute Pain

Following a CABG, pain is experienced due to both the thoracic incision and removal of the saphenous vein from the leg. Dissection of the internal mammary artery (usually the left IMA) from the chest wall also causes chest pain on the affected side. Chest tube sites are also uncomfortable. The leg from which the saphenous vein graft was obtained may be more painful than the chest incision.

- Frequently assess for pain, including its location and character. Document its intensity using a standard pain scale. Assess for verbal and nonverbal indicators of pain. Validate pain cues with the client. *Pain is subjective, and differs among individuals. Incisional pain is expected; however, anginal pain also may develop. It is important to differentiate the type of pain.*

### PRACTICE ALERT *Promptly report anginal or cardiac pain. Cardiac pain may indicate a perioperative or postoperative myocardial infarction.* ■

- Administer analgesics on a scheduled basis, by PCA, or by continuous infusion for the first 24 to 48 hours. *Research demonstrates that adequate pain management in the immediate postoperative period reduces complications from sympathetic stimulation and allows faster recovery. Pain causes muscle tension and vasoconstriction, impairing circulation and tissue perfusion, slowing wound healing, and increasing cardiac work.*
- Premedicate 30 minutes before activities or planned procedures. *Premedication and the subsequent reduction of pain improves client participation and cooperation with care.*

### Ineffective Airway Clearance/Impaired Gas Exchange

Atelectasis due to impaired ventilation and airway clearance is a common pulmonary complication of cardiac surgery. Gas exchange may also be affected by blood loss and decreased oxygen-carrying capacity following surgery. Phrenic nerve paralysis is a potential complication of cardiac surgery which may also contribute to impaired ventilation and gas exchange.

- Evaluate respiratory rate, depth, effort, symmetry of chest expansion, and breath sounds frequently. *Pain, anxiety, excess fluid volume, surgical injury, narcotics and anesthesia, and altered homeostasis can affect respiratory rate, depth, and effort postoper-* *atively. Decreased chest expansion or asymmetrical movement may indicate impaired ventilation of one lung, and needs further evaluation.*
- Note endotracheal tube (ETT) placement on chest X-ray. Mark tube position and secure in place. Insert an oral airway if an oral ETT is used. *The chest X-ray documents correct ETT placement above the bifurcation to the right and left mainstem bronchus. Marking its appropriate placement allows evaluation of potential tube movement. Secure the tube firmly in place to prevent slippage or inadvertent removal. An oral airway helps prevent obstruction of an oral ETT by biting.*
- Maintain ventilator settings as ordered. Monitor arterial blood gases (ABGs) as ordered. *Mechanical ventilation promotes optimal lung expansion and oxygenation postoperatively. ABGs are used to evaluate oxygenation and acid-base balance.*
- Suction as needed. *Suctioning is performed only as indicated to clear airway secretions.*
- Prepare for ventilator weaning and extubation, as appropriate. *The client is removed from the ventilator and extubated as soon as possible to reduce complications associated with mechanical ventilation and intubation.*
- After extubation, teach use of the incentive spirometer, and encourage use every 2 hours. Encourage deep breathing; advise against vigorous coughing. Teach use of a "cough pillow" to splint chest incision and decrease pain. Frequently turn and encourage movement. Dangle on postoperative day 1. *Deep breathing, controlled coughing, and position changes improve ventilation and airway clearance and help prevent complications. Vigorous coughing may excessively increase intrathoracic pressure and cause sternal instability.*

### Risk for Infection

Following an open chest procedure, a sternal infection may develop that can progress to involve the mediastinum. Clients with IMA grafts, who are diabetic, are older, or malnourished are at high risk: Harvesting of IMA disrupts blood supply to the sternum, and these clients have impaired immune responses and healing.

- Assess sternal wound every shift. Document redness, warmth, swelling, and/or drainage from the site. Note wound approximation. *These assessments provide indicators of inflammation and healing.*
- Maintain a sterile dressing for the first 48 hours, then leave the incision open to air. Use Steri-Strips as needed to maintain approximation of the wound edges. *The sterile dressing prevents early contamination of the wound, whereas exposing the incision after 48 hours promotes healing.*
- Report signs of wound infection: a swollen, reddened area that is hot and painful to the touch; drainage from the wound; impaired healing, or healed areas that reopen. *Evidence of infection or impaired healing requires further evaluation and treatment.*
- Culture wound drainage as indicated. *Identifying the infective organism facilitates appropriate antibiotic therapy.*
- Collaborate with the dietitian to promote nutrition and fluid intake. *Good nutritional status is vital to healing and immune function.*

*continued on page 825*

## NURSING CARE OF THE CLIENT HAVING A CORONARY ARTERY BYPASS GRAFT (continued)

### Disturbed Thought Processes

Many factors affect neuropsychologic function after CABG, including the length of cardiopulmonary bypass, age, presurgery organic brain dysfunction, severity of illness, and decreased cardiac output. Sensory overload and deprivation, sleep disruption, and numerous drugs also affect thinking and mental clarity.

- Frequently reorient during initial recovery period. State that surgery is over and that the client is in the recovery area. *Frequent reorientation provides emotional support and reality checks.*
- Explain all procedures before performing them. Speak in a clear, calm voice. Encourage questions, and give honest answers. *These measures provide information, decrease anxiety, and establish trust.*
- Secure all intravenous lines and invasive catheters/tubes (e.g., ETT, Foley catheter, nasogastric tube). *Disoriented clients may tug or pull at invasive equipment, disrupting them and increasing the risk of injury.*
- Note verbal responses to questions. Correct misconceptions immediately (e.g., "Mr. Snow, look at all the special equipment in this room. Does this room look like your bedroom at home?"). *Helping the client recognize differences in the hospital environment offers a basis for continual reality checks.*
- Maintain a calendar and clock within the client's view. *This provides current information regarding day, date, and time.*
- Involve family members in providing reorientation. Place familiar objects and photographs within view. Encourage family presence. *The family provides reassurance and contact with the familiar, assisting with orientation.*
- Promote client participation in care and decision making as appropriate. *This allows the client to maintain a degree of power and control and enables the client to take an active role in recovery.*
- Report signs of hallucinations, delusions, depression, or agitation. *These may indicate progressive deterioration of mental status.*
- Administer sedatives cautiously. *Mild sedation may help prevent injury. Some sedatives may, however, have adverse effects, increasing confusion and disorientation.*
- Reevaluate neurologic status every shift. *These data allow evaluation of the effect of interventions.*

- Assess knowledge and understanding of angina. *Assessment allows tailoring of teaching and interventions to the needs of the client.*
- Teach about angina and atherosclerosis as needed, building on current knowledge base. *This can help the client understand that angina is a manageable disease and that pain can usually be controlled and the disease progress slowed.*
- Provide written and verbal instructions about prescribed medications and their use. *Written instructions reinforce teaching and are available to the client for future reference.*
- Stress the importance of taking chest pains seriously while maintaining a positive attitude. *Although it is vital to recog-* *nize the significance of chest pain and deal with it appropriately, it is also important to maintain a positive outlook.*
- Refer to a cardiac rehabilitation program or other organized activities and support groups for clients with coronary artery disease. *Programs such as these help the client develop risk factor management strategies, maintain a program of supervised activity, and gain coping skills.*

## Using NANDA, NIC, and NOC

Chart 29–1 shows links between NANDA nursing diagnoses, NIC, and NOC when caring for the client with angina.

### CHART 29–1 NANDA, NIC, AND NOC LINKAGES

#### The Client with CHD and Angina

| NURSING DIAGNOSES | NURSING INTERVENTIONS | NURSING OUTCOMES |
|---|---|---|
| • Activity Intolerance | • Cardiac Care: Rehabilitative | • Activity Tolerance |
| • Ineffective Coping | • Coping Enhancement | • Coping |
| | • Emotional Support | • Role Performance |
| • Ineffective Health Maintenance | • Health Education | • Health-Promoting Behavior |
| | • Risk Identification | • Risk Detection |
| | • Self-Responsibility Facilitation | • Health-Seeking Behavior |
| • Ineffective Sexuality Patterns | • Anticipatory Guidance | • Role Performance |
| • Ineffective Tissue Perfusion: Cardiopulmonary | • Cardiac Care | • Cardiac Pump Effectiveness |
| | • Cardiac Precautions | • Circulation Status |
| | • Medication Administration | • Tissue Perfusion: Cardiac |

*Note. Data from Nursing Outcomes Classification (NOC) by M. Johnson & M. Maas (Eds.), 1997, St. Louis: Mosby; Nursing Diagnoses: Definitions & Classification 2001–2002 by North American Nursing Diagnosis Association, 2001, Philadelphia: NANDA; Nursing Interventions Classification (NIC) by J.C. McCloskey & G. M. Bulechek (Eds.), 2000, St. Louis: Mosby. Reprinted by permission.*

## Home Care

Many clients with stable angina manage their pain effectively, continuing to live active and productive lives. To promote effective management of this disorder, include the following topics in teaching for home care.

- Coronary heart disease and the processes that cause chest pain, including the relationship between the pain and reduced blood flow to the heart muscle
- Use and effects (desired and adverse) of prescribed medications; importance of not discontinuing medications abruptly
- Nitroglycerine use for acute angina: Always carry several tablets (not the entire supply); prophylactic use before activities that often cause chest pain; take tablet at first indication of pain rather than waiting to see if the pain develops; seek immediate medical assistance if three nitroglycerin tablets over 15 to 20 minutes do not relieve the pain
- The importance of calling 911 or going to the emergency department immediately for unrelieved chest pain
- Appropriate storage of nitroglycerin: This unstable compound needs to be stored in a cool, dry, dark place; no more than a 6-month supply should be kept on hand

For the client who has undergone cardiac surgery, also include the following:

- Respiratory care, activity, and pain management
- The importance of actively participating in rehabilitation
- Manifestations of infection or other potential complications and their management

## Nursing Care Plan
## A Client with Coronary Artery Bypass Surgery

Six weeks ago, John Clements, age 50, was discharged from the hospital after emergency triple bypass surgery. Despite having emergency surgery, his postoperative recovery was uneventful, and he was discharged 6 days after admission. He returns to the clinic for a postoperative stress test and to discuss his cardiac rehabilitation program. Anne Wagner, RN, CNS, a cardiac clinical nurse specialist and the program coordinator, meets Mr. Clements to obtain specific information regarding his medical status.

### ASSESSMENT

Mr. Clements's medical history reveals significant CHD, an anterior wall myocardial infarction that led to his emergency triple bypass, and hyperlipidemia. Current medications include Cardizem, Isordil, Ecotrin, and Transderm-Nitro 5. The ECG reveals sinus rhythm with some ST segment and T wave flattening. Resting heart rate 68, and blood pressure 136/84.

Mr. Clements has a strong family history of CHD. He does not smoke and uses alcohol occasionally in social situations. He enjoys "good Southern-style cooking" and watching television. Mr. Clements states his only regular exercise used to be an evening of dancing with his wife and friends about once a month, "But I get short of breath walking around the block now, so I guess I can't go dancing anymore!"

Mr. Clements owns his own contracting business and states that he typically works about 50 to 60 hours per week. He tells Ms. Wagner, "I don't know what this program is supposed to do for me. I have got to get back to work! You just can't sit around in my business—you have to make sure that the work is getting done on time, and you have to check on supplies and equipment and the like. But I feel like a weakling—I need to get my energy back!"

### DIAGNOSES

- Activity intolerance related to general weakness and fatigue
- Ineffective role performance related to health crisis

### EXPECTED OUTCOMES

- Verbalize an understanding of the definition and components of his structured cardiac rehabilitation program.
- Verbalize a desire to make lifestyle changes.
- Identify resources available in the community to assist with lifestyle changes.
- Participate in his activity program without suffering any complications.
- Verbalize an increase in energy after 6 weeks on the program.
- Accept the reality of the temporary change in his usual work responsibilities.

### PLANNING AND IMPLEMENTATION

- Define the purpose and components of a cardiac rehabilitation program.
- Enroll in "heart health" classes, including cardiac anatomy, physiology, and coronary heart disease; exercise and activity prescriptions; lifestyle modifications, including diet counseling and stress management; emotional reactions to CAD; sexual activity; use of cardiac medications; and self-responsibility for health.
- Plan an exercise program based on stress test results, physical examination, and interview.
- Encourage to schedule rest periods before and after activity/exercise.
- Review signs and symptoms of overexertion.
- Provide information about community resources for emotional and educational support.
- Assist to identify strategies for dealing with concerns about his business role.

### EVALUATION

Mr. Clements decides to "give the rehab program a try." Ms. Wagner and an exercise physiologist work with him to plan an individualized exercise/activity program. A registered dietitian provides dietary counseling. Ms. Wagner emphasizes stress management strategies. Mr. Clements is able to list manifestations of overexertion and states that he realizes the need for gradual activity progression.

After 6 weeks, Mr. Clements has reported a significant increase in energy and strength. "I am feeling much stronger, and have been sleeping better. Mary and I are taking evening walks around the neighborhood. My chest soreness is also gone." He has completed the 12-week cardiac rehabilitation program, and another stress test indicates that his cardiac function is adequate. Mr.

## Nursing Care Plan

## A Client with Coronary Artery Bypass Surgery (continued)

Clements has joined the local Mended Hearts support group and states that he is now incorporating "heart-healthy" considerations into his daily routines.

### Critical Thinking in the Nursing Process

1. Develop a personalized risk factor reduction plan for Mr. Clements.
2. How might denial affect Mr. Clements's ability to (a) accept the need for cardiac rehabilitation, (b) comply with the proposed lifestyle changes, and (c) make permanent adjustments to his daily life?

3. How does spousal support influence a client's compliance with a structured cardiac rehabilitation program?
4. Mr. Clements tells you that since the surgery, his wife has been afraid that sexual activity will induce another heart attack. How would you respond to these concerns?

See Evaluating Your Response in Appendix C.

# THE CLIENT WITH ACUTE MYOCARDIAL INFARCTION

An **acute myocardial infarction (AMI),** necrosis (death) of myocardial cells, is a life-threatening event. If circulation to the affected myocardium is not promptly restored, loss of functional myocardium affects the heart's ability to maintain an effective cardiac output. This may ultimately lead to cardiogenic shock and death.

Heart disease remains the leading cause of death in the United States. Of the major heart diseases, myocardial infarction (MI) or *heart attack,* and other forms of ischemic heart disease cause the majority of deaths. Annually, approximately 650,000 people in the United States experience their first MI; another 450,000 suffer an MI subsequent to the initial one. Nearly 530,000 people died of coronary heart disease in 2000, with most of these deaths related to MI (NHLBI, 2002).

The majority of deaths from MI occur during the initial period after symptoms begin: approximately 60% within the first hour, and 40% prior to hospitalization. Heightening public awareness of the manifestations of MI, the importance of seeking immediate medical assistance, and training in cardiopulmonary resuscitation (CPR) techniques are vital to decrease deaths due to MI.

Myocardial infarction rarely occurs in clients without preexisting coronary heart disease. While no specific cause has been identified, the risk factors for MI are those for coronary heart disease: age, gender, heredity, race; smoking, obesity, hyperlipidemia, hypertension, diabetes, sedentary lifestyle, diet, and others. See the previous section of this chapter on coronary heart disease for further discussion of these risk factors.

## PATHOPHYSIOLOGY

Atherosclerotic plaque may form stable or unstable lesions. *Stable* lesions progress by gradually occluding the vessel lumen, whereas *unstable* (or *complicated*) lesions are prone to

rupture and thrombus formation. Stable lesions often cause angina (discussed in the previous section); unstable lesions often lead to **acute coronary syndromes,** or acute ischemic heart diseases. Acute coronary syndromes include unstable angina, myocardial infarction, and sudden cardiac death (McCance & Huether, 2002).

Myocardial infarction occurs when blood flow to a portion of cardiac muscle is blocked, resulting in prolonged tissue ischemia and irreversible cell damage. Coronary occlusion is usually caused by ulceration or rupture of a complicated atherosclerotic lesion. When an atherosclerotic lesion ruptures or ulcerates, substances are released that stimulate platelet aggregation, thrombin generation, and local vasomotor tone. As a result, a thrombus (clot) forms, occluding the vessel and interrupting blood flow to the myocardium distal to the obstruction.

Cellular injury occurs when the cells are denied adequate oxygen and nutrients. When ischemia is prolonged, lasting more than 20 to 45 minutes, irreversible hypoxemic damage causes cellular death and tissue necrosis. Oxygen, glycogen, and ATP stores of ischemic cells are rapidly depleted. Cellular metabolism shifts to an anaerobic process, producing hydrogen ions and lactic acid. Cellular acidosis increases cells' vulnerability to further damage. Intracellular enzymes are released through damaged cell membranes into interstitial spaces.

Cellular acidosis, electrolyte imbalances, and hormones released in response to cellular ischemia affect impulse conduction and myocardial contractility. The risk of dysrhythmias increases, and myocardial contractility decreases, reducing stroke volume, cardiac output, blood pressure, and tissue perfusion.

The subendocardium suffers the initial damage, within 20 minutes of injury, because this area is the most susceptible to changes in coronary blood flow. If blood flow is restored at this point, the infarction is limited to subendocardial tissue (a *subendocardial* or *non Q wave infarction*). The damage progresses to the epicardium within 1 to 6 hours. When all layers of the myocardium are affected, it is known as a *transmural infarction.* A significant Q wave develops with a transmural infarction, so this also may be called a *Q wave MI.* Complications such as heart failure are more frequently associated with Q wave MIs; however, clients with non Q wave MIs frequently experience recurrent ischemia or subsequent MI within weeks or months of the event (Woods et al., 2000).

The necrotic, infarcted tissue is surrounded by regions of injured and ischemic tissues. Tissue in this ischemic area is potentially viable; restoration of blood flow minimizes the amount of tissue lost. This surrounding tissue also undergoes metabolic changes. It may be *stunned,* its contractility impaired for hours to days following reperfusion, or *hibernating,* a process that protects myocytes until perfusion is restored. *Myocardial remodeling* also may occur, with cellular hypertrophy and loss of contractility in regions distant from the infarction. Rapid restoration of blood flow limits these changes (McCance & Huether, 2002).

When a larger artery is compromised, *collateral vessels* connecting smaller arteries in the coronary system dilate to maintain blood flow to the cardiac muscle. The degree of collateral circulation helps determine the extent of myocardial damage from ischemia. Acute occlusion of a coronary artery without any collateral flow results in massive tissue damage and possible death. Progressive narrowing of the larger coronary arteries allows collateral vessels to develop and enlarge, meeting the demand for blood flow. Good collateral circulation can limit the size of an MI.

Myocardial infarction usually affects the left ventricle because it is the major "workhorse" of the heart; its muscle mass is greater, as are its oxygen demands.

Myocardial infarctions are described by the damaged area of the heart. The coronary artery that is occluded determines the area of damage. Occlusion of the left anterior descending (LAD) artery affects blood flow to the anterior wall of the left ventricle (an *anterior MI*) and part of the interventricular septum. Occlusion of the left circumflex artery (LCA) causes a *lateral MI. Right ventricular, inferior,* and *posterior infarcts* involve occlusions of the right coronary artery (RCA) and posterior descending artery (PDA). Occlusion of the left main coronary artery is the most devastating, causing ischemia of the entire left ventricle, and a grave prognosis. Identifying the infarct site helps predict possible complications and determine appropriate therapy.

## Cocaine-Induced MI

Acute myocardial infarction may develop due to cocaine intoxication. Cocaine increases sympathetic nervous system activity by both increasing the release of catecholamines from central and peripheral stores and interfering with the reuptake of catecholamines. This increased catecholamine concentration stimulates the heart rate and increases its contractility, increases the automaticity of cardiac tissues and the risk of dysrhythmias, and causes vasoconstriction and hypertension. The client with cocaine-induced MI may present with an altered level of consciousness, confusion and restlessness, seizure activity, tachycardia, hypotension, increased respiratory rate, and respiratory crackles.

## MANIFESTATIONS

Pain is a classic manifestation of myocardial infarction. Chest pain due to MI is more severe than anginal pain. However, it is not the intensity of the chest pain that distinguishes MI from angina, but its duration and its continuous nature. The onset of pain is sudden and usually is not associated with activity. In fact, most MIs occur in the early morning. Clients with a history of angina may have more frequent anginal attacks in the days or weeks prior to an MI. Chest pain may be described as crushing and severe; as a pressure, heavy, or squeezing sensation; or as chest tightness or burning. The pain often begins in the center of the chest (*substernal*), and may radiate to the shoulders, neck, jaw, or arms. It lasts more than 15 to 20 minutes and is not relieved by rest or nitroglycerin.

Women and older adults often experience atypical chest pain, presenting with complaints of indigestion, heartburn, nausea, and vomiting (see the box below). Up to 25% of clients with acute MI deny chest discomfort (Woods et al., 2000).

Compensatory mechanisms cause many of the other symptoms of MI. Sympathetic nervous system stimulation causes anxiety, tachycardia, and vasoconstriction. This results in cool, clammy, mottled skin. Pain and blood chemistry changes stimulate the respiratory center, causing tachypnea. The client often has a sense of impending doom and death. Tissue necrosis causes an inflammatory reaction that increases the white blood cell count and elevates the temperature. Serum cardiac enzyme levels rise as enzymes are released from necrotic cardiac cells.

## Meeting Individualized Needs

### RECOGNIZING A MYOCARDIAL INFARCTION IN WOMEN AND OLDER ADULTS

Women and older adults often present with atypical manifestations of MI. However, heart disease is the number one cause of death in both groups, making early recognition and aggressive treatment vital.

Women are more likely than men to have a "silent" or unrecognized heart attack. They often experience epigastric pain and nausea, causing them to blame their discomfort on heartburn. Shortness of breath is common, as is fatigue and weakness of the shoulders and upper arms.

Older people often seek treatment for vague complaints of difficulty breathing, confusion, fainting, dizziness, abdominal pain, or cough. They often attribute their symptoms to a stroke. The prevalence of silent ischemia is greater in older adults.

Stress the importance of seeking medical help promptly for atypical manifestations of MI. Prompt diagnosis and intervention reduces the mortality and morbidity of MI in women and older adults, just as it does in men. Despite this fact, both women and older adults are more likely to delay seeking treatment and are less likely to be accurately diagnosed and aggressively treated for CHD.

## Manifestations of Acute Myocardial Infarction

- Chest pain: substernal or precordial (across the entire chest wall); may radiate to neck, jaw, shoulder(s), or left arm
- Tachycardia, tachypnea
- Dyspnea, shortness of breath
- Nausea and vomiting
- Anxiety, sense of impending doom
- Diaphoresis
- Cool, mottled skin; diminished peripheral pulses
- Hypotension or hypertension
- Palpitations, dysrhythmias
- Signs of left heart failure
- Decreased level of consciousness

Other manifestations may vary, depending on the location and amount of infarcted tissue. Hypertension, hypotension, or signs of heart failure may develop. Vagal stimulation may cause nausea and vomiting, bradycardia, and hypotension. Hiccuping may develop due to diaphagmatic irritation. If a large vessel is occluded, the first sign of MI may be sudden death. Typical manifestations of MI are listed in the box above.

The risk of complications associated with myocardial infarction is related to the size and location of the MI.

### Dysrhythmias

**Dysrhythmias,** disturbances or irregularities of heart rhythm, are the most frequent complication of MI. Dysrhythmias are discussed in detail in the next section of this chapter.

Infarcted tissue is *arrhythmogenic;* that is, it affects the generation and conduction of electrical impulses in the heart, increasing the risk of dysrhythmias. Premature ventricular contractions (PVCs) are common following an MI, developing in more than 90% of clients with an acute MI. While not dangerous in themselves, they may be predictive of more dangerous dysrhythmias such as ventricular tachycardia or ventricular fibrillation (Woods et al., 2000). The risk of ventricular fibrillation is greatest the first hour after MI; it is a frequent cause of sudden cardiac death associated with acute MI. Its incidence declines with time. If the infarct affects a conduction pathway, electrical conduction may be affected. Any degree of atrioventricular (AV) block may occur following MI, especially when the anterior wall is infarcted. First-degree and Mobitz I (Wenckebach) blocks are most common, although complete heart block may develop. Bradydysrhythmias (abnormal slow rhythms) also may develop, particularly when the inferior wall of the ventricle is affected.

### Pump Failure

Myocardial infarction reduces myocardial contractility, ventricular wall motion, and compliance. Impaired contractility and filling may produce heart failure. The risk of heart failure is greatest when large portions of the left ventricle are infarcted. Heart failure may be more severe with an anterior infarction. Loss of 20% to 30% of the left ventricular muscle mass may cause manifestations of left-sided heart failure, including dyspnea, fatigue, weakness, and respiratory crackles on auscultation. Inferior or right ventricular MI may lead to right-sided heart failure with manifestations such as neck vein distention and peripheral edema. Hemodynamic monitoring is often initiated for clients with evidence of heart failure. Heart failure and its manifestations are discussed in greater depth in Chapter 30.

**CARDIOGENIC SHOCK.** *Cardiogenic shock,* impaired tissue perfusion due to pump failure, results when functioning myocardial muscle mass decreases by more than 40%. The heart is unable to pump enough blood to meet the needs of the body and maintain organ function. Low cardiac output due to cardiogenic shock also impairs perfusion of the coronary arteries and myocardium, further increasing tissue damage. Mortality from cardiogenic shock is greater than 70%, although this can be reduced by prompt intervention with revascularization procedures. See Chapter 6 for a more extensive discussion of cardiogenic shock.

### Infarct Extension

Approximately 10% of clients experience extension or reinfarction in the area of the original infarction during the first 10 to 14 days after an MI. *Extension* of the MI is characterized by increased myocardial necrosis from continued blood flow impairment and ongoing injury. *Expansion* of the MI is described as a permanent expansion of the infarcted area from thinning and dilation of the muscle. Infarct extension and expansion may cause manifestations such as continuing chest pain, hemodynamic compromise, and worsening heart failure.

### Structural Defects

Necrotic muscle is replaced by scar tissue that is thinner than the ventricular muscle mass. This can lead to such complications as ventricular aneurysm, rupture of the interventricular septum or papillary muscle, and myocardial rupture. A *ventricular aneurysm* is an outpouching of the ventricular wall. It may develop when a large section of the ventricle is replaced by scar tissue. Because it does not contract during systole, stroke volume decreases. Blood may pool within the aneurysm, causing clots to form. Ischemia of the papillary muscle or chordae tendineae may cause structural damage leading to papillary muscle dysfunction or rupture. This affects AV valve function (usually the mitral valve), causing *regurgitation,* backflow of blood into the atria during systole. The interventricular septum may perforate or rupture due to ischemia and infarction. Myocardial rupture is a risk between days 4 and 7 after MI, when the injured tissue is soft and weak. This potential complication of MI is often fatal.

### Pericarditis

Tissue necrosis prompts an inflammatory response. *Pericarditis,* inflammation of the pericardial tissue surrounding the heart, may complicate AMI, usually within 2 to 3 days. Pericarditis causes chest pain that may be aching or sharp and stabbing, aggravated by movement or deep breathing. A *pericardial friction rub* may be heard on auscultation of heart sounds.

*Dressler's syndrome,* thought to be a hypersensitivity response to necrotic tissue or an autoimmune disorder, may develop days to weeks after AMI. It is a symptom complex characterized by fever, chest pain, and dyspnea. Dressler's syndrome may spontaneously resolve or recur over several months, causing significant discomfort and distress.

## COLLABORATIVE CARE

Immediate treatment goals for the MI client are to:

* Relieve chest pain.
* Reduce the extent of myocardial damage.
* Maintain cardiovascular stability.
* Decrease cardiac workload.
* Prevent complications.

Slowing the process of coronary heart disease and reducing the risk of future MI is a major long-term management goal for the client.

Rapid assessment and early diagnosis is important in treating AMI. "Time is muscle" is a medical truism for the client with AMI. The evolution of an AMI is dynamic: The quicker the artery is reopened (medically, surgically, or spontaneously), the more myocardium can be salvaged. Survival and long-term outcomes following AMI are improved by rapidly restoring blood flow to the "stunned" myocardium surrounding the infracted tissue, reducing myocardial oxygen demand and limiting the accumulation of toxic by-products of necrosis and reperfusion (Braunwald et al., 2001). The American Heart Association (AHA) recommends initiation of definitive treatment within 1 hour of entry into the health care system.

The major problem interfering with timely reperfusion is delay in seeking medical care following the onset of symptoms. Up to 44% of clients with symptoms of chest discomfort or pain wait more than 4 hours before seeking treatment. Many factors are cited as reasons for treatment delay, including advanced age, the perception of the seriousness of symptoms, denial, access to medical care, the availability of an emergency response system, and in-hospital delays (see the Nursing Research box below). Immediate evaluation of the client presenting with manifestations of myocardial infarction is essential to early diagnosis and treatment.

### Diagnostic Tests

Diagnostic testing is used to establish the diagnosis of AMI.

### Serum Cardiac Markers

*Serum cardiac markers* are proteins released from necrotic heart muscle. The proteins most specific for diagnosis of MI are the creatine phosphokinase (CK or CPK) and cardiac-specific troponins (see Table 29–5).

## Nursing Research

### Evidence-Based Practice for the Client Experiencing Acute Myocardial Infarction

Delay in seeking treatment significantly affects the mortality and morbidity of clients experiencing AMI. Research indicates that the sooner clients seek treatment after the onset of symptoms the greater the degree of myocardial salvage. However, many clients with AMI do not receive prompt treatment because they delay seeking medical care. In one study, researchers used the Health Belief Model as a framework for their study of variables associated with treatment delay in clients experiencing cardiac symptomatology (Dracup & Moser, 1997).

These researchers were interested in internal and/or external motivators that affected the client's decision to seek medical care. Seventy-seven subjects with a diagnosis of suspected or confirmed MI made up the sample. The study sample consisted of mainly white (82%) males (71%) with a mean age of 58.6 (+11.7) years; ages ranged from 35 to 80. Data were collected via a client questionnaire and chart review.

In this study, 60% of the sample delayed seeking treatment for longer than 3 hours. The median delay for the entire sample was 5 hours. Findings revealed that (1) clients over the age of 60 were more likely to delay treatment than younger clients, (2) the presence of family members increased the delay time, possibly because of a "shared denial" of the seriousness of the symptoms, and (3) the client's interpretation of the symptoms as not serious added to the delay.

#### IMPLICATIONS FOR NURSING

Efforts to educate the public in the seriousness of cardiac symptomatology must be continued and expanded. Programs should emphasize the warning signs of myocardial ischemia and infarction, the negative consequences of delay in seeking treatment, the benefits associated with early treatment of acute MI, and how and when to access the emergency response system.

Nurses should recognize that clients over age 60 may need extra attention and reinforcement of emergency information. Teaching individualized to the cardiac history and other existing disease processes may help the client to distinguish manifestations that require treatment from those that are associated with chronic problems. Refusal to acknowledge the warnings of cardiac disease was shown to correlate with treatment delay. Therefore, every opportunity must be taken to educate the public to make appropriate decisions during a potential cardiac event. Including the family in this teaching is encouraged. This data showed that clients who had family members present during the cardiac event delayed an average of 9 hours, compared to a 2-hour delay for clients who were alone during the experience.

#### Critical Thinking in Client Care

1. In what settings, other than the hospital, can nurses provide cardiac education classes to the public?
2. How does the concept of denial affect the client's decision to seek medical care?
3. How does the Health Belief Model offer a framework for the purposes of this study?
4. What is the extent of the emergency response system in your area, and how is it accessed?
5. What is the average length of time from activation of the system to arrival at the emergency center? How does this affect the overall onset-to-treatment goal of 60 minutes?

## TABLE 29–5  Cardiac Markers

| Marker | Normal Level | Primary Tissue Location | Significance of Elevation | Changes Occuring with MI | | |
| --- | --- | --- | --- | --- | --- | --- |
| | | | | Appears | Peaks | Duration |
| CK (CPK) | Male: 12 to 80 U/L Female: 10 to 70 U/L | Cardiac muscle, skeletal muscle, brain | Injury to muscle cells | 3 to 6 hours | 12 to 24 hours | 24 to 48 hours |
| CK-MB | 0% to 3% of total CK | Cardiac muscle | MI, cardiac ischemia, myocarditis, cardiac contusion, defibrillation | 4 to 8 hours | 18 to 24 hours | 72 hours |
| $cT_nT$ | < 0.2 mcg/L | Cardiac muscle | Acute MI, unstable angina | 2 to 4 hours | 24 to 36 hours | 10 to 14 days |
| $cT_nI$ | < 3.1 mcg/L | Cardiac muscle | Acute MI, unstable angina | 2 to 4 hours | 24 to 36 hours | 7 to 10 days |

- *Creatine phosphokinase* is an important enzyme for cellular function found principally in cardiac and skeletal muscle and the brain. CK levels rise rapidly with damage to these tissues, appearing in the serum 4 to 6 hours after AMI, peaking within 12 to 24 hours, and then declining over the next 48 to 72 hours. The CK level correlates with the size of the infarction; the greater the amount of infarcted tissue, the higher the serum CK level.

- *CK-MB* (also called MB-bands) is a subset of CK specific to cardiac muscle. This isoenzyme of CK is considered the most sensitive indicator of MI. Elevated CK alone is not specific for MI; elevated CK-MB greater than 5% is considered a positive indicator of MI. CK-MB levels do not normally rise with chest pain from angina or causes other than MI.

- Cardiac muscle troponins, *cardiac-specific troponin T ($cT_nT$)* and *cardiac-specific troponin I ($cT_nI$)*, are proteins released during myocardial infarction that are sensitive indicators of myocardial damage. These proteins are part of the actin-myocin unit in cardiac muscle and normally are not detectable in the blood. With necrosis of cardiac muscle, troponins are released and blood levels rise. The specificity of $cT_nT$ and $cT_nI$ to cardiac muscle necrosis makes these markers particularly useful when skeletal muscle trauma contributes to elevated CK levels (e.g., when CPR has been performed or traumatic injury occurred at the time of the MI). They are sensitive enough to detect very small infarctions that do not cause significant CK elevation. Both $cT_nT$ and $cT_nI$ remain in the blood for 10 to 14 days after an MI, making them useful to diagnose MI when medical treatment is delayed.

Serum levels of cardiac markers are ordered on admission and for 3 succeeding days. Serial blood levels help establish the diagnosis and determine the extent of myocardial damage.

Other laboratory tests may include the following:

- *Myoglobin* is one of the first cardiac markers to be detectable in the blood after an MI. It is released within a few hours of symptom onset. Its lack of specificity to cardiac muscle and rapid excretion (blood levels return to normal within 24 hours) limit its use, however (Braunwald et al., 2001).

- *Complete blood count (CBC)* shows an elevated white blood cell (WBC) count due to inflammation of the injured myocardium. The *erythrocyte sedimentation rate (ESR)* also rises because of inflammation.

- *Arterial blood gases (ABGs)* may be ordered to assess blood oxygen levels and acid-base balance.

Electrocardiography, echocardiography, and myocardial nuclear scans are the most common diagnostic tests performed when AMI is suspected. With the exception of the ECG, the timing of these tests depends on the client's immediate condition. Hemodynamic monitoring may be initiated in the unstable client following MI.

- The *electrocardiogram* reflects changes in conduction due to myocardial ischemia and necrosis. Characteristic ECG changes seen in AMI include T wave inversion, elevation of the ST segment, and formation of a Q wave. Ischemic changes in the heart are seen as depression of the ST segment or inversion of the T wave (see Figure 29–2). With myocardial injury, elevation of the ST segment occurs (Figure 29–6A ■). Significant Q wave development (Figure 29–6B) indicates a transmural, or full-thickness infarction. Myocardial damage can be localized using the 12-lead ECG. See the next section of this chapter for more information about ECGs.

- *Echocardiography* is a noninvasive test to evaluate cardiac wall motion and left ventricular function. Images are produced as ultrasound waves strike cardiac structures and are reflected back through a transducer. Echocardiography can be done at the bedside.

- *Radionuclide imaging* may be done to evaluate myocardial perfusion. These studies cannot differentiate between an acute MI and old scar tissue, but do help identify the specific area of myocardial ischemia and damage. Several isotopes may be used. Thallium-201 collects in normally perfused myocardium; ischemic areas appear blue or as "cold" spots when the heart is scanned for radioactivity. In contrast, technetium-99m pyrophosphate, another commonly used radioisotope, accumulates in ischemic tissue and appears red, or "hot."

- *Hemodynamic monitoring* may be initiated when AMI significantly affects cardiac output and hemodynamic status. These invasive procedures are described in Chapter 30.

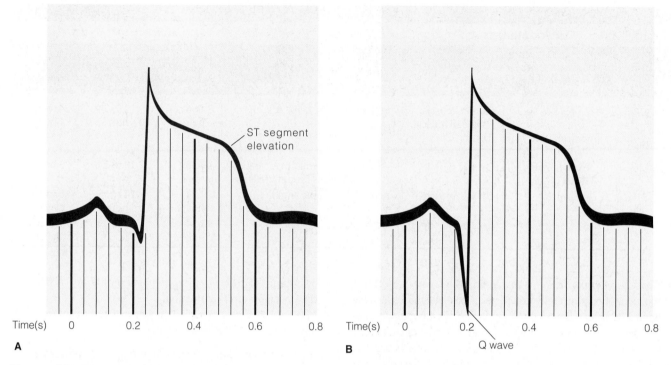

**Figure 29–6** ■ ECG changes characteristic of MI. *A*, ST segment elevation characteristic of myocardial injury. *B*, Clinically significant Q wave characteristic of a transmural infarction.

## Medications

Aspirin, a platelet inhibitor, is now considered an essential part of treating AMI. A 160 to 325 mg aspirin tablet is given by emergency personnel, with the instructions that it is to be chewed (for buccal absorption). This initial dose is followed by a daily oral dose of 160 to 325 mg of aspirin.

Other medications are used to help reduce oxygen demand and increase oxygen supply. Thrombolytic agents, analgesics, and antidysrhythmic agents are among the principal classes of drugs used.

### Thrombolytic Therapy

Thrombolytic agents, drugs that dissolve or break up blood clots, are first-line drugs used to treat acute MI. These drugs activate the fibrinolytic system to lyse or destroy the clot, restoring blood flow to the obstructed artery. Early thrombolytic administration (within the first 6 hours of MI onset) limits infarct size, reduces heart damage, and improves outcomes. Activation of the fibrinolytic system can cause multiple complications; approximately 0.5% to 5% of clients receiving thrombolytic drugs experience serious bleeding complications. Not every client is a candidate for thrombolytic therapy; for example, it is contraindicated in clients with known bleeding disorders, history of cerebrovascular disease, uncontrolled hypertension, pregnancy, or recent trauma or surgery of the head or spine (Tierney et al., 2001).

Four thrombolytic agents are commonly used today. Among the four, little difference in effectiveness has been demonstrated; there are, however, big differences in cost. Streptokinase, a biologic agent derived from group C *Streptococcus* organisms, is the least expensive of the drugs. Its primary drawback is the risk of a severe hypersensitivity reaction, in-

cluding anaphylaxis. Streptokinase is administered by intravenous infusion. Anisoylated plasminogen streptokinase activator complex (APSAC) is a related drug that can be administered by bolus over 2 to 5 minutes. It has many of the same effects as streptokinase, but is considerably more expensive. Tissue plasminogen activator (t-PA) and reteplase are more effective in reestablishing myocardial perfusion, especially when the pain developed more than 3 hours previously. These drugs, however, are the most expensive. Nursing care of the client receiving a thrombolytic agent is outlined on the next page.

### Analgesia

Pain relief is vital in treating the client with AMI. Pain stimulates the sympathetic nervous system, increasing the heart rate and blood pressure and, in turn, myocardial workload. Sublingual nitroglycerin may be given (up to three 0.4-mg doses at 5-minute intervals). In addition to pain relief, nitroglycerin may decrease myocardial oxygen demand and increase the supply of oxygen to the myocardium by dilating collateral vessels. Morphine sulfate is the drug of choice for pain and sedation. Following an initial intravenous dose of 4 to 8 mg, small doses (2 to 4 mg) may be repeated intravenously every 5 minutes until pain is relieved. It is important to assess frequently for pain relief and possible adverse effects of analgesia, such as excessive sedation. See Chapter 4 ⊙ for more details about morphine administration. Antianxiety agents such as diazepam (Valium) may also be administered to promote rest.

### Antidysrhythmics

Dysrhythmias are a common complication of AMI, particularly in the first 12 to 24 hours. Antidysrhythmic medications are used as needed to treat dysrhythmias. They also may be given

# NURSING CARE OF THE CLIENT RECEIVING THROMBOLYTIC THERAPY

## PREINFUSION CARE

- Obtain nursing history, and perform a physical assessment. *Information obtained from the history and physical exam helps determine whether thrombolytic therapy is appropriate. The goal is to initiate thrombolytic therapy within 30 minutes of arrival.*
- Evaluate for contraindications to thrombolytic therapy: recent surgery or trauma (including prolonged CPR), bleeding disorders or active bleeding, cerebral vascular accident, neurosurgery within the last 2 months, gastrointestinal ulcers, diabetic hemorrhagic retinopathy, and uncontrolled hypertension. *Thrombolytic agents dissolve clots and therefore may precipitate intracranial, internal, or peripheral bleeding.*
- Inform the client of the purpose of the therapy. Discuss the risk of bleeding and the need to keep the extremity immobile during and after the infusion. *Minimal movement of the extremity is necessary to prevent bleeding from the infusion site.*

## DURING THE INFUSION

- Assess and record vital signs and the infusion site for hematoma or bleeding every 15 minutes for the first hour, every 30 minutes for the next 2 hours, and then hourly until the intravenous catheter is discontinued. Assess pulses, color, sensation, and temperature of both extremities with each vital sign check. *Vital signs and the site are frequently assessed to detect possible complications.*
- Remind the client to keep the extremity still and straight. Do not elevate head of bed above 15 degrees. *Extremity immobilization helps prevent infusion site trauma and bleeding. Hypotension may develop; keeping the bed flat helps maintain cerebral perfusion.*
- Maintain continuous cardiac monitoring during the infusion. Keep antidysrhythmic drugs and the emergency cart readily available for treatment of significant dysrhythmias. *Ventricular dysrhythmias commonly occur with reperfusion of the ischemic myocardium.*

## POSTINFUSION CARE

- Assess vital signs, distal pulses, and infusion site frequently as needed. *The client remains at high risk for bleeding following thrombolytic therapy.*
- Evaluate response to therapy: normalization of ST segment, relief of chest pain, reperfusion dysrhythmias, early peaking of the CK and CK-MB. *These are signs that the clot has been dissolved and the myocardium is being reperfused.*
- Maintain bed rest for 6 hours. Keep the head of the bed at or below 15 degrees. Reinforce the need to keep the extremity straight and immobile. Avoid any injections for 24 hours after catheter removal. *Precautions such as these are important to prevent bleeding.*
- Assess puncture sites for bleeding. On catheter removal hold direct pressure over the site for at least 30 minutes. Apply a pressure dressing to any venous or arterial sites as needed. Perform routine care in a gentle manner to avoid bruising or injury. *Thrombolytic therapy disrupts normal coagulation. Peripheral bleeding may occur at puncture sites, and there may not be sufficient fibrin to form a clot. Direct or indirect pressure may be needed to control the bleeding.*
- Assess body fluids, including urine, vomitus, and feces, for evidence of bleeding; frequently assess for changes in level of consciousness and manifestations of increased intracranial pressure, which may indicate intracranial bleeding. Assess surgical sites for bleeding. Monitor hemoglobin and hematocrit levels, prothrombin time (PT), and partial thromboplastin time (PTT). *These provide additional means of assessing for bleeding.*
- Administer platelet-modifying drugs (e.g., aspirin, dipyridamole) as ordered. *Platelet inhibitors decrease platelet aggregation and adhesion and are used to prevent reocclusion of the artery.*
- Report manifestations of reocclusion, including changes in the ST segment, chest pain, or dysrhythmias. *Early recognition of reocclusion is vital to save myocardial tissue.*

prophylactically to prevent dysrhythmias. Ventricular dysrhythmias are treated with a class I or class III antidysrhythmic drug (see the Medication Administration box on page 854). Symptomatic bradycardia (bradycardia with associated hypotension and other signs of low cardiac output) is treated with intravenous atropine, 0.5 to 1 mg. Intravenous verapamil or the short-acting beta blocker esmolol (Brevibloc) may be ordered to treat atrial fibrillation or other supraventricular tachydysrhythmias.

## Other Medications

Beta blockers such as propranolol (Inderal), atenolol (Tenormin), and metoprolol (Lopressor) reduce pain, limit infarct size, and decrease the incidence of serious ventricular dysrhythmias in AMI. These drugs decrease the heart rate, reducing cardiac work and myocardial oxygen demand. Initial doses are given intravenously. Oral beta blocker therapy is continued to reduce the risk of reinfarction and death related to cardiovascular causes (Braunwald et al., 2001).

Angiotensin-converting enzyme (ACE) inhibitors also reduce mortality associated with AMI. These drugs reduce ventricular remodeling following an MI, reducing the risk for subsequent heart failure. They also may reduce the risk of reinfarction (Braunwald et al., 2001).

Intravenous nitroglycerin may be administered for the first 24 to 48 hours to reduce myocardial work. Nitroglycerin is a peripheral and arterial vasodilator that reduces afterload. It dilates coronary arteries and collateral channels in the heart, increasing coronary blood flow to save myocardial tissue at risk. Nitrates may, however, cause reflex tachycardia or excessive hypotension, so close monitoring is necessary during administration. See the Medication Administration box on page 818 for the nursing implications of these drugs.

Anticoagulants and other antiplatelet medications often are prescribed to maintain coronary artery patency following thrombolysis or a revascularization procedure. Abciximab (ReoPro) suppresses platelet aggregation and reduces the risk of reocclusion following angioplasty. It also improves vessel opening with thrombolytic therapy, permitting lower doses of thrombolytic drugs (Lehne, 2001). Standard or low-molecular-weight heparin preparations often are given to clients with AMI. Heparin helps establish and maintain patency of the affected coronary artery. It also is used, along with long-term warfarin, to prevent systemic or pulmonary embolism in clients with significant left ventricular impairment or atrial fibrillation following AMI. See Chapter 33 ⮂ for more information about anticoagulant therapy.

Clients with pump failure and hypotension may receive intravenous dopamine, a vasopressor. At low doses (less than 5 mg/kg/min), it improves blood flow to the kidneys, preventing renal ischemia and possible acute renal failure (see Chapter 27). With increasing doses, dopamine increases myocardial contractility and causes vasoconstriction, improving blood pressure and cardiac output.

Antilipemic agents are used for the client with hyperlipidemia. A stool softener such as docusate sodium is prescribed to maintain normal bowel function and reduce straining.

## Medical Management

The client with a suspected or confirmed MI is monitored continuously. Care is provided in the intensive coronary care unit for the first 24 to 48 hours, after which time less intensive monitoring (e.g., telemetry) may be required. An intravenous line is established to allow rapid administration of emergency medications.

Bed rest is prescribed for the first 12 hours to reduce the cardiac workload. The bedside commode generally is allowed; studies have shown this to be less stressful than using a bedpan. If the client's condition is stable, sitting in a chair at the bedside is permitted after 12 hours. Activities are gradually increased as tolerated. A quiet, calm environment with limited outside stimuli is preferred. Visitors are limited to promote rest. Oxygen is administered by nasal cannula at 2 to 5 L/min to improve oxygenation of the myocardium and other tissues.

A liquid diet is often prescribed for the first 4 to 12 hours to reduce gastric distention and myocardial work. Following that, a low-fat, low-cholesterol, reduced-sodium diet is allowed. Sodium restrictions may be lifted after 2 to 3 days if no evidence of heart failure is present. Small, frequent feedings are often recommended. Drinks containing caffeine, and very hot and cold foods may also be limited.

## Revascularization Procedures

Many clients with AMI are treated with immediate or early percutaneous coronary revascularization (PCR) such as angioplasty and stent placement. PCR may follow thrombolytic therapy or be used in place of thrombolytic therapy to restore blood flow to ischemic myocardium. When compared with thrombolytic therapy, prompt PCR reduces hospital mortality (Braunwald et al., 2001). In some cases, CABG surgery may be performed. The choice of procedure depends on the client's age and immediate condition, the time elapsed from the onset of manifestations, and the extent of myocardial disease and dam-

age. These procedures and related nursing care are covered in more depth in the preceding section on angina.

## Other Invasive Procedures

For clients with large MIs and evidence of pump failure, invasive devices may be used to temporarily take over the function of the heart, allowing the injured myocardium to heal. The intra-aortic balloon pump is widely used to augment cardiac output. Ventricular assist devices are indicated for clients requiring more or longer term artificial support than the intra-aortic balloon pump provides.

### Intra-Aortic Balloon Pump

The *intra-aortic balloon pump (IABP)*, also called intra-aortic balloon counterpulsation, is a mechanical circulatory support device that may be used after cardiac surgery or to treat cardiogenic shock following AMI. The IABP temporarily supports cardiac function, allowing the heart gradually to recover by decreasing myocardial workload and oxygen demand and increasing perfusion of the coronary arteries.

A catheter with a 30 to 40 mL balloon is introduced into the aorta, usually via the femoral artery. The balloon catheter is connected to a console that regulates the inflation and deflation of the balloon. The IABP catheter inflates during diastole, increasing perfusion of the coronary and renal arteries, and deflates during systole, decreasing afterload and cardiac workload (Figure 29–7 ■). The inflation–deflation sequence is triggered by the ECG pattern. During the most acute period, the balloon inflates and deflates with each heart beat (1:1 ratio), providing maximal assistance to the heart. As the client's condition improves, the IABP is weaned to inflate–deflate at varying intervals (e.g., 1:2, 1:4, 1:8). This provides a continually decreasing amount of support as the heart muscle recovers. When mechanical assistance is no longer required, the IABP catheter is removed.

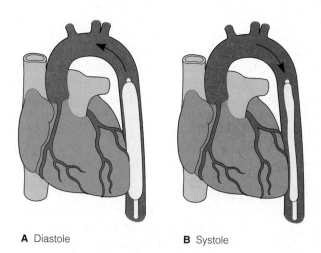

**A** Diastole          **B** Systole

**Figure 29–7 ■** The intra-aortic balloon pump. *A,* When inflated during diastole, the balloon supports cerebral, renal, and coronary artery perfusion. *B,* The balloon deflates during systole, so cardiac output is unimpeded.

## Ventricular Assist Devices

Use of *ventricular assist devices (VADs)* to aid the failing heart is becoming more common with advances in technology. Whereas the IABP can supplement cardiac output by approximately 10% to 15%, the VAD temporarily takes partial or complete control of cardiac function, depending on the type of device used. VADs may be used as temporary or complete assist in AMI and cardiogenic shock when there is a chance for recovery of normal heart function after a period of cardiac rest. The device also may be used as a bridge to heart transplant. Nursing care for the client with a VAD is supportive and includes assessing hemodynamic status and for complications associated with the device. Clients with VAD are at considerable risk for infection; strict aseptic technique is used with all invasive catheters and dressing changes. Pneumonia also is a risk due to immobility and ventilatory support. Mechanical failure of the VAD is a life-threatening event that requires immediate intervention (Urden, Stacy, & Lough 2002).

## Cardiac Rehabilitation

**Cardiac rehabilitation** is a long-term program of medical evaluation, exercise, risk factor modification, education, and counseling designed to limit the physical and psychological effects of cardiac illness and improve the client's quality of life (Woods et al., 2000). Cardiac rehabilitation begins with admission for a cardiac event such as AMI or a revascularization procedure. Phase 1 of the program is the inpatient phase. A thorough assessment of the client's history, current status, risk factors, and motivation is obtained. During this phase, activity progresses from bed rest to independent performance of activities of daily living (ADLs) and ambulation within the facility. Both subjective and objective responses to increasing activity levels are evaluated. Excess fatigue, shortness of breath, chest pain, tachypnea, tachycardia, or cool, clammy skin indicate activity intolerance. Phase 2, immediate outpatient cardiac rehabilitation, begins within 3 weeks of the cardiac event. The goals for the outpatient program are to increase activity level, participation, and capacity; improve psychosocial status and treat anxiety or depression; and provide education and support for risk factor reduction. Continuation programs, phase 3 of cardiac rehabilitation, are directed at providing a transition to independent exercise and exercise maintenance. During this final phase, the client may "check in" every 3 months to evaluate risk factors, quality of life, and exercise habits (Woods et al., 2000).

## NURSING CARE

## Health Promotion

Health promotion activities to prevent acute myocardial infarction are those outlined for coronary heart disease and angina in previous sections of this chapter. In addition, discuss risk factor management, use of prescribed medications, and cardiac rehabilitation to reduce the risk of complications or future infarctions.

## Assessment

Nursing assessment for the client with AMI must be both timely and ongoing. Assessment data related to AMI includes the following:

- Health history: complaints of chest pain, including its location, intensity, character, radiation, and timing; associated symptoms such as nausea, heartburn, shortness of breath, and anxiety; treatment measures taken since onset of pain; past medical history, especially cardiac related; chronic diseases; current medications and any known allergies to medications; smoking history and use of recreational drugs and alcohol
- Physical examination: general appearance including obvious signs of distress; vital signs; peripheral pulses; skin color, temperature, moisture; level of consciousness; heart and breath sounds; cardiac rhythm (on beside monitor); bowel sounds, abdominal tenderness

## Nursing Diagnoses and Interventions

Priorities of nursing care include relieving chest pain, reducing cardiac work, and promoting oxygenation. Psychosocial support is especially important, because an acute myocardial infarction can be devastating, bringing the client face-to-face with his or her own mortality for the first time.

### Acute Pain

Chest pain occurs when the oxygen supply to the heart muscle does not meet the demand. Myocardial ischemia and infarction cause pain, as does reperfusion of an ischemic area following thrombolytic therapy or emergent PTCA. Pain stimulates the sympathetic nervous system, increasing cardiac work. Pain relief is a priority of care for the client with AMI.

- Assess for verbal and nonverbal signs of pain. Document characteristics and the intensity of the pain, using a standard pain scale. Verify nonverbal indicators of pain with the client. *Frequent, careful pain assessment allows early intervention to reduce the risk of further damage. Pain is a subjective experience; its expression may vary with location and intensity, previous experiences, and cultural and social background. Pain scales provide an objective tool for measuring pain and a way to assess pain relief or reduction.*
- Administer oxygen at 2 to 5 L/min per nasal cannula. *Supplemental oxygen increases oxygen supply to the myocardium, decreasing ischemia and pain.*
- Promote physical and psychologic rest. Provide information and emotional support. *Rest decreases cardiac workload and sympathetic nervous system stimulation, promoting comfort. Information and emotional support help decrease anxiety and provide psychologic rest.*
- Titrate intravenous nitroglycerin as ordered to relieve chest pain, maintaining a systolic blood pressure greater than 100 mmHg. *Nitroglycerin decreases chest pain by dilating peripheral vessels, reducing cardiac work, and dilating coronary vessels, including collateral channels, improving blood flow to ischemic tissue.*

*Intravenous nitroglycerine causes peripheral vasodilation, which may lead to hypotension, reduced coronary blood flow, and tachycardia. Reduce the nitro flow rate and notify the physician if this occurs.* ■

- Administer 2 to 4 mg morphine by intravenous push for chest pain as needed. *Morphine is an effective narcotic analgesic for chest pain. It decreases pain and anxiety, acts as a venodilator, and decreases the respiratory rate. The resulting reduction in preload and sympathetic nervous system stimulation reduces cardiac work and oxygen consumption.*

*Reassess for relief of chest pain. The goal of care is to achieve pain relief, not simply a reduction in pain to a "manageable" level.* ■

## Ineffective Tissue Perfusion

Cardiac muscle damage affects its compliance, contractility, and the cardiac output. The extent of the effect on tissue perfusion depends on the location and amount of damage. Anterior wall infarcts have a greater effect on cardiac output than do right ventricular infarcts. Infarcted muscle also increases the risk for cardiac dysrhythmias, which can also affect the delivery of blood and oxygen to the tissues.

- Assess and document vital signs. Report increases in heart rate and changes in rhythm, blood pressure, and respiratory rate. *Decreased cardiac output activates compensatory mechanisms that may cause tachycardia and vasoconstriction, increasing cardiac work.*
- Assess for changes in level of consciousness (LOC); decreased urine output; moist, cool, pale, mottled or cyanotic skin; dusky or cyanotic mucous membranes and nail beds; diminished to absent peripheral pulses; delayed capillary refill. *These are manifestations of impaired tissue perfusion. A change in LOC is often the first manifestation of altered perfusion because brain tissue and cerebral function depends on a continuous supply of oxygen.*
- Auscultate heart and breath sounds. Note abnormal heart sounds (e.g., an $S_3$ or $S_4$ gallop or a murmur) or adventitious lung sounds. *Abnormal heart sounds or adventitious lung sounds may indicate impaired cardiac filling or output, increasing the risk for decreased tissue perfusion.*
- Monitor ECG rhythm continuously. *Dysrhythmias can further impair cardiac output and tissue perfusion.*

*Obtain a 12-lead ECG to assess complaints of chest pain. Report marked changes to the physician. Continued or unrelieved chest pain may indicate further mycoardial ischemia and extension of the infarct; an ECG during episodes of chest pain provides a valuable diagnostic tool to assess myocardial perfusion.* ■

- Monitor oxygen saturation levels. Administer oxygen as ordered. Obtain and assess ABGs as indicated. *Oxygen saturation is an indicator of gas exchange, tissue perfusion, and the*

*effectiveness of oxygen administration. ABGs provide a more precise measurement of blood oxygen levels and allow assessment of acid-base balance.*
- Administer antidysrhythmic medications as needed. *Dysrhythmias affect tissue perfusion by altering cardiac output.*
- Obtain serial CK, isoenzyme, and troponin levels as ordered. *Levels of cardiac markers, CK isoenzymes in particular, correlate with the extent of myocardial damage.*
- Plan for invasive hemodynamic monitoring. *Hemodynamic monitoring facilitates AMI management and treatment evaluation by providing a means of assessing pressures in the systemic and pulmonary arteries, the relationship between oxygen supply and demand, cardiac output, and cardiac index.*

*Continuously evaluate the response to interventions such as thrombolytic therapy, drugs to improve cardiac output and tissue perfusion, and drugs to reduce cardiac work. Adverse effects of therapy may reduce the effectiveness of treatment. Bleeding due to thrombolytic therapy may affect vascular volume and cardiac output; reperfusion dysrhythmias also may affect cardiac output. Drugs used to improve cardiac output may also increase cardiac work, whereas those given to reduce cardiac work may significantly affect contractility and cardiac output.* ■

## Ineffective Coping

Coping mechanisms help a person deal with a life-threatening event or with acute changes in health. However, certain coping mechanisms may be detrimental to restoring health, particularly if the client relies on them for a prolonged period. Denial, for example, is a common coping mechanism among post–MI clients. In the initial stages, denial can reduce anxiety. Continued denial, however, can interfere with learning and compliance with treatment.

- Establish an environment of caring and trust. Encourage the client to express feelings. *Establishing a trusting nurse–client relationship provides a safe environment for the client to discuss feelings of helplessness, powerlessness, anxiety, and hopelessness. The nurse may then be able to provide additional resources to meet the client's needs.*
- Accept denial as a coping mechanism, but do not reinforce it. *Denial may initially help by diminishing the psychological threat to health, decreasing anxiety. However, its prolonged use can interfere with acceptance of reality and cooperation, possibly delaying treatment and hindering recovery.*
- Note aggressive behaviors, hostility, or anger. Document any failure to comply with treatments. *These signs can indicate anxiety and denial.*
- Help the client identify positive coping skills used in the past (e.g., problem-solving skills, verbalization of feelings, asking for help, prayer). Reinforce use of positive coping behaviors. *Coping behaviors that have been successful in the past can help the client deal with the current situation. These familiar methods can decrease feelings of powerlessness.*
- Provide opportunities for the client to make decisions about the plan of care, as possible. *This promotes self-confidence*

*and independence. Participating in care planning gives the client a sense of control and the opportunity to use positive coping skills.*

- Provide privacy for the client and significant other to share their questions and concerns. *Privacy provides an opportunity for the client and partner to share their feelings and fears, offer support and encouragement to one another, relieve anxiety, and establish effective coping methods.*

## Fear

The fear of death and disability can be a paralyzing emotion that adversely affects the client's recovery from acute myocardial infarction.

- Identify the client's level of fear, noting verbal and nonverbal signs. *This information enables the nurse to plan appropriate interventions. Clients may not voice concerns; attention to nonverbal indicators is important. Controlling fear helps decrease sympathetic nervous system responses and catecholamine release that may increase feelings of fear and anxiety.*
- Acknowledge the client's perception of the situation. Allow to verbalize concerns. *A sudden change in health status causes anxiety and fear of the unknown. Verbalizing these fears may help the client cope with change and allow the health care team to provide information and correct misconceptions.*
- Encourage questions and provide consistent, factual answers. Repeat information as needed. *Accurate and consistent information can reduce fear. Honest explanations help strengthen the client-nurse relationship and help the client develop realistic expectations. Anxiety and fear decrease the ability to concentrate and retain information; therefore, information may need to be repeated.*
- Encourage self-care. Allow the client to make decisions regarding the plan of care. *This promotes personal responsibility for health and allows some control over the situation. Clients' confidence increases as their dependence decreases.*
- Administer antianxiety medications as ordered. *These medications promote rest and relaxation and decrease feelings of anxiety, which may act as barriers to health restoration.*
- Teach nonpharmacologic methods of stress reduction (e.g., relaxation techniques, mental imagery, music therapy, breathing exercises, meditation, massage). *Stress management techniques can help reduce tension and anxiety, provide a sense of control, and enhance coping skills.*

## Using NANDA, NIC, and NOC

Chart 29–2 shows links between NANDA nursing diagnoses, NIC, and NOC for the client with acute myocardial infarction.

## Home Care

Cardiac rehabilitation begins with admission to the health care facility and continues through the inpatient stay and after discharge into the rehabilitative period. The emphasis is on realistic application of information to maintain lifestyle changes.

Assessing readiness to learn is an important first step in preparing for home care. The client in strong denial may not identify any relevance to the information being taught. Evaluate ability to learn, assessing physiologic and psychologic health, beliefs regarding personal responsibility for health, and expectations of the health care system. Also assess developmental level, ability to perform psychomotor skills, cognitive function, learning disabilities, existing knowledge base, and the influence of previous learning experiences. Provide written material to supplement teaching and encourage questions.

Include the following topics in teaching for home care.

- The normal anatomy and physiology of the heart, and the specific area of heart damage

---

## CHART 29–2 NANDA, NIC, AND NOC LINKAGES

### The Client with Acute Myocardial Infarction

| NURSING DIAGNOSES | NURSING INTERVENTIONS | NURSING OUTCOMES |
|---|---|---|
| • Acute Pain | • Analgesic Administration<br>• Medication Management | • Pain Control<br>• Pain: Disruptive Effects |
| • Anxiety | • Anxiety Reduction<br>• Coping Enhancement | • Anxiety Control<br>• Coping |
| • Decreased Cardiac Output | • Cardiac Care: Acute<br>• Hemodynamic Regulation<br>• Shock Management: Cardiac | • Cardiac Pump Effectiveness<br>• Circulation Status<br>• Tissue Perfusion: Peripheral<br>• Vital Signs Status |
| • Ineffective Family Coping | • Coping Enhancement<br>• Family Involvement Promotion | • Family Coping |
| • Ineffective Tissue Perfusion: Cardiopulmonary | • Bleeding Precautions<br>• Dysrhythmia Management<br>• Cardiac Care: Rehabilitative | • Cardiac Pump Effectiveness<br>• Tissue Perfusion: Cardiac |

*Note. Data from Nursing Outcomes Classification (NOC) by M. Johnson & M. Maas (Eds.), 1997, St. Louis: Mosby; Nursing Diagnoses: Definitions & Classification 2001–2002 by North American Nursing Diagnosis Association, 2001, Philadelphia: NANDA; Nursing Interventions Classification (NIC) by J.C. McCloskey & G. M. Bulechek (Eds.), 2000, St. Louis: Mosby. Reprinted by permission.*

- The process of CHD and implications of MI
- Purposes and side effects of prescribed medications
- The importance of complying with the medical regimen and cardiac rehabilitation program and of keeping follow-up appointments
- Information about community resources, such as the local chapter of the American Heart Association

After discharge, follow up by telephone within 1 week and periodically thereafter during the recovery period. Provide telephone numbers of resource personnel who are available to respond to questions and concerns after discharge. Because the client who has had an MI is at high risk for sudden cardiac death; encourage family members to learn CPR and provide information about community resources for CPR training.

## Nursing Care Plan
## A Client with Acute Myocardial Infarction

Betty Williams, a 62-year-old psychologist, is admitted to the emergency department with complaints of severe substernal chest pain. Mrs. Williams states that the pain began after lunch, about 4 hours ago. She initially attributed the pain to indigestion. She described the pain, which now radiates to her jaw and left arm, as "really severe heartburn." It is accompanied by a "choking feeling," severe shortness of breath, and diaphoresis. The pain is unrelieved by rest, antacids, or three sublingual nitroglycerin tablets (0.4 mg).

Oxygen is started per nasal cannula at 5 L/min. Central and peripheral intravenous lines are inserted. A 12-lead ECG and the following labwork are obtained: cardiac troponins, CK and CK isoenzymes, ABGs, CBC, and a chemistry panel. Morphine sulfate relieves Mrs. Williams's pain.

Mrs. Williams's medical history includes type 2 diabetes, angina, and hypertension. She has a 45-year history of cigarette smoking, averaging 1.5 to 2 packs per day. Family history reveals that Mrs. Williams's father died at age 42 of AMI, and her paternal grandfather died at age 65 of AMI. Mrs. Williams is taking the following medications: tolbutamide (Orinase), hydrochlorothiazide, and isosorbide (Isordil).

Based on ECG changes and cardiac markers, an acute anterior MI is diagnosed. Mrs. Williams has no contraindications to thrombolytic therapy and is deemed a good candidate. Intravenous alteplase (t-PA, Activase) is given by bolus followed by intravenous infusions of alteplase and heparin. She is transferred to the coronary care unit (CCU).

### ASSESSMENT

Dan Morales, RN, is Mrs. Williams's primary care nurse. Mrs. Williams is alert and oriented to person, place, and time. Vital signs are T 99.6° F (37.5° C), P 118, R 24 with adequate depth, and BP 172/92. Auscultation reveals an $S_4$ and fine crackles in the bases of both lungs. The ECG shows sinus tachycardia with occasional PVCs. Her skin is cool and slightly diaphoretic. Capillary refill is less than 3 seconds, and peripheral pulses are strong and equal. Her nail beds are pink.

A triple-lumen central line is in place. Nitroglycerin is infusing at 200 mcg/min in the distal lumen; the alteplase infusion is in the middle lumen; and a heparin infusion is in the proximal lumen. The peripheral intravenous line has a saline lock. Mrs. Williams states, "The pain is better since the nurse in the ER gave me a shot. But it has been coming and going. I would rate it a 4 right now, but it was terrible before. The doctor told me that this drug I'm getting will quickly open up the artery that is blocked. I hope it works! Do many people get this drug?"

### DIAGNOSES

- *Acute pain* related to ischemic myocardial tissue
- *Anxiety and fear* related to change in health status
- *Ineffective protection* related to the risk of bleeding secondary to thrombolytic therapy
- *Risk for decreased cardiac output* related to altered cardiac rate and rhythm

### EXPECTED OUTCOMES

- Rate chest pain as 2 or lower on a pain scale of 0 to 10.
- Verbalize reduced anxiety and fear.
- Demonstrate no signs of internal or external bleeding.
- Maintain an adequate cardiac output during and following reperfusion therapy.

### PLANNING AND IMPLEMENTATION

The following interventions are planned and implemented during the immediate phase of Mrs. Williams's hospitalization.

- Instruct to report all chest pain. Monitor and evaluate pain using a scale of 0 to 10. Titrate intravenous nitroglycerin infusion for chest pain; stop infusion if systolic BP is below 100 mmHg. Administer 2 to 4 mg morphine intravenously for chest pain unrelieved by nitroglycerin infusion.
- Encourage verbalization of fears and concerns. Respond honestly, and correct misconceptions about the disease, therapeutic interventions, or prognosis.
- Assess knowledge of CHD. Explain the purpose of thrombolytic therapy to dissolve the fresh clot and reperfuse the heart muscle, limiting heart damage.
- Explain the need for frequent monitoring of vital signs and potential bleeding.
- Assess for manifestations of internal or intracranial bleeding: complaints of back or abdominal pain, headache, decreased level of consciousness, dizziness, bloody secretions or excretions, or pallor. Test all stools, urine, and vomitus for occult blood. Notify physician immediately of any abnormal findings.
- Monitor for signs of reperfusion: decreased chest pain, return of ST segment to baseline, reperfusion dysrhythmias (e.g., PVCs, bradycardia, and heart block).
- Continuously monitor ECG for changes in cardiac rate, rhythm, and conduction. Assess vital signs.
- Treat dangerous dysrhythmias or other cardiac events per protocol. Notify the physician.
- Discuss continuing cardiac care and rehabilitation.

## Nursing Care Plan

### A Client with Acute Myocardial Infarction *(continued)*

**EVALUATION**

The initial morphine dose reduces Mrs. Williams's chest pain from a rating of 8 to 4. The nitroglycerin infusion and thrombolytic therapy further reduce her pain to 2. The nitroglycerin infusion is gradually discontinued after 24 hours. As her pain subsides, Mrs. Williams states that she feels "much better now that the pain is gone. I was afraid it would just get worse." She verbalizes an understanding of thrombolytic therapy to limit myocardial damage. No indication of bleeding problems are noted. Reperfusion is indicated by relief of chest pain, return of the ST segment to baseline on the ECG, early peaking of CK levels; and increased frequency of PVCs but no significant dysrhythmias. Mrs. Williams remains in CCU for 36 hours and is transferred to the floor.

**Critical Thinking in the Nursing Process**

1. How would the initial plan of care have changed if Mrs. Williams were not a candidate for thrombolytic therapy?
2. Two days after her initial therapy, Mrs. Williams complains of palpitations. You notice frequent PVCs on the ECG monitor. What do you do?
3. What health promotion topics would you teach Mrs. Williams before discharge?
4. Mrs. Williams states, "I've been smoking for over 45 years, and I'm not going to stop now! Besides, it calms me down when I'm anxious." How would you respond to this statement?

See Evaluating Your Response in Appendix C.

# CARDIAC RHYTHM DISORDERS

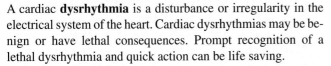

Heart muscle contracts in response to electrical stimulation. In the normal heart, electrical stimulation produces a synchronized, rhythmic heart muscle contraction that propels blood into the vascular system. Changes in cardiac rhythm affect this synchronized activity and the heart's ability to effectively pump blood to body tissues.

## THE CLIENT WITH A CARDIAC DYSRHYTHMIA

A cardiac **dysrhythmia** is a disturbance or irregularity in the electrical system of the heart. Cardiac dysrhythmias may be benign or have lethal consequences. Prompt recognition of a lethal dysrhythmia and quick action can be life saving.

Dysrhythmias develop for many reasons. Not all are pathologic; some alterations in cardiac rhythm occur in response to events such as exercise or fear. For example, a rapid heart rate due to exercise, fever, or excitement is a normal response to the body's demand for oxygen or to stimulation of the sympathetic nervous system. Slow heart rates also may be normal. *Athletic heart syndrome,* which results from long-term training on the heart muscle, allows the heart to beat more slowly and forcefully while maintaining cardiac output and tissue perfusion. Many athletes have a heart rate of less than 60 beats per minute. Aging affects cardiac rhythm as well (see the box on page 840).

Regardless of cause, a dysrhythmia can significantly affect cardiac performance, depending on heart muscle health. The client's response to the dysrhythmia is key in determining the urgency and type of treatment needed.

## PHYSIOLOGY REVIEW

Cardiac muscle is unique. Unlike skeletal muscle tissue, cardiac muscle can generate an electrical impulse and contraction independent of the nervous system.

## Conduction Pathways

Electrical activity of the heart is normally controlled by the *cardiac conduction system,* a network of specialized cells and conduction pathways that initiate and spread electrical impulses that cause the heart to beat (see Figure 28–7). *Pacemaker cells* spontaneously generate electrical impulses at a regular rate. Specialized conduction tissue rapidly transmits these impulses to myocardial cells. Myocardial muscle cells contract in response to the impulse. Electrical stimulation of heart muscle always precedes mechanical contraction.

Pacemaker cells are found throughout the heart. The *sinoatrial (SA)* or *sinus node* is the primary pacemaker of the heart. It usually fires at a regular rate of 60 to 100 BPM, initiating impulses that are conducted throughout the heart. The sinus node impulse spreads through the atria via the *interatrial pathways.* Conduction fibers narrow through the *atrioventricular (AV) node,* briefly delaying impulse conduction. This delay allows atrial muscle to contract, delivering an extra bolus of blood to the ventricles before they contract (the **atrial kick**). The AV node also controls the number of impulses that reach the ventricles, preventing extremely rapid heart rates. From the AV node, the impulse travels down the *bundle of His,* the *right* and *left bundle branches,* and to the *Purkinje fibers* of the ventricular conduction system. The Purkinje fibers terminate in ventricular muscle, prompting mechanical contraction, or *systole.*

If the sinus node fails, secondary pacemakers in the AV node (with an intrinsic rate of 40 to 60 BPM), and the Purkinje fibers (intrinsic rate of 15 to 40 BPM) take over as the pacemaker at a slower rate. This provides backup mechanism for electrical stimulation of the heart.

## Electrophysiologic Properties

Four unique properties of cardiac cells allow effective heart function. Three properties are electrical; the fourth is cardiac muscle's mechanical response to electrical stimulation.

## Nursing Care of the Older Adult

### CARDIAC DYSRHYTHMIAS

Aging affects the heart and the cardiac conduction system, increasing the incidence of dysrhythmias and conduction defects. Older adults may experience dysrhythmias even when no evidence of heart disease is found.

Older adults have a higher incidence of both ventricular and supraventricular dysrhythmias without detrimental effects than younger people. Ectopic beats, including short runs of ventricular tachycardia, occur more commonly during exercise in older adults. These dysrhythmias do not affect cardiac morbidity or mortality. Fibrosis of the bundle branches can lead to atrioventricular blocks; a prolonged PR interval is common in clients over the age of 65. Older adults also have a higher incidence of diseases that may affect heart rhythm. An elderly client with hyperthyroidism, for example, may present with atrial fibrillation, syncope, and confusion instead of the usual manifestations of goiter, tremor, and exophthalmos.

### ASSESSING FOR HOME CARE

Assessing older adults for problems related to cardiac dysrhythmias focuses on the effect of the dysrhythmia on functional health status.

- Ask about a history of cardiovascular disease and current medications.
- Inquire about symptoms such as episodes of dizziness, lightheadedness, fainting, palpitations, chest pain, or shortness of breath.
- Ask about relationship of symptoms such as palpitations to intake of certain foods and caffeine-containing beverages.
- Evaluate for other contributing factors such as smoking or alcohol intake.
- Inquire about a history of falls, particularly those occurring without apparent reason.

### TEACHING FOR HOME CARE

Teach measures to reduce the risk of cardiac dysrhythmias and potential adverse consequences of dysrhythmias,

- Emphasize the importance of taking medications as prescribed. Discuss possible effects of over-the-counter medications on the heart.
- Encourage reducing or eliminating caffeine intake. Caffeine increases the risk of ectopic beats and rapid heart rates.
- Encourage participation in a smoking cessation program and reduce or eliminate alcohol intake if appropriate.
- Encourage engaging in regular exercise. Discuss the beneficial effects of exercise to maintain muscle mass, including cardiac muscle, and cardiovascular health.
- Instruct to contact primary care provider for evaluation of symptoms such as dizziness, fainting, frequent palpitations, shortness of breath, unexplained falls, or chest pain.

- *Automaticity* is the ability of pacemaker cells to spontaneously initiate an electrical impulse. The SA node, the dominant pacemaker, normally generates impulses at the fastest rate, 60 to 100 times a minute. Myocardial muscle cells do not possess this ability.
- *Excitability* is the ability of myocardial cells to respond to stimuli generated by pacemaker cells.
- *Conductivity* is the ability to transmit an impulse from cell to cell. When one cell is stimulated, the impulse rapidly spreads throughout the heart muscle.
- *Contractility* is the ability of myocardial fibers to shorten in response to a stimulus. Heart muscle responds in an *all-or-nothing* manner: Stimulation of one muscle fiber causes the entire muscle mass to contract to its fullest extent as one unit.

### The Action Potential

Movement of ions across cell membranes causes the electrical impulse that stimulates muscle contraction. This electrical activity, called the *action potential*, produces the waveforms represented on ECG strips.

In the resting state, positive and negative ions align on either side of the cell membrane, producing a relatively negative charge within the cell and a positive extracellular charge (Figure 29–8 ■). The cell is said to be *polarized*. The negative resting membrane potential is maintained at about −90 millivolts (mV) by the sodium-potassium pump in the cell membrane.

When the resting cell is stimulated by an electrical charge from a neighboring cell or by a spontaneous event, its cell membrane permeability changes. Sodium ions enter the cell rapidly through openings called *fast sodium channels*. *Slow calcium-sodium channels* also open, allowing calcium into the cell. The membrane becomes less permeable to potassium ions. Addition of these positively charged ions to intracellular fluid changes the membrane potential from negative to slightly positive at +20 to +30 mV. This change in the electrical charge across the cell membrane is called **depolarization.**

As the cell becomes more positive, it reaches a point called the *threshold potential*. When the threshold potential is reached, an action potential is generated. The action potential causes a chemical reaction of calcium within the cell. This, in turn, causes actin and myosin filaments to slide together, producing cardiac muscle contraction. The action potential spreads to surrounding cells, causing a coordinated muscle contraction. As soon as the myocardium is completely depolarized, repolarization begins.

**Repolarization** returns the cell to its resting, polarized state. During *rapid repolarization*, fast sodium channels close abruptly, and the cell begins to regain its negative charge. During the *plateau phase*, muscle contraction is prolonged as slow calcium-sodium channels remain open. When these channels close, the sodium-potassium pump restores ion concentration to normal resting levels. The cell membrane is then polarized, ready for the cycle to start again. Each heartbeat represents one

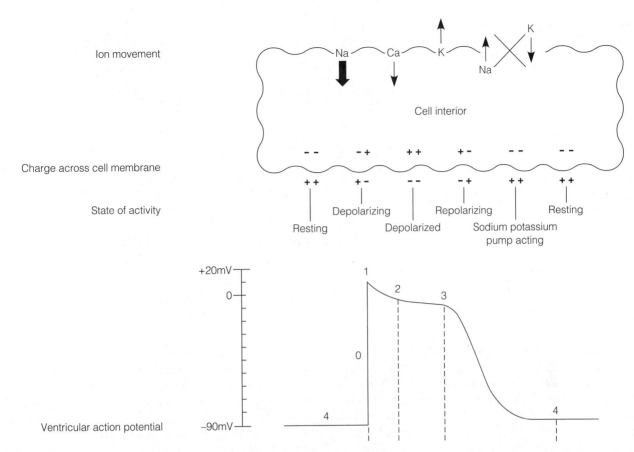

Ion movement

Cell interior

Charge across cell membrane

State of activity

Resting   Depolarizing   Depolarized   Repolarizing   Sodium potassium pump acting   Resting

Ventricular action potential

+20mV
0
−90mV

**Figure 29–8** ■ Action potential of a cardiac cell. In the resting state (phase 4), the cell membrane is polarized: the cell's interior has a negative charge compared to that of extracellular fluid. On depolarization (phase 0), sodium ions diffuse rapidly across the cell membrane into the cell, and calcium channels open. In the fully depolarized state (phase 1), the cell's interior has a net positive charge compared to its exterior. During the plateau period (phase 2), calcium moves into the cell and potassium diffusion slows, prolonging the action potential. In phase 3, calcium channels close, the sodium-potassium pump removes sodium from the cell, and the cell membrane again becomes polarized with a net negative charge.

cardiac cycle, with one depolarization and repolarization cycle and one complete cardiac muscle contraction and relaxation (systole and diastole).

Normally, only pacemaker cells demonstrate automaticity. Pacemaker cells have a resting potential that is much less negative ($-70$ to $-50$ mV) than other cardiac muscle cells. Their threshold potential also is lower than that of other myocardial cells. These differences result from constant leakage of sodium and potassium ions into the cell.

Myocardial cells have a unique protective property, the **refractory period,** during which they resist stimulation. This property protects cardiac muscle from spasm and tetany. During the *absolute refractory period,* depolarization will not occur no matter how strongly the cell is stimulated. It is followed by the *relative refractory period,* during which a greater than normal stimulus is required to generate another action potential. During the *supernormal period* that follows, a mild stimulus will cause depolarization. Many cardiac dysrhythmias are triggered during the relative refractory and supernormal periods.

## Electrocardiography

**Electrocardiography** is the graphic recording of the heart's electrical activity detected through electrodes placed on the surface of the body. Electrical activity is shown as a series of waveforms on a visual display, a strip recorder (graphic record), or both. ECG waveforms and patterns are examined to detect dysrhythmias as well as myocardial damage, the effects of drugs, and electrolyte imbalances.

The *electrocardiogram (ECG)* is a graphic record of this activity. *Electrodes* applied to the body surface are used to obtain a graphic representation of cardiac electrical activity. These electrodes detect the magnitude and direction of electrical currents produced in the heart. They attach to the electrocardiograph by an insulated wire called a *lead.* The electrocardiograph converts the electrical impulses it receives into a series of waveforms which represent cardiac depolarization and repolarization. Placement of electrodes on different parts of the body allows different views of this electrical activity, much like turning the head while holding a camera provides different views of the scenery.

Both bipolar and unipolar leads are used in recording the ECG. A *bipolar lead* uses two electrodes of opposite polarity (negative and positive). In a *unipolar* lead, one positive electrode and a negative reference point at the center of the heart are used. The electrical potential between the two monitoring points is graphically recorded as the ECG waveform.

**Figure 29–9** ■ Planes of the heart. *A,* the frontal plane. *B,* the horizontal plane.

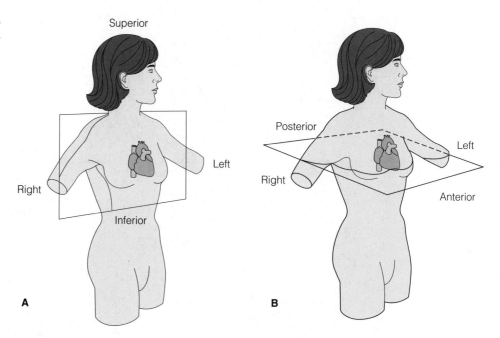

A

B

The heart can be viewed from both the *frontal plane* and the *horizontal plane* (Figure 29–9 ■). Each plane provides a unique perspective of the heart muscle. The frontal plane is an imaginary cut through the body that views the heart from top to bottom (superior–inferior) and side to side (right–left). This perspective of the heart is analogous to a paper doll cutout. It provides information about the inferior and lateral walls of the heart. The horizontal plane is a cross-sectional view of the heart from front to back (anterior–posterior) and side to side (right–left). Information regarding the anterior, septal, and lateral walls of the heart, as well as the posterior wall, are obtained from this view.

A standard 12-lead ECG provides a simultaneous recording of six limb leads and six precordial leads (Figure 29–10 ■). The *limb leads* provide information about the heart in the frontal plane and include three bipolar leads (I, II, III) and three unipolar leads (aV$_R$, aV$_L$, and aV$_F$). The bipolar limb leads measure electrical activity between a negative lead on one extremity and a positive lead on another. The unipolar limb leads (called *augmented leads*) measure the electrical activity between a single positive electrode on a limb (right arm [R], left arm [L], or left leg [F for foot]), and the center of the heart.

The *precordial leads,* also known as chest leads or V leads, view the heart in the horizontal plane. They include six unipolar leads (V$_1$, V$_2$, V$_3$, V$_4$, V$_5$, and V$_6$), which measure electrical activity between the center of the heart and a positive electrode on the chest wall.

ECG waveforms reflect the direction of electrical flow in relation to a positive electrode. Current flowing toward the positive electrode produces an upward (positive) waveform; current flowing away from the positive electrode produces a downward (negative) waveform. Current flowing perpendicular to the positive pole produces a *biphasic* (both positive and negative) waveform. Absence of electrical activity is represented by a straight line called the *isoelectric line.*

ECG waveforms are recorded by a heated stylus on heat-sensitive paper. The paper is marked at standard intervals that represent time and voltage or amplitude (Figure 29–11 ■). Each small box is 1 mm². The recording speed of the standard ECG is 25 mm/second, so each small box represents 0.04 second. Five small boxes horizontally and vertically make one large box, equivalent to 0.20 second. Five large boxes represent 1 full second. Measured vertically, each small box represents 0.1 millivolt (mV).

The cardiac cycle is depicted as a series of waveforms, the P, Q, R, S, and T waves (Figure 29–12 ■). The *P wave* represents atrial depolarization and contraction. The impulse is from the sinus node. The P wave precedes the QRS complex and is normally smooth, round, and upright. P waves may be absent when the SA node is not acting as the pacemaker. Atrial repolarization occurs during ventricular depolarization and usually is not seen on the ECG.

The *PR interval* represents the time required for the sinus impulse to travel to the AV node and into the bundle branches. This

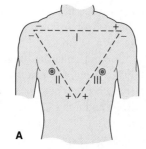

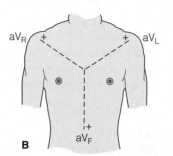

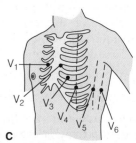

**Figure 29–10** ■ Leads of the 12-lead ECG. *A,* Bipolar limb leads I, II, III. *B,* Unipolar limb leads aV$_R$, aV$_L$, aV$_F$. *C,* Unipolar precordial leads V$_1$ to V$_6$.

A

B

C

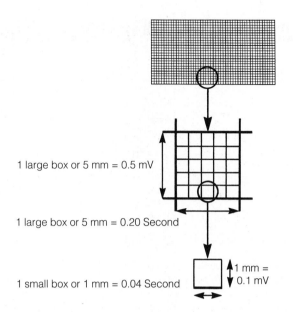

**Figure 29-11** ■ Time and voltage measurements on ECG paper at a recording speed of 25 mm/second.

interval is measured from beginning of P wave to beginning of QRS complex. If no Q wave is seen, the beginning of the R wave is used. The PR interval is normally 0.12 to 0.20 second (up to 0.24 second is considered normal in clients over age 65). PR intervals greater than 0.20 second indicate a delay in conduction from the SA node to the ventricles.

The *QRS complex* represents ventricular depolarization and contraction. The QRS complex includes three separate waves: The Q wave is the first negative deflection, the R wave is the

positive or upright deflection, and the S wave is the first negative deflection after the R wave. Not all QRS complexes have all three waves; nonetheless, the complex is called a QRS complex. The normal duration of a QRS complex is from 0.06 to 0.10 second. QRS complexes greater than 0.10 second indicate delays in transmitting the impulse through the ventricular conduction system.

The *ST segment* signifies the beginning of ventricular repolarization. The ST segment, the period from the end of the QRS complex to the beginning of the T wave, should be isoelectric. An abnormal ST segment is displaced (elevated or depressed) from the isoelectric line.

The *T wave* represents ventricular repolarization. It normally has a smooth, rounded shape that is usually less than 10 mm tall. It usually points in the same direction as the QRS complex. Abnormalities of the T wave may indicate myocardial ischemia or injury, or electrolyte imbalances.

The *QT interval* is measured from the beginning of the QRS complex to the end of the T wave. It represents the total time of ventricular depolarization and repolarization. Its duration varies with gender, age, and heart rate; usually, it is 0.32 to 0.44 second long. Prolonged QT intervals indicate a prolonged relative refractory period and a greater risk of dysrhythmias. Shortened QT intervals may result from medications or electrolyte imbalances.

The *U wave* is not normally seen. It is thought to signify repolarization of the terminal Purkinje fibers. If present, the U wave follows the same direction as the T wave. It is most commonly seen in hypokalemia.

Interpreting an ECG strip to determine the cardiac rhythm is a skill that takes practice to learn and master. Many methods are used to analyze ECGs. One sequence of steps to evaluate an ECG strip is listed in Box 29-3. It is important to use a consistent method for ECG analysis. The data obtained can then be used to determine cardiac rhythm. Identifying and interpreting complex dysrhythmias requires advanced skills and knowledge obtained through further training.

## PATHOPHYSIOLOGY

Dysrhythmias arise through two major mechanisms: altered impulse formation (automaticity) and altered conductivity.

Dysrhythmias due to altered impulse formation include changes in rate and rhythm and the development of ectopic beats. This category includes *tachydysrhythmias* (rapid heart rates), *bradydysrhythmias* (slow heart rates), and ectopic rhythms. These dysrhythmias result from a change in the automaticity of cardiac cells. Impulse formation may abnormally increase or decrease. Aberrant (abnormal) impulses may originate outside normal conduction pathways, causing **ectopic beats.** Ectopic beats interrupt the normal conduction sequence; depending on the site and of abnormal impulses, they may have little effect on the client or pose a significant threat.

Conduction abnormalities result from failure or delay of impulse transmission. They cause varying degrees of **heart block,** a block in the normal conduction pathways. Myocardial injury or infarction can obstruct or delay impulse conduction. Bundle branch blocks are common in acute myocardial infarction.

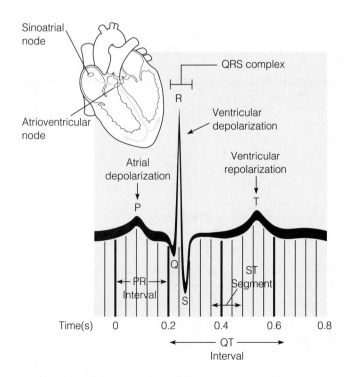

**Figure 29-12** ■ Normal ECG waveform and intervals.

## BOX 29–3   ■ ECG Rhythm Analysis

■ *Step 1: Determine rate.* Assess heart rate. Use P waves to determine the atrial rate and R waves for the ventricular rate. Several approaches can determine the heart rate.

•  Count the number of complexes in a 6-second rhythm strip (the top margin of ECG paper is marked at 3-second intervals), and multiply by 10. This provides an estimate of the rate and is particularly valuable if rhythms are irregular.

•  Count the number of large boxes between two consecutive complexes, and divide 300 (the number of large boxes in 1 minute) by this number. For example, there are 6 large boxes between two R waves; 300 divided by 6 equals a ventricular rate of 50 BPM. Memorize the following sequence for rapid rate determination: 300, 150, 100, 75, 60, 50, 43. One large box between complexes equals a rate of 300; two, a rate of 150; three, a rate of 100; and so on.

•  Count the number of small boxes between two consecutive complexes, and divide 1500 (the number of small boxes in 1 minute) by this number. For example, there are 19 small boxes between two R waves; 1500 divided by 19 equals a ventricular rate of 79 BPM. This is the most precise measurement of heart rate.

■ *Step 2: Determine regularity.* Regularity is the consistency with which the P waves or QRS complexes occur. In a regular rhythm, all waves occur at a consistent rate. Rhythm regularity is determined by measuring the interval between consecutive waves. Place one point of an ECG caliper (a measuring device) on the peak of the P wave (for atrial rhythm) or the R wave (for ventricular rhythm). Adjust the other point to the peak of the next wave, P to P or R to R (see the figure in this box). Keeping the calipers set at this distance, evaluate intervals between consecutive waves. The rhythm is *regular* if all caliper points fall on succeeding wave peaks. Alternately, use a strip of blank paper on top of the ECG strip, marking the peaks of two or three consecutive waves. Then move the paper along the strip to consecutive waves. Wave peaks that vary by more than one to three small boxes (depending on the rate) are *irregular*. Irregular rhythms may be *irregularly irregular* (if the intervals have no pattern) or *regularly irregular* (if a consistent pattern to the irregularity can be identified).

■ *Step 3: Assess P wave.* The presence or absence of P waves helps determine origin of the rhythm. All the P waves should be alike

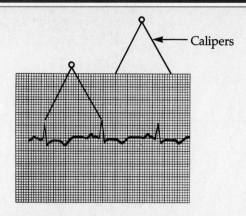

Calipers

in size and shape (*morphology*). If P waves are not seen or they differ in shape, the rhythm may not originate in the sinus node.

■ *Step 4: Assess P to QRS relationship.* Determine the relationship between P waves and QRS complexes. There should be one and only one P wave for every QRS complex, because the normal stimulus for ventricular contraction originates in the sinus node.

■ *Step 5: Determine interval durations.* To evaluate impulse transmission through the cardiac conduction system, measure the PR interval, QRS duration, and QT interval. To measure, count the number of small boxes from the beginning of the interval to the end, and multiply by 0.04 second. Then determine whether the interval duration is within its normal limits. For example, the PR interval is 3.5 small boxes wide, or 0.14 second. This is within the normal limits of 0.12 to 0.20 second. This interval should be consistent, not varying from beat to beat. A PR interval greater than 0.20 second or one that varies from beat to beat is abnormal.

The QRS complex duration is normally between 0.06 and 0.10 second. A QRS complex greater than 0.12 second indicates delayed ventricular conduction.

The QT interval is normally 0.32 to 0.44 second. It varies inversely with the heart rate: The faster the heart rate, the shorter the QT interval. As a general rule, the QT interval should be no more than half the previous R–R interval. A prolonged QT interval indicates a prolonged relative refractory period of the heart.

■ *Step 6: Identify abnormalities.* Note the presence and frequency of *ectopic* (extra) beats, deviation of the ST segment above or below the baseline, and abnormalities in waveform shape and duration.

---

The *reentry phenomenon,* a phenomenon of normal and slow conduction, is a major cause of tachydysrhythmias. A stimulus such as an ectopic beat triggers the reentry phenomenon. The impulse is delayed in one area of the heart but conducted normally through the rest. Muscle that has been depolarized by the normally conducted impulse is repolarized by the time the impulse traveling through the area of slow conduction reaches it, thus initiating another cycle of depolarization (Porth, 2002). The result is a dysrhythmia that propagates itself.

Cardiac rhythms are classified according to the site of impulse formation or the site and degree of conduction block. *Supraventricular rhythms* arise above the ventricles. These rhythms usually produce a QRS complex within the normal range. Sinus rhythms, atrial rhythms, and junctional (arising from the AV junction) rhythms are all supraventricular rhythms. *Ventricular rhythms* originate in the ventricles and may prove fatal if left un-

treated. *AV conduction blocks* result from a defect in impulse transmission from the atria to the ventricles. The major normal and abnormal cardiac rhythms are summarized in Table 29–6.

## Supraventricular Rhythms

### Normal Sinus Rhythm

**Normal sinus rhythm (NSR)** is the normal heart rhythm, in which impulses originate in the SA (sinus) node and travel through all normal conduction pathways without delay. All waveforms are of normal configuration, look alike, and have consistent (fixed) durations. The rate is between 60 and 100 BPM.

### Sinus Node Dysrhythmias

Sinus node dysrhythmias may occur as a normal compensatory response (e.g., to exercise) or because of altered automaticity. In these rhythms, as in NSR, the initiating impulse is from the

TABLE 29–6  Characteristics of Selected Cardiac Rhythms and Dysrhythmias

| Rhythm/ECG Appearance | ECG Characteristics | Management |
|---|---|---|
| **Supraventricular Rhythms**<br>*Normal sinus rhythm (NSR)*<br>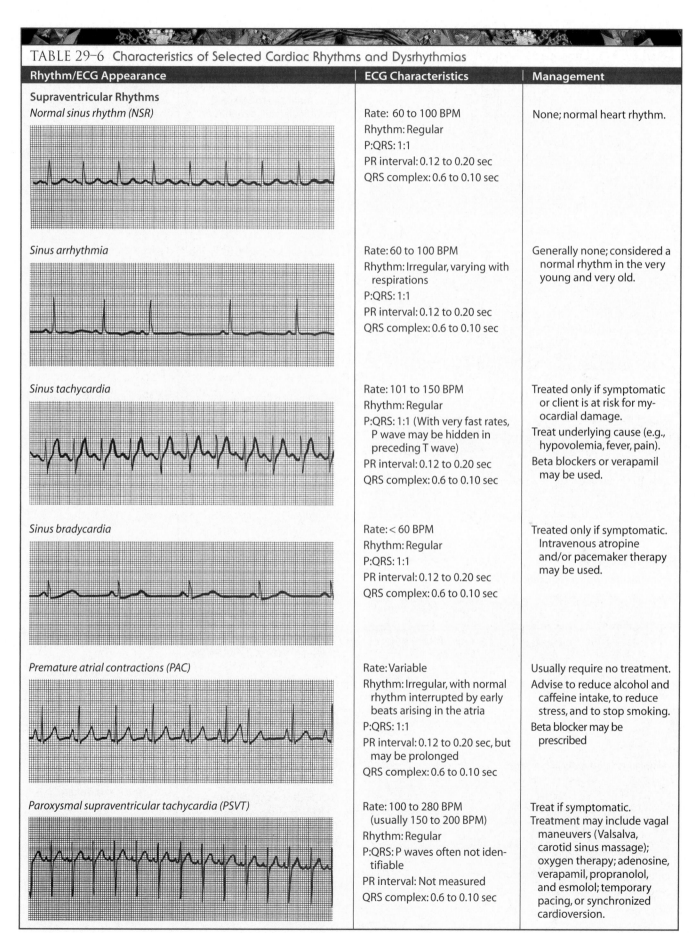 | Rate: 60 to 100 BPM<br>Rhythm: Regular<br>P:QRS: 1:1<br>PR interval: 0.12 to 0.20 sec<br>QRS complex: 0.6 to 0.10 sec | None; normal heart rhythm. |
| *Sinus arrhythmia* | Rate: 60 to 100 BPM<br>Rhythm: Irregular, varying with respirations<br>P:QRS: 1:1<br>PR interval: 0.12 to 0.20 sec<br>QRS complex: 0.6 to 0.10 sec | Generally none; considered a normal rhythm in the very young and very old. |
| *Sinus tachycardia* | Rate: 101 to 150 BPM<br>Rhythm: Regular<br>P:QRS: 1:1 (With very fast rates, P wave may be hidden in preceding T wave)<br>PR interval: 0.12 to 0.20 sec<br>QRS complex: 0.6 to 0.10 sec | Treated only if symptomatic or client is at risk for my-ocardial damage.<br>Treat underlying cause (e.g., hypovolemia, fever, pain).<br>Beta blockers or verapamil may be used. |
| *Sinus bradycardia* | Rate: < 60 BPM<br>Rhythm: Regular<br>P:QRS: 1:1<br>PR interval: 0.12 to 0.20 sec<br>QRS complex: 0.6 to 0.10 sec | Treated only if symptomatic. Intravenous atropine and/or pacemaker therapy may be used. |
| *Premature atrial contractions (PAC)* | Rate: Variable<br>Rhythm: Irregular, with normal rhythm interrupted by early beats arising in the atria<br>P:QRS: 1:1<br>PR interval: 0.12 to 0.20 sec, but may be prolonged<br>QRS complex: 0.6 to 0.10 sec | Usually require no treatment.<br>Advise to reduce alcohol and caffeine intake, to reduce stress, and to stop smoking.<br>Beta blocker may be prescribed |
| *Paroxysmal supraventricular tachycardia (PSVT)* | Rate: 100 to 280 BPM (usually 150 to 200 BPM)<br>Rhythm: Regular<br>P:QRS: P waves often not iden-tifiable<br>PR interval: Not measured<br>QRS complex: 0.6 to 0.10 sec | Treat if symptomatic.<br>Treatment may include vagal maneuvers (Valsalva, carotid sinus massage); oxygen therapy; adenosine, verapamil, propranolol, and esmolol; temporary pacing, or synchronized cardioversion. |

*(continued on page 846)*

## TABLE 29-6 Characteristics of Selected Cardiac Rhythms and Dysrhythmias (continued)

| Rhythm/ECG Appearance | ECG Characteristics | Management |
|---|---|---|
| *Atrial flutter* | Rate: Atrial 240 to 360 BPM; ventricular rate depends on degree of AV block and usually is <150 BPM<br>Rhythm: Atrial regular; ventricular usually regular<br>P:QRS: 2:1, 4:1, 6:1; may vary<br>PR interval: Not measured<br>QRS complex: 0.6 to 0.10 sec. | Synchronized cardioversion; medications to slow ventricular response such as a beta blocker or calcium channel blocker (verapamil), followed by ibutilide, quinidine, procainamide, flecainide, or amiodarone. |
| *Atrial fibrillation* | Rate: Atrial 300 to 600 BPM (too rapid to count); ventricular 100 to 180 BPM in untreated clients<br>Rhythm: Irregularly irregular<br>P:QRS: Variable<br>PR interval: Not measured<br>QRS complex: 0.06 to 0.10 sec | Synchronized cardioversion; medications to reduce ventricular response rate: verapamil, propranolol, or digoxin; anticoagulant therapy to reduce risk of clot formation and stroke. |
| *Junctional escape rhythm* | Rate: 40 to 60 BPM; junctional tachycardia 60 to 140 BPM<br>Rhythm: Regular<br>P:QRS: P waves may be absent, inverted and immediately preceding or succeeding QRS complex, or hidden in QRS complex<br>PR interval: <0.10 sec<br>QRS complex: 0.06 to 0.10 sec | Treat cause if symptomatic. |
| **Ventricular Rhythms**<br>*Premature ventricular contractions (PVC)* | Rate: Variable<br>Rhythm: Irregular, with PVC interrupting underlying rhythm and followed by a compensatory pause<br>P:QRS: No P wave noted before PVC<br>PR interval: Absent with PVC<br>QRS complex: Wide (>0.12 sec) and bizarre in appearance; differs from normal QRS complex | Treat if symptomatic or in presence of severe heart disease. Advise against stimulant use (caffeine, nicotine). Beta blockers, or class I of II antidysrhythmic agents (see the box on page 854) may be used. |
| *Ventricular tachycardia (VT or V tach)* | Rate: 100 to 250 BPM<br>Rhythm: Regular<br>P:QRS: P waves usually not identifiable<br>PR interval: Not measured<br>QRS complex: 0.12 sec or greater; bizarre shape | Treat if VT is sustained, symptomatic, or associated with organic heart disease. Treatment includes intravenous procainamide or lidocaine and/or immediate cardioversion if unconscious or unstable. Surgical ablation or antitachycardia pacing with an implanted cardioverter/defibrilator (ICD) for repeated episodes. |

## TABLE 29-6 Characteristics of Selected Cardiac Rhythms and Dysrhythmias (continued)

| Rhythm/ECG Appearance | ECG Characteristics | Management |
|---|---|---|
| *Ventricular fibrillation (VF, V fib)* 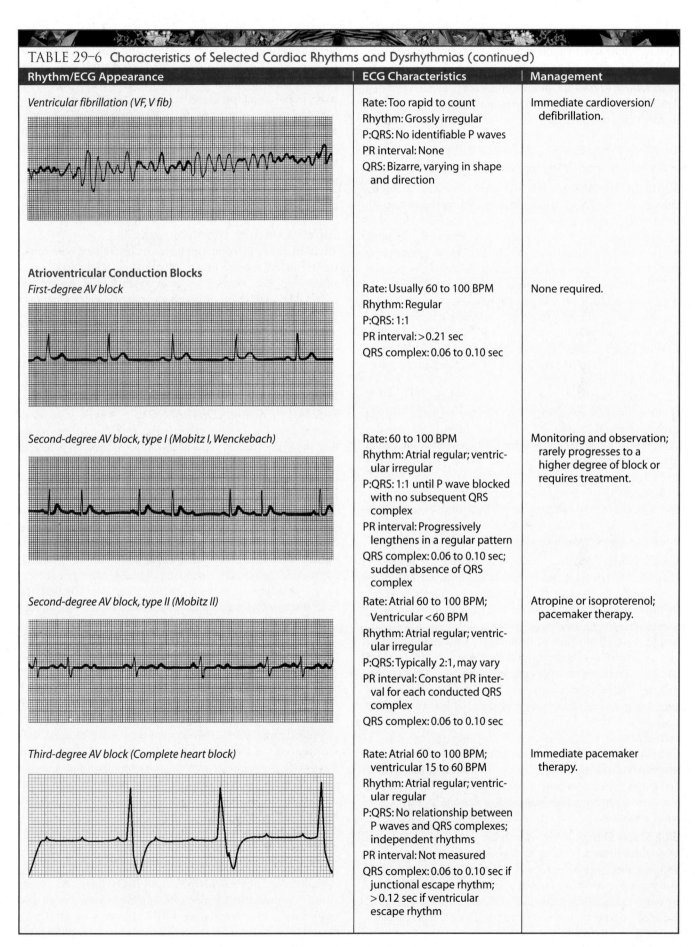 | Rate: Too rapid to count<br>Rhythm: Grossly irregular<br>P:QRS: No identifiable P waves<br>PR interval: None<br>QRS: Bizarre, varying in shape and direction | Immediate cardioversion/ defibrillation. |
| **Atrioventricular Conduction Blocks**<br>*First-degree AV block* | Rate: Usually 60 to 100 BPM<br>Rhythm: Regular<br>P:QRS: 1:1<br>PR interval: >0.21 sec<br>QRS complex: 0.06 to 0.10 sec | None required. |
| *Second-degree AV block, type I (Mobitz I, Wenckebach)* | Rate: 60 to 100 BPM<br>Rhythm: Atrial regular; ventricular irregular<br>P:QRS: 1:1 until P wave blocked with no subsequent QRS complex<br>PR interval: Progressively lengthens in a regular pattern<br>QRS complex: 0.06 to 0.10 sec; sudden absence of QRS complex | Monitoring and observation; rarely progresses to a higher degree of block or requires treatment. |
| *Second-degree AV block, type II (Mobitz II)* | Rate: Atrial 60 to 100 BPM; Ventricular <60 BPM<br>Rhythm: Atrial regular; ventricular irregular<br>P:QRS: Typically 2:1, may vary<br>PR interval: Constant PR interval for each conducted QRS complex<br>QRS complex: 0.06 to 0.10 sec | Atropine or isoproterenol; pacemaker therapy. |
| *Third-degree AV block (Complete heart block)* | Rate: Atrial 60 to 100 BPM; ventricular 15 to 60 BPM<br>Rhythm: Atrial regular; ventricular regular<br>P:QRS: No relationship between P waves and QRS complexes; independent rhythms<br>PR interval: Not measured<br>QRS complex: 0.06 to 0.10 sec if junctional escape rhythm; >0.12 sec if ventricular escape rhythm | Immediate pacemaker therapy. |

sinus node. They differ from NSR in rate or regularity of the rhythm. Sinus dysrhythmias include sinus arrhythmia, sinus tachycardia, and sinus bradycardia.

**SINUS ARRHYTHMIA.** *Sinus arrhythmia* is a sinus rhythm in which the rate varies with respirations, causing an irregular rhythm. The rate increases during inspiration and decreases with expiration. Sinus arrhythmia is common in the very young and the very old. It can be caused by an increase in vagal tone, by digitalis toxicity, or by morphine administration.

**SINUS TACHYCARDIA.** *Sinus tachycardia* has all of the characteristics of NSR, except that the rate is greater than 100 BPM. Tachycardia arises from enhanced automaticity in response to changes in the internal environment. Sympathetic nervous system stimulation or blocked vagal (parasympathetic) activity increases the heart rate. Tachycardia is a normal response to any condition or event that increases the body's demand for oxygen and nutrients, such as exercise or hypoxia. In the client on bed rest, tachycardia is an ominous sign. Sinus tachycardia may be an early sign of cardiac dysfunction, such as heart failure. Tachycardia is detrimental in clients with cardiac disease because it increases cardiac work and oxygen use.

Common causes of sinus tachycardia include exercise, excitement, anxiety, pain, fever, hypoxia, hypovolemia, anemia, hyperthyroidism, myocardial infarction, heart failure, cardiogenic shock, pulmonary embolism, caffeine intake, and certain drugs, such as atropine, epinephrine (Adrenalin), or isoproterenol (Isuprel).

Manifestations of sinus tachycardia include a rapid pulse rate. The client may complain of feeling that the heart is "racing," shortness of breath, and dizziness. In the presence of heart disease, sinus tachycardia may precipitate chest pain.

**SINUS BRADYCARDIA.** *Sinus bradycardia* has all of the characteristics of NSR, but the rate is less than 60 BPM. Sinus bradycardia may result from increased vagal (parasympathetic) activity or from depressed automaticity due to injury or ischemia to the sinus node. Sinus bradycardia may be normal (e.g., in clients with athletic heart syndrome). The heart rate also normally slows during sleep because the parasympathetic nervous system is dominant at this time. Other causes of sinus bradycardia include pain, increased intracranial pressure, sinus node disease, acute myocardial infarction (especially with inferior wall damage), hypothermia, acidosis, and certain drugs.

Sinus bradycardia may be asymptomatic; it is important to assess the client before treating the rhythm. Manifestations of decreased cardiac output, such as decreased level of consciousness, syncope (faintness), or hypotension indicate a need for intervention.

**SICK SINUS SYNDROME.** *Sick sinus syndrome (SSS)* results from sinus node disease or dysfunction that causes problems with impulse formation, transmission, and conduction. Sick sinus syndrome is often found in older adults. It may be caused by direct injury to sinus tissue, fibrosis of conduction fibers associated with aging, and such drugs as digitalis, beta blockers, and calcium channel blockers.

ECG characteristics of SSS include sinus bradycardia, sinus arrhythmia, sinus pauses or arrest, and atrial tachydysrhythmias such as atrial fibrillation, atrial flutter, or atrial tachycardia. Bradycardia-tachycardia syndrome, characterized either by **paroxysmal** (abrupt onset and termination) atrial tachycardia followed by prolonged sinus pauses or alternating periods of bradycardia and tachycardia also may indicate sinus node dysfunction.

Manifestations of sinus node dysfunction often are intermittent, related to a drop in cardiac output caused by the irregular rhythm. Fatigue, dizziness, lightheadedness, and syncope are common. The heart rate may not increase in response to stressors such as exercise or fever.

### Supraventricular Dysrhythmias

When an action potential originates in atrial tissue outside the sinus node, the resulting rhythm is classified as a *supraventricular rhythm.* In these dysrhythmias, an ectopic pacemaker takes over, or overrides, the SA node. They may also occur when the SA node fails; an *escape rhythm* develops as a fail-safe mechanism to maintain the heart rate. The most common supraventricular dysrhythmias are premature atrial contractions, paroxysmal supraventricular tachycardia, atrial flutter, and atrial fibrillation. These rhythms may be paroxysmal, that is, occur in bursts with an abrupt beginning and end.

**PREMATURE ATRIAL CONTRACTIONS.** A *premature atrial contraction (PAC)* is an ectopic atrial beat that occurs earlier than the next expected sinus beat. PACs can arise anywhere in the atria. They are usually asymptomatic and benign, but they may initiate paroxysmal supraventricular tachycardia in susceptible individuals. PACs are common in older adults, often occurring without an obvious cause. Strong emotions, excessive alcohol intake, tobacco, and stimulants such as caffeine can precipitate PACs. They also may be associated with myocardial infarction, heart failure and other cardiac disorders, hypoxemia, pulmonary embolism, digitalis toxicity, and electrolyte or acid-base imbalances. In clients with underlying heart disease, PACs may precede a more serious dysrhythmia.

The ECG tracing shows interruption of the underlying rhythm by a premature complex that looks similar to the underlying beats. The ectopic impulse of the PAC is usually conducted normally, leading to depolarization of cardiac muscle and a normal QRS complex. Because the impulse arises above the ventricles, it follows normal conduction pathways through the ventricles. The QRS complex is narrow or matches those of the underlying rhythm. The shape of the P wave of a PAC differs from normal P waves because its impulse arises outside the sinus node. A *noncompensatory pause* usually follows, as the PAC resets the SA node rhythm. Occasionally, the ectopic impulse may not be conducted through the heart, resulting in a lone P wave without a QRS, or a nonconducted PAC.

PACs cause few manifestations. If frequent, they may cause palpitations or a fluttering sensation in the chest. Early beats may be noted on auscultating or palpating the pulse.

**PAROXYSMAL SUPRAVENTRICULAR TACHYCARDIA.** *Paroxysmal supraventricular tachycardia (PSVT)* is tachycardia of sudden onset and termination. PSVT is usually initiated by a reentry loop in or around the AV node; that is, an impulse reenters the same section of tissue over and over, causing repeated depolarizations.

PSVT occurs more frequently in women. Sympathetic nervous system stimulation and stressors such as fever, sepsis, and hyperthyroidism may precipitate PSVT. It also may be associated with heart diseases such as CHD, myocardial infarction, rheumatic heart disease, myocarditis, or acute pericarditis. Abnormal conduction pathways associated with Wolff-Parkinson-White (WPW) syndrome may account for PSVT.

PSVT affects ventricular filling and cardiac output, and decreases coronary artery perfusion. Its manifestations include complaints of palpitations and a "racing" heart, anxiety, dizziness, dyspnea, anginal pain, diaphoresis, extreme fatigue, and polyuria (urine output may reach up to 3 L in the first few hours after PSVT onset).

**ATRIAL FLUTTER.** *Atrial flutter* is a rapid and regular atrial rhythm thought to result from an intra-atrial reentry mechanism. Causes include sympathetic nervous system stimulation due to anxiety, caffeine and alcohol intake; thyrotoxicosis; coronary heart disease or myocardial infarction; pulmonary embolism; and abnormal conduction syndromes, such as WPW syndrome. Older persons with rheumatic heart disease and/or valvular disease are especially vulnerable.

Clients with atrial flutter may complain of palpitations or a fluttering sensation in the chest or throat. If the ventricular rate is rapid, manifestations of decreased cardiac output, such as decreased level of consciousness, hypotension, decreased urinary output, and cool clammy skin, may be noted. The atrial kick (additional ventricular filling with atrial contraction) is lost because of inadequate atrial filling.

ECG characteristics include a "sawtooth" or "picket fence" appearance of P waves, which are labeled flutter (F) waves. The atrial rate is rapid, usually around 300 BPM. As a protective mechanism, many impulses are blocked at the AV node, and the ventricular rate is rarely greater than 150 to 170 BPM. Usually, atrial impulses are evenly conducted through the AV node, for example, two impulses to one QRS complex (2:1), four impulses to one QRS complex (4:1), or six impulses to one QRS complex (6:1). A constant conduction ratio results in a regular ventricular rhythm; the ventricular rhythm is irregular if the conduction ratio varies. The ventricular rate usually ranges from 150 to 170 BPM in 2:1 conduction and 60 to 75 BPM for lower conduction ratios. The T wave is usually hidden by overriding F waves; some F waves may be hidden in the QRS complex.

**ATRIAL FIBRILLATION.** *Atrial fibrillation* is a common dysrhythmia characterized by disorganized atrial activity without discrete atrial contractions. Extremely rapid atrial impulses bombard the AV node, resulting in an irregularly irregular ventricular response. Atrial fibrillation may occur suddenly and recur, or it may persist as a chronic dysrhythmia. Atrial fibrillation is commonly associated with heart failure, rheumatic heart disease, coronary heart disease, hypertension, and hyperthyroidism.

Manifestations of atrial fibrillation relate to the rate of the ventricular response. With rapid response rates, manifestations of decreased cardiac output such as hypotension, shortness of breath, fatigue, and angina may develop. Clients with extensive heart disease may develop syncope or heart failure. Peripheral pulses are irregular and of variable amplitude (strength).

The specific ECG characteristics of atrial fibrillation include an irregularly irregular rhythm and the absence of identifiable P waves. The atrial rate is so rapid that it is not measurable. The ventricular rate varies.

Atrial fibrillation increases the risk for formation of thromboemboli. Organ infarction may occur as a result; the incidence of stroke is high.

## Junctional Dysrhythmias

Rhythms that originate in AV nodal tissue are termed *junctional.* The AV junction includes the AV node and the bundle of His, which branches into the right and left bundle branches. An impulse arising from the AV junction may occur in response to failure of higher pacemakers, as in a *junctional escape rhythm,* or it may result from an abnormal mechanism, such as altered automaticity. An impulse arising from the AV junction may or may not be conducted back up to the atria. This conduction against the normal flow or pattern is called *retrograde conduction.* The resulting atrial wave, called a P′ wave, may be found before, during, or after the QRS complex, depending on the speed of conduction. The P′ wave is inverted in some ECG leads because the impulse moves from the AV node up to the atria instead of from the SA node down toward the AV node. In addition, the P′R interval is shorter than normal (less than 0.12 sec). The QRS complex is typically narrow.

A junctional rhythm may be due to drug toxicity (e.g., digitalis, beta blockers, or calcium channel blockers), or other causes such as hypoxemia, hyperkalemia, increased vagal tone or damage to the AV node, myocardial infarction, and heart failure. Loss of synchronized atrial contraction and the atrial kick may affect cardiac output, leading to manifestations of decreased cardiac output and impaired myocardial tissue perfusion. Heart failure may develop.

*Premature junctional contractions (PJCs)* occur before the next expected beat of the underlying rhythm. Isolated PJCs may occur in healthy people and are insignificant. *Junctional tachycardia* is a junctional rhythm with a rate greater than 60 BPM. It is caused by increased automaticity of AV nodal tissue. The ventricular rate is usually less than 140 BPM. Both rhythms are most commonly associated with digitalis toxicity, hypoxia, ischemia, or electrolyte imbalances.

## Ventricular Dysrhythmias

Ventricular dysrhythmias originate in the ventricles. Because the ventricles pump blood into the pulmonary and systemic vasculature, any disruption of their rhythm can affect cardiac output and tissue perfusion. A wide and bizarre QRS complex (greater than 0.12 sec) is a characteristic feature of ventricular dysrhythmias. This occurs because ventricular ectopic impulses begin and travel outside normal conduction pathways. Other characteristics include no relationship of the QRS complex to a P wave, increased amplitude of the QRS complex, an abnormal ST segment, and a T wave deflected in the opposite direction from the QRS complex.

## Premature Ventricular Contractions

*Premature ventricular contractions (PVCs)* are ectopic ventricular beats that occur before the next expected beat of the underlying rhythm. They usually do not reset the atrial rhythm and are followed by a full compensatory pause. PVCs often have no significance in people without heart disease. Frequent, recurrent, or multifocal PVCs may be associated with an increased risk for lethal dysrhythmias. PVCs result from either enhanced automaticity or a reentry phenomenon. They may be triggered by anxiety or stress; tobacco, alcohol, or caffeine use; hypoxia, acidosis, and electrolyte imbalances; sympathomimetic drugs; coronary heart disease; heart failure; and mechanical stimulation of the heart (e.g., the insertion of a cardiac catheter); or reperfusion after thrombolytic therapy. The incidence and significance of PVCs is greatest after myocardial infarction.

PVCs may be isolated or occur in a specific pattern. Two PVCs in a row are called a *couplet* or *paired* PVCs. Three consecutive PVCs (a *triplet* or *salvo*) is a short run of ventricular tachycardia. *Ventricular bigeminy* is characterized by a PVC following each normal beat; a PVC noted every third beat is called *ventricular trigeminy*. When the ventricular impulse arises from one ectopic site, all PVCs look the same (*monomorphic*) and are called *unifocal* PVCs. *Multifocal* PVCs arise from different ectopic sites and appear different from one another on the ECG (*polymorphic*).

The frequency and patterns of PVCs can be indicative of myocardial irritability and the risk for a lethal dysrhythmia. The following are considered warning signs in the client with acute heart disease (e.g., an acute MI).

- PVCs that develop within the first 4 hours of an MI
- Frequent PVCs (six or more per minute)
- Couplets or triplets
- Multifocal PVCs
- R-on-T phenomenon (PVCs falling on the T wave)

In people without heart disease, isolated PVCs usually are insignificant and do not require treatment. Clients may complain of feeling their hearts "skip a beat" or of palpitations. In clients with preexisting heart disease, PVCs may indicate a drug toxicity or an increased risk for lethal dysrhythmias and cardiac arrest. The risk is greatest following acute MI.

## Ventricular Tachycardia

*Ventricular tachycardia (VT; V tach)* is a rapid ventricular rhythm defined as three or more consecutive PVCs. Ventricular tachycardia may occur in short bursts, or "runs," or may persist for more than 30 seconds (sustained ventricular tachycardia). The rate is greater than 100 BPM, and the rhythm is usually regular. Reentry is the usual electrophysiologic mechanism responsible for VT. Myocardial ischemia and infarction are the most common predisposing factors for VT. It also is associated with cardiac structural disorders such as valvular disease, rheumatic heart disease, or cardiomyopathy. It may occur in the absence of heart disease, and with anorexia nervosa, metabolic disorders, and drug toxicity.

Nonsustained VT may occur paroxysmally and convert back to an effective rhythm spontaneously. The client may experience a fluttering sensation in the chest or complain of palpitations and brief shortness of breath. Clients in sustained VT generally develop signs and symptoms of decreased cardiac output and hemodynamic instability, including severe hypotension, a weak or nonpalpable pulse, and loss of consciousness. Allowed to continue, VT can deteriorate into ventricular fibrillation. Sustained ventricular tachycardia is a medical emergency that requires immediate intervention, particularly in clients with cardiac disease.

## Ventricular Fibrillation

*Ventricular fibrillation (VF; V fib)* is extremely rapid, chaotic ventricular depolarization causing the ventricles to quiver and cease contracting; the heart does not pump. This is known as **cardiac arrest;** it is a medical emergency requiring immediate intervention with cardiopulmonary resuscitation (CPR). Death will follow the onset of VF within 4 minutes if the rhythm is not recognized and terminated and an effective perfusing rhythm reestablished.

Ventricular fibrillation is usually triggered by severe myocardial ischemia or infarction. It occurs without warning 50% of the time. It is the terminal event in many disease processes or traumatic conditions. Ventricular fibrillation may be precipitated by a single PVC or may follow VT. Other causes of VF include digitalis toxicity, reperfusion therapy, antidysrhythmic drugs, hypokalemia and hyperkalemia, hypothermia, metabolic acidosis, mechanical stimulation (as with the insertion of cardiac catheters or pacing wires), and electric shock.

Clinically, loss of ventricular contractions results in absence of a palpable or audible pulse. The client loses consciousness and stops breathing as perfusion ceases. The ECG shows grossly irregular, bizarre complexes with no discernable rate or rhythm.

## Atrioventricular Conduction Blocks

Conduction defects that delay or block transmission of the sinus impulse through the AV node are called *atrioventricular (AV) conduction blocks.* Impaired conduction may result from tissue injury or disease, increased vagal (parasympathetic) tone, drug effects, or a congenital defect. AV conduction blocks vary in severity from benign to severe.

### First-Degree AV Block

*First-degree AV block* is a benign conduction delay that generally poses no threat, has no symptoms, and requires no treatment. Impulse conduction through the AV node is slowed, but all atrial impulses are conducted to the ventricles. It may result from injury or infarct of the AV node, other cardiac diseases, or drug effects. The ECG shows all characteristics of NSR, except the PR interval is greater than 0.20 second.

### Second-Degree AV Block

*Second-degree AV block* is characterized by failure to conduct one or more impulses from the atria to the ventricles. Two patterns of second-degree AV block are seen, identified as type I and type II.

***SECOND-DEGREE AV BLOCK—TYPE I.*** *Type I second-degree AV block (Mobitz type I or Wenckebach phenomenon)* is characterized by a repeating pattern of increasing AV conduction delays until an impulse fails to conduct to the ventricles. On the ECG, PR intervals progressively lengthen until one QRS complex is not conducted, or dropped. The ventricular rate remains adequate to maintain cardiac output, and the client usually is asymptomatic. Mobitz type I AV block usually is transient, associated with acute MI or drug intoxication (e.g., digitalis, beta blockers, or calcium channel blockers). It rarely progresses to complete heart block.

**SECOND-DEGREE AV BLOCK—TYPE II.** *Type II second-degree AV block (Mobitz type II)* involves intermittent failure of the AV node to conduct an impulse to the ventricles without preceding delays in conduction. The PR interval remains constant, but not all P waves are followed by QRS complexes (e.g., there may be two P waves for every QRS). Conduction through the His-Purkinje system usually is delayed as well, causing a widened QRS complex (Braunwald et al., 2001). Mobitz type II block is frequently associated with acute anterior wall MI and a high rate of mortality (Porth, 2002). Manifestations of Mobitz type II block depend on the ventricular rate. Pacemaker therapy may be required to maintain the cardiac output

### Third-Degree AV Block

*Third-degree AV block (complete heart block)* occurs when atrial impulses are completely blocked at the AV node, and fail to reach the ventricles. As a result, the atria and ventricles are controlled by different and independent pacemakers, with separate rates and rhythms. The ventricular impulse arises from either junctional fibers (with a rate of 40 to 60 BPM) or a ventricular pacemaker at a rate of less than 40 BPM. The width of the QRS complex depends on the location of the escape pacemaker. The QRS is wide and the rate is slow when the rhythm arises distal to the bundle of His.

Third-degree block is frequently associated with an inferior or anteroseptal myocardial infarction. Other causes include congenital conditions, acute or degenerative cardiac disease or damage, drug effects, and electrolyte imbalances. The slow escape rhythm significantly affects cardiac output, causing manifestations such as syncope (known as a *Stokes-Adams attack*), dizziness, fatigue, exercise intolerance, and heart failure. Third-degree AV block is life threatening and requires immediate intervention to maintain adequate cardiac output.

### AV Dissociation

Complete dissociation of atrial and ventricular rhythms can occur in conditions other than third-degree AV block. The two primary factors leading to AV dissociation are severe sinus bradycardia and a lower pacemaker (junctional or ventricular) that competes with or exceeds the normal sinus rhythm (Braunwald et al., 2001). AV dissociation may result from acute myocardial ischemia or infarction, cardiac surgery, or drug effects. The ECG shows separate and competing atrial (P waves) and ventricular (QRS complexes) rhythms.

### Ventricular Conduction Blocks

Once the impulse enters the ventricles, its conduction through the right and left bundle branches may be impaired (*bundle branch block*). As a result, the impulse is conducted more slowly than normal through the ventricles. On the ECG, the QRS complex is prolonged. Its appearance varies, depending on the affected bundle (right or left). Typically, no clinical manifestations are associated with bundle branch block unless it occurs in conjunction with an AV block.

## COLLABORATIVE CARE

Cardiac dysrhythmias may be either benign or critical: Recognizing lethal dysrhythmias is a matter of life and death. Major goals of care include identifying the dysrhythmia, evaluating its effect on physical and psychosocial well-being, and treating underlying causes. This may involve correcting fluid and electrolyte or acid-base imbalances; treating hypoxia, pain, or anxiety; administering antidysrhythmic medications; or mechanical and surgical interventions.

### Diagnostic Tests

Diagnostic tests for dysrhythmias include the electrocardiogram, cardiac monitoring, and electrophysiology studies. Laboratory tests such as serum electrolytes, drug levels, and arterial blood gases may be done to help identify the cause of the dysrhythmia.

#### Electrocardiogram

The 12-lead ECG may be required to accurately diagnose a dysrhythmia. It also provides information about underlying disease processes, such as myocardial infarction or other cardiac disease. The ECG may also be used to monitor the effects of treatment.

#### Cardiac Monitoring

Cardiac monitoring allows continuous observation of the cardiac rhythm. It is used in many different circumstances (Box 29–4). Different types of ECG monitoring are employed for different situations.

---

**BOX 29–4 ■ Indications for Cardiac Monitoring**

- Perioperative monitoring of heart rate and rhythm
- Detecting and identifying dysrhythmias
- Monitoring the effects of cardiac and noncardiac diseases on the heart
- Monitoring clients with potentially life-threatening conditions:
  a. Major trauma (especially cardiac trauma)
  b. Dissecting aneurysm
  c. Acute myocardial infarction
  d. Heart failure
  e. Shock
  f. Other emergency conditions
- Evaluating responses to procedures and interventions:
  a. Drug therapies
  b. Diagnostic procedures
  c. Ablative techniques
  d. Angioplasty or cardiac catheterization
  e. Cardiac surgery
  f. Pacemaker function
  g. Automatic implantable cardioverter-defibrillator function

***CONTINUOUS CARDIAC MONITORING.*** Continuous monitoring of the cardiac rhythm is provided by bedside and central monitoring stations. Electrodes placed on the client's chest attach to cables connected to a monitor. The heart rate and rhythm is visually displayed on a bedside monitor connected to a central monitoring station. The central station allows simultaneous monitoring of multiple clients within a nursing unit. Alarms on both bedside and central monitors warn of potential problems such as very rapid or very slow heart rates. Alarm limits are preset by the nurse for the individual client. Procedure 29–1 describes how to place a client on cardiac monitoring.

*Telemetry* may be used in acute care settings when the client is ambulatory. Chest electrodes are connected to a portable transmitter worn around the neck or waist; the ECG is transmitted electronically to a central monitoring station for continuous monitoring.

***HOME MONITORING.*** Clients often complain of palpitations or other heart symptoms but are asymptomatic during evaluation in a hospital or community-based setting. Ambulatory or Holter monitoring may be used to identify intermittent dysrhythmias, to detect silent ischemia, to monitor the effects of treatment, and to assess pacemaker or automatic cardioverter-defibrillator function. Electrodes are applied and the leads attached to the portable telemetry monitor that records and stores all electrical activity. Clients are instructed to leave the electrode pads in place during monitoring, record any cardiac symptoms or events in a journal (such as chest pain, palpitations, syncope), and are told when to return to the clinic. After the prescribed period, usu-

---

## Procedure 29–1 — Initiating Cardiac Monitoring

### SUPPLIES

- Bedside monitor and cable or telemetry unit with fresh battery
- Electrodes—self-adherent, pregelled, disposable
- Lead wires
- Washcloth, soap, and towel
- Alcohol prep pads
- Dry gauze pads or ECG prep pads

### BEFORE THE PROCEDURE

Explain the reason for ECG monitoring. Reassure client that changes in heart rhythm can be noted and immediately treated if necessary. Explain that loose or disconnected lead wires, poor electrode contact, excessive movement, electrical interference, or equipment malfunction may trigger alarms and alert the staff, allowing correction of the problem. Reassure that movement allowed, within activity restrictions, while on the monitor. Explain skin preparation procedure. Provide for privacy, and drape appropriately.

### PROCEDURE

1. Follow standard precautions
2. Check equipment for damage (i.e., fraying, bent, or broken wires). Connect lead wires to cable, and secure connections.
3. Select electrode sites on the chest wall, avoiding areas of excessive movement, joints, skin creases, scar tissue, or other lesions.
4. Clean sites with soap and water, and dry thoroughly. Alcohol may be used to remove skin oils; allow the skin to dry for 60 seconds after use.
5. Gently rub the site with a dry gauze pad or ECG prep pad to remove dead skin cells, debris, and residue.
6. Open the electrode package; peel the backing from the electrode, and check to ensure that the center of the pad is moist with conductive gel.
7. Apply electrode pads, pressing firmly to ensure contact (see figure).
8. Attach leads and position cable with sufficient slack for comfort. Place the telemetry unit (if used) in gown pouch or pocket.
9. Assess ECG tracing on the monitor, adjusting settings as needed.
10. Set monitor alarm limits typically at 20 BPM higher and lower than the client's baseline rate. Turn alarms on, and leave on at all times. Assess immediately if an alarm is triggered.
11. Time and date pads with every change.

### AFTER THE PROCEDURE

Monitor periodically for comfort. Assess electrode and lead wire connections as needed. Remove and apply new pads every 24 to 48 hours or whenever the pad becomes dislodged or nonadherent. Clean gel residue from previous site, and document skin condition under the pads. Choose an alternative site if the skin appears irritated or blistered. Document ECG strips according to unit policy and/or physician's order, as well 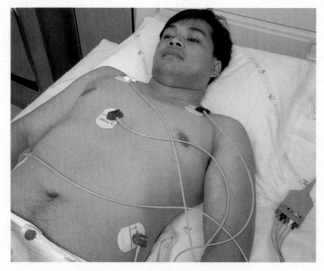 when the cardiac rhythm or the client's condition changes (especially with complaints of chest pain, decreased level of consciousness, or changes in vital signs). Note the date, time, client identification, monitor lead, duration of PR and QT intervals, and rhythm interpretation on each ECG strip.

ally 48 to 72 hours, the client returns and the monitor is removed. Diary entries are compared to the recorded heart rhythms to identify the effects of dysrhythmias.

### Electrophysiology Studies

Diagnostic cardiac *electrophysiology (EP) procedures* are used to identify dysrhythmias and their causes. EP studies are used to analyze components of the conduction system, identify sites of ectopic stimulation, and evaluate the effectiveness of treatment. EP procedures can be used for both diagnosis and as a therapeutic intervention.

In the electrophysiology laboratory, electrode catheters are guided by fluoroscopy into the heart through the femoral or brachial vein. The timing and sequence of electrical activation during normal and abnormal (aberrant) rhythms is observed and measured. Electrical stimulation may be used to induce dysrhythmias similar to the client's clinical dysrhythmia (Woods et al., 2000). Following diagnosis, an EP procedure may be used to treat the dysrhythmia, for example, by overdrive pacing (stimulating the client's heart rate to a rate faster than that of the tachydysrhythmia) to break the dysrhythmia's cycle, or to perform ablative therapy to destroy the ectopic site. See the section on ablative techniques for further information.

Nursing care for the client undergoing an EP procedure is similar to that for a coronary angiogram (see the box on page 817). The procedure and expected sensations are explained. The client remains awake during the procedure; antianxiety medications or sedatives are given to reduce apprehension. Intravenous heparin may be given during the procedure to reduce the risk of thromboembolism.

Complications of EP procedures are infrequent, but include fatal ventricular fibrillation, cardiac perforation, and major venous thrombosis (Woods et al., 2000). Careful postprocedure monitoring is vital.

## Medications

The goal of drug therapy is to suppress dysrhythmia formation. No drug has been found to be completely safe and effective. Antidysrhythmic drugs may be used for acute treatment of dysrhythmias or to manage chronic conditions. The overall goal of therapy is to maintain an effective cardiac output by stabilizing cardiac rhythm.

It is important to remember that virtually all antidysrhythmic drugs also have *prodysrhythmic* effects; that is, they can worsen existing dysrhythmias and precipitate new ones. Because of this tendency, studies that demonstrate higher mortality rates in clients receiving antidysrhythmic medications, and the increasing safety and availability of interventional techniques, the use of antidysrhythmic medications is declining.

Most antidysrhythmic drugs are classified by their effects on the cardiac action potential. Most are class I drugs, or fast sodium channel blockers. By blocking sodium channels, these drugs slow impulse conduction in the atria and ventricles. This class is further divided into subclasses A, B, and C. Class II drugs are beta blockers, which decrease SA node automaticity, AV conduction velocity, and myocardial contractility. Class III agents block potassium channels, delaying repolarization and prolong-

ing the relative refractory period. Class IV drugs are calcium channel blockers. Their effect is similar to that of beta blockers. Adenosine and digoxin do not fit within the major classes. Both drugs reduce SA node automaticity and slow AV conduction. Ibutilide and magnesium also fall outside the major classes, but are used to treat dysrhythmias. See the Medication Administration box on page 854 for identifies common antidysrhythmic drugs within each class and the nursing implications in caring for clients receiving antidysrhythmic drugs.

Drugs that affect the autonomic nervous system may also be used to treat dysrhythmias. Sympathomimetics, such as epinephrine, stimulate the heart, increasing both heart rate and contractility. Anticholinergic agents such as atropine are used to decrease vagal tone and increase the heart rate. Magnesium sulfate is an unclassified drug that has been shown to be safe and effective in treating ventricular tachycardias.

## Countershock

*Countershock* is used to interrupt cardiac rhythms that compromise cardiac output and the client's welfare. Delivery of a direct current charge depolarizes all cardiac cells at the same time. This simultaneous depolarization may stop a tachydysrhythmia and allow the sinus node to recover control of impulse formation. There are two types of countershock: synchronized cardioversion and defibrillation.

### Synchronized Cardioversion

*Synchronized cardioversion* delivers direct electrical current synchronized with the client's heart rhythm. Synchronization of the shock with the QRS complex prevents ventricular fibrillation by avoiding current delivery during the vulnerable period of repolarization. Cardioversion is usually done as an elective procedure to treat supraventricular tachycardia, atrial fibrillation, atrial flutter, or even a hemodynamically stable ventricular tachycardia.

The nurse assists with cardioversion by preparing the client before the procedure; obtaining any laboratory tests ordered; obtaining and documenting ECG strips prior to, during, and after treatment; setting up the equipment; and monitoring the client's response. Procedure 29–2 describes synchronized cardioversion.

Clients in atrial fibrillation are at high risk for thromboembolism following cardioversion. Loss of atrial contractions with atrial fibrillation leads to blood pooling in the atria, increasing the risk of clot formation. When the atria begin to contract following successful cardioversion, clots may be dislodged, embolizing to the pulmonary or systemic circulation. If possible, anticoagulants are given for several weeks before cardioversion is attempted.

### Defibrillation

Unlike carefully synchronized cardioversion, *defibrillation* is an emergency procedure that delivers direct current without regard to the cardiac cycle. Ventricular fibrillation is immediately treated as soon as the dysrhythmia is recognized. Early defibrillation has been shown to improve survival in clients experiencing VF.

Defibrillation can be delivered by external or internal paddles or pads. Conductive gel pads or paste is applied, and external paddles or pads are placed on the chest wall at the apex and

# Medication Administration

## Antidysrhythmic Drugs

### CLASS I DRUGS: SODIUM CHANNEL BLOCKERS

#### Class IA

Quinidine (Cardioquin, Quinidex, Quinaglute)
Procainamide (Pronestyl, Procan SR)
Disopyramide (Norpace, Norpace CR)

Class IA decrease the flow of sodium into the cell and prolong the action potential. This decreases automaticity, slows the rate of impulse conduction, and prolongs refractoriness. They are used to treat both supraventricular and ventricular tachycardias.

#### Class IB

Lidocaine (Xylocaine)          Tocainide (Tonocard)
Mexiletine (Mexitil)           Phenytoin (Dilantin)

Class IB, or lidocaine-like, drugs decrease the refractory period but have little effect on automaticity. Drugs in this class are used primarily to treat ventricular dysrhythmias, including PVCs and ventricular tachycardia.

#### Class IC

Flecainide (Tambocor)          Propafenone (Rythmol)

Class IC drugs slow impulse conduction velocity but have little effect on refractoriness. They are used to reduce or eliminate tachydysrhythmias associated with reentry. Their significant prodysrhythmic effects limit their usefulness, but they may be used to treat supraventricular tachycardia.

### CLASS II DRUGS: BETA-BLOCKERS

Esmolol (Brevibloc)
Propranolol (Inderal)
Acebutolol (Sectral)

Class II drugs are beta blockers that decrease automaticity and conduction through the AV node. They also reduce the heart rate and myocardial contractility. They are used to treat supraventricular tacycardia and to slow the ventricular response rate to atrial fibrillation. These drugs may cause bronchospasm and are contraindicated for clients with asthma, chronic obstructive pulmonary disease (COPD), or other restrictive or obstructive lung diseases.

### CLASS III DRUGS: POTASSIUM CHANNEL BLOCKERS

Sotalol (Betapace)             Bretylium (Bretylol)
Amiodarone (Cordarone)         Ibutilide (Corvert)

Class III drugs block potassium channels, prolonging repolarization and the refractory period. Drugs in this class are used primarily to treat ventricular tachycardia and ventricular fibrillation. Amiodarone may also be used for supraventricular tachycardias.

### CLASS IV DRUGS: CALCIUM CHANNEL BLOCKERS

Verapamil (Calan, Isoptin, Verelan)
Diltiazem (Cardizem, Dilacor XR)

Calcium channel blockers decrease automaticity and AV nodal conduction. They are used to manage supraventricular tachycardias. Like the beta blockers, calcium channel blockers reduce myocardial contractility.

### OTHER DRUGS

Adenosine (Adenocard)              Digoxin

Adenosine and digoxin decrease conduction through the AV node and are used to treat supraventricular tachycardias.

### Nursing Responsibilities

- Obtain baseline data including vital signs, cardiac rhythm (including rate, PR and QT intervals, and QRS duration), and physical assessment (especially cardiac, neurologic, and respiratory status).
- Assess medication regimen to identify drugs that may interfere with antidysrhythmic therapy.
- Monitor ECG to evaluate the effectiveness of therapy and to assess for possible dysrhythmias precipitated by treatment.
- Immediately report manifestations of drug toxicity:
  - Procainimide—signs of heart failure; conduction delays or ventricular dysrhythmias; skin rash, myalgias or arthralgias, flulike symptoms.
  - Disopyramide—urinary retention, heart failure, eye pain
  - Lidocaine—changes in neurologic status, such as agitation, confusion, dizziness, nervousness
  - Amiodarone—pulmonary fibrosis (increasing dyspnea, cough, hepatic dysfunction—changes in liver function tests, jaundice); vision changes, photosensitivity
  - Digoxin—anorexia, nausea, vomiting; blurred, or double vision; yellow green halos; new-onset dysrhythmias
- Use an infusion pump to administer intravenous infusions. Monitor the dose and assess its appropriateness (in mg/min or µg/kg/min).

### Client and Family Teaching

- Take the drug exactly as prescribed. Do not skip or double doses. Check with your physician if a dose is missed.
- Take your pulse and record the rate daily before rising. Count the pulse for 1 full minute. Bring the record with you to each office or clinic visit
- Report the following to the physician: irregular pulse rate or rhythm, dizziness, eye pain, changes in vision, skin rashes or color changes, wheezing or other respiratory problems, changes in behavior.

---

base of the heart (Figure 29–13 ■). Internal paddles are applied directly on the heart, and may be used in surgery, the emergency department, or critical care. Internal defibrillation is done only by a physician; external defibrillation may be performed by any health care provider who has been trained in the procedure. Automatic external defibrillators (AEDs) are available on most hospital units to allow early defibrillation for cardiac arrest. (See Procedure 29–3.)

## Pacemaker Therapy

A **pacemaker** is a pulse generator used to provide an electrical stimulus to the heart when the heart fails to generate or conduct its own at a rate that maintains the cardiac output. The pulse generator is connected to *leads* (insulated wires) passed intravenously into the heart or sutured directly to the epicardium. The leads sense intrinsic electrical activity of the heart and provide an electrical stimulus to the heart when necessary (pacing).

## Procedure 29–2 | Elective Synchronized Cardioversion

### SUPPLIES

- Cardioverter-defibrillator with ECG cable and monitor
- Conductive gel pads or paste
- Dry gauze pads
- Emergency drug kit and resuscitation equipment
- IV Supplies (catheter, solution, administration set)

### PREPROCEDURE

Explain the purpose of the procedure (to restore an effective cardiac rhythm). Describe the procedure in simple, non-threatening terms. Advise that some discomfort may be felt with each countershock, but a sedative will be given to minimize discomfort. Witness the signature on an informed consent form for this procedure. Document preprocedure rhythm on an ECG strip. Ensure a patent intravenous access site for emergency drug administration. Keep NPO as specified prior to the procedure. Assess acid-base and electrolyte levels (especially potassium, magnesium, and calcium) and drug levels if appropriate. Report abnormalities to the physician prior to the procedure. Document vital signs, level of consciousness, and peripheral pulses. Administer the prescribed sedative, and provide for safety. Remove any medication patches from the chest and all metallic objects. Place in supine position, and provide for privacy.

### PROCEDURE

1. Use standard precautions.
2. Turn on the cardioverter-defibrillator and ECG monitor.
3. Connect the client's ECG cable to the cardioverter. Select a lead with prominent R waves for monitoring.
4. Set cardioverter to "synchronize" mode. Observe the ECG waveform on the monitor for indications of synchronization, such as a flashing bold line or a blip. Many units also display the message "synchronized mode" on the monitor.
5. Place conductive pads on the chest below the right clavicle to the right of the sternum and in the midaxillary line on the left. If using conductive paste, spread it evenly on the defibrillator paddles.
6. Turn on the ECG recording strip for a continuous printout during the procedure.
7. Charge the paddles to the prescribed energy dose. The machine will beep to indicate that the selected energy level has been reached and that the paddles are ready for discharge.
8. The paddles are applied firmly to the chest over the conductive pads by the physician.
9. Turn oxygen off and remove it.
10. Ensure that no one is touching the client or the bed prior to discharge of the electrical shock. There may be a slight delay in shock delivery as the machine synchronizes with the R wave.
11. Assess client status and ECG rhythm. Assure a patent airway and the presence of a pulse.
12. The procedure may be repeated if unsuccessful. The energy level may be increased with each attempt.
13. Remove conductive pads. Using a dry gauze pad, clean paste from the chest and the paddles.

### POSTPROCEDURE

Assess client for return of consciousness from sedative or cardioversion. Evaluate neurologic, cardiovascular, and respiratory status. Assess for possible complications, including emboli (especially cerebral), respiratory depression, and dysrhythmias. Document postcardioversion rhythm strip. Assess skin for burns. Document the procedure and the client's response in the medical record.

---

Pacemakers are used to treat both acute and chronic conduction defects such as third-degree AV block. They also may be used to treat bradydysrhythmias and tachydysrhythmias.

*Temporary pacemakers* use an external pulse generator (Figure 29–14 ■) attached to a lead threaded intravenously into the right ventricle, to temporary pacing wires implanted during cardiac surgery, or to external conductive pads placed on the chest wall for emergency pacing.

*Permanent pacemakers* use an internal pulse generator placed in a subcutaneous pocket in the subclavian space or abdominal wall. The generator connects to leads sewn directly onto the heart (*epicardial*) or passed transvenously into the heart (*endocardial*). Epicardial pacemakers (Figure 29–15 ■) require surgical exposure of the heart. Leads may be placed during cardiac surgery, or using a small subxiphoid incision to expose on the heart. Transvenous pacemaker leads are positioned in the right heart via the cephalic, subclavian, or jugular vein (Figure 29–16 ■). Local anesthesia can be used for permanent pacer insertion.

Pacemakers are programmed to stimulate the atria or the ventricles (*single-chamber pacing*), or both (*dual-chamber pacing*). Table 29–7 defines terms used to describe pacemaker modes and functions. The most commonly used pacemakers either: (a) sense activity in and pace the ventricles only; or (b) sense activity in and pace both the atria and the ventricles. Dual-chamber or *atrioventricular sequential pacing* stimulates both chambers of the heart in sequence. AV pacing imitates the normal sequence of atrial contraction followed by ventricular contraction, improving cardiac output.

Pacing is detected on the ECG strip by the presence of pacing artifact (Figure 29–17 ■ on page 858). A sharp spike is noted before the P wave with atrial pacing, and before the QRS complex with ventricular pacing. Pacing spikes are seen before both the P wave and QRS complex in AV sequential pacing. Capture is noted if there is a contraction of the chamber immediately following the pacer spike. Problems in sensing, pacing, and capture are noted in Table 29–8 (on page 859).

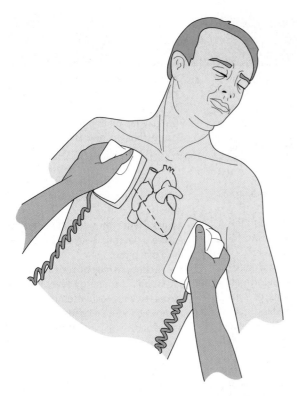

**Figure 29–13** ■ Placement of paddles for defibrillation.

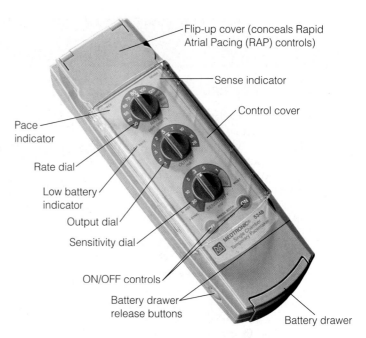

Flip-up cover (conceals Rapid Atrial Pacing (RAP) controls)

Sense indicator

Control cover

Pace indicator

Rate dial

Low battery indicator

Output dial

Sensitivity dial

ON/OFF controls

Battery drawer release buttons

Battery drawer

**Figure 29–14** ■ Programmable settings on a temporary pacemaker.

*Courtesy of Medtronics, Inc.*

Care of the client with a temporary or permanent pacemaker focuses on monitoring for pacemaker malfunctioning, maintaining safety (Box 29–5), and preventing infection and postoperative complications. Nursing care for the client having a pacemaker implant is outlined on page 860.

## Implantable Cardioverter-Defibrillator

Sudden cardiac death claims more than 300,000 lives per year in the United States (Woods et al., 2000). The *implantable cardioverter-defibrillator (ICD)* detects life-threatening changes in the cardiac rhythm and automatically delivers an electric shock to convert the dysrhythmia back

---

| Procedure 29–3 | **Emergency External Defibrillation** |
| --- | --- |

### SUPPLIES

- Automatic external defibrillator or defibrillator with ECG cable and monitor
- Conductive gel pads or paste
- Dry gauze pads
- Emergency medications and cart with pacemaker, airway management equipment, and oxygen supplies.

### PREPROCEDURE

Verify the lethal dysrhythmia, such as pulseless VT, VF, or asystole. Initiate the cardiac arrest (code) procedure, and obtain the defibrillator. If one is not immediately available, begin CPR until the emergency cart and defibrillator are brought to the bedside. Place client in supine position on a firm surface.

### PROCEDURE

1. Turn on the defibrillator. Set it in *defibrillation* mode.
2. Turn ECG recording on for a continuous printout of events during the procedure.
3. Set the energy level and charge the paddles. Initial defibrillation is usually performed at 200 joules.
4. Place conductive pads on the chest, or spread conductive paste evenly on the paddles.
5. Position the paddles, holding them firmly on the chest wall.
6. **Ensure that no one is touching the client or the bed. State, "All clear."**
7. Depress the button on each paddle simultaneously to discharge the energy.
8. Evaluate cardiac rhythm and for a pulse after each defibrillation attempt.

9. If the first attempt is unsuccessful, repeat the procedure, increasing the energy level to 300 joules and 360 joulesfor successive attempts. Reapply conductive paste as necessary.
10. If unsuccessful after three defibrillation attempts, implement ACLS protocols.

### POSTPROCEDURE

If the dysrhythmia is successfully converted, evaluate and support neurologic, cardiovascular, and respiratory status. Monitor and titrate any intravenous infusions as ordered. Maintain ventilatory support as needed. Evaluate skin for burns. Obtain blood for laboratory analysis as ordered. Monitor vital signs and ECG continuously. Transfer to the intensive care unit (ICU) as indicated. Provide support and information to the client and family.

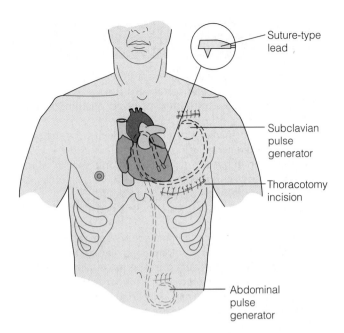

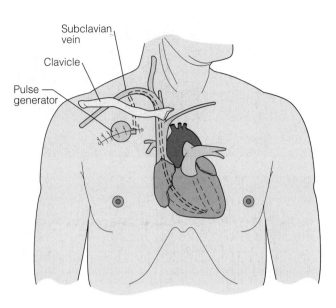

**Figure 29–15** ■ A permanent epicardial pacemaker. The pulse generator may be placed in subcutaneous pockets in the subclavian or abdominal regions.

**Figure 29–16** ■ A permanent transvenous (endocardial) pacemaker with the lead placed in the right ventricle via the subclavian vein.

into a normal rhythm. ICDs are used for sudden death survivors, clients with recurrent ventricular tachycardia, and clients with demonstrated risk factors for sudden death. ICDs can deliver a shock as needed, provide pacing on demand, and can store ECG records of tachycardic episodes (Woods et al., 2000).

A pulse generator connected to lead electrodes for rhythm detection and current delivery is implanted in the left pectoral region. The lead is threaded transvenously to the apex of the right ventricle. The ICD is programmed to sense a change in heart rate or rhythm. When it detects a potentially lethal rhythm, it shocks the heart to convert the rhythm. The device can be programmed or reprogrammed at the bedside as necessary. The ICD may be tested prior to discharge.

Local or general anesthesia is used, and the client may be discharged within 24 hours. The lithium-powered battery must be surgically replaced every 5 years. Complications and nursing care are similar to that for a client having a permanent pacemaker implant (see the Nursing Care box on page 860).

## Cardiac Mapping and Catheter Ablation

Cardiac mapping and catheter ablation are used to locate and destroy an ectopic focus. These diagnostic and therapeutic measures use electrophysiology techniques, and can be performed in the cardiac catheterization laboratory. *Cardiac mapping* is used to identify the site of earliest impulse formation in the atria or the ventricles. Intracardiac and extracardiac catheter electrodes and computer technology are used to pinpoint the ectopic site on a map of the heart. These same catheters can be used to deliver the ablative intervention.

*Ablation* destroys, removes, or isolates an ectopic focus. In most instances, radio frequency energy produced by high-frequency alternating current is used to create heat as it

## TABLE 29–7  Terms Used to Describe Pacemaker Functions

| Term | Definition |
| --- | --- |
| Asynchronous pacing | Pacemaker delivers a pacing stimulus at a set rate regardless of intrinsic cardiac activity. |
| Base rate | Rate at which the pacemaker paces when no cardiac activity is sensed. |
| Capture | The ability of the pacing stimulus to generate a cardiac depolarization. |
| Demand pacing | Pacemaker delivers a pacing stimulus only when the intrinsic rate falls below the pacemaker's base rate. |
| Dual-chamber pacing | Allows both the atria and the ventricles to be paced; most frequently used permanent pacing mode. |
| Lead | An insulated wire that senses intrinsic cardiac activity and delivers a pacing stimulus as programmed. |
| Output | The electrical stimulus delivered by the pulse generator. |
| Pacing spike | A small vertical spike noted on the ECG with every pacemaker stimulus. |
| Sensing | The pacemaker's ability to identify and respond to intrinsic cardiac activity. |
| Single-chamber pacing | Pacing of only the atria or the ventricles, not both; most common temporary pacing mode used. |

*Note. Adapted from Cardiac Nursing (4th ed.) by S. L. Woods, E. S. S. Froelicher, & S. U. Motzer, 2000, Philadelphia: Lippincott.*

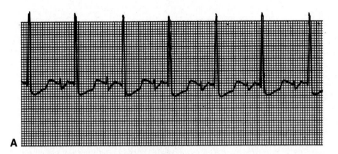

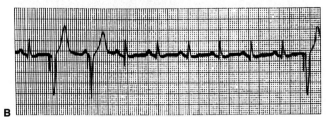

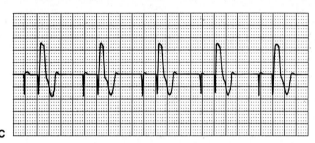

**Figure 29–17** ■ Pacing artifacts. *A,* Atrial pacing and ventricular sensing. Note the pacer spike preceding the P wave. *B,* Ventricular demand pacing. Note the absence of pacer spikes when the client's natural rhythm predominates. *C,* Atrioventricular pacing. Note the pacer spikes preceding both P waves and QRS complexes.

passes through tissue. Catheter ablation is used to treat supraventricular tachycardias, atrial fibrillation and flutter, and, in some cases, paroxysmal ventricular tachycardia (Woods et al., 2000).

Anticoagulant therapy may be started after catheter ablation to reduce the risk of clot formation at the ablation site.

## Other Therapies

In addition to medications and interventional techniques, other measures may be used to treat selected dysrhythmias. Vagal maneuvers that stimulate the parasympathetic nervous system may be used to slow the heart rate in supraventricular tachycardias. These maneuvers include *carotid sinus massage* and the *Valsalva maneuver.* Carotid sinus massage is performed only by a physician during continuous cardiac monitoring. Excessive slowing of the heart rate may result. The Valsalva maneuver, forced exhalation against a closed glottis (e.g., bearing down) increases intrathoracic pressure and vagal tone, slowing the pulse rate.

## NURSING CARE

Caring for the client with cardiac dysrhythmias requires the ability to recognize, identify, and, in some cases, promptly treat the dysrhythmia. The urgency of intervention is determined by

### BOX 29–5   ■ Safety Measures for Clients with a Temporary Pacemaker

■ Ensure that all electrical equipment in use has a grounded plug; do not use adapters or extension cords.
■ Encourage the use of battery-powered equipment (e.g., electric razor).
■ Remove any damaged electrical equipment from the unit, including equipment that
   a. Has been abused (e.g., has been dropped or in which liquid has been spilled).
   b. From which anyone has received a shock.
   c. Has frayed, worn, or otherwise damaged electrical cords or plugs.
   d. Has other evidence of impaired function, such as a hot smell during use or control knobs that are loose or do not consistently produce the expected response.
■ Wear gloves when handling pacer electrodes or wires.
■ Insulate pacemaker terminals and pacing wires with nonconductive, moistureproof material (e.g., a rubber glove).
■ Test the pacemaker battery prior to use.
■ Keep a spare pacemaker, cable, batteries, and battery tester available at all times.
■ Immediately report any apparent deviation from expected pacemaker function.

the effects of the dysrhythmia on the client. Nursing care focuses on maintaining cardiac output, monitoring the response to therapy, and teaching.

### Health Promotion

Health promotion measures to prevent coronary heart disease also reduce the risk for dysrhythmias. In most cases, dysrhythmias develop as a result of ischemic or structural changes in the heart, rather than in isolation. Advise clients who are at risk or who complain of occasional palpitations or "flutters" in their chest to reduce their intake of caffeine and other sympathetic nervous system stimulants, such as excess chocolate.

### Assessment

Assessment is vital before treating any suspected dysrhythmia. What appears to be ventricular tachycardia on the monitor may be the client scratching or brushing the teeth. Apparent asystole on the monitor may be due to a loose electrode patch. Similarly, a heart rate of 52 BPM may not affect the overall cardiac output in some clients. Review Chapter 28 for complete assessment of the client with a cardiac problem.

- Health history: complaints of palpitations (ask for further definition of palpitations), "fluttering" sensations, or a sensation of the heart racing; episodes of dizziness, lightheadedness, or syncope (fainting); timing (duration, time of day); correlation with food or beverage intake, activity; presence of chest pain, shortness of breath, or other associated symptoms; history of heart or endocrine disease (such as hyperthyroidism); current medications
- Physical examination: level of consciousness (LOC); vital signs, including apical pulse for a full minute; regularity and

## TABLE 29-8  Potential Pacemaker Problems and Corrective Strategies

| Problem | Possible Causes | Corrective Measures |
|---|---|---|
| **Undersensing**<br>Device fails to detect existing cardiac depolarizations, therefore competes with the native rhythms.<br><br>Undetected R waves<br><br>Competing pacer spikes | Lead disconnected from pacer or from viable myocardium.<br>Sensitivity set too low.<br>Lead fracture.<br>Low battery. | Check connection of lead to pacer.<br>Increase sensitivity.<br>Reposition or change lead.<br>Change battery. |
| **Oversensing**<br>Device detects noncardiac electrical events and interprets them as cardiac depolarizations, therefore is wrongly inhibited from pacing.<br><br>When artifact ceases, pacing resumes<br><br>Pacer interprets artifact as cardiac activity and fails to fire | Sensitivity set too high.<br><br>Interference from electrical sources (ungrounded equipment, short circuits) is detected and misinterpreted by the device.<br>Lead disconnected from pacer or from viable myocardium. | Decrease sensitivity (turn sensing control to a LARGER number).<br>Remove all ungrounded electrical equipment or have it evaluated by hospital engineers.<br>Check connection of lead to pacer. |
| **Noncapture**<br>Device emits stimuli which fail to depolarize the myocardium.<br><br>Pacer stimuli which fail to initiate myocardial depolarization | Output set too low in the noncaptured chamber.<br>Lead fracture.<br>High pacing threshold due to medication or metabolic changes.<br>Low battery. | Increase output in the noncaptured chamber.<br>Reposition or change lead.<br>Alter medication regimen, correct metabolic changes.<br>Change battery. |

Note. From "Cardiac Rhythm Control Devices" (p. 92) by C. L. Witherell, 1994, *Critical Care Nursing Clinics of North America, 6*(1).

PERIOPERATIVE PACEMAKER CARE PLAN

MediaLink

# NURSING CARE OF THE CLIENT HAVING A PERMANENT PACEMAKER IMPLANT

## PREOPERATIVE CARE

- Provide routine preoperative care and teaching as outlined in Chapter 7. ⊖⊃
- Assess knowledge and understanding of the procedure, clarifying and expanding on existing knowledge as needed. *Clarifying knowledge, providing information, and conveying emotional support reduces anxiety and fear and allows the client to develop a realistic outlook regarding pacer therapy.*
- Place ECG monitor electrodes away from potential incision sites. *This helps preserve skin integrity.*
- Teach range-of-motion (ROM) exercises for the affected side. *ROM exercises of the affected arm and shoulder prevent stiffness and impaired function following pacemaker insertion.*

## POSTOPERATIVE CARE

- Provide postoperative monitoring, analgesia, and care as outlined in Chapter 7.
- Obtain a chest X-ray as ordered. *A postoperative chest X-ray is used to identify lead location and detect possible complications, such as pneumothorax or pleural effusion.*
- Position for comfort. Minimize movement of the affected arm and shoulder during the initial postoperative period. *Restricting movement minimizes discomfort on the operative side and allows the leads to become anchored, reducing the risk of dislodging.*
- Assist with gentle ROM exercises at least three times daily, beginning 24 hours after pacemaker implantation. *ROM exercises help restore normal shoulder movement and prevent contractures on the affected side.*
- Monitor pacemaker function with cardiac monitoring or intermittent ECGs. Report pacemaker problems to the physician:
  - Failure to pace. *This may indicate battery depletion, damage or dislodgement of pacer wires, or inappropriate sensing.*
  - Failure to capture (the pacemaker stimulus is not followed by ventricular depolarization). *The electrical output of the pacemaker may not be adequate, or the lead may be dislodged.*
  - Improper sensing (the pacemaker is firing or not firing, regardless of the intrinsic rate). *This increases the risk for decreased cardiac output and dysrhythmias.*
  - Runaway pacemaker (a pacemaker firing at a rapid rate). *This may by due to generator malfunction or problems with sensing.*
  - Hiccups. *A lead positioned near the diaphragm can stimulate it, causing hiccups. Hiccups may occur in extremely thin clients or may indicate a medical emergency with perforation of the right ventricle by the pacing electrode tip.*
- Assess for dysrhythmias and treat as indicated. *Until the catheter is "seated" or adheres to the myocardium, its movement*

*may cause myocardial irritability and dysrhythmias. Fibrotic tissue develops within 2 to 3 days.*

- Document the date of pacemaker insertion, the model and type, and settings. *This information is important for future reference.*
- Immediately report signs of potential complications, including myocardial perforation, cardiac tamponade, pneumothorax or hemothorax, emboli, skin breakdown, bleeding, infection, endocarditis, or poor wound healing (see Chapter 30 for more information about cardiac tamponade and endocarditis, and Chapter 36 for pneumothorax and hemothorax ). *Early identification of complications allows for aggressive intervention.*
- Provide a pacemaker identification card including the manufacturer's name, model number, mode of operation, rate parameters, and expected battery life. *This card provides a reference for the client and future health care providers.*

## HOME CARE

Provide appropriate teaching for the client and family about:

- Placement of the pacemaker generator and leads in relation to the heart.
- How the pacemaker works and the rate at which it is set.
- Battery replacement. Most pacemaker batteries last 6 to 12 years. Replacement requires a outpatient surgery to open the subcutaneous pocket and replace the battery.
- How to take and record the pulse rate. Instruct to assess pulse daily before arising and notify the physician if 5 or more BPM slower than the preset pacemaker rate.
- Incision care and signs of infection. Bruising may be present following surgery.
- Signs of pacemaker malfunction to report, including dizziness, fainting, fatigue, weakness, chest pain, or palpitations.
- Activity restrictions as ordered. This usually is limited to contact sports (which may damage the generator) and avoiding heavy lifting for 2 months after surgery.
- Resume sexual activity as recommended by the physician. Avoid positions that cause pressure on the site.
- Avoid tight-fitting clothing over the pacemaker site to reduce irritation and avoid skin breakdown.
- Carry the pacemaker identification card at all times, and wear a MedicAlert bracelet or tag.
- Notify all care providers of the pacemaker.
- Do not hold or use certain electrical devices over the pacemaker site, including household appliances or tools, garage door openers, antitheft devices, or burglar alarms. Pacemakers will set off airport security detectors; notify security officials of its presence.
- Maintain follow-up care with the physician as recommended.

---

amplitude of peripheral pulses; color; presence of dyspnea, adventitious lung sounds; ECG rhythm analysis; oxygen saturation levels

## Nursing Diagnoses and Interventions

The effect of the dysrhythmia on cardiac output is the priority of nursing care. Other potential nursing diagnoses related to

dysrhythmias may include *Ineffective tissue perfusion, Activity intolerance,* and *Fear* or *Anxiety.*

## Decreased Cardiac Output

Dysrhythmias can affect cardiac output. Bradycardias decrease cardiac output if the stroke volume does not increase to compensate for the slow heart rate. Tachycardia reduces diastolic filling time, affecting stroke volume and coronary artery perfusion. Loss of the atrial kick in junctional rhythms, atrial fibrillation, and AV blocks also decreases ventricular filling and cardiac output. In ventricular fibrillation, loss of ventricular contractions causes cardiac arrest and no cardiac output.

**PRACTICE ALERT** *Before treating any dysrhythmia, assess the client, not just the monitor! Loose electrode pads, disconnected leads or cables, and muscle movement can simulate critical dysrhythmias. The client's condition is the best indicator of the need for treatment.* ■

- Assess for decreased cardiac output: decreased LOC; tachycardia; tachypnea; hypotension; low oxygen saturation; diaphoresis; low urine output; cool, clammy, mottled skin; pallor or cyanosis; diminished peripheral pulses. *Initial signs of decreased cardiac output may be subtle, such as decreased LOC. Early recognition of the dysrhythmia's effect on cardiac output facilitates appropriate treatment and may prevent further adverse effects.*
- Monitor ECG; post ECG strip every shift and when rhythm changes occur. *Documenting cardiac rhythm provides a record of disease progression and treatment effectiveness.*

**PRACTICE ALERT** *Assess vital signs, ECG, and oxygen saturation every 5 to 15 minutes during acute dysrhythmic episodes and during antidysrhythmic drug infusions. These data provide a record of cardiac output during the dysrhythmia. Antidysrhythmic drugs can adversely affect heart rate, rhythm, and blood pressure, further decreasing cardiac output.* ■

- Assess for underlying causes of dysrhythmias, such as hypovolemia, hypoxia, anemia, vagal stimulation, or medications. *Sinus tachycardia often develops in response to tissue hypoxia. Vagal stimulation (such as the Valsalva maneuver) can precipitate bradycardia.*
- Assess serum electrolytes (especially potassium, calcium, and magnesium) and digitalis and antidysrhythmic drug levels as indicated. Report abnormal values. *Electrolyte imbalances affect cardiac depolarization and repolarization and may cause dysrhythmias. Toxic levels of digitalis and antidysrhythmic drugs can precipitate further dysrhythmias. Impaired renal or hepatic function increases the risk for toxicity, as does aging.*
- Be prepared to administer antidysrhythmic medications as indicated. Implement Advanced Cardiac Life Support (ACLS) protocols as needed. *Emergency drugs should be readily available, especially on units with high-risk clients. See Table 29-6 and the Medication Administration box on page 854 for drugs used to treat common dysrhythmias that may affect cardiac output.*
- If appropriate, instruct to perform the Valsalva maneuver (bear down as if straining or coughing) for supraventricular tachycardia or ventricular tachycardia without angina. *Vagal maneuvers stimulate the parasympathetic system and may terminate some dysrhythmias. The Valsalva maneuver is contraindicated if chest pain occurs with the dysrhythmia.*

- Prepare to assist with cardioversion. Prepare the client per orders or hospital protocol (see Procedure 29–2). Explain the procedure to reduce anxiety. Have emergency equipment readily available. *Elective or emergency cardioversion is a treatment of choice for certain dysrhythmias.*

**PRACTICE ALERT** *On recognizing ventricular fibrillation and cardiac arrest, begin emergency procedures. Call for help. Obtain defibrillator and immediately defibrillate. If the defibrillator will be brought by another health care provider, begin CPR. Initiate ACLS protocols and assist with resuscitation measures as directed. Cardiac output ceases with ventricular fibrillation. Immediate or early defibrillation has been shown to have the greatest impact on survival following cardiac arrest.* ■

- After cardiac arrest, transfer to critical care. Perform and document head-to-toe assessment; obtain laboratory tests, 12-lead ECG, and chest X-ray as ordered; monitor and maintain oxygenation and intravenous infusions; and monitor vital signs and cardiac rhythm. *The period following resuscitation is critical, necessitating careful monitoring. Postarrest assessment allows comparison of the client's condition with prearrest status and may identify CPR-related injuries. Correcting electrolyte disturbances, hypoxia, and acid-base imbalances is important to prevent further dysrhythmias and potential adverse effects on cardiac output. Intravenous access is crucial to maintain drug infusions. Hemodynamic monitoring may be instituted. The 12-lead ECG documents myocardial status, and the chest X-ray provides information about pulmonary status and and possible thoracic injury due to CPR.*
- Notify the family of significant changes in the client's condition or cardiac arrest, providing up-to-date information. Prepare family members prior to visits by explaining interventions (such as invasive tubes, a ventilator, or additional equipment) implemented since the last visit. *Concern for the family and significant others is part of holistic nursing. Researchers studying the needs of families have found that one of the most important needs was information about their loved one's condition. Clients and families need and appreciate honest communication and compassionate care. Preparing the family for critical changes in the client's condition and plan of care helps them to cope with a situational crisis.*

## Using NANDA, NIC, and NOC

Chart 29–3 shows links between NANDA nursing diagnoses, NIC, and NOC when caring for the client with a dysrhythmia.

## Home Care

Dysrhythmias have a significant physical and psychologic impact on the client and all family members. Many of these clients and their families are under a great deal of stress from frequent hospitalizations, experimentation with therapies, frustration, and the fear of sudden cardiac death. A major teaching effort focuses on coping strategies and lifestyle changes, as

## CHART 29–3 NANDA, NIC, AND NOC LINKAGES

### The Client with a Dysrhythmia

| NURSING DIAGNOSIS | NURSING INTERVENTIONS | NURSING OUTCOMES |
| --- | --- | --- |
| • Activity Intolerance | • Energy Management<br>• Self-Care Assistance | • Activity Tolerance<br>• Self-Care: ADL |
| • Anxiety | • Anxiety Reduction | • Anxiety Control |
| • Decreased Cardiac Output | • Cardiac Care: Acute<br>• Cardiac Precautions | • Cardiac Pump Effectiveness<br>• Circulation Status |
| • Deficient Knowledge | • Teaching: Disease Process<br>• Teaching: Procedure/Treatment | • Knowledge: Disease Process<br>• Knowledge: Treatment Procedure(s) |
| • Ineffective Tissue Perfusion | • Dysrhythmia Management<br>• Vital Signs Monitoring | • Cardiac Pump Effectiveness<br>• Vital Signs Status |

*Note. Data from Nursing Outcomes Classification (NOC) by M. Johnson & M. Maas (Eds.), 1997, St. Louis: Mosby; Nursing Diagnoses: Definitions & Classification 2001–2002 by North American Nursing Diagnosis Association, 2001, Philadelphia: NANDA; Nursing Interventions Classification (NIC) by J.C. McCloskey & G. M. Bulechek (Eds.), 2000, St. Louis: Mosby. Reprinted by permission.*

well as specific management of prescribed therapies. Include the following topics as appropriate when teaching the client and family for home care.

- Function, maintenance, precautions, and signs of malfunction or complications of any implanted device such as a pacemaker or ICD
- Monitoring pulse rate and rhythm
- Activity or dietary restrictions, and any potential effects of the dysrhythmia or its treatment on lifestyle
- Medication management to reduce the risk of dysrhythmias, including the desired and potential adverse effects of antidysrhythmic drugs

- Specific instructions related to planned diagnostic tests or procedures
- The importance of follow-up visits with the cardiologist
- The importance of and where to obtain CPR training for the client and family members

In addition, discuss fears related to treatment or implanted devices, such as that of shocking a significant other during close contact or sexual activity. Explain that if a shock occurs, the partner may feel a slight buzz or tingling but should not be harmed. Refer to and encourage the client and family to attend a peer support group for the specific condition.

## Nursing Care Plan
## A Client with Supraventricular Tachycardia

Elisa Vasquez, 53 years old, is admitted to the cardiac unit with complaints of palpitations, lightheadedness, and shortness of breath. Her history reveals rheumatic fever at age 12 with subsequent rheumatic heart disease and mitral stenosis. An intravenous line is in place and she is receiving oxygen. Marcia Lewin, RN, is assigned to Ms. Vasquez.

### ASSESSMENT

Ms. Lewin's assessment reveals that Ms. Vasquez is moderately anxious. Her ECG shows supraventricular tachycardia (SVT) with a rate of 154. Vital signs: T 98.8° F (37.1° C), R 26, BP 95/60. Peripheral pulses weak but equal, mucous membranes pale pink, skin cool and dry. Fine crackles noted in both lung bases. A loud $S_3$ gallop and a diastolic murmur are noted. Ms. Vasquez is still complaining of palpitations and tells Ms. Lewin, "I feel so nervous and weak and dizzy." Ms. Vasquez's cardiologist orders 2.5 mg of verapamil to be given slowly via intravenous push and tells Ms. Lewin to prepare to assist with synchronized cardioversion if drug therapy does not control the ventricular rate.

### DIAGNOSIS

- *Decreased cardiac output* related to inadequate ventricular filling associated with rapid tachycardia
- *Ineffective tissue perfusion: cerebral/cardiopulmonary/peripheral* related to decreased cardiac output
- *Anxiety* related to unknown outcome of altered health state

### EXPECTED OUTCOMES

- Maintain adequate cardiac output and tissue perfusion.
- Demonstrate a ventricular rate within normal limits and stable vital signs.
- Verbalize reduced anxiety.
- Verbalize an understanding of the rationale for the treatment measures to control the heart rate.

### PLANNING AND IMPLEMENTATION

- Provide oxygen per nasal cannula at 4 L/min.
- Continuously monitor ECG for rate, rhythm, and conduction. Assess vital signs and associated symptoms with changes in ECG. Report findings to physician.

## Nursing Care Plan

### A Client with Supraventricular Tachycardia *(continued)*

- Explain the importance of rapidly reducing the heart rate. Explain the cardioversion procedure and encourage questions.
- Encourage verbalization of fears and concerns. Answer questions honestly, correcting misconceptions about the disease process, treatment, or prognosis.
- Administer intravenous diazepam as ordered before cardioversion.
- Document pretreatment vital signs, level of consciousness, and peripheral pulses.
- Place emergency cart with drugs and airway management supplies in client unit.
- Assist with cardioversion as indicated.
- Assess LOC, level of sedation, cardiovascular and respiratory status, and skin condition following cardioversion.
- Document procedure and postcardioversion rhythm, and response to intervention.

### EVALUATION

Intravenous verapamil lowers Ms. Vasquez's heart rate to 138 for a short time, after which it increases to 164 with BP of 82/64. Her cardiologist, Dr. Mullins, performs carotid sinus massage. The ventricular rate slows to 126 for 2 minutes, revealing atrial flutter waves, and then returns to a rate of 150. Dr. Mullins explains the treatment options, including synchronized cardioversion. Ms. Vasquez agrees to the procedure.

Ms. Vasquez is lightly sedated and synchronized cardioversion is performed. One countershock converts Ms. Vasquez to regular sinus rhythm at 96 BPM with BP 112/60.

Ms. Vasquez is sleepy from the sedation but recovers without incident. She states that she feels "much better," and her vital signs return to her normal levels. She remains in NSR with a rate of 86 to 92 for the remainder of her hospital stay. Dr. Mullins places Ms. Vasquez on furosemide to treat manifestations of mild heart failure.

### Critical Thinking in the Nursing Process

1. What is the scientific basis for using carotid massage to treat supraventricular tachycardias? Was this an appropriate maneuver in the case of Ms. Vasquez?
2. What other treatment options might the physician have used to treat Ms. Vasquez's supraventricular tachycardia if she had been asymptomatic with stable vital signs?
3. Develop a teaching plan for Ms. Vasquez related to her prescription for furosemide.

See Evaluating Your Response in Appendix C.

## THE CLIENT WITH SUDDEN CARDIAC DEATH

**Sudden cardiac death (SCD)** is defined as unexpected death occurring within 1 hour of the onset of cardiovascular symptoms. It usually is caused by ventricular fibrillation and cardiac arrest. *Cardiac arrest* is the sudden collapse, loss of consciousness, and cessation of effective circulation that precedes biologic death. Nearly half of all cardiac arrest victims die before reaching the hospital; only 25% to 30% of out-of-hospital cardiac arrest victims survive to be discharged (Woods et al., 2000).

Almost 50% of all deaths due to coronary heart disease are attributed to SCD. Coronary heart disease causes up to 80% of all sudden cardiac deaths in the United States. Other cardiac pathologies such as cardiomyopathy and valvular disorders also may lead to SCD. Noncardiac causes of sudden death include electrocution, pulmonary embolism, and rapid blood loss from a ruptured aortic aneurysm.

Ventricular fibrillation is the most common dysrhythmia associated with sudden cardiac death, accounting for 65% to 80% of cardiac arrests. Sustained severe bradydysrhythmias, *asystole* or cardiac standstill, and pulseless electrical activity (organized cardiac electrical activity without a mechanical response) are responsible for most remaining SCDs (Braunwald

et al., 2001). Selected cardiac and noncardiac causes of sudden cardiac death are listed in Box 29–6.

Risk factors for SCD are those associated with coronary heart disease (see the first section of this chapter). Advancing age and male gender are powerful risk factors. After age 65, the gap between male and female incidence of SCD narrows (Braunwald et al., 2001). Clients with dysrhythmias such as recurrent VT may have a higher risk of SCD.

### PATHOPHYSIOLOGY

Evidence of coronary heart disease with significant atherosclerosis and narrowing of two or more major coronary arteries is found in 75% of SCD victims. Although most have had prior myocardial infarction, only 20% to 30% have recent acute myocardial infarction. An acute change in cardiovascular status precedes cardiac arrest by up to 1 hour; however, often the onset is instantaneous or abrupt. Tachycardia develops, and the number of PVCs increase. This is followed by a run of ventricular tachycardia that deteriorates into ventricular fibrillation (Braunwald et al., 2001).

Abnormalities of myocardial structure or function also contribute. Structural abnormalities include infarction, hypertrophy, myopathy, and electrical anomalies. Functional deviations are caused by such factors as ischemia followed by reperfusion, altered homeostasis, autonomic nervous system

## NURSING CARE

Nursing care of the client experiencing sudden cardiac death requires prompt recognition of the event and immediate initiation of BLS and ALS protocols. As noted before, early defibrillation of unstable VT and VF is the most important key to survival of cardiac arrest victims. Important concepts of emergency cardiac care follow.

- Treat the client, not the monitor. Recognize signs and symptoms of cardiac compromise early.
- Activate the emergency medical services system (i.e., call a code or call 911).
- Begin and continue basic cardiac life support principles throughout the resuscitation effort.
- Continually assess the effectiveness of emergency interventions.
- Defibrillate pulseless VT or VF as soon as possible.
- Initiate ALS protocols early.

The family is not forgotten during resuscitation. If the family is present, they are usually offered a private consultation room in which to await the outcome. If the family is not present, they are notified that their family member is not doing well and asked to come to the hospital as soon as possible. The situation is presented in a careful manner to prevent the family from racing to the hospital, precipitating an automobile crash. Pastoral care or the family's choice of spiritual support is offered to help during this difficult time. Attendance of family members during resuscitation efforts is controversial, and depends on institutional protocols and family desires.

After successful resuscitation, the nurse provides care specific to the client's underlying disease processes and needs. Intravenous infusions such as lidocaine, bretylium, or dopamine may be ordered to prevent further dysrhythmias and maintain hemodynamic stability.

If the client does not survive the arrest, the nurse provides postmortem care and emotional and spiritual support to the family.

Nursing diagnoses to consider for the client experiencing SCD include the following:

- *Ineffective tissue perfusion: Cerebral* related to ineffective cardiac output
- *Impaired spontaneous ventilation* related to cardiac arrest
- *Spiritual distress* related to unexplained sudden cardiac death
- *Disturbed thought processes* related to compromised cerebral circulation
- *Fear* related to risk for future episodes of sudden cardiac death

The risk for a future episode of sudden cardiac death requires careful and effective teaching for home care prior to discharge. Discuss the following topics with the client and family.

- Risk factor reduction for coronary heart disease
- Planned diagnostic studies to identify the cause of SCD, and possible interventions
- The risks and benefits of an ICD if appropriate
- The importance of carrying a card at all times listing all current medications and the health care provider
- Early manifestations or warning signs of cardiac arrest

- The importance of CPR training and maintaining proficiency in performing CPR (Provide referral to local CPR training providers or scheduled classes through the American Heart Association or American Red Cross.)

Nurses can impact death rates from cardiac arrest through community teaching as well. Survival rates from sudden cardiac death improve in communities in which a significant portion of the population is trained in CPR and early response by EMS agencies is stressed. Work with community groups and individuals can help create a population of people able to perform effective CPR.

## SPECIAL FOCUS: ADVANCE DIRECTIVES AND THE DO-NOT-RESUSCITATE ORDER

Most if not all hospitals have formal policies and procedures for resuscitation of clients who experience cardiac or respiratory arrest. *Advance directives* provide for the client's right to self-determination, that is, the client's right to make treatment decisions and to be responsible for the outcomes of those decisions. The living will and the durable power of attorney for health care are types of available advance directives. Both enable the client to state his or her wishes for medical treatments in end-of-life decisions. Nurses can assist clients to understand the purpose of advance directives.

Classification systems identifying the extent of resuscitative measures employed for clients who suffer a cardiac or respiratory arrest may include the following:

- *Full code:* Involves all resuscitative measures necessary to revive the client: defibrillation, CPR, respiratory, and pharmacologic support.
- *Partial code (varies by institution and client preference):* May involve full resuscitative measures with daily reassessment of code status, or may limit measures to be used in case of cardiac arrest.
- *No code:* The third classification may prohibit all resuscitative measures or limit measures to drug treatment without defibrillation, CPR, or intubation.
- *Comfort care:* Some institutions have a fourth class that allows discontinuation of all treatment except for pain and comfort measures.

Clients are usually considered a full code on hospital admission, unless an advance directive is in place. Without a written DNR order or advance directive, the nurse is obligated to begin resuscitation measures if indicated by the client's condition. This can create an ethical dilemma for nurses caring for critically ill or terminal clients should cardiac arrest ensue. Nurses should be aware of institutional policies and procedures regarding code status and advance directives.

DNR orders do not mean withdrawing care. Optimal nursing care is provided to these clients and their families. Health care providers collaborate to design an individualized plan of care for the client. The team approach, encouraging discussion of these issues between clients, families, and health care providers, allows information sharing and facilitates compassionate care planning. More information on DNRs, advance directives, and care of the family experiencing a loss is provided in Chapter 11.

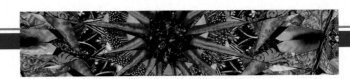

 ## EXPLORE MediaLink

NCLEX review questions, case studies, care plan activities, MediaLink applications, and other interactive resources for this chapter can be found on the Companion Website at www.prenhall.com/lemone.

Click on Chapter 29 to select the activities for this chapter. For animations, video clips, more NCLEX review questions, and an audio glossary, access the Student CD-ROM accompanying this textbook.

## TEST YOURSELF

1. The nurse evaluates her teaching as effective when a client identifies which of the following modifiable risk factors for coronary heart disease (CHD) as contributing to the greatest extent?

   a. Obesity
   b. Diet
   c. Smoking
   d. Stress

2. When assessing a client with stable angina, the nurse would expect to find:

   a. Persistent ECG changes
   b. Correlation between activity level and pain
   c. Increasing nocturnal pain
   d. Evidence of impaired cardiac output such as weak peripheral pulses

3. In planning care for the client with acute myocardial infarction, (AMI) the nurse identifies the highest priority goal of care as:

   a. Stable ECG rhythm
   b. Ability to verbalize causes and effects of CHD

   c. Compliance with prescribed bed rest
   d. Relief of pain

4. Which of the following nursing diagnoses is of highest priority for the client undergoing thrombolytic therapy?

   a. *Ineffective protection*
   b. *Ineffective health maintenance*
   c. *Risk for powerlessness*
   d. *Anxiety*

5. The nurse recognizes second-degree AV block, type II (Mobitz II), and intervenes appropriately when he:

   a. Records the finding in the chart
   b. Prepares for temporary pacemaker insertion
   c. Administers a class IB antidysrhythmic drug
   d. Places the client in Fowler's position

See Test Yourself answers in Appendix C.

## BIBLIOGRAPHY

Ackley, B. J., & Ladwig, G. B. (2002). *Nursing diagnosis handbook: A guide to planning care* (5th ed.). St. Louis: Mosby.

Artinian, N. T. (2001). Perceived benefits and barriers of eating heart healthy. *MEDSURG Nursing, 10*(3), 129–138

Ayers, D. M. M. (2002). EBCT: Beaming in on coronary artery disease. *Nursing, 32*(4), 81.

Beattie, S. (2000). A portrait of postop a-fib. *RN, 63*(3), 26–29.

Braunwald, E., Fauci, A. S., Kasper, D. L., Hauser, S. L., Longo, D. L., & Jameson, J. L. (2001). *Harrison's Principles of internal medicine* (15th ed.). New York: McGraw-Hill.

Bubien, R. S. (2000). A new beat on an old rhythm. *American Journal of Nursing, 100*(1), 42–50.

Bullock, B. A., & Henze, R. L. (2000). *Focus on pathophysiology.* Philadelphia: Lippincott.

Copstead, L. C., and Banasik, J. L. (2000). *Pathophysiology: Biological and behavioral perspectives* (2nd ed.). Philadelphia: Saunders.

Cowan, M. J., Pike, K. C., & Budzynski, H. K. (2001). Psychosocial nursing therapy following sudden cardiac arrest: Impact on

two-year survival. *Nursing Research, 50*(2), 68–76.

Crumlish, C. M., Bracken, J., Hand, M. M., Keenan, K., Ruggiero, H., & Simmons, D. (2000). When time is muscle. *American Journal of Nursing, 100*(1), 26–33.

Deglin, J. H., & Vallerand, A. H. (2003). *Davis's drug guide for nurses* (8th ed.). Philadelphia: F.A. Davis.

Dracup, K., & Moser, D. K. (1997). Beyond sociodemographics: Factors influencing the decision to seek treatment for symptoms of acute myocardial infarction. *Heart & Lung, 26*(4), 253–262.

Fontaine, K. L. (2000). *Healing practices: Alternative therapies for nursing.* Upper Saddle River, NJ: Prentice Hall Health.

Gallo, J. J., Busby-Whitehead, J., Rabins, P. V., Silliman, R. A., & Murphy, J. B. (Eds.). (1999). *Reichel's care of the elderly: Clinical aspects of aging* (5th ed.). Philadelphia: Lippincott Williams & Wilkins.

Glessner, T. M., & Walker, M. K. (2001). Standardized measures: Documenting processes and

outcomes of care for patients undergoing coronary artery bypass grafting. *MEDSURG Nursing, 10*(1), 23–29.

Goodman, D. (2001). Automatic external defibrillation. *MEDSURG Nursing, 10*(5), 251–253, 276, 278.

Granger, B. B., & Miller, C. M. (2001). Acute coronary syndrome. *Nursing, 31*(11), 36–43.

Humphreys, D. R. (2001). Enhanced external counter pulsation: Beating angina. *Nursing, 31*(10), 54–55.

Incredibly easy! Understanding chest pain. (2001). *Nursing, 31*(12), 28.

Johnson, M., Bulechek, G., Dochterman, J. M., Maas, M., & Moorhead, S. (2001). *Nursing diagnoses, outcomes, & interventions.* St. Louis: Mosby.

Johnson, M., Maas, M., & Moorhead, S. (Eds.). (2000). *Nursing outcomes classification (NOC)* (2nd ed.). St. Louis: Mosby.

Kuhn, M. A. (1999). *Complementary therapies for health care providers.* Philadelphia: Lippincott.

Lehne, R. A. (2001). *Pharmacology for nursing care* (4th ed.). Philadelphia: Saunders.

Malarkey, L. M., & McMorrow, M. E. (2000). *Nurse's manual of laboratory tests and diagnostic procedures* (2nd ed.). Philadelphia: Saunders.

Mancini, M. E., & Kaye, W. (1999). AEDs: Changing the way you respond to cardiac arrest. *American Journal of Nursing, 99*(5), 26–30.

McAvoy, J. A. (2000). Cardiac pain: Discover the unexpected. *Nursing, 30*(1), 34–39.

McCance, K. L., & Huether, S. E. (2002). *Pathophysiology: The biologic basis for disease in adults and children* (4th ed.). St. Louis: Mosby.

McCloskey, J. C., & Bulechek, G. M. (Eds.) (2000). *Nursing interventions classification (NIC)* (3rd ed.). St. Louis: Mosby.

Meeker, M. H., & Rothrock, J. C. (1999). *Alexander's care of the patient in surgery* (11th ed.). St. Louis: Mosby.

National Cholesterol Education Program. (2001). *Adult treatment panel III report.* National Cholesterol Education Program Expert Panel on Detection, Evaluation, and Treatment of High Blood Cholesterol in Adults.

National Heart, Lung, and Blood Institute. National Institutes of Health. (2002). *Morbidity & mortality: 2002 chart book of cardiovascular, lung, and blood diseases.* Bethesda, MD: Author.

Navuluri, R. (2001). Antiplatelet and fibrinolytic therapy. *American Journal of Nursing, 101*(10), Hospital Extra 24A, 24D.

North American Nursing Diagnosis Association. (2001). *NANDA nursing diagnoses: Definitions & classification 2001–2002.* Philadelphia: NANDA.

Palatnik, A. M. (2001). Critical care. Acute coronary syndrome: New advances and nursing strategies. *Nursing, 31*(5), 32cc1–32cc2, 32cc4, 32cc6.

Photo guide. How to perform 3- or 5-lead monitoring. (2002). *Nursing, 32*(4), 50–52.

Porth, C. M. (2002). *Pathophysiology: Concepts of altered health states* (6th ed.). Philadelphia: Lippincott.

Robinson, A. W. (1999). Getting to the heart of denial. *American Journal of Nursing, 99*(5), 38–42.

Shaffer, R. S. (2002). ICD therapy: The patient's perspective. *American Journal of Nursing, 102*(2), 46–49.

Siomko, A. J. (2000). Demystifying cardiac markers. *American Journal of Nursing, 100*(1), 36–40.

Snowberger, P. (2001). VT or SVT? You can tell at the bedside. *RN, 64*(2), 26–31.

Steinke, E. E. (2000). Sexual counseling after myocardial infarction. *American Journal of Nursing, 100*(12), 38–43.

Sullivan, C. (2000). Critical care. Easing severe angina with laser surgery. *Nursing, 30*(4), 32cc1–32cc2, 32cc4

Tierney, L. M., McPhee, S. J., & Papadakis, M. A. (2001). *Current medical diagnosis & treatment* (40th ed.). New York: Lange Medical Books/McGraw-Hill.

Urden, L. D., Stacy, K. M., & Lough, M. E. (2002). *Thelan's critical care nursing: Diagnosis and management* (4th ed.). St. Louis: Mosby.

U. S. Preventive Services Task Force. (2002). Aspirin for the primary prevention of cardiovascular events: Recommendations and rationale. *American Journal of Nursing, 102*(3), 67, 69–70.

———. (2002). Screening for lipid disorders in adults: Recommendations and rationale. *American Journal of Nursing, 102*(6), 91, 93, 95.

Whitney, E. N., & Rolfes, S. R. (2002). *Understanding nutrition* (9th ed.). Belmont, CA: Wadsworth.

Wilkinson, J. M. (2000). *Nursing diagnosis handbook with NIC interventions and NOC outcomes* (7th ed.). Upper Saddle River, NJ: Prentice Hall Health.

Woods, S. L., Froelicher, E. S. S., & Motzer, S. U. (2000). *Cardiac nursing* (4th ed.). Philadelphia: Lippincott.

Writing Group for the Women's Health Initiative Investigators. (2002). Risks and benefits of estrogen plus progestin in healthy postmenopausal women. [On-line]. *JAMA, 288*(3). Available: http://jama.ama-assn.org/issues/v288n3/fffull/joc21036.html

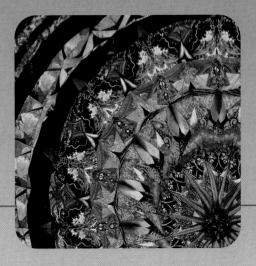

### CHAPTER 30

# Nursing Care of Clients with Cardiac Disorders

 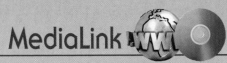
## LEARNING OUTCOMES

After completing this chapter, you will be able to:

■ Apply knowledge of normal cardiac anatomy and physiology and assessment techniques in caring for clients with cardiac disorders.

■ Compare and contrast the pathophysiology and manifestations of common cardiac disorders, including heart failure, structural disorders, and inflammatory disorders.

■ Identify common diagnostic tests used for cardiac disorders and their nursing implications.

■ Discuss indications for and management of clients with hemodynamic monitoring.

■ Discuss nursing implications for medications commonly prescribed for clients with cardiac disorders.

■ Describe nursing care for the client undergoing cardiac surgery or cardiac transplant.

■ Use the nursing process to provide individualized care for clients with cardiac disorders.

■ Provide appropriate teaching and home care for clients with cardiac disorders and their families.

Cardiac disorders affect the structure and/or function of the heart. These disorders interfere with the heart's primary purpose: to pump enough blood to meet the body's demand for oxygen and nutrients. Disruptions in cardiac function affect the functioning of other organs and tissues, potentially leading to organ system failure and death.

Heart failure is the most common cardiac disorder. Other cardiac disorders discussed in this chapter include structural cardiac disorders, such as valve disorders and cardiomyopathy, and inflammatory cardiac disorders, such as endocarditis and pericarditis. Before continuing with this chapter, please review the heart's anatomy and physiology and nursing assessment in Chapter 28.

# HEART FAILURE

**Heart failure,** the inability of the heart to pump enough blood to meet the metabolic demands of the body, is the end result of many conditions. Frequently, it is a long-term effect of coronary heart disease and myocardial infarction when left ventricular damage is extensive enough to impair cardiac output (see Chapter 29). Other diseases of the heart also may cause heart failure, including structural and inflammatory disorders. In normal hearts, failure can result from excessive demands placed on the heart. Heart failure may be acute or chronic.

## THE CLIENT WITH HEART FAILURE

As mentioned, heart failure is the inability of the heart to function as a pump to meet the needs of the body. As a result, cardiac output falls, leading to decreased tissue perfusion. The body initially adjusts to reduced cardiac output by activating inherent compensatory mechanisms to restore tissue perfusion. These normal mechanisms may result in vascular congestion— and hence, the commonly used term *congestive heart failure (CHF)*. As these mechanisms are exhausted, heart failure ensues, with increased morbidity and mortality.

Heart failure is a disorder of cardiac function. It frequently is due to *impaired myocardial contraction,* which may result from coronary heart disease and myocardial ischemia or infarct or from a primary cardiac muscle disorder such as cardiomyopathy or myocarditis. Structural cardiac disorders, such as valve disorders or congenital heart defects, and hypertension also can lead to heart failure when the heart muscle is damaged by the long-standing *excessive workload* associated with these conditions. Other clients without a primary abnormality of myocardial function may present with manifestations of heart failure due to *acute excess demands* placed on the myocardium,

such as volume overload, hyperthyroidism, and massive pulmonary embolus (Table 30–1). Hypertension and coronary heart disease are the leading causes of heart failure in the United States. The high prevalence of hypertension in African Americans contributes significantly to their risk for and incidence of heart failure.

Nearly 5 million people in the United States are currently living with heart failure; approximately 550,000 new cases of heart failure are diagnosed annually (American Heart Association [AHA], 2001). Its incidence and prevalence increase with age: Less than 5% of people between ages 55 and 64 have heart failure, whereas 6% to 10% of people older than 65 are affected (see the box on the following page) (Hunt et al., 2001). The prognosis for a client with heart failure depends on its underlying cause and how effectively precipitating factors can be treated. Most clients with heart failure die within 8 years of the diagnosis. The risk for sudden cardiac death is dramatically increased, occurring at a rate 6 to 9 times that of the general population (AHA, 2001).

### PHYSIOLOGY REVIEW

The mechanical pumping action of cardiac muscle propels the blood it receives to the pulmonary and systemic vascular systems for reoxygenation and delivery to the tissues. *Cardiac output (CO)* is the amount of blood pumped from the ventricles in 1 minute. Cardiac output is used to assess cardiac performance, especially left ventricular function. Effective cardiac output depends on adequate functional muscle mass and the ability of the ventricles to work together. Cardiac output normally is regulated by the oxygen needs of the body: As oxygen use increases, cardiac output increases to maintain cellular function. *Cardiac reserve* is the ability of the heart to increase CO to meet metabolic demand. Ventricular damage reduces the cardiac reserve.

| TABLE 30–1   Selected Causes of Heart Failure | | |
|---|---|---|
| **Impaired Myocardial Function** | **Increased Cardiac Workload** | **Acute Noncardiac Conditions** |
| • Coronary heart disease | • Hypertension | • Volume overload |
| • Cardiomyopathies | • Valve disorders | • Hyperthyroidism |
| • Rheumatic fever | • Anemias | • Fever, infection |
| • Infective endocarditis | • Congenital heart defects | • Massive pulmonary embolus |

## Nursing Care of the Older Adult

### HEART FAILURE

Heart failure is common in older adults, affecting nearly 10% of people over the age of 75 years.

Aging affects cardiac function. Diastolic filling is impaired by decreased ventricular compliance. With aging, the heart is less responsive to sympathetic nervous system stimulation. As a result, maximal heart rate, cardiac reserve, and exercise tolerance are reduced. Concurrent health problems such as arthritis that affect stamina or mobility often contribute to a more sedentary lifestyle, further decreasing the heart's ability to respond to increased stress.

### Assessing for Home Care

The older adult with heart failure may not be dyspneic, instead presenting with weakness and fatigue, somnolence, confusion, disorientation, or worsening dementia. Dependent edema and respiratory crackles may or may not indicate heart failure in older adults.

Assess the diet of the older adult. Decreased taste may lead to increased use of salt to bring out food flavors. Limited mobility or visual acuity may cause the older adult to rely on prepared foods that are high in sodium such as canned soups and frozen meals. Discuss normal daily activities and assess sleep and rest patterns. It is also important to assess the environment for:

- Safe roads or neighborhoods for walking
- Access to pharmacy, medical care, and assistive services such as a cardiac rehabilitation program or structured exercise programs designed for older adults

### Client and Family Teaching

Teaching for the older adult with heart failure focuses on maintaining function and promptly identifying and treating episodes of heart failure. Teach clients how to adapt to changes in cardiovascular function associated with aging, such as:

- Allowing longer warm-up and cool-down periods during exercise
- Engaging in regular exercise such as walking 3 to 4 times a week
- Resting with feet elevated (e.g., in a recliner) when fatigued
- Maintaining adequate fluid intake
- Preventing infection through pneumococcal and influenza immunizations

---

Cardiac output is a product of heart rate and stroke volume. *Heart rate* affects cardiac output by controlling the number of ventricular contractions per minute. It is influenced by the autonomic nervous system, catecholamines, and thyroid hormones. Activation of a stress response (e.g., hypovolemia or fear) stimulates the sympathetic nervous system, increasing the heart rate and its contractility. Elevated heart rates increase cardiac output. Very rapid heart rates, however, shorten ventricular filling time (diastole), reducing stroke volume and cardiac output. On the other hand, a slow heart rate reduces cardiac output simply because of fewer cardiac cycles.

*Stroke volume* is the volume of blood ejected with each heartbeat; it is determined by preload, afterload, and myocardial contractility. *Preload* is the volume of blood in the ventricles at end-diastole (just prior to contraction). The blood in the ventricles exerts pressure on the ventricle walls, stretching muscle fibers. The greater the blood volume, the greater force with which the ventricle contracts to expel the blood. End-diastolic volume (EDV) depends on the amount of blood returning to the ventricles (*venous return*), and the distensibility or stiffness of the ventricles (*compliance*). See Box 30–1.

*Afterload* is the force needed to eject blood into the circulation. This force must be great enough to overcome arterial pressures within the pulmonary and systemic vascular systems. The right ventricle must generate enough force to open the pulmonary valve and eject its blood into the pulmonary artery. The left ventricle ejects its blood into the systemic circulation by overcoming the arterial resistance behind the aortic valve. Increased systemic vascular resistance increases afterload, impairing stroke volume and increasing myocardial work.

*Contractility* is the natural ability of cardiac muscle fibers to shorten during systole. Contractility is necessary to overcome arterial pressures and eject blood during systole. Impaired contractility affects cardiac output, by reducing stroke volume.

### BOX 30–1 ■ Explaining Physiologic Terms Using Practical Examples

The concepts of preload, the Frank-Starling mechanism, compliance, and afterload can be difficult to understand and to explain to clients. Use common analogies to make these concepts easier to understand.

- *Preload:* Think about a new rubber band. As you stretch the rubber band further, it snaps back into shape with greater force.
- *Frank-Starling mechanism:* When you repeatedly stretch that rubber band beyond a certain limit, it loses some elasticity and fails to return to its original shape and size.
- *Compliance:* Use a new rubber balloon to illustrate this concept. A new balloon is not very compliant—it takes a lot of work (force) to inflate it. As the balloon is repeatedly stretched, it becomes more compliant, expanding easily with less force.
- *Afterload:* When a hose is crimped or plugged, more force is required to eject a stream of water out its end.

The *ejection fraction (EF)* is the percentage of blood in the ventricle that is ejected during systole. A normal ejection fraction is approximately 60%.

## PATHOPHYSIOLOGY

When the heart begins to fail, mechanisms are activated to compensate for the impaired function and maintain the cardiac output. The primary compensatory mechanisms are (1) the Frank-Starling mechanism; (2) neuroendocrine responses including activation of the sympathetic nervous system and the renin-angiotensin system; and (3) myocardial hypertrophy. These mechanisms and their effects are summarized in Table 30–2.

| TABLE 30-2 | Compensatory Mechanisms For Heart Failure | | |
| --- | --- | --- | --- |
| **Mechanism** | **Physiology** | **Effect on Body Systems** | **Complications** |
| Frank-Starling mechanism | The greater the stretch of cardiac muscle fibers, the greater the force of contraction. | • Increased contractile force leading to increased CO | • Increased myocardial oxygen demand<br>• Limited by overstretching |
| Neuroendocrine response | Decreased CO stimulates the sympathetic nervous system and catecholamine release. | • Increased HR, BP, and contractility<br>• Increased vascular resistance<br>• Increased venous return | • Tachycardia with decreased filling time and decreased CO<br>• Increased vascular resistance<br>• Increased myocardial work and oxygen demand |
| | Decreased CO and decreased renal perfusion stimulate renin/angiotensin system. | • Vasoconstriction and increased BP | • Increased myocardial work<br>• Renal vasoconstriction and decreased renal perfusion |
| | Angiotensin stimulates aldosterone release from adrenal cortex. | • Salt and water retention by the kidneys<br>• Increased vascular volume | • Increased preload and afterload<br>• Pulmonary congestion |
| | ADH is released from posterior pituitary. | • Water excretion inhibited | • Fluid retention and increased preload and afterload<br>• Pulmonary congestion |
| | Atrial natriuretic factor is released. | • Increased sodium excretion<br>• Diuresis | |
| | Blood flow is redistributed to vital organs (heart and brain). | • Decreased perfusion of other organ systems<br>• Decreased perfusion of skin and muscles | • Renal failure<br>• Anaerobic metabolism and lactic acidosis |
| Ventricular hypertrophy | Increased cardiac workload causes myocardial muscle to hypertrophy and ventricles to dilate. | • Increased contractile force to maintain CO | • Increased myocardial oxygen demand<br>• Cellular enlargement |

Decreased cardiac output initially stimulates aortic baroreceptors, which in turn stimulate the sympathetic nervous system (SNS). SNS stimulation produces both cardiac and vascular responses through the release of norepinephrine. Norepinephrine increases heart rate and contractility by stimulating cardiac beta receptors. Cardiac output improves as both heart rate and stroke volume increase. Norepinephrine also causes arterial and venous vasoconstriction, increasing venous return to the heart. Increased venous return increases ventricular filling and myocardial stretch, increasing the force of contraction (the Frank-Starling mechanism). Overstretching the muscle fibers past their physiologic limit results in an ineffective contraction.

Blood flow is redistributed to the brain and the heart to maintain perfusion of these vital organs. Decreased renal perfusion causes renin to be released from the kidneys. Activation of the renin-angiotensin system produces additional vasoconstriction and stimulates the adrenal cortex to produce aldosterone and the posterior pituitary to release antidiuretic hormone (ADH). Aldosterone stimulates sodium reabsorption in renal tubules, promoting water retention. ADH acts on the distal tubule to inhibit water excretion and causes vasoconstriction. The effect of these hormones is significant vasoconstriction and salt and water retention, with a resulting increase in vascular volume. Increased ventricular filling increases the force of contraction, improving cardiac output. The increased vascular volume and venous return also increase atrial pressures, stimulating the release of an additional hormone, *atrial natriuretic factor (ANF)* or *atriopeptin.* Atrial natriuetic factor balances the effects of the other

hormones to a certain extent, promoting sodium and water excretion and inhibiting the release of norepinephrine, renin, and ADH. This hormone is thought to be a natural preventive that delays severe cardiac decompensation.

*Ventricular remodeling* occurs as the heart chambers and myocardium adapt to fluid volume and pressure increases. The chambers dilate to accommodate excess fluid resulting from increased vascular volume and incomplete emptying. Initially, this additional stretch causes more effective contractions. *Ventricular hypertrophy* occurs as existing cardiac muscle cells enlarge, increasing their contractile elements (actin and myosin) and force of contraction.

Although these responses may help in the short-term regulation of cardiac output, it is now recognized that they hasten the deterioration of cardiac function. The onset of heart failure is heralded by *decompensation,* the loss of effective compensation. Heart failure progresses due to the very mechanisms that initially maintained circulatory stability.

The rapid heart rate shortens diastolic filling time, compromises coronary artery perfusion, and increases myocardial oxygen demand. Resulting ischemia further impairs cardiac output. Beta-receptors in the heart become less sensitive to continued SNS stimulation, decreasing heart rate and contractility. As the beta-receptors become less sensitive, norepinephrine stores in the cardiac muscle become depleted. In contrast, alpha-receptors on peripheral blood vessels become increasingly sensitive to persistent stimulation, promoting vasoconstriction and increasing afterload and cardiac work.

Initially, ventricular hypertrophy and dilation increase cardiac output, but chronic distention causes the ventricular wall eventually to thin and degenerate. The purpose of hypertrophy is thus defeated. In addition, chronic overloading of the dilated ventricle eventually stretches the fibers beyond the optimal point for effective contraction. The ventricles continue to dilate to accommodate the excess fluid, but the heart loses the ability to contract forcefully. The heart muscle may eventually become so large that the coronary blood supply is inadequate, causing ischemia.

Chronic distention exhausts atrial stores of ANF. The effects of norepinephrine, renin, and ADH prevail, and the renin-angiotensin pathway is continually stimulated. This mechanism ultimately raises the hemodynamic stress on the heart by increasing both preload and afterload. As heart function deteriorates, less blood is delivered to the tissues and to the heart itself. Ischemia and necrosis of the myocardium further weaken the already failing heart, and the cycle repeats.

In normal hearts, the cardiac reserve allows the heart to adjust its output to meet metabolic needs of the body, increasing the cardiac output by up to 5 times the basal level during exercise. Clients with heart failure have minimal to no cardiac reserve. At rest, they may be unaffected; however, any stressor (e.g., exercise, illness) taxes their ability to meet the demand for oxygen and nutrients. Manifestations of activity intolerance when the person is at rest indicate a critical level of cardiac decompensation.

## Classifications

Heart failure is commonly classified in several different ways, depending on the underlying pathology. Classifications include systolic versus diastolic failure, left-sided versus right-sided failure, high-output versus low-output failure, and acute versus chronic failure.

### Systolic Versus Diastolic Failure

*Systolic failure* occurs when the ventricle fails to contract adequately to eject a sufficient blood volume into the arterial system. Systolic function is affected by loss of myocardial cells due to ischemia and infarction, cardiomyopathy, or inflammation. The manifestations of systolic failure are those of decreased cardiac output: weakness, fatigue, and decreased exercise tolerance.

*Diastolic failure* results when the heart cannot completely relax in diastole, disrupting normal filling. Passive diastolic filling decreases, increasing the importance of atrial contraction to preload. Diastolic dysfunction results from decreased ventricular compliance due to hypertrophic and cellular changes and impaired relaxation of the heart muscle. Its manifestations result from increased pressure and congestion behind the ventricle: shortness of breath, tachypnea, and respiratory crackles if the left ventricle is affected; distended neck veins, liver enlargement, anorexia, and nausea if the right ventricle is affected. Many clients have components of both systolic and diastolic failure.

### Left-Sided Versus Right-Sided Failure

Depending on the pathophysiology involved, either the left or the right ventricle may be primarily affected. In chronic heart failure, however, both ventricles typically are impaired to some degree. Coronary heart disease and hypertension are common causes of *left-sided heart failure,* whereas *right-sided heart failure* often is caused by conditions that restrict blood flow to the lungs, such as acute or chronic pulmonary disease. Left-sided heart failure also can lead to right-sided failure as pressures in the pulmonary vascular system increase with congestion behind the failing left ventricle.

As left ventricular function fails, cardiac output falls. Pressures in the left ventricle and atrium increase as the amount of blood remaining in the ventricle after systole increases. These increased pressures impair filling, causing congestion and increased pressures in the pulmonary vascular system. Increased pressures in this normally low-pressure system increase fluid movement from the blood vessels into interstitial tissues and the alveoli (Figure 30–1 ■).

The manifestations of left-sided heart failure result from pulmonary congestion and decreased cardiac output. Fatigue and activity intolerance are common early manifestations. Dizziness and syncope also may result from decreased cardiac output. Pulmonary congestion causes dyspnea, shortness of breath, and cough. The client may develop **orthopnea** (difficulty breathing while lying down), prompting use of two or

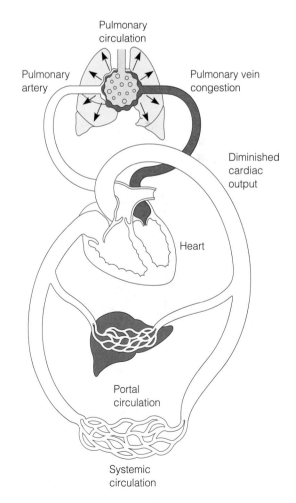

**Figure 30–1 ■** The hemodynamic effects of left-sided heart failure.

three pillows or a recliner for sleeping. Cyanosis from impaired gas exchange may be noted. On auscultation of the lungs, inspiratory crackles (rales) and wheezes may be heard in lung bases. An $S_3$ gallop may be present, reflecting the heart's attempts to fill an already distended ventricle.

In right-sided heart failure, increased pressures in the pulmonary vasculature or right ventricular muscle damage impair the right venticle's ability to pump blood into the pulmonary circulation. The right ventricle and atrium become distended, and blood accumulates in the systemic venous system. Increased venous pressures cause abdominal organs to become congested and peripheral tissue edema to develop (Figure 30–2 ■).

Dependent tissues tend to be affected because of the effects of gravity; edema develops in the feet and legs, or if the client is bedridden, in the sacrum. Congestion of gastrointestinal tract vessels causes anorexia and nausea. Right upper quadrant pain may result from liver engorgement. Neck veins distend and become visible even when the client is upright due to increased venous pressure.

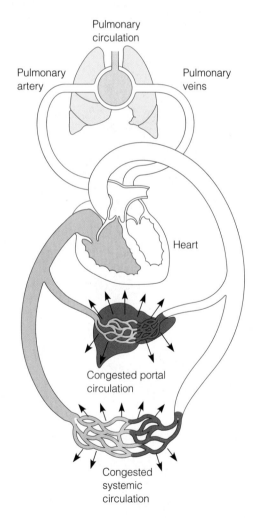

**Figure 30–2 ■** The hemodynamic effects of right-sided heart failure.

### High-Output Failure

Clients in hypermetabolic states (e.g., hyperthyroidism, infection, anemia, or pregnancy) require increased cardiac output to maintain blood flow and oxygen to the tissues. If the increased blood flow cannot meet the oxygen demands of the tissues, compensatory mechanisms are activated to further increase cardiac output, which in turn further increases oxygen demand. Thus, even though cardiac output is high, the heart is unable to meet increased oxygen demands. This condition is known as *high-output failure.*

### Acute Versus Chronic Failure

*Acute failure* is the abrupt onset of a myocardial injury (such as a massive MI) resulting in suddenly decreased cardiac function and signs of decreased cardiac output. *Chronic failure* is a progressive deterioration of the heart muscle due to cardiomyopathies, valvular disease, or CHD.

## MANIFESTATIONS AND COMPLICATIONS

In addition to the previous manifestations for the various classifications of heart failure, other signs and symptoms commonly are seen.

A fall in cardiac output activates mechanisms that cause increased salt and water retention. This causes weight gain and further increases pressures in the capillaries, resulting in edema. *Nocturia,* voiding more than one time at night, develops as edema fluid from dependent tissues is reabsorbed when the client is supine. **Paroxysmal nocturnal dyspnea (PND),** a frightening condition in which the client awakens at night acutely short of breath, also may develop. Paroxysmal nocturnal dyspnea occurs when edema fluid that has accumulated during the day is reabsorbed into the circulation at night, causing fluid overload and pulmonary congestion. Severe heart failure may cause dyspnea at rest as well as with activity, signifying little or no cardiac reserve. Both an $S_3$ and an $S_4$ gallop may be heard on auscultation.

The compensatory mechanisms initiated in heart failure can lead to complications in other body systems. Congestive hepatomegaly and splenomegaly caused by engorgement of the portal venous system results in increased abdominal pressure, ascites, and gastrointestinal problems. With prolonged right-sided heart failure, liver function may be impaired. Myocardial distention can precipitate dysrhythmias, futher impairing cardiac output. Pleural effusions and other pulmonary problems may develop. Major complications of severe heart failure are cardiogenic shock (described in Chapter 6) 🔗 and acute pulmonary edema, a medical emergency described in the next section of this chapter.

See page 875 for the *Multisystem Effects of Heart Failure.*

### COLLABORATIVE CARE

The main goals for care of heart failure are to slow its progression, reduce cardiac workload, improve cardiac function, and control fluid retention. Treatment strategies are based on the evolution and progression of heart failure (Table 30–3).

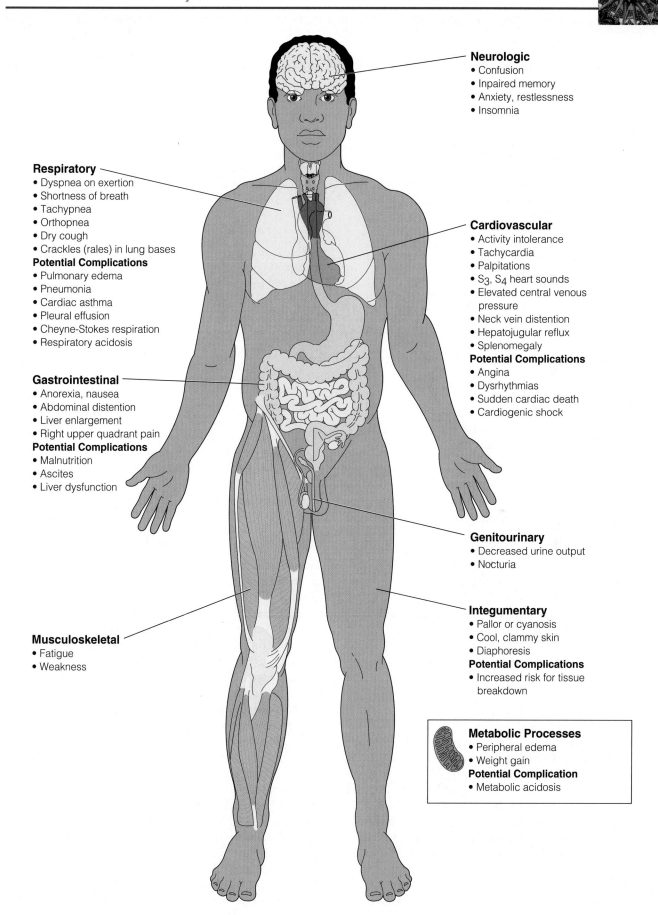

**Neurologic**
- Confusion
- Inpaired memory
- Anxiety, restlessness
- Insomnia

**Respiratory**
- Dyspnea on exertion
- Shortness of breath
- Tachypnea
- Orthopnea
- Dry cough
- Crackles (rales) in lung bases

**Potential Complications**
- Pulmonary edema
- Pneumonia
- Cardiac asthma
- Pleural effusion
- Cheyne-Stokes respiration
- Respiratory acidosis

**Cardiovascular**
- Activity intolerance
- Tachycardia
- Palpitations
- $S_3$, $S_4$ heart sounds
- Elevated central venous pressure
- Neck vein distention
- Hepatojugular reflux
- Splenomegaly

**Potential Complications**
- Angina
- Dysrhythmias
- Sudden cardiac death
- Cardiogenic shock

**Gastrointestinal**
- Anorexia, nausea
- Abdominal distention
- Liver enlargement
- Right upper quadrant pain

**Potential Complications**
- Malnutrition
- Ascites
- Liver dysfunction

**Genitourinary**
- Decreased urine output
- Nocturia

**Integumentary**
- Pallor or cyanosis
- Cool, clammy skin
- Diaphoresis

**Potential Complications**
- Increased risk for tissue breakdown

**Musculoskeletal**
- Fatigue
- Weakness

**Metabolic Processes**
- Peripheral edema
- Weight gain

**Potential Complication**
- Metabolic acidosis

| TABLE 30–3 | Stages of Heart Failure | |
|---|---|---|
| Stage | Description | Selected Treatment Measures |
| A | Clients at high risk for developing heart failure, but without identified structural or functional impairment | Treat underlying risk factors (e.g., hypertension, CHD) ACE inhibitor therapy Exercise Salt restriction |
| B | Clients with structural heart disease but no manifestations of heart failure | As for stage A ACE inhibitor or beta-blocker therapy Valve replacement if indicated |
| C | Clients with current or prior symptoms of heart failure associated with underlying structural heart disease | As for stages A and B Drug therapy with a diuretic, ACE inhibitor, beta blocker, and (usually) digitalis |
| D | Clients with advanced structural heart disease and manifestations of heart failure at rest despite aggressive treatment (end-stage heart failure) | As for stages A, B, and C as appropriate Hemodynamic monitoring Infusion of positive inotropic agents Valve replacement, cardiac transplant, partial left ventriculectomy as indicated |

*Note. Adapted from "ACC/AHA Guidelines for the Evaluation and Management of Chronic Heart Failure in the Adult: Executive Summary: A Report of the American College of Cardiology/American Heart Association Task Force on Practice Guidelines (Committee to Revise the 1995 Guidelines) for the Evaluation and Management of Heart Failure" by S. A. Hunt, D. W. Baker, M. H. Chin, M. P. Ciquegrani, A. M. Feldman, G. S. Francis, T. G. Ganiats, S. Goldstein, G. Gregoratos, M. L. Jessup, R. J. Noble, M. Packer, M. A. Silver, and L. W. Stevenson, 2001 Circulation, 104, pp. 2996–3007.*

## Diagnostic Tests

Diagnosis of heart failure is based on the history, physical examination, and diagnostic findings.

- *Atrial natriuretic factor (ANF),* also called *atrial natriuretic hormone (ANH),* and *B-type natriuretic peptide (BNP)* are hormones released by the heart muscle in response to changes in blood volume. Blood levels of these hormones increase in heart failure.
- *Serum electrolytes* are measured to evaluate fluid and electrolyte status. Serum osmolarity may be low due to fluid retention. Sodium, potassium, and chloride levels provide a baseline for evaluating the effects of treatment.
- *Urinalysis, blood urea nitrogen (BUN),* and *serum creatinine* are obtained to evaluate renal function.
- *Liver function tests* including ALT, AST, LDH, serum bilirubin, and total protein and albumin levels, are obtained to evaluate possible effects of heart failure on liver function.
- In acute heart failure, *arterial blood gases (ABGs)* are drawn to evaluate gas exchange in the lungs and tissues.
- *Chest X-ray* may show pulmonary vascular congestion and cardiomegaly in heart failure.
- *Electrocardiography* is used to identify ECG changes associated with ventricular enlargement and to detect dysrhythmias, myocardial ischemia, or infarction.
- *Echocardiography with Doppler flow studies* are performed to evaluate left ventricular function. Echocardiography uses ultrasound waves reflected off cardiac structures to produce images of the heart. The transducer which generates and receives the reflected waves may be placed on the chest wall (*transthoracic echocardiography*). For more accurate evaluation of the posterior surface of the heart, the transducer may

be on the distal end of an endoscope inserted into the esophagus (*transesophageal echocardiography*). Doppler flow studies use ultrasound waves reflecting off red blood cells to measure the velocity of blood flow across valves, within cardiac chambers, and through the great vessels.
- *Radionuclide imaging* is used to evaluate ventricular function and size (see Chapter 29).

## Hemodynamic Monitoring

**Hemodynamics** is the study of forces involved in blood circulation. Hemodynamic monitoring is used to assess cardiovascular function in the critically ill or unstable client. The main goals of invasive hemodynamic monitoring are to evaluate cardiac and circulatory function and the response to interventions.

Hemodynamic parameters include heart rate, arterial blood pressure, central venous pressure, pulmonary pressures, and cardiac output. *Direct* hemodynamic parameters are obtained straight from the monitoring device (e.g., heart rate, arterial and venous pressures). *Indirect* or *derived* measurements are calculated using the direct data (e.g., the cardiac index, mean arterial blood pressure [MAP], and stroke volume). Invasive hemodynamic monitoring is routinely used in critical care units.

Hemodynamic monitoring systems measure the pressure within a vessel and convert this signal into an electrical waveform that is amplified and displayed. The electrical signal may be graphically recorded on graph paper and displayed digitally on the monitor. System components include an invasive catheter threaded into an artery or vein connected to a transducer by stiff, high-pressure tubing. The pressure transducer translates pressures into an electrical signal that is relayed to the monitor. Additional components of the system include

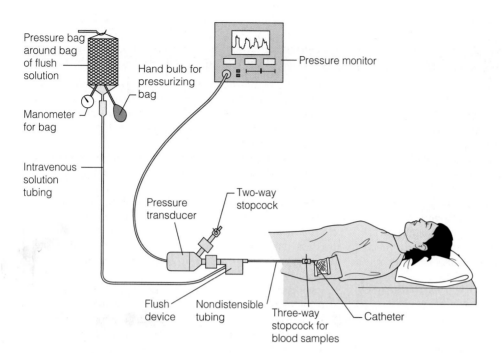

**Figure 30–3** ■ A hemodynamic monitoring setup.

stopcocks and a continuous flush system with normal saline or heparinized saline and an infusion pressure bag to prevent clots from forming in the catheter. Figure 30–3 ■ illustrates a pressure transducer and typical hemodynamic monitoring system.

Hemodynamic pressure monitoring may be used to measure peripheral arterial pressures, or central pressures, such as central venous pressure (CVP) and pulmonary artery pressure (PAP). Although the information obtained from invasive monitoring is valuable, the procedure is not without risk. Nursing care of the client undergoing hemodynamic monitoring is outlined on page 878. Box 30–2 lists potential complications of central pressure monitoring.

### Intra-Arterial Pressure Monitoring

Intra-arterial pressure monitoring is commonly used in intensive and coronary care units. An indwelling arterial line, commonly called an *art line* or an *A line*, allows direct and continuous monitoring of systolic, diastolic, and mean arterial blood pressure and provides easy access for arterial blood sampling. Arterial lines are used to assess blood volume, monitor the effects of vasoactive drugs, and to obtain frequent arterial blood gas determinations. Because the invasive catheter is inserted directly into the artery, it offers immediate access for blood gas measurements and blood testing.

| BOX 30–2 ■ Potential Complications of Central Catheters | |
| --- | --- |
| ■ Bleeding | ■ Venospasm |
| ■ Hematoma | ■ Infection |
| ■ Pneumothorax | ■ Air embolism |
| ■ Hemothorax | ■ Thromboembolism |
| ■ Arterial puncture | ■ Brachial nerve injury |
| ■ Dysrhythmias | ■ Thoracic duct injury |

The arterial blood pressure reflects the cardiac output and the resistance to blood flow created by the elastic arterial walls (*systemic vascular resistance, SVR*). Cardiac output is determined by the blood volume and the ability of the ventricles to fill and effectively pump that blood. Systemic vascular resistance is primarily determined by vessel diameter and distensibility (compliance). Factors such as sympathetic nervous system input, circulating hormones (e.g., epinephrine, norepinephrine, atrial natiuretic factor, and vasopressin), and the renin-angiotensin system affect SVR.

The systolic blood pressure, normally about 120 mmHg in healthy adults, reflects the pressure generated during ventricular systole. During diastole, elastic arterial walls keep a minimum pressure within the vessel (diastolic blood pressure) to maintain blood flow through the capillary beds. The average diastolic pressure in a healthy adult is 80 mmHg. The **mean arterial pressure (MAP)** is the average pressure in the arterial circulation throughout the cardiac cycle. It reflects the driving pressure, or perfusion pressure, an indicator of tissue perfusion. The formula MAP = CO × SVR often is used to show the relationships between factors determining the blood pressure. Mean arterial pressures of 70 to 90 mmHg are desirable. Perfusion to vital organs is severely jeopardized at MAPs of 50 or less; MAPs greater than 105 mmHg may indicate hypertension or vasoconstriction.

### Central Venous Pressure Monitoring

*Central venous pressure (CVP)* is a measure of blood volume and venous return. CVP also reflects right heart filling pressures. It is elevated in right-sided heart failure. CVP is primarily used to monitor fluid volume status. To measure CVP, a catheter is inserted in the internal jugular or subclavian vein. The distal tip of the catheter is positioned in the superior vena cava just above the right atrium. CVP may be measured in either centimeters of water (cm $H_2O$) or in millimeters of mercury

## NURSING CARE OF THE CLIENT UNDERGOING HEMODYNAMIC MONITORING

- Calibrate and level the system at least once a shift using the right atrium as a constant reference level. Relevel the transducer after a change in position. Mark the right atrial position (at the fourth intercostal space, midaxillary line) on the chest wall, and use this as a reference point for all readings. *Calibration and leveling ensure that accurate pressures are recorded. Marking the right atrial level provides a consistent reference point for all caregivers.*
- Measure all pressures between breaths. *This ensures that intrathoracic pressure does not influence pressure readings.*
- Maintain 300 mmHg of pressure on the flush solution at all times. *This ensures a continuous flow of flush solution through the pressure tubing and catheter to prevent clot formation and catheter occlusion.*
- Monitor pressure trends rather than individual readings. *Individual readings may not reflect the client's true status. Trends in pressure readings along with clinical observations provide a better overall picture of the client's status.*
- Obtain a chest X-ray before infusing intravenous fluid into any newly placed central line. *Chest X-ray verifies the location of the catheter and helps prevent pulmonary complications of incorrect catheter placement such as pneumothorax.*
- Set alarm limits for monitored hemodynamic variables. Turn alarms on. *Alarms warn of hemodynamic instability. Always investigate alarms. They may be temporarily silenced to change tubing or draw blood but should never be turned off.*
- Use aseptic technique during catheter insertion and site care. *Aseptic technique is important to prevent infection.*

- Assess and document appearance of the insertion site at least every shift; observe for signs of infiltration, infection, or phlebitis. *Frequent assessment allows early detection and prompt treatment of complications.*
- Change intravenous solutions every 24 hours, site dressing every 48 hours, and tubing to the insertion site every 72 hours. Label solution, tubing, and dressing with date and time of change. *These measures help prevent infection.*
- Thoroughly flush stopcock ports after drawing blood samples from the pressure line. *Flushing prevents colonization of bacteria and occlusion of the catheter.*
- Assess pulse and perfusion distal to the monitoring site. *Frequent assessment is vital to ensure perfusion of the distal extremity.*
- When discontinuing the pressure line, apply manual pressure to the insertion site as soon as the catheter tip is out. Hold pressure for 5 to 15 minutes or until the bleeding stops. *This is particularly important for arterial lines to prevent bleeding and hematoma formation.*
- Secure all connections and stopcocks. *This is done to prevent disconnection of the invasive line and potential hemorrhage.*
- Ensure that electrical equipment is grounded, intact, and operating as expected. *This helps prevent electrical injury.*
- Loosely restrain the affected extremity if the client pulls on the catheter or connections. *Restraints may be necessary to prevent injury from accidental or intentional disconnection or discontinuation of invasive lines (i.e., if the client has dementia or is agitated).*
- Keep tubing free of kinks and tension. *This prevents the catheter from becoming clotted or inadvertently dislodged.*

---

(mmHg). A water manometer is a clear tube with calibrated markings that is attached between a central catheter and the intravenous fluid bag. Pressure in the venous system causes fluid in the manometer to rise or fall. The CVP is recorded by noting the fluid level in the manometer. If the central line is connected to a pressure transducer, venous pressure is displayed digitally in millimeters of mercury.

The normal range for CVP is 2 to 8 cm $H_2O$ or 2 to 6 mmHg, but CVP varies in individual clients. Hypovolemia and shock decrease the CVP; fluid overload, vasoconstriction, and cardiac tamponade increase CVP.

### Pulmonary Artery Pressure Monitoring

The pulmonary artery (PA) catheter is a flow-directed, balloon-tipped catheter first used in the early 1970s. The PA catheter is often called a *Swan-Ganz catheter,* after the physicians who developed it. The PA catheter is used to evaluate left ventricular and overall cardiac function. The PA catheter is inserted into a central vein, usually the internal jugular or subclavian vein, and threaded into the right atrium. A small balloon at the tip of the catheter allows the catheter to be drawn into the right ventricle and from there into the pulmonary artery. The inflated balloon carries the catheter forward until the balloon wedges in a small branch of pulmonary vasculature. Once in place, the balloon is deflated, and multiple lumens of the

catheter allow measurement of pressures in the right atrium, pulmonary artery, and left ventricle. The normal PA pressure is around 25/10 mmHg; normal mean pulmonary artery pressure is about 15 mmHg. Pulmonary artery pressure is increased in left-sided heart failure.

Inflation of the balloon effectively blocks pressure from behind the balloon and allows measurement of pressures generated by the left ventricle. This is known as pulmonary artery wedge pressure (PAWP or PWP) and is used to assess left ventricular function. The normal pulmonary artery wedge pressure is 8 to 12 mmHg. PAWP is increased in left ventricular failure and pericardial tamponade, and decreased in hypovolemia.

Cardiac output also can be measured with the PA catheter using a technique called thermodilution. Cardiac output and the cardiac index are used to assess the heart's ability to meet the body's oxygen demands. Because body size affects overall cardiac output, the cardiac index is a more precise measure of heart function. The *cardiac index* is a calculation of cardiac output per square meter of body surface area. The normal cardiac index is 2.8 to 4.2 L/min/m².

### Medications

Clients with heart failure often receive multiple medications to reduce cardiac work and improve cardiac function. The

main drug classes used to treat heart failure are the angiotensin-converting enzyme (ACE) inhibitors, beta blockers, diuretics, inotropic medications (including digitalis, sympathomimetic agents, and phosphodiesterase inhibitors), direct vasodilators, and antidysrhythmic drugs. Nursing implications for ACE inhibitors, diuretics, and inotropic medications are found in the Medication Administration box below.

ACE inhibitors and beta blockers interfere with the neurohormonal mechanisms of sympathetic activation and the renin-angiotensin system. ACE inhibitors interrupt the conversion of angiotensin I to angiotensin II by inhibiting the enzyme that mediates the conversion (angiotensin-converting enzyme). Angiotensin II causes intense vasoconstriction, increasing afterload and ventricular wall stress and increasing preload and ventricular dilation. It also stimulates aldosterone and ADH production, causing fluid retention. ACE inhibitors block this renin-angiotensin system activity, decreasing cardiac work and increasing cardiac output. They reduce the progression and manifestations of heart failure, thus reducing the number and frequency of hospital admissions, decreasing mortality rates, and preventing cardiac complications (Braunwald et al., 2001).

## Medication Administration

### Heart Failure

#### ANGIOTENSIN-CONVERTING ENZYME (ACE) INHIBITORS

Enalapril (Vasotec)          Lisinopril (Prinivil, Zestril)
Captopril (Capoten)          Fosinopril (Monopril)
Moexipril (Univasc)          Quinapril (Accupril)
Ramipril (Altace)            Trandolapril (Mavik)

ACE inhibitors prevent acute coronary events and reduce mortality in heart failure. ACE inhibitors interfere with production of angiotensin II, resulting in vasodilation, reduced blood volume, and prevention of its effects in the heart and blood vessels. In heart failure, ACE inhibitors reduce afterload and improve cardiac output and renal blood flow. They also reduce pulmonary congestion and peripheral edema. ACE inhibitors suppress myocyte growth and reduce ventricular remodeling in heart failure.

##### Nursing Responsibilities
- Do not give these drugs to women in the second and third trimesters of pregnancy.
- Carefully monitor clients who are volume depleted or who have impaired renal function.
- Use an infusion pump when administering ACE inhibitors intravenously.
- Monitor blood pressure closely for 2 hours following first dose and as indicated thereafter.
- Monitor serum potassium levels; ACE inhibitors can cause hyperkalemia.
- Monitor white blood cell (WBC) count for potential neutropenia. Report to the physician.

##### Client and Family Teaching
- Take the drug at the same time every day to ensure a stable blood level.
- Monitor your blood pressure and weight weekly. Report significant changes to your doctor.
- Avoid making sudden position changes; for example, rise from bed slowly. Lie down if you become dizzy or lightheaded, particularly after the first dose.
- Report any signs of easy bruising and bleeding, sore throat or fever, edema, or skin rash. Immediately report swelling of the face, lips, or eyelids, and itching or breathing problems.
- A persistent, dry cough may develop. Contact your doctor if this becomes a problem.
- Take captopril or moexipril 1 hour before meals.

#### DIURETICS

Chlorothiazide (Diuril)             Spironolactone (Aldactone)
Furosemide (Lasix)                  Triamterene (Dyrenium)
Ethacrynic acid (Edecrin)           Amiloride (Midamor)
Bumetanide (Bumex)                  Acetazolamide (Diamox)
Hydrochlorothiazide (HydroDIURIL)

Diuretics act on different portions of the kidney tubule to inhibit the reabsorption of sodium and water and promote their excretion. With the exception of the potassium-sparing diuretics—spironolactone, triamterene, and amiloride—diuretics also promote potassium excretion, increasing the risk of hypokalemia. Spironolactone, an aldosterone receptor blocker, reduces symptoms and slows progression of heart failure. Aldosterone receptors in the heart and blood vessels promote myocardial remodeling and fibrosis, activate the sympathetic nervous system, and promote vascular fibrosis (which decreases compliance) and baroreceptor dysfunction (Lehne, 2001).

##### Nursing Responsibilities
- Obtain baseline weight and vital signs.
- Monitor blood pressure, intake and output, weight, skin turgor, and edema as indicators of fluid volume status.
- Assess for volume depletion, particularly with loop diuretics (furosemide, ethacrynic acid, and bumetanide): dizziness, orthostatic hypotension, tachycardia, muscle cramping.
- Report abnormal serum electrolyte levels to the physician. Replace electrolytes as indicated.
- Do not administer potassium replacements to clients receiving a potassium-sparing diuretic.
- Evaluate renal function by assessing urine output, BUN, and serum creatinine.
- Administer intravenous furosemide slowly, no faster than 20 mg/minute. Evaluate for signs of ototoxicity. Do not administer this drug or ethacrynic acid concurrently with aminoglycoside antibiotics (e.g., gentamycin) which are also ototoxic.

##### Client and Family Teaching
- Drink at least 6 to 8 glasses of water per day.
- Take your diuretic at times that will be the least disruptive to your lifestyle, usually in the morning and early afternoon if a second dose is ordered. Take with meals to decrease gastric upset.

*(continued on page 880)*

## Medication Administration

### Heart Failure (continued)

- Monitor your blood pressure, pulse, and weight weekly. Report significant weight changes to your doctor.
- Report any of the following to your doctor: severe abdominal pain, jaundice, dark urine, abnormal bleeding or bruising, flulike symptoms, signs of hypokalemia, hyponatremia, and dehydration (thirst, salt craving, dizziness, weakness, rapid pulse). See Chapter 5 ⊖⊃ for manifestations of electrolyte imbalances.
- Avoid sudden position changes. You may experience dizziness, lightheadedness, or feelings of faintness.
- Unless you are taking a potassium-sparing diuretic, integrate foods rich in potassium into your diet (see Chapter 5 ). ⊖⊃ Limit sodium use.

### POSITIVE INOTROPIC AGENTS

#### Digitalis Glycosides

Digoxin (Lanoxin)

Digitalis improves myocardial contractility by interfering with ATPase in the myocardial cell membrane and increasing the amount of calcium available for contraction. The increased force of contraction causes the heart to empty more completely, increasing stroke volume and cardiac output. Improved cardiac output improves renal perfusion, decreasing renin secretion. This decreases preload and afterload, reducing cardiac work. Digitalis also has electrophysiologic effects, slowing conduction through the AV node. This decreases the heart rate and reduces oxygen consumption.

#### Nursing Responsibilities

- Assess apical pulse before administering. Withhold digitalis and notify the physician if heart rate is below 60 BPM and/or manifestations of decreased cardiac output are noted. Record apical rate on medication record.
- Evaluate ECG for scooped (spoon-shaped) ST segment, AV block, bradycardia, and other dysrhythmias (especially PVCs and atrial tachycardias).
- Report manifestations of digitalis toxicity: anorexia, nausea, vomiting, abdominal pain, weakness, vision changes (diplopia, blurred vision, yellow-green or white halos seen around objects), and new-onset dysrhythmias.
- Assess potassium, magnesium, calcium, and serum digoxin levels before giving digitalis. Hypokalemia can precipitate toxicity even when the serum digitalis level is in the "normal" range.
- Monitor clients with renal insufficiency or renal failure and older adults carefully for digitalis toxicity.
- Prepare to administer digoxin immune fab (Digibind) for digoxin toxicity.

#### Client and Family Teaching

- Take your pulse daily before taking your digoxin. Do not take the digoxin if your pulse is below 60 or if you are weak, fatigued, lightheadeded, dizzy, short of breath, or having chest pain. Notify your physician immediately.
- Contact your doctor if you develop manifestations of digitalis toxicity: palpitations, weakness, loss of appetite, nausea, vomiting, abdominal pain, blurred or colored vision, double vision.
- Avoid using antacids and laxatives; they decrease digoxin absorption.
- Notify your physician immediately if you develop manifestations of potassium deficiency: weakness, lethargy, thirst, depression, muscle cramps, or vomiting.
- Incorporate foods high in potassium into your diet: fresh orange or tomato juice, bananas, raisins, dates, figs, prunes, apricots, spinach, cauliflower, and potatoes.

### Sympathomimetic Agents

Dopamine (Inotropin)          Dobutamine (Dobutrex)

Sympathomimetic agents stimulate the heart, improving the force of contraction. Dobutamine is preferred in managing heart failure because it does not increase the heart rate as much as dopamine, and it has a mild vasodilatory effect. These drugs are given by intravenous infusion and may be titrated to obtain their optimal effects.

### Phosphodiesterase Inhibitors

Amrinone (Inocor)          Milrinone (Primacor)

Phosphodiesterase inhibitors are used in treating acute heart failure to increase myocardial contractility and cause vasodilation. The net effects are an increase in cardiac output and a decrease in afterload.

### Nursing Responsibilities

- Use an infusion pump to administer these agents. Monitor hemodynamic parameters carefully.
- Avoid discontinuing these drugs abruptly.
- Change solutions and tubing every 24 hours.
- Amrinone is given as an intravenous bolus over 2 to 3 minutes, followed by an infusion of 5 to 10 mg/kg/min.
- Amrinone may be infused full strength or diluted in normal saline or half-strength saline. Do not mix this drug with dextrose solutions. After dilution, amrinone can be piggybacked into a line containing a dextrose solution.
- Monitor liver function and platelet counts; amrinone may cause hepatotoxicity and thrombocytopenia.

### Client and Family Teaching

- Notify the nursing staff if you experience abdominal pain or notice a skin rash or bruising.

Beta blockers improve cardiac function in heart failure by inhibiting SNS activity. This prevents the long-term deleterious effects of sympathetic stimulation. Because beta blockers reduce the force of myocardial contraction and may actually worsen symptoms, they are used in low doses. The combination of ACE inhibitors and beta blockers improves client outcomes. Beta blockers are discussed on page 818.

Clients with symptomatic heart failure often are treated with diuretics as well. Diuretics relieve symptoms related to fluid retention. They may, however, cause significant electrolyte imbalances and rapid fluid loss. Clients with severe heart failure are often treated with a loop, or high-ceiling, diuretic such as furosemide (Lasix), bumetanide (Bumex), torsemide (Demadex), or ethacrynic acid (Edecrin). These drugs have a

rapid onset of action, inhibiting chloride reabsorption in the ascending loop of Henle, prompting sodium and water excretion. Their major drawback is their efficacy in promoting diuresis; loss of vascular volume can stimulate the SNS. Thiazide diuretics may be used for clients with less severe manifestations of heart failure. These agents promote fluid excretion by blocking sodium reabsorption in the terminal loop of Henle and the distal tubule.

Vasodilators relax smooth muscle in blood vessels, causing dilation. Arterial dilation reduces peripheral vascular resistance and afterload, reducing myocardial work. Venous dilation reduces venous return and preload. Pulmonary vascular relaxation reduces pulmonary capillary pressure, allowing reabsorption of fluid from interstitial tissues and the alveoli. Vasodilators include nitrates, hydralazine, and prazosin, an alpha-adrenergic blocker. See Chapter 33 ⟨⟩ for more information about vasodilators.

Nitrates produce both arterial and venous vasodilation. They may be given by nasal spray or the sublingual, oral, or intravenous route. Sodium nitroprusside is a potent vasodilator that may be used to treat acute heart failure. It can cause excessive hypotension, so is often given along with dopamine or dobutamine to maintain the blood pressure. Isosorbide or nitroglycerin ointment may be used in long-term management of heart failure. See page 818.

Digitalis glycosides are used judiciously in symptomatic heart failure. Digitalis has a *positive inotropic effect* on the heart, increasing the strength of myocardial contraction by increasing the intracellular calcium concentrations. Digitalis also decreases SA node automaticity and slows conduction through the AV node, increasing ventricular filling time.

Digitalis has a narrow therapeutic index; in other words, therapeutic levels are very close to toxic levels. Early manifestations of digitalis toxicity include anorexia, nausea and vomiting, headache, altered vision, and confusion. A number of cardiac dysrhythmias are also associated with digitalis toxicity, including sinus arrest, supraventricular and ventricular tachycardias, and high levels of AV block. Low serum potassium levels increase the risk of digitalis toxicity, as do low magnesium and high calcium levels. Older adults are at particular risk for digitalis toxicity.

Digitalis levels may be affected by a number of other drugs; check for potential interactions.

Dysrhythmias are common in clients with heart failure. Although PVCs are may be frequent, they are often not associated with an increased risk of ventricular tachycardia and fibrillation. Because many antidysrhythmic medications depress left ventricular function, PVCs are frequently left untreated in heart failure. Amiodarone is the drug of choice to treat nonsustained ventricular tachycardia, which is associated with a poor prognosis. See page 854.

## Diet and Activity

A sodium-restricted diet is recommended to minimize sodium and water retention. Intake is generally limited to 1.5 to 2 g of sodium per day, a moderate restriction. Box 5–4 lists high-sodium foods to avoid; Box 5–5 includes client teaching regarding sodium-restricted diet. Activity may be restricted to bed rest during acute episodes of heart failure to reduce cardiac workload and allow the heart to recompensate. Prolonged bed rest and continued activity limitations, however, are not recommended. A moderate, progressive activity program is prescribed to improve myocardial function.

## Other Treatments

In end-stage heart failure, devices to provide circulatory assistance or surgery may be required. Surgery may be used to treat the underlying cause of failure (e.g., replacement of diseased valves) or to improve quality of life. Valve replacement is discussed later in this chapter. Heart transplant is currently the only clearly effective surgical treatment for end-stage heart failure; its use is limited by the availability of donor hearts.

### Circulatory Assistance

Devices such as the intra-aortic balloon pump or a left-ventricular assist device may be used when the client is expected to recover or as a bridge to transplant. (see Chapter 29). Newer devices that will allow longer term support outside the hospital are in the developmental stages. These devices will serve either as a bridge to transplant or allow the myocardium to heal over an extended period of time.

### Cardiac Transplantation

Heart transplant is the treatment of choice for end-stage heart disease. Survival rates are good: 85% at 1 year and 70% at 5 years (Braunwald et al., 2001). The most frequently used transplant procedure leaves posterior walls of the atria, the superior and inferior vena cavae, and pulmonary veins of the recipient intact (Figure 30–4A ■). The atrial walls of the donor heart are then anatomosed to the recipient's atria (Figure 30–4B). The donor pulmonary artery and aorta are anatomosed to the recipient vessels (Figure 30–4C). Care is taken to avoid damaging the sinus node of the donor heart. Donor organs typically are obtained from young accident victims with no evidence of cardiac trauma.

Nursing care of the heart transplant client is similar to care of any cardiac surgery client (see page 823). Infection and rejection are major postoperative concerns; these are the chief causes of mortality in transplant clients. Immunosuppressive drugs are given to prevent rejection of the transplanted organ, even when the tissue match is good (see Chapter 9). ⟨⟩ Although immunosuppressive medications help prevent organ rejection, they impair the client's defenses against infection. The donor heart is also denervated during the transplant procedure. Lack of innervation by the autonomic nervous system affects its response to position changes, stress, exercise, and certain drugs.

### Other Procedures

Other surgical procedures such as cardiomyoplasty and ventricular reduction surgery do not improve the prognosis or quality of life in clients with end-stage heart failure. *Cardiomyoplasty* involves wrapping the latissimus dorsi muscle around the heart to support the failing myocardium. The muscle is stimulated in synchrony with the heart, providing a more

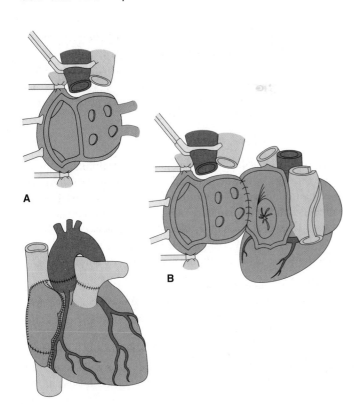

**Figure 30–4** ■ Cardiac transplantation. *A*, The heart is removed, leaving the posterior walls of the atria intact. The donor heart is anastomosed to the atria, *B*, and the great vessels, *C*.

forceful contraction and increasing cardiac output. In ventricular reduction surgery (or *partial ventriculectomy*), a portion of the anteriolateral left ventricular wall is resected to improve cardiac function (Tierney et al., 2001).

## Complementary Therapies

Strong evidence supports the use of several complementary therapies for heart failure. Hawthorn, a shrubby tree, contains natural cardiotonic ingredients in its blossoms, leaves, and fruit. It increases the force of myocardial contraction, dilates blood vessels, and has a natural ACE inhibitor. Hawthorn should never be used without consulting an experienced herb practitioner and advising the physician (Fontaine, 2000). Nutritional supplements of coenzyme Q10, magnesium, and thiamine may be used in conjunction with other treatments. Coenzyme Q10 improves mitochrondria function and energy production. Researchers in Japan linked lower levels of coenzyme Q10 with a higher mortality rate in clients with heart failure (Kuhn, 1999).

## End of Life Care

Unless a cardiac transplant is performed, chronic heart failure is ultimately a terminal disease. The client and family need honest discussions about the anticipated course of the disease and treatment options. It is important to discuss advance directives such as the living will and medical power of attorney, differentiating potential acute events from which recovery would be anticipated (e.g., reversible exacerbation of heart failure,

sudden cardiac arrest) from prolonged life support without reasonable expectation of functional recovery. Hospice services are available for clients with heart failure, and should be offered when appropriate. Severe dyspnea is common in the final stages of the disease. It may be managed with narcotic analgesics or with frequent intravenous diuretics and continuous infusion of a positive inotropic agent (Hunt et al., 2001).

## NURSING CARE

### Health Promotion

Health promotion activities to reduce the risk for and incidence of heart failure are directed at the risk factors. Teach clients about coronary heart disease, the primary underlying cause of heart failure. Discuss CHD risk factors, and ways to reduce those risk factors (see Chapter 29).

Hypertension also is a major cause of heart failure. Routinely screen clients for elevated blood pressure, and refer clients to a primary care provider as indicated. Discuss the importance of effectively managing hypertension to reduce the future risk for heart failure. Likewise, stress the relationship between effective diabetes management and reduced risk of heart failure.

### Assessment

Obtain both subjective and objective data when assessing the client with heart failure.

- Health history: complaints of increasing shortness of breath, dyspnea with exertion, decreasing activity tolerance, or paroxysmal nocturnal dyspnea; number of pillows used for sleeping; recent weight gain; presence of a cough; chest or abdominal pain; anorexia or nausea; history of cardiac disease, previous episodes of heart failure; other risk factors such as hypertension or diabetes; current medications; usual diet and activity and recent changes
- Physical examination: general appearance; ease of breathing, conversing, changing positions; apparent anxiety; vital signs including apical pulse; color of skin and mucous membranes; neck vein distension, peripheral pulses, capillary refill, presence and degree of edema; heart and breath sounds; abdominal contour, bowel sounds, tenderness; right upper abdominal tenderness, liver enlargement

### Nursing Diagnoses and Interventions

Heart failure impacts quality of life, interfering with such daily activities as self-care and role performance. Reducing the oxygen demand of the heart is a major nursing care goal for the client in acute heart failure. This includes providing rest and carrying out prescribed treatment measures to reduce cardiac work, improve contractility, and manage symptoms.

#### Decreased Cardiac Output

As the heart fails as a pump, stroke volume and tissue perfusion decrease.

- Monitor vital signs and oxygen saturation as indicated. *Decreased cardiac output stimulates the SNS to increase*

the heart rate in an attempt to restore CO. Tachycardia at rest is common. Diastolic blood pressure may initially be elevated because of vasoconstriction; in late stages, compensatory mechanisms fail, and BP falls. Oxygen saturation levels provide a measure of gas exchange and tissue perfusion.

- Auscultate heart and breath sounds regularly. $S_1$ and $S_2$ may be diminished if cardiac function is poor. A ventricular gallop ($S_3$) is an early sign of heart failure; atrial gallop ($S_4$) may also be present. Crackles are often heard in the lung bases; increasing crackles, dyspnea, and shortness of breath indicate worsening failure.

**PRACTICE ALERT** *Report manifestations of decreased cardiac output and tissue perfusion: changes in mentation; decreased urine output; cool, clammy skin; diminished pulses; pallor or cyanosis; dysrhythmias. These are manifestations of decreased tissue perfusion to organ systems. ■*

- Administer supplemental oxygen as needed. *This improves oxygenation of the blood, decreasing the effects of hypoxia and ischemia.*
- Administer prescribed medications as ordered. *Drugs are used to decrease the cardiac workload and increase the effectiveness of contractions.*
- Encourage rest, explaining the rationale. Elevate the head of the bed to reduce the work of breathing. Provide a bedside commode, and assist with ADLs. Instruct to avoid the Valsalva maneuver. *These measures reduce cardiac workload.*

**PRACTICE ALERT** *Promote psychologic rest and decrease anxiety. Maintain a quiet environment, encourage expression of fears and feelings. Explain care measures and their purpose. Psychologic rest decreases oxygen consumption and improves cardiac function. ■*

## Excess Fluid Volume

As cardiac output falls, compensatory mechanisms cause salt and water retention, increasing blood volume. This increased fluid volume places additional stress on the already failing ventricles, making them work harder to move the fluid load.

- Assess respiratory status and auscultate lung sounds at least every 4 hours. Notify the physician of significant changes in condition. *Declining respiratory status indicates worsening left heart failure.*

**PRACTICE ALERT** *Immediately notify the physician if the client develops air hunger, an overwhelming sense of impending doom or panic, tachypnea, severe orthopnea, or a cough productive of large amounts of pink, frothy sputum. Acute pulmonary edema, a medical emergency, can develop rapidly, necessitating immediate intervention to preserve life. ■*

- Monitor intake and output. Notify the physician if urine output is less than 30 mL/h. Weigh daily. *Careful monitoring of fluid volume is important during treatment of heart failure. Diuretics may reduce circulating volume, producing hypovolemia despite persistent peripheral edema. A fall in urine output may indicate significantly reduced cardiac output and renal ischemia. Weight is an objective measure of fluid status: 1 L of fluid is equal to 2.2 lb of weight.*
- Record abdominal girth every shift. Note complaints of a loss of appetite, abdominal discomfort, or nausea. *Venous congestion can lead to ascites and may affect gastrointestinal function and nutritional status.*
- Monitor and record hemodynamic measurements. Report significant changes and negative trends. *Hemodynamic measurements provide a means of monitoring condition and response to treatment.*
- Restrict fluids as ordered. Allow choices of fluid type and timing of intake, scheduling most fluid intake during morning and afternoon hours. Offer ice chips and frequent mouth care; provide hard candies if allowed. *Providing choices increases the client's sense of control. Ice chips, hard candies, and mouth care relieve dry mouth and thirst and promote comfort.*

## Activity Intolerance

Clients with heart failure have little or no cardiac reserve to meet increased oxygen demands. As the disease progresses and cardiac function is further compromised, activity intolerance increases. The low cardiac output and inability to participate in activities may hinder self-care.

**PRACTICE ALERT** *Monitor vital signs and cardiac rhythm during and after activities. Tachycardia, dysrhythmias, increasing dyspnea, changes in blood pressure, diaphoresis, pallor, complaints of chest pain, excessive fatigue, or palpitations indicate activity intolerance. Instruct to rest if manifestations are noted. The failing heart is unable to increase cardiac output to meet increased oxygen demands associated with activity. Assessing response to activities helps evaluate cardiac function. Decreasing activity tolerance may signal deterioration of cardiac function, not overexertion. ■*

- Organize nursing care to allow rest periods. *Grouping activities together allows adequate time to "recharge."*
- Assist with ADLs as needed. Encourage independence within prescribed limits. *Assisting with ADLs helps ensure that care needs are met while reducing cardiac workload. Involving the client promotes a sense of control and reduces helplessness.*
- Plan and implement progressive activities. Use passive and active ROM exercises as appropriate. Consult with physical therapist on activity plan. *Progressive activity slowly increases exercise capacity by strengthening and improving cardiac function without strain. Activity also helps prevent skeletal muscle atrophy. ROM exercises prevent complications of immobility in severely compromised clients.*

- Provide written and verbal information about activity after discharge. *Written information provides a reference for important information. Verbal information allows clarification and validation of the material.*

### Deficient Knowledge: Low-Sodium Diet

Diet is an important part of long-term management of heart failure to manage fluid retention.

- Discuss the rationale for sodium restrictions. *Understanding fosters compliance with the prescribed diet.*
- Consult with dietitian to plan and teach a low-sodium and, if necessary for weight control, low-kcal diet. Provide a list of high-sodium, high-fat, high-cholesterol foods to avoid. Provide American Heart Association materials. *Dietary planning and teaching increases the client's sense of control and participation in disease management. Food lists are useful memory aids.*

**PRACTICE ALERT** *Teach how to read food labels for nutritional information. Many processed foods contain "hidden" sodium, which can be identified by careful label reading.* ■

- Assist the client to construct a 2-day meal plan choosing foods low in sodium. *This allows learning assessment, clarification of misunderstandings, and reinforcement of teaching.*
- Encourage small, frequent meals rather than three heavy meals per day. *Small, frequent meals provide continuing energy resources and decrease the work required to digest a large meal.*

## Using NANDA, NIC, and NOC

Chart 30–1 shows links between NANDA nursing diagnoses, NIC, and NOC for the client with heart failure.

## Home Care

Heart failure is a chronic condition requiring active participation by the client and family for effective management. In teaching for home care, include the following topics:

- The disease process and its effects on the client's life
- Warning signals of cardiac decompensation that require treatment
- Desired and adverse effects of prescribed drugs; monitoring for effects; importance of compliance with drug regimen to prevent acute and long-term complications of heart failure
- Prescribed diet and sodium restriction; practical suggestions for reducing salt intake; recommend American Heart Association materials and recipes
- Exercise recommendations to strengthen the heart muscle and improve aerobic capacity (Box 30–3)
- The importance of keeping scheduled follow-up appointments to monitor disease progression and effects of therapy.

Provide referrals for home health care and household assistance (shopping, transportation, personal needs, and housekeeping) as indicated. Referrals to community agencies, such as local cardiac rehabilitation programs, heart support groups, or the AHA, can provide with additional materials and psychosocial support.

---

### CHART 30–1 NANDA, NIC, AND NOC LINKAGES

#### The Client with Heart Failure

| NURSING DIAGNOSES | NURSING INTERVENTIONS | NURSING OUTCOMES |
|---|---|---|
| • Activity Intolerance | • Cardiac Care: Rehabilitative<br>• Energy Management<br>• Self-Care Assistance | • Activity Tolerance<br>• Energy Conservation<br>• Self-Care: Activities of Daily Living (ADLs) |
| • Decreased Cardiac Output | • Cardiac Care: Acute<br>• Hemodynamic Regulation<br>• Vital Signs Monitoring | • Cardiac Pump Effectiveness<br>• Circulation Status<br>• Vital Signs Status |
| • Fatigue | • Activity Therapy<br>• Environmental Management<br>• Nutrition Management | • Endurance<br>• Energy Conservation<br>• Nutritional Status: Energy |
| • Excess Fluid Volume | • Fluid Management<br>• Invasive Hemodynamic Monitoring<br>• Medication Management | • Electrolyte and Acid-Base Balance<br>• Fluid Balance |
| • Ineffective Health Maintenance | • Discharge Planning<br>• Teaching: Prescribed Activity/Exercise<br>• Teaching: Prescribed Diet<br>• Decision-Making Support | • Knowledge: Health Resources<br>• Knowledge: Treatment Regimen<br>• Participation: Health Care Decisions |

*Note. Data from Nursing Outcomes Classification (NOC) by M. Johnson & M. Maas (Eds.), 1997, St. Louis: Mosby; Nursing Diagnoses: Definitions & Classifications 2001–2002 by North American Nursing Diagnosis Association, 2001, Philadelphia: NANDA; Nursing Interventions Classification (NIC) by J.C. McCloskey & G. M. Bulechek (Eds.), 2000, St. Louis: Mosby. Reprinted by permission.*

## BOX 30–3 ■ Home Activity Guidelines for the Client with Heart Failure

■ Perform as many activities as independently as you can.

■ Space your meals and activities.
  a. Eat six small meals a day.
  b. Allow time during the day for periods of rest and relaxation.

■ Perform all activities at a comfortable pace.
  a. If you get tired during any activity, stop what you are doing and rest for 15 minutes.
  b. Resume activity only if you feel up to it.

■ Stop any activity that causes chest pain, shortness of breath, dizziness, faintness, excessive weakness, or sweating. Rest. Notify your physician if your activity tolerance changes and if symptoms continue after rest.

■ Avoid straining. Do not lift heavy objects. Eat a high-fiber diet and drink plenty of water to prevent constipation. Use laxatives or stool softeners, as approved by your physician, to avoid constipation and straining during bowel movements.

■ Begin a graded exercise program. Walking is good exercise that does not require any special equipment (except a good pair of walking shoes). Plan to walk twice a day at a comfortable, slow pace for the first couple of weeks at home, and then gradually increase the distance and pace. Below is a suggested schedule—but progress at your own speed. Take your time. Aim for walking at least 3 times per week (every other day).

| | | |
|---|---|---|
| Week 1 | 200 to 400 ft (1/4 mile) | Twice a day, slow leisurely pace |
| Week 2 | 1/4 mile | 15 min, minimum of 3 times per week |
| Weeks 2 to 3 | 1/2 mile | 30 min, minimum of 3 times per week |
| Weeks 3 to 4 | 1 mile | 30 min, minimum of 3 times per week |
| Weeks 4 to 5 | 1 1/2 mile | 30 min, minimum of 3 times per week |
| Weeks 5 to 6 | 2 miles | 40 min, minimum of 3 times per week |

## Nursing Care Plan
### A Client with Heart Failure

One year ago, Arthur Jackson, 67 years old, had a large anterior wall MI and underwent subsequent coronary artery bypass surgery. On discharge, he was started on a regimen of enalapril (Vasotec), digoxin, furosemide (Lasix), coumadin, and a potassium chloride supplement. He is now in the cardiac unit complaining of severe shortness of breath, hemoptysis, and poor appetite for 1 week. He is diagnosed with acute heart failure.

### ASSESSMENT

Mr. Jackson refuses to settle in bed, preferring to sit in the bedside recliner in high Fowler's position. He states, "Lately, this is the only way I can breathe." Mr. Jackson states that he has not been able to work in his garden without getting short of breath. He complains of his shoes and belt being too tight.

When Ms. Takashi, RN, Mr. Jackson's nurse, obtains his nursing history, Mr. Jackson insists that he takes his medications regularly. He states that he normally works in his garden for light exercise. In his diet history, Mr. Jackson admits fondness for bacon and Chinese food and sheepishly admits to snacking between meals "even though I need to lose weight."

Mr. Jackson's vital signs are: BP 95/72 mmHg, HR 124 and irregular, R 28 and labored, and T 97.5°F (36.5°C). The cardiac monitor shows atrial fibrillation. An $S_3$ is noted on auscultation; the cardiac impulse is left of the midclavicular line. He has crackles and diminished breath sounds in the bases of both lungs. Significant jugular venous distention, 3+ pitting edema of feet and ankles, and abdominal distention are noted. Liver size is within normal limits by percussion. Skin cool and diaphoretic. Chest X-ray shows cardiomegaly and pulmonary infiltrates.

### DIAGNOSES

• *Excess fluid volume* related to impaired cardiac pump and salt and water retention

• *Activity intolerance* related to impaired cardiac output

• *Impaired health maintenance* related to lack of knowledge about diet restrictions

### EXPECTED OUTCOMES

• Demonstrate loss of excess fluid by weight loss and decreases in edema, jugular venous distention, and abdominal distention.

• Demonstrate improved activity tolerance.

• Verbalize understanding of diet restrictions.

### PLANNING AND IMPLEMENTATION

• Hourly vital signs and hemodynamic pressure measurements.

• Administer and monitor effects of prescribed diuretics and vasodilators.

• Weigh daily; strict intake and output.

• Enforce fluid restriction of 1500 mL/24 hours: 600 mL day shift, 600 mL evening shift, 300 mL at night.

• Auscultate heart and breath sounds every 4 hours and as indicated.

• Administer oxygen per nasal cannula at 2 L/min. Monitor oxygen satururation continuously. Notify physician if less than 94%.

• High Fowler's or position of comfort.

• Notify physician of significant changes in laboratory values.

• Teach about all medications and how to take and record pulse. Provide information about anticoagulant therapy and signs of bleeding.

• Design an activity plan with Mr. Jackson that incorporates preferred activities and scheduled rest periods.

• Instruct about sodium-restricted diet. Allow meal choices within allowed limits.

*(continued on page 886)*

## Nursing Care Plan
## A Client with Heart Failure *(continued)*

• Consult dietitian for planning and teaching Mr. and Mrs. Jackson about low-sodium diet.

### EVALUATION

Mr. Jackson is discharged after 3 days in the cardiac unit. He has lost 8 pounds during his stay and states it is much easier to breathe and his shoes fit better. He is able to sleep in semi-Fowler's position with only one pillow. His peripheral edema has resolved. Mr. and Mrs. Jackson met with the dietitian, who helped them develop a realistic eating plan to limit sodium, sugar, and fats. The dietitian also provided a list of high-sodium foods to avoid. Mr. Jackson is relieved to know that he can still enjoy Chinese food prepared without monosodium glutamate (MSG) or added salt. Ms. Takashi and the physical therapist designed a progressive activity plan with Mr. Jackson that he will continue at home. He remains in atrial fibrillation, a chronic condition. His knowledge of digoxin and coumadin has been assessed and reinforced. Ms. Takashi confirms that he is able to accurately check his pulse and can list signs of digoxin toxicity and excessive bleeding.

### Critical Thinking in the Nursing Process

1. Mr. Jackson's medication regimen remains the same after discharge. What specific teaching does he need related to potential interactions of these drugs?
2. Mr. Jackson tells you, "Talk to my wife about my medications—she's Tarzan and I'm Jane now." How would you respond?
3. Design an exercise plan for Mr. Jackson to prevent deconditioning and conserve energy.
4. Mr. Jackson tells you, "Sometimes I forget whether I have taken my aspirin, so I'll take another just to be sure. After all, they are only baby aspirin. One or two extra a day shouldn't hurt, right?" What is your response?
5. Mr. Jackson is admitted to the neuro unit 6 months later with a cerebral vascular accident (CVA). What is the probable cause of his stroke?

See Evaluating Your Response in Appendix C.

---

## THE CLIENT WITH PULMONARY EDEMA

**Pulmonary edema** is an abnormal accumulation of fluid in the interstitial tissue and alveoli of the lung. Both cardiac and noncardiac disorders can cause pulmonary edema. Cardiac causes include acute myocardial infarction, acute heart failure, and valvular disease. *Cardiogenic pulmonary edema,* the focus of this section, is a sign of severe cardiac decompensation. Noncardiac causes of pulmonary edema include primary pulmonary disorders, such as acute respiratory distress syndrome (ARDS), trauma, sepsis, drug overdose, or neurologic sequelae. Pulmonary edema due to ARDS is discussed in Chapter 36. ∞

Pulmonary edema is a medical emergency: The client is literally drowning in the fluid in the alveolar and interstitial pulmonary spaces. Its onset may be acute or gradual, progressing to severe respiratory distress. Immediate treatment is necessary.

### PATHOPHYSIOLOGY

In cardiogenic pulmonary edema, the contractility of the left ventricle is severely impaired. The ejection fraction falls as the ventricle is unable to eject the blood that enters it, causing a sharp rise in end-diastolic volume and pressure. Pulmonary hydrostatic pressures rise, ultimately exceeding the osmotic pressure of the blood. As a result, fluid leaking from the pulmonary capillaries congests interstitial tissues, decreasing lung compliance, and interfering with gas exchange. As capillary and interstitial pressures increase further, the tight junctions of the alveolar walls are disrupted, and the fluid enters the alveoli, along with large red blood cells and protein molecules. Ventilation and gas exchange are severely disrupted, and hypoxia worsens.

## MANIFESTATIONS

The client with acute pulmonary edema presents with classic manifestations (see box below). Dyspnea, shortness of breath, and labored respirations are acute and severe, accompanied by orthopnea, inability to breathe when lying down. Cyanosis is present, and the skin is cool, clammy, and diaphoretic. A productive cough with pink, frothy sputum develops due to fluid, RBCs, and plasma proteins in the alveoli and airways. Crackles are heard throughout the lung fields on auscultation. As the condition worsens, lung sounds become harsher. The client often is restless and highly anxious, although severe hypoxia may cause confusion or lethargy.

As noted earlier, pulmonary edema is a medical emergency. Without rapid and effective intervention, severe tissue hypoxia and acidosis will lead to organ system failure and death.

### Manifestations of Pulmonary Edema

**RESPIRATORY**
- Tachypnea
- Labored respirations
- Dyspnea
- Orthopnea
- Paroxysmal nocturnal dyspnea
- Cough productive of frothy, pink sputum
- Crackles, wheezes

**CARDIOVASCULAR**
- Tachycardia
- Hypotension
- Cyanosis
- Cool, clammy skin
- Hypoxemia
- Ventricular gallop

**NEUROLOGIC**
- Restlessness
- Anxiety
- Feeling of impending doom

## COLLABORATIVE CARE

Immediate treatment for acute pulmonary edema focuses on restoring effective gas exchange and reducing fluid and pressure in the pulmonary vascular system. The client is placed in an upright sitting position with the legs dangling to reduce venous return by trapping some excess fluid in the lower extremities. This position also facilitates breathing.

Diagnostic testing is limited to assessment of the acute situation. *Arterial blood gases (ABGs)* are drawn to assess gas exchange and acid-base balance. Oxygen tension (Pao$_2$) is usually low. Initially, carbon dioxide levels (Paco$_2$) may also be reduced because of rapid respirations. As the condition progresses, the Paco$_2$ rises and respiratory acidosis develops (see Chapter 5). *Oxygen saturation* levels also are continuously monitored. The *chest X-ray* shows pulmonary vascular congestion and alveolar edema. Provided the client's condition allows, *hemodynamic monitoring* is instituted. In cardiogenic pulmonary edema, the pulmonary artery wedge pressure (PAWP) is elevated, usually over 25 mmHg. Cardiac output may be decreased.

Morphine is administered intravenously to relieve anxiety and improve the efficacy of breathing. It also is a vasodilator that reduces venous return and lowers left atrial pressure. Although morphine is very effective for clients with cardiogenic pulmonary edema, naloxone, its antidote, is kept readily available in case respiratory depression occurs.

Oxygen is administered using a positive pressure system that can achieve a 100% oxygen concentration. A continuous positive airway pressure (CPAP) mask system may be used, or the client may be intubated and mechanical ventilation employed (see Chapter 36). Positive pressure increases alveolar pressures and gas exchange while decreasing fluid diffusion into the alveoli.

Potent loop diuretics such as furosemide, ethacrynic acid, or bumetanide are administered intravenously to promote rapid diuresis. Furosemide is also a venous dilator, reducing venous return to the heart. Vasodilators such as intravenous nitroprusside are given to improve cardiac output by reducing afterload. Dopamine or dobutamine and possibly digoxin are administered to improve the myocardial contractility and cardiac output. Intravenous aminophylline may be used cautiously to reduce bronchospasm and decrease wheezing.

When the client's condition has stabilized, further diagnostic tests may be done to determine the underlying cause of pulmonary edema, and specific treatment measures directed at the cause instituted.

## NURSING CARE

Nursing care of the client with acute pulmonary edema focuses on relieving the pulmonary effects of the disorder. Interventions are directed toward improving oxygenation, reducing fluid volume, and providing emotional support.

The nurse often is instrumental in recognizing early manifestations of pulmonary edema and initiating treatment. As with many critical conditions, emergent care is directed toward the ABCs: airway, breathing, and circulation.

## Nursing Diagnoses and Interventions

### Impaired Gas Exchange

Accumulated fluid in the alveoli and airways interfere with ventilation of and gas exchange within the alveoli.

- Ensure airway patency.

**PRACTICE ALERT** *Assess the effectiveness of respiratory efforts and airway clearance. Pulmonary edema increases the work of breathing. This increased effort can lead to fatigue and decreased respiratory effort.* ■

- Assess respiratory status frequently, including rate, effort, use of accessory muscles, sputum characteristics, lung sounds, and skin color. *The status of a client in acute pulmonary edema can change rapidly for the better or worse.*
- Place in high-Fowler's position with the legs dangling. *The upright position facilitates breathing and decreases venous return.*
- Administer oxygen as ordered by mask, CPAP mask, or ventilator. *Supplemental oxygen promotes gas exchange; positive pressure increases the pressure within the alveoli, airways, and thoracic cavity, decreasing venous return, pulmonary capillary pressure, and fluid leak into the alveoli.*
- Encourage to cough up secretions; provide nasotracheal suctioning if necessary. *Coughing moves secretions from smaller airways into larger airways where they can be suctioned out if necessary.*

**PRACTICE ALERT** *Have emergency equipment readily available in case of respiratory arrest. Be prepared to assist with intubation and initiation of mechanical ventilation. Fatigue, impaired gas exchange, and respiratory acidosis can lead to respiratory and cardiac arrest.* ■

### Decreased Cardiac Output

Cardiogenic pulmonary edema usually is caused by either an acute decrease in myocardial contractility or increased workload that exceeds the ability of the left ventricle.

- Monitor vital signs, hemodynamic status, and rhythm continuously. *Acute pulmonary edema is a critical condition, and cardiovascular status can change rapidly.*
- Assess heart sounds for possible S$_3$, S$_4$, or murmurs. *These abnormal heart sounds may be due to excess work or may indicate the cause of the acute pulmonary edema.*
- Initiate an intravenous line for medication administration. Administer morphine, diuretics, vasodilators, bronchodilators, and positive inotropic medications (e.g., digoxin) as ordered. *These drugs reduce cardiac work and improve contractility.*

**PRACTICE ALERT** *Insert an indwelling catheter; record output hourly. Urine output of less than 30 mL/hr indicates severely impaired cardiac output and a risk for renal failure or other complications.* ■

MediaLink | ACUTE PULMONARY EDEMA CARE PLAN

- Keep accurate intake and output records. Restrict fluids as ordered. *Fluids may be restricted to reduce vascular volume and cardiac work.*

### Fear

Acute pulmonary edema is a very frightening experience for everyone (including the nurse).

- Provide emotional support for the client and family members. *Fear and anxiety stimulate the sympathetic nervous system, which can lead to ineffective respiratory patterns and interfere with cooperation with care measures.*
- Explain all procedures and the reasons to the client and family members. Keep information brief and to the point. Use short sentences and a reassuring tone. *Anxiety and fear interfere with the ability to assimilate information; brief, factual information and reassurance reduce anxiety and fear.*

- Maintain close contact with the client and family, providing reassurance that recovery from acute pulmonary edema is often as dramatic as its onset.
- Answer questions, and provide accurate information in a caring manner. *Knowledge reduces anxiety and psychologic stress associated with this critical condition.*

### Home Care

During the acute period, teaching is limited to immediate care measures. Once the acute episode of pulmonary edema has resolved, teach the client and family about its underlying cause and prevention of future episodes. If pulmonary edema follows an acute MI, include information related to CHD and the AMI, as well as information related to heart failure. Review the teaching and home care for clients with these disorders for further information.

# INFLAMMATORY HEART DISORDERS

Any layer of cardiac tissue—the endocardium, myocardium, or pericardium—can become inflamed, thus damaging the heart valves, heart muscle, or pericardial lining. Manifestations of inflammatory heart disorders range from very mild to life threatening. This section discusses the causes and management of rheumatic heart disease, endocarditis, myocarditis, and pericarditis.

## THE CLIENT WITH RHEUMATIC FEVER AND RHEUMATIC HEART DISEASE

**Rheumatic fever** is a systemic inflammatory disease caused by an abnormal immune response to pharyngeal infection by group A beta-hemolytic streptococci. The peak incidence of rheumatic fever is between ages 5 and 15; although it is rare after age 40, it may affect people of any age. Rheumatic fever usually is a self-limiting disorder, although it may become recurrent or chronic. Although the heart commonly is involved in the acute inflammatory process, only about 10% of people with rheumatic fever develop rheumatic heart disease (Porth, 2002). Rheumatic heart disease frequently damages the heart valves and is a major cause of mitral and aortic valve disorders discussed in the next section of this chapter.

In the United States and other industrialized nations, rheumatic fever and its sequelae are rare. About 3% of people with untreated group A streptococcal pharyngitis develop rheumatic fever (Braunwald et al., 2001). Rheumatic fever and rheumatic heart disease remain significant public health problems in many developing countries. Highly virulent strains of group A streptococci have caused scattered outbreaks in the United States in recent years (McCance & Huether, 2002).

Risk factors for streptococcal infections of the pharynx include environmental and economic factors such as crowded living conditions, malnutrition, immunodeficiency, and poor access to health care. Evidence also suggests an unknown genetic factor in susceptibility to rheumatic fever.

## PATHOPHYSIOLOGY

The pathophysiology of rheumatic fever is not yet totally understood. It is thought to result from an abnormal immune response to M proteins on group A β-hemolytic streptococcal bacteria. These antigens can bind to cells in the heart, muscles, and brain. They also bind with receptors in synovial joints, provoking an autoimmune response (McCance & Huether, 2002). The resulting immune response to the bacteria also leads to inflammation in tissues containing these M proteins. Inflammatory lesions develop in connective tissues on the heart, joints, and skin. The antibodies may remain in the serum for up to 6 months following the initiating event. See Chapters 8 and 9 ⊙⊙ for more information about the immune system and inflammatory response.

*Carditis,* inflammation of the heart, develops in about 50% of people with rheumatic fever. The inflammatory process usually involves all three layers of the heart—the pericardium, myocardium, and endocardium. *Aschoff bodies,* localized areas of tissue necrosis surrounded by immune cells, develop in cardiac tissues. Pericardial and myocardial inflammation tends to be mild and self-limiting. Endocardial inflammation, however, causes swelling and erythema of valve structures and small vegetative lesions on valve leaflets. As the inflammatory process resolves, fibrous scarring occurs, causing deformity.

**Rheumatic heart disease (RHD)** is slowly progressive valvular deformity that may follow acute or repeated attacks of rheumatic fever. Valve leaflets become rigid and deformed; commissures (openings) fuse, and the chordae tendineae fibrose and shorten. This results in stenosis or regurgitation of the valve. In **stenosis,** a narrowed fused valve obstructs forward blood flow. **Regurgitation** occurs when the valve fails to close properly (an *incompetent* valve), allowing blood to flow

## Manifestations of Rheumatic Fever

### CARDIAC

- Chest pain
- Friction rub
- Heart murmur

### MUSCULOSKELETAL

- *Migratory polyarthritis*: redness, heat, swelling, pain, and tenderness of more than one joint
- Usually affects large joints of extremities

### SKIN

- *Erythema marginatum*: transitory pink, nonpruritic, macular lesions on trunk or inner aspect of upper arms or thighs
- *Subcutaneous nodules* over extensors of wrist, elbow, ankle, and knee joints

### NEUROLOGIC

- *Sydenham's chorea*: irritability, behavior changes; sudden, jerky, involuntary movements

back through it. Valves on the left side of the heart are usually affected; the mitral valve is most frequently involved.

## MANIFESTATIONS

Manifestations of rheumatic fever typically follow the initial streptococcal infection by about 2 to 3 weeks. Fever and migratory joint pain are often initial manifestations. The knees, ankles, hips, and elbows are common sites of swelling and inflammation. *Erythema marginatum* is a temporary nonpruritic skin rash characterized by red lesions with clear borders and blanched centers usually found on the trunk and proximal extremities. Neurologic symptoms of rheumatic fever, although rare in adults, may range from irritability and an inability to concentrate to clumsiness and involuntary muscle spasms.

Manifestations of carditis include chest pain, tachycardia, a pericardial friction rub, or evidence of heart failure. On auscultation, an $S_3$, $S_4$, or a heart murmur may be heard. Cardiomegaly or pericardial effusion may develop. Other manifestations of rheumatic fever are listed in the box above.

## COLLABORATIVE CARE

Management of the client with rheumatic heart disease focuses on eradicating the streptococcal infection and managing the manifestations of the disease. Carditis and resulting heart failure are treated with measures to reduce the inflammatory process and manage the heart failure. Activities are limited, but bed rest is not generally ordered.

### Diagnostic Tests

In addition to the history and physical examination, a number of laboratory and diagnostic tests may be ordered for the client with suspected rheumatic fever. Table 30–4 identifies tests and values indicative of carditis associated with rheumatic fever.

| TABLE 30–4 | Diagnostic Tests for Rheumatic Heart Disease |
| --- | --- |
| **Test** | **Values Characteristic of Rheumatic Heart Disease** |
| White blood cell count (WBC) | Greater than 10,000/mm³ |
| Red blood cell count (RBC) | Less than 4 million/mm³ |
| Erythrocyte sedimentation rate (ESR) | More than 20 mm/h |
| C-reactive protein | Positive |
| Antistreptolysin (ASO) titer | Above 250 IU/mL |
| Throat culture | Usually positive for group A beta-hemolytic streptococci |
| Cardiac enzymes | Elevated in severe carditis |
| ECG changes | Prolonged PR interval |
| Chest X-ray | May show cardiac enlargement |
| Echocardiogram | May show valvular damage, enlarged chambers, decreased ventricular function, or pericardial effusion |

- *Complete blood count (CBC)* and *erythrocyte sedimentation rate (ESR)* are indicators of the inflammatory process. The white blood cell count is elevated, and the number of red blood cells may be low due to the inflammatory inhibition of erythropoiesis. The ESR, a general indicator of inflammation, is elevated.
- *C-reactive protein (CRP)* is positive in an active inflammatory process.
- *Antistreptolysin (ASO) titer* is a test for streptococcal antibodies. It rises within 2 months of the onset and is positive in most clients with rheumatic fever.
- Throat culture is positive for group A β-hemolytic streptococcus in only 25% to 40% of clients with acute rheumatic fever (Braunwald et al., 2001).

### Medications

As soon as rheumatic fever is diagnosed, antibiotics are started to eliminate the streptococcal infection. Penicillin is the antibiotic of choice to treat group A streptococci. Antibiotics are prescribed for at least 10 days. Erythromycin or clindamycin is used if the client is allergic to penicillin. Prophylactic antibiotic therapy is continued for 5 to 10 years to prevent recurrences. Recurrences after 5 years or age 25 are rare (Tierney et al., 2001). Penicillin G, 1.2 million units injected intramuscularly every 3 to 4 weeks, is the prophylaxis of choice. Oral penicillin, amoxicillin, sulfadiazine, or erythromycin may also be used.

Joint pain and fever are treated with salicylates (e.g., aspirin), ibuprofen, or another nonsteroidal anti-inflammatory drug (NSAID); corticosteroids may be used for severe pain due to inflammation or carditis. See Chapter 9 ∞ for information about the use of these anti-inflammatory medications.

# NURSING CARE

## Health Promotion

Rheumatic fever is preventable. Prompt identification and treatment of streptococcal throat infections helps decrease spread of the pathogen and the risk for rheumatic fever. Characteristics of streptococcal sore throat include a red, fiery-looking throat, pain with swallowing, enlarged and tender cervical lymph nodes, fever range of 101° to 104°F (38.3° to 40.0°C), and headache. Emphasize the importance of finishing the complete course of medication to eradicate the pathogen.

## Assessment

Assess clients at risk for rheumatic fever (prolonged, untreated or recurrent pharyngitis) for possible manifestations.

- Health history: complaints of recent sore throat with fever, difficulty swallowing, and general malaise; treatment measures; previous history of strep throat or rheumatic fever; history of heart murmur or other cardiac problems; current medications
- Physical examination: vital signs including temperature; skin color, presence of rash on trunk or proximal extremities; mental status; evidence of inflamed joints; heart and lung sounds

## Nursing Diagnoses and Interventions

The nursing care focus for the client with RHD is on providing supportive care and preventing complications. Teaching to prevent recurrence of rheumatic fever is extremely important. *Pain* and *Activity intolerance* are priority nursing diagnoses for the client with rheumatic fever and RHD.

### Acute Pain

Joint and chest pain due to acute inflammation is common in rheumatic fever. Pain and inflammation may interfere with rest and healing.

- Administer anti-inflammatory drugs as ordered. Promptly report manifestations of aspirin toxicity, including tinnitus, vomiting, and gastrointestinal bleeding. Give aspirin and other NSAIDs with food, milk, or antacids to minimize gastric irritation. *Joint pain and fever may be treated with anti-inflammatory agents such as aspirin and NSAIDs. When used for its anti-inflammatory effect, aspirin doses may be high, and it is given around the clock (e.g., every 4 hours). Steroids may be prescribed for severe carditis.*
- Provide warm, moist compresses for local pain relief of acutely inflamed joints. *Moist heat helps relieve pain associated with inflamed joints by reducing inflammation.*
- Auscultate heart sounds as indicated (every shift or each home visit). Notify the physician if a pericardial friction rub or a new murmur develops. *A friction rub is produced as inflamed pericardial surfaces rub against each other. This also stimulates pain receptors, and may increase discomfort.*

### Activity Intolerance

The client with acute carditis or RHD may develop heart failure if the heart is unable to supply enough oxygen to meet the body's demand. Manifestations of fatigue, weakness, and dyspnea on exertion may result.

- Explain the importance of activity limitations and reinforce teaching as needed. *Activities are limited during the acute phase of carditis to reduce the workload of the heart. Understanding the rationale improves cooperation with the limitations.*
- Encourage social and diversional activities such as visits with friends and family, reading, playing cards or board games, watching television, and listening to music or talking books. *Diversional activities provide a focus for the client whose physical activities must be limited.*
- Encourage gradual increases in activity, monitoring for evidence of intolerance or heart failure. Consult a cardiac rehabilitation specialist to help design an activity progression schedule. *Gradual activity progression is encouraged as the client's condition improves. Activity tolerance is monitored and activities modified as needed.*

## Home Care

Most clients with rheumatic fever and carditis do not require hospitalization. Teaching for home care focuses on both acute care and preventing recurrences and further tissue damage. Include the following topics.

- The importance of completing the full course of antibiotic therapy and continuing antibiotic prophylaxis as prescribed For the client with chronic RHD, include the importance of antibiotic prophylaxis for invasive procedures (e.g., dental care, endoscopy, or surgery) to prevent bacterial endocarditis. Pamphlets on endocarditis prevention are helpful reminders, and are available from the American Heart Association.
- Preventive dental care and good oral hygiene to maintain oral health and prevent gingival infections, which can lead to recurrence of the disease
- Early recognition of streptococcal sore throat and appropriate treatment for both the client and family members
- Early manifestations of heart failure to report to the physician
- Prescribed medications, including their dosage, route, intended and potential adverse effects, and manifestations to report to the physician
- Dietary sodium restriction if ordered or recommended. A high-carbohydrate, high-protein diet may be recommended to facilitate healing and combat fatigue.

Refer for home health services or household assistance as indicated.

# THE CLIENT WITH INFECTIVE ENDOCARDITIS

**Endocarditis,** inflammation of the endocardium, can involve any portion of the endothelial lining of the heart. The valves usually are affected. Endocarditis is usually infectious in nature, characterized by colonization or invasion of the endocardium and heart valves by a pathogen.

| TABLE 30-5 | Classifications of Infective Endocarditis | |
| --- | --- | --- |
| | **Acute Infective Endocarditis** | **Subacute Infective Endocarditis** |
| Onset | Sudden | Gradual |
| Usual organism | *Staphylococcus aureus* | *Streptococcus viridans*, enterococci, gram-negative and gram-positive bacilli, fungi, yeasts |
| Risk factors | Usually occurs in previously normal heart; intravenous drug use, infected intravenous sites | Usually occurs in damaged or deformed hearts; dental work, invasive procedures, and infections |
| Pathologic process | Rapid valve destruction | Valve destruction leading to regurgitation; embolization of friable vegetations |
| Presentation | Abrupt onset with spiking fever and chills; manifestations of heart failure | Gradual onset of febrile illness with cough, dyspnea, arthralgias, abdominal pain |

Endocarditis is relatively uncommon, with an incidence of 1.5 to 6.2 cases per 100,000 people in developed countries (Braunwald et al., 2001). The greatest risk factor for endocarditis is previous heart damage. Lesions develop on deformed valves, on valve prostheses, or in areas of tissue damage due to congential deformities or ischemic disease. The left side of the heart, the mitral valve in particular, is usually affected. Intravenous drug use also is a significant risk factor. The right side of the heart usually is affected in these clients. Other risk factors include invasive catheters (e.g., a central venous catheter, hemodynamic monitoring, or an indwelling urinary catheter), dental procedures or poor dental health, and recent heart surgery.

Endocarditis is classified by its acuity and disease course (Table 30–5). *Acute infective endocarditis* has an abrupt onset and is a rapidly progressive, severe disease. Although almost any organism can cause infective endocarditis, virulent organisms such as *Staphylococcus aureus* cause a more abrupt onset and destructive course. *S. aureus* is commonly the infective organism in acute endocarditis. In contrast, *subacute infective endocarditis* has a more gradual onset, with predominant systemic manifestations. It is more likely to occur in clients with preexisting heart disease. *Streptococcus viridans,* enterococci, other gram-negative and gram-positive bacilli, yeasts, and fungi tend to cause the subacute forms of endocarditis (Porth, 2002).

*Prosthetic valve endocarditis (PVE)* may occur in clients with a mechanical or tissue valve replacement. This infection may develop in the early postoperative period (within 2 months after surgery) or late. Prosthetic valve endocarditis accounts for 10% to 20% of endocarditis cases. It usually affects males over the age of 60, and is more frequently associated with aortic valve prostheses than with mitral valve replacements. Early PVE is usually due to prosthetic valve contamination during surgery or perioperative bacteremia. Its course often is rapid, and mortality is high. Late-onset PVE more closely resembles subacute endocarditis.

## PATHOPHYSIOLOGY

Entry of pathogens into the bloodstream is required for infective endocarditis to develop. Bacteria may enter through oral lesions, during dental work or invasive procedures, such as intravenous catheter insertion, surgery, or urinary

catheterization; during intravenous drug use; or as a result of infectious processes such as urinary tract or upper respiratory infection.

The initial lesion is a sterile platelet-fibrin vegetation formed on damaged endothelium (Figure 30–5 ■). In acute infective endocarditis, these lesions develop on healthy valve structures, although the mechanism is unknown. In subacute endocarditis, they usually develop on already damaged valves or in endocardial tissue that has been damaged by abnormal pressures or blood flow within the heart.

Organisms that have invaded the blood colonize these vegetations. The vegetation enlarges as more platelets and fibrin are attracted to the site and cover the infecting organism. This covering "protects" the bacteria from quick removal by immune defenses such as phagocytosis by neutrophils, antibodies, and complement. Vegetations may be singular or multiple. They expand while loosely attached to edges of the valve. Friable vegetations can break or shear off, embolizing and traveling through the bloodstream to other organ systems. When they lodge in small vessels, they may cause hemorrhages, infarcts, or abscesses. Ultimately, the vegetations scar and deform the valves and cause turbulence of blood flowing through the heart. Heart valve function is affected, either obstructing forward blood flow, or closing incompletely.

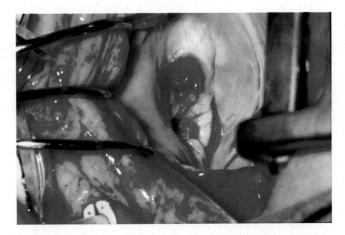

**Figure 30–5** ■ A vegetative lesion of bacterial endocarditis.

*Source: M. English/Custom Medical Stock Photo, Inc.*

## Manifestations of Infective Endocarditis

- Chills and fever
- General malaise, fatigue
- Arthralgias
- Cough, dyspnea
- Heart murmur
- Anorexia, abdominal pain
- Petechiae, splinter hemorrhages
- Splenomegaly

## MANIFESTATIONS AND COMPLICATIONS

The manifestations of infective endocarditis often are nonspecific (see the box above). A temperature above 101.5°F (39.4°C) and flulike symptoms develop, accompanied by cough, shortness of breath, and joint pain. The presentation of acute staphylococcal endocarditis is more severe, with a sudden onset, chills, and a high fever. Heart murmurs are heard in 90% of persons with infective endocarditis. An existing murmur may worsen, or a new murmur may develop.

Embolic complications may affect any organ system, particularly the lungs, brain, kidneys, and the skin and mucous membranes. Splenomegaly is common in chronic disease. Peripheral manifestations of infective endocarditis result from microemboli or circulating immune complexes. These manifestations include:

- *Petechiae,* small, purplish-red hemorrhagic spots on the trunk, conjunctiva, and mucous membranes.
- *Splinter hemorrhages,* hemorrhagic streaks under the fingernails or toenails.
- *Osler's nodes,* small, reddened, painful raised growths on finger and toe pads.
- *Janeway lesions,* small, nontender, purplish-red macular lesions on the palms of the hands and soles of the feet.
- *Roth's spots,* small, whitish spots (cotton-wool spots) seen on the retina.

Infective endocarditis often causes complications such as heart failure, infarction of other organs from embolization of vegetative fragments, abscess, and aneurysms due to infiltration of the arterial wall by organisms. Without treatment, endocarditis is almost universally fatal; fortunately, antibiotic therapy is usually effective to treat this disease.

## COLLABORATIVE CARE

Eradicating the infecting organism and minimizing valve damage and other adverse consequences of infective endocarditis are the priorities of care.

### Diagnostic Tests

There are no definitive tests for infective endocarditis, but diagnostic tests help establish the diagnosis.

- *Blood cultures* usually are positive for bacteria or other pathogens. Blood cultures are considered positive when a typical infecting organism is identified from two or more separate blood cultures (drawn from different sites and/or at different times, e.g., 12-hour intervals).
- *Echocardiography* allows visualization of vegetations and evaluation of valve function. Transthoracic echocardiography (TTE) is noninvasive and can be done at the client's bedside; however, it is less sensitive than transesophageal echocardiography (TEE). The ultrasound transducer is combined with an endoscope in TEE. See page 548 for nursing care of the client undergoing an upper endoscopy. Echocardiography can be diagnostic for infective endocarditis when combined with positive blood cultures.
- *Serologic immune testing* for circulating antigens to typical infective organisms may be done.

Other diagnostic tests may include the CBC, ESR, serum creatinine, chest X-ray, and an electrocardiogram.

### Medications

Preventing endocarditis in clients at high risk is important. Antibiotics are commonly prescribed for clients with preexisting valve damage or heart disease prior to high risk procedures (Table 30–6).

| TABLE 30–6 Antibiotic Prophylaxis for Infective Endocarditis | | |
| --- | --- | --- |
| **Indications for Prophylaxis** | **Selected Procedures for Which Prophylaxis Is Recommended** | **Suggested Antibiotics** |
| Prosthetic valves | Dental procedures in which bleeding is likely, including cleaning | Amoxicillin |
| Previous episode(s) of infective endocarditis | Most surgeries | Erythromycin |
| Rheumatic heart disease | Bronchoscopy | Ampicillin |
| Hypertrophic cardiomyopathy | Cystoscopy | Clindamycin |
| Mitral valve prolapse with regurgitation and murmur | Urinary catheterization when infection is present | Vancomycin |
| Sclerotic aortic valve | Incision and drainage of infected tissue | (*Note:* choice of antibiotic depends on procedure) |
| Most congenital heart malformations | Vaginal delivery if infection is present | |

Antibiotic therapy effectively treats infective endocarditis in most cases. The goal of therapy is to eradicate the infecting organism from the blood and vegetative lesions in the heart. The fibrin covering that protects colonies of organisms from immune defenses also protects them from antibiotic therapy. Therefore, an extended course of multiple intravenous antibiotics is required.

Following blood cultures, antibiotic therapy is initiated with drugs known to be effective against the most common infecting organisms: staphylococci, streptococci, and enterococci. The initial regimen may include nafcillin or oxacillin, penicillin or ampicillin, and gentamicin. Once the organism has been identified, therapy is tailored to that organism. Streptococcal and enterococcal infections are treated with a combination of penicillin and gentamicin. If the client is allergic to penicillin, ceftriaxone, cefazolin, or vancomycin may be used. Staphyloccoal infections are treated with nafcillin or oxacillin and gentamicin; cefazolin or vancomycin may be used if penicillin allergy is present. Intravenous drug therapy is continued for 2 to 8 weeks, depending on the infecting organism, the drugs used, and the results of repeat blood cultures. See Chapter 8 for the nursing implications for antibiotic therapy. ⊖⊙

The client with prosthetic valve endocarditis requires extended treatment, usually 6 to 8 weeks. Combination therapy using vancomycin, rifampin, and gentamicin is used to treat these resistant infections.

## Surgery

Some clients with infective endocarditis require surgery to:

- Replace severely damaged valves.
- Remove large vegetations at risk for embolization
- Remove a valve that is a continuing source of infection that does not respond to antibiotic therapy.

The most common indication for surgery is valvular regurgitation that causes heart failure and does not respond to medical therapy. When the infection has not responded to antibiotic therapy within 7 to 10 days, the infected valve may be replaced to facilitate eradication of the organism. Clients with fungal endocarditis usually require surgical intervention. More information on valve replacement surgery is provided in the section on valve disorders.

## NURSING CARE

### Health Promotion

Prevention of endocarditis is vital in susceptible people. Education is a key part of prevention. Use every opportunity to educate individuals and the public about the risks of intravenous drug use, including endocarditis. Discuss preventive measures with all clients with specific risk factors, such as a heart murmur or known heart disease.

### Assessment

Assessment related to ineffective endocarditis includes identifying risk factors and manifestations of the disease.

- Health history: complaints of persistent flulike symptoms, fatigue, shortness of breath, and activity intolerance; history of recent dental work or other invasive procedures; known heart murmur, valve or other heart disorder; recent intravenous drug use
- Physical examination: Vital signs including temperature; apical pulse and heart sounds; rate and ease of respirations, lung sounds; skin color, temperature, and presence of petechiae or splinter hemorrhages

## Nursing Diagnoses and Interventions

Nursing care focuses on managing the manifestations of endocarditis, administering antibiotics, and teaching the client and family members about the disorder. In addition to the diagnoses identified below, nursing diagnoses and interventions for heart failure also may be appropriate for clients with infective endocarditis.

### Risk for Imbalanced Body Temperature

Fever is common in clients with infective endocarditis. It may be acutely elevated and accompanied by chills, particularly with acute infective endocarditis. The inflammatory process initiates a cycle of events that affects the regulation of temperature and causes discomfort.

- Record temperature every 2 to 4 hours. Report temperature above 101.5°F (39.4°C). Assess for complaints of discomfort. *Fever is usually low grade (below 101.5°F [39.4°C]) in infective endocarditis; higher temperatures may cause discomfort. The temperature usually returns to normal within 1 week after initiation of antibiotic therapy. Continued fever may indicate a need to modify the treatment regimen.*
- Obtain blood cultures as ordered, before initial antibiotic dose. *Initial blood cultures are obtained before antibiotic therapy is started to obtain adequate organisms to culture and identify. Follow-up cultures are used to assess the effectiveness of therapy.*
- Provide anti-inflammatory or antipyretic agents as prescribed. *Fever may be treated with anti-inflammatory or antipyretic agents such as aspirin, ibuprofen, or acetaminophen.*
- Administer antibiotics as ordered; obtain peak and trough drug levels as indicated. *Intravenous antibiotics are given to eradicate the pathogen. Peak and trough levels are used to evaluate the dose effectiveness in maintaining a therapeutic blood level.*

### Risk for Ineffective Tissue Perfusion

Embolization of vegetative lesions can threaten tissue and organ perfusion. Vegetations from the left heart may lodge in arterioles or capillaries of the brain, kidneys, or peripheral tissues, causing infarction or abscess. A large embolism can cause manifestations of stroke or transient ischemic attack, renal failure, or tissue ischemia. Emboli from the right side of the heart become entrapped in pulmonary vasculature, causing manifestations of pulmonary embolism.

- Assess for, document, and report manifestations of decreased organ system perfusion:
  a. Neurologic: changes in level of consciousness, numbness or tingling in extremities, hemiplegia, visual disturbances, or manifestations of stroke

b. Renal: decreased urine output, hematuria, elevated BUN or creatinine
c. Pulmonary: dyspnea, hemoptysis, shortness of breath, diminished breath sounds, restlessness, sudden chest or shoulder pain
d. Cardiovascular: chest pain radiating to jaw or arms, tachycardia, anxiety, tachypnea, hypotension

*All major organs and tissues, and the microcirculation may be affected by emboli when vegetations break off due to turbulent blood flow. Emboli may cause manifestations of organ dysfunction. The most devastating effects of emboli are in the brain and the myocardium, with resulting infarctions. Intravenous drug users have a high risk of pulmonary emboli as a result of right-sided endocardial fragments.*

- Assess and document skin color and temperature, quality of peripheral pulses, and capillary refill. *Peripheral emboli affect tissue perfusion, with a risk for tissue necrosis and possible extremity loss.*

### Ineffective Health Maintenance

The client with endocarditis often is treated in the community. Teaching about disease management and prevention of possible recurrences of endocarditis is vital.

- Demonstrate intravenous catheter site care and intermittent antibiotic administration if the client and family will manage therapy. Have the client and/or significant other redemonstrate appropriate techniques. *Intermittent antibiotic infusions may be managed by the client or family members, or the client may go to an outpatient facility to receive the infusions. Appropriate site care is necessary to reduce the risk of trauma and infection.*
- Explain the actions, doses, administration, and desired and adverse effects of prescribed drugs. Identify manifestations to be reported to the physician. Provide practical information about measures to reduce the risk of superinfection (e.g., consuming 8 oz of yogurt or buttermilk containing live bacterial cultures daily). *Careful compliance with prescribed drug therapy is vital to eradicate the infecting organism. Antibiotic therapy can, however, cause superinfections such as candidiasis due to elimination of normal body flora.*
- Teach about the function of heart valves and the effects of endocarditis on heart function. Include a simple definition of endocarditis, and explain the risk for its recurrence. *Information helps the client and family understand endocarditis, its treatment, and its effects. Understanding increases compliance.*
- Describe the manifestations of heart failure to be reported to the physician. *Evidence of heart failure may necessitate modification of the treatment regimen or replacement of infected valves.*

**PRACTICE ALERT** *Stress the importance of notifying all care providers of valve disease, heart murmur, or valve replacement before undergoing invasive procedures. Invasive procedures provide a portal of entry for bacteria. A history of valve disease increases the risk for the development or recurrence of endocarditis.* ▪

- Encourage good dental hygiene and mouth care and regular dental checkups. Teach how to prevent bleeding from the gums and avoid developing mouth ulcers (e.g., gentle toothbrushing, ensuring that dentures fit properly, and avoiding toothpicks, dental floss, and high-flow water devices). *The oropharynx harbors streptococci, which are common causes of endocarditis. Bleeding gums offer an opportunity for bacteria to enter the bloodstream.*
- Encourage the client to avoid people with upper respiratory infections. *Streptococci are normal pathogens in the upper respiratory tract; exposure to people with upper respiratory infections may increase the risk of infection.*
- If anticoagulant therapy is ordered, explain its actions, administration, and major side effects. Identify manifestations of bleeding to be promptly reported to the physician. *Clients with valve disease or a prosthetic valve following infective endocarditis may require continued anticoagulant therapy to prevent thrombi and emboli. Knowledge is vital for appropriate management of anticoagulant therapy and prevention of complications.*

### Home Care

When preparing the client with infective endocarditis for home care, provide teaching as outlined for the nursing diagnosis, *Ineffective health maintenance.* In addition, discuss the following topics.

- Although serious and frightening, infective endocarditis can usually be treated effectively with intravenous antibiotics.
- The importance of promptly reporting any unusual manifestation, such as a change in vision, sudden pain, or weakness, so that interventions to control complications can be promptly implemented.
- The rationale for all treatments and procedures.
- Preventing recurrences of infective endocarditis.
- The importance of maintaining contact with the physician for follow-up care and monitoring for long-term effects such as progressive valve damage and dysfunction.
- If appropriate, explain the risks associated with intravenous drug use.

Provide educational materials on infective endocarditis from the American Heart Association. Refer as appropriate to home health or home intravenous therapy services. Refer the client and family members or significant others as appropriate to a drug or substance abuse treatment program or facility. Provide follow-up care to ensure compliance with the referral and treatment plan.

## THE CLIENT WITH MYOCARDITIS

**Myocarditis** is inflammation of the heart muscle. It usually results from an infectious process, but also may occur as an immunologic response, or due to the effects of radiation, toxins, or drugs. In the United States, myocarditis is usually viral, caused by coxsackievirus B. Approximately 10% of people with HIV disease develop myocarditis due to infiltration of the myocardium by the virus. Bacterial myocarditis, much less common, may be associated with endocarditis caused by *Staphylococcus aureus,* or with diphtheria. Parasitic infections caused by *Trypanosoma cruzi* (Chagas' disease) are common in Central and South America (Braunwald et al., 2001).

Myocarditis may occur at any age, and it is more common in men than women. Factors that alter immune response (e.g., malnutrition, alcohol use, immunosuppressive drugs, exposure to radiation, stress, and advanced age) increase the risk for myocarditis. It also is a common complication of rheumatic fever and pericarditis. Viral myocarditis usually is self-limited; it may progress, however, to become chronic, leading to dilated cardiomyopathy (see the section of this chapter that follows).

## PATHOPHYSIOLOGY AND MANIFESTATIONS

In myocarditis, myocardial cells are damaged by an inflammatory process that causes local or diffuse swelling and damage. Infectious agents infiltrate interstitial tissues, forming abscesses. Autoimmune injury may occur when the immune system destroys not only the invading pathogen but also myocardial cells. The extent of damage to cardiac muscle ultimately determines the long-term outcome of the disease.

The manifestations of myocarditis depend on the degree of myocardial damage. The client may be asymptomatic. Nonspecific manifestations of inflammation such as fever, fatigue, general malaise, dyspnea, palpitations, and arthralgias may be present. A nonspecific febrile illness or upper respiratory infection often precedes the onset of myocarditis symptoms. Abnormal heart sounds such as muffled $S_1$, an $S_3$, murmur, and pericardial friction rub may be heard. Severe myocarditis may lead to heart failure. In some cases, manifestations of myocardial infarction, including chest pain, may occur.

## COLLABORATIVE CARE

Myocarditis treatment focuses on resolving the inflammatory process to prevent further damage to the myocardium.

Diagnostic studies may be ordered to help diagnose myocarditis.

- *Electrocardiography* may show transient ST segment and T wave changes, as well as dysrhythmias and possible heart block.
- *Cardiac markers,* such as the creatinine kinase, troponin T, and troponin I, may be elevated, indicating myocardial cell damage.
- *Endomyocardial biopsy* to examine myocardial cells is necessary to establish a definitive diagnosis; patchy cell necrosis and the inflammatory process can be identified.

If appropriate, antimicrobial therapy is used to eradicate the infecting organism. Antiviral therapy with interferon-α may be instituted. Immunosuppressive therapy with corticosteroids or other immunosuppressive agents (see Chapter 9 ⊂⊃ ) may be used to minimize the inflammatory response. Heart failure is treated as needed, using ACE inhibitors and drugs. Clients with myocarditis often are particularly sensitive to the effects of dig-

italis, so it is used with caution. Other medications used in treating myocarditis include antidysrhythmic agents as to control dysrhythmias and anticoagulants to prevent emboli.

Bed rest and activity restrictions are ordered during the acute inflammatory process to reduce myocardial work and prevent myocardial damage. Activities may be limited for as long as 6 months to a year (Porth, 2002).

## NURSING CARE

Nursing care is directed at decreasing myocardial work and maintaining cardiac output. Both physical and emotional rest are indicated, because anxiety increases myocardial oxygen demand. Hemodynamic parameters and the ECG are monitored closely, especially during the acute phase of the illness. Activity tolerance, urine output, and heart and breath sounds are frequently assessed for manifestations of heart failure. Consider the following nursing diagnoses for the client with myocarditis.

- *Activity intolerance* related to impaired cardiac muscle function
- *Decreased cardiac output* related to myocardial inflammation
- *Fatigue* related to inflammation and impaired cardiac output
- *Anxiety* related to possible long-term effects of the disorder
- *Excess fluid volume* related to compensatory mechanisms for decreased cardiac output

### Home Care

Include the following topics when preparing the client with myocarditis for home care.

- Activity restrictions and other prescribed measures to reduce cardiac workload
- Early manifestations of heart failure to report to the physician
- The importance of following the prescribed treatment regimen
- Any recommended dietary modifications (such as a low-sodium diet for heart failure)
- Prescribed medications, their purpose, doses, and possible adverse effects
- The importance of adhering to the treatment plan and recommended follow-up appointments to reduce the risk of long-term consequences such as cardiomyopathy

## THE CLIENT WITH PERICARDITIS

The pericardium is the outermost layer of the heart. It is a two-layered membranous sac with a thin layer of serous fluid (normally no more than 30 to 50 mL) separating the layers. It protects and cushions the heart and the great vessels, provides a barrier to infectious processes in adjacent structures, prevents displacement of the myocardium and blood vessels, and prevents sudden distention of the heart.

**Pericarditis** is the inflammation of the pericardium. Pericarditis may be a primary disorder or develop secondarily to another cardiac or systemic disorder. Some possible causes of

| BOX 30–4 | ■ Selected Causes of Pericarditis |
|---|---|

**INFECTIOUS**

- Viruses
- Bacteria
- Tuberculosis
- Fungi
- Syphilis
- Parasites

**NONINFECTIOUS**

- Myocardial and pericardial injury
- Uremia
- Neoplasms
- Radiation
- Trauma or surgery
- Myxedema
- Autoimmune disorders
- Rheumatic fever
- Connective tissue diseases
- Prescription and nonprescription drugs
- Postcardiac injury

pericarditis are listed in Box 30–4. Acute pericarditis is usually viral and affects men (usually under the age of 50) more frequently than women (Tierney et al., 2001). Pericarditis affects 40% to 50% of clients with end-stage renal disease and uremia. Postmyocardial infarction pericarditis and postcardiotomy (following open-heart surgery) pericarditis also are common.

## PATHOPHYSIOLOGY

Pericardial tissue damage triggers an inflammatory response. Inflammatory mediators released from the injured tissue cause vasodilation, hyperemia, and edema. Capillary permeability increases, allowing plasma proteins, including fibrinogen, to escape into the pericardial space. White blood cells amass at the site of injury to destroy the causative agent. Exudate is formed, usually fibrinous or serofibrinous (a mixture of serous fluid and fibrinous exudate). In some cases, the exudate may contain red blood cells or, if infectious, purulent material. The inflammatory process may resolve without long-term effects, or scar tissue and adhesions may form between the pericardial layers.

Fibrosis and scarring of the pericardium may restrict cardiac function. Pericardial effusions may develop as serous or purulent exudate (depending on the causative agent) collects in the pericardial sac. Pericardial effusion may be recurrent. Chronic inflammation causes the pericardium to become rigid.

## MANIFESTATIONS AND COMPLICATIONS

Classic manifestations of acute pericarditis include chest pain, a pericardial friction rub, and fever. Chest pain, the most common symptom, has an abrupt onset. It is caused by inflammation of nerve fibers in the lower parietal pericardium and pleura covering the diaphragm. The pain is usually sharp, may be steady or intermittent, and may radiate to the back or neck. The pain can mimic myocardial ischemia; careful assessment is important to rule out myocardial infarction. Pericardial pain is aggravated by respiratory movements (i.e., deep inspiration and/or coughing), changes in body position, or swallowing. Sitting upright and leaning forward reduces the discomfort by moving the heart away from the diaphragmatic side of the lung pleura.

Although not always present, a *pericardial friction rub* is the characteristic sign of pericarditis. A pericardial friction rub is a leathery, grating sound produced by the inflamed pericardial layers rubbing against the chest wall or pleura. It is heard most clearly at the left lower sternal border with the client sitting up or leaning forward. The rub is usually heard on expiration and may be constant or intermittent.

A low-grade fever (below 100°F [38.4°C]) often develops due to the inflammatory process. Dyspnea and tachycardia are common.

Pericardial effusion, cardiac tamponade, and constrictive pericarditis are possible complications of acute pericarditis.

### Pericardial Effusion

A *pericardial effusion* is an abnormal collection of fluid between the pericardial layers that threatens normal cardiac function. The fluid may consist of pus, blood, serum, lymph, or a combination. The manifestations of a pericardial effusion depend on the rate at which the fluid collects. Although the pericardium normally contains about 30 to 50 mL of fluid, the sac can stretch to accommodate a gradual accumulation of fluid. Over time, the pericardial sac can accommodate up to 2 L of fluid without immediate adverse effects. Conversely, a rapid buildup of pericardial fluid (as little as 100 mL) does not allow the sac to stretch and can compress the heart, interfering with myocardial function. This compression of the heart is known as **cardiac tamponade.** Slowly developing pericardial effusion is often painless and has few manifestations. Heart sounds may be distant or muffled. The client may have a cough or mild dyspnea.

### Cardiac Tamponade

Cardiac tamponade is a medical emergency that must be aggressively treated to preserve life. Cardiac tamponade may result from pericardial effusion, trauma, cardiac rupture, or hemorrhage. Rapid collection of fluid in the pericardial sac interferes with ventricular filling and pumping, critically reducing cardiac output.

Classic manifestations of cardiac tamponade result from rising intracardiac pressures, decreased diastolic filling, and decreased cardiac output. A hallmark of cardiac tamponade is a paradoxical pulse, or *pulsus paradoxus*. A parodoxical pulse markedly decreases in amplitude during inspiration. Intrathoracic pressure normally drops during inspiration, enhancing venous return to the right heart. This draws more blood into the right side of the heart than the left, causing the interventricular septum to bulge slightly into the left ventricle. When ventricular filling is impaired by excess fluid in the pericardial sac, this bulging of the interventricular septum decreases cardiac output during inspiration. On palpation of the carotid or femoral artery, the pulse is diminished or absent during inspiration. A drop in systolic blood pressure of more than 10 mmHg during inspiration also indicates pulsus paradoxus.

Other manifestations of cardiac tamponade include muffled heart sounds, dyspnea and tachypnea, tachycardia, a narrowed pulse pressure, and distended neck veins (see the box on the next page).

## Manifestations of Cardiac Tamponade

- Paradoxical pulse
- Narrowed pulse pressure, hypotension
- Tachycardia
- Weak peripheral pulses
- Distant, muffled heart sounds
- Jugular venous distention
- High central venous pressure
- Decreased level of consciousness
- Low urine output
- Cool, mottled skin

## Chronic Constrictive Pericarditis

Chronic pericardial inflammation can lead to scar tissue formation between the pericardial layers. This scar tissue eventually contracts, restricting diastolic filling and elevating venous pressure. Constrictive pericarditis may follow viral infection, radiation therapy, or heart surgery. Its manifestations include progressive dyspnea, fatigue, and weakness. Ascites is common; peripheral edema may develop. Neck veins are distended, and may be particularly noticeable during inspiration (*Kussmaul's sign*). This occurs because the right atrium is unable to dilate to accommodate increased venous return during inspiration.

## COLLABORATIVE CARE

Care for the client with pericarditis focuses on identifying its cause if possible, reducing inflammation, relieving symptoms, and preventing complications. The client is closely monitored for early manifestations of cardiac tamponade so that it can be treated promptly.

## Diagnostic Tests

There are no specific laboratory tests to diagnose pericarditis, but tests are often performed to differentiate pericarditis from myocardial infarction.

- *CBC* shows elevated WBCs and an ESR greater than 20 mm/h indicating acute inflammation.
- *Cardiac enzymes* may be slightly elevated because the inflammatory process extends to involve the epicardial surface of the heart. Cardiac enzymes are typically much lower in pericarditis than in myocardial infarction.
- *Electrocardiography* shows typical changes associated with pericarditis, such as diffuse ST segment elevation in all leads. This resolves more quickly than changes of acute MI and is not associated with the QRS complex and T wave changes typically seen in MI. With a large pericardial effusion, the QRS amplitude may be decreased. Atrial dysrhythmias may occur in acute pericarditis.
- *Echocardiography* is used to assess heart motion, for pericardial effusion, and the extent of restriction.
- *Hemodynamic monitoring* may be used in acute pericarditis or pericardial effusion to assess pressures and cardiac output.

Elevated pulmonary artery pressures and venous pressures occur with impaired filling due to pericardial effusion or constrictive pericarditis.

- *Chest X-ray* may show cardiac enlargement if a pericardial effusion is present.
- *Computed tomography (CT scan)* or *magnetic resonance imaging (MRI)* may be used to identify pericardial effusion or constrictive pericarditis.

## Medications

Drug treatment for pericarditis addresses its manifestations. Aspirin and acetaminophen may be used to reduce fever. Nonsteroidal anti-inflammatory drugs (NSAIDs) are used to reduce inflammation and promote comfort. In severe cases or with recurrent pericarditis, corticosteroids may be given to suppress the inflammatory response.

## Pericardiocentesis

*Pericardiocentesis* may be done to remove fluid from the pericardial sac for diagnostic or therapeutic purposes (Figure 30–6 ■). The physician inserts a large (16 to 18 gauge) needle to the left of the xiphoid process into the pericardial sac and withdraws excess fluid. The needle is attached to an ECG monitoring lead to help determine if the needle is touching the epicardial surface, which helps prevent piercing the myocardium. Pericardiocentesis may be an emergency procedure for the client with cardiac tamponade. Nursing implications for pericardiocentesis are outlined in the box on page 898.

## Surgery

For recurrent pericarditis or recurrent pericardial effusion, a rectangular piece of the pericardium, or "window," may be excised to allow collected fluid to drain into the pleural space. Constrictive pericarditis may necessitate a partial or total *pericardiectomy,* removal of part or all of the pericardium, to relieve the ventricular compression and allow adequate filling.

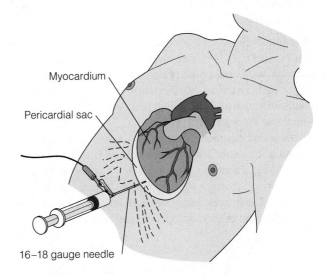

Myocardium

Pericardial sac

16–18 gauge needle

**Figure 30–6** ■ Pericardiocentesis.

## Nursing Implications for Diagnostic Tests
### Pericardiocentesis

**BEFORE THE PROCEDURE**
- Gather all supplies:
  a. Pericardiocentesis tray
  b. ECG machine and electrode patches
  c. Emergency cart with defibrillator
  d. Dressing
  e. Culture bottles (if indicated)
- Reinforce teaching and answer questions about the procedure or associated care. Provide emotional support.
- Ensure that informed consent has been obtained.
- Provide for privacy.
- Obtain and document baseline vital signs.
- Connect the client to a cardiac monitor; obtain a baseline rhythm strip for comparison during and after the procedure.
- Connect the precordial ECG lead to the hub of the aspiration needle using an alligator clamp.

**PROCEDURE**
- Follow standard precautions.
- Position seated at a 45- to 60-degree angle. Place a dry towel under the rib cage to catch blood or fluid leakage.

- Observe the ST segment for elevation and the ECG monitor for signs of myocardial irritability (PVCs) during the procedure; these indicate that the needle is touching the myocardium and should be withdrawn slightly.
- Notify the physician of changes in cardiac rhythm, blood pressure, heart rate, level of consciousness, and urine output. These may indicate cardiac complications.
- Monitor central venous pressure (CVP) and blood pressure closely. As the effusion is relieved, CVP will decrease, and BP will increase.

**AFTER THE PROCEDURE**
- Document the procedure and the client's response to and tolerance of the procedure.
- Continue to monitor vital signs and cardiac rhythm every 15 min during the first hour, every 30 min during the next hour, every hour for the next 24 hours.
- Record the amount of fluid removed as output on the intake and output record.
- If indicated, send a sample of aspirated fluid for culture and sensitivity and laboratory analysis.
- Assess heart and breath sounds.

## NURSING CARE

### Health Promotion

While it may not yet be possible to identify many clients at risk for and to prevent acute pericarditis, early identification and treatment of the disorder can reduce the risk of complications. Promptly report a pericardial friction rub or other manifestations of pericarditis in clients with recent AMI, cardiac surgery, or systemic diseases associated with a risk for pericarditis.

### Assessment

Assessment data to collect from the client with suspected pericarditis includes:

- Health history: complaints of acute substernal or precordial chest pain, effect of movement and breathing on discomfort, pain radiation, associated symptoms; recent AMI, heart surgery, or other cardiac disorder; current medications; chronic conditions such as renal failure or a connective tissue or autoimmune disorder
- Physical examination: vital signs including temperature, variation in systolic BP with respirations; strength of peripheral pulses, variations with respiratory movement; apical pulse, clarity, changes with respiratory movement, presence of a friction rub; neck vein distension; level of consciousness, skin color, and other indicators of cardiac output

### Nursing Diagnoses and Interventions

Nursing care for the client with pericarditis may occur in the acute or community setting. Closely observe for early manifestations of increasing effusion or cardiac tamponade. Priority nursing diagnoses relate to comfort, the risk for tamponade, and effects of the acute inflammatory process.

### Acute Pain

Inflamed pericardial layers rubbing against each other and the lung pleura stimulate phrenic nerve pain fibers in the lower portion of the parietal pericardium. Pain is usually acute and may be severe until inflammation resolves.

- Assess chest pain using a standard pain scale and noting the quality and radiation of the pain. Note nonverbal cues of pain (grimacing, guarding behaviors), and validate with the client. *Careful assessment helps identify the cause of pain. The pain of pericarditis may radiate to the neck or back and is aggravated by movement, coughing, or deep breathing. A pain scale allows evaluation of the effectiveness of interventions.*
- Auscultate heart sounds every 4 hours. *Presence of a pericardial friction rub often correlates with the location and severity of the pain.*
- Administer NSAIDs on a regular basis as prescribed with food. Document effectiveness. *NSAIDs reduce fever, inflammation, and pericardial pain. They are most effective when administered around the clock on a consistent basis. Administering the medications with food helps decrease gastric distress.*
- Maintain a quiet, calm environment, and position of comfort. Offer back rubs, heat/cold therapy, diversional activity, and emotional support. *Supportive interventions enhance the effects of the medication, may decrease pain perception, and convey a sense of caring.*

## Ineffective Breathing Pattern

Respiratory movement intensifies pericardial pain. In an effort to decrease pain, the client often breathes shallowly, increasing the risk for pulmonary complications.

**PRACTICE ALERT** *Document respiratory rate, effort, and breath sounds every 2 to 4 hours. Report adventitious or diminished breath sounds. Shallow, guarded respirations may lead to increased respiratory rate and effort. Poor ventilation of peripheral alveoli may lead to congestion or atelectasis.* ■

- Encourage deep breathing and use of the incentive spirometer. Provide pain medication before respiratory therapy, as needed. *Deep breathing and an incentive spirometer promote alveolar ventilation and prevent atelectasis. Analgesia prior to respiratory treatments improves their effectiveness by decreasing guarding.*
- Administer oxygen as needed. *Supplementary oxygen promotes optimal gas exchange and tissue oxygenation.*
- Place in Fowler's or high-Fowler's position. Assist to a position of comfort. *Appropriate positioning reduces the work of breathing and decreases chest pain due to pericarditis.*

## Risk for Decreased Cardiac Output

The acute inflammatory process of pericarditis can lead to significant pericardial effusion and cardiac tamponade. This potentially fatal complication can also occur with chronic pericardial effusion if the amount of fluid exceeds the ability of the pericardial sac to expand. Constrictive pericarditis increases the risk for decreased cardiac output because of restricted cardiac filling.

- Document vital signs hourly during the acute inflammatory processes. *Frequent assessment allows early recognition of manifestations of decreased cardiac output, such as tachycardia, hypotension, or changes in pulse pressure.*

**PRACTICE ALERT** *Assess heart sounds and peripheral pulses, and observe for neck vein distention and paradoxical pulse hourly. Promptly report distant, muffled heart sounds, new murmurs or extra heart sounds, decreasing quality of peripheral pulses, and distended neck veins. Acute pericardial effusion interferes with normal cardiac filling and pumping, causing venous congestion and decreased cardiac output. As the amount of fluid increases in the pericardial sac, heart sounds are obscured. A drop in systolic blood pressure of more than 10 mmHg on inspiration signifies an abnormal response to changes in intrathoracic pressure.* ■

- Report significant changes or trends in hemodynamic parameters and dysrhythmias. *Compression of the heart interferes with venous return, increasing CVP and right atrial pressures; dysrhythmias may also occur.*
- Promptly report other signs of decreased cardiac output: decreased level of consciousness; decreased urine output; cold, clammy, mottled skin; delayed capillary refill; and weak peripheral pulses. *These signs of decreased organ and tissue perfusion indicate a significant drop in cardiac output.*

- Maintain at least one patent intravenous access site. *The client in cardiac tamponade may require rapid intravenous fluid infusion to restore blood volume and administration of emergency drugs to support the circulation.*
- Prepare for emergency pericardiocentesis and/or surgery as necessary. Provide appropriate explanations and reassurance. Observe for adverse responses during pericardiocentesis. *Excess pericardial fluid must be rapidly evacuated to prevent further compromise of cardiac output and death. Emotional support and explanations reduce the client's and family's anxiety and promote a caring atmosphere.*

## Activity Intolerance

In chronic constrictive pericarditis, pericardial adhesions and scarring restrict pericardial compliance, restricting heart filling and movement. Restricted filling and ineffective cardiac contraction decrease the cardiac output. The heart cannot compensate for increased metabolic demands by increasing cardiac output, and cardiac reserve falls significantly.

- Document vital signs, cardiac rhythm, skin color, and temperature before and after activity. Note any subjective complaints of fatigue, shortness of breath, chest pain, palpitations, or other symptoms with activity. *These parameters help determine the response to increased cardiac work. Increased heart rate and respiratory rate and effort, decreased blood pressure, and dysrhythmias are indicators of activity intolerance. Pallor or cyanosis and cool, clammy, mottled skin are signs of decreased tissue perfusion. Complaints of weakness, shortness of breath, fatigue, dizziness, or palpitations are further evidence of activity intolerance.*
- Work with the client and physical therapist to develop a realistic, progressive activity plan. Monitor response. Encourage independence, but provide assistance as needed. *Client involvement in planning increases the likelihood of success, as well as the client's self-esteem and sense of control. Promoting self-care provides additional control and independence and enhances self-image. Activity that significantly increases the heart rate (more than 20 BPM over resting) should be stopped and reassessed for intensity.*
- Plan interventions and care activities to allow uninterrupted rest and sleep. *This supports healing and restoration of physical and emotional health.*

## Using NANDA, NIC, and NOC

Chart 30–2 shows links between NANDA nursing diagnoses, NIC, and NOC for the client with pericarditis.

## Home Care

Include the following topics when teaching the client and family in preparation for home care.

- The importance of continuing anti-inflammatory medications as ordered Advise to take NSAIDs with food, milk, or antacids to minimize gastric distress, and to notify the physician if unable to tolerate the drug. Instruct to avoid aspirin or preparations containing aspirin while taking NSAIDs because it may interfere with activity.

- Prescribed medications, including dose, desired and possible adverse effects, and interactions with other drugs or food
- Monitoring weight twice weekly because NSAIDs may cause fluid retention.
- Maintaining fluid intake of at least 2500 mL per day to minimize the risk of renal toxicity due to NSAID use.

- Measures to maintain activity restriction if ordered. Activity will be gradually increased once the inflammatory process has resolved.
- Manifestations of recurrent pericarditis, and the importance of reporting these manifestations promptly to the physician.

## CHART 30–2  NANDA, NIC, AND NOC LINKAGES

### The Client with Pericarditis

| NURSING DIAGNOSES | NURSING INTERVENTIONS | NURSING OUTCOMES |
| --- | --- | --- |
| • Activity Intolerance | • Energy Management<br>• Nutrition Management<br>• Self-Care Assistance | • Endurance<br>• Energy Conservation<br>• Self-Care: Activities of Daily Living (ADLs) |
| • Acute Pain | • Medication Management<br>• Positioning | • Comfort Level<br>• Pain: Disruptive Effects |
| • Deficient Knowledge | • Teaching: Disease Process<br>• Teaching: Procedure/Treatment | • Knowledge: Disease Process<br>• Knowledge: Treatment Regimen |
| • Risk for Decreased Cardiac Output | • Cardiac Care: Acute<br>• Invasive Hemodynamic Monitoring<br>• Vital Signs Monitoring | • Cardiac Pump Effectiveness<br>• Circulation Status<br>• Vital Signs Status |

Note. Data from Nursing Outcomes Classification (NOC) by M. Johnson & M. Maas (Eds.), 1997, St. Louis: Mosby; Nursing Diagnoses: Definitions & Classification 2001–2002 by North American Nursing Diagnosis Association, 2001, Philadelphia: NANDA; Nursing Interventions Classification (NIC) by J.C. McCloskey & G. M. Bulechek (Eds.), 2000, St. Louis: Mosby. Reprinted by permission.

# DISORDERS OF CARDIAC STRUCTURE

## THE CLIENT WITH VALVULAR HEART DISEASE

Proper heart valve function ensures one-way blood flow through the heart and vascular system. **Valvular heart disease** interferes with blood flow to and from the heart. Acquired valvular disorders can result from acute conditions, such as infective endocarditis, or from chronic conditions, such as rheumatic heart disease. Rheumatic heart disease is the most common cause of valvular disease (McCance & Huether, 2002). Acute myocardial infarction also can damage heart valves, causing tearing, ischemia, or damage to the papillary muscles that affects valve leaflet function. Congenital heart defects may affect the heart valves, often with no manifestations until adulthood. Aging affects heart structure and function, and also increases the risk for valvular disease.

## PHYSIOLOGY REVIEW

The heart valves direct blood flow within and out of the heart. The valves are fibroelastic tissue supported by a ring of fibrous tissue (the annulus) which provides support.

The atrioventricular (AV) valves, the **mitral** (or *bicuspid*) **valve** on the left and the **tricuspid valve** on the right, separate the atria from the ventricles. These valves normally are fully open during diastole, allowing blood to flow freely from the atria into the ventricles. Rising pressure within the ventricles at the onset of systole (contraction) closes the AV valves, creating the $S_1$ heart sound ("lub"). The leaflets of the AV valves are connected to ventricular papillary muscles by fibrous *chordae tendineae*. The chordae tendineae prevent the valve leaflets from bulging back into the atria during systole.

The semilunar valves, the **aortic** and **pulmonic valves,** separate the ventricles from the great vessels. They open during systole, allowing blood to flow out of the heart with ventricular contraction. As the ventricle relaxes and intraventricular pressure falls at the beginning of diastole, the higher pressure within the great vessels (the aorta and pulmonary artery) closes these valves, creating the $S_2$ heart sound ("dup").

## PATHOPHYSIOLOGY AND MANIFESTATIONS

Valvular heart disease occurs as two major types of disorders: stenosis and regurgitation. **Stenosis** occurs when valve leaflets fuse together and cannot fully open or close. The valve open-

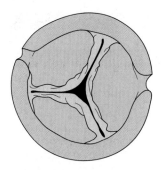 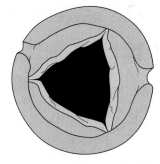

**A.** Thickened and stenotic valve leaflets

**B.** Retracted fibrosed valve openings

**Figure 30–7** ■ Valvular heart disorders. *A,* Stenosis of a heart valve. *B,* An incompetent or regurgitant heart valve.

ing narrows and becomes rigid (Figure 30–7A ■). Scarring of the valves from endocarditis or infarction, and calcium deposits can lead to stenosis. Stenotic valves impede the forward flow of blood, decreasing cardiac output because of impaired ventricular filling or ejection and stroke volume. Because stenotic valves also do not close completely, some backflow of blood occurs when the valve should be fully closed.

Regurgitant valves (also called *insufficient* or *incompetent* valves) do not close completely (Figure 30–7B). This allows **regurgitation,** or backflow of blood, through the valve into the area it just left. Regurgitation can result from deformity or erosion of valve cusps caused by the vegetative lesions of bacterial endocarditis, by scarring or tearing from myocardial infarction, or by cardiac dilation. As the heart enlarges, the valve *annulus* (supporting ring of the valve) is stretched, and the valve edges no longer meet to allow complete closure.

Valvular disease causes hemodynamic changes both in front of and behind the affected valve. Blood volume and pressures are reduced in front of the valve, because flow is obstructed through a stenotic valve and backflow occurs through a regurgitant valve. By contrast, volumes and pressures characteristically increase behind the diseased valve. These hemodynamic changes may lead to pulmonary complications or heart failure. Higher pressures and compensatory changes to maintain cardiac output lead to remodeling and hypertrophy of the heart muscle.

Stenosis increases the work of the chamber behind the affected valve as the heart attempts to move blood through the narrowed opening. Excess blood volume behind regurgitant valves causes dilation of the chamber. In mitral stenosis, for example, the left atrium hypertrophies to generate enough pressure to open and deliver its blood through the narrowed mitral valve. Not all of the blood is delivered before the valve closes, leaving blood to accumulate in the left atrium. This chamber dilates to accommodate the excess volume.

Eventually, cardiac output falls as compensatory mechanisms become less effective. The normal balance of oxygen supply and demand is upset, and the heart begins to fail. In-creased muscle mass and size increase myocardial oxygen consumption. The size and workload of the heart exceed its blood supply, causing ischemia and chest pain. Eventually, necrosis occurs and functional muscle is lost. Contractile force, stroke volume, and cardiac output decrease. High pressures on the left side of the heart are reflected backward into the pulmonary system, causing pulmonary edema, pulmonary hypertension, and, eventually, right ventricular failure.

Valvular disorders interfere with the smooth flow of blood through the heart. The flow becomes turbulent, causing a **murmur,** a characteristic manifestation of valvular disease. Table 30–7 describes the murmurs associated with various types of valvular disorders.

Blood forced through the narrowed opening of a stenotic valve or regurgitated from a higher pressure chamber through an incompetent valve creates a jet stream effect (much like water spurting out of a partially occluded hose opening). The physical force of this jet stream damages the endocardium of the receiving chamber, increasing the risk for infective endocarditis.

The higher pressures on the left side of the heart subject its valves (the mitral and aortic valves) to more stress and damage than those on the right side of the heart (the tricuspid and pulmonic). Pulmonic valve disease is the least common of the valvular disorders.

## Mitral Stenosis

*Mitral stenosis* narrows the mitral valve, obstructing blood flow from the left atrium into the left ventricle during diastole. It is usually caused by rheumatic heart disease or bacterial endocarditis; it rarely results from congenital defects. It affects females more frequently (66%) than males (Braunwald et al., 2001). Mitral stenosis is chronic and progressive.

In mitral valve stenosis, fibrous tissue replaces normal valve tissue, causing valve leaflets to stiffen and fuse. Resulting changes in blood flow through the valve lead to calcification of the valve leaflets. As calcium is deposited in and on the valve, the leaflets become more rigid and narrow the opening further. As the valve leaflets become less mobile, the chordae tendineae fuse, thicken, and shorten. Thromboemboli may form on the calcified leaflets.

The narrowed mitral opening impairs blood flow into the left ventricle, reducing end-diastolic volume and pressure, and decreasing stroke volume. The narrowed opening also forces the left atrium to generate higher pressure to deliver blood to the left ventricle. This leads to left atrial hypertrophy. The left atrium also dilates as obstructed blood flow increases its volume. As the resistance to blood flow increases, high atrial pressures are reflected back into the pulmonary vessels, increasing pulmonary pressures (Figure 30–8 ■). Pulmonary hypertension increases the workload of the right ventricle, causing it to dilate and hypertrophy. Eventually, heart failure occurs.

Mitral stenosis may be asymptomatic or cause severe impairment. Its manifestations depend on cardiac output and

TABLE 30-7  Heart Murmurs Timing and Characteristics

| Murmur | Cardiac Cycle Timing | Auscultation Site | Configuration of Sound | Continuity |
|---|---|---|---|---|
| Mitral stenosis | Diastole | Apical | $S_2$ ... $S_1$ | Rumble that increases in sound toward the end, continuous |
| Mitral regurgitation | Systole | Apex | $S_1$ ... $S_2$ | Holosystolic (occurs throughout systole), continuous |
| Aortic stenosis | Midsystolic | Right sternal border (RSB) 2nd intercostal space (ICS) | $S_1$ ... $S_2$ | Crescendo-decrescendo, continuous |
| Aortic regurgitation | Diastole (early) | 3rd ICS, LSB | $S_2$ ... $S_1$ | Decrescendo, continuous |
| Tricuspid stenosis | Diastole | Lower LSB | $S_2$ ... $S_1$ | Rumble that increases in sound toward the end, continuous |
| Tricuspid regurgitation | Systole | 4th ICS, LSB | $S_1$ ... $S_2$ | Holosystolic, continuous |

pulmonary vascular pressures. Dyspnea on exertion (DOE) is typically the earliest manifestation. Others include cough, hemoptysis, frequent pulmonary infections such as bronchitis and pneumonia, paroxysmal nocturnal dyspnea, orthopnea, weakness, fatigue, and palpitations. As the stenosis worsens, manifestations of right heart failure, including jugular venous distension, hepatomegaly, ascites, and peripheral edema develop. Crackles may be heard in the lung bases. In severe mitral stenosis, cyanosis of the face and extremities may be noted. Chest pain is rare but may occur.

On auscultation, a loud $S_1$, a split $S_2$, and a mitral opening snap may be heard. The opening snap reflects high left atrial pressure. The murmur of mitral stenosis occurs during diastole, and is typically low-pitched, rumbling, crescendo-decrescendo. It is heard best with the bell of the stethoscope in the apical region. It may be accompanied by a palpable thrill (vibration).

Atrial dysrhythmias, particularly atrial fibrillation, are common due to chronic atrial distention. Thrombi may form and subsequently embolize to the brain, coronary arteries, kidneys, spleen, and extremities—potentially devastating complications.

Women with mitral stenosis may be asymptomatic until pregnancy. As the heart tries to compensate for increased circulating volume (30% more in pregnancy) by increasing cardiac output, left atrial pressures rise, tachycardia reduces ventricular filling and stroke volume, and pulmonary pressures increase. Sudden pulmonary edema and heart failure may threaten the lives of the mother and fetus.

## Mitral Regurgitation

*Mitral regurgitation* or *insufficiency* allows blood to flow back into the left atrium during systole because the valve does not close fully. Rheumatic heart disease is a common cause of mitral regurgitation. Men develop mitral regurgitation more frequently than women. Degenerative calcification of the mitral annulus may cause mitral regurgitation in older women. Processes that dilate the mitral annulus or affect the supporting structures, papillary muscles, or the chordae tendineae may cause mitral regurgitation (e.g., left ventricular hypertrophy and MI). Congenital defects also may cause mitral regurgitation.

In mitral regurgitation, blood flows into both the systemic circulation and back into the left atrium through the deformed valve during systole. This increases left atrial volume (Figure 30-9 ■). The left atrium dilates to accommodate its extra volume, pulling the posterior valve leaflet further away from the valve opening and worsening the defect. The left ventricle dilates to accommodate its increased preload and low cardiac output, further aggravating the problem.

Mitral regurgitation may be asymptomatic or cause symptoms such as fatigue, weakness, exertional dyspnea, and orthopnea. In severe or acute regurgitation, manifestations of left-sided heart failure develop, including pulmonary congestion and edema. High pulmonary pressures may lead to manifestations of right-sided heart failure.

The murmur of mitral regurgitation is usually loud, high pitched, rumbling, and holosystolic (occurring throughout sys-

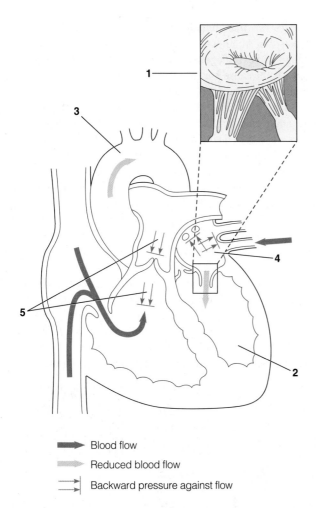

Blood flow

Reduced blood flow

Backward pressure against flow

**Figure 30–8** ■ Mitral stenosis. Narrowing of the mitral valve orifice (1), reduces blood volume to left ventricle (2), reducing cardiac output (3). Rising pressure in the left atrium (4) causes left atrial hypertrophy and pulmonary congestion. Increased pressure in pulmonary vessels (5), causes hypertrophy of the right ventricle and right atrium.

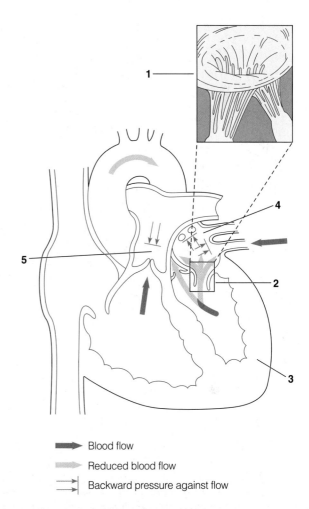

Blood flow

Reduced blood flow

Backward pressure against flow

**Figure 30–9** ■ Mitral regurgitation. The mitral valve closes incompletely (1), allowing blood to regurgitate during systole from the left ventricle to the left atrium (2). Cardiac output falls; to compensate, the left ventricle hypertrophies (3). Rising left atrial pressure (4) causes left atrial hypertrophy and pulmonary congestion. Elevated pulmonary artery pressure (5) causes slight enlargement of the right ventricle.

tole). It is often accompanied by a palpable thrill and is heard most clearly at the cardiac apex. It may be characterized as a cooing or gull-like sound or have a musical quality (Braunwald et al., 2001).

## Mitral Valve Prolapse

*Mitral valve prolapse (MVP)* is a type of mitral insufficiency that occurs when one or both mitral valve cusps billow into the atrium during ventricular systole. MVP is more common in young women between ages 14 and 30; its incidence declines with age. Its cause often is unclear. It also can result from acute or chronic rheumatic damage, ischemic heart disease, or other cardiac disorders. It commonly affects people with inherited connective tissue disorders such as Marfan syndrome (see the Meeting Individual Needs box to the right). Mitral valve prolapse usually is benign, but about 0.01% to 0.02% of people with MVP have thickened mitral leaflets and a significant risk of morbidity and sudden death.

### Meeting Individualized Needs

#### CLIENTS WITH MARFAN SYNDROME

Marfan syndrome is a genetic (autosomal dominant) connective tissue disorder that affects the skeleton, eyes, and cardiovascular system. Skeletal characteristics include a long, thin body, with long extremities and long, tapering fingers, sometimes called *arachnodactyly* (spider fingers) (Copstead & Banasik, 2000). Joints are hyperextensible, and skeletal deformities such as kyphosis, scoliosis, pigeon chest, or pectus excavatum are common. The potentially life-threatening cardiovascular effects of Marfan syndrome include mitral valve prolapse, progressive dilation of the aortic valve ring, and weakness of arterial walls. People with Marfan syndrome frequently die young, between 30 and 40 years, often due to dissection and rupture of the aorta (Porth, 2002).

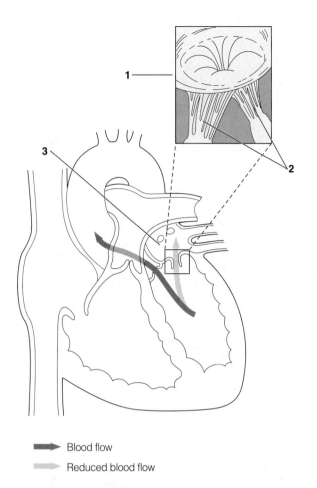

Blood flow

Reduced blood flow

**Figure 30–10** ■ Mitral valve prolapse. Excess tissue in the valve leaflets (1) and elongated cordae tendineae (2) impair mitral valve closure during systole. Some ventricular blood regurgitates into the left atrium (3).

Excess collagen tissue in the valve leaflets and elongated cordae tendineae impair closure of the mitral valve, allowing the leaflets to billow into the left atrium during systole. Some ventricular blood volume regurgitates into the left atrium (Figure 30–10 ■).

Mitral valve prolapse usually is asymptomatic. A midsystolic ejection click or murmur may be audible. A high-pitched late systolic murmur, sometimes described as a "whoop" or "honk," due to the regurgitation of blood through the valve, may develop in MVP. Atypical chest pain is the most common symptom of MVP. It may be left sided or substernal, and is frequently related to fatigue, not exertion. Tachydysrhythmias may develop with MVP, causing palpitations, lightheadedness, and syncope. Increased sympathetic nervous system tone may cause a sense of anxiety (Woods et al., 2000).

Mitral valve prolapse increases the risk for bacterial endocarditis. Progressive worsening of regurgitation can lead to heart failure. Thrombi may form on prolapsed valve leaflets; embolization may cause transient ischemic attacks (TIAs).

## Aortic Stenosis

*Aortic stenosis* obstructs blood flow from the left ventricle into the aorta during systole. Aortic stenosis is more common in

males (80%) than females (Braunwald et al., 2001). Aortic stenosis may be idiopathic, or due to a congenital defect, rheumatic damage, or degenerative changes. When rheumatic heart disease is the cause, mitral valve deformity is also often present. Rheumatic heart disease destroys aortic valve leaflets, with fibrosis and calcification causing rigidity and scarring. In the older adult, calcific aortic stenosis may result from degenerative changes associated with aging. Constant "wear and tear" on this valve can lead to fibrosis and calcification. Idiopathic calcific stenosis generally is mild and does not impair cardiac output.

As aortic stenosis progresses, the valve annulus decreases in size, increasing the work of the left ventricle to eject its volume through the narrowed opening into the aorta. To compensate, the ventricle hypertrophies to maintain an adequate stroke volume and cardiac output (Figure 30–11 ■). Left ventricular compliance also decreases. The additional workload increases myocardial oxygen consumption, which can precipitate myocardial ischemia. Coronary blood flow may also decrease in aortic stenosis. As left ventricular end-diastolic pressure increases because of reduced stroke volume, left atrial pressures increase. These pressures also affect the pulmonary vascular system; pulmonary vascular congestion and pulmonary edema may result.

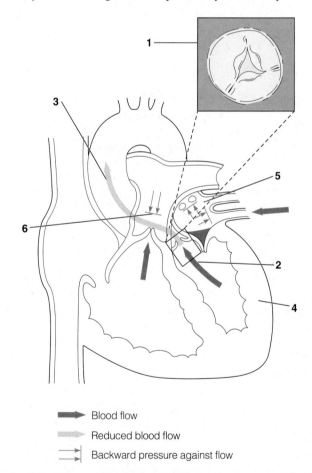

Blood flow

Reduced blood flow

Backward pressure against flow

**Figure 30–11** ■ Aortic stenosis. The narrowed aortic valve orifice (1), decreases the left ventricular ejection fraction during systole (2), and cardiac output (3). The left ventricle hypertrophies (4). Incomplete emptying of left atrium (5) causes backward pressure through pulmonary veins and pulmonary hypertension. Elevated pulmonary artery pressure (6) causes right ventricular strain.

Aortic stenosis may be asymptomatic for many years. As the disease progresses and compensation fails, usually between age 50 and 70 years, obstructed cardiac output causes manifestations of left ventricular failure. Dyspnea on exertion, angina pectoris, and exertional syncope are classic manifestations of aortic stenosis. Pulse pressure, an indicator of stroke volume, narrows to 30 mmHg or less. Hemodynamic monitors show increased left atrial pressure and pulmonary artery wedge pressure, as well as decreased stroke volume and cardiac output.

Aortic stenosis produces a harsh systolic murmur best heard in the second intercostal space to the right of the sternum. This crescendo-decrescendo murmur is produced by turbulence of blood entering the aorta through the stenotic valve. A palpable thrill is often felt. The murmur may radiate to the carotid arteries. Ventricular hypertrophy displaces the cardiac impulse to the left of the midclavicular line. As aortic stenosis progresses, $S_3$ and $S_4$ heart sounds may be heard, indicating heart failure and reduced left ventricular compliance.

As cardiac output falls, tissue perfusion decreases. Late in the disease, pulmonary hypertension and right ventricular failure develop. Untreated, symptomatic aortic stenosis has a poor prognosis; 10% to 20% of these clients experience sudden cardiac death (Braunwald et al., 2001).

## Aortic Regurgitation

*Aortic regurgitation,* also called *aortic insufficiency,* allows blood to flow back into the left ventricle from the aorta during diastole. It is more common in males (75%) in its "pure" form; in females, it is commonly associated with coexisting mitral valve disease. Most aortic regurgitation (67%) results from rheumatic heart disease (Braunwald et al., 2001). Other causes include congenital disorders, infective endocarditis, blunt chest trauma, aortic aneurysm, syphilis, Marfan syndrome, and chronic hypertension.

In aortic regurgitation, thickened and contracted valve cusps, scarring, fibrosis, and calcification impede complete valve closure. Chronic hypertension and aortic aneurysm may dilate and stretch the aortic valve opening, increasing the degree of regurgitation.

In aortic regurgitation, volume overload affects the left ventricle as blood from the aorta adds to blood received from the atrium during diastole. This increases diastolic left ventricular pressure. Increased preload causes more forceful contractions and a high stroke volume (Figure 30–12 ■). With time, muscle cells hypertrophy to compensate for increased cardiac work and afterload; eventually this hypertrophy compromises cardiac output and increases regurgitation.

High left-ventricular pressures increase left atrial workload and pressure. This pressure is transmitted to the pulmonary vessels causing pulmonary congestion. The workload of the right ventricle increases as a result, and right-sided heart failure may develop. Acute aortic regurgitation from traumatic injury or infective endocarditis causes a rapid decline in hemodynamic status from acute heart failure and pulmonary edema, because compensatory mechanisms do not have time to develop.

Aortic regurgitation may be asymptomatic for many years, even when severe. The increased stroke volume may cause

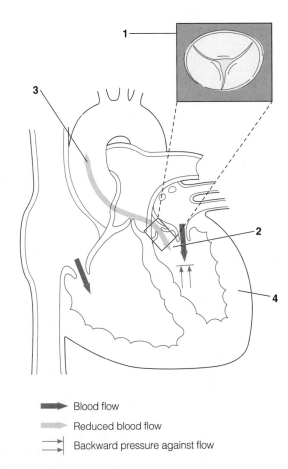

Blood flow

Reduced blood flow

Backward pressure against flow

**Figure 30–12** ■ Aortic regurgitation. The cusps of the aortic valve widen and fail to close during diastole (1). Blood regurgitates from the aorta into the left ventricle (2) increasing left ventricular volume and decreasing cardiac output (3). The left ventricle dilates and hypertrophies (4) in response to the increase in blood volume and workload.

complaints of persistent palpitations, especially when recumbent. A throbbing pulse may be visible in arteries of the neck; the force of contraction may cause a characteristic head bob (Musset's sign) and shake the whole body. Other symptoms include dizziness, and exercise intolerance.

Fatigue, exertional dyspnea, orthopnea, and paroxysmal nocturnal dyspnea are common in aortic regurgitation. Anginal pain may result from excessive cardiac work and decreased coronary perfusion. Unlike CAD, angina often occurs at night and may not respond to conventional therapy.

The murmur of aortic regurgitation is heard during diastole as blood flows back into the left ventricle from the aorta. It is a "blowing," high-pitched sound heard most clearly at the third left intercostal space. A palpable thrill and ventricular heave may be noted. An $S_3$ and $S_4$ may be heard as the heart fails and ventricular compliance diminishes. The apical impulse is displaced to the left.

High systolic and low diastolic pressures cause a widened pulse pressure. The arterial pressure waveform has a rapid upstroke and quickly collapsing downstroke, known as a *water-hammer pulse.* It is caused by the force of rapid and early delivery of the stroke volume into the aorta.

## Tricuspid Valve Disorders

*Tricuspid stenosis* obstructs blood flow from the right atrium to the right ventricle. It usually results from rheumatic heart disease; mitral stenosis often occurs concurrently with tricuspid stenosis.

Fibrosed, retracted tricuspid valve cusps and fused leaflets narrow the valve orifice and prevent complete closure. Right ventricular filling is impaired during diastole, and during systole, some blood regurgitates back into the right atrium. Pressure in the right atrium increases, and it enlarges in response to the increased pressure and workload. This increased right atrial pressure is reflected backward into the systemic circulation. Right ventricular stroke volume decreases, reducing the volume delivered to the pulmonary system and left heart. Stroke volume, cardiac output, and tissue perfusion fall.

Manifestations of tricuspid stenosis relate to systemic congestion and right-sided heart failure. They include increased central venous pressure, jugular venous distention, ascites, hepatomegaly, and peripheral edema. Low cardiac output causes fatigue and weakness. The low-pitched, rumbling diastolic murmur of tricuspid stenosis is most clearly heard in the fourth intercostal space at the left sternal border or over the xiphoid process.

*Tricuspid regurgitation* usually occurs secondarily to right ventricular dilation. Stretching distorts the valve and its supporting structures, preventing complete valve closure. Left ventricular failure is the usual cause of right ventricular overload; pulmonary hypertension is another cause. The valve may also be damaged by rheumatic heart disease, infective endocarditis, inferior MI, trauma, or other conditions.

Tricuspid regurgitation allows blood to flow back into the right atrium during systole, increasing right atrial pressures. Increased right atrial pressure causes manifestations of right-sided heart failure, including systemic venous congestion and low cardiac output. Atrial fibrillation due to atrial distention is common. The retrograde flow of blood over the deformed tricuspid valve causes a high-pitched, blowing systolic murmur heard over the tricuspid or xiphoid area.

## Pulmonic Valve Disorders

*Pulmonic stenosis* obstructs blood flow from the right ventricle into the pulmonary system. It usually is a congenital disorder, although rheumatic heart disease or cancer also may cause pulmonic stenosis. The right ventricle hypertrophies to generate the pressure needed to pump blood into the pulmonary system. The right atrium also hypertrophies to overcome the high pressures generated in the right ventricle. Right-sided heart failure occurs when the ventricle can no longer generate adequate pressure to force blood past the narrowed valve opening.

Pulmonic stenosis typically is asymptomatic unless severe. Dyspnea on exertion and fatigue are early signs. As the condition progresses, right-sided heart failure develops, with peripheral edema, ascites, hepatomegaly, and increased venous pressures. Turbulent blood flow caused by the narrowed valve generates a harsh, systolic crescendo-decrescendo murmur heard in the pulmonic area, the second left intercostal space.

*Pulmonic regurgitation* is more common than pulmonary stenosis. It is a complication of pulmonary hypertension, which stretches and dilates the pulmonary orifice, causing incomplete valve closure. Infective endocarditis, pulmonary artery aneurysm, and syphilis also may cause pulmonic regurgitation.

Incomplete valve closure allows blood to flow back into the right ventricle during diastole, decreasing blood flow to the pulmonary circuit. The extra blood increases right ventricular end-diastolic volume. When the ventricle can no longer compensate for the increased volume, right-sided heart failure develops. The murmur of pulmonic regurgitation is a high-pitched, decrescendo, blowing sound heard along the left sternal border during diastole.

## COLLABORATIVE CARE

A heart murmur identified during routine physical examination often is the initial indication of valvular disease. If no symptoms are present, close observation for disease progression and prophylactic therapy to prevent infection of the diseased heart may be the only treatment.

Manifestations of heart failure are treated with diet and medications (see the preceding section on heart failure). When medical management is no longer effective, surgery is considered.

### Diagnostic Tests

The following diagnostic tests help to identify and diagnose valvular disease.

- *Echocardiography* is used routinely to diagnose valvular disease. Thickened valve leaflets, vegetations or growths on valve leaflets, myocardial function, and chamber size can be determined, and pressure gradients across valves and pulmonary artery pressures can be estimated. Either transthoracic or transesophageal echocardiography may be used.
- *Chest X-ray* can identify cardiac hypertrophy, chamber and great vessel enlargement, and dilation of the pulmonary vasculature. Calcification of the valve leaflets and annular openings may also be visible.
- *Electrocardiography* can demonstrate atrial and ventricular hypertrophy, conduction defects, and dysrhythmias associated with valvular disease.
- *Cardiac catheterization* may be used to assess contractility and to determine the pressure gradients across the heart valves, in the heart chambers, and in the pulmonary system.

### Medications

Heart failure resulting from valvular disease is treated with diuretics, ACE inhibitors, vasodilators, and possibly digitalis glycosides. Digitalis increases the force of myocardial contraction to maintain cardiac output. Diuretics, ACE inhibitors, and vasodilators reduce preload and afterload. (See the Medication Administration box on page 879).

In clients with valvular disorders, atrial distention often causes atrial fibrillation. Digitalis or small doses of beta blockers are given to slow the ventricular response (see Chapter 29 for more information about atrial fibrillation and its treatment). Anticoagulant therapy is added to prevent clot and embolus formation, a common complication of atrial fibrillation as blood pools in the noncontracting atria. Anticoagulant therapy also is required following insertion of a mechanical heart valve. See Chapter 33 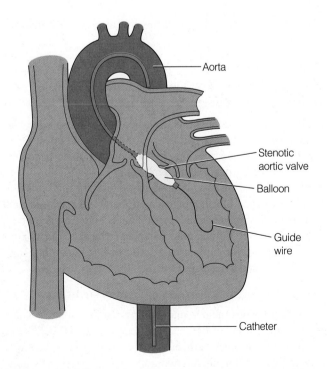 for more information about anticoagulant therapy.

Valvular damage increases the risk for infective endocarditis as altered blood flow allows bacterial colonization. Antibiotics are prescribed prophylactically prior to any dental work, invasive procedures, or surgery to minimize the risk of bacteremia (bacteria in the blood) and subsequent endocarditis.

## Percutaneous Balloon Valvuloplasty

*Percutaneous balloon valvuloplasty* is an invasive procedure performed in the cardiac catheterization laboratory. A balloon catheter similar to that used in coronary angioplasty procedures is inserted into the femoral vein or artery. Guided by fluoroscopy, the catheter is advanced into the heart and positioned with the balloon straddling the stenotic valve. The balloon is then inflated for approximately 90 seconds to divide the fused leaflets and enlarge the valve orifice (Figure 30–13 ■). Balloon valvuloplasty is the treatment of choice for symptomatic mitral valve stenosis. It is used to treat children and young adults with aortic stenosis, and may be indicated for older adults who are poor surgical risks, and as a "bridge to surgery" when heart function is severely compromised (Braunwald et al., 2001). Nursing care of the client with a balloon valvuloplasty is similar to that of the client following coronary revascularization (see page 820).

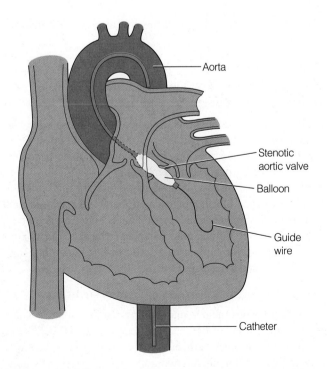

**Figure 30–13** ■ Balloon valvuloplasty. The balloon catheter is guided into position straddling the stenosed valve. The balloon is then inflated to increase the size of the valve opening.

*Labels: Aorta; Stenotic aortic valve; Balloon; Guide wire; Catheter*

## Surgery

Surgery to repair or replace the diseased valve may be done to restore valve function, alleviate symptoms, and prevent complications and death. Ideally, diseased valves are repaired or replaced before cardiopulmonary function is severely compromised. The diseased valve is repaired when possible, because the risk for surgical mortality and complications is lower than with valve replacement.

### Reconstructive Surgery

*Valvuloplasty* is a general term for reconstruction or repair of a heart valve. Methods include "patching" the perforated portion of the leaflet, resecting excess tissue, debriding vegetations or calcification, and other techniques. Valvuloplasty may be used for stenotic or regurgitant mitral and tricuspid valves, mitral valve prolapse, and aortic stenosis. Common valvuloplasty procedures include the following:

- *Open commissurotomy,* surgical division of fused valve leaflets, is done to open stenotic valves. Fused commissures (junctions between valve leaflets or cusps) are incised, and calcium deposits are debrided as needed.
- *Annuloplasty* repairs a narrowed or an enlarged or dilated valve annulus, the supporting ring of the valve. A prosthetic ring may be used to resize the opening, or stitches and purse-string sutures may be used to reduce and gather excess tissue. Annuloplasty may be used for either stenotic or regurgitant valves.

### Valve Replacement

Valve replacement is indicated when manifestations of valve dysfunction develop, preferably before left heart function is seriously impaired. In general, three factors determine the outcome of valve replacement surgery: (1) heart function at the time of surgery: (2) intraoperative and postoperative care, and (3) characteristics and durability of the replacement valve.

Many different prosthetic heart valves are available, including mechanical and biologic tissue valves. Selection depends on the valve hemodynamics, resistance to clot formation, ease of insertion, anatomic suitability, and client acceptance (Meeker & Rothrock, 1999). The client's age, underlying condition, and contraindications to anticoagulation (such as a desire to become pregnant) also are considered in selecting the appropriate prosthesis. Table 30–8 lists the advantages and disadvantages of biologic and mechanical valves.

Biologic tissue valves may be *heterografts,* excised from a pig (Figure 30–14A ■) or made of calf pericardium, or *homografts* from a human (obtained from a cadaver or during heart transplant). Biologic valves allow more normal blood flow and have a low risk of thrombus formation. As a result, long-term anticoagulation rarely is necessary. They are less durable, however, than mechanical valves. Up to 50% of biologic valves must be replaced by 15 years.

Mechanical prosthetic valves have the major advantage of long-term durability. These valves are frequently used when life expectancy exceeds 10 years. Their major disadvantage is the need for lifetime anticoagulation to prevent the development of clots on the valve.

TABLE 30–8    Advantages and Disadvantages of Prosthetic Heart Valves

| Category | Types | Advantages | Disadvantages |
|---|---|---|---|
| Mechanical valves | Ball-and-cage<br>Tilting disc | Long-term durability<br>Good hemodynamics | Lifetime anticoagulation<br>Audible click<br>Risk of thromboembolism<br>Infections are harder to treat |
| Biologic tissue valves | Porcine heterograft<br>Bovine heterograft<br>Human aortic homograft | Low incidence of<br>  thromboembolism<br>No long-term anticoagulation<br>Good hemodynamics<br>Quiet<br>Infections are easier to treat | Prone to deterioration<br>Frequent replacement is<br>  required |

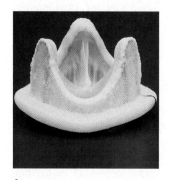
A

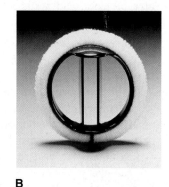
B

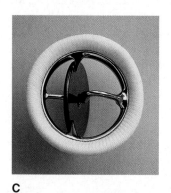
C

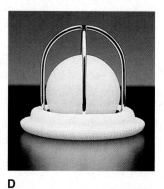
D

**Figure 30–14** ■ Prosthetic heart valves. *A,* Carpentier-Edwards porcine xenograft. *B,* St. Jude Medical valve. *C,* Medtronic Hall prosthetic valve. *D,* Starr-Edwards prosthetic valve.

*Courtesy of Baxter (A and D); St. Jude Medical (B); and Medtronics, Inc. (C).*

Most mechanical valves are either a tilting disk or a ball and cage design (Figures 30–14B, C, and D). The tilting-disc valve designs are frequently used because they have a lower profile than the caged-ball types, allowing blood to flow through the valve with less obstruction. The St. Jude bileaflet design has good hemodynamics and low risk for clot formation. Both biologic and mechanical valves increase the risk of endocarditis, although its incidence is fairly low.

## NURSING CARE

### Health Promotion

Preventing rheumatic heart disease is a key element in preventing heart valve disorders. Rheumatic heart disease is a consequence of rheumatic fever (see the previous section of this chapter), an immune process that may be a sequela to β-hemolytic streptococcal infection of the pharynx (strep throat). Early treatment of strep throat prevents rheumatic fever. Teach individual clients, families, and communities about the importance of timely and effective treatment of strep throat. Emphasize the importance of completing the full prescription of antibiotics to prevent development of resistant bacteria. Prophylactic antibiotic therapy before invasive procedures to prevent infectious endocarditis is an important health promotion measure for clients with preexisting heart disease.

### Assessment

Assessment data related to valvular heart disease includes the following:

- Health history: complaints of decreasing exercise tolerance, dyspnea on exertion, palpitations; history of frequent respiratory infections; previous history of rheumatic heart disease, endocarditis, or a heart murmur
- Physical examination: vital signs; skin color and temperature, evidence of clubbing or peripheral edema; neck vein distention; breath sounds; heart sounds and presence of $S_3$, $S_4$, or murmur; timing, grade, and characteristics of any murmur; palpate for cardiac heave and thrills; abdominal contour, liver and spleen size

### Nursing Diagnoses and Interventions

Nursing priorities include maintaining cardiac output, managing manifestations of the disorder, teaching about the disease process and its management, and preventing complications. Nursing care of the client undergoing valve surgery is similar to that of the client having other types of open-heart surgery (see page 823), with increased attention to anticoagulation and preventing endocarditis.

## Decreased Cardiac Output

Nearly all valve disorders affect ventricular filling and/or emptying, reducing cardiac output. Stenosis of the AV valves impairs ventricular filling and increases atrial pressures. Regurgitation of these valves reduces cardiac output as a portion of the blood in the ventricle regurgitates into the atria during systole. Stenosis of the semilunar valves obstructs ventricular outflow to the great vessels; regurgitation allows blood to flow back into the ventricles, creating higher filling pressures. When compensatory measures fail, heart failure develops.

- Monitor vital signs and hemodynamic parameters, reporting changes from the baseline. *A fall in systolic blood pressure and tachycardia may indicate decreased cardiac output. Increasing pulmonary artery and pulmonary wedge pressures may also indicate decreased cardiac output, causing increased congestion and pressure in the pulmonary vascular system.*

**PRACTICE ALERT** *Promptly report changes in level of consciousness; distended neck veins; dyspnea or respiratory crackles; urine output less than 30 mL/h; cool, clammy, or cyanotic skin; diminished peripheral pulses; or slow capillary refill. These findings indicate decreased cardiac output and impaired tissue and organ perfusion.* ▪

- Monitor intake and output; weigh daily. Report weight gain of 3 to 5 lb within 24 hours. *Fluid retention is a compensatory mechanism that occurs when cardiac output decreases; 2.2 lb (1 kg) of weight equals 1 L of fluid.*
- Restrict fluids as ordered. *Fluid intake may be restricted to reduce cardiac workload and pressures within the heart and pulmonary circuit.*
- Monitor oxygen saturation continuously and arterial blood gases as ordered. Report oxygen saturation less than 95% (or as specified) and abnormal ABG results. *Oxygen saturation levels and ABGs allow assessment of oxygenation.*
- Elevate the head of the bed. Administer supplemental oxygen as ordered. *These measures improve alveolar ventilation and oxygenation.*
- Provide for physical, emotional, and mental rest. *Physical and psychologic rest decreases the cardiac workload.*
- Administer prescribed medications as ordered to reduce cardiac workload. *Diuretics, ACE inhibitors, and direct vasodilators may be prescribed to reduce fluid volume and afterload, reducing cardiac work.*

## Activity Intolerance

Altered blood flow through the heart impairs delivery of oxygen and nutrients to the tissues. As the heart muscle fails and is unable to compensate for altered blood flow, tissue perfusion is further compromised. Dyspnea on exertion is often an early symptom of valvular disease.

- Monitor vital signs before and during activities. *A change in heart rate of more than 20 BPM, a change of 20 mmHg or more in systolic BP, and complaints of dyspnea, shortness of breath, excessive fatigue, chest pain, diaphoresis, dizziness, or syncope may indicate activity intolerance.*

- Encourage self-care and gradually increasing activities as allowed and tolerated. Provide for rest periods, uninterrupted sleep, and adequate nutritional intake. *Gradual progression of activities avoids excessive cardiac stress. Encouraging self-care increases the client's self-esteem and sense of power. Adequate rest and nutrition facilitate healing, decrease fatigue, and increase energy reserves.*
- Provide assistance as needed. Suggest use of a shower chair, sitting while brushing hair or teeth, and other energy-saving measures. *Reducing energy expenditure helps maintain a balance of oxygen supply and demand.*
- Consult with cardiac rehabilitation specialist or physical therapist for in-bed exercises and an activity plan. *In-bed exercises may help improve strength.*
- Discuss ways to conserve energy at home. *Information provides practical ways to deal with activity limitations and empowers the client to manage these limitations.*

## Risk for Infection

Damaged and deformed valve leaflets and turbulent blood flow through the heart significantly increase the risk of infective endocarditis. Invasive diagnostic and monitoring lines (e.g., cardiac catheterization, hemodynamic monitoring) and disrupted skin with surgery also increase the risk of infection.

- Use aseptic technique for all invasive procedures. *Invasive procedures breach the body's protective mechanisms, potentially allowing bacteria to enter. Aseptic technique reduces this risk.*

**PRACTICE ALERT** *Record temperature every 4 hours; notify physician if temperature exceeds 100.5°F (38.5°C). Fever may be an early indication of infection.* ▪

- Assess wounds and catheter sites for redness, swelling, warmth, pain, or evidence of drainage. *These signs of inflammation may signal infection.*
- Administer antibiotics as ordered. Ensure completion of the full course. *Antibiotics are used to prevent and treat infection. Completion of the full course of therapy prevents drug-resistant organisms from multiplying.*
- Monitor WBC and differential. Notify physician of leukocytosis or leukopenia. *A high WBC and increased percentage of immature WBCs (bands) may indicate bacterial infection; a low WBC count may indicate an impaired immune response and increased susceptibility to infection.*

## Ineffective Protection

Anticoagulant therapy commonly is prescribed for clients with chronic atrial fibrillation, a history of emboli, and following valve replacement surgery. Although chronic anticoagulant therapy decreases the risk of clots and emboli, it increases the risk for bleeding and hemorrhage.

**PRACTICE ALERT** *Monitor the International Normalized Ratio (INR) or prothrombin time (PT or protime). Report an INR > 3.5 or a PT > 2.5 times the normal to the physician. An excessively high INR or PT indicate excessive anticoagulation and an increased risk for bleeding.* ▪

- Test stools and vomitus for occult blood. *Bleeding due to excessive anticoagulation may not be apparent.*
- Instruct to avoid using aspirin or other nonsteroidal anti-inflammatory drugs (NSAIDs). Encourage reading ingredient labels on over-the-counter drugs; many contain aspirin. *Aspirin and other NSAIDs interfere with clotting and may potentiate the effects of the anticoagulant therapy.*
- Advise using a soft-bristled toothbrush, electric razor, and gentle touch when cleaning fragile skin. *These measures decrease the risk of skin or gum trauma and bleeding.*

**PRACTICE ALERT** *Monitor hemoglobin, hematocrit, and platelet count as ordered. Notify the physician of decreasing hemoglobin and hematocrit levels or if the platelet count falls below 50,000/mm³. Low hemoglobin and hematocrit indicate blood loss. Platelet counts below 50,000/mm³ significantly increase the risk of bleeding.* ∎

## Using NANDA, NIC, and NOC

Chart 30–3 shows links between NANDA nursing diagnoses, NIC, and NOC for the client with valvular heart disease.

## Home Care

For most clients, valvular disease is a chronic condition. The client has primary responsibility for managing effects of the disorder. To prepare the client and family for home care, discuss the following topics.

- Management of symptoms, including any necessary activity restrictions or lifestyle changes
- The importance of adequate rest to prevent fatigue
- Diet restrictions to reduce fluid retention and symptoms of heart failure

- Information about prescribed medications, including purpose, desired and possible adverse effects, scheduling, and possible interactions with other drugs
- The importance of keeping follow-up appointments to monitor the disease and its treatment
- Notifying all health care providers about valve disease or surgery to facilitate prescription of prophylactic antibiotics before invasive procedures or dental work
- Manifestations to immediately report to the health care provider: increasing severity of symptoms, especially of worsening heart failure or pulmonary edema; signs of transient ischemic attacks or other embolic events; evidence of bleeding, such as joint pain, easy bruising, black and tarry stools, bleeding gums, or blood in the urine or sputum

Provide referrals to community resources such as home maintenance services, home health services, and structured cardiac rehabilitation programs. Refer the client and family (especially the primary food preparer) to a dietitian or nutritionist for teaching and assistance with menu planning.

## THE CLIENT WITH CARDIOMYOPATHY

The **cardiomyopathies** are disorders that affect the heart muscle itself. They are a diverse group of disorders that affect both systolic and diastolic functions. Cardiomyopathies may be either primary or secondary in origin. Primary cardiomyopathies are idiopathic; their cause is unknown. Secondary cardiomyopathies occur as a result of other processes, such as ischemia, infectious disease, exposure to toxins, connective tissue disorders, metabolic disorders, or nutritional deficiencies. In many cases, the cause of cardiomyopathy is

---

**CHART 30–3  NANDA, NIC, AND NOC LINKAGES**

### The Client with Valvular Heart Disease

| NURSING DIAGNOSES | NURSING INTERVENTIONS | NURSING OUTCOMES |
|---|---|---|
| • Activity Intolerance | • Energy Management<br>• Self-Care Assistance | • Activity Tolerance<br>• Energy Conservation |
| • Decreased Cardiac Output | • Cardiac Care: Rehabilitative<br>• Hemodynamic Regulation<br>• Fluid Management | • Cardiac Pump Effectiveness<br>• Tissue Perfusion: Peripheral |
| • Fatigue | • Teaching: Prescribed Activity / Exercise<br>• Energy Management<br>• Nutrition Management | • Endurance<br>• Energy Conservation<br>• Nutritional Status: Energy |
| • Ineffective Health Maintenance | • Teaching: Disease Process<br>• Coping Enhancement<br>• Decision-Making Support | • Treatment Behavior: Illness or Injury<br>• Participation: Health Care Decisions |

*Note. Data from Nursing Outcomes Classification (NOC) by M. Johnson & M. Maas (Eds.), 1997, St. Louis: Mosby; Nursing Diagnoses: Definitions & Classification 2001–2002 by North American Nursing Diagnosis Association, 2001, Philadelphia: NANDA; Nursing Interventions Classification (NIC) by J.C. McCloskey & G. M. Bulechek (Eds.), 2000, St. Louis: Mosby. Reprinted by permission.*

## Nursing Care Plan
## A Client with Mitral Valve Prolapse

Julie Snow, a 22-year-old college student, sees a nurse practitioner at the college health clinic for a physical examination after experiencing palpitations, fatigue, and a headache during midterm examinations. Ms. Snow tells Lakisha Johnson, FNP, "I'm scared that something is wrong with me."

Over the last few months, Ms. Snow has had occasional palpitations that she describes as "feeling like my heart is doing flip-flops." Rarely, these palpitations have been accompanied by a sharp, stabbing pain in her chest that lasts only a few seconds. She initially attributed her symptoms to stress, but she is increasingly concerned because the "attacks" are becoming more frequent. Ms. Snow states that she has "always been healthy," does not smoke, uses alcohol socially, and exercises, albeit intermittently. Ms. Snow admits that she has been drinking a lot of coffee and cola and eating a lot of "junk food" lately.

### ASSESSMENT

Ms. Johnson's assessment of Ms. Snow documents the following: height 66 in. (168 cm), weight 140 lb (63.6 kg), T 99.3, BP 118/64, P 82, and R 18. Slightly anxious but in no acute distress. Systolic click and soft crescendo murmur grade II/VI noted on auscultation. Apical impulse at fifth ICS left MCL. Lungs clear to auscultation. Review of remaining systems reveals no apparent abnormalities. An ECG shows sinus rhythm with occasional PACs. Based on the admission history, manifestations, and physical assessment, Ms. Johnson suspects mitral valve prolapse (MVP).

### DIAGNOSES

- *Anxiety* related to fear of heart disease and implications for lifestyle
- *Powerlessness* related to unpredictability of symptoms
- *Risk of infection (endocarditis)* related to altered valve function

### EXPECTED OUTCOMES

- Verbalize an understanding of MVP and its management.
- Discuss ways to decrease or relieve MVP symptoms.
- Acknowledge the risk for endocarditis and identify precautions to prevent it.

### PLANNING AND IMPLEMENTATION

- Consult with and refer to cardiologist for continued monitoring and follow-up.
- Teach about MVP, including heart valve anatomy, physiology, and function, common manifestations of MVP, and treatment rationale.
- Discuss symptoms of progressive mitral regurgitation, and the need to report these to the cardiologist.
- Discuss recommended follow-up care and its rationale.
- Allow to verbalize feelings and share concerns about MVP. Encourage to attend an MVP support group meeting.

- Discuss the prognosis for MVP, emphasizing that most clients live normal lives using diet and lifestyle management.
- Instruct to keep a weekly record of symptoms and their frequency for 1 month.
- Discuss lifestyle changes to manage symptoms: aerobic exercise with warmup and cooldown periods; maintaining adequate fluid intake, especially during hot weather or exercise; relaxation techniques (e.g., meditation, deep-breathing exercises, music therapy, yoga, guided imagery, heat therapy, or progressive muscle relaxation) to perform daily; avoiding caffeine and crash diets; forming healthy eating habits.
- Teach about infective endocarditis risk and prevention with prophylactic antibiotics. Encourage notifying dentist and other health care providers of MVP before dental or any invasive procedure.

### EVALUATION

After several educational sessions at the college health clinic, Ms. Snow verbalizes an understanding of MVP by explaining heart valve function, listing common manifestations of MVP, and describing indications of deteriorating heart function. She states she will report these manifestations to her cardiologist if they occur. She is given a booklet on MVP for additional reading. She also verbalizes understanding of the risk of endocarditis, and states that she will notify her doctors of her MVP and the need for antibiotics before invasive procedures. Ms. Snow is attending a monthly MVP support group (led by a cardiology clinical nurse specialist) on campus and states, "I am so glad to know I'm not alone! It really helps to know that others are living well with MVP." Her weekly symptom log shows her symptoms are associated with late-night studying and drinking large amounts of coffee and cola. Ms. Snow has moderated her caffeine intake and increased her fluids, relieving her symptoms. In addition, Ms. Snow is taking a relaxation music therapy class. Ms. Snow states that she realizes that she has "the ability to control my life through the choices I make."

### Critical Thinking in the Nursing Process

1. Develop an action plan for Ms. Snow that outlines specific activities she can use to manage symptoms of MVP.
2. Why are clients with symptomatic MVP encouraged to include regular exercise in their health habits?
3. How does the support of family, friends, and other people with MVP assist MVP clients in managing their condition?
4. What manifestations would indicate a progressive worsening of Ms. Snow's mitral regurgitation?

See Evaluating Your Response in Appendix C.

unknown. In 1999, more than 27,000 deaths were directly attributed to cardiomyopathy. Mortality associated with cardiomyopathy is higher in older adults, men, and African Americans (AHA, 2001).

## PATHOPHYSIOLOGY AND MANIFESTATIONS

The cardiomyopathies are categorized by their pathophysiology and presentation into three groups: dilated, hypertrophic, and restrictive. Table 30–9 compares the causes, pathophysiology, manifestations, and management of the cardiomyopathies.

### Dilated Cardiomyopathy

*Dilated cardiomyopathy* is the most common type of cardiomyopathy, accounting for 87% of cases (AHA, 2001). The cause of dilated cardiomyopathy is unknown, although alcohol and cocaine abuse, chemotherapeutic drugs, pregnancy, and

systemic hypertension may contribute to its development. Some cases of dilated cardiomyopathy are genetic; it can be transmitted in an autosomal dominant, autosomal recessive, or X-linked pattern (Porth, 2002).

In dilated cardiomyopathy, heart chambers dilate and ventricular contraction is impaired. Both end-diastolic and end-systolic volumes increase, and the left ventricular ejection fraction is substantially reduced, decreasing cardiac output. Left ventricular dilation is prominent; left ventricular hypertrophy is usually minimal. The right ventricle also may be enlarged. Extensive interstitial fibrosis (scarring) is evident; necrotic myocardial cells also may be seen (Braunwald et al., 2001).

Manifestations of dilated cardiomyopathy develop gradually. Heart failure often presents years after the onset of dilation and pump failure. Both right- and left-sided failure occur, with dyspnea on exertion, orthopnea, paroxysmal nocturnal dys-

| TABLE 30-9 | Classifications of Cardiomyopathy | | |
|---|---|---|---|
| | **Dilated** | **Hypertrophic** | **Restrictive** |
| | | | |
| Causes | Usually idiopathic; may be secondary to chronic alcoholism or myocarditis | Hereditary; may be secondary to chronic hypertension | Usually secondary to amyloidosis, radiation, or myocardial fibrosis |
| Pathophysiology | Scarring and atrophy of myocardial cells<br>Thickening of ventricular wall<br>Dilation of heart chambers<br>Impaired ventricular pumping<br>Increased end-diastolic and end-systolic volumes<br>Mural thrombi common | Hypertrophy of ventricular muscle mass<br>Small left ventricular volume<br>Septal hypertrophy may obstruct left ventricular outflow<br>Left atrial dilation | Excess rigidity of ventricular walls restricts filling<br>Myocardial contractility remains relatively normal |
| Manifestations | Heart failure<br>Cardiomegaly<br>Dysrhythmias<br>$S_3$ and $S_4$ gallop; murmur of mitral regurgitation | Dyspnea, anginal pain, syncope<br>Left ventricular hypertrophy<br>Dysrhythmias<br>Loud $S_4$<br>Sudden death | Dyspnea, fatigue<br>Right-sided heart failure<br>Mild to moderate cardiomegaly<br>$S_3$ and $S_4$<br>Mitral regurgitation murmur |
| Management | Management of heart failure<br>Implantable cardioverter-defibrillator (ICD) as needed<br>Cardiac transplantation | Beta-blockers<br>Calcium channel blockers<br>Antidysrhythmic agents<br>ICD, dual-chamber pacing<br>Surgical excision of part of the ventricular septum | Management of heart failure<br>Exercise restriction |

pnea, weakness, fatigue, peripheral edema, and ascites. Both $S_3$ and $S_4$ heart sounds are commonly heard, as well as an AV regurgitation murmur. Dysrhythmias are common, including supraventricular tachycardias, atrial fibrillation, and complex ventricular tachycardias. Untreated dysrhythmias can lead to sudden death (Porth, 2002). Mural thrombi (blood clots in the heart wall) may form in the left ventricular apex and embolize to other parts of the body.

The prognosis of dilated cardiomyopathy is grim; most clients get progressively worse and 50% die within 5 years after the diagnosis; 75% die within 10 years (AHA, 2001).

## Hypertrophic Cardiomyopathy

*Hypertrophic cardiomyopathy* is characterized by decreased compliance of the left ventricle and hypertrophy of the ventricular muscle mass. This impairs ventricular filling, leading to small end-diastolic volumes, and low cardiac output. About half of all clients with hypertrophic cardiomyopathy have a family history of the disease. It is genetically transmitted in an autosomal dominant pattern (Braunwald et al., 2001).

The pattern of left ventricular hypertrophy is unique in that the muscle may not hypertrophy "equally." In a majority of clients, the interventricular septal mass, especially the upper portion, increases to a greater extent than the free wall of the ventricle. The enlarged upper septum narrows the passageway of blood into the aorta, impairing ventricular outflow. For this reason, this disorder is also known as *idiopathic hypertrophic subaortic stenosis (IHSS)* or *hypertrophic obstructive cardiomyopathy (HOCM)*.

Hypertrophic cardiomyopathy may be asymptomatic for many years. Symptoms typically occur when increased oxygen demand causes increased ventricular contractility. They may develop suddenly during or after physical activity; in children and young adults, sudden cardiac death may be the first sign of the disorder. Hypertrophic cardiomyopathy is the probable or definite cause of death in 36% of young athletes who die suddenly (AHA, 2001). It is hypothesized that sudden cardiac death is due to ventricular dysrhythmias or hemodynamic factors. Predictors of sudden cardiac death in this population include age of less than 30 years, a family history of sudden death, syncopal episodes, severe ventricular hypertrophy, and ventricular tachycardia seen on ambulatory ECG monitoring (Braunwald et al., 2001). For a brief synopsis of a nursing research study regarding family presence during CPR and invasive procedures, see the box below.

The usual manifestations of hypertrophic cardiomyopathy are dyspnea, angina, and syncope. Angina may result from ischemia due to overgrowth of the ventricular muscle, coronary artery abnormalities, or decreased coronary artery perfusion. Syncope may occur when the outflow tract obstruction severely decreases cardiac output and blood flow to the brain. Ventricular dysrhythmias are common; atrial fibrillation also may develop. Other manifestations of hypertrophic cardiomyopathy include fatigue, dizziness, and palpitations. A harsh, crescendo-decrescendo systolic murmur of variable intensity heard best at the lower left sternal border and apex is characteristic in hypertrophic cardiomyopathy. An $S_4$ may also be noted on auscultation.

---

## Nursing Research

### Evidence-Based Practice for Sudden Cardiac Death

When cardiac arrest occurs or invasive procedures are performed, family members typically are asked to leave the client's care unit. The traditional rationale for this practice is fear of disrupted clinical interventions, trauma of the witnesses, and risk for increased hospital liability. However, in 1995, the Emergency Nurses Association (ENA) adopted a position supporting family presence during invasive procedures, including resuscitation efforts (CPR), as a means of "preserving the wholeness, dignity, and integrity of the family unit from birth to death" (Myers et al., 2000, p. 33). This study evaluated the responses of families, nurses, and physicians to family presence during invasive procedures and CPR.

Results of the study showed that families saw their presence as a positive experience and their right. They viewed themselves as active care partners, and being present met their needs for information and providing comfort and connection with the client. Nurses overwhelmingly supported family presence; attending physicians also demonstrated a positive response. Physician residents were the least supportive of family presence.

### IMPLICATIONS FOR NURSING

Family members often are asked to leave the client's side during invasive procedures and CPR with the intention of protecting them from the trauma of witnessing painful or distressing events.

This study clearly showed being present as a positive experience, even when the ultimate outcome was the client's death.

Offering the opportunity to be present and providing information, psychologic and emotional support to an appropriate family member during invasive procedures and CPR supports the family unit and the client during times of crisis. Screening is important: People who are combative, emotionally unstable, or have altered mental status (e.g., dementia, alcohol intoxication) probably are not appropriate. It also is important to allow families to decline the invitation without guilt.

### Critical Thinking In Client Care

1. Identify procedures and situations in which family members are often asked to leave the client's side. When would it be appropriate to allow at least one significant other to remain with the client?

2. How would you present the option and prepare a family member for being present during a traumatic event such as CPR following the sudden death of a young adult with undiagnosed hypertrophic cardiomyopathy?

3. You support family presence during traumatic events and procedures, but your charge nurse does not. What steps might you use to effect a change in policy on your unit?

## Restrictive Cardiomyopathy

The least common form of cardiomyopathy, *restrictive cardiomyopathy* is characterized by rigid ventricular walls that impair diastolic filling. Causes of restrictive cardiomyopathy include myocardial fibrosis and infiltrative processes, such as amyloidosis. Fibrosis of the myocardium and endocardium causes excessive stiffness and rigidity of the ventricles. Decreased ventricular compliance impairs filling, with decreased ventricular size, elevated end-diastolic pressures, and decreased cardiac output. Contractility is unaffected, and the ejection fraction is normal.

The manifestations of restrictive cardiomyopathy are those of heart failure and decreased tissue perfusion. Dyspnea on exertion and exercise intolerance are common. Jugular venous pressure is elevated, and $S_3$ and $S_4$ are common. The prognosis for restrictive cardiomyopathy is poor. Most clients die within 3 years, and the systemic nature of the underlying disease process precludes effective treatment.

## COLLABORATIVE CARE

With the exception of treating an underlying cause, little can be done to treat either dilated or restrictive cardiomyopathies. For these disorders, treatment focuses on managing heart failure and treating dysrhythmias. Refer to the section of this chapter on heart failure and Chapter 29 for specific treatment strategies. Treatment of hypertrophic cardiomyopathy focuses on reducing contractility and preventing sudden cardiac death. Strenuous physical exertion is restricted, as it may precipitate dysrhythmias or sudden cardiac death. Dietary and sodium restrictions may help diminish the manifestations.

### Diagnostic Tests

Diagnosis begins with a history and physical assessment to rule out known causes of heart failure. Other tests may include the following:

- *Echocardiography* is done to assess chamber size and thickness, ventricular wall motion, valvular function, and systolic and diastolic function of the heart.
- *Electrocardiography* and *ambulatory ECG monitoring* demonstrate cardiac enlargement and detect dysrhythmias.
- *Chest X-ray* shows cardiomegaly, enlargement of the heart, and any pulmonary congestion or edema.
- *Hemodynamic studies* are used to assess cardiac output and pressures in the cardiac chambers and pulmonary vascular system.
- *Radionuclear scans* help identify changes in ventricular volume and mass, as well as perfusion deficits.
- *Cardiac catheterization* and *coronary angiography* may be done to evaluate coronary perfusion, the cardiac chambers, valves, and great vessels for function and structure, pressure relationships, and cardiac output.
- *Myocardial biopsy* uses the tranvenous route to obtain myocardial tissue for biopsy. The cells are examined for infiltration, fibrosis, or inflammation.

## Medications

The drug regimen used to treat heart failure also is used for dilated or restrictive cardiomyopathy. This includes ACE inhibitors, vasodilators, and digitalis (see the previous section of this chapter). Beta blockers also may be used with caution in clients with dilated cardiomyopathy. Anticoagulants are given to reduce the risk of thrombus formation and embolization. Antidysrhythmic drugs are avoided if possible due to their tendency to precipitate further dysrhythmias (Braunwald et al., 2001).

Beta blockers are the drugs of choice to reduce anginal symptoms and syncopal episodes associated with hypertrophic cardiomyopathy. The negative inotropic effects of beta blockers and calcium channel blockers decrease the myocardial contractility, decreasing obstruction of the outflow tract. Beta blockers also decrease heart rate and increase ventricular compliance, increasing diastolic filling time and cardiac output. Vasodilators, digitalis, nitrates, and diuretics are contraindicated. Amiodarone may be used to treat ventricular dysrhythmias (Braunwald et al., 2001).

## Surgery

Without definitive treatment, clients with cardiomyopathy develop end-stage heart failure. Cardiac transplant is the definitive treatment for dilated cardiomyopathy. Ventricular assist devices may be used to support cardiac output until a donor heart is available. Transplantation is not a viable option for restrictive cardiomyopathy, because transplantation does not eliminate the underlying process causing infiltration or fibrosis, and eventually the transplanted organ is affected as well. See the section on heart failure for more information about cardiac transplantation.

In severely symptomatic clients with obstructive hypertrophic cardiomyopathy, excess muscle may be surgically resected from the aortic valve outflow tract. The septum is incised, and tissue is removed. This procedure provides lasting improvement in about 75% of clients (Braunwald et al., 2001).

An implantable cardioverter-defibrillator (ICD) often is inserted to treat potentially lethal dysrhythmias, reducing the need for antidyrhythmic medications. A dual-chamber pacemaker also may be used for to treat hypertrophic cardiomyopathy.

## NURSING CARE

Nursing assessment and care for clients with dilated and restrictive cardiomyopathy is similar to that for clients with heart failure. Teaching about the disease process and its management is vital. Some degree of activity restriction often is necessary; assist to conserve energy while encouraging self-care. Support coping skills and adaptation to required lifestyle changes. Provide information and support for decision making about cardiac transplantation if that is an option. Discuss the toxic and vasodilator effects of alcohol, and encourage abstinence. See the nursing care section for heart failure for nursing diagnoses and suggested interventions.

The client with hypertrophic cardiomyopathy requires care similar to that provided for myocardial ischemia; nitrates and other vasodilators, however, are avoided. If surgery is performed, nursing care is similar to that for any client undergoing open-heart surgery or cardiac transplant. Discuss the genetic transmission of hypertrophic cardiomyopathy, and suggest screening of close relatives (parents and siblings).

Provide pre- and postoperative care and teaching as appropriate for clients undergoing invasive procedures or surgery for cardiomyopathy.

Nursing diagnoses that may be appropriate for clients with cardiomyoapathy include:

- *Decreased cardiac output* related to impaired left ventricular filling, contractility, or outflow obstruction
- *Fatigue* related to decreased cardiac output
- *Ineffective breathing pattern* related to heart failure
- *Fear* related to risk for sudden cardiac death
- *Ineffective role performance* related to decreasing cardiac function and activity restrictions
- *Anticipatory grieving* related to poor prognosis

## Home Care

Cardiomyopathies are chronic, progressive disorders generally managed in home and community care settings unless surgery or transplant are planned or end-stage heart failure develops. When teaching the client and family for home care, include the following topics.

- Activity restrictions and dietary changes to reduce manifestations and prevent complications
- Prescribed drug regimen, its rationale, intended and possible adverse effects
- The disease process, its expected ultimate outcome, and treatment options
- Cardiac transplantation, including the procedure, the need for lifetime immunosuppression to prevent transplant rejection, and the risks of postoperative infection and long-term immunosuppression
- Symptoms to report to the physician or for which immediate care is needed.
- Cardiopulmonary rescusitation procedures and available training sites

Refer the client and family for home and social services and counseling as indicated. Provide community resources such as support groups or the AHA.

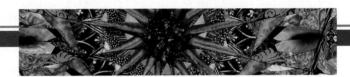

 **EXPLORE MediaLink**

# TEST YOURSELF

1. In reviewing the physician's admitting notes for a client with heart failure, the nurse notes that the client has an ejection fraction of 25%. The nurse recognizes this as meaning:

   a. Ventricular function is severely impaired
   b. The amount of blood being ejected from the ventricles is within normal limits
   c. 25% of the blood entering the ventricle remains in the ventricle after systole
   d. Cardiac output is greater than normal, overtaxing the heart

2. In assessing a client admitted 24 hours previously with heart failure, the nurse notes that the client has lost 2.5 lb (1 kg) of weight, his heart rate is 88 (HR was 105 on admission), and he now has crackles in the bases of his lung fields only. The nurse correctly interprets this data as indicating:

   a. The client's condition is unchanged from admission
   b. A need for more aggressive treatment

   c. The treatment regimen is achieving the desired effect
   d. No further treatment is required at this time as the failure has resolved

3. Morphine 2 to 5 mg IV as needed for pain and dyspnea is ordered for a client in acute pulmonary edema. The nurse appropriately:

   a. Questions this order because no time intervals have been specified
   b. Administers the drug as ordered, monitoring respiratory status
   c. Withholds the drug until the client's respiratory status improves
   d. Administers the drug only when the client complains of chest pain

4. An appropriate goal of nursing care for the client with acute infective endocarditis would be:
   a. "Will resume usual activities within 1 week of treatment."
   b. "Will relate the benign and self-limiting nature of the disease."
   c. "Will consider cardiac transplantation as a viable treatment option."
   d. "Will state the importance of continuing intravenous antibiotic therapy as ordered."

5. An expected assessment finding in a client with mitral stenosis being admitted for a valve replacement would be:
   a. Muffled heart sounds
   b. $S_3$ and $S_4$ heart sounds
   c. Diastolic murmur heard at the apex
   d. Cardiac heave

See Test Yourself answers in Appendix C.

# BIBLIOGRAPHY

Ackley, B. J., & Ladwig, G. B. (2002). *Nursing diagnosis handbook: A guide to planning care* (5th ed.). St. Louis: Mosby.

American Heart Association. (2001). *2002 heart and stroke statistical update.* Dallas, TX: Author.

Ammon, S. (2001). Managing patients with heart failure. *American Journal of Nursing, 101*(12), 34–40.

Baptiste, M. M. (2001). Aortic valve replacement. *RN, 64*(1), 58–63.

Bither, C. J., & Apple, S. (2001). Home management of the failing heart. *American Journal of Nursing, 101*(12), 41–45.

Braunwald, E., Fauci, A. S., Kasper, D. L., Hauser, S. L., Longo, D. L., & Jameson, J. L. (2001). *Harrison's principles of internal medicine* (15th ed.). New York: McGraw-Hill.

Bullock, B. A., & Henze, R. L. (2000). *Focus on pathophysiology.* Philadelphia: Lippincott.

Capriotti, T. (2002). Current concepts and pharmacologic treatment of heart failure. *MEDSURG Nursing, 11*(2), 71–83.

Carelock, J., & Clark, A. P. (2001). Heart failure: Pathophysiologic mechanisms. *American Journal of Nursing, 101*(12), 26–33.

Copstead, L. C., and Bansik, J. L. (2000). *Pathophysiology: Biological and behavioral perspectives* (2nd ed.). Philadelphia: Saunders.

Deglin, J. H., & Vallerand, A. H. (2003). *Davis's drug guide for nurses* (8th ed.). Philadelphia: F.A. Davis.

Fontaine, K. L. (2000). *Healing practices: Alternative therapies for nursing.* Upper Saddle River, NJ: Prentice Hall Health.

Gallo, J. J., Busby-Whitehead, J., Rabins, P. V., Silliman, R. A., & Murphy, J. B. (Eds.). (1999). *Reichel's care of the elderly: Clinical aspects of aging* (5th ed.). Philadelphia: Lippincott Williams & Wilkins.

Hunt, S. A., Baker, D. W., Chin, M. H., Ciquegrani, M. P., Feldman, A. M., Francis, G. S., Ganiats, T. G., Goldstein, S., Gregoratos, G.,

Jessup, M. L., Noble, R. J., Packer, M., Silver, M. A., and Stevenson, L. W. (2001) ACC/AHA guidelines for the evaluation and management of chronic heart failure in the adult: Executive summary: A report of the American College of Cardiology / American Heart Association Task Force on Practice Guidelines (Committee to Revise the 1995 Guidelines for the Evaluation and Management of Heart Failure). *Circulation, 104,* 2996–3007.

Johnson, M., Bulechek, G., Dochterman, J. M., Maas, M., & Moorhead, S. (2001). *Nursing diagnoses, outcomes, & interventions.* St. Louis: Mosby.

Johnson, M., Maas, M., & Moorhead, S. (Eds.). (2000). *Nursing outcomes classification (NOC)* (2nd ed.). St. Louis: Mosby.

Kearney, K. (2000). Emergency. Digitalis toxicity. *American Journal of Nursing, 100*(6), 51–52.

Kuhn, M. A. (1999). *Complementary therapies for health care providers.* Philadelphia: Lippincott.

Lehne, R. A. (2001). *Pharmacology for nursing care* (4th ed.). Philadelphia: Saunders.

Malarkey, L.M., & McMorrow, M.E. (2000). *Nurse's manual of laboratory tests and diagnostic procedures* (2nd ed.). Philadelphia: Saunders.

McCance, K. L., & Huether, S. E. (2002). *Pathophysiology: The biologic basis for disease in adults and children* (4th ed.). St. Louis: Mosby.

McCloskey, J. C., & Bulechek, G. M. (Eds.) (2000). *Nursing interventions classification (NIC)* (3rd ed.). St. Louis: Mosby.

Meeker, M. H., & Rothrock, J. C. (1999). *Alexander's care of the patient in surgery* (11th ed.). St. Louis: Mosby.

Miracle, V. A. (2001). Put the brakes on pericarditis. *Nursing, 31*(4), 44–45.

Myers, T. A., Eichhorn, D. J., Guzzetta, C. E., Clark, A. P., Klein, J. D., Taliaferro, E., & Calvin, A. (2000). Family presence during invasive procedures and resuscitation: The experi-

ence of family members, nurses, and physicians. *American Journal of Nursing, 100*(2), 32–42.

National Heart, Lung, and Blood Institute. National Institutes of Health. (2002). *Morbidity & mortality: 2002 chart book of cardiovascular, lung, and blood diseases.* Bethesda, MD: Author.

North American Nursing Diagnosis Association. (2001). *NANDA nursing diagnoses: Definitions & classification 2001–2002.* Philadelphia: NANDA.

Porth, C. M. (2002). *Pathophysiology: Concepts of altered health states* (6th ed.). Philadelphia: Lippincott.

Pugh, L. C., Havens, D. S., Xie, S., Robinson, J. M., & Blaha, C. (2001). Case management for elderly persons with heart failure: The quality of life and cost outcomes. *MEDSURG Nursing, 10*(2), 71–75.

Springhouse. (1999). *Nurse's handbook of alternative & complementary therapies.* Springhouse, PA: Author.

Tierney, L. M., McPhee, S. J., & Papadakis, M. A. (2001). *Current medical diagnosis & treatment* (40th ed.). New York: Lange Medical Books/McGraw-Hill.

Urden, L. D., Stacy, K. M., & Lough, M. E. (2002). *Thelan's critical care nursing: Diagnosis and management* (4th ed.). St. Louis: Mosby

Way, L. W., & Dahoerty, G. M. (2003). *Current surgical diagnosis & treatment* (11th ed.). New York: Lange Medical/McGraw-Hill.

Wilkinson, J. M. (2000). *Nursing diagnosis handbook with NIC interventions and NOC outcomes* (7th ed.). Upper Saddle River, NJ: Prentice Hall Health.

Woods, S. L., Froelicher, E. S. S., & Motzer, S. U. (2000). *Cardiac nursing* (4th ed.). Philadelphia: Lippincott.

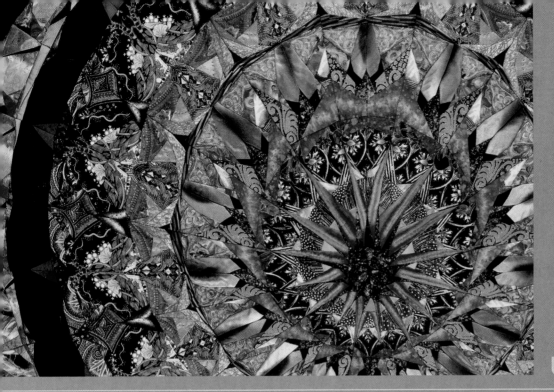

UNIT 9

# RESPONSES TO ALTERED PERIPHERAL TISSUE PERFUSION

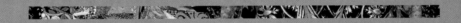

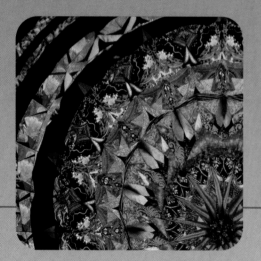

# Assessing Clients with Hematologic, Peripheral Vascular, and Lymphatic Disorders

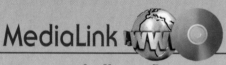

## MediaLink

### www.prenhall.com/lemone

Additional resources for this chapter can be found on the Student CD-ROM accompanying this textbook, and on the Companion Website at www.prenhall.com/lemone. Click on Chapter 31 to select the activities for this chapter.

**CD-ROM**
- Audio Glossary
- NCLEX Review

*Animations*
- Lymphatic System
- The Immune Response

**Companion Website**
- More NCLEX Review
- Functional Health Pattern Assessment
- Case Study
  Arterial Blood Pressure

## LEARNING OUTCOMES

After completing this chapter, you will be able to:

- Review the structures and functions of the arterial and venous networks of the peripheral vascular system and the lymphatic system.

- Describe the physiologic dynamics of blood flow, peripheral resistance, and blood pressure.

- Describe the major factors influencing arterial blood pressure.

- Identify interview questions pertinent to the assessment of the peripheral vascular and lymphatic systems.

- Describe physical assessment techniques for peripheral vascular and lymphatic function.

- Identify manifestations of impairment in the function of the peripheral vascular and lymphatic systems.

As the heart ejects blood with each beat, a closed system of blood vessels transports oxygenated blood to all body organs and tissues and then returns it to the heart for reoxygenation in the lungs. This branching network of vessels is called the peripheral vascular system. Systemic circulation is made possible by the vessels of the peripheral vascular system: the arteries, veins, and capillaries. The lymphatic system is a special vascular system that helps maintain sufficient blood volume in the cardiovascular system by picking up excess tissue fluid and returning it to the bloodstream.

## REVIEW OF ANATOMY AND PHYSIOLOGY
### Arterial and Venous Networks

The two main components of the peripheral vascular system are the arterial network and the venous network. The arterial network begins with the major arteries that branch from the aorta. The major arteries of the systemic circulation are illustrated in Figure 31–1 ■. These major arteries branch into successively smaller arteries, which in turn subdivide into the smallest of the arterial vessels, called arterioles. The smallest arterioles feed into beds of hairlike capillaries in the body's organs and tissues.

In the capillary beds, oxygen and nutrients are exchanged for metabolic wastes, and deoxygenated blood begins its journey back to the heart through venules, the smallest vessels of the venous network. Venules join the smallest of veins, which in turn join larger and larger veins. The blood transported by the veins empties into the superior and inferior venae cavae entering the right side of the heart. The major veins of the systemic circulation are shown in Figure 31–2 ■.

### Structure of Blood Vessels

The structure of blood vessels reflects their different functions within the circulatory system (Figure 31–3 ■). Except for the tiniest vessels, blood vessel walls have three layers: the tunica intima, the tunica media, and the tunica adventitia. The tunica intima, the innermost layer, is made of simple squamous epithelium (the endothelium); this provides a slick surface to facilitate the flow of blood. In arteries, the middle layer, or tunica media, is made of smooth muscle and is thicker than the tunica media of veins. This makes arteries more elastic than veins and allows the arteries to alternately expand and recoil as the heart contracts and relaxes with each beat, producing a pressure wave, which can be felt as a **pulse** over an artery. The smaller arterioles are less elastic than arteries but contain more smooth muscle, which promotes their constriction (narrowing) and dilation (widening). In fact, arterioles rather than arteries exert the major control over arterial blood pressure. The tunica adventitia, or outermost layer, is made of connective tissue and serves to protect and anchor the vessel. Veins have a thicker tunica adventitia than do arteries.

Blood in the veins travels at a much lower pressure than blood in the arteries. Veins have thinner walls, a larger lumen, and greater capacity, and many are supplied with valves that help blood flow against gravity back to the heart (see Figure 31–3). The "milking" action of skeletal muscle contraction (called the *muscular pump*) also supports venous return. When skeletal muscles contract against veins, the valves proximal to the contraction open, and blood is propelled toward the heart. The abdominal and thoracic pressure changes that occur with breathing (called the *respiratory pump*) also propel blood toward the heart.

The tiny capillaries, which connect the arterioles and venules, contain only one thin layer of tunica intima that is permeable to the gases and molecules exchanged between blood and tissue cells. Capillaries typically are found in interwoven networks. They filter and shunt blood from terminal arterioles to postcapillary venules.

### Physiology of Arterial Circulation

The factors that affect arterial circulation are blood flow, peripheral vascular resistance, and blood pressure. **Blood flow** refers to the volume of blood transported in a vessel, in an organ, or throughout the entire circulation over a given period of time. It is commonly expressed as liters or milliliters per minute or cubic centimeters per second.

**Peripheral vascular resistance (PVR)** refers to the opposing forces or impedance to blood flow as the arterial channels become more and more distant from the heart. Peripheral vascular resistance is determined by three factors:

- *Blood viscosity:* The greater the viscosity, or thickness, of the blood, the greater its resistance to moving and flowing.
- *Length of the vessel:* The longer the vessel, the greater the resistance to blood flow.
- *Diameter of the vessel:* The smaller the diameter of a vessel, the greater the friction against the walls of the vessel and, thus, the greater the impedance to blood flow.

Blood pressure is the force exerted against the walls of the arteries by the blood as it is pumped from the heart. It is most accurately referred to as mean arterial pressure (MAP). The highest pressure exerted against the arterial walls at the peak of ventricular contraction (systole) is called the systolic blood pressure. The lowest pressure exerted during ventricular relaxation (diastole) is the diastolic blood pressure.

Mean arterial blood pressure is regulated mainly by cardiac output (CO) and peripheral vascular resistance (PVR), as represented in this formula: $MAP = CO \times PVR$. For clinical use, the MAP may be estimated by calculating the diastolic blood pressure plus one-third of the pulse pressure (the difference between the systolic and diastolic blood pressure).

### Factors Influencing Arterial Blood Pressure

Blood flow, peripheral vascular resistance, and blood pressure, which influence arterial circulation, are in turn influenced by various factors. The sympathetic and parasympathetic nervous systems are the primary mechanisms that regulate blood pressure. Stimulation of the sympathetic nervous system exerts a major effect on peripheral resistance by causing vasoconstriction of the arterioles, thereby increasing blood pressure. Parasympathetic stimulation causes vasodilation of the arterioles, lowering blood pressure. Baroreceptors and chemoreceptors in the aortic arch, carotid sinus, and other large vessels are sensitive to pressure and chemical changes and cause reflex

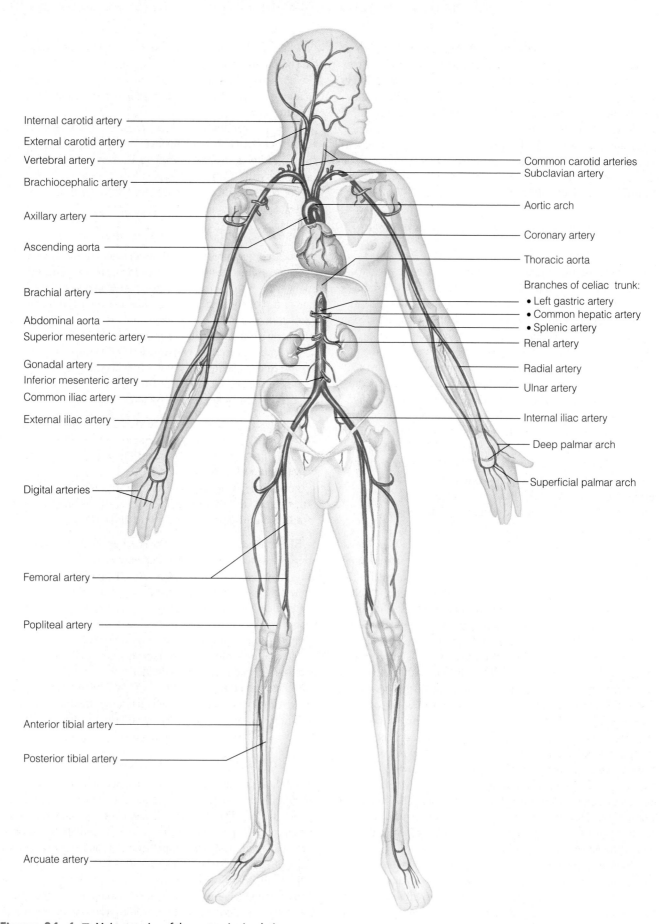

Internal carotid artery

External carotid artery

Vertebral artery

Brachiocephalic artery

Axillary artery

Ascending aorta

Brachial artery

Abdominal aorta

Superior mesenteric artery

Gonadal artery

Inferior mesenteric artery

Common iliac artery

External iliac artery

Digital arteries

Femoral artery

Popliteal artery

Anterior tibial artery

Posterior tibial artery

Arcuate artery

Common carotid arteries

Subclavian artery

Aortic arch

Coronary artery

Thoracic aorta

Branches of celiac trunk:
• Left gastric artery
• Common hepatic artery
• Splenic artery

Renal artery

Radial artery

Ulnar artery

Internal iliac artery

Deep palmar arch

Superficial palmar arch

**Figure 31–1** ■ Major arteries of the systemic circulation.

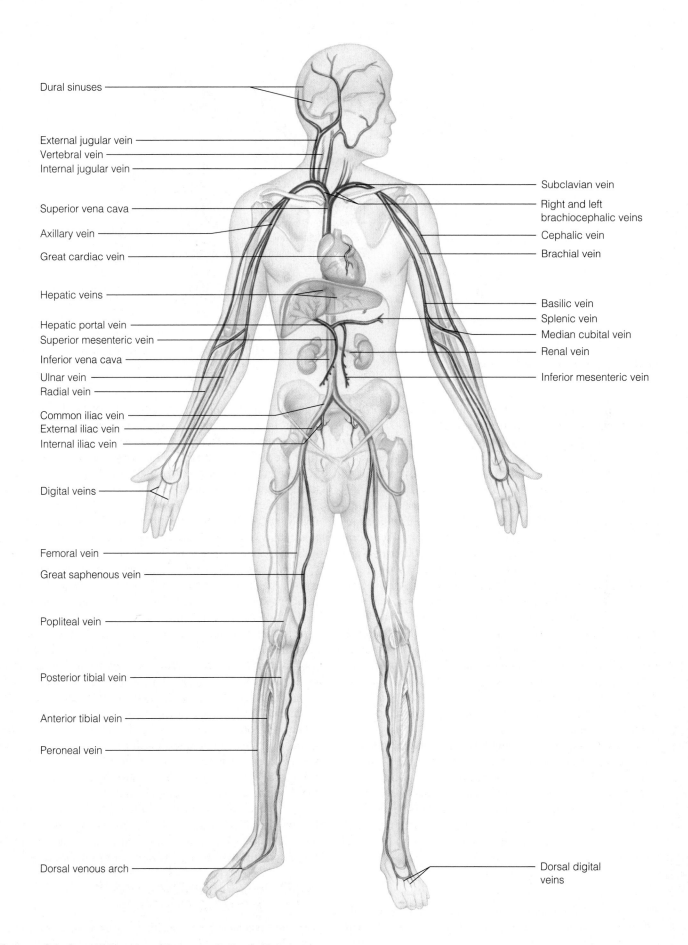

Dural sinuses

External jugular vein
Vertebral vein
Internal jugular vein

Superior vena cava

Axillary vein

Great cardiac vein

Hepatic veins

Hepatic portal vein
Superior mesenteric vein
Inferior vena cava
Ulnar vein
Radial vein

Common iliac vein
External iliac vein
Internal iliac vein

Digital veins

Femoral vein
Great saphenous vein

Popliteal vein

Posterior tibial vein

Anterior tibial vein

Peroneal vein

Dorsal venous arch

Subclavian vein
Right and left
brachiocephalic veins
Cephalic vein
Brachial vein

Basilic vein
Splenic vein
Median cubital vein
Renal vein

Inferior mesenteric vein

Dorsal digital
veins

**Figure 31–2** ■ Major veins of the systemic circulation.

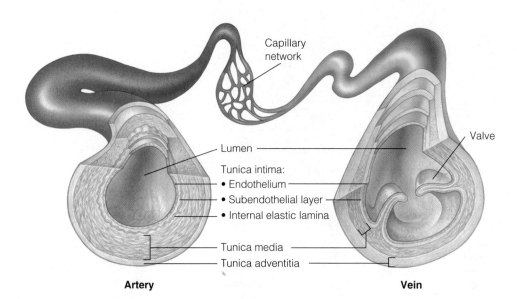

**Figure 31–3** ■ Structure of arteries, veins, and capillaries. Capillaries are composed of only a fine tunica intima. Notice that the tunica media is thicker in arteries than in veins.

sympathetic stimulation, resulting in vasoconstriction, increased heart rate, and increased blood pressure.

The kidneys help maintain blood pressure by excreting or conserving sodium and water. When blood pressure decreases, the kidneys initiate the renin-angiotensin mechanism. This stimulates vasoconstriction, resulting in the release of the hormone aldosterone from the adrenal cortex, increasing sodium ion reabsorption and water retention. In addition, pituitary release of antidiuretic hormone (ADH) promotes renal reabsorption of water. The net result is an increase in blood volume and a consequent increase in cardiac output and blood pressure.

Temperatures may also affect peripheral resistance: Cold causes vasoconstriction, whereas warmth produces vasodilation. Many chemicals, hormones, and drugs influence blood pressure by affecting cardiac output and/or peripheral vascular resistance. For example, epinephrine causes vasoconstriction and increased heart rate; prostaglandins dilate blood vessel diameter (by relaxing vascular smooth muscle); endothelin, a chemical released by the inner lining of vessels, is a potent vasoconstrictor; nicotine causes vasoconstriction; and alcohol and histamine cause vasodilation.

Dietary factors, such as intake of salt, saturated fats, and cholesterol, elevate blood pressure by affecting blood volume and vessel diameter. Race, gender, age, weight, time of day, position, exercise, and emotional state may also affect blood pressure. These factors influence the arterial pressure; systemic venous pressure, though it is much lower, is also influenced by such factors as blood volume, venous tone, and right atrial pressure.

## The Lymphatic System

The structures of the lymphatic system include the lymphatic vessels and several lymphoid organs (Figure 31–4 ■). The lymphatic vessels, or lymphatics, form a network around the arterial and venous channels and interweave at the capillary beds.

They collect and drain excess tissue fluid, called lymph, that "leaks" from the cardiovascular system and accumulates at the venous end of the capillary bed. The lymphatics return this fluid to the heart through a one-way system of lymphatic venules and veins that eventually drain into the right lymphatic duct and left thoracic duct, both of which empty into their respective subclavian veins. Lymphatics are a low-pressure system without a pump; their fluid transport depends on the rhythmic contraction of their smooth muscle and the muscular and respiratory pumps that assist venous circulation.

The organs of the lymphatic system are the lymph nodes, the spleen, the thymus, the tonsils, and the Peyer's patches of the small intestine. Lymph nodes are small aggregates of specialized cells that assist the body's immune system by removing foreign material, infectious organisms, and tumor cells from lymph. Lymph nodes are distributed along the lymphatic vessels, forming clusters in certain body regions such as the neck, axilla, and groin (see Figure 31–4). The spleen, the largest lymphoid organ, is in the upper left quadrant of the abdomen under the thorax. The main function of the spleen is to filter the blood by breaking down old red blood cells and storing or releasing to the liver their by-products (such as iron). The spleen also synthesizes lymphocytes, stores platelets for blood clotting, and serves as a reservoir of blood. The thymus gland is in the lower throat and is most active in childhood, producing hormones (such as thymosin) that facilitate the immune action of lymphocytes. The tonsils of the pharynx and Peyer's patches of the small intestine are lymphoid organs that protect the upper respiratory and digestive tracts from foreign pathogens.

## ASSESSING PERIPHERAL VASCULAR AND LYMPHATIC FUNCTION

The nurse conducts both a health assessment interview to collect subjective data and a physical assessment to collect objective data.

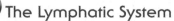

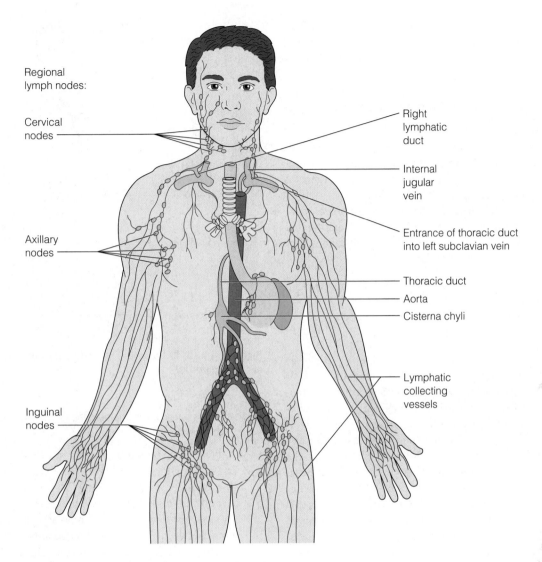

Regional lymph nodes:

Cervical nodes

Axillary nodes

Inguinal nodes

Right lymphatic duct

Internal jugular vein

Entrance of thoracic duct into left subclavian vein

Thoracic duct

Aorta

Cisterna chyli

Lymphatic collecting vessels

**Figure 31–4** ■ The lymphatic system.

## The Health Assessment Interview

This section provides guidelines for collecting subjective data through a health assessment interview specific to the functions of the peripheral vascular system and the lymphatic system.

### The Peripheral Vascular System

The health assessment of the peripheral vascular system may focus on the client's chief complaint (such as swelling or pain in the legs), or it may be part of a full cardiovascular assessment. If the client has a chief complaint, analyze its onset, characteristics and course, severity, precipitating and relieving factors, and any associated symptoms, noting the timing and circumstances. For example, ask the client the following:

- Does the leg pain occur only with activities such as walking, or also during rest?
- Do your ankles swell at the end of the day, after sitting for prolonged periods, or after sleeping all night?
- Does temperature or the position of your body affect the symptoms?

Next explore the client's medical and family history for any cardiovascular disorders, such as heart disease, arteriosclerosis, peripheral vascular disease (PVD), stroke, hypertension (HTN), hyperlipidemia (elevated fat in blood) and blood clots, or other chronic illnesses (e.g., diabetes). Ask about past surgery of the heart or blood vessels or tests to evaluate their function and about any medications that affect circulation or blood pressure.

Continue the assessment interview with a review of symptoms. Ask the client about past or present pain, burning, numbness, or tingling in the limbs or digits; leg fatigue or cramps; changes in skin color or temperature, texture of hair, ulcers or skin irritation, varicose veins, phlebitis (inflamed veins) or edema (swelling). Explore the client's nutritional history for intake of protein, vitamins and minerals, salt, fats, and fluid. Quantify any consumption of caffeine and alcohol and history of smoking (in pack years) or other tobacco use. Assess the client's activity level for exercise habits and tolerance.

It is important to consider socioeconomic factors that may precipitate or aggravate circulatory problems (e.g., inadequate clothing, shoes, or shelter) and occupational factors, such as prolonged standing or sitting or exposure to temperature extremes. Also assess psychosocial factors that may affect the client's stress level and emotional state.

Other questions and leading statements, categorized by functional health patterns, can be found on the Companion Website.

### The Lymphatic System

The health assessment of the lymphatic system includes a review of specific lymphatic findings, such as lymph node enlargement or swollen glands, as well as other more general complaints about infection or impaired immunity, such as fever, fatigue, or weight loss. If a health problem exists, analyze its onset, characteristics, severity, and precipitating and relieving factors, noting the timing and circumstances. For example, ask the client the following:

- Did you notice that the glands in your neck became swollen after an infection?
- Have you noticed increased fatigue or weakness?
- Have you ever been exposed to radiation?

Explore the client's history for chronic illnesses (e.g., cardiovascular disease, renal disease, cancer, tuberculosis, HIV infection), predisposing factors (e.g., surgery, trauma, infection, blood transfusions, intravenous drug use), and environmental exposure (e.g., radiation, toxic chemicals, travel-related infectious disease). Review the family history for any incidence of cancer, anemia, or blood dyscrasias. Ask the client about past or present bleeding (e.g., from the nose, gums, or mouth; from vomiting; from the rectum; bruising) and associated symptoms (e.g., pallor, dizziness, fatigue, difficulty breathing); lymph node changes (e.g., enlargement, pain or tenderness, itching, warmth); swelling of extremities; and recurrent irritations or infections. Lastly, an assessment of the client's socioeconomic status, lifestyle, intravenous drug use, and sexual practices may be significant in determining risk for diseases associated with impaired lymphatic function.

Other questions and leading statements, categorized by functional health patterns, can be found on the Companion Website.

### Physical Assessment:
### The Peripheral Vascular System

Physical assessment of the peripheral vascular system can be performed as part of the full cardiovascular assessment or alone for clients who have known or suspected peripheral vascular disease or who are at risk for circulatory complications (e.g., clients who have undergone surgery or are immobile). The techniques used to assess the peripheral vascular system include auscultation of blood pressure, palpation of the major pulse points of the body (Figure 31–5 ■), and inspection of the skin for such changes as edema, ulcerations, or alterations in color and temperature. Recommended equipment for this assessment includes a stethoscope, a tape measure, and a metric ruler. The client may be assessed in the supine, sitting, and standing positions. Box 31–1 reviews guidelines for blood pressure measurement.

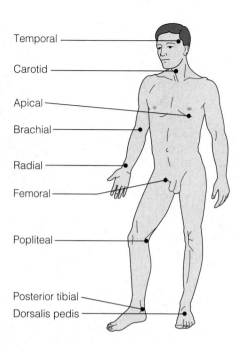

**Figure 31–5** ■ Body sites at which peripheral pulses are most easily palpated.

### Blood Pressure and Pulse Pressure Assessment with Abnormal Findings (✓)

- Auscultate blood pressure in each arm with the client seated.
  - ✓ Consistent BP readings over 140/90 in adults under age 40 is considered hypertension.
  - ✓ BP under 90/60 is considered hypotension.
  - ✓ An **auscultatory gap**—a temporary disappearance of sound between the systolic and diastolic BP—may be a normal variation, or it may be associated with systolic HTN or a drop in diastolic BP due to aortic stenosis.
  - ✓ **Korotkoff's sounds** (see Box 31–1) may be heard down to zero with cardiac valve replacements, hyperkinetic states, thyrotoxicosis, and severe anemia, as well as after vigorous exercise.
  - ✓ The sounds of aortic regurgitation may obscure the diastolic BP.
  - ✓ A difference of over 10 mmHg between arms suggests arterial compression on the side of the lower reading, aortic dissection, or coarctation of the aorta.
- Auscultate blood pressure in each arm with the client standing. If orthostatic changes occur, measure the BP with the client supine, legs dangling, and again with the client standing, 1 to 3 minutes apart.
  - ✓ A decrease in systolic BP of over 10 to 15 mmHg and a drop in diastolic BP on standing is called **orthostatic hypotension.** Causes include antihypertensive medications, volume depletion, peripheral neurovascular disease, prolonged bed rest, and aging.
- Observe the pulse pressure. The **pulse pressure** is the difference between the systolic and diastolic BP. For example, if the BP is 140/80, the pulse pressure is 60. A normal pulse pressure is one-third the systolic measurement.

## BOX 31–1 ■ Guidelines for Blood Pressure Measurement

### REVIEW OF KOROTKOFF'S SOUNDS

The first sound heard is the systolic pressure; at least two consecutive sounds should be clear. If the sound disappears and then is heard again 10 to 15 mm later, an auscultatory gap is present; this may be a normal variant, or it may be associated with hypertension. The first diastolic sound is heard as a muffling of the Korotkoff's sound and is considered the best approximation of the true diastolic pressure. The second diastolic sound is the level at which sounds are no longer heard.

The American Heart Association recommends documenting all three readings when measuring blood pressure, for example, 120/72/64. If only two readings are documented, the systolic and the second diastolic pressure are taken, for example, 120/64.

### TECHNIQUE REMINDERS

- Choose a cuff of an appropriate size: The cuff should snugly cover two-thirds of the upper arm, and the bladder should completely encircle the arm. The bladder should be centered over the brachial artery, with the lower edge 2 to 3 cm above the antecubital space.
- The client's arm should be slightly flexed and supported (on a table or by the examiner) at heart level.
- To determine how high to inflate the cuff, palpate the brachial pulse, and inflate the cuff to the point on the manometer at which the pulse is no longer felt; then, add 30 mmHg to this reading, and use the sum as the target for inflation. Wait 15 seconds before reinflating the cuff to auscultate the BP.
- To recheck a BP, wait at least 30 seconds before attempting another inflation.
- Always inflate the cuff completely, then deflate it. Once deflation begins, allow it to continue; do not try to reinflate the cuff if the first systolic sound is not heard or if the cuff inadvertently deflates.
- The bell of the stethoscope more effectively transmits the low-pitched sounds of BP.

### SOURCES OF ERROR

- Falsely high readings can occur if the cuff is too small, too loose, or if the client supports his or her own arm.
- Falsely low readings can occur if a standard cuff is used on a client with thin arms.

- Inadequate inflation may result in underestimation of the systolic pressure or overestimation of the diastolic pressure if an auscultatory gap is present.
- Rapid deflation and repeated or slow inflations (causing venous congestion) can lead to underestimation of the systolic BP and overestimation of the diastolic BP.

### FACTORS ALTERING BLOOD PRESSURE

- A change from the horizontal to upright position causes a slight decrease (5 to 10 mm) in systolic BP; the diastolic BP remains unchanged or rises slightly.
- BP taken in the arm is lower when the client is standing.
- If the BP is taken with the client in the lateral recumbent position, a lower BP reading may be obtained in both arms; this is especially apparent in the right arm with the client in the left lateral position.
- Factors that increase BP include exercise, caffeine, cold environment, eating a large meal, painful stimuli, and emotions.
- Factors that lower BP include sleep (by 20 mmHg) and very fast, slow, or irregular heart rates.
- BP tends to be higher in taller or heavier clients.

### ALTERNATIVE METHODS OF BLOOD PRESSURE MEASUREMENT

- The palpatory method may be necessary if severe hypotension is present and the BP is inaudible. Palpate the brachial pulse, and inflate the cuff 30 mm above the point where the pulse disappears; deflate the cuff, and note the point on the manometer where the pulse becomes palpable again. Record this as the palpatory systolic BP.
- Leg BP measurement may be needed when there is injury of the arms or to rule out coarctation of the aorta or aortic insufficiency when arm diastolic BP is over 90 mmHg. Place the client in the prone or supine position with the leg slightly flexed. Place a large leg cuff on the thigh with the bladder centered over the popliteal artery. Place the bell of the stethoscope over the popliteal space. Normal leg systolic BP is higher than arm BP; diastolic BP should be equal to or lower than arm BP. Abnormally low leg BP occurs with aortic insufficiency and coarctation of the aorta.

---

✓ A widened pulse pressure with an elevated systolic BP occurs with exercise, arteriosclerosis, severe anemia, thyrotoxicosis, and increased intracranial pressure.

✓ A narrowed pulse pressure with a decreased systolic BP occurs with shock, cardiac failure, and pulmonary embolus.

### Skin Assessment with Abnormal Findings (✓)

- Inspect the color of the skin.
  - ✓ Pallor reflects constriction of peripheral blood flow (e.g., due to syncope or shock) or decreased circulating oxyhemoglobin (e.g., due to anemia).
  - ✓ Central cyanosis of the lips, earlobes, oral mucosa, and tongue suggests chronic cardiopulmonary disease. (See Box 31–2 for abnormal findings associated with peripheral vascular and lymphatic assessment.)

### Artery and Vein Assessment with Abnormal Findings (✓)

- Palpate the temporal arteries.
  - ✓ Redness, swelling, nodularity, and variations in pulse amplitude may occur with temporal arteritis.
- Inspect and palpate the carotid arteries. Note symmetry, the pulse rate, rhythm, volume, and amplitude. Note any variation with respiration. Describe all pulses as increased, normal, diminished, or absent. Scales ranging from 0 to 4+ are sometimes used as follows:

0 = Absent
1+ = Diminished
2+ = Normal
3+ = Increased
4+ = Bounding

## BOX 31–2 ■ Abnormal Findings Associated with Peripheral Vascular and Lymphatic Assessment

- *Pallor* is an absence of color of the skin. The degree of pallor depends on the client's normal skin color and health status. Dark skin may appear ashen or have a yellowish tinge.
- *Cyanosis* is a bluish discoloration of the skin and mucous membranes in people with light skin. In people with dark skin, cyanosis may be difficult to observe. Inspect the nail beds and conjunctiva.
- *Edema* is an abnormal accumulation of fluid in the interstitial spaces of body tissues. It is often most apparent in the lower extremities.
- *Varicose veins* are tortuous and dilated veins that have incompetent valves. The saphenous veins of the legs are most commonly affected.
- *Enlarged lymph nodes* result from infection or malignancy.
- *Atrophic changes* are changes in size or activity of body tissues as the result of pathology or injury. Decreased blood flow and oxygenation of the lower extremities often cause atrophic changes of loss of hair, thickened toe nails, changes in pigmentation, and ulcerations.
- *Gangrene* is the necrosis (or death) of tissue, most often the result of loss of blood supply and infection. Gangrene often begins in the most distal of the tissues of the extremities.
- *Pressure ulcers,* also called decubitus ulcers or bed sores, are the result of ischemia and hypoxia of tissue following prolonged pressure. These ulcers often are located over bony prominences. If untreated, the tissue changes proceed from red skin to deep, craterlike ulcers.

## BOX 31–3 ■ Types of Pulse Patterns

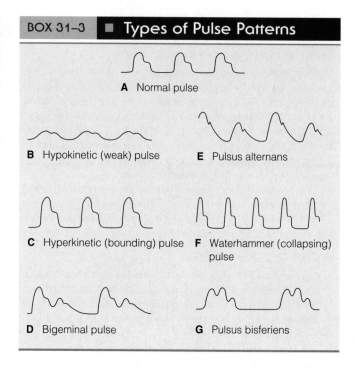

A  Normal pulse

B  Hypokinetic (weak) pulse

C  Hyperkinetic (bounding) pulse

D  Bigeminal pulse

E  Pulsus alternans

F  Waterhammer (collapsing) pulse

G  Pulsus bisferiens

Pulse waveforms are shown in Box 31–3.

✓ A unilateral pulsating bulge is seen with a tortuous or kinked carotid artery.

✓ Alterations in pulse rate or rhythm are due to cardiac dysrhythmias.

✓ An absent pulse indicates arterial occlusion.

✓ A hypokinetic (weak) pulse is associated with decreased stroke volume (Box 31–3B). This may be due to congestive heart failure (CHF), aortic stenosis, or hypovolemia; to increased peripheral resistance, which may result from cold temperatures; or to arterial narrowing, commonly found with atherosclerosis.

✓ A hyperkinetic (bounding) pulse occurs with increased stroke volume and/or decreased peripheral resistance (Box 31–3C). This may result from states in which cardiac output is high or from aortic regurgitation. It also may occur with anemia, hyperthyroidism, bradycardia, or reduced compliance, as with atherosclerosis.

✓ A bigeminal pulse is marked by decreased amplitude of every second beat (Box 31–3D). This may be due to premature contractions (usually ventricular).

✓ Pulsus alternans is a regular pulse with alternating strong and weak beats (Box 31–3E). This may be due to left ventricular failure and severe HTN.

✓ The waterhammer pulse (collapsing pulse) has a greater than normal amplitude with a sharp rise and fall (Box 31–3F). It occurs with aortic insufficiency.

✓ Pulsus bisferiens has two main peaks in amplitude ("double beat") and occurs with combined aortic stenosis and regurgitation, pericardial effusion, and constrictive pericarditis (Box 31–3G).

✓ Pulsus paradoxus is a pulse in which the amplitude is diminished or absent during inspiration and exaggerated during expiration. Pulsus paradoxus occurs with cardiac tamponade, constrictive pericarditis, and severe chronic lung disease.

✓ A palpable thrill over the carotid artery suggests arterial narrowing, as with atherosclerosis.

- Auscultate the carotid arteries, using the bell of the stethoscope.

✓ A murmuring or blowing sound heard over stenosed peripheral vessels is known as a bruit. A bruit heard over the middle to upper carotid artery suggests atherosclerosis.

- Inspect and palpate the internal and external jugular veins for venous pressure. See Box 31–4 for guidelines for assessing jugular venous pressure.

✓ An increase in jugular venous pressure over 3 cm and located above the sternal angle reflects increased right atrial pressure. This occurs with right ventricular failure or, less commonly, with constrictive pericarditis, tricuspid stenosis, and superior venae cavae obstruction.

- If venous pressure is elevated, assess the hepatojugular reflex. (Compress the liver in the right upper abdominal quadrant with the palm of the hand for 30 to 60 seconds while observing the jugular veins.)

✓ A decrease in venous pressure reflects reduced left ventricular output or blood volume.

## BOX 31–4 ■ Assessing Jugular Venous Pressure

When a client with normal venous pressure lies in the supine position, full neck veins are normally visible, but as the head of the bed is elevated, the pulsations disappear. In the client with greatly elevated venous pressure, visible pulsations of the jugular vein are present even in the upright position. To conduct the inspection:

1. Remove clothing from the client's neck and chest. Elevate the head of the the bed 30 to 45 degrees, and turn the client's head to the opposite side. Shine a light tangentially across the neck to increase shadows. If the external jugular veins are distended, they will be visible vertically between the mandible and outer clavicle.

2. If jugular distention is present, assess the jugular venous pressure (JVP) by measuring from the highest point of visible distention to the sternal angle (the point at which the clavicles meet) on both sides of the neck (see the accompanying figure). Bilateral measurements above 3 cm are considered elevated and indicate increased venous pressure; distention on only one side may indicate obstruction.

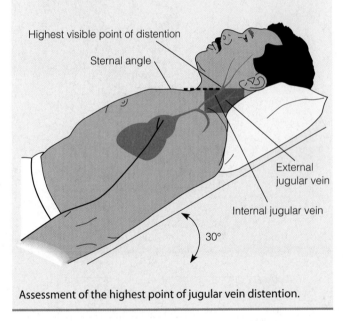

Assessment of the highest point of jugular vein distention.

✓ Unilateral neck vein distention suggests local compression or anatomic anomaly.

✓ A rise in the column of neck vein distention over 1 cm with liver compression indicates right heart failure.

## Upper Extremity Assessment
## with Abnormal Findings (✓)

• Inspect and palpate the arms, noting size and symmetry, skin color, and temperature.

 ✓ Unilateral swelling with venous prominence occurs with venous obstruction.

 ✓ Extreme localized pallor of the fingers is seen with Raynaud's disease.

 ✓ Cyanosis of the nailbeds reflects chronic cardiopulmonary disease.

 ✓ Cold temperature of the hands and fingers occurs with vasoconstriction.

• Palpate the nail beds for capillary refill. (Apply pressure to the client's fingertips. Watch for blanching of the nail beds. Release the pressure. Note the time it takes for capillary refill, indicated by the return of pink color on release of the pressure.)

 ✓ Capillary refill that takes more than 2 seconds reflects circulatory compromise, such as hypovolemia or anemia.

• Assess venous pattern and pressure. (Elevate one of the client's arms over the head for a few seconds. Slowly lower the arm. Observe the filling of the client's hand veins.)

 ✓ Distention of hand veins at elevations over 9 cm above heart level reflects an increase in systemic venous pressure.

• Palpate the radial and brachial pulses. Note rate, rhythm, volume amplitude, symmetry, variations with respiration.

 ✓ Alterations in pulse rate or rhythm are due to cardiac dysrhythmias (such as atrial fibrillation, atrial flutter, and premature ventricular contractions). A pulse rate over 100 beats per minute is tachycardia; a pulse rate below 60 BPM is bradycardia.

 ✓ A pulse deficit (slower radial rate than apical rate) occurs with dysrhythmias and CHF.

 ✓ Irregularities of rhythm produce early beats and pauses (skipped beats) in the pulse, which may be regular in pattern, sporadic, or grossly irregular.

 ✓ Diminished or absent radial pulses may be due to thromboangitis obliterans (Buerger's disease) or acute arterial occlusion.

 ✓ A weak and thready pulse, often with tachycardia, reflects decreased cardiac output.

 ✓ A bounding pulse occurs with hyperkinetic states and atherosclerosis.

 ✓ Unequal pulses between extremities suggest arterial narrowing or obstruction on one side.

 ✓ In sinus dysrhythmia (a normal variant, especially in young adults), the pulse rate increases with inspiration and decreases with expiration.

• If arterial insufficiency is suspected, palpate the ulnar pulse and perform the Allen test:

 • Have the client make a tight fist.

 • Compress both the radial and ulnar arteries.

 • Have the client open the hand to a slightly flexed position.

 • Observe for pallor and manifestations of pain.

 • Release the ulnar artery and observe for the return of pink color within 3 to 5 seconds.

 • Repeat the procedure on the radial artery.

 ✓ The normal ulnar artery may or may not have a palpable pulse.

 ✓ Persistent pallor with the Allen test suggests ulnar artery occlusion.

• Inspect and palpate each leg, noting size, shape, and symmetry; arterial pattern; skin color, temperature, and texture; hair pattern; pigmentation; rashes; ulcers, sensation; and capillary refill.

✓ Chronic arterial insufficiency may be due to arteriosclerosis or autonomic dysfunction, or to acute occlusion resulting from thrombosis, embolus, or aneurysm.

✓ Signs of arterial disruption include pallor, dependent rubor (dusky redness); cool to cold temperature; and atrophic changes, such as hair loss with shiny and smooth texture, thickened nails, sensory loss, slow capillary refill, and muscle atrophy.

✓ Ulcers with symmetric margins, a deep base, black or necrotic tissue, and absence of bleeding may occur at pressure points on or between the toes, on the heel, on the lateral malleolar or tibial area, over the metatarsal heads, or along the side or sole of the foot.

✓ Gangrene due to complete arterial occlusion presents as black, dry, hard skin; pregangrenous color changes include deep cyanosis and purple-black discoloration.

## Lower Extremity Assessment with Abnormal Findings (✓)

• With the client supine, assess the venous pattern of the legs. Repeat with the client standing.

✓ Signs of venous insufficiency include swelling, thickened skin, cyanosis, stasis dermatitis (brown pigmentation, erythema, and scaling), and superficial ankle ulcers located predominantly at the medial malleolus with uneven margins, ruddy granulation tissue, and bleeding. Varicose veins appear as dilated, tortuous, and thickened veins, which are more prominent in a dependent position.

• Palpate the femoral, popliteal, posterior tibial, and dorsalis pedis pulses for volume, amplitude, and symmetry.

✓ Diminished or absent leg pulses suggest partial or complete arterial occlusion of the proximal vessel and are often due to arteriosclerosis obliterans.

✓ Increased and widened femoral and popliteal pulsations suggest aneurysm.

✓ Absence of a posterior tibial pulse with signs and symptoms of arterial insufficiency is usually due to acute occlusion by thrombosis or embolus.

✓ Diminished or absent pedal pulses are often due to popliteal occlusion associated with diabetes mellitus.

• If pulses are diminished, observe for postural color changes. Elevate both legs 60 degrees, and observe the color of the soles of the feet. Have the client sit and dangle the legs; note the return of color to the feet.

✓ Extensive pallor on elevation is suggestive of arterial insufficiency.

✓ Rubor (dusky redness) of the toes and feet along with delayed venous return (over 45 seconds) suggests arterial insufficiency.

• If arterial insufficiency is suspected, auscultate the femoral arteries.

✓ Femoral bruits suggest arterial narrowing due to arteriosclerosis.

• Inspect and gently palpate the calves.

✓ Redness, warmth, swelling, tenderness, and cords along a superficial vein suggest thrombophlebitis or deep vein thrombosis (DVT).

• Inspect and palpate for edema. Use your thumb to compress the dorsum of the client's foot, around the ankles, and along the tibia (Figure 31–6A ■). A depression in the skin that does not immediately refill is called pitting edema. Edema can be graded on a scale of from 1+ to 4+ (Figure 31–6B):

| | |
|---|---|
| 1+ (−2mm depression) | No visible change in the leg; slight pitting |
| 2+ (−4mm depression) | No marked change in the shape of the leg; pitting slightly deeper |
| 3+ (−6mm depression) | Leg visibly swollen; pitting deep |
| 4+ (−8mm depression) | Leg very swollen; pitting very deep |

✓ Edema may be caused by disease of the cardiovascular system such as CHF; by renal, hepatic, or lymphatic problems; or by infection.

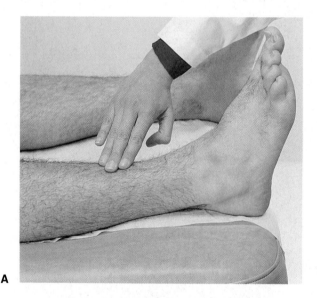

A

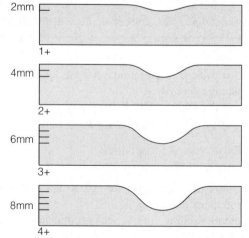

B

**Figure 31–6 ■** Evaluation of edema. *A,* Palpating for edema over the tibia. *B,* Four-point scale for grading edema.

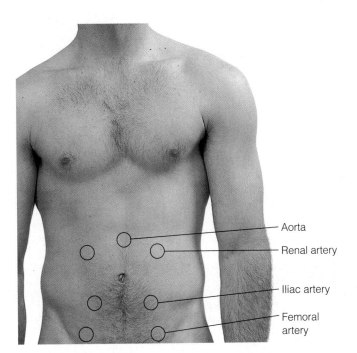

**Figure 31–7** ■ Auscultation sites of the abdominal aorta and its branches.

Aorta

Renal artery

Iliac artery

Femoral artery

✓ Venous distention suggests venous insufficiency or incompetence.

## Abdominal Assessment with Abnormal Findings (✓)

- Inspect and palpate the abdominal aorta. Note size, width, and any visible pulsations or bulging.
  - ✓ A pulsating mass in the upper abdomen suggests an aortic aneurysm, particularly in the older adult.
  - ✓ An aorta greater than 2.5 to 3 cm in width reflects pathologic dilation, most likely due to arteriosclerosis.
- Auscultate the epigastrium and each abdominal quadrant, using the bell of the stethoscope (Figure 31–7 ■).
  - ✓ Abdominal bruits reflect turbulent blood flow associated with partial arterial occlusion.
  - ✓ A bruit heard over the aorta suggests an aneurysm.
  - ✓ A bruit heard over the epigastrium and radiating laterally, especially with HTN, suggests renal artery stenosis.
  - ✓ Bruits heard in the lower abdominal quadrants suggest partial occlusion of the iliac arteries.

## Physical Assessment: The Lymphatic System

Physical assessment of the lymphatic system is usually integrated into the assessment of other body systems. For example, the tonsils are observed with the pharynx during the head and neck assessment; the regional lymph nodes are evaluated with corresponding body regions (e.g., occipital, auricular, and cervical nodes are evaluated with assessment of the head and neck, axillary nodes with assessment of the breast or thorax, epitrochlear node with assessment of the peripheral vascular exam of the arms, and inguinal nodes with assessment of the

abdomen); the spleen can be palpated during the abdominal assessment. The techniques of inspection and palpation are used for the lymphatic examination; a tape measure and metric ruler may be helpful.

## Skin Assessment with Abnormal Findings (✓)

- Inspect the skin of the extremities and over the regional lymph nodes, noting any edema, erythema, red streaks, or skin lesions.
  - ✓ **Lymphangitis** (inflammation of a lymphatic vessel) may produce a red streak with induration (hardness) following the course of the lymphatic collecting duct; infected skin lesions may be present, particularly between the digits.
  - ✓ **Lymphedema** (swelling due to lymphatic obstruction) occurs with congenital lymphatic anomaly (Milroy's disease) or with trauma to the regional lymphatic ducts from surgery or metastasis (e.g., arm lymphedema after radical mastectomy with axillary node removal).
  - ✓ Edema of lymphatic origin is usually not pitting, and the skin may be thickened; one example is the taut swelling of the face and body that occurs with myxedema, associated with hypothyroidism.

## Lymph Node Assessment with Abnormal Findings (✓)

- Palpate the regional lymph nodes of the head and neck, axillae, arms, and groin.
     Use firm, circular movements of the finger pads and note size, shape, symmetry, consistency, delineation, mobility, tenderness, sensation, and condition of overlying skin.
  - ✓ **Lymphadenopathy** refers to the enlargement of lymph nodes (over 1 cm) with or without tenderness. It may be caused by inflammation, infection, or malignancy of the nodes or the regions drained by the nodes.
  - ✓ Lymph node enlargement with tenderness suggests inflammation (lymphadenitis). With bacterial infection, the nodes may be warm and matted with localized swelling.
  - ✓ Malignant or metastatic nodes may be hard, indicating lymphoma; rubbery, indicating Hodgkin's disease; or fixed to adjacent structures. Usually they are not tender.
  - ✓ Ear infections and scalp and facial lesions, such as acne, may cause enlargement of the preauricular and cervical nodes.
  - ✓ Anterior cervical nodes are enlarged and infected with streptococcal pharyngitis and mononucleosis.
  - ✓ Lymphadenitis of the cervical and submandibular nodes occurs with herpes simplex lesions.
  - ✓ Brain tumors may metastasize to the occipital nodes.
  - ✓ Enlargement of supraclavicular nodes, especially the left, is highly suggestive of metastatic disease from abdominal and thoracic cancer.
  - ✓ Axillary lymphadenopathy is associated with breast cancer.
  - ✓ Lesions of the genitals may produce enlargement of the inguinal nodes.
  - ✓ Persistent generalized lymphadenopathy is associated with acquired immune deficiency syndrome (AIDS) and AIDS-related complex (ARC).

## Spleen Assessment with Abnormal Findings (✓)

- Palpate for the spleen, in the upper left quadrant of the abdomen.
  - ✓ A palpable spleen in the left upper abdominal quadrant of an adult may indicate abnormal enlargement (splenomegaly) and may be associated with cancer, blood dyscrasias, and viral infection, such as mononucleosis.
- Percuss for splenic dullness in the lowest left intercostal space (ICS) at the anterior axillary line or in the ninth to tenth ICS at the midaxillary line (Figure 31–8 ■).
  - ✓ A dull percussion note in the lowest left ICS at the anterior axillary line or below the tenth rib at the midaxillary line suggests splenic enlargement.

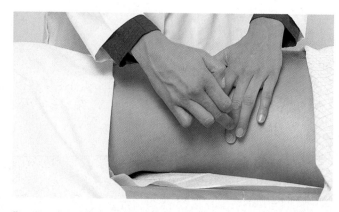

**Figure 31–8** ■ Percussing the spleen.

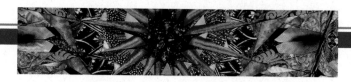

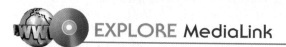 EXPLORE MediaLink

NCLEX review questions, case studies, care plan activities, MediaLink applications, and other interactive resources for this chapter can be found on the Companion Website at www.prenhall.com/lemone.

Click on Chapter 31 to select the activities for this chapter. For animations, video clips, more NCLEX review questions, and an audio glossary, access the Student CD-ROM accompanying this textbook.

## TEST YOURSELF

1. What part of the peripheral vascular system has the major control of blood pressure?

   a. Veins
   b. Capillaries
   c. Arteries
   d. Arterioles

2. Which of the following components of the lymphatic system is/are the largest?

   a. Spleen
   b. Tonsils
   c. Thymus
   d. Peyer's patches

3. What method would be most appropriate to assess the carotid arteries?

   a. Inspect for absence of movement
   b. Auscultate with the bell of the stethoscope

   c. Palpate with firm pressure
   d. Percuss lightly over each artery

4. When auscultating the abdominal aorta, you hear a murmuring or blowing sound. You would document this sound as a:

   a. Hypokinetic pulse
   b. Bigeminal pulse
   c. Bruit
   d. Dysrhythmia

5. Swelling of a body part as a result of lymphatic obstruction is labeled:

   a. Lymphedema
   b. Lymphadenopathy
   c. Atrophic change
   d. Central cyanosis

See Test Yourself answers in Appendix C.

## BIBLIOGRAPHY

Andresen, G. (1998). Assessing the older patient. *RN, 61*(3), 46–56.

Ayello, E. (2000). On the lookout for peripheral vascular disease. *Nursing, 30*(6 Home Health), 64hh1–2, 64hh4.

Ayello, E. (2001). Why is pressure ulcer risk assessment so important? *Nursing, 31*(11), 74–80.

Faria, S. (1999). Assessment of peripheral arterial pulses. *Home Care Provider, 4*(4), 140–141.

Hoskins, M. (1997). Using dopplers. *Community Nurse, 3*(3), 17–18.

MacLaren, J. (2001). Skin changes in lymphoedema: Pathophysiology and management options. *International Journal of Palliative Nursing, 7*(8), 381–382, 384–388.

McConnell, E. A. (1997). Performing Allen's test . . . whether ulnar and radial arteries are patent. *Nursing, 17*(11), 26.

Watson, R. (2000). Assessing cardiovascular functioning in older people. *Nursing Older People, 12*(6), 27–28.

Weber, J., & Kelley, J. (2002). *Health assessment in nursing* (2nd ed.). Philadelphia: Lippincott.

Willis, K. (2001). Gaining perspective on peripheral vascular disease. *Nursing, 31*(2 Hospital Nursing), 32hn1–4.

Wilson, S., & Giddens, J. (2001). *Health assessment for nursing practice.* St. Louis: Mosby.

Young, T. (2001). Leg ulcer assessment. *Practice Nurse, 21*(7), 50, 52.

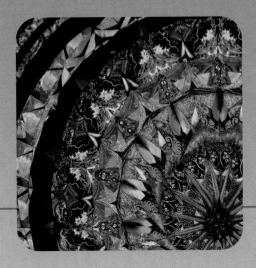

CHAPTER 32

# Nursing Care of Clients with Hematologic Disorders

## LEARNING OUTCOMES

After completing this chapter, you will be able to:

- Relate the physiology and assessment of the hematologic system and related systems (see Chapter 31) to commonly occurring hematologic disorders.

- Describe the pathophysiology of common hematologic disorders.

- Identify diagnostic tests commonly used for hematologic disorders.

- Discuss nursing implications for medications prescribed for hematologic disorders.

- Discuss nursing implications for bone marrow transplantation, chemotherapy, and radiation for hematologic disorders.

- Compare and contrast bleeding disorders.

- Describe the major types of leukemia and the most common treatment modalities and nursing interventions.

- Differentiate Hodgkin's disease from non-Hodgkin's lymphomas.

- Use the nursing process to provide individualized care to clients with hematologic disorders.

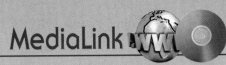

## www.prenhall.com/lemone

Additional resources for this chapter can be found on the Student CD-ROM accompanying this textbook, and on the Companion Website at www.prenhall.com/lemone. Click on Chapter 32 to select the activities for this chapter.

**CD-ROM**
- Audio Glossary
- NCLEX Review

*Animation*
- Sickle Cell Anemia

**Companion Website**
- More NCLEX Review
- Case Study
    Immune Thrombocytopenic Purpura
- Care Plan Activity
    Acute Myelocytic Leukemia
- MediaLink Applications
    Stem Cell Transplant
    Sickle Cell Anemia

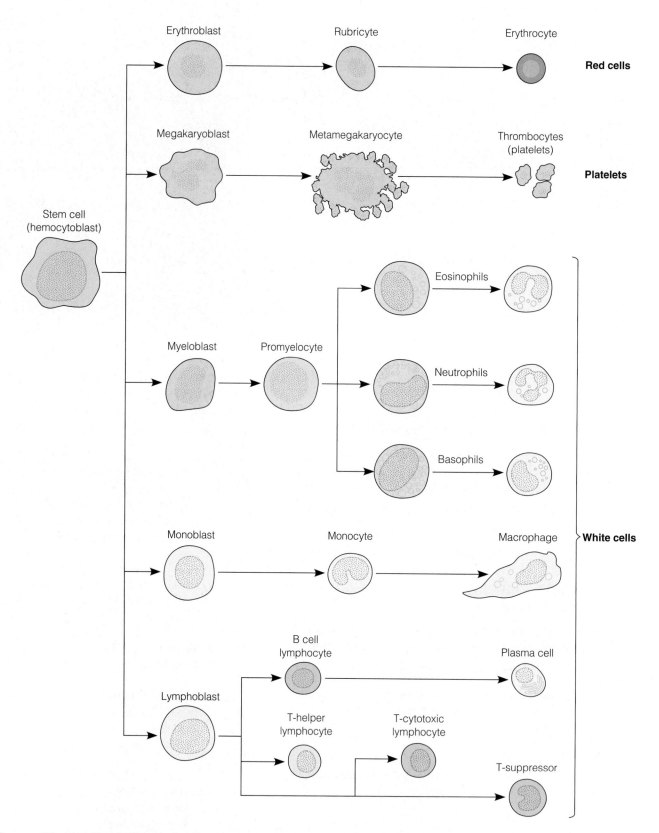

**Figure 32–1** ■ Blood cell formation from stem cells. Regulatory factors control the differentiation of stem cells into blasts. Each of the five kinds of blasts is committed to producing one type of mature blood cell. Erythroblasts, for example, can differentiate only into RBCs; megakaryoblasts can differentiate only into platelets.

Disorders affecting the blood and blood-forming organs have effects that range from minor disruptions in daily activities to major life-threatening crises. Clients with hematologic disorders need holistic nursing care, including emotional support and care for problems involving major body systems.

Blood is an exchange medium between the external environment and the body's cells. Blood consists of plasma, solutes (e.g., proteins, electrolytes, and organic constituents), red blood cells, white blood cells, and platelets, which are fragments of cells.

The *hematopoietic* (blood-forming) system includes the bone marrow (myeloid) tissues, where blood cells form, and the lymphoid tissues of the lymph nodes, where white blood cells mature and circulate. All blood cells originate from cells in the bone marrow called **stem cells,** or *hemocytoblasts.* Regulatory mechanisms cause stem cells to differentiate into families of parent cells, each of which gives rise to one of the formed elements of the blood (red blood cells, platelets, and white cells). The origin of the cellular components of blood is illustrated in Figure 32–1 ■.

This chapter focuses on health changes resulting from changes in red cells, white cells, platelets, and clotting factors. An overview of each type of blood cell is provided before the disorders are presented to facilitate understanding the effects of, responses to, and care of clients with hematologic disorders.

# RED BLOOD CELL DISORDERS

**Red blood cells (RBCs)** and the hemoglobin molecules they contain are required for oxygen transport to body tissues. Hemoglobin also binds with some carbon dioxide, carrying it to the lungs for excretion. Abnormal numbers of RBCs, changes in their size and shape, or altered hemoglobin content or structure can adversely affect health. Anemia, the most common RBC disorder, is an abnormally low RBC count or reduced hemoglobin content. Polycythemia is an abnormally high RBC count.

## PHYSIOLOGY REVIEW OF RED BLOOD CELLS

The red blood cell (**erythrocyte**) is shaped like a biconcave disk (Figure 32–2 ■). This unique shape increases the surface area of the cell and allows the cell to pass through very small capillaries without disrupting the cell membrane. RBCs are the most common type of blood cell.

Hemoglobin is the oxygen-carrying protein within RBCs. It consists of the heme molecule and globin, a protein molecule. Globin is made of four polypeptide chains—two alpha chains and two beta chains (Figure 32–3 ■). Each of the four polypeptide chains contains a heme unit containing an iron atom. The iron atom binds reversibly with oxygen, allowing it to transport oxygen as *oxyhemoglobin* to the cells. Hemoglobin is synthesized within the RBC. The rate of synthesis depends on the availability of iron (Porth, 2002).

Normal adult laboratory values for red blood cells are defined and identified in Table 32–1. The size, color, and shape of stained RBCs also may be analyzed. RBCs may be *normocytic* (normal size), smaller than normal (*microcytic*), or

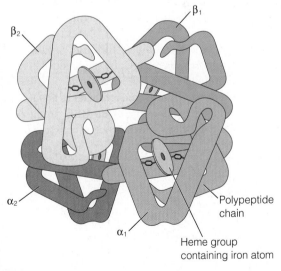

**Figure 32–3** ■ The hemoglobin molecule includes globin (a protein) and heme, which contains iron. Globin is made of four subunits, two alpha and two beta polypeptide chains. A heme disk containing an iron atom (red dot) nests within the folds of each protein subunit. The iron atoms combine reversibly with oxygen, transporting it to the cells.

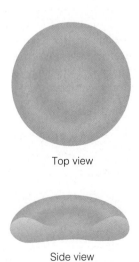

Top view

Side view

**Figure 32–2** ■ Top and side view of a red blood cell (erythrocyte). Note the distinctive concave shape.

## TABLE 32–1 Normal Laboratory Values for Red Blood Cells

| Laboratory Test | Normal Range | Definition |
| --- | --- | --- |
| Red blood cell (RBC) count | | Number of circulating RBCs per mm³ of blood |
| • Men | 4.2–5.4 million/mm³ | |
| • Women | 3.6–5.0 million/mm³ | |
| Reticulocytes | 1.0%–1.5% of total RBC | Number of immature RBCs per mm³ of blood |
| Hemoglobin (Hgb) | | Amount of hemoglobin per dL (100 mL) of blood |
| • Men | 14–16.5 g/dL | |
| • Women | 12–15 g/dL | |
| Hematocrit (Hct) | | Packed volume of RBCs in 100 mL of blood |
| • Men | 40%–50% | expressed as a percentage |
| • Women | 37%–47% | |
| Mean corpuscular volume (MCV) | 85–100 fL/cell | Average volume of individual RBCs |
| Mean corpuscular hemoglobin concentration (MCHC) | 31–35 g/dL | Average concentration or percentage of hemoglobin per RBC |
| Mean corpuscular hemoglobin (MCH) | 27–34 pg/cell | Calculated average weight of hemoglobin per RBC |

larger than normal (*macrocytic*). Their color may be normal (*normochromic*) or diminished (*hypochromic*).

## Red Blood Cell Production and Regulation

In adults, RBC production (**erythropoiesis**) (Figure 32–4 ■) begins in red bone marrow of the vertebrae, sternum, ribs, and pelvis, and is completed in the blood or spleen. *Erythroblasts* begin forming hemoglobin while they are in the bone marrow, a process that continues throughout RBC lifespan. Erythroblasts differentiate into *normoblasts*. As these slightly smaller cells mature, their nucleus and most organelles are ejected, eventually causing normoblasts to collapse inward and assume the characteristic biconcave shape of RBCs. The cells enter the circulation as *reticulocytes,* which fully mature in about 48 hours. The complete sequence from stem cell to RBC takes 3 to 5 days.

Tissue hypoxia is the stimulus for RBC production. The hormone *erythropoietin* is released by the kidneys in response to hypoxia. It stimulates the bone marrow to produce RBCs. However, the process of RBC production takes about 5 days to maximize. During periods of increased RBC production, the percentage of reticulocytes in the blood exceeds that of mature cells.

## Red Blood Cell Destruction

RBCs have a life span of about 120 days. Old or damaged RBCs are *lysed* (destroyed) by phagocytes in the spleen, liver, bone marrow, and lymph nodes. The process of RBC destruction is called **hemolysis.** Phagocytes save and reuse amino acids and iron from heme units in the lysed RBCs. Most of the heme unit is converted to bilirubin, an orange-yellow pigment that is removed from the blood by the liver and excreted in the bile.

During disease processes causing increased hemolysis or impaired liver function, bilirubin accumulates in the serum, causing a yellowish appearance of the skin and sclera (*jaundice*).

## THE CLIENT WITH ANEMIA

**Anemia** is an abnormally low number of circulating RBCs, low hemoglobin concentration, or both. Decreased numbers of circulating RBCs is the usual cause of anemia. This may result from blood loss, inadequate RBC production, or increased RBC destruction. Insufficient or defective hemoglobin within RBCs contributes to anemia. Depending on its severity, anemia may affect all major organ systems.

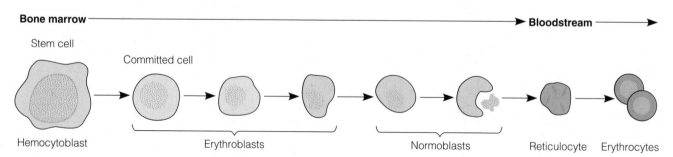

**Figure 32–4** ■ Erythropoiesis. RBCs begin as erythroblasts within the bone marrow, maturing into normoblasts, which eventually eject their nucleus and organelles to become reticulocytes. Reticulocytes mature within the blood or spleen to become erythrocytes.

## PATHOPHYSIOLOGY AND MANIFESTATIONS

A number of different pathologic mechanisms can lead to anemia (Box 32–1). Regardless of the cause, every type of anemia reduces the oxygen-carrying capacity of the blood, leading to tissue hypoxia. The resulting manifestations depend on the severity of the anemia, how quickly it develops, and other factors such as age and health status.

When anemia develops gradually and the RBC reduction is moderate, successful compensatory mechanisms may result in few symptoms except when the oxygen needs of the body increase due to exercise or infection. Symptoms develop as RBCs are further reduced. Pallor of the skin, mucous membranes, conjunctiva, and nail beds develops as a result of blood redistribution to vital organs and lack of hemoglobin. As tissue oxygenation decreases, the heart and respiratory rates rise. Tissue hypoxia may cause angina, fatigue, dyspnea on exertion, and night cramps. It also stimulates erythropoietin release; increased erythropoietin activity may cause bone pain. Cerebral hypoxia can lead to headache, dizziness, and dim vision. Heart failure may develop in severe anemia.

With rapid blood loss, blood volume is decreased as well as the oxygen-carrying capacity of the blood. Signs of circulatory shock may occur. With chronic bleeding, fluid shifts from the interstitial spaces into the vessels, maintaining blood volume. Blood viscosity is reduced, which may result in a systolic heart murmur. See page 936 for *Multisystem Effects of Anemia*.

Anemia is categorized by cause: blood loss, nutritional, hemolytic, and bone marrow suppression. The pathophysiology of these types of anemias follows.

## Blood Loss Anemia

When anemia results from acute or chronic bleeding, RBCs and other blood components are lost from the body. With acute blood loss, circulating volume decreases, increasing the risk for shock and circulatory failure (see Chapter 6). Fluid shifts from the interstitial spaces into the vascular compartment to maintain blood volume, diluting the cellular components of the blood and reducing its viscosity. In acute blood loss, circulating RBCs are of normal size and shape, but the hemoglobin and hematocrit are reduced. If sufficient iron is available, the number of circulating RBCs returns to normal within 3 to 4 weeks after the bleeding episode. Chronic blood loss, on the other hand, depletes iron stores as RBC production attempts to maintain the RBC supply. The resulting RBCs are microcytic (small) and hypochromic (pale).

## Nutritional Anemias

Nutritional anemias result from nutrient deficits that affect RBC formation (erythropoiesis) or hemoglobin synthesis. The nutrient deficit may be caused by inadequate diet, malabsorption, or an increased need for the nutrient. The most common types of nutritional anemias are iron deficiency anemia, vitamin $B_{12}$ anemia, and folic acid deficiency anemia. Vitamin $B_{12}$ and folic acid anemias are sometimes called megaloblastic anemias, as enlarged nucleated RBCs called megaloblasts are seen in these anemias.

### Iron Deficiency Anemia

**Iron deficiency anemia** is the most common type of anemia. It develops when the supply of iron is inadequate for optimal RBC formation. The body cannot synthesize hemoglobin without iron. Iron deficiency anemia results in fewer numbers of RBCs, microcytic and hypochromic RBCs, as well as malformed RBCs (poikilocytosis).

Excessive iron loss due to chronic bleeding is the usual cause of iron deficiency anemia in adults. Menstrual blood loss is the most common cause in adult females. Iron deficiency anemia also may result from inadequate dietary iron intake (less than 1 mg/day), malabsorption, or the increased iron requirements associated with pregnancy and lactation. Box 32–2 summarizes common causes of iron deficiency anemia.

Iron deficiency anemia is particularly common in older adults. Chronic, occult (hidden) blood loss may occur from slowly bleeding ulcers, gastrointestinal inflammation, hemorrhoids, and cancer. Inadequate dietary iron intake also contributes to anemia in the older adult. Access to transportation may limit fresh food consumption, a factor contributing to poor iron intake among all adults, especially people with limited or fixed incomes.

---

| BOX 32–1 | ■ Pathophysiologic Mechanisms of Anemia |
| --- | --- |

### DECREASED RBC PRODUCTION

■ Altered hemoglobin synthesis
- Iron deficiency
- Thalassemias
- Chronic inflammation

■ Altered DNA synthesis
- Vitamin $B_{12}$ or folic acid malabsorption or deficiency

■ Bone marrow failure
- Aplastic anemia (stem cell dysfunction)
- Red cell aplasia
- Myeloproliferative leukemias
- Cancer metastasis, lymphoma
- Chronic infection or inflammation, physical and emotional fatigue

### INCREASED RBC LOSS OR DESTRUCTION

■ Acute or chronic blood loss
- Hemorrhage or trauma
- Chronic gastrointesinal bleeding, menorrhagia

■ Increased hemolysis
- Hereditary cell membrane disorders
- Defective hemoglobin—Sickle cell anemia or trait
- Pyruvate kinase (PK) or G6PD deficiency affecting glycolysis or cell oxidation
- Immune mechanisms and disorders (e.g., blood reaction, hypersensitivity responses, autoimmune disorders)
- Splenomegaly and hypersplenism
- Infection
- Erythrocyte trauma (e.g., due to cardiopulmonary bypass, hemolytic uremic syndrome)

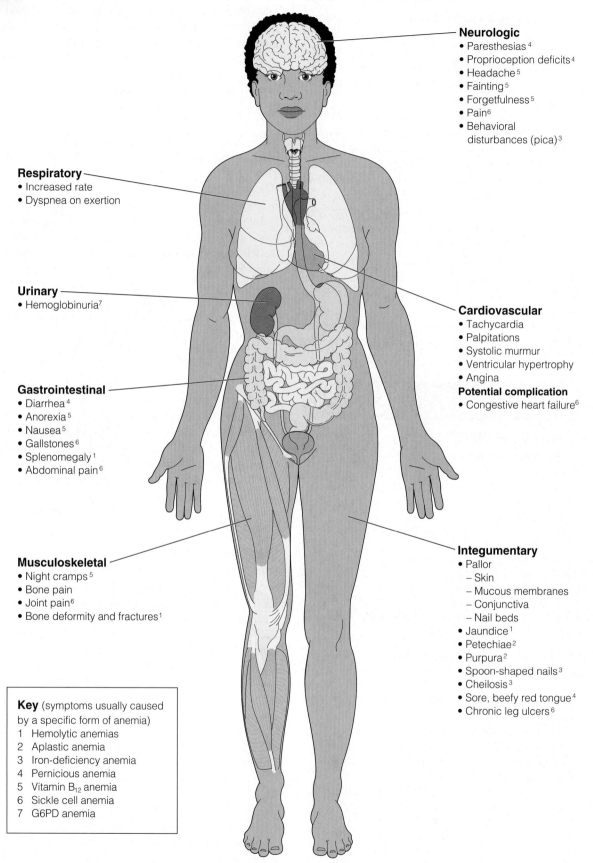

**Neurologic**
- Paresthesias [4]
- Proprioception deficits [4]
- Headache [5]
- Fainting [5]
- Forgetfulness [5]
- Pain [6]
- Behavioral disturbances (pica) [3]

**Respiratory**
- Increased rate
- Dyspnea on exertion

**Urinary**
- Hemoglobinuria [7]

**Cardiovascular**
- Tachycardia
- Palpitations
- Systolic murmur
- Ventricular hypertrophy
- Angina

**Potential complication**
- Congestive heart failure [6]

**Gastrointestinal**
- Diarrhea [4]
- Anorexia [5]
- Nausea [5]
- Gallstones [6]
- Splenomegaly [1]
- Abdominal pain [6]

**Musculoskeletal**
- Night cramps [5]
- Bone pain
- Joint pain [6]
- Bone deformity and fractures [1]

**Integumentary**
- Pallor
  – Skin
  – Mucous membranes
  – Conjunctiva
  – Nail beds
- Jaundice [1]
- Petechiae [2]
- Purpura [2]
- Spoon-shaped nails [3]
- Cheilosis [3]
- Sore, beefy red tongue [4]
- Chronic leg ulcers [6]

**Key** (symptoms usually caused by a specific form of anemia)
1. Hemolytic anemias
2. Aplastic anemia
3. Iron-deficiency anemia
4. Pernicious anemia
5. Vitamin $B_{12}$ anemia
6. Sickle cell anemia
7. G6PD anemia

BOX 32–2   ■ Causes of Iron Deficiency Anemia

- Dietary deficiencies
- Decreased absorption
  a. Partial or total gastrectomy
  b. Chronic diarrhea
  c. Malabsorption syndromes
- Increased metabolic requirements
  a. Pregnancy
  b. Lactation
- Blood loss
  a. Gastrointestinal bleeding (especially due to ulcers or chronic aspirin use)
  b. Menstrual losses
- Chronic hemoglobinuria

In addition to the general manifestations of anemia described earlier, chronic iron deficiency may lead to brittle, spoon-shaped nails; cheilosis (cracks at the corners of the mouth); a smooth, sore tongue; and pica (a craving for unusual substances, such as clay or starch).

The primary treatment for iron deficiency anemia is increased dietary intake of iron-rich foods and oral or parenteral iron supplements.

## Vitamin $B_{12}$ Deficiency Anemia

Vitamin $B_{12}$ is necessary for DNA synthesis and is almost exclusively found in foods derived from animals. **Vitamin $B_{12}$ deficiency** occurs when inadequate vitamin $B_{12}$ is consumed, or, more commonly, when it is poorly absorbed from the gastrointestinal tract. Deficiency of this vitamin impairs cell division and maturation, especially in rapidly proliferating red blood cells. As a result, macrocytic, misshapen (oval rather than concave) RBCs with thin membranes are produced. Great numbers of these large, immature RBCs enter the circulation. These cells are fragile, incapable of carrying adequate amounts of oxygen, and have a shortened life span.

Failure to absorb dietary vitamin $B_{12}$ is called **pernicious anemia.** It develops due to lack of *intrinsic factor,* a substance secreted by the gastric mucosa. Intrinsic factor binds with vitamin $B_{12}$ and travels with it to the ileum, where the vitamin is absorbed. In the absence of intrinsic factor, vitamin $B_{12}$ cannot be absorbed into the body.

Vitamin $B_{12}$ deficiency may also result from other malabsorption disorders and dietary factors. Resection of the stomach or ileum, loss of pancreatic secretions, and chronic gastritis can affect vitamin $B_{12}$ absorption. Dietary deficiencies of vitamin $B_{12}$ are rare, usually occurring only among strict vegetarians.

Manifestations of vitamin $B_{12}$ deficiency anemia develop gradually as bodily stores of the vitamin are depleted. Pallor or slight jaundice and weakness develop. In pernicious anemia, a smooth, sore, beefy red tongue and diarrhea may occur. Because vitamin $B_{12}$ is important for neurologic function, *paresthesias* (altered sensations, such as numbness or tingling) in the ex-

tremities and problems with *proprioception* (the sense of one's position in space) develop. These manifestations may progress to difficulty maintaining balance due to spinal cord damage. Central nervous system manifestations of relatively short duration (6 months or less) are reversible with treatment, but may be permanent if treatment is delayed (Tierney et al, 2001).

When the anemia results from insufficient dietary intake of vitamin $B_{12}$, clients are instructed to increase their intake of foods containing the vitamin, such as meats, eggs, and dairy products. Vitamin $B_{12}$ supplements may be ordered for severe anemia or for clients who are strict vegetarians. Parenteral vitamin $B_{12}$ replacement is required when malabsorption disorders or lack of intrinsic factor is the cause. Parenteral replacement therapy must be continued for life.

## Folic Acid Deficiency Anemia

Like vitamin $B_{12}$, folic acid is required for DNA synthesis and normal maturation of red blood cells. **Folic acid deficiency anemia** is characterized by fragile, megaloblastic cells. Folic acid is found in green leafy vegetables, fruits, cereals, and meats, and is absorbed from the intestines.

Folic acid deficiency anemia due to inadequate intake is more common among people who are chronically undernourished. This includes older adults, alcoholics, and the drug addicted. Alcoholics are especially at risk because alcohol suppresses folate metabolism, which forms folic acid. Increased folic acid requirements also may lead to anemia. Pregnant women are at the greatest risk. Infants and teenagers can develop temporary folic acid deficiencies during periods of rapid growth. Impaired folic acid absorption and metabolism can cause folic acid deficiency anemia. Malabsorption disorders such as celiac sprue (a hereditary gastrointestinal disorder characterized by inability to metabolize amino acids found in gluten), and certain medications, such as methotrexate and some chemotherapeutic agents, may be implicated. Causes of folic acid deficiency anemia are summarized in Box 32–3.

BOX 32–3   ■ Causes of Folic Acid Deficiency Anemia

- Inadequate dietary intake
  *At risk:*
  a. Older adults
  b. Alcoholics
  c. Clients receiving total parenteral nutrition
- Increased metabolic requirements
  *At risk:*
  a. Pregnant women
  b. Infants and teenagers
  c. Clients undergoing hemodialysis
  d. Clients with forms of hemolytic anemia
- Folic acid malabsorption and impaired metabolism
  a. Celiac sprue
  b. Chemotherapeutic agents, folate antagonists (methotrexate, pentamidine), or anticonvulsants
  c. Alcoholism

The manifestations develop gradually as folic acid stores are depleted. Signs and symptoms may include pallor, progressive weakness and fatigue, shortness of breath, and heart palpitations. Manifestations similar to those associated with vitamin $B_{12}$ anemia, such as glossitis, cheilosis, and diarrhea, are common. No neurologic symptoms occur with folic acid deficiency anemia, helping differentiate it from vitamin $B_{12}$ deficiency anemia. These two nutritional anemias do, however, sometimes coexist.

Among the undernourished, adding foods containing folic acid to the diet usually corrects the anemia. Other clients often require oral folic acid supplements. Depending on the cause of the deficiency, folate replacement may continue for a short or an expended period of time. Folate supplements are recommended for all women who can become pregnant and during pregnancy. Folate deficiency is strongly associated with neural tube defects such as meningomyelocele. The neural tube develops early in the process of fetal development, often before pregnancy is recognized.

## Hemolytic Anemias

**Hemolytic anemias** are characterized by premature destruction (*lysis*) of RBCs. When RBCs break down, iron and other by-products of their destruction remain in the plasma. RBC lysis may occur within the circulatory system or due to phagocytosis by cells of the reticuloendothelial system. In response to hemolysis, the hematopoietic activity of bone marrow increases, leading to increased reticulocytes in circulating blood. Most types of hemolytic anemia are characterized by normocytic and normochromic RBCs.

There are many different causes of hemolytic anemias (Box 32–4). The cause may be *intrinsic,* arising from disorders within the RBC itself, or *extrinsic,* originating outside the RBC. Intrinsic disorders include cell membrane defects, defects in hemoglobin structure and function, and inherited enzyme deficiencies. Extrinsic causes of hemolytic anemia include drugs, bacterial and other toxins, and trauma. This section discusses sickle cell anemia, thalassemia, acquired hemolytic anemia, and glucose-6-phosphate dehydrogenase anemia.

| BOX 32–4 ■ Causes of Hemolytic Anemia |
| --- |

**INTRINSIC**

- RBC cell-membrane defects
- Hemoglobin structure defects (e.g., sickle cell anemia, thalassemia)
- Inherited enzyme defects (e.g., G6PD deficiency)

**EXTRINSIC**

- Drugs, chemicals
- Toxins and venoms
- Bacterial and other infections
- Trauma, burns
- Mechanical damage (prosthetic heart valves)

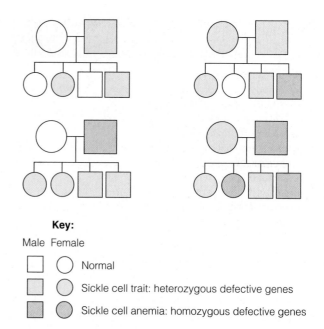

**Key:**

Male   Female

☐ ◯   Normal

☐ ◯   Sickle cell trait: heterozygous defective genes

☐ ◯   Sickle cell anemia: homozygous defective genes

**Figure 32–5** ■ Inheritance pattern for sickle cell anemia.

## Sickle Cell Anemia

**Sickle cell anemia** is a hereditary, chronic hemolytic anemia. It is characterized by episodes of *sickling,* during which RBCs become abnormally crescent shaped. The disorder is transmitted as an autosomal recessive genetic defect (Figure 32–5 ■). This defect causes synthesis of an abnormal form of hemoglobin (HbS) within red blood cells. Sickle cell anemia can significantly shorten life span, with most deaths occurring due to infection (McCance & Huether, 2002).

The disease is most common among people of African descent (see Focus on Diversity box on page 939). In the United States, 7% to 13% of blacks carry the defective gene, having inherited it from one parent (McCance & Huether, 2002). These people have *sickle cell trait.* About 40% of their hemoglobin is HbS (Porth, 2002). They are likely to remain asymptomatic unless stressed by severe hypoxia. Less than 1% of African Americans are homozygous for the disorder; that is, they have inherited a defective gene from both parents. These people have *sickle cell disease;* nearly all their hemoglobin is HbS (Porth, 2002). They are at risk for **sickle cell crisis,** severe episodes of fever and intense pain that are the hallmark of this disorder.

The HbS gene changes the structure of the beta chain of the hemoglobin molecule. When hypoxemia develops and HbS is deoxygenated, it crystallizes into rodlike structures. Clusters of these rods form long chains that deform the erythrocyte into a crescent or sickle shape. The sickled cells tend to clump together and obstruct capillary blood flow, causing ischemia and possible infarction of surrounding tissue. See *Pathophysiology Illustrated* on page 940.

When normal oxygen tension is restored, the sickled RBCs resume their normal shape; that is, they "unsickle." Repeated episodes of sickling and unsickling weaken RBC cell mem-

## Focus on Diversity

### SICKLE CELL ANEMIA

Sickle cell anemia tends to affect people whose origins are in equatorial countries, particularly those in central Africa, the Near East, the Mediterranean region, and parts of India. Hispanics from the Caribbean and Central and South America also may have the HbS gene. This gene may protect against lethal forms of malaria, an endemic disease in many equatorial regions.

The gene for HbS is transmitted in an autosomal recessive pattern from parent to offspring. A parent with one HbS gene (heterozygous) has a 50% risk of transmitting the gene to each child (see Figure 32–5). If both parents carry the gene, each child has a 25% risk of inheriting the gene from both parents. A person who carries both HbS genes (homozygous) is likely to develop sickle cell disease.

Sickle cell anemia is a serious chronic and recurrent disease. The stress of the disease is compounded by the risk for its transmission to offspring. Recommend that all clients with sickle cell trait or disease obtain genetic counseling as part of their family planning process.

branes. The weakened RBCs are hemolyzed and removed. Consequently, the normal life span of RBCs is greatly reduced in sickle cell anemia, increasing the demand for RBC production. Conditions likely to trigger sickling include hypoxia, low environmental or body temperature, excessive exercise, anesthesia, dehydration, infections, or acidosis.

The acute and chronic manifestations of sickle cell anemia arise from episodes of RBC sickling. Sickling causes general manifestations of hemolytic anemia, including pallor, fatigue, jaundice, and irritability. Extensive sickling can precipitate a crisis due to occluded circulation, impaired erythropoiesis, or sequestration of large amounts of blood in the liver or spleen.

A vasoocclusive or thrombotic crisis occurs when sickling develops in the microcirculation. Obstruction of blood flow triggers vasospasm that halts all blood flow in the vessel. Lack of blood flow leads to tissue ischemia and infarction. Vasoocclusive crises are painful and last an average of 4 to 6 days. Infarction of small vessels in the extremities causes painful swelling of the hands and feet; large joints also may be affected. Priapism (persistent, painful erection of the penis) may develop. Abdominal pain may signal infarction of abdominal organs and structures. Stroke may result from cerebral vessel occlusion (McCance & Huether, 2002). Repeated infarcts associated with sickling can affect the structure and function of nearly every organ system.

Compromised erythropoiesis can lead to profound *aplastic anemia* in sickle cell disease due to the shortened RBC life span. *Sequestration crises* are marked by pooling of large amounts of blood in the liver and spleen. This sickle cell crisis only occurs in children.

There is no cure for this disease; treatment is primarily supportive. Treatment for sickle cell crisis includes rest, oxygen,

and analgesics for pain. Adequate hydration is essential to improve blood flow, reduce pain, and prevent renal damage. Precipitating factors are treated, and folic acid supplements may be given to meet the increased demands for RBC production. Blood transfusions may be necessary during surgery or pregnancy. Genetic counseling is recommended for people at risk for sickle cell anemia.

### Thalassemia

**Thalassemia** is an inherited disorder of hemoglobin synthesis in which either the alpha or beta chains of the hemoglobin molecule are missing or defective. This leads to deficient hemoglobin production and fragile hypochromic, microcytic RBCs called *target cells* because of their distinctive bull's-eye appearance.

Thalassemia usually affects certain populations. People of Mediterranean descent (southern Italy and Greece) are more likely to have beta-defect thalassemias (often called *Cooley's anemia* or Mediterranean anemia). People of Asian ancestry, especially from Thailand, the Philippines, and China, more often have alpha-defect thalassemia. Africans and African Americans may have both alpha- and beta-defect thalassemia. As with sickle cell anemia, only one defective beta chain-forming gene may be present (*beta-thalassemia minor*), causing mild symptoms or both may be defective (*beta-thalassemia major*), leading to more severe symptoms. Children with thalassemia major rarely reach adulthood, although repeated blood transfusions may extend their lifespan (McCance & Huether, 2002). Four genes are responsible for alpha chain formation; one, two, three, or all four may be defective. In the latter case (*alpha-thalassemia major*), death is inevitable and usually occurs in utero. Genetic studies and counseling are recommended for people at risk for this illness.

People with thalassemia minor often are asymptomatic. When manifestations do occur, they include mild to moderate anemia, mild splenomegaly, bronze skin coloring, and bone marrow hyperplasia. The major form of the disease causes severe anemia, heart failure, and liver and spleen enlargement from increased red cell destruction. Fractures of the long bones, ribs, and vertebrae may result from bone marrow expansion and thinning due to increased hematopoiesis. Accumulation of iron in the heart, liver, and pancreas following repeated transfusions for treatment may eventually cause failure of these organs.

### Acquired Hemolytic Anemia

*Acquired hemolytic anemia* results from hemolysis due to factors outside of the RBC. Causes of acquired hemolytic anemias include:

- Mechanical trauma to RBCs produced by prosthetic heart valves, severe burns, hemodialysis, or radiation
- Autoimmune disorders
- Bacterial or protozoal infection
- Immune-system-mediated responses, such as transfusion reactions
- Drugs, toxins, chemical agents, or venoms

### Hemoglobin S and Red Blood Cell Sickling

Sickle cell anemia is caused by an inherited autosomal recessive defect in Hb synthesis. Sickle cell hemoglobin (HbS) differs from normal hemoglobin only in the substitution of the amino acid valine for glutamine in both beta chains of the hemoglobin molecule.

When HbS is oxygenated, it has the same globular shape as normal hemoglobin. However, when HbS off-loads oxygen, it becomes insoluble in intracellular fluid and crystallizes into rodlike structures. Clusters of rods form polymers (long chains) that bend the erythrocyte into the characteristic crescent shape of the sickle cell.

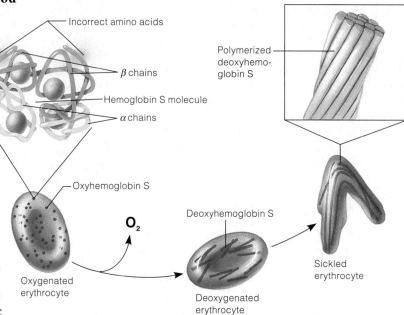

### The Sickle Cell Disease Process

Sickle cell disease is characterized by episodes of acute painful crises. Sickling crises are triggered by conditions causing high tissue oxygen demands or that affect cellular pH. As the crisis begins, sickled erythrocytes adhere to capillary walls and to each other, obstructing blood flow and causing cellular hypoxia. The crisis accelerates as tissue hypoxia and acidic metabolic waste products cause further sickling and cell damage.

Sickle cell crises cause microinfarcts in joints and organs, and repeated crises slowly destroy organs and tissues. The spleen and kidneys are especially prone to sickling damage.

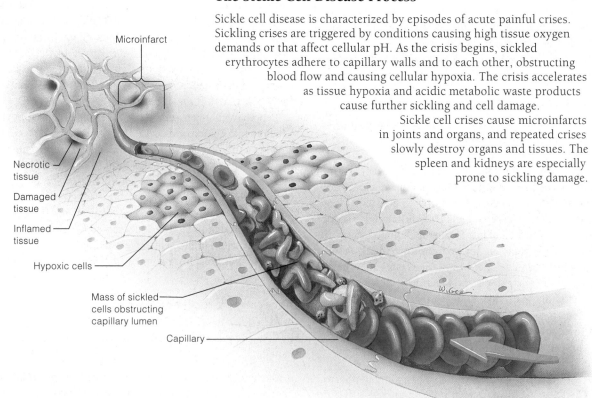

The manifestations of acquired hemolytic anemia depend on the extent of hemolysis and the body's ability to replace destroyed RBCs. The anemia itself often is mild to moderate as erythropoiesis increases to replace the destroyed RBCs. The spleen enlarges as it removes damaged or destroyed RBCs. If the breakdown of heme units exceeds the liver's ability to conjugate and excrete bilirubin, jaundice develops. When the condition is severe, bone marrow expands, and bones may be deformed or may develop pathologic fractures. The severity of generalized manifestations of anemia (tachycardia, pallor, etc.) depends on the degree of anemia and deficiency of tissue oxygenation.

### Glucose-6-Phosphate Dehydrogenase (G6PD) Anemia

*Glucose-6-phosphate dehydrogenase (G6PD) anemia* is caused by a hereditary defect in RBC metabolism. It is relatively common in people of African and Mediterranean descent. The defective gene is located on the X chromosome and therefore affects more males than females. There are many variations of this genetic defect.

G6PD is an enzyme that catalyzes glycolysis, the process in which an RBC derives cellular energy. A defect in G6PD action causes direct oxidation of hemoglobin, damaging the RBC. Hemolysis usually occurs only when the affected person is exposed to stressors (e.g., drugs such as aspirin, sulfonamides, or vitamin K derivatives) that increase the metabolic demands on RBCs. The G6PD deficiency impairs the necessary compensatory increase in glucose metabolism and causes cellular damage. Damaged RBCs are destroyed over a period of 7 to 12 days.

When exposed to a stressor triggering G6PD anemia, symptoms develop within several days. These may include pallor, jaundice, hemoglobinuria (hemoglobin in the urine), and an elevated reticulocyte count. As new RBCs develop, counts return to normal.

### Aplastic Anemia

In **aplastic anemia,** the bone marrow fails to produce all three types of blood cells, leading to *pancytopenia.* Normal bone marrow is replaced by fat. Fortunately, aplastic anemia is rare. *Fanconi anemia* is a rare aplastic anemia caused by defects of DNA repair. The underlying cause of about 50% of acquired aplastic anemia is unknown (*idiopathic aplastic anemia*). Other cases follow stem cell damage caused by exposure to radiation or certain chemical substances such as benzene, arsenic, nitrogen mustard, certain antibiotics (especially chloramphenicol), and chemotherapeutic drugs (McCance & Huether, 2002). Aplastic anemia also may occur with viral infections such as mononucleosis, hepatitis C, and HIV disease (Porth, 2002). Anemia develops as the bone marrow fails to replace RBCs that have reached the end of their life span. Remaining RBCs are normochromic and normocytic.

Manifestations of aplastic anemia vary with the severity of the pancytopenia. Its onset usually is insidious, but may be sudden. Manifestations include fatigue, pallor, progressive weakness, exertional dyspnea, headache, and ultimately tachycardia

and heart failure. Platelet deficiency leads to bleeding problems. A deficiency of white blood cells increases the risk of infection, causing manifestations such as fever.

Treatment focuses on removing the causative agent, if known, and using blood transfusions. Transfusions may be discontinued as soon as the bone marrow resumes blood cell production. Complete recovery may take months. Bone marrow transplant may be the treatment of choice in some instances.

## COLLABORATIVE CARE

Ensuring adequate tissue oxygenation is the priority of care in treating anemia. Specific therapy is determined by the underlying cause of the disorder. Usual treatments include medications, dietary modifications, blood replacement, or supportive interventions.

### Diagnostic Tests

When anemia is suspected, the following laboratory and diagnostic tests may be ordered.

- *Complete blood count (CBC)* is done to determine blood cell counts, hemoglobin, hematocrit, and red blood cell indices (see Table 32–1).
- *Iron levels* and *total iron-binding capacity* are performed to detect iron deficiency anemia. A low serum iron concentration and elevated total iron-binding capacity are indicative of iron deficiency anemia.
- *Serum ferritin* is low due to depletion of the total iron reserves available for hemoglobin synthesis. Ferritin is an iron-storage protein produced by the liver, spleen, and bone marrow. Ferritin mobilizes stored iron when metabolic needs are higher than dietary intake.
- *Sickle cell test* is a screening test to evaluate hemolytic anemia and detect HbS.
- *Hemoglobin electrophoresis* separates normal hemoglobin from abnormal forms. It is used to evaluate hemolytic anemia, diagnose thalassemia, and differentiate sickle cell trait from sickle cell disease (Malarkey & McMorrow, 2000).
- *Schilling test* measures vitamin $B_{12}$ absorption before and after intrinsic factor administration to differentiate between pernicious anemia and intestinal malabsorption of the vitamin. A 24-hour urine sample is collected following administration of radioactive vitamin $B_{12}$. Lower than normal levels of the tagged $B_{12}$ when intrinsic factor is given concurrently indicate malabsorption rather than pernicious anemia.
- *Bone marrow examination* is done to diagnose aplastic anemia. In aplastic anemia, normal marrow elements are significantly decreased as they are replaced by fat cells. Nursing implications for bone marrow collection are described on page 942.
- *Quantitative assay of G6PD* may be performed to confirm a diagnosis of glucose-6-phosphate dehydrogenase deficiency.

## Nursing Implications for Diagnostic Tests

### Bone Marrow Studies

Bone marrow specimens are obtained by either aspiration or biopsy. The preferred site for bone marrow aspiration is the posterior iliac crest; the sternum may also be used. The procedure is performed by inserting a needle into the bone and drawing out a sample of the blood in the marrow. A bone marrow biopsy is performed by making a small incision over the bone and screwing a core biopsy instrument into the bone to obtain a specimen. Bone marrow studies are used to diagnose leukemias, metastatic cancer, lymphoma, aplastic anemia, and Hodgkin's disease.

#### Preparation of the Client
- Explain the purpose and procedure of the test.
- Record vital signs. Assure presence of a signed consent for the procedure.
- Ask the client to void.
- Place in supine position if the specimen will be obtained from the sternum or anterior iliac crest; prone position if the posterior iliac crest will be used.
- Assist in remaining still during the procedure.

#### After the Procedure
- Apply pressure to the puncture site for 5 to 10 minutes.
- Assess vital signs, and compare results to preprocedure readings.
- Apply a dressing to the puncture site, and monitor for bleeding and infection for 24 hours.

#### Client and Family Teaching
- The procedure (either aspiration or biopsy) takes about 20 minutes.
- A sedative may be given prior to the procedure.
- It is important to remain very still during the procedure to prevent accidental injury.
- Although the area will be anesthetized with a local anesthetic, insertion of the needle will be painful for a short time. Taking deep breaths may make this part of the procedure less painful.
- The aspiration site may ache for 1 or 2 days.
- Report any unusual bleeding immediately.

## Medications

Medications used to treat anemia depend on its cause. Iron replacement therapy is ordered for iron deficiency anemia. Supplemental iron may be given by mouth or intramuscularly. Parenteral vitamin $B_{12}$ is given when malabsorption or lack of intrinsic factor leads to vitamin $B_{12}$ deficiency anemia. Folic acid is ordered for women of childbearing age, pregnant women, and clients with folic acid deficiency or sickle cell anemia to meet the increased demands of the bone marrow. Hydroxyurea, a drug that promotes fetal hemoglobin production, may be prescribed for clients with sickle cell disease. Resulting increased levels of fetal hemoglobin interfere with the sickling process and reduce the incidence of painful crises (Braunwald et al., 2001). Nursing implications for clients receiving iron, vitamin $B_{12}$, and folic acid are found in the Medication Administration box on page 943.

Immunosuppressive therapy with antithymocyte globulin (ATG), corticosteroids, and cyclosporine may be used to treat aplastic anemia. Androgens may stimulate blood cell production in some clients with aplastic anemia. See Chapter 9 for more information about immunosuppression.

## Dietary Therapy

Dietary modifications are recommended for nutritional deficiency anemias, such as iron deficiency anemia, vitamin $B_{12}$ deficiency anemia, or folic acid deficiency anemia. Box 32–5 identifies good sources of dietary iron, vitamin $B_{12}$, and folic acid.

## Blood Transfusion

Blood transfusions may be indicated to treat anemias resulting from major blood loss, such as from trauma or major surgery, and severe anemia regardless of cause. Blood transfusions are fully discussed in Chapter 6.

---

### BOX 32–5 ■ Dietary Sources of Iron, Folic Acid, and Vitamin $B_{12}$

#### IRON
Iron in the diet comes from two sources. *Heme iron* makes up about one-half of the iron from animal sources. *Nonheme iron* includes the remaining iron from animal sources and all the iron from plants, legumes, and nuts. Heme iron promotes absorption of nonheme iron from other foods when both forms are consumed at the same time. Absorption of nonheme iron is also enhanced by vitamin C and inhibited by tea and coffee.

#### SOURCES OF HEME IRON
- Beef
- Chicken
- Egg yolk
- Clams, oysters
- Pork loin
- Turkey
- Veal

#### SOURCES OF NONHEME IRON
- Bran flakes
- Brown rice
- Whole-grain breads
- Dried beans
- Dried fruits
- Greens
- Oatmeal

#### SOURCES OF FOLIC ACID
- Green leafy vegetables
- Broccoli
- Organ meats
- Eggs
- Wheat germ
- Asparagus
- Liver
- Milk
- Yeast
- Kidney beans

#### SOURCES OF VITAMIN $B_{12}$
- Liver
- Fresh shrimp and oysters
- Eggs
- Milk
- Kidney
- Meats (muscle)
- Cheese

# Medication Administration

## Drugs to Treat Anemia

### IRON SOURCES

Ferrous sulfate (Feosol, Fer-in-sol)
Ferrous gluconate (Fergon, Ferralet, Fertinic)
Iron dextran injection (Imferon)
Iron polysaccharide

Iron preparations are normally taken by mouth and are absorbed from the gastrointestinal tract. They are given to treat anemias resulting from iron deficiency or blood loss. When absorbed, iron combines with transferrin. This complex then is transported to the bone marrow and incorporated into hemoglobin.

### Nursing Responsibilities

- Prior to giving the drug, assess for use of drugs that might interact with iron (e.g., antacids, allopurinol, chloramphenicol, tetracyclines, vitamin E), gastrointestinal bleeding, and manifestations of anemia.
- Administer iron preparations with orange juice to enhance absorption.
- If using an elixir, give it through a straw to prevent staining the teeth.
- Monitor for manifestations of iron toxicity: nausea, diarrhea, or constipation; symptoms of anaphylactic shock (extreme cases).
- Monitor hemoglobin and reticulocyte counts.
- If the client is also taking tetracyclines, schedule the dose of iron 2 hours before tetracycline (iron reduces the absorption of tetracycline).

### Client and Family Teaching

- Gastrointestinal side effects may be reduced by taking iron with food (but not milk, which decreases absorption).
- Stools may be dark green or black; this is harmless.
- Increase fluids and fiber in diet to decrease constipation.

### VITAMIN B$_{12}$ SOURCES

Cyanocobalamin (Kaybovite [oral], Anacobin [parenteral], Bedoz)

Cyanocobalamin is used to treat vitamin B$_{12}$ deficiencies or malabsorption and pernicious anemia. It is rapidly absorbed when administered orally or by injection, and it is stored in the liver. Intrinsic factor is necessary for absorption from the gastrointestinal tract.

### Nursing Responsibilities

- Do not expose crystalline injection to light.
- Assess for other drugs that might interfere with the therapeutic response: chloramphenicol, cimetidine, colchicine, and timed-release potassium decrease its effectiveness.
- Do not mix cyanocobalamin in a syringe with other medications.
- Administer parenteral doses intramuscularly or deep subcutaneously to decrease local irritation.
- Monitor hemoglobin, RBC counts, reticulocyte counts, and potassium levels.

### Client and Family Teaching

- A burning sensation with injection is temporary.
- Avoid alcohol, which interferes with absorption.
- If used to treat pernicious anemia, the medication must be taken for life.

### FOLIC ACID SOURCES

Folic acid (Folvite, novofolacid)

Synthetic folic acid is used to treat folic acid deficiency and megaloblastic or macrocytic anemia. It is absorbed from the gastrointestinal tract and stored in the liver.

### Nursing Responsibilities

- Prior to giving the medication, assess for use of drugs that alter its effect: corticosteroids, methotrexate, oral contraceptives, phenytoin, sulfonamides.
- Do not mix folic acid with other medications in the same syringe.
- Monitor for possible hypersensitivity response of skin rash.

### Client and Family Teaching

- Large doses of folic acid may cause the urine to become darker yellow.
- Excess alcohol intake increases folic acid requirements.

## Complementary Therapies

Complementary health care practitioners may recommend specific plant enzymes to treat nutritional anemias. Plant enzymes are believed to aid digestion of proteins, fats, and carbohydrates, facilitating absorption of their nutrients. Therapy is determined by the specific type of anemia. Plant enzymes should not be used alone to treat anemia, and it is important to check for possible interactions with prescribed medications before starting therapy.

## NURSING CARE

## Health Promotion

Nursing measures to prevent anemia focus on teaching good dietary habits to all clients, regardless of age. Stress the impor-
tance of consuming adequate amounts of iron, folate, and the B vitamins. Provide a list of dietary sources of these nutrients. Discuss alternate iron sources with vegetarian clients, and teach them that foods high in vitamin C enhance the absorption of iron from grains, legumes, and other sources. Emphasize the importance of adequate iron intake in women of childbearing age and older adults. Stress the increased need for these nutrients during pregnancy, and discuss strategies to ensure an adequate intake.

## Assessment

Assessment data to collect for clients with suspected anemia includes:

- Health history: complaints of shortness of breath with activity, fatigue, weakness, dizziness or fainting, palpitations; history of previous anemia, bleeding episodes;

menstrual history (if appropriate); medications; chronic diseases; usual diet and patterns of alcohol intake or cigarette smoking

- Physical examination: general appearance, skin color; vital signs including temperature; heart and lung sounds; peripheral pulses, capillary refill; abdominal tenderness; obvious bleeding or bruising

## Nursing Diagnoses and Interventions

Anemia affects circulating oxygen levels and tissue oxygenation. Priority nursing diagnoses include activity intolerance, altered oral mucous membranes, and self-care deficits. With acute blood-loss anemia, risk for insufficient cardiac output also is a priority. Clients with sickle cell disease have specific needs related to the effects of the disease on tissue perfusion; see the section on disseminated intravascular coagulation (DIC) later in this chapter for nursing interventions appropriate to ineffective tissue perfusion, associated pain, and maintaining oxygenation.

### Activity Intolerance

Anemia causes weakness and shortness of breath on exertion. These symptoms are due to decreased circulating oxygen levels secondary to low hemoglobin levels. Weakness, fatigue, and/or vertigo may occur even during activities of daily living, including those associated with self-care, home life, job performance, and social roles.

- Help identify ways to conserve energy when performing necessary or desired activities. *Modifying the approach to a particular activity may reduce cardiorespiratory symptoms and activity-related fatigue. Alternative ways of performing tasks (e.g., sitting when performing hygiene care and kitchen tasks) may reduce oxygen demands. In some cases, assistance from others is necessary to conserve energy and reduce symptoms.*
- Help the client and family establish priorities for tasks and activities. *Because family members may need to assume responsibility for additional tasks, the plan's success depends on mutually established goals.*
- Assist to develop a schedule of alternating activity and rest periods throughout the day. *Rest periods decrease oxygen needs, reducing strain on the heart and lungs, and allowing restoration of homeostasis before further activities.*
- Encourage 8 to 10 hours of sleep at night. *Rest decreases oxygen demands and increases available energy for morning activities.*
- Monitor vital signs before and after activity. *Vital signs provide a measure of activity tolerance. Increased heart and respiratory rates or a change in blood pressure may indicate intolerance of the activity.*
- Discontinue activity if any of the following occurs.
  a. Complaints of chest pain, breathlessness, or vertigo
  b. Palpitations or tachycardia that does not return to normal within 4 minutes of resting
  c. Bradycardia
  d. Tachypnea or dyspnea
  e. Decreased systolic blood pressure

*These changes may signify cardiac decompensation due to insufficient oxygenation. The intensity, duration, or frequency of the activity needs to be reduced.*
- Instruct the client not to smoke. *Smoking causes vasoconstriction and increases carbon monoxide levels in the blood, interfering with tissue oxygenation.*

### Impaired Oral Mucous Membrane

Glossitis and cheilosis may occur with nutritional deficiencies of iron, folate, and vitamin $B_{12}$. The tongue and lips become very red, and fissures or cracks may form at the corners of the mouth.

- Monitor condition of lips and tongue daily. *Glossitis and cheilosis increase the risk for bleeding and infection and may require medical treatment. Pain and discomfort may interfere with oral intake, further worsening the nutritional deficiency.*
- Use a mouthwash of saline, saltwater, or half-strength peroxide and water to rinse the mouth every 2 to 4 hours. Avoid alcohol-based mouthwashes. *This cleanses and soothes oral mucous membranes. Alcohol-based mouthwashes further irritate and dry oral tissues.*
- Provide frequent oral hygiene (after each meal and at bedtime) with a soft bristle toothbrush or sponge. *Removing food debris from painful fissures promotes comfort. A soft toothbrush reduces irritation or bleeding of oral mucosa. Keeping the oral cavity clean also reduces the risk of infection.*
- Apply a petroleum-based lubricating jelly or ointment to the lips after oral care. *Lubricating ointment helps to retain moisture, facilitate healing, and protect the lips from other drying agents.*
- Instruct to avoid hot, spicy, or acidic foods. *Such foods may further irritate and dry mucous membranes.*
- Encourage soft, cool, bland foods. *Foods that are soothing to the mucous membranes promote comfort and help maintain adequate food and fluid intake. Minimizing oral pain may also promote compliance with oral care routines.*
- Encourage eating four to six small meals daily with high protein and vitamin content. *Small, frequent meals may be better tolerated, increasing intake. Nutrient-rich meals promote healing of the mucous membranes.*

### Risk for Decreased Cardiac Output

Cardiac output may be affected by acute bleeding and volume loss or by heart failure resulting from severe anemia. In addition, impaired tissue oxygenation leads to an increased respiratory rate and dyspnea.

- Monitor vital signs, breath sounds, and apical pulse. *Increased cardiac workload can affect the blood pressure, heart, and respiratory rates. Increased blood flow can lead to heart murmur or abnormal heart sounds such as $S_3$ or $S_4$. Tachypnea and dyspnea may affect the depth of respirations, alveolar ventilation, and blood and tissue oxygenation.*
- Assess for pallor, cyanosis, and dependent edema. *Blood is shunted to the vital organs, causing vasoconstriction of skin vessels. This, in addition to lower levels of hemoglobin, cause pallor. Cyanosis, especially of the lips and nail beds, indicates inadequate oxygenation of blood. Dependent edema occurs in response to right ventricular failure.*

**PRACTICE ALERT** *Report signs of decreased cardiac output to the physician. Severe anemia can lead to heart failure, necessitating additional treatment.* ■

### Self-Care Deficit

Energy expenditures for activities of daily living (ADLs) may cause oxygen demands to exceed supply in the client with severe anemia.

- Assist with ADLs, such as bathing, grooming, and eating, as needed. *Assistance decreases energy expenditures and tissue requirements for oxygen, reducing cardiac workload.*
- Discuss the importance of rest periods prior to such activities as dressing. *Rest reduces oxygen demand and cardiac workload. The person who is able to perform self-care in activities of daily living maintains independence, self-esteem, and morale.*

### Using NANDA, NIC, and NOC

Chart 32–1 shows links between NANDA nursing diagnoses, NIC, and NOC for the client with anemia.

### Home Care

With the exception of anemia resulting from acute hemorrhage, most clients with anemia are treated in the home and community setting. Include the following topics when preparing the client and family for home care.

- Nutritional strategies to address deficiencies
- Prescribed medications, vitamins, or mineral supplements and their appropriate use, intended effect, possible adverse effects, and interactions with food or other medications
- Energy conservation strategies
- Other recommended treatment measures and follow-up
- If the anemia is genetically transmitted, such as sickle cell anemia, include inheritance patterns of the disorder, symptoms of crisis, and manifestations to report to the physician

Provide referrals for counseling to facilitate decisions about pregnancy as indicated. Also refer for nutritional assistance and teaching, home health care, or assistance with self-care and home maintenance activities as indicated. Older adults with nutritional anemias may benefit from community services such as senior meals or Meals-on-Wheels.

---

## CHART 32–1   NANDA, NIC, AND NOC LINKAGES

### The Client with Anemia

| NURSING DIAGNOSES | NURSING INTERVENTIONS | NURSING OUTCOMES |
|---|---|---|
| • Activity Intolerance | • Energy Management<br>• Nutrition Management | • Activity Tolerance<br>• Endurance |
| • Fatigue | • Environmental Management | • Energy Conservation |
| • Ineffective Health Maintenance | • Health Education<br>• Self-Responsibility Facilitation<br>• Teaching: Procedure/Treatment | • Health-Seeking Behavior<br>• Knowledge: Health Behaviors<br>• Knowledge: Treatment Regimen |
| • Impaired Oral Mucous Membrane | • Oral Health Restoration<br>• Oral Health Maintenance | • Oral Health<br>• Tissue Integrity: Skin and Mucous Membranes |

*Note. Data from Nursing Outcomes Classification (NOC) by M. Johnson & M. Maas (Eds.), 1997, St. Louis: Mosby; Nursing Diagnoses: Definitions & Classification 2001–2002 by North American Nursing Diagnosis Association, 2001, Philadelphia: NANDA; Nursing Interventions Classification (NIC) by J.C. McCloskey & G. M. Bulechek (Eds.), 2000, St. Louis: Mosby. Reprinted by permission.*

---

## THE CLIENT WITH POLYCYTHEMIA

**Polycythemia,** or *erythrocytosis,* is an excess of red blood cells characterized by a hematocrit higher than 55%. The two major types of polycythemia are primary and secondary. *Primary polycythemia,* also called *polycythemia vera,* is an uncommon disorder of increased RBC production. This condition more commonly affects men of European Jewish ancestry between age 40 and 70. *Secondary polycythemia* occurs in response to elevated erythropoietin levels. This commonly is a compensatory response to hypoxia, often due to living at a high altitude, smoking, or chronic lung disease. A third type of polycythemia, *relative polycythemia,* is not due to an excess of RBCs but to fluid deficit. The total red blood cell count is normal, but fluid loss increases cell concentration, thus raising the hematocrit. Relative polycythemia is corrected by rehydration.

## Nursing Care Plan
## A Client with Folic Acid Deficiency Anemia

Sheri Matthews is a 76-year-old widow who lives alone. She tells Lisa Apana, RN, the nurse in her care provider's office, that she liked to cook when her husband was alive, but preparing an entire meal just for herself seems senseless. She relates that her typical day's menu includes coffee for breakfast, a bologna sandwich and coffee for lunch, and a hot dog or two, a few cookies, and a glass of milk for dinner.

### ASSESSMENT

Mrs. Matthews's nursing history includes a 20 lb (9 kg) weight loss since her husband died 8 months ago. She states that she sometimes has heart palpitations and always feels weak. Physical assessment shows: T 98.8°F (37.1°C), P 110, R 22, BP 90/52. Skin warm, pale, and dry. Diagnostic tests indicate folic acid deficiency anemia, and Mrs. Matthews is started on an oral folic acid supplement and instructed about foods containing folic acid.

### DIAGNOSES

- *Activity intolerance* related to weakness secondary to decreased tissue oxygenation
- *Imbalanced nutrition: Less than body requirements* related to lack of motivation to cook and understanding of nutritional needs, as manifested by weight loss of 20 lb, and folic acid deficiency
- *Deficient knowledge* related to lack of information about a well-balanced diet and foods containing folic acid

### EXPECTED OUTCOMES

- Verbalize the importance of taking folic acid supplements and eating a balanced diet.
- Gain at least 1 lb (0.45 kg) per week.
- Return to previous level of physical energy.
- Consume a balanced diet, including foods containing folic acid.

### PLANNING AND IMPLEMENTATION

- Discuss foods required for a well-balanced diet, as well as dietary sources of folic acid.

- Develop a dietary plan with Mrs. Matthews which includes food preferences and foods that are easy and quick to prepare.
- Discuss the importance of taking the folic acid supplement. Advise to continue taking it even after she begins to feel better.
- Help Mrs. Matthews develop a schedule of activities that provides adequate rest and energy for cooking.

### EVALUATION

Mrs. Matthews gained 1 lb (0.45 kg) during the first week of treatment. She has met with a nutritionist and has a better understanding of nutritional needs. She states that she can prepare hot meals when she schedules a rest period before and after lunch. Ms. Apana has provided written and verbal information about the folic acid supplement and diet. Mrs. Matthews verbalizes understanding, stating, "I will continue to take the folic acid until the doctor tells me to stop. I'm beginning to enjoy cooking again, now that I have a reason to cook!" Ms. Apana contacts the local senior services representative to determine if Mrs. Matthews is able to participate in the local Meals-on-Wheels program.

### Critical Thinking in the Nursing Process

1. What is the pathophysiologic basis for Mrs. Matthews's abnormal vital signs during her initial assessment?
2. Design a week's menu that includes foods high in folic acid.
3. Why was Mrs. Matthews placed on a folic acid supplement in addition to dietary modifications?
4. Why is the older adult at increased risk for developing folic acid deficiency anemia? Consider physiologic, economic, and social factors.

See Evaluating Your Response in Appendix C.

## PATHOPHYSIOLOGY AND MANIFESTATIONS

### Primary Polycythemia

Primary polycythemia, or polycythemia vera (PV), is a neoplastic stem cell disorder characterized by overproduction of RBCs and, to a lesser extent, white blood cells and platelets. It is classified as a myeloproliferative disorder. Its cause is unknown. In PV, colonies of endogenous erythroid stem cells develop. These colonies produce RBCs in the absence of erythropoietin, leading to excess RBC production.

Initially, PV is asymptomatic, and the diagnosis may be made during routine blood tests. Its manifestations are caused by increased blood volume and viscosity. Hypertension is common, and may lead to complaints of headaches, dizziness, and vision and hearing disruptions. Venous stasis causes *plethora,* a ruddy, red color of the face, hands, feet, and mucous

membranes. This often is accompanied by severe, painful itching of the fingers and toes. Retinal and cerebral vessels may be engorged. Hypermetabolism develops, causing weight loss and night sweats. Mental status may be altered, leading to drowsiness or delirium.

Thrombosis and hemorrhage are potential complications of PV. Thrombosis may cause transient ischemic attacks, angina, or manifestations of peripheral vascular disease. Gastrointestinal bleeding may occur, and portal hypertension may develop.

### Secondary Polycythemia

Secondary polycythemia, or erythrocytosis, is increased numbers of RBCs in response to excess erythropoietin secretion or prolonged hypoxia. Secondary polycythemia is the most common form of polycythemia.

## Manifestations of Polycythemia

- Hypertension
- Headache, tinnitus, blurred vision
- Plethora: dark redness of the lips, feet, ears, fingernails, and mucous membranes
- Splenomegaly (polycythemia vera)
- Severe pruritus, extremity pain
- Weight loss, night sweats
- Gastrointestinal bleeding
- Intermittent claudication
- Symptoms from thrombosis within various organs

Abnormally high erythropoietin levels can result from kidney disease or erythropoietin-secreting tumors (e.g., renal cell carcinoma). Chronic hypoxia that stimulates erythropoietin release is a more common cause of secondary polycythemia. People living at high altitudes where the atmospheric oxygen pressure is lower develop a degree of polycythemia, as do people with chronic heart or lung disease and smokers. Abnormal hemoglobin that forms tighter bonds with oxygen also may lead to secondary polycythemia.

The manifestations of secondary polycythemia are similar to those of primary polycythemia. Splenomegaly, however, does not develop. Early symptoms often are overshadowed by the manifestations of the underlying disorder. For the manifestations of polycythemia see the box above.

## COLLABORATIVE CARE

In PV, serum erythropoietin levels are low. Bone marrow studies show hyperplasia of all hematopoietic elements. With secondary polycythemia, serum erythropoietin levels usually are high, and bone marrow studies show only red stem cell hyperplasia.

For secondary polycythemia, treatment focuses on the underlying cause of the disorder. It is a physiologic response in people living at high altitudes, and unless the hematocrit is too high or oxygen saturation levels are low, no treatment is usu-ally necessary. Smokers are urged to quit. Measures to raise oxygen saturation levels and reduce tissue hypoxia often will relieve the polycythemia. Clients with both primary and secondary polycythemia benefit from periodic phlebotomy, removing 300 to 500 mL of blood, to keep blood volume and viscosity within normal levels. For PV, chemotherapeutic agents such as hydroxyurea may be used to suppress marrow function but may increase the risk of developing leukemia (discussed later in this chapter). Pruritus may be relieved by antihistamines, or may require more aggressive treatment with interferon alpha or other treatments. One 325 mg aspirin tablet daily may be ordered to control thrombosis without increasing the risk of bleeding.

## NURSING CARE

Preventing polycythemia begins with educating children and adults about the dangers of smoking. Measures to reduce risk factors for cardiovascular disease also may be beneficial.

This chronic condition is managed in community-based settings unless a complication develops. Teach the client and family the importance of maintaining adequate hydration, increasing fluid intake during hot weather and when exercising. Discuss measures to prevent blood stasis: elevating legs and feet when sitting, using support stockings, and continuing treatment measures. Instruct to report manifestations of thrombosis (leg or calf pain, chest pain, neurologic symptoms) or bleeding (black, tarry stools, vomiting blood or coffee-ground emesis) immediately. Monitor the hematocrit and cell counts throughout treatment.

Examples of nursing diagnoses appropriate for the client with polycythemia follow:

- *Decisional conflict regarding smoking cessation* related to addictive effects
- *Pain* related to effects of altered blood flow in distal extremities
- *Risk for ineffective tissue perfusion* related to sluggish blood flow and increased risk for thrombosis

# PLATELET AND COAGULATION DISORDERS

Platelet and coagulation disorders affect **hemostasis,** control of bleeding. Hemostasis is a series of complex interactions between platelets and clotting mechanisms that maintains a relatively steady state of blood volume, blood pressure, and blood flow through injured vessels.

## PHYSIOLOGY REVIEW
### Platelets

**Platelets,** or **thrombocytes,** are cell fragments that have no nucleus and cannot replicate. They are metabolically active, however, producing ATP and releasing mediators required for clotting. Platelets are formed in the bone marrow as pinched-off portions of large megakaryocytes (see Figure 32–1). Platelet production is controlled by *thrombopoietin,* a protein produced by the liver, kidney, smooth muscle, and bone marrow. The number of circulating platelets controls thrombopoietin release. Once released from the bone marrow, platelets remain in the spleen for about 8 hours before entering the circulation. Platelets live up to 10 days in circulation. There are about 250,000 to 400,000 platelets in each milliliter of blood. An excess of platelets is *thrombocytosis.* A deficit of platelets is *thrombocytopenia.*

## Hemostasis

**Hemostasis,** or blood clotting, is a complex process that controls bleeding and clotting. The five stages to hemostasis are (1) vessel spasm, (2) formation of the platelet plug, (3) development of an insoluble fibrin clot, (4) clot retraction, and (5) clot dissolution.

### Vessel Spasm

When a blood vessel is damaged, thromboxane $A_2$ ($TXA_2$) is released from platelets and cells, causing *vessel spasm.* This spasm constricts the damaged vessel for about 1 minute.

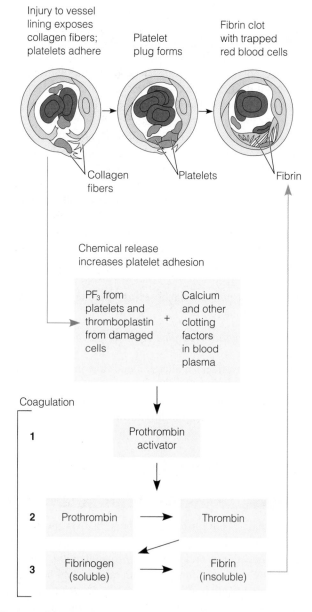

**Figure 32–6** ■ Platelet plug formation and blood clotting. The flow diagram summarizes the events leading to fibrin clot formation. $PF_3$ (blue arrow) released from damaged tissue combines with other clotting factors to release prothrombin activator, the first step of coagulation. Second, prothrombin is converted into thrombin. Finally, thrombin transforms soluble fibrinogen into insoluble fibrin (red arrow) to form a clot.

### Formation of the Platelet Plug

Platelets attracted to the damaged vessel wall change from smooth disks to spiny spheres. Receptors on the activated platelets bind with *von Willebrand's factor,* a protein molecule, and exposed collagen fibers at the site of injury to form the *platelet plug* (Figure 32–6 ■). The platelets release adenosine diphosphate (ADP) and $TXA_2$ to activate nearby platelets, adhering them to the developing plug. Activation of the clotting pathway on the platelet surface converts fibrinogen to fibrin. Fibrin, in turn, forms a meshwork that binds the platelets and other blood cells to form a stable plug (Figure 32–7 ■).

### Blood Coagulation

The process of **coagulation** creates a meshwork of fibrin strands that cements the blood components to form an insoluble clot. Coagulation requires many interactive reactions and two clotting pathways (Figure 32–8 ■). The slower intrinsic pathway is activated when blood contacts collagen in the injured vessel wall; the faster extrinsic pathway is activated when blood is exposed to tissues. The final outcome of both pathways is fibrin clot formation. Each procoagulation substance is activated in sequence; the activation of one coagulation factor activates another in turn. Table 32–2 lists known factors, their origin, and their function or pathway. A deficiency of one or more factors or inappropriate inactivation of any factor alters normal coagulation.

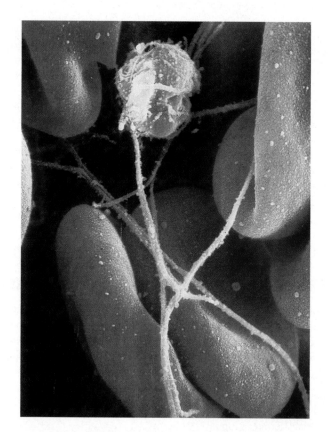

**Figure 32–7** ■ Scanning electron micrograph of a RBC trapped in a fibrin mesh. The spherical gray object at top is a platelet.

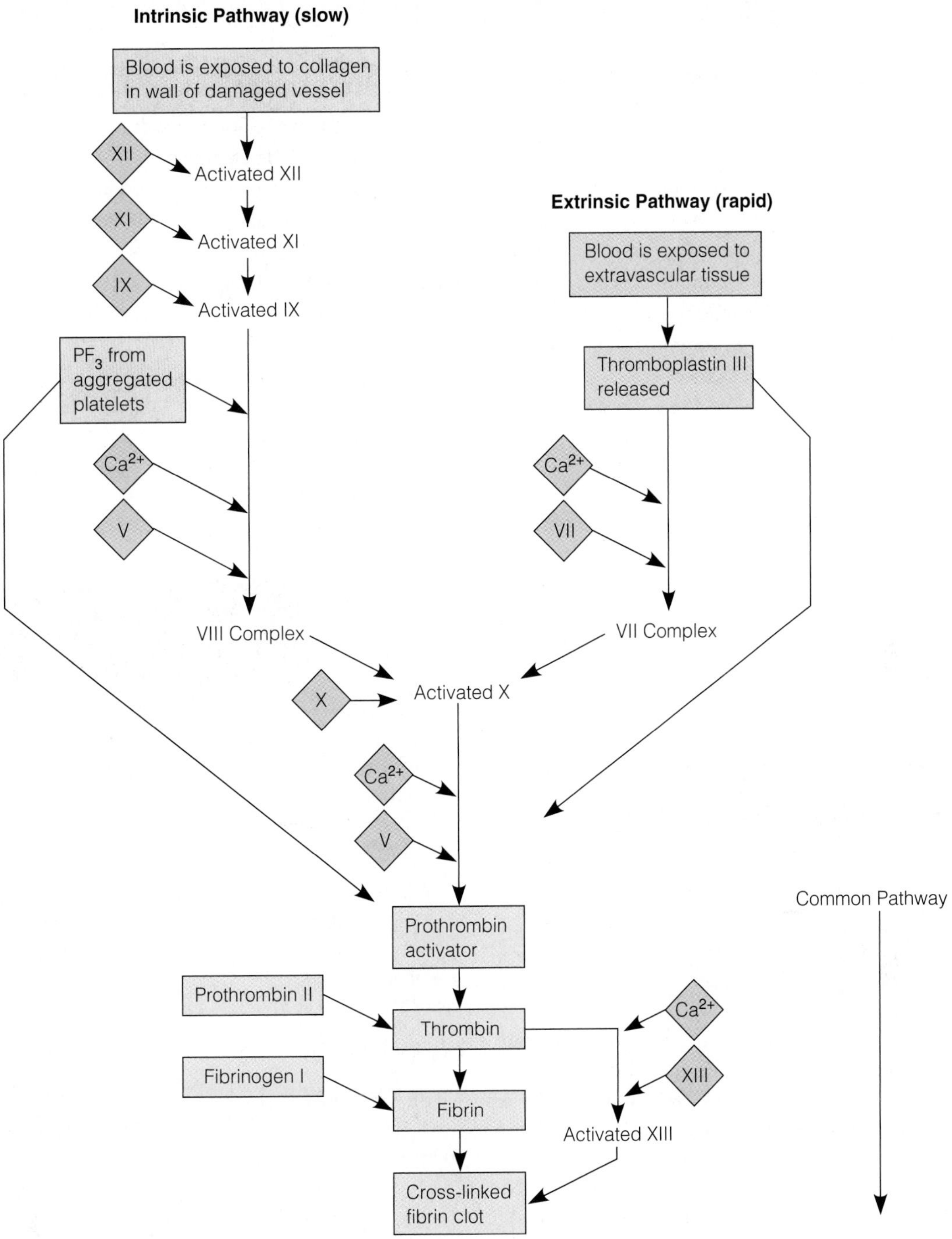

**Figure 32–8** ■ Clot formation. Both the slower intrinsic pathway and the more rapid extrinsic pathway activate factor X. Factor X then combines with other factors to form prothrombin activator. Prothrombin activator transforms prothrombin into thrombin, which then transforms fibrinogen into long fibrin strands. Thrombin also activates factor XIII, which draws the fibrin strands together into a dense meshwork. The complete process of clot formation occurs within 3 to 6 minutes after blood vessel damage.

## Clot Retraction

After the clot is stabilized (within about 30 minutes), trapped platelets contract, much like muscle cells. Platelet contraction squeezes the fibrin strands, pulling the broken portions of the ruptured blood vessel closer together. Growth factors released by the platelets stimulate cell division and tissue repair of the damaged vessel.

## Clot Dissolution

*Fibrinolysis,* the process of clot dissolution, begins shortly after the clot has formed, restoring blood flow and promoting tissue repair. Like coagulation, fibrinolysis requires a sequence of interactions between activator and inhibitor substances. Plasminogen, an enzyme that promotes fibrinolysis, is converted into plasmin, its active form, by chemical mediators released

| TABLE 32–2 | Blood Coagulation Factors | |
|---|---|---|
| **Factor** | **Name** | **Function or Pathway** |
| I | Fibrinogen | Converted to fibrin strands |
| II | Prothrombin | Converted to thrombin |
| III | Thromboplastin | Catalyzes conversion of thrombin |
| IV | Calcium ions | Needed for all steps of coagulation |
| V | Proaccelerin | Extrinsic/intrinsic pathways |
| VII | Serum prothrombin conversion accelerator | Extrinsic pathway |
| VIII | Antihemophilic factor | Intrinsic pathway |
| IX | Plasma prothrombin component | Intrinsic pathway |
| X | Stuart factor | Extrinsic/intrinsic pathways |
| XI | Plasma prothrombin antecedent | Intrinsic pathway |
| XII | Hageman factor | Intrinsic pathway |
| XIII | Fibrin stabilizing factor | Cross-links fibrin strands to form insoluble clot |

from vessel walls and the liver. Plasmin dissolves the clot's fibrin strands and certain coagulation factors. Stimuli such as exercise, fever, and vasoactive drugs promote plasminogen activator release. The liver and endothelium also produce fibrinolytic inhibitors.

## THE CLIENT WITH THROMBOCYTOPENIA

**Thrombocytopenia** is a platelet count of less than 100,000 per milliliter of blood. It can lead to abnormal bleeding. A continuing decline in circulating platelets to less than 20,000/mL can lead to spontaneous bleeding and hemorrhage from minor trauma. Bleeding due to platelet deficiency usually occurs in small vessels, causing manifestations such as *petechiae* (small red or purple spots that do not blanch with pressure) and *purpura* (purple bruising). The mucous membranes of the nose, mouth, GI tract, and vagina often bleed. Serious and potentially fatal bleeding occurs when the platelet count is less than 10,000/mL.

Thrombocytopenia results from one of three mechanisms: decreased production, increased sequestration in the spleen, or accelerated destruction. Primary thrombocytopenia that leads to increased platelet destruction is discussed below. Secondary thrombocytopenia may be caused by aplastic anemia, bone marrow malignancy, infection, radiation therapy, or drug therapy (Box 32–6). Platelet sequestration usually is due to an enlarged spleen. Up to 80% of platelets may be removed from circulation with significant splenomegaly (Porth, 2002). Finally, thrombocytopenia may result from premature platelet destruction associated with disseminated intravascular coagulation (DIC).

## PATHOPHYSIOLOGY AND MANIFESTATIONS

The two types of primary thrombocytopenia are immune thrombocytopenic purpura and thrombotic thrombocytopenic purpura.

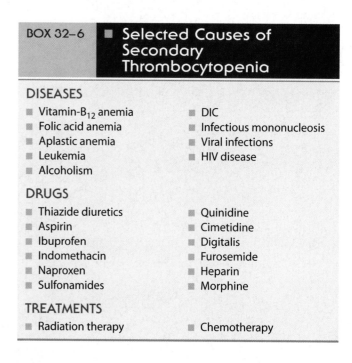

BOX 32–6  ■  **Selected Causes of Secondary Thrombocytopenia**

**DISEASES**

- Vitamin-B$_{12}$ anemia
- Folic acid anemia
- Aplastic anemia
- Leukemia
- Alcoholism
- DIC
- Infectious mononucleosis
- Viral infections
- HIV disease

**DRUGS**

- Thiazide diuretics
- Aspirin
- Ibuprofen
- Indomethacin
- Naproxen
- Sulfonamides
- Quinidine
- Cimetidine
- Digitalis
- Furosemide
- Heparin
- Morphine

**TREATMENTS**

- Radiation therapy
- Chemotherapy

### Immune Thrombocytopenic Purpura

*Immune thrombocytopenic purpura (ITP),* also known as *idiopathic thrombocytopenic purpura,* is an autoimmune disorder in which platelet destruction is accelerated. In its chronic form, ITP typically affects young adults between age 20 and 40; women are affected more often than men. Acute ITP is more common in children, and often follows a viral illness. Acute ITP typically lasts only 1 to 2 months (McCance & Huether, 2002).

In ITP, proteins on the platelet cell membrane stimulate autoantibody production, usually IgG antibodies. These autoantibodies adhere to the platelet membrane. Although the platelets function normally, the spleen reacts to them as being foreign and destroys the altered platelets after only 1 to 3 days of circulation.

The manifestations of ITP are due to bleeding from small vessels and mucous membranes. Petechiae and purpura develop, often on the anterior chest, arms, neck, and oral mucous membranes. Bruising also may be apparent. As bleeding progresses, epistaxis (nosebleed), hematuria, excess menstrual bleeding, and bleeding gums occur. Spontaneous intracranial bleeding is rare but does occur. Associated symptoms include weight loss, fever, and headache.

## Thrombotic Thrombocytopenic Purpura

*Thrombotic thrombocytopenic purpura (TTP)* is a rare disorder in which thrombi occlude arterioles and capillaries of the microcirculation. Many organs are affected, including the heart, kidneys, and brain. The incidence of TTP is increasing (McCance & Huether, 2002). Its cause is unknown. Platelet aggregation is a key feature of the disorder. As RBCs circulate through partially occluded vessels, they fragment, leading to hemolytic anemia (Porth, 2002).

TTP may be acute, the more common and severe form, or chronic. Acute idiopathic TTP may be fatal within months if untreated. The manifestations of TTP include purpura and petechiae, and neurologic symptoms such as headache, seizures, and altered consciousness.

## COLLABORATIVE CARE

The diagnosis of thrombocytopenia is based on history, manifestations, and diagnostic test results. Management focuses on treating or removing any causative factors and treating the platelet deficiency.

### Diagnostic Tests

The following diagnostic tests are used to identify thrombocytopenia.

- *CBC* evaluates all cellular components of the blood, as well as the hemoglobin and hematocrit.
- *Platelet count* is decreased.
- *Antinuclear antibodies (ANA)* are measured to assess for autoantibodies.
- *Serologic studies* for hepatitis viruses, cytomegalovirus (CMV), Epstein-Barr virus, toxoplasma, and HIV may be done.
- *Bone marrow examination* evaluates for aplastic anemia and megakaryocyte production.

### Medications

Oral glucocorticoids, such as prednisone, are prescribed to suppress the autoimmune response. Many clients who respond to glucocorticoid treatment relapse when the drug is withdrawn, however. Immunosuppressive drugs such as azathioprine, cyclophosphamide, and cyclosporine may be used.

### Treatments

*Platelet transfusions* may be required to treat acute bleeding due to thrombocytopenia. Platelets are prepared from fresh whole blood; one unit contains 30 to 60 mL of platelet concen-

trate. The expected increase in platelets after one unit is infused is 10,000/mL. *Plasmapheresis,* or *plasma exchange therapy,* is the primary treatment for acute thrombotic thrombocytopenic purpura. The client's plasma is removed and replaced with fresh frozen plasma to remove autoantibodies, immune complexes, and toxins.

### Surgery

A *splenectomy* (surgical removal of the spleen) is the treatment of choice if the client with ITP relapses when glucocorticoids are discontinued. The spleen is the site of platelet destruction and antibody production. This surgery often cures the disorder, although relapse may occur years after splenectomy.

## NURSING CARE

### Assessment

- Health history: complaints of bruising with minor or no trauma, bleeding gums, nosebleed, heavy or prolonged menstrual periods, black, tarry, or bloody stools, hematemesis, headache, fever, or neurologic symptoms; recent weight loss; recent viral or other illness; current and recent medications; exposure to toxins
- Physical examination: skin and mucous membranes for color, temperature, petechiae, purpura, or bruises; vital signs; weight; mental status and level of consciousness; heart and breath sounds; abdominal exam; body fluids for occult blood

### Nursing Diagnoses and Interventions

Inadequate platelets impair hemostasis, placing the client at risk for bleeding. Bleeding gums, an early sign of the disorder, affects oral mucous membrane integrity as well.

### Ineffective Protection

Bleeding is a serious complication associated with thrombocytopenia. As platelet counts (measured in cubic millimeters) decrease, the risk of bleeding increases: The risk is minimal with counts greater than 50,000 mm$^3$; moderate when the count is between 20,000 and 50,000 mm$^3$; and significant when the count falls below 20,000 mm$^3$.

- Monitor vital signs, heart and breath sounds every 4 hours. Frequently assess for other manifestations of bleeding:
  a. Skin and mucous membranes for petechiae, ecchymoses, and hematoma formation
  b. Gums, nasal membranes, and conjunctiva for bleeding
  c. Overt or occult blood in emesis, urine, or stool
  d. Vaginal bleeding
  e. Prolonged bleeding from puncture sites
  f. Neurologic changes: headache, visual changes, altered mental status, decreasing level of consciousness, seizures
  g. Abdominal: epigastric pain, absence of bowel sounds, increasing abdominal girth, abdominal guarding or rigidity

*Early identification of bleeding is important to prevent serious blood loss and shock.*

**PRACTICE ALERT** *Avoid invasive procedures such as rectal temperatures, urinary catheterization, and parenteral injections to the extent possible. Diagnostic procedures such as biopsy or lumbar puncture should be avoided if the platelet count is less than 50,000 mm³. Invasive procedures can cause tissue trauma and bleeding. Procedures that use large-bore needles should be delayed until the platelet count is increased.* ■

- Apply pressure to puncture sites for 3 to 5 minutes; apply pressure to arterial blood gas sites for 15 to 20 minutes. *Pressure promotes hemostasis and clot formation.*
- Instruct to avoid forcefully blowing the nose or picking crusts from the nose, straining to have a bowel movement, and forceful coughing or sneezing. *These activities increase the risk of external and internal bleeding.*

### Impaired Oral Mucous Membranes

Thrombocytopenia frequently leads to bleeding of the gums and oral mucosa. As a result, risk for infection and impaired nutrition increases.

- Frequently assess the mouth for bleeding. Inquire about oral pain or tenderness. *Breakdown of oral mucous membranes increases the risk of infection and bleeding, and causes discomfort with eating.*
- Encourage use of a soft-bristle toothbrush or sponge to clean teeth and gums. *Hard bristles may abrade oral mucosa, causing bleeding and increasing the risk of infection.*
- Instruct to rinse the mouth with saline every 2 to 4 hours. Apply petroleum jelly to lips as needed to prevent dryness and cracking. *Saline mouth rinses and petroleum jelly help maintain oral tissue integrity and promote cleansing and healing.*
- Instruct to avoid alcohol-based mouthwashes, very hot foods, alcohol, and crusty foods. Teach to drink cool liquids at least every 2 hours. *Avoiding foods and liquids that traumatize oral mucosa increases comfort; fluid intake prevents dehydration and helps maintain mucous membrane integrity.*

### Home Care

In the adult, ITP often is a chronic disorder that the client and family must learn to manage. Secondary thrombocytopenia may be either acute or chronic. Discuss the following topics when preparing the client and family for home care.

- Nature of the disorder, its usual course, and the treatment plan
- Use, desired and potential adverse effects of prescribed medications
- Risks and benefits of surgery or treatments such as plasma replacement therapy
- The importance of follow-up tests and visits for care
- Measures to reduce the risk of bleeding: safety measures such as a soft-bristle toothbrush, electric razor, avoidance of contact sports and hazardous activities, and avoiding medications that further interfere with platelet function (Box 32–7)

Refer for home health or other community services (e.g., housekeeping, shopping) as indicated.

---

**BOX 32–7 ■ Medications That May Interfere with Platelet Function**

#### OVER-THE-COUNTER MEDICATIONS

- Aspirin and salicylates, including:
  - Alka-Seltzer
  - Bufferin
  - Doan's Pills
  - Ecotrin
  - Excedrin
  - Midol
  - Pepto-Bismol
  - Vanquish
- NSAIDS such as
  - Advil
  - Aleve
  - Nuprin
  - Pamprin IB

#### PRESCRIPTION MEDICATIONS

- Aspirin-containing analgesics
- Chemotherapy drugs
- Antibiotics such as penicillin
- Carbamazapine (Tegretol)
- Colchicine
- Dipyridamole (Persantine)
- Gold salts
- Heparin
- Quinine derivatives
- Sulfonamides
- Thiazide diuretics

---

## THE CLIENT WITH DISSEMINATED INTRAVASCULAR COAGULATION

**Disseminated intravascular coagulation (DIC)** is a disruption of hemostasis characterized by widespread intravascular clotting and bleeding. It may be acute and life threatening or relatively mild. DIC is a clinical syndrome that develops as a complication of a wide variety of other disorders (Box 32–8). Sepsis is the most common cause of DIC. Gram-negative and gram-positive bacteria as well as viruses, fungi, and protozoal infections may lead to DIC (McCance & Huether, 2002).

---

**BOX 32–8 ■ Conditions That May Precipitate Disseminated Intravascular Coagulation**

#### TISSUE DAMAGE

- Trauma: burns, gunshot wounds, frostbite, head injury
- Obstetric complications: septic abortion, abruptio placentae, amniotic fluid embolus, retained dead fetus
- Neoplasms: acute leukemia, adenocarcinomas
- Hemolysis
- Fat embolism

#### VESSEL DAMAGE

- Aortic aneurysm
- Acute glomerulonephritis
- Hemolytic uremic syndrome

#### INFECTIONS

- Bacterial infection or sepsis
- Viral or mycotic infections
- Parasitic or rickettsial infection

## PATHOPHYSIOLOGY

DIC is triggered by endothelial damage, release of tissue factors into the circulation, or inappropriate activation of the clotting cascade by an endotoxin. Both the intrinsic and the extrinsic clotting cascade may be activated, although the extrinsic cascade usually is the one activated. Extensive thrombin entering the systemic circulation overwhelms natural anticoagulants, leading to unrestricted clot formation (McCance & Huether, 2002). Clotting may be localized to an individual organ, or widespread with deposition of small thrombi and emboli throughout the microvasculature (Braunwald et al., 2001). The widespread clotting consumes clotting factors and activates fibrinolytic processes with anticoagulant production. As a result, hemorrhage occurs (Figure 32–9 ■).

The sequence of DIC follows:

1. Endothelial damage, tissue factors, or toxins stimulate the clotting cascade.
2. Excess thrombin within the circulation overwhelms naturally occurring anticoagulants.
3. Widespread clotting occurs within the microvasculature.
4. Thrombi and emboli impair tissue perfusion, leading to ischemia, infarction, and necrosis.
5. Clotting factors (including platelets) are consumed faster than they can be replaced.
6. Clotting activates fibrinolytic processes which begin to break down clots.
7. Fibrin degradation products (*FDPs,* potent anticoagulants) are released, contributing to bleeding.
8. Clotting factors are depleted, the ability to form clots is lost, and hemorrhage occurs.

## MANIFESTATIONS

The manifestations of DIC result from both clotting and bleeding, although bleeding is more obvious, especially in acute DIC. Bleeding ranges from oozing blood following an injection to frank hemorrhage from every body orifice (see box below). Chronic DIC may be asymptomatic, or may present with peripheral cyanosis, thrombosis, and pregangrenous changes in the fingers and toes, nose, and genitalia (Braunwald et al., 2001).

### Manifestations of DIC

- Frank hemorrhage from incisions
- Oozing of blood from punctures, intravenous catheter sites
- Purpura, petechiae, bruising
- Cyanosis of extremities
- Gastrointestinal bleeding or hemorrhage
- Dyspnea, tachypnea, bloody sputum
- Tachycardia, hypotension
- Hematuria, oliguria, acute renal failure
- Manifestations of increased intracranial pressure: decreased level of consciousness, papillary, motor, and sensory changes
- Mental status changes

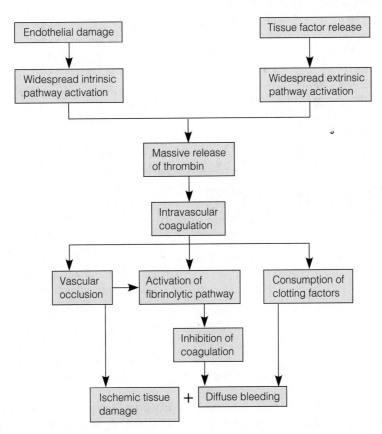

**Figure 32–9** ■ Disseminated intravascular coagulation (DIC). Endothelial cell injury or release of tissue factors activate the intrinsic or extrinsic clotting pathway (or both). As a result, numerous microthrombi form throughout the vasculature, causing ischemic tissue damage. Simultaneously, rapid consumption of clotting factors and activation of fibrinolytic mechanisms trigger widespread bleeding.

## COLLABORATIVE CARE

Treatment of DIC is directed toward treating the underlying disorder and preventing further bleeding or massive thrombosis. Treatment stabilizes the client, reduces complications, and allows recovery to occur; it does not cure DIC (Braunwald et al., 2001).

### Diagnostic Tests

Diagnostic tests are used to confirm the diagnosis of DIC and evaluate the risk for hemorrhage.

- *CBC* and *platelet count* are used to evaluate the hemoglobin, hematocrit, and number of circulating platelets. *Schistocytes,* fragmented RBCs, may be noted due to cell trapping and damage within fibrin thrombi. The platelet count is decreased.
- *Coagulation studies* show prolonged *prothrombin time (PT), partial thromboplastin time (PTT),* and *thrombin time,* and a low *fibrinogen level* due to depletion of clotting factors. The fibrinogen level helps predict bleeding in DIC: As it falls, the risk of bleeding increases (Braunwald et al., 2001).
- *Fibrin degradation products (FDPs)* or *fibrin split products (FSPs)* are increased due to the fibinolysis that occurs with DIC.

### Treatments

When bleeding is the major manifestation of DIC, fresh frozen plasma and platelet concentrates are given to restore clotting factors and platelets. Heparin, although controversial, may be administered. Heparin interferes with the clotting cascade and may prevent further clotting factor consumption due to uncontrolled thrombosis. It is used when bleeding is not controlled by plasma and platelets, as well as when the client has manifestations of thrombotic problems such as acrocyanosis and possible gangrene. Long-term heparin therapy (administered by injection or continuous infusion using a portable pump) may be necessary for clients with chronic DIC

## NURSING CARE

### Assessment

Nurses can be instrumental in identifying early manifestations of DIC, facilitating timely intervention. Focused nursing assessment for DIC includes:

- Health history: recent abortion (spontaneous or therapeutic) or current pregnancy; presence of a known malignant tumor; history of abnormal bleeding episodes or a hematologic disorder
- Physical examination: bleeding from puncture wounds (e.g., injections), IV sites, incisions; hematuria, obvious or occult blood in emesis or stool, epistaxis, other abnormal bleeding; vital signs; heart and breath sounds; abdominal assessment including girth, contour, bowel sounds, tenderness or guarding to palpation; color, temperature, skin condition of hands, feet, and digits; petechiae or purpura of skin, mucous membranes

### Nursing Diagnoses and Interventions

Clients with acute DIC often are critically ill, with multiple nursing care needs. Priority nursing diagnoses discussed in this section focus on impaired tissue perfusion and gas exchange, pain, and fear. Septic shock may precipitate DIC; hemorrhagic shock may occur as a complication of DIC. See Chapter 6 ⊂⊃ for nursing diagnoses and interventions related to these problems.

#### Ineffective Tissue Perfusion

Thrombi and emboli forming throughout the microcirculation affect the perfusion of multiple organs and tissues. Additionally, bleeding due to clotting factor consumption affects cardiac output and blood flow to these tissues.

- Assess extremity pulses, warmth, and capillary refill. Monitor level of consciousness (LOC) and mental status. *Monitoring central and peripheral tissue perfusion facilitates early treatment of impaired perfusion.*

**PRACTICE ALERT**   *Promptly report complaints of chest pain, changes in mental status, LOC, tissue perfusion, respirations, gastrointestinal function, and urinary output. Chest pain or respiratory changes (tachypnea, dyspnea, orthopnea) may be due to angina, pulmonary embolism, or bleeding into lung tissue. Changes in mentation or LOC can indicate cerebral ischemia. A painful, pale, and cold extremity with no or diminished pulses indicates arterial occlusion. Prompt intervention is critical to save the extremity. Acute abdominal pain, decreased bowel sounds, and GI bleeding may indicate mesenteric occlusion, a surgical emergency. Decreased urine output may signify renal artery thrombosis; renal failure may develop.* ■

- Carefully reposition at least every 2 hours. *Position changes facilitate circulation and tissue perfusion, as well as provide an opportunity to assess for purpura, pallor, and bleeding.*
- Discourage crossing the legs, and do not elevate the knees on the bed or with a pillow. *These positions may impair arterial and venous flow to the lower legs and feet, increasing vascular stasis and the risk for thrombosis.*
- Minimize use of tape on the skin, using binders, nonadhesive dressings, and other devices as needed. *Preventing skin trauma reduces the risk for bleeding and potential infection.*

#### Impaired Gas Exchange

Microclots in the pulmonary vasculature are likely to interfere with gas exchange in the client with DIC.

- Monitor oxygen saturation continuously. Administer oxygen as ordered. *Oxygen saturation levels are a noninvasive means of assessing gas exchange. Supplemental oxygen promotes gas exchange and reduces cardiac work, relieving dyspnea.*
- Place in Fowler's or high-Fowler's position as tolerated. *Elevating the head of the bed improves diaphragmatic excursion and alveolar ventilation.*
- Maintain bed rest. *Bed rest reduces oxygen demands and cardiac work.*

- Encourage deep breathing and effective coughing. *Increased respiratory depth and clearance of secretions from airways improves alveolar ventilation and oxygenation.*
- Cautious nasotracheal suctioning may be instituted if cough is ineffective or an endotracheal tube is in place. *Removal of secretions facilitates ventilation and oxygenation. However, care must be used to minimize suction-induced hypoxia and airway trauma.*

> **PRACTICE ALERT** *Monitor arterial blood gas results; report abnormal results to the physician. Low $Pa_{O_2}$ and rising $Pa_{CO_2}$ levels indicate impaired gas exchange and may signify the need for additional treatment.* ■

- Administer analgesics and antianxiety drugs as needed to control pain and anxiety. Provide reassurance and comfort measures. *Pain and anxiety increase the respiratory rate and decrease the depth of respirations, reducing effective ventilation and gas exchange.*

### Pain

Both the underlying cause of DIC and tissue ischemia from microvascular clots can cause pain. Identifying the etiology of pain is important to identify potential complications or harmful effects of DIC and to institute effective treatment.

- Use a standard pain scale chart to evaluate and monitor pain and analgesic effectiveness. *Monitoring pain and response to medication facilitates development of an appropriate and effective treatment plan.*

> **PRACTICE ALERT** *Notify the physician promptly of new or a sudden increase in pain, especially when accompanied by changes in assessment findings. New or increased complaints of pain may signify increased circulatory impairment and ischemic changes in tissues such as the heart, bowel, or extremities. Circulation to a painful, pale or cyanotic, or cold extremity may be occluded by an arterial clot. Prompt intervention is necessary to save the extremity. Acute abdominal pain may signify mesenteric occlusion, a surgical emergency. Anginal pain may indicate occlusion of coronary arteries.* ■

- Handle extremities gently. *Gentle handling reduces the risk of further injury to and pain in ischemic tissues.*
- Apply cool compresses to painful joints. *Application of cold decreases pain through the gate-control mechanism, inhibiting the dorsal horn of the spinal cord and reducing the sensation of pain.*

> **PRACTICE ALERT** *Continuously monitor effects of analgesics, mental and respiratory status. Analgesics may mask manifestations of neurologic impairment due to thromboembolism, and may depress the respiratory center, further impairing gas exchange. Judicious analgesic administration with careful monitoring is vital to safely provide effective pain relief.* ■

### Fear

The underlying serious illness and a complication such as DIC results in an uncertain prognosis, often accompanied by fear.

- Encourage the client and family to verbalize concerns. *This helps the client and family identify their concerns and frame questions.*
- Answer questions truthfully. *Providing honest answers is vital to developing a therapeutic nurse-client relationship. Accurate responses allow the client and family to set priorities as they plan for an uncertain future.*
- Help the client and family identify coping strategies to manage this significant situational stressor. *Implementing past effective coping methods may provide the skills to manage the current crisis.*
- Provide emotional support. *The presence of a caring nurse helps reduce the fear and anxiety associated with a crisis.*
- Maintain a calm environment. *A calm environment provides reassurance that the situation is in control, reduces anxiety, and promotes rest.*
- Respond promptly when the client calls for help. *Prompt responses to expressed needs helps develop a trusting relationship and a sense of security that assistance is readily available.*
- Teach relaxation techniques. *Relaxation techniques can reduce muscle tension and other signs of anxiety. Gaining control over physical responses can help the client gain a sense of control over the situation.*

### Home Care

Although the immediate crisis of acute DIC is resolved prior to discharge, the client may have some continuing effects of the disorder, such as impaired tissue integrity of distal extremities. Teach the client and family about specific care needs, such as foot care (see Box 33–4) or dressing changes. Provide instruction about any continuing medications and follow-up care. ⌘

Clients with chronic DIC may require continuing heparin therapy, using either intermittent subcutaneous injections or a portable infusion pump. Teach the client and family members how to administer the injection or manage the infusion pump. Provide a referral to home health care or a home intravenous management service for assistance. Discuss the manifestations of excessive bleeding or recurrent clotting that need to be reported to the physician.

## THE CLIENT WITH HEMOPHILIA

**Hemophilia** is a group of hereditary clotting factor disorders that lead to persistent and sometimes severe bleeding. Although often considered a disease of children, hemophilia may be diagnosed in adults. Deficiencies of three clotting factors, VIII, IX, and XI, account for 90% to 95% of the bleeding disorders collectively called hemophilia (McCance & Huether, 2002).

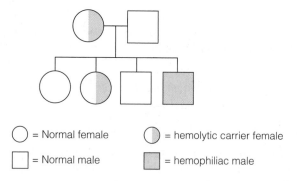

○ = Normal female     ◑ = hemolytic carrier female

□ = Normal male     ▨ = hemophiliac male

**Figure 32–10** ■ The inheritance pattern of hemophilia A and B. Both are transmitted as X-linked recessive disorders. Females may be carriers, but only males develop these disorders.

## PATHOPHYSIOLOGY

**Hemophilia A** (or *classic hemophilia*) is the most common type of hemophilia, caused by deficiency or dysfunction of clotting factor VIII. The estimated incidence of hemophilia A is 1 in 10,000 male births. It is transmitted as an X-linked recessive disorder from mothers to sons (Figure 32–10 ■). The genetic defect of hemophilia A on the X chromosome may cause deficient factor VIII production or a defective form of the protein. When the concentration of the clotting factor is 5% to 35% of normal, the disease is *mild*. Bleeding is infrequent, and usually associated with trauma. Concentrations of 1% to 5% of normal result in *moderate* disease. Again, bleeding usually occurs secondarily to trauma. *Severe* hemophilia occurs when concentrations are less than 1% of normal. Bleeding is frequent, often occurring without trauma (Braunwald et al., 2001; McCance & Huether, 2002).

**Hemophilia B** (also called *Christmas disease*), accounts for about 15% of cases, and is caused by a deficiency in factor IX. Despite the difference in clotting factor deficits, hemophilia A and B are clinically identical. Hemophilia B also is transmitted from mother to son as an X-linked recessive disorder.

**Von Willebrand's disease**, often considered as a type of hemophilia, is the most common hereditary bleeding disorder (Porth, 2002). It is caused by a deficit of or defective von Willebrand (vW) factor, a protein that mediates platelet adhesion (Tierney et al., 2001). Reduced levels of factor VIII often also are present, because vW factor carries factor VIII. This clotting disorder is transmitted in an autosomal dominant pattern, and affects men and women equally. Bleeding associated with von Willebrand's disease rarely is severe. It often is diagnosed when prolonged bleeding follows surgery or a dental extraction.

*Factor XI deficiency* (or *hemophilia C*) is inherited in an autosomal recessive pattern, and most often affects Ashkenazi Jews (Braunwald et al., 2001). It is usually a mild disorder, identified when postoperative bleeding is prolonged. A comparison of the types of hemophilia is found in Table 32–3.

People with hemophilia form a platelet plug at the site of bleeding, but the clotting factor deficit impairs formation of a stable fibrin clot. The effect of vW factor deficiency is somewhat different, in that platelet aggregation at the site of injury is impaired. In either case, prolonged or extensive bleeding may result. Often bleeding occurs in response to injury or as a result of surgery. However, a severe clotting factor deficit can lead to spontaneous bleeding into the joints (*hemarthrosis*), deep tissues, and central nervous system. Hemarthrosis often causes joint deformity and disability, usually of the elbows, hips, knees, and ankles.

## MANIFESTATIONS

The following are manifestations of hemophilia.

- Hemarthrosis
- Easy bruising and cutaneous hematoma formation with minor trauma (e.g., an injection)
- Bleeding from the gums and prolonged bleeding following minor injuries or cuts
- Gastrointestinal bleeding, with hematemesis (vomiting blood), occult blood in the stools, gastric pain, or abdominal pain
- Spontaneous hematuria or epistaxis (nosebleed)
- Pain or paralysis due to the pressure of hematomas on nerves

Intracranial hemorrhage is a potentially life-threatening manifestation of hemophilia.

TABLE 32–3    Types of Hemophilia

| Type/Name | Deficiency | Characteristics | Treatment |
|---|---|---|---|
| Hemophilia A (Classic hemophilia) | Factor VIII | Transmitted by females; occurs primarily in males; bleeding time normal; coagulation time prolonged | Factor VIII concentrate or cryoprecipitate |
| Hemophilia B | Factor IX | Transmitted by females; occurs primarily in males; bleeding time normal; coagulation time prolonged | Factor IX (Christmas disease concentrate) |
| von Willebrand's disease | vW factor Factor VIII | Occurs in both females and males; bleeding time and coagulation time are both prolonged | Cryoprecipitate and DDAVP |
| Factor XI deficiency | Factor XI | Occurs in both males and females; the activated partial thromboplastin time is prolonged | Fresh frozen plasma |

## COLLABORATIVE CARE

Treatment of hemophilia focuses on preventing and/or treating bleeding, primarily by replacing deficient clotting factors. Specific treatment depends on the severity of the disorder and the specific factor deficiency. Care may be complicated by hepatitis or HIV disease in people with hemophilia treated with clotting factor concentrates prepared from multiple units of donated blood. Today, routine testing of all blood, improved blood donor screening, and current methods of treating hemophilia have significantly reduced the risk for these bloodborne diseases.

### Diagnostic Tests

The following laboratory tests may be ordered.

- *Serum platelet levels* are measured and are usually normal.
- *Coagulation studies* such as APTT, bleeding time, and prothrombin time are used to screen for hemophilia when abnormal bleeding occurs. APTT is increased in all types of hemophilia. Prothrombin time is unaffected in these disorders but may be measured to rule out other disorders. Bleeding time is prolonged in von Willebrand's disease but normal in hemophilia A and B.
- *Factor assays* are performed; factor VIII is decreased in hemophilia A and often in von Willebrand's disease, factor IX is decreased in hemophilia B, and factor XI in hemophilia C.
- *Amniocentesis* or *chorionic villus sampling* are used to identify the genetic defect of hemophilia when there is a known family history of the disease.

### Medications

Deficient clotting factors are replaced regularly, as a prophylactic measure before surgery and dental procedures, and to control bleeding. Clotting factors may be given as fresh-frozen plasma, cryoprecipitates, or concentrates. Factor levels are measured on a regular basis to determine whether the treatment is adequate. Clotting factors are often self-administered and may be taken either on a regular or intermittent schedule.

Fresh-frozen plasma replaces all clotting factors (including both factor VIII and factor IX) except platelets. When the cause of bleeding is not yet determined, fresh-frozen plasma may be administered intravenously until a definitive diagnosis is made.

Hemophilia A is usually treated with either heat-treated factor VIII concentrate (heat treating reduces the risk of transmitting disease) or recombinant factor VIII. Although recombinant factor VIII, produced using recombinant DNA technology, eliminates the risk of viral disease transmission, its use is limited by cost. The dose of factor VIII is determined by the severity of the deficit and the presence or prospect of active bleeding (e.g., planned surgery).

Desmopressin acetate (DDAVP, Stimate) may be given to people with mild hemophilia A or von Willebrand's disease prior to minor surgeries. This drug causes release of factor VIII and will raise blood levels by two- or threefold for several hours, reducing the risk of bleeding and the need for clotting factor concentrate (Tierney et al., 2001).

Factor IX concentrate (administered intravenously) is used to treat hemophilia B. Because factor IX concentrates also contain a number of other proteins, there is risk of thrombosis with recurrent use. They are used judiciously, only when needed. Products produced by recombinant technology or that are monoclonally purified carry a lower risk of stimulating thrombus formation (Braunwald et al., 2001). Fresh-frozen plasma replaces factor XI and is used when necessary. It may be given daily until the risk for bleeding decreases.

Factor VIII concentrates contain functional vW factor, and may be used to treat von Willebrand's disease. Aspirin is avoided in all types of hemophilia.

## NURSING CARE

### Health Promotion

Encourage clients with a family history of hemophilia or bleeding disorders to seek genetic counseling during their family planning process. Although tests are available for the hemophilia gene, the technology to correct the disorder in utero does not yet exist.

### Assessment

While severe hemophilia usually is diagnosed in childhood, milder cases may not be identified until surgery, invasive dental work, or a traumatic injury causes extensive or prolonged bleeding. Focused assessment related to hemophilia includes the following:

- Health history: previous bleeding episodes with or without trauma; history of easy bruising, hematomas, epistaxis, bleeding gums, hematuria, vomiting blood, or joint pain; aspirin use; family history of hemophilia or bleeding disorders
- Physical examination: vital signs; bruising or bleeding of skin or mucous membranes; mental status; abdominal assessment; presence of joint deformity, decreased range of motion

### Nursing Diagnoses and Interventions

Impaired blood clotting, the need for continuing care and disease management, and the risk for genetic transmission of hemophilia are priority problems for the client with hemophilia.

#### Ineffective Protection

The inability to form stable clots and stem bleeding from injured blood vessels creates a significant risk for the client with hemophilia. Nursing care measures focus on preventing injury and protecting the skin from damage.

- Monitor for signs of bleeding, including hematomas, ecchymoses, and purpura, as well as surface oozing or bleeding. Check emesis and stool for occult blood. *Bleeding may occur in cutaneous tissues as well as internal organs. Bleeding in the upper gastrointestinal tract may not be readily apparent in the stool.*
- Notify the physician of any apparent bleeding. *Prompt intervention with administration of clotting factor concentrate decreases the risk of hemorrhage and subsequent hypovolemia.*

- Avoid intramuscular injections, rectal temperatures, and enemas. *These can pose a risk of tissue and vascular trauma, which can precipitate bleeding.*
- Use safety measures in personal care. For example, use an electric razor rather than a razor blade to shave. *Use of an electric razor minimizes the opportunity to develop superficial cuts that may result in bleeding.*
- If bleeding occurs, control blood loss using gentle pressure, ice, or a topical hemostatic agent, such as absorbable gelatin sponge, microfibrillar collagen hemostat, or topical thrombin. *Direct pressure occludes bleeding vessels. Ice, a vasoconstrictor, may facilitate bleeding control, as do topical hemostatic agents.*
- Instruct to avoid activities that increase the risk of trauma, including contact sports, physical exertion associated with job performance, and to eliminate safety hazards in the home. *Depending on the severity of the clotting factor deficit, even minor trauma can lead to serious bleeding episodes. Safer activities such as noncontact sports (e.g., swimming, golf) and occupations that do not require physical labor may be substituted.*

### Risk for Ineffective Health Maintenance

Hemophilia is a chronic disorder, requiring active management to prevent and control bleeding and complications. Frequent visits to the physician or clinic may be necessary. In addition, the client may need to learn to self-administer clotting factors and measures to prevent complications. The lifelong nature of the disorder may interfere with compliance, especially during early adulthood.

- Assess knowledge of disorder and the related treatments. *Assessment allows identification of knowledge gaps and provides a basis on which to provide additional information. Impaired disease management may be due to lack of knowledge or a conscious decision not to follow the recommendations of the health care provider.*
- Provide information about the bleeding disorder and prescribed medications and treatments. *Individualized instruction is more effective than general, possibly irrelevant information.*
- Provide emotional support, expressing confidence in the client's self-care abilities. *Emotional support helps the client incorporate the care regimen into his or her lifestyle.*
- Provide supervised learning and practice opportunities for administering clotting factors and topical hemostatic agents. *Successful practice sessions instill confidence in the ability to manage care and provide an opportunity for questions and exploring alternatives.*

### Using NANDA, NIC, and NOC

Chart 32–2 shows links between NANDA nursing diagnoses, NIC, and NOC for the client with hemophilia.

### Home Care

Discuss the following topics when preparing the client with a bleeding disorder and the family for home care.

- Recognizing the manifestations of internal bleeding: pallor, weakness, restlessness, headache, disorientation, pain, swelling. These manifestations require emergency medical care and should be reported immediately.
- Applying cold packs and immobilizing the joint for 24 to 48 hours if hemarthrosis occurs
- Using analgesics for pain; avoiding prescription and over-the-counter drugs containing aspirin
- Ensuring a safe home environment (e.g., padding sharp edges of furniture, using transition lighting or a night light; avoiding scatter rugs, and wearing protective gloves when working in the house or yard)
- Using safe grooming practices such as electric razors
- Wearing a MedicAlert bracelet in case of accident
- Practicing good dental hygiene to decrease potential tooth decay and extractions. If dental procedures are necessary, discuss the need for prophylactic factor administration with the dentist and physician.

---

## CHART 32–2  NANDA, NIC, AND NOC LINKAGES

### The Client with Hemophilia

| NURSING DIAGNOSES | NURSING INTERVENTIONS | NURSING OUTCOMES |
| --- | --- | --- |
| • Impaired Physical Mobility | • Exercise Therapy: Joint Mobility<br>• Pain Management | • Joint Movement: Active<br>• Mobility Level |
| • Ineffective Health Maintenance | • Health Education<br>• Self-Responsibility Facilitation<br>• Teaching: Procedure/Treatment | • Health-Seeking Behavior<br>• Knowledge: Health Behaviors<br>• Knowledge: Treatment Regimen |
| • Ineffective Protection | • Bleeding Precautions<br>• Blood Products Administration | • Coagulation Status |
| • Pain | • Medication Management<br>• Positioning | • Comfort Level |

*Note. Data from Nursing Outcomes Classification (NOC) by M. Johnson & M. Maas (Eds.), 1997, St. Louis: Mosby; Nursing Diagnoses: Definitions & Classification 2001–2002 by North American Nursing Diagnosis Association, 2001, Philadelphia: NANDA; Nursing Interventions Classification (NIC) by J.C. McCloskey & G. M. Bulechek (Eds.), 2000, St. Louis: Mosby. Reprinted by permission.*

- Following safer-sex practices
- Preparing and administering intravenous medications

Refer the client and family to a local hemophilia or bleeding disorders support group. Provide contact information for national organizations and information clearinghouses, such as:

National Hemophilia Foundation
112 West 32nd Street
New York, NY 10001
1-800-42-handi
www.hemophilia.org

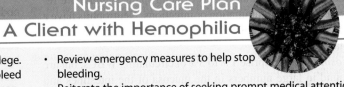

## Nursing Care Plan
## A Client with Hemophilia

Jermiel Cruise is a 20-year-old student at the community college. He is admitted to the emergency department with a nosebleed that began when he fell during a touch football game. It has continued to bleed for over an hour.

### ASSESSMENT

Mr. Cruise states that he has hemophilia and realizes that playing contact sports "is probably a dumb thing to do." He adds that he has not had any recent bleeding episodes. An icebag and manual pressure are applied in the emergency department. The physician orders factor VIII concentrate to be administered. Physical assessment findings are: T 97.2°F (36.2°C), BP 118/64, R 18. Skin pale but warm. Laboratory tests reveal a prolonged APTT and a normal bleeding time and PT. Following treatment, Mr. Cruise's bleeding subsides.

### DIAGNOSES

- *Risk for aspiration* related to uncontrolled nosebleed
- *Noncompliance* with activity recommendations
- *Ineffective protection* related to lack of clotting factor VIII

### EXPECTED OUTCOMES

- Exhibit no further signs of bleeding.
- Maintain vital signs within his usual range.
- Maintain an open airway.
- Identify sports and recreation activities in which he can safely participate.
- Verbalize self-care measures to control bleeding.

### PLANNING AND IMPLEMENTATION

- Monitor vital signs and for further signs of bleeding.
- Assess airway and auscultate breath sounds.

- Review emergency measures to help stop bleeding.
- Reiterate the importance of seeking prompt medical attention if bleeding should occur.
- Advise regarding the importance of wearing a MedicAlert bracelet identifying him as a hemophiliac.
- Discuss alternative noncontact sports and recreational activities.

### EVALUATION

On discharge, Mr. Cruise has no further signs of bleeding, shock, or aspiration. He is able to verbalize methods to help stop local bleeding and the importance of seeking medical attention promptly when bleeding continues. Mr. Cruise agrees to stop at a local drug store on the way home to order a MedicAlert bracelet. In addition, Mr. Cruise verbalizes an understanding of the importance of avoiding contact sports and has identified swimming and golf as alternative leisure activities that he might enjoy.

### Critical Thinking in the Nursing Process

1. What is the pathophysiologic basis for the bleeding that occurs in hemophilia A and B?
2. What was Mr. Cruise's priority nursing diagnosis? Why?
3. Why is family planning a special consideration with a client who has hemophilia?
4. Outline a plan to teach the family of a client diagnosed with hemophilia how to administer an intravenous infusion.
5. Develop a care plan for Mr. Cruise for the nursing diagnosis, *Impaired social interaction.* Consider Mr. Cruise's age and developmental level in creating the plan.

See Evaluating Your Response in Appendix C.

# WHITE BLOOD CELL AND LYMPHOID TISSUE DISORDERS

Disorders of the white blood cells and lymphoid tissue include infectious mononucleosis, the leukemias, multiple myeloma, and malignant lymphomas (Hodgkin's disease and non-Hodgkin's lymphoma). A review of the physiology of white blood cells and lymphoid tissues precedes discussion of the diseases.

## PHYSIOLOGY REVIEW

### White Blood Cells

**White blood cells (WBCs),** also called leukocytes, are a part of the body's defense against microorganisms. On average, there are 5,000 to 10,000 WBCs per cubic millimeter of blood,

accounting for about 1% of total blood volume. **Leukocytosis** is a higher than normal WBC count; **leukopenia** is a WBC count that is lower than normal.

WBCs originate from hemopoietic stem cells in the bone marrow. These stem cells differentiate into the various types of white blood cells (see Figure 32–1).

The two basic types of WBCs are granular leukocytes (or *granulocytes*) and nongranular leukocytes. Granulocytes have horseshoe-shaped nuclei and contain large granules in the cytoplasm. Stimulated by granulocyte-macrophage colony-stimulating factor (GM-CSF) and granulocyte colony-stimulating factor (G-CSF), granulocytes mature fully in the bone marrow before

### TABLE 32–5   FAB Classification of Acute Leukemia

| Type | Class | Predominant Cells | Prognosis |
|------|-------|-------------------|-----------|
| Acute Lymphocytic Leukemia (ALL) | $L_1$ | Immature lymphoblasts | >90% remission rate in children |
| | $L_2$ | Mature lymphoblasts | Relapse common after 2 or more years of remission |
| Acute Myelocytic Leukemia | $M_0$ | Undifferentiated cells | Poor |
| | $M_1$ | Immature myeloblasts | Good; complete response in 65% or more |
| | $M_2$ | Mature myeloblasts | Good for 2 or more years of remission |
| | $M_3$ | Promyelocytes | Good in adults |
| | $M_4$ | Myelocytes and monocytes | Poorest in adults |
| | $M_5$ | Poorly or well-differentiated monocytes | Poor |
| | $M_6$ | Predominant eythroblasts | Variable |
| | $M_7$ | Megakaryocytes | |

The general manifestations of leukemia (regardless of type) result from anemia, infection, and bleeding. These include pallor, fatigue, tachycardia, malaise, lethargy, and dyspnea on exertion. Infection may cause fever, night sweats, oral ulcerations, and frequent or recurrent respiratory, urinary, integumentary, or other infections. Increased bleeding due to thrombocytopenia leads to bruising; petechiae; bleeding gums; and bleeding within specific organs and tissues. *Multisystem Effects of Leukemia* can be seen on page 963.

Other manifestations result from leukemic cell infiltration, increased metabolism, and increased leukocyte destruction. Infiltration of the liver, spleen, lymph nodes, and bone marrow causes pain and tissue swelling in the involved areas. Meningeal infiltration may cause manifestations of increased intracranial pressure, such as headache, altered level of consciousness, cranial nerve impairment, nausea, and vomiting. Infiltration of the kidneys may affect renal function, with decreased urine output and increased blood urea nitrogen and creatinine. Increased metabolism causes heat intolerance, weight loss, dyspnea on exertion, and tachycardia. Destruction of large numbers of WBCs releases substantial amounts of uric acid into the circulation; uric acid crystals may obstruct renal tubules, causing renal insufficiency.

## Acute Myelocytic Leukemia

**Acute myelocytic leukemia (AML)** is characterized by uncontrolled proliferation of myeloblasts (the precursors of granulocytes) and hyperplasia of the bone marrow and spleen. AML accounts for most acute leukemia in adults. Treatment induces complete remission in 70% of clients, although only about 25% achieve cure or long-term remission (Porth, 2002).

The manifestations of AML result from neutropenia and thrombocytopenia. Decreased neutrophils lead to recurrent severe infections, such as pneumonia, septicemia, abscesses, and mucous membrane ulceration. The manifestations of thrombocytopenia include petechiae, purpura, and ecchymoses (bruising), epistaxis (nosebleeds), hematomas, hematuria, and gastrointestinal bleeding. Bone infarctions or subperiosteal infiltrates of

### TABLE 32–6   Major Types of Leukemia

| Classification | Characteristics | Manifestations | Treatment |
|----------------|-----------------|----------------|-----------|
| Acute lymphoblastic leukemia (ALL) | Primarily affects children and young adults; leukemic cells may infiltrate CNS | Recurrent infections; bleeding; pallor, bone pain, weight loss, sore throat, fatigue, night sweats, weakness | Chemotherapy; bone marrow transplant (BMT), or stem cell transplant (SCT) |
| Chronic lymphocytic leukemia (CLL) | Primarily affects older adults; insidious onset and slow, chronic course | Fatigue; exercise intolerance; lymphadenopathy and splenomegaly; recurrent infections, pallor, edema, thrombophlebitis | Often requires no treatment; chemotherapy; BMT |
| Acute myelocytic leukemia (AML) | Common in older adults, may affect children and young adults. Strongly associated with toxins, genetic disorders, and treatment of other cancers | Fatigue, weakness, fever; anemia; headache, bone and joint pain; abnormal bleeding and bruising; recurrent infection; lymphadenopathy, splenomegaly, and hepatomegaly | Chemotherapy; SCT |
| Chronic myelocytic leukemia (CML) | Primarily affects adults; early course slow and stable, progressing to aggressive phase in 3–4 years | Early: Weakness, fatigue, dyspnea on exertion; possible splenomegaly. Later: fever, weight loss, night sweats | Interferon-α; chemotherapy, SCT |

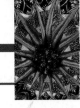

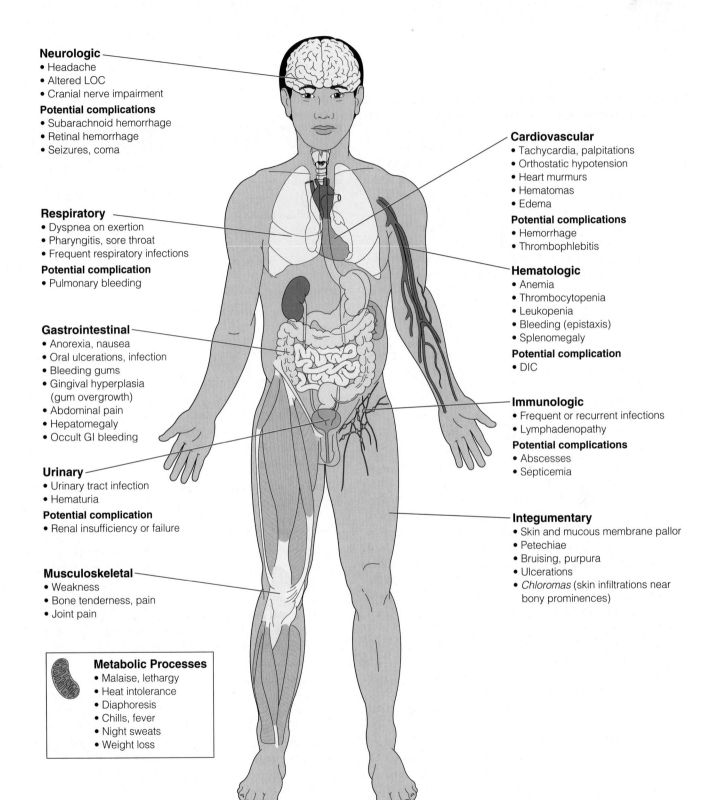

**Neurologic**
- Headache
- Altered LOC
- Cranial nerve impairment

**Potential complications**
- Subarachnoid hemorrhage
- Retinal hemorrhage
- Seizures, coma

**Respiratory**
- Dyspnea on exertion
- Pharyngitis, sore throat
- Frequent respiratory infections

**Potential complication**
- Pulmonary bleeding

**Gastrointestinal**
- Anorexia, nausea
- Oral ulcerations, infection
- Bleeding gums
- Gingival hyperplasia
  (gum overgrowth)
- Abdominal pain
- Hepatomegaly
- Occult GI bleeding

**Urinary**
- Urinary tract infection
- Hematuria

**Potential complication**
- Renal insufficiency or failure

**Musculoskeletal**
- Weakness
- Bone tenderness, pain
- Joint pain

**Metabolic Processes**
- Malaise, lethargy
- Heat intolerance
- Diaphoresis
- Chills, fever
- Night sweats
- Weight loss

**Cardiovascular**
- Tachycardia, palpitations
- Orthostatic hypotension
- Heart murmurs
- Hematomas
- Edema

**Potential complications**
- Hemorrhage
- Thrombophlebitis

**Hematologic**
- Anemia
- Thrombocytopenia
- Leukopenia
- Bleeding (epistaxis)
- Splenomegaly

**Potential complication**
- DIC

**Immunologic**
- Frequent or recurrent infections
- Lymphadenopathy

**Potential complications**
- Abscesses
- Septicemia

**Integumentary**
- Skin and mucous membrane pallor
- Petechiae
- Bruising, purpura
- Ulcerations
- *Chloromas* (skin infiltrations near
  bony prominences)

leukemic cells may cause bone pain. Anemia is a late manifestation, causing fatigue, headaches, pallor, and dyspnea on exertion. Death usually results from infection or hemorrhage.

Bone marrow aspiration shows a proliferation of immature WBCs. The CBC shows thrombocytopenia and normocytic, normochromic anemia.

## Chronic Myelocytic Leukemia

**Chronic myelocytic leukemia (CML)** is characterized by abnormal proliferation of all bone marrow elements. CML is usually associated with a chromosome abnormality called the Philadelphia chromosome, a translocation of chromosome 22 to chromosome 9. This type of leukemia constitutes approximately 20% of adult leukemias. It usually affects clients over age 50; its incidence is higher in men than in women. Ionizing radiation and exposure to chemicals are implicated as causes of CML.

People with CML are often asymptomatic in the early stages and, in fact, are often diagnosed when a routine blood test reveals abnormal cell counts. Anemia causes weakness, fatigue, and dyspnea on exertion. The spleen often is enlarged, causing abdominal discomfort. Within 3 to 4 years, disease progresses to a more aggressive phase. Rapid cell proliferation and hypermetabolism cause fatigue, weight loss, sweating, and heat intolerance. Finally, the disease evolves to acute leukemia, with blast cell proliferation and constitutional symptoms. Survival following the onset of this final stage averages only 2 to 4 months (Porth, 2002).

## Acute Lymphocytic Leukemia

**Acute lymphocytic leukemia (ALL)** is the most common type of leukemia in children and young adults. ALL causes abnormal proliferation of lymphoblasts in the bone marrow, lymph nodes, and spleen.

The onset of ALL is usually rapid. Lymphoblasts proliferating in bone marrow and peripheral tissues crowd the growth of normal cells. Normal hematopoiesis is suppressed, leading to thrombocytopenia, leukopenia, and anemia. Manifestations of infections, bleeding, and anemia develop. Bone pain resulting from rapid generation of marrow elements, lymphadenopathy, and liver enlargement are also common. Infiltration of the central nervous system causes headaches, visual disturbances, vomiting, and seizures.

The CBC shows an elevated WBC count with increased lymphocytes on the differential. RBC and platelet counts are decreased. Bone marrow studies reveal a hypercellular marrow with growth of lymphoblasts. Combination chemotherapy produces complete remission in 80% to 90% of adults with ALL.

## Chronic Lymphocytic Leukemia

**Chronic lymphocytic leukemia (CLL)** is characterized by proliferation and accumulation of small, abnormal, mature lymphocytes in the bone marrow, peripheral blood, and body tissues. The abnormal cells are usually B-lymphocytes that are unable to produce adequate antibodies to maintain normal immune function. CLL occurs more commonly in adults, especially in older adults (median age 65). CLL is the least common type of the major leukemias.

CLL has a slow onset and is often diagnosed during a routine physical examination. If symptoms are present, they usually include vague complaints of weakness or malaise. Possible clinical findings include anemia, infection, and enlarged lymph nodes, spleen, and liver. As in other leukemias, bone marrow hyperplasia is present. Erythrocyte and platelet counts are reduced. Leukocyte counts may either be elevated or reduced, but abnormal cells are always present. In CLL, years may elapse before treatment is required. Survival of this disease averages approximately 7 years.

## COLLABORATIVE CARE

Treatment for leukemia focuses on achieving remission or cure and relieving symptoms. The methods of treatment may include chemotherapy, radiation therapy, and bone marrow or stem cell transplantation. Cure is more often achieved in children with acute leukemia than in adults, although long-term remissions (disease-free periods with no signs or symptoms) often can be achieved.

### Diagnostic Tests

The following diagnostic tests are ordered when leukemia is suspected.

- *CBC* with differential is done to evaluate cell counts, hemoglobin and hematocrit levels, and the number, distribution, and morphology (size and shape) of WBCs.
- *Platelets* are measured to identify possible thrombocytopenia secondary to the leukemia and the risk of bleeding.
- *Bone marrow examination* provides information about cells within the marrow, the type of erythropoiesis, and the maturity of erythropoietic and leukopoietic cells.

Table 32–7 outlines usual diagnostic test results in the various forms of leukemia.

### Chemotherapy

Single agent or combination chemotherapy is used to treat most types of leukemia, with the goal of eradicating leukemic cells and producing remission. Table 32–8 outlines typical chemotherapy regimens for different types of leukemia. Combination chemotherapy reduces drug resistance and toxicity, and interrupts cell growth at various stages of the cell cycle, producing complimentary effect of the drugs used. Cancer treatment with chemotherapy is discussed in detail in Chapter 10.

Chemotherapy for leukemia generally is divided into the induction phase and postremission therapy. During *induction,* drug doses are high to eradicate leukemic cells from the bone marrow. These high doses often also damage stem cells and interfere with production of normal blood cells. Circulating mature blood cells are not affected because they are no longer dividing. The degree of bone marrow suppression is influenced by a number of factors, including age, nutritional status, concurrent chronic diseases such as impaired liver or renal function, the drug and drug dose, and prior treatment.

*Colony-stimulating factors (CSFs),* also called hematopoietic growth factors, often are administered to "rescue" the bone marrow following induction chemotherapy. CSFs are cytokines

TABLE 32-7  Diagnostic Findings by Type of Leukemia

| Test | AML | CML | ALL | CLL |
|---|---|---|---|---|
| RBC count | Low | Low | Low | Low |
| Hemoglobin | Low | Low | Low | Low |
| Hematocrit | Low | Low | Low | Low |
| Platelet count | Very low | High early, low late | Low | Low |
| WBC count | Varies | Increased | Varies | Increased |
|   Myeloblasts | Present | | | |
|   Neutrophils | Decreased | Increased | Decreased | Normal |
|   Lymphocytes | | Normal | | Increased |
|   Monocytes | | Normal/low | | |
|   Blasts | Present | Present (crisis) | Present | |
| Bone marrow | Hypercellular | | Hypercellular | |
|   Myeloblasts | Present | | | |
|   Lymphoblasts | | | Present | |
|   Lymphocytes | | | | Present |

that regulate the growth and differentiation of blood cells. Factors that support neutrophil maturation, *granulocyte-macrophage CSF (GM-CSF)* and *granulocyte CSF (G-CSF)* are commonly used. Bone pain is a common side effect of therapy with these agents. Clients also may experience fevers, chills, anorexia, muscle aches, and lethargy (Braunwald et al., 2001).

Once remission has been achieved, postremission chemotherapy is continued to eradicate any additional leukemic cells, prevent relapse, and prolong survival. A single chemotherapeutic agent, combination therapy, or bone marrow transplant may be used for postremission treatment.

TABLE 32-8  Chemotherapeutic Regimens Used to Treat Leukemia

| | |
|---|---|
| Acute myelocytic leukemia | • Cytarabine (Cytoxan, an alkylating agent), *with* daunorubicin (Cerubidine, an antitumor antibiotic), or idarubicin (Idamycin, an antitumor antibiotic)<br>• All-*trans* retinoic acid (ATRA) added for clients with promyelocytic leukemia |
| Chronic myelocytic leukemia | • Imatinib mesylate (STI571, Gleevec), a Bcr-Abl tyrosine kinase (enzyme) inhibitor<br>• Hydroxyurea (a DNA inhibitor) *or* homoharringtonine (HHT, a plant alkaloid) |
| Acute lymphocytic leukemia | • Daunorubicin (Cerubidine, an antitumor antibiotic) *with* vincristine (Oncovin, a plant alkaloid) *with* prednisone *with* asparaginase (Elspar) |
| Chronic lymphocytic leukemia | • Fludarabine (Fludara, an antimetabolite) *or* chlorambucil (Chloromycetin, an antitumor antibiotic)<br>• Cyclophosphamide (Cytoxan, an alkylating agent), vincristine, and prednisone<br>• Cyclophosphamide, doxorubicin (Adriamycin, an antitumor antibiotic), vincristine, and prednisone |

## Radiation Therapy

Radiation therapy damages cellular DNA. While the cell continues to function, it cannot divide and multiply. Cells that divide rapidly, such as bone marrow and cancer cells (radiosensitive cells), respond quickly to radiation therapy. Although normal cells are affected, they are better able to recover from the damage caused by the radiation than are cancer cells. The types of delivery, effects, and toxicities of radiation are discussed in greater detail in Chapter 10.

## Bone Marrow Transplant

**Bone marrow transplant (BMT)** is the treatment of choice for some types of leukemia (see Table 32–6). BMT often is used in conjunction with or following chemotherapy or radiation. There are two major categories of BMT: In allogeneic BMT, the bone marrow of a healthy donor is infused into the client with the illness; in autologous BMT, the client is infused with his or her own bone marrow.

### Allogeneic BMT

*Allogeneic BMT* uses bone marrow cells from a donor (often from a sibling with closely matched tissue antigens; closely matched unrelated donors also may be used). Prior to allogeneic BMT, high doses of chemotherapy and/or total body irradiation are used to destroy leukemic cells in the bone marrow. Then donor marrow is infused through a central venous line. Prior to BMT and reestablishment of bone marrow function, the client is critically ill and at significant risk for infection and bleeding due to depletion of WBCs and platelets.

Allogeneic BMT may precipitate *graft-versus-host disease (GVHD)*, which develops in 25% to 60% of all clients receiving an allogeneic BMT. In GVHD, immune cells of the donated bone marrow identify the recipient's body tissue as foreign. Consequently, T lymphocytes in the donated marrow attack the liver, skin, and gastrointestinal tract, causing skin rashes progressing to desquamation (loss of skin), diarrhea, gastrointestinal bleeding, and liver damage. GVHD is treated with antibiotics and steroids; immunosuppressant drugs such as thalidomide and immunotoxin (Xomazyme) may be used if necessary.

## Autologous BMT

*Autologous BMT* uses the client's own bone marrow to restore bone marrow function after chemotherapy or radiation. This procedure is often called *bone marrow rescue*. In autologous BMT, about 1 L of bone marrow is aspirated (usually from the iliac crests) during a period of disease remission. The bone marrow is then frozen and stored for use after treatment. If relapse occurs, lethal doses of chemotherapy or radiation are given to destroy the immune system and malignant cells, and to prepare space in the bone marrow for new cells. The filtered bone marrow is then thawed and infused intravenously through a central line. The infused marrow cells slowly become a part of the client's bone marrow, the neutrophil count increases, and normal hematopoiesis takes place.

As in allogeneic BMT, the client is critically ill during the period of bone marrow destruction and immunosuppression. The client is hospitalized in a private room for 6 to 8 weeks or more. Potential complications include malnutrition, infection, and bleeding.

## Stem Cell Transplant

Allogeneic **stem cell transplant (SCT)** is an alternative to bone marrow transplant. SCT results in complete and sustained replacement of the recipient's blood cell lines (WBCs, RBCs, and platelets) with cells derived from the donor stem cells.

Donors must have tissue that is closely matched with that of the recipient. Prior to harvesting, hematopoietic growth factors, including G-CSF and GM-CSF, are administered to the donor for 4 to 5 days. This increases the concentration of stem cells in peripheral blood, allowing it to be used for the transplant instead of bone marrow. Peripheral blood is removed and white cells are separated from the plasma, then administered via a large central venous catheter. Large concentrations of stem cells also are present in umbilical cord blood. This may be stored and used in some cases (Braunwald et al., 2001).

The recipient undergoes similar treatment prior to SCT as for BMT. The risks for infection and other complications, as well as GVHD, are similar.

## Biologic Therapy

Cytokines such as interferons and interleukins are biologic agents that may be used to treat some leukemias. These agents modify the body's response to cancer cells; in some cases they are cytotoxic as well. Interferons are a complex group of messenger proteins normally produced in response to antigens such as viruses (see Chapter 9). ☜ They have multiple effects, including moderating immune function and inhibiting abnormal cell proliferation and growth. Interferon-α may be used to treat some leukemias, particularly CML. Side effects commonly associated with interferon therapy include flulike symptoms, persistent fatigue and lethargy, weight loss, and muscle and joint pain.

## Complementary Therapies

Although many complementary and alternative medicine therapies have been purported to treat cancer in general, at this time none have been shown to have sustained benefit in treating leukemia.

# NURSING CARE

## Health Promotion

Health promotion activities related to leukemia include teaching about leukemia risk factors, particularly those that can be controlled. Discuss the potential dangers of exposure to ionizing radiation and certain chemicals such as benzene. Encourage all clients to avoid smoking cigarettes. Discuss genetic counseling with clients at high risk for having a child with Down syndrome (over age 35).

## Assessment

Focused assessment data related to leukemia includes:

- Health history: complaints of fatigue, weakness, dyspnea on exertion, frequent infections, sore throat, night sweats, bleeding gums, or nose bleeds; recent weight loss; exposure to ionizing radiation (multiple X-rays, residence near a site of radiation or atomic testing) or chemicals (occupational); prior treatment for cancer; history of an immune disorder
- Physical examination: skin and mucous membranes for bruising, purpura, petechiae, ulcers or lesions; pallor; vital signs including orthostatic vitals; heart and lung sounds; abdominal examination; stool for occult blood

## Nursing Diagnoses and Interventions

When caring for the client with leukemia, the nurse considers the chronic and life-threatening nature of the disease as well as the effects of treatment. See the Nursing Research box on the following page. Priority nursing problems may include *Risk for infection, Imbalanced nutrition, Impaired oral mucous membranes, Impaired protection (bleeding),* and *Grieving.*

### Risk for Infection

Changes in white blood cell function impair the immune and inflammatory responses in leukemia, increasing the risk for infection. WBCs may be immature and ineffective, or, in some cases, deficient. Chemotherapy or radiation therapy further depresses bone marrow function, and increases the risk for infection.

- Promptly report manifestations of infection: fever, chills, throat pain, cough, chest pain, burning on urination, purulent drainage, and itching and burning in vaginal or rectal areas. *Prompt reporting allows timely intervention to prevent overwhelming infection and sepsis.*
- Institute infection protection measures.
  a. Maintain protective isolation as indicated.
  b. Ensure meticulous handwashing among all people in contact with the client.
  c. Assist as needed with appropriate hygiene measures.
  d. Restrict visitors with colds, flu, or infections.
  e. Provide oral hygiene after every meal.
  f. Avoid invasive procedures when possible, including injections, intravenous catheters, catheterizations, and rectal and vaginal procedures. When necessary, use strict aseptic technique for all invasive procedures and monitor carefully for infection.

## Nursing Research

### Evidence-Based Practice for Clients with Acute Leukemia and Lymphoma

Clients with acute leukemia and malignant lymphoma experience a number of distressing manifestations of their disease, including malaise and fatigue, fever, night sweats, infections, and possible hemorrhage. Treatments such as radiation therapy and chemotherapy often have numerous adverse effects as well, including anorexia and nausea, stomatitis, lethargy, malaise, and fatigue. In this study, clients in remission from acute leukemia or malignant lymphoma were surveyed regarding physical problems, their view of help they received and who was of most help during treatment, and the impact of the disease and treatment on their current life (Persson, Hallberg, & Ohlsson, 1997).

Clients identified energy loss and nutritional problems as being most troublesome during disease treatment. In general, clients with more physical problems were less satisfied with the nursing care they received, suggesting that nurses were less effective in meeting the needs of the sickest clients. Clients continued to experience reduced psychological and sexual energy and a significant need for intimate help and counseling during remission. While family relationships improved, work and finances were negatively impacted by their disease.

#### IMPLICATIONS FOR NURSING

This study points out the need for nurses to actively focus their care on the physical problems experienced during treatment,

especially energy loss and nutritional problems. Overwhelming fatigue interferes with the client's ability to provide self-care, but its effects may not be readily apparent to nurses. The long-term effects of reduced psychological and sexual energy, as well as continued susceptibility to infections, indicate a need for continued follow-up care, teaching, and possibly referral to counseling services.

#### Critical Thinking in Client Care

1. Explain the physiologic responses to malignancies and cancer treatments that cause fatigue, malaise, and nutritional problems.
2. Clients undergoing treatment for leukemia, malignant lymphoma, and other cancers may have few outward manifestations of their disease or responses to treatment. Discuss how this apparent well-being may affect the nurses' perception of care needs.
3. How may continued problems of fatigue and lack of psychologic and sexual energy affect family relations?
4. Develop a nursing care plan for a client with acute leukemia to address the problem: Ineffective sexuality patterns related to fatigue and lack of energy.

---

*These precautions minimize exposure to bacterial, viral, and fungal pathogens. Infection is the major cause of death in clients with leukemia. Mucous membranes are especially susceptible to breakdown and infection as a result of tissue damage from chemotherapy or radiation.*

- Monitor vital signs including temperature and oxygen saturation every 4 hours. Report temperature spikes with chilling, tachypnea, tachycardia, restlessness, change in $PaO_2$, and hypotension. *The inflammatory response may be impaired in leukemia, masking signs of infection until sepsis develops, indicated by manifestations such as those above.*

- Monitor neutrophil levels (measured in cubic millimeters) for relative risk for infection:

  2000 to 2500: no risk
  1000 to 2000: minimal risk
  500 to 1000: moderate risk
  Below 500: severe risk

  *Neutrophils are the first line of defense against infection. As levels decrease, the risk for infection increases.*

- Explain infection precautions and restrictions and their rationale; explain that these measures are usually temporary. *Client and family understanding increases compliance and lowers the risk of infection.*

### Imbalanced Nutrition:
### Less Than Body Requirements

The client with leukemia may have difficulty meeting nutritional needs due to increased metabolism, fatigue, loss of appetite from radiation, nausea and vomiting from chemotherapy,

or painful oral mucous membranes that make chewing and swallowing difficult and/or painful.

- Weigh regularly and evaluate weight loss over time to determine degree of malnutrition. A weight loss of 10% to 20% may indicate malnutrition. *A minimum intake of nutrients is necessary for health and tissue repair; cancer increases metabolic needs over this basal requirement. Weight loss occurs when metabolic requirements are not met. Both the disease process and its treatment can interfere with nutrient intake.*

- Address causative or contributing factors to inadequate food and fluid intake.
  a. Provide mouth care before and after meals; use a soft toothbrush or sponges as necessary.
  b. Provide liquids with different textures and tastes.
  c. Increase liquid intake with meals.
  d. Reduce intake of milk and milk products, which makes mucus more tenacious.
  e. Assist to a sitting position for eating.
  f. Ensure that the environment is clean and odor-free.
  g. Provide medications for pain or nausea 30 minutes before meals, if prescribed.
  h. Provide rest periods before meals.
  i. Offer small, frequent meals including low-fat, high kcal foods throughout the day.
  j. Provide commercial supplements, such as Ensure.
  k. Avoid painful or unpleasant procedures immediately before or after meals.

MediaLink | ACUTE MYELOCYTIC LEUKEMIA CARE PLAN

l. Suggest measures to improve food tolerance, such as eating dry foods when arising, consuming salty foods if allowed, and avoiding very sweet, rich, or greasy foods. *Anorexia, nausea and vomiting, diarrhea, stomatitis, taste changes, and dysphagia often make eating difficult during cancer treatment when good nutrition is most important. Maintaining nutritional status decreases morbidity and mortality by preventing weight loss, improving the response to treatment, minimizing adverse effects, and improving quality of life. Small, frequent meals are often better tolerated, especially high-protein, high-kcal foods.*

## Impaired Oral Mucous Membrane

*Stomatitis,* inflammation and ulceration of the oral mucous membrane, is common in leukemia. Chemotherapy can further impair the integrity of constantly dividing oral tissues.

- Inspect the buccal region, gums, sublingual area, and the throat daily for swelling or lesions. Ask about oral pain or burning. *Breakdown of the oral mucous membrane increases the risk of infection and bleeding, causes pain and discomfort with eating and swallowing, and may cause swelling that interferes with the airway.*
- Culture any oral lesions. *Herpes simplex virus and* Candida *(yeast) are more common in clients with neutropenia. Herpes lesions are usually red, raised, fluid-filled blisters;* Candida *causes a white coating and patches of white plaque.*
- Assist with mouth care and oral rinses with saline or a solution of hydrogen peroxide and water (1:1 or 1:3 hydrogen peroxide and water) every 2 to 4 hours. Apply petroleum jelly to the lips to prevent dryness and cracking. *These measures help prevent infection and increase comfort.*
- Encourage use of soft-bristle toothbrush or sponge to clean teeth and gums. *Toothbrushes with hard bristles may abrade inflamed mucosa, causing bleeding and increasing the risk of infection.*
- Administer medications as ordered to treat infection or relieve pain. *Topical antifungal agents such as nystatin may be prescribed to treat* Candida *infections. Topical anesthetics such as lidocaine may be prescribed to relieve comfort and facilitate good oral care.*
- Instruct to avoid alcohol-based mouthwashes, citrus fruit juices, spicy foods, very hot or very cold foods, alcohol, and crusty foods. Suggest bland, cool foods and cool liquids at least every 2 hours. *Avoiding mucosa-traumatizing foods and liquids increases comfort; bland, cool foods and liquids cause the least pain. Intake of adequate fluids is necessary to prevent dehydration.*

## Ineffective Protection

Bleeding is the second most common cause of leukemia deaths. As platelet counts decrease, the risk of bleeding increases (see the preceding section on thrombocytopenia).

- Assess vital signs every 4 hours and body systems every shift for bleeding.
  a. Skin and mucous membranes for petechiae, ecchymoses, and purpura
  b. Gums, nasal membranes, and conjunctiva for bleeding
  c. Vomitus, stool, and urine for visible or occult blood
  d. Vaginal bleeding
  e. Prolonged bleeding from puncture sites
  f. Neurologic changes such as headache, visual changes, altered mentation, decreased level of consciousness, seizures
  g. Abdomen for complaints of epigastric pain, diminished bowel sounds, increasing abdominal girth, rigidity or guarding

*Early identification of bleeding helps prevent significant blood loss and potential shock. Internal hemorrhage may lead to tachycardia, hypotension, pallor, and diaphoresis. Bleeding into the lungs may cause dyspnea; bleeding into the abdomen causes increased girth, pain, and guarding. Intracranial bleeding affects mental status and level of consciousness.*

- Avoid invasive procedures such as rectal temperatures and suppositories, vaginal douches, suppositories, or tampons, urinary catheterization, and parenteral injections if possible. Diagnostic procedures such as biopsy or lumbar puncture should not be done if the platelet count is less than 50,000. *Invasive procedures can cause tissue trauma and bleeding. Procedures that use large-bore needles should be delayed until the platelet count is increased.*
- Apply pressure to injection sites for 3 to 5 minutes, and to arterial punctures for 15 to 20 minutes. *Pressure prevents prolonged bleeding by prompting hemostasis and clot formation.*
- Instruct to avoid forcefully blowing or picking the nose, forceful coughing or sneezing, and straining to have a bowel movement. *These activities can damage mucous membranes, increasing the risk for bleeding.*

## Anticipatory Grieving

The diagnosis of cancer and a potentially life-threatening illness causes actual or perceived losses, such as loss of function, independence, normal appearance, friends, self-esteem, and self. Grieving is the emotional response to those losses. The adaptive process of mourning a loss and resolving grief is called grief work; grief work cannot begin until a loss is acknowledged. See Chapter 11 ⊂⊃ for a detailed discussion of grief and loss.

- Discuss roles of the client and family and ways in which they managed stressful situations in the past. Assess coping strategies and their effectiveness. Help identify sources of strength and support. Discuss changing roles resulting from leukemia diagnosis, and its effect on spiritual, social, and economic status, and usual lifestyle. Evaluate cultural or ethnic factors that affect grief reactions. *Grieving is a normal response to a real or potential loss that begins at the time of diagnosis. The timing, duration, and intensity of grief and responses to grief may differ among family members. Share information on diagnosis, role change, and physical loss among all family members to build the foundation for mutual understanding and trust.*
- Use therapeutic communication skills to facilitate open discussion of losses and provide permission to grieve. *Encouraging discussion of the meaning of the loss helps decrease some of the anxiety associated with loss. This in turn allows*

## CHART 32–3   NANDA, NIC, AND NOC LINKAGES

### The Client with Leukemia

| NURSING DIAGNOSES | NURSING INTERVENTIONS | NURSING OUTCOMES |
|---|---|---|
| • Fatigue | • Energy Management<br>• Nutrition Management<br>• Self-Care Assistance | • Endurance<br>• Energy Conservation<br>• Nutritional Status: Energy |
| • Ineffective Protection | • Bleeding Precautions<br>• Infection Protection<br>• Neurologic Monitoring | • Coagulation Status<br>• Immune Status<br>• Neurological Status: Consciousness |
| • Imbalanced Nutrition: Less than Body Requirements<br>• Impaired Oral Mucous Membrane | • Nutrition Management<br>• Nutrition Monitoring<br>• Oral Health Restoration<br>• Oral Health Maintenance | • Nutritional Status<br>• Nutritional Status: Food and Fluid Intake<br>• Oral Health<br>• Tissue Integrity: Skin and Mucous Membranes |

*Note. Data from* Nursing Outcomes Classification (NOC) *by M. Johnson & M. Maas (Eds.), 1997, St. Louis: Mosby;* Nursing Diagnoses: Definitions & Classification 2001–2002 *by North American Nursing Diagnosis Association, 2001, Philadelphia: NANDA;* Nursing Interventions Classification (NIC) *by J.C. McCloskey & G. M. Bulechek (Eds.), 2000, St. Louis: Mosby. Reprinted by permission.*

*the client and family to examine the current situation and compare it with past situations that they have coped with successfully.*

- Provide information about agencies that may help in resolving grief, and make referrals as indicated. Consider self-help groups, cancer support groups, and bereavement groups. *Participating in support groups with others who are anticipating or experiencing a similar loss can decrease feelings of isolation.*

## Using NANDA, NIC, and NOC

Chart 32–3 shows links between NANDA nursing diagnoses, NIC, and NOC for the client with leukemia.

## Home Care

Client and family teaching for home care after treatment for leukemia focuses on encouraging self-care, providing information about the disease and the treatment, preventing infection and injury, and promoting nutrition. Teaching topics for each of these areas are as follows.

### Encouraging Self-Care

- Hygiene measures and energy conservation during self-care activities
- Oral hygiene including using a soft-bristle toothbrush several times daily; avoid flossing
- Reporting lesions, bleeding, or signs of infection promptly
- Maintaining a balance of rest and activity

### Information about Leukemia and Treatment

- Bone marrow function, the pathophysiology of leukemia, and potential complications of leukemia
- Prognosis for the specific type of leukemia
- Treatment measures such as chemotherapy, radiation, bone marrow or stem cell transplant, their purpose and effects,

where treatment is available, and potential adverse effects or risks
- Community, regional, and national resources for people with leukemia

### Preventing Infection and Injury

- Handwashing and other measures to reduce exposure to pathogens such as avoiding people who are ill and avoiding crowds
- Avoiding foodborne illnesses by washing fruits and vegetables, proper food storage
- Dental hygiene measures
- Avoiding immunizations
- Manifestations to report: fever, chills, burning on urination, foul-smelling urine, vaginal or rectal discharge, skin lesions
- Avoiding contact sports or strenuous exercise if platelet count is low
- Using an electric razor for shaving, avoiding rectal or vaginal suppositories, vaginal tampons, or enemas
- Increasing dietary fiber and using a bulk-forming laxative as needed to prevent straining
- Avoiding over-the-counter or prescription drugs that interfere with platelet function (see Box 32–6)
- The importance of reporting any bleeding (nosebleeds, rectal bleeding, vomiting blood, excessive menstrual periods, blood in the urine, bleeding gums, bruises, or collections of blood under the skin) or changes in behavior to the health care provider

### Promoting Nutrition

- Eating several small, low-fat, high-calorie meals and drinking five to eight glasses of water daily
- Reporting continued weight loss, loss of appetite, or inability to eat for 24 hours
- Discussing dietary needs with the dietitian

## Nursing Care Plan
## A Client with Acute Myelocytic Leukemia

Catherine Cole is a 37-year-old secretary who lives with her husband, Ray, and teenage daughter, Amy, in an apartment in a large metropolitan area. About 2 months ago, Mrs. Cole began to tire easily and experience night sweats several times a week. She also noted that she was pale, bruised easily, and was having heavier menstrual periods. Blood tests ordered by her primary care provider are abnormal. She is admitted for a bone marrow biopsy.

### ASSESSMENT

Mary Losapio, RN, obtains a nursing history and physical assessment for Mrs. Cole. Mrs. Cole tells her, "I'm so tired, and I have these bruises all over me. I'm so afraid of the results of the bone marrow examination. I don't know what we will do if I have cancer." Mrs. Cole clutches her husband's hand and then begins to cry. Physical assessment data include: Height 64 inches (156 cm), weight 106 lb (48.1 kg); vital signs T 100°F, P 102, R 22, BP 130/82. Numerous petechiae scattered over trunk and arms; ecchymoses noted on lower right arm and right calf. Oral mucosa is red, with several small ulcerations in buccal areas.

Blood count shows reduced RBCs, hemoglobin, and hematocrit levels. The WBC is high, with myeloblasts seen on differential. The platelet count is very low. A tentative diagnosis of acute myelogenous leukemia is made.

### DIAGNOSES

- *Risk for infection* related to altered WBC production and immune function
- *Ineffective protection* related to reduced platelet count and risk for bleeding
- *Impaired oral mucous membrane* secondary to anemia and reduced platelets
- *Fatigue* related to anemia
- *Anxiety* related to fear of leukemia diagnosis

### EXPECTED OUTCOMES

- Remain free of infection.
- Experience no significant bleeding.
- Have intact oral mucous membranes.
- Manage self-care activities despite fatigue.
- Verbalize decreased anxiety.

### PLANNING AND IMPLEMENTATION

- Place in a private room.
- Limit visitors to immediate family for the present.

- Instruct all staff, the family, and client to carefully wash hands. Post a sign over the washbasin in the room as a reminder.
- Record vital signs every 4 hours.
- Avoid invasive procedures unless absolutely necessary.
- Monitor for bleeding every 4 hours, including skin, oral mucosa, abdominal assessment, body fluids, and menstrual pad count.
- Instruct to perform oral hygiene every 2 to 4 hours, using a soft-bristle toothbrush.
- Ask the dietitian to work with Mrs. Cole to identify preferred foods. Instruct to avoid foods that may damage oral mucosa, such as very hot, very cold, or highly acidic or spicy foods.
- Provide for periods of rest alternating with activity.
- Teach about the bone marrow biopsy. Allow time for questions and to verbalize fears.
- Refer to the oncology nurse specialist for further teaching and support.

### EVALUATION

The bone marrow biopsy confirms the diagnosis of acute myelogenous leukemia. Mrs. Cole is very upset, but calms as the physician and the oncology nurse discuss treatment plans and the possibility of remission. She decides to have outpatient chemotherapy. During her hospital stay, Mrs. Cole remained free of infection or further bleeding. She tells Ms. Losapio that her mouth feels better, although it is still painful. During routine assessment, Mrs. Cole remarks, "You know, I was so scared when I came here, but I think I am a little less so now. Sometimes not knowing what is wrong is worse than knowing."

### Critical Thinking in the Nursing Process

1. Describe how alterations in WBCs can increase a person's susceptibility to infection.
2. List sources of potential infection for the hospitalized client.
3. What is the rationale for having the client do her own oral and physical hygiene?
4. Outline a teaching plan for this client and her family for home care to prevent infection.
5. Develop a care plan for Mrs. Cole for the nursing diagnosis, *Activity intolerance*.

See Evaluating Your Response in Appendix C.

---

Assistance with physical care, finances, and transportation may be required following discharge. Refer the client and family to social services, support groups, home care services as needed, and other agencies that can provide needed services (such as local chapters of the American Cancer Society, which can provide hospital beds and transportation for outpatient cancer treatment).

## THE CLIENT WITH MULTIPLE MYELOMA

**Multiple myeloma** is a malignancy in which plasma cells multiply uncontrollably and infiltrate the bone marrow, lymph nodes, spleen, and other tissues. *Plasma cells* are B-cell lymphocytes that develop to produce antibodies (immunoglobins).

The incidence of multiple myeloma is increasing, with an estimated 48,100 cases diagnosed annually. It affects blacks more than twice as often as whites, and men more frequently than women. The incidence of multiple myeloma increases with age, rarely occurring before age 40. Its cause is unknown (McCance & Huether, 2002). Possible contributing factors include genetic predisposition, oncogenic virus, inflammatory stimuli, and chronic antigenic stimulation.

## PATHOPHYSIOLOGY AND MANIFESTATIONS

Malignant plasma cells arise from one clone of B cells that produce abnormally large amounts of a particular immunoglobin called the *M protein.* This abnormal protein interferes with normal antibody production and impairs the humoral immune response. It also increases blood viscosity and may damage kidney tubules. As myeloma cells proliferate, they replace the bone marrow and infiltrate the bone itself. Cortical bone is progressively destroyed by tumor growth and enzymes produced by myeloma cells. These enzymes facilitate bone destruction, its infiltration by tumor cells, development of new blood vessels to sustain the tumor, and growth of myeloma cells (McCance & Huether, 2002). Affected bones (primarily the vertebrae, ribs, skull, pelvis, femur, clavicle, and scapula) are weakened and may break without trauma (*pathologic fracture*).

The disease develops slowly. Manifestations of multiple myeloma are due to its effects on the bone and the impaired immune response due to M protein production. Bone pain is the most common presenting symptom. With progression of the disease, the pain may increase in severity and become more localized. Rapid bone destruction releases calcium from the bone, leading to hypercalcemia and manifestations of neurologic dysfunction, such as lethargy, confusion, and weakness.

As functional antibody formation decreases and the humoral immune response is suppressed, recurrent infections develop. Cell-mediated immunity remains intact. *Bence Jones proteins* are found in the urine in multiple myeloma. These proteins are toxic to the renal tubules, and may lead to renal failure with azotemia and uremia (see Chapter 27 ⊖ for more information about renal failure).

About 15% of clients with multiple myeloma die within 3 months of the diagnosis. More frequently, the disease course is chronic, progressing more rapidly with each relapse after remission. The acute terminal stage of the disease is marked by pancytopenia and widespread organ infiltration by myeloma cells (Braunwald et al., 2001).

## COLLABORATIVE CARE

Diagnostic tests for multiple myeloma include the following:

- *X-rays* and other radiologic studies of the bone may reveal multiple punched-out lesions.
- *Bone marrow examination* shows an abnormal number of immature plasma cells.
- *CBC* shows moderate to severe anemia.

- *Urinalysis* shows Bence Jones protein in the urine.
- *Biopsy* of myeloma lesions confirms the diagnosis of multiple myeloma.

There is no cure for multiple myeloma. Treatment includes systemic chemotherapy to control progression of the disease and supportive care to reduce complications of the disease and their effects.

Combination chemotherapy with an alkylating agent (melphalan [Alkeran], cyclophosphamide [Cytoxan], or chlorambucil [Chloromycetin]) and prednisone administered for 4 to 7 days every 4 to 6 weeks is commonly used. Chemotherapy typically reduces bone pain, hypercalcemia, anemia, and the number of infections (Braunwald et al., 2001). Localized radiation therapy may be used to treat painful bone lesions.

Supportive care may include treatment of hypercalcemia with hydration, possible biphosphonate therapy to reduce bone loss (see Chapter 39 ⊖), and calcium, vitamin D, and fluoride supplements to support bone structure. Plasma exchange therapy (plasmapheresis) to remove circulating M proteins is used as needed to treat acute renal failure. Infections are treated promptly when they develop.

## NURSING CARE

### Assessment

Focused assessment data for the client with multiple myeloma includes the following:

- Health history: complaints of back or bone pain, onset, duration, and intensity; complaints of weakness, fatigue, anorexia; history of frequent or recurrent infections; neurologic symptoms such as numbness and tingling or clumsiness
- Physical examination: level of consciousness and mental status; mobility, gait; localized tenderness or pain, bony crepitus with movement or palpation; movement and sensation in extremities

### Nursing Diagnoses and Interventions

Nursing care of the client with multiple myeloma focuses on problems of chronic pain, impaired mobility, and the risk for injury. Risk for infection is a major nursing care focus; see the previous section on leukemia for specific interventions to reduce this risk. Other nursing care needs are similar to those of clients with other cancers and chronic pain. See Chapters 4 and 10 ⊖ for additional specific nursing interventions for these problems.

### Chronic Pain

Clients with multiple myeloma typically experience chronic back pain and deep bone pain as myeloma cells saturate the bone marrow and invade the bone structure. Pathologic fractures are a common and reoccurring problem.

- Assess pain, including intensity (use a standard pain scale), onset, duration, precipitating factors, and effective relief measures. *Identifying the intensity, causes, and precipitating factors of pain helps determine and evaluate effective pain relief measures.*

- Determine position of greatest comfort, and assist as needed into this position. *The client is best able to identify positions that minimize pain, but may need assistance with repositioning.*
- Support position with pillows. *Bony prominences may be painful due to infiltrates. Pillows can help relieve pressure on these prominences, thus reducing pain.*
- Provide uninterrupted rest periods. *Adequate rest facilitates pain relief and improves pain tolerance.*
- Teach adjunctive pain relief strategies such as relaxation or guided imagery. *A combination of pharmacologic and non-pharmacologic methods provides better management of chronic pain, especially bone pain.*
- Teach effective analgesic use, including the family in instruction. *Analgesics are most effective when taken before pain becomes severe. Clients and their families may be reluctant to use prescription analgesics on a regular basis.*
- Report unrelieved pain to the physician. *A different analgesic or addition of an adjunctive medication such as a nonsteroidal anti-inflammatory drug (NSAID) may be needed to effectively control pain.*

### Impaired Physical Mobility

Painful bony infiltrates and pathologic fractures may limit mobility. A brace or splint may be used to protect extremities or support the back. In addition, persistent weakness associated with the cancer and anemia may limit the client's ability to participate in usual activities.

**PRACTICE ALERT** *Gently support extremities during repositioning. Weakened extremities due to infiltration of bone by myeloma cells and muscle atrophy from lack of use increase the risk for pathologic fractures.* ■

- Assist to change position at least every 2 hours. *Assistance with repositioning is necessary due to weakness. Frequent repositioning improves comfort and reduces the risk for impaired skin and tissue integrity.*
- Provide a trapeze to assist in repositioning. *A trapeze provides better leverage, allowing the client to assist with repositioning and providing a degree of independence. The ability to participate in self-care improves self-esteem.*

### Risk for Injury

The bone involvement of multiple myeloma places the client at high risk for pathologic and traumatic fractures. Pathologic fractures can occur with simple activities such as turning or reaching for an item. The spine usually is affected; the ribs and bones of the extremities also may be at risk for fracture.

- Place needed items close at hand. *Straining to reach objects increases the risk of falling or sustaining other injury.*
- Provide safety measures to prevent falls from bed: Place the bed in a low position, use side rails as indicated, and place the call bell within reach. *Safety measures help prevent accidental injury. A secure environment minimizes risk and helps prevent falls.*

- Provide shoes with nonskid soles, a clear pathway, adequate lighting, and a level surface free of scatter rugs or other hazards when ambulating. Provide a walker as needed for support and security. *Weightbearing exercise promotes bone repair. Safety measures, such as an unobstructed pathway and a firm walking surface, help prevent falls.*

### Home Care

When teaching clients and their families for home care, include the following topics.

- Strategies for home maintenance management
- Signs and symptoms of complications to be reported to the physician (e.g., symptoms of vertebral and extremity fractures)
- Manifestations of infection to report: fever and chills; increased malaise, fatigue, or weakness; cough with or without sputum; sore throat; dysuria, nocturia, frequency, urgency, or malodorous urine

Provide referrals for home health and home maintenance services, physical or occupational therapy, social services, and hospice care as appropriate.

## THE CLIENT WITH MALIGNANT LYMPHOMA

**Lymphomas** are malignancies of lymphoid tissue. They are characterized by the proliferation of lymphocytes, histiocytes (resident monocytes or macrophages), and their precursors or derivatives. Although there are many types of malignant lymphoid cells, at this time lymphomas commonly are identified as Hodgkin's disease or non-Hodgkin's lymphoma.

Malignant lymphomas are the sixth leading cause of cancer deaths in the United States. Approximately 60,900 new cases of lymphoma were diagnosed in 2002, and 25,800 deaths were attributed to the disease. The incidence of non-Hodgkin's lymphoma has nearly doubled since 1970, but currently has stabilized except among black females. The incidence of Hodgkin's disease has declined since the late 1980s (ACS, 2002a).

While the cause of lymphoma is unknown, some risk factors have been identified. Immunosuppression due to drug therapy following organ transplant or to HIV disease increases the risk for non-Hodgkin's lymphoma. Infectious agents such as human T-cell leukemia/lymphoma virus-1 (HTLV-1) and the Epstein-Barr virus (EBV) also have been identified as risk factors. Others may include occupational herbicide or chemical exposure (ACS, 2002a).

## PATHOPHYSIOLOGY
### Hodgkin's Disease

*Hodgkin's disease* is a lymphatic cancer, occurring most often in people between the ages of 15 and 35 or over age 50. It is somewhat more common in men than women. Approximately 7000 new cases of Hodgkin's disease were diagnosed in 2002 (ACS, 2002). The exact cause of Hodgkin's disease is unknown, but both EBV infection and genetic factors appear to play a role

TABLE 32–9    Subtypes of Hodgkin's Disease

| Subtype | Incidence | Prognosis |
|---------|-----------|-----------|
| Lymphocyte predominant | More common in adults and in males | Disease usually localized at diagnosis; excellent prognosis |
| Nodular sclerosing | Most common form; usually affects adolescents and young adults; more common in females | Good if diagnosed early |
| Mixed cellularity | Common in adults; more common in males | Poorer prognosis with 50% to 60% 5-year survival |
| Lymphocyte depleted | Least common form; usually affects older adults and people with HIV disease | Poor prognosis with 5-year survival rate of less than 50% |

in its development. Hodgkin's disease is one of the most curable cancers. As many as 60% to 90% of people with localized disease achieve cure with a normal life span (Porth, 2002).

Hodgkin's disease develops in a single lymph node or chain of nodes, spreading to adjoining nodes. Involved lymph nodes contain *Reed-Sternberg cells* (malignant cells) surrounded by host inflammatory cells. These malignant cells secrete inflammatory mediator substances, attracting inflammatory cells to the tumor site. They may invade almost any tissue in the body. The spleen often is involved; as the disease progresses, the liver, lungs, digestive tract, and CNS may be affected (Porth, 2002). Rapid proliferation of abnormal lymphocytes impairs the immune response, especially cell-mediated immune responses. Infections are common. Four subtypes of Hodgkin's disease have been identified, based on the predominant cells. Table 32–9 outlines these subtypes.

## Manifestations

The most common symptom of Hodgkin's disease is one or more painlessly enlarged lymph nodes, usually in the cervical or subclavicular region. Systemic manifestations such as persistent fever, night sweats, fatigue, and weight loss are associated with a poorer prognosis for the disease. Late symptoms such as malaise, pruritus, and anemia indicate spread of the disease (Porth, 2002). The spleen may be enlarged, and other organ systems such as the lungs and gastrointestinal tract are occasionally involved.

## Non-Hodgkin's Lymphoma

*Non-Hodgkin's lymphoma* is a diverse group of lymphoid tissue malignancies that do not contain Reed-Sternberg cells. Non-Hodgkin's lymphomas tend to arise in peripheral lymph nodes and spread early to tissues throughout the body. Non-Hodgkin's lymphoma is more common than Hodgkin's disease, affecting an estimated 53,900 people annually and causing about 24,400 deaths in 2002 (ACS, 2002). Older adults are more often affected, and it occurs more frequently in men than in women. Like Hodgkin's disease, its cause is unknown, although both genetic and environmental factors (e.g., viral infections such as EBV, HTLV-1 and HTLV-2, and HIV) are thought to play a role.

As in most malignancies, non-Hodgkin's lymphoma begins as a single transformed cell; it may arise from T cells, B cells, or tissue macrophages (histocytes). Different cell types of non-Hodgkin's lymphoma develop in different regions of the lymph node. It tends to spread early and unpredictably to other lymphoid tissues and organs. Extranodal spread may involve the nasopharynx, gastrointestinal tract, bone, CNS, thyroid, testes, and soft tissue.

The prognosis for non-Hodgkin's lymphoma ranges from excellent to poor, depending on the identified cell type and grade of differentiation. Low grade tumors (better differentiated) tend to be less aggressive and more curable. Higher grade tumors often are disseminated at the time of diagnoses, and have a poorer prognosis (Copstead & Banasik, 2000).

## Manifestations

The early manifestations of non-Hodgkin's lymphoma are similar to those for Hodgkin's disease. Painless lymphadenopathy may be localized or widespread. Systemic manifestations such as fever, night sweats, fatigue, and weight loss may be present, but are less common in non-Hodgkin's lymphoma. Organ system involvement may cause symptoms such as abdominal pain, nausea, and vomiting. Headaches, peripheral or cranial nerve symptoms, altered mental status, or seizures may signal CNS involvement.

The manifestations and clinical features of Hodgkin's disease and non-Hodgkin's lymphoma are compared in Table 32–10.

## COLLABORATIVE CARE

Chemotherapy and radiation therapy, either alone or in combination, are the primary treatments for Hodgkin's and non-Hodgkin's lymphomas. Use of monoclonal antibodies to the lymphoma cells, and bone marrow and peripheral stem cell transplants are under investigation for treating lymphomas as well. See the previous section on treatment of leukemia for more information about these transplants.

## Diagnostic Tests

The following diagnostic tests may be ordered for lymphomas.

- *CBC* often shows a mild normochromic, normocytic anemia in Hodgkin's disease; other findings in Hodgkin's disease may include leukocytosis with high neutrophil and eosinophil counts, and an elevated sed rate. In non-Hodgkin's lymphoma, the CBC typically remains normal until late in the disease, when pancytopenia may develop.

TABLE 32–10  Features and Manifestations of Hodgkin's Disease and Non-Hodgkin's Lymphoma

| Feature or Manifestation | Hodgkin's Disease | Non-Hodgkin's Lymphoma |
|---|---|---|
| Lymphadenopathy | Localized to a single node or chain, often cervical, subclavicular, or mediastinal | Multiple peripheral nodes, nodes of the mesentery often involved |
| Spread | Orderly and continuous | Diffuse and unpredictable |
| Extranodal involvement | Rare | Early and common |
| Bone marrow involvement | Uncommon | Common |
| Fever, night sweats, weight loss | Common | Uncommon until disease is extensive |
| Other manifestations | Fatigue, pruritus, splenomegaly; anemia, neutrophilia | Abdominal pain, nausea, vomiting; dyspnea, cough; CNS symptoms; lymphocytopenia |

- *Chest X-ray* is done to identify possible enlarged mediastinal lymph nodes and pulmonary involvement.
- *Chest* or *abdominal CT scan* may be done to identify abnormal or enlarged nodes.
- *Bipedal lymphangiography* uses radiographic dye injected into the lymphatic channels of the lower legs to identify the extent of iliac, para-aortic, and abdominal lymph node involvement.
- *Biopsy* of the largest, most central enlarged lymph node is done to establish the diagnosis for both Hodgkin's disease and non-Hodgkin's lymphoma. The presence of Reed-Sternberg cells confirms the diagnosis of Hodgkin's disease.

## Staging

Staging is used to determine the extent of the disease and appropriate treatment. The Ann Arbor Staging System may be used to assess the extent and severity of lymphomas. The newer Cotswold Staging Classification System is used for Hodgkin's disease. The stages are similar in both systems:

Stage I: involvement of a single lymph node region, lymphoid structure, or extralymphatic site

Stage II: involvement of two or more lymph node regions on the same side of the diaphragm, or localized extralymphatic involvement

Stage III: involvement of lymph node regions or structures on both sides of the diaphragm; may involve the spleen or localized extranodal disease

Stage IV: diffuse or disseminated extralymphatic disease

The presence or absence of systemic symptoms is indicated by either an A (no systemic symptoms) or B (systemic symptoms of fever, night sweats, weight loss).

## Chemotherapy

Combination chemotherapy is used to treat both Hodgkin's disease and non-Hodgkin's lymphoma. In both cases, chemotherapy often is followed by radiation therapy to involved lymph node regions. The choice of drug combination depends on the stage of the disease as well as the client's age and general condition. The usual combination used in the United States is the ABVD regimen (doxorubicin, bleomycin, vinbalstine, and deacarbazine). The MOPP regimen (nitrogen mustard, vincristine, procarbazine, and prednisone) also is commonly used.

More than 75% of clients with Hodgkin's disease who do not have systemic symptoms achieve complete remission with treatment. A number of other combination regimens also are effective in treating lymphoma, some of which produce fewer adverse effects.

## Radiation Therapy

Radiation therapy is the primary treatment for early-stage Hodgkin's disease. In later stages and in non-Hodgkin's lymphoma it usually is combined with chemotherapy. Many lymphomas are highly responsive to radiation. The involved lymph node region is treated, with careful shielding to protect unaffected areas and minimize the extent of radiation burn and normal cell destruction. If the disease is advanced, total nodal irradiation may be done (Figure 32–11 ■).

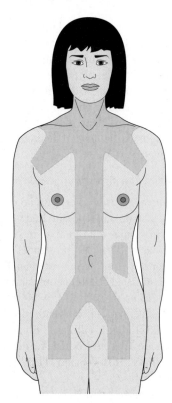

**Figure 32–11** ■ Total nodal or extended field radiation for lymphoma.

## Complications of Treatment

Both chemotherapy and radiation therapy may have long-term effects. Permanent sterility is common, especially in older adults. Bone marrow depression can lead to immunosuppression, anemia, and bleeding. Secondary cancers and cardiac injury are the most serious late adverse effects of treatment. Chemotherapy regimens using the MOPP or a related protocol carry a risk of acute leukemia. Cancers such as breast or lung cancer may develop 10 or more years after thoracic radiation. Thoracic radiation also increases the risk for coronary heart disease and hypothyroidism (Braunwald et al., 2001).

## NURSING CARE

### Assessment

Focused assessment of the client with Hodgkin's disease or non-Hodgkin's lymphoma includes:

- Nursing history: complaints of enlarged lymph node(s), fever, night sweats, weight loss, fatigue or general malaise, abdominal pain, respiratory symptoms, numbness or tingling of extremities, visual changes, or changes in mentation; history of infectious mononucleosis, HIV disease, or other immunosuppressive disorders
- Physical examination: mental status exam; inspect and palpate lymph nodes (cervical, subclavicular, axillary, and inguinal) for enlargement, tenderness; heart and lung sounds; abdominal examination for tenderness, masses, liver or spleen enlargement

### Nursing Diagnoses and Interventions

Nursing care of the client with malignant lymphoma involves both physical and emotional support during diagnosis and treatment. Common nursing care problems include impaired protection due to bone marrow suppression, fatigue, nausea, and altered body image. See the nursing care section for leukemia for specific nursing interventions for *Ineffective protection.*

### Fatigue

General malaise and fatigue may accompany malignant lymphoma and are side effects of chemotherapy. In addition, the physical and psychologic stress of dealing with a chronic, debilitating disease and its treatment may cause fatigue.

- Inquire about feelings of malaise (a vague feeling of body weakness or discomfort) and fatigue (a pervasive, drained feeling that cannot be eliminated). *Both malaise and fatigue are subjective experiences with physiologic, situational, and psychologic components.*
- Encourage verbalization of feelings about the impact of the disease and fatigue on lifestyle. *Discussion of feelings helps the client clarify values and may assist in identifying priorities.*
- Encourage enjoyable but quiet activities, such as reading, listening to music, or hobbies. *Enjoyable activities help decrease feelings of fatigue. Quiet activities conserve energy while yielding a sense of accomplishment.*

- Encourage to establish priorities and include rest periods or naps when scheduling daily activities. *This provides a sense of control over activities and helps maintain self-esteem. Scheduled rest periods help restore energy and decrease fatigue.*
- Encourage delegation of some responsibilities to family members. *Delegation helps maintain the client's involvement and role in family decisions and responsibilities, while conserving energy for those activities identified as high priority by the client.*
- Identify and encourage the client to use energy-saving equipment. *Performing tasks with less exertion and in less time helps conserve energy.*
- Encourage a diet high in carbohydrates and fluids. *A high-carbohydrate diet helps maintain muscle glycogen stores. A liberal fluid intake promotes excretion of metabolic by-products that may contribute to malaise and fatigue.*

### Nausea

The effects of malignant lymphoma and its treatment with chemotherapy and/or radiation therapy can contribute to nausea and interfere with nutritional status. Nausea, a sensation of abdominal fullness, and fear of vomiting often limit food intake. See also the nursing diagnosis, *Imbalanced nutrition,* in the section on leukemia for additional interventions.

- Assess precipitating factors for nausea and/or vomiting, the frequency of vomiting, and relief measures used by the client. *Careful assessment allows development of interventions tailored to the client's situation and needs.*

**PRACTICE ALERT**  *Provide ordered antiemetics before chemotherapy is started. Administering prescribed antiemetics before chemotherapy helps prevent nausea and the psychological association of nausea with chemotherapy.* ■

- Teach measures to prevent or relieve nausea and vomiting.
  a. Eat soda crackers and suck on hard candy.
  b. Eat soft, bland foods that are cold or at room temperature.
  c. Avoid unpleasant odors, and get fresh air.
  d. Eat prior to but not immediately before chemotherapy.
  e. Use distraction or progressive muscle relaxation when nauseated.
  f. If vomiting occurs, gradually resume oral intake with frequent sips of clear liquids or ice, progressing to bland foods.
  *Crackers and hard candy often relieve queasiness, whereas hot, spicy, sweet, or strong smelling foods may increase nausea. Alternative nausea relief measures may be effective.*
- Provide small feedings of high-kcal, high-protein foods and fluids. *This increases nutritional intake.*
- Assist with oral care, general hygiene, and environmental control of temperature, appearance, and odors. *These measures enhance appetite.*
- Identify and provide preferred foods. *This promotes nutritional intake.*
- Assist to a sitting position during and immediately after meals. *The sitting position helps decrease early feelings of fullness.*

## Disturbed Body Image

The diagnosis of cancer is often devastating to the sense of trust in and the perception of one's body. Radiation and chemotherapy lead to changes in appearance and body function (e.g., hair loss, reduced libido, and infertility), further altering body image. Reactions to this diagnosis vary and may include refusal to look in a mirror, discuss the effects of the disease or treatment, unwillingness to participate in rehabilitation, inappropriate treatment decisions, increasing dependence on others or refusal to provide self-care, hostility, withdrawal, and signs of grieving.

- Assess perception of body image through subjective information such as:
  What the client likes most and least about his or her body.
  Pre-illness perception of sick or disabled people.
  Current understanding of health and limitations imposed by illness or treatment.
  Feelings about the illness and its effect on perception of self and others.
  *Body image is one's mental idea or picture of the body. It is based on past and present experiences and includes components of one's actual body and emotional responses to that body. Body image changes constantly. There is often a time lag between an actual body change and the changed body image; during this time, the diagnosis, teaching, and treatment may be rejected.*
- Discuss the risk for and measures to cope with alopecia. Suggest wearing wigs, scarves, hats, or caps. Teach proper scalp care using baby shampoo or mild soap, a soft brush, sunscreen, and mineral oil to reduce itching. If eyelashes and eyebrows are lost, teach eye protection, such as wearing eyeglasses and caps with wide brims. *Chemotherapeutic agents attack rapidly dividing cells such as those responsible for hair growth. Hair loss usually begins 1 to 2 weeks after initiation of chemotherapy, with maximum loss 1 to 2 months later. Alopecia may range from thinning to total hair loss.*

*Regrowth depends on the treatment schedule and doses; however, it usually begins 2 to 3 months after treatment ends. New hair may be softer, more curly, and slightly different in color. Teaching and emotional support help the client anticipate hair loss, discuss its potential effect on body image, and learn self-care techniques.*
- Discuss available resources for financial assistance with purchase of wigs, including local American Cancer Society chapters and insurance plans. *A well-matched wig (or one the color the client has always wished for!) can help maintain a positive body image.*

## Sexual Dysfunction

Sexual dysfunction may result from the malignancy and the effects of radiation and chemotherapy. Reproductive tissues are made of rapidly dividing cells, and cancer treatment may cause temporary or permanent sterility, changes in menstruation, and changes in libido.

- Encourage discussion of actual or potential sexual dysfunction or sterility with the client and significant other. *Clients may be reluctant to discuss this unintended effect of treatment unless encouraged.*
- Assess knowledge, provide information, and clarify misconceptions. Discuss realistic measures for coping (e.g., sperm banking prior to chemotherapy or radiation therapy). *Clients and their partners may be unclear about expected effects on sexuality, reproduction, and the permanency of these effects.*
- Refer for counseling as indicated. *Sexual counseling can help the client and partner develop alternative strategies for expressing their sexuality.*

## Risk for Impaired Skin Integrity

Malignant lymphomas may cause significant pruritus and drenching night sweats. As a result, skin integrity may be impaired. In addition, radiation therapy can cause superficial burns, which also may affect skin integrity.

---

### CHART 32–4  NANDA, NIC, AND NOC LINKAGES

#### The Client with Malignant Lymphoma

| NURSING DIAGNOSES | NURSING INTERVENTIONS | NURSING OUTCOMES |
|---|---|---|
| • Disturbed Body Image | • Active Listening<br>• Emotional Support<br>• Spiritual Support | • Body Image<br>• Psychosocial Adjustment: Life Change |
| • Impaired Skin Integrity | • Radiation Therapy Management<br>• Skin Surveillance | • Tissue Integrity: Skin and Mucous Membranes |
| • Nausea | • Medication Management<br>• Nausea Management | • Comfort Level<br>• Nutritional Status: Food and Fluid Intake |
| • Sexual Dysfunction | • Coping Enhancement<br>• Sexual Counseling | • Self-Esteem<br>• Sexual Functioning |

*Note. Data from Nursing Outcomes Classification (NOC) by M. Johnson & M. Maas (Eds.), 1997, St. Louis: Mosby; Nursing Diagnoses: Definitions & Classification 2001–2002 by North American Nursing Diagnosis Association, 2001, Philadelphia: NANDA; Nursing Interventions Classification (NIC) by J.C. McCloskey & G. M. Bulechek (Eds.), 2000, St. Louis: Mosby. Reprinted by permission.*

- Frequently assess skin, especially in areas undergoing radiation. *Early identification of lesions allows timely treatment and can prevent further disruption of this important line of defense against infection.*
- Provide and teach measures to promote comfort and relieve itching: Use cool water and a mild soap to bathe; blot (rather than rub) dry skin; apply plain cornstarch or non-perfumed lotion or powder to the skin unless contraindicated; use lightweight blankets and clothing; maintain adequate humidity and a cool room temperature; wash bedding and clothes in mild detergent, and put them through second rinse cycle. *Pruritus is aggravated by excessive warmth, excessive dryness, rough fabrics, fatigue, and stress. Lotions and some powders may be contraindicated during radiation therapy.*

## Using NANDA, NIC, and NOC

Chart 32–4 shows links between NANDA nursing diagnoses, NIC, and NOC for the client with malignant lymphoma.

## Home Care

When teaching the client and family for home care, include the following topics in addition to those previously identified for specific nursing diagnoses.

- Information about the illness, planned treatment, and anticipated side effects of treatment
- Skin care and measures to relieve itching and protect areas of radiation
- Symptoms to report to the physician, including those of vertebral compression (decreased sensation or strength in lower extremities)

---

# Nursing Care Plan
# A Client with Hodgkin's Disease

Albin Quito, age 28, is the nurse manager of a thoracic intensive care unit in a large teaching hospital. Lately he has been more tired than usual, often wakes up at night covered with sweat, and just does not feel well. He had thought that his symptoms were due to a viral illness and his busy work schedule. However, yesterday morning Albin noticed a large swollen area on the right side of his neck. He made an appointment with his primary health provider who found a large cervical lymph node. A biopsy of the node and a CT scan of the chest were scheduled.

## ASSESSMENT

David Herzog, the nurse in charge of the outpatient clinic, obtains a nursing history and assessment on Mr. Quito. His physical examination is essentially normal, with the exception of the enlarged node, which is not tender to palpation. When Mr. Quito is weighed, he tells Mr. Herzog that he has lost 7 lb (3.2 kg) in the past 2 months. In reviewing the results of the blood studies, Mr. Herzog notes mild anemia and an increased neutrophil count. The lymph node biopsy shows Reed-Sternberg cells. The clinic physician and Mr. Herzog tell Mr. Quito that the findings indicate stage 1-B Hodgkin's disease but that the prognosis is very good. The physician recommends a short course of combination chemotherapy followed by radiation therapy to involved sites.

## DIAGNOSES

- *Anxiety* related to the diagnosis of Hodgkin's disease and effects of treatment on job performance
- *Risk for infection* related to potential bone marrow depression due to chemotherapy
- *Fatigue* related to effects of cancer, chemotherapy, and radiation therapy

## EXPECTED OUTCOMES

- Verbalize reduced anxiety.
- Remain free of infection.
- Identify and use methods to preserve energy.

## PLANNING AND IMPLEMENTATION

- Encourage to consider a leave of absence from work during course of treatment.
- Discuss joining a support group for people with cancer.
- Provide information about the illness, combination chemotherapy, and radiation therapy.
- Reinforce knowledge of actions to decrease the risk of infection.
- Discuss ways to decrease fatigue and maintain energy:
  - Take a 1- to 2-hour nap once or twice a day.
  - Avoid overexertion during weekends and time off.
  - Maintain a well-balanced diet.

## EVALUATION

When Mr. Quito returns the following week to begin chemotherapy, he brings his friend Nancy to meet Mr. Herzog and asks him to discuss his treatment with her. Mr. Quito says, "I am still really scared, but being able to talk about this with Nancy will help a lot." Mr. Quito has made arrangements to take a 4-month leave from work, with the understanding that his job will be held for him. He states that he will have some problems with money but is working them out. He also says he feels that taking a nap is silly but that he will rest to maintain his energy level. Mr. Quito and Nancy express confidence that he will be cured and say they plan to be active members of the cancer support group—even after recovery.

## Critical Thinking in the Nursing Process

1. Discuss the rationale for treating Hodgkin's disease with chemotherapy and radiation.
2. Design a teaching plan to help Mr. Quito prevent infection while he is at home.
3. What effect does the diagnosis of cancer have on the developmental tasks of a young adult?
4. Develop a care plan for Mr. Quito for the diagnosis, *Ineffective role performance.*

See Evaluating Your Response in Appendix C.

- Use of analgesics and alternative relief strategies for abdominal pain and peripheral neuropathies
- Respiratory care if mediastinal nodes are enlarged or lungs or pleurae are involved
- Planning activities of daily living to ensure adequate rest and exercise
- Measures to relieve nausea and maintain adequate nutrition

Refer clients and family members to the local chapter of the American Cancer Society for information, assistance, and counseling. A list of state and local agencies that offer information about malignant lymphoma and financial assistance can be obtained from the Leukemia Society of America.

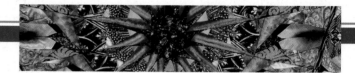

 **EXPLORE MediaLink**

NCLEX review questions, case studies, care plan activities, MediaLink applications, and other interactive resources for this chapter can be found on the Companion Website at www.prenhall.com/lemone.

Click on Chapter 32 to select the activities for this chapter. For animations, video clips, more NCLEX review questions, and an audio glossary, access the Student CD-ROM accompanying this textbook.

## TEST YOURSELF

1. In assessing a female client with moderate anemia, the nurse would expect to find which of the following?

   a. Hematocrit 45%
   b. Pulse rate 140
   c. Complains of shortness of breath with exercise
   d. WBC 14,000/μL

2. The nurse administering platelets to a client with disseminated intravascular coagulation (DIC) understands that the intended effect of this treatment is to:

   a. Replace specific clotting factors
   b. Promote intravascular clotting
   c. Restore tissue oxygenation
   d. Replace depleted platelets

3. A client whose husband has hemophilia asks if her newborn baby girl could have the disease. The nurse's response is based on the knowledge that:

   a. The most common forms of hemophilia are transmitted as sex-linked recessive disorders; her daughter is at risk for carrying the defective gene
   b. Because hemophilia is a sex-linked recessive disorder carried on the Y chromosome, her daughter has no risk of having or carrying the disease
   c. Hemophilia is an autosomal dominant disorder; therefore, her daughter has a 50% chance of having the disorder

   d. Although hemophilia is genetically transmitted, its pattern of inheritance is unknown, and her daughter will need to be tested for the defective gene

4. Which of the following nursing diagnoses would be of highest priority for the client hospitalized for a bone marrow transplant to treat relapse of acute myelocytic leukemia?

   a. *Disturbed body image*
   b. *Ineffective protection*
   c. *Anxiety*
   d. *Imbalanced nutrition: Less than body requirements*

5. A client with non-Hodgkin's lymphoma tells the nurse, "I might as well give up on dating. No woman will want me now." What is the most appropriate response?

   a. "It sounds like you are concerned about the effects of this disease and the proposed treatment plan."
   b. "Don't worry. Malignant lymphomas are very treatable when caught in an early state of the disease."
   c. "Well, you may never be able to have children all right, but there are other ways to have a satisfying relationship with a woman."
   d. "Lots of women find bald men attractive; besides, your hair may grow back soft and curly."

See Test Yourself answers in Appendix C.

## BIBLIOGRAPHY

Ackley, B. J., & Ladwig, G. B. (2002). *Nursing diagnosis handbook: A guide to planning care* (5th ed.). St. Louis: Mosby.

Alcoser, P. W., & Burchett, S. (1999). Bone marrow transplantation: Immune system suppression and reconstitution. *American Journal of Nursing, 99*(6), 26–31.

American Cancer Society. (2002a). *Cancer facts and figures 2002.* Atlanta: Author.

_____ . (2002b). *Gleevec's new successes show growing promise of targeted therapies.* Available: www.cancer.org/eprise/main/docroot/NWS/content/NWS_1_1x_Gleevec

Braunwald, E., Fauci, A. S., Kasper, D. L., Hauser, S. L., Longo, D. L., & Jameson, J. L. (2001). *Harrison's principles of internal medicine* (15th ed.). New York: McGraw-Hill.

Bullock, B. A., & Henze, R. L. (2000). *Focus on pathophysiology.* Philadelphia: Lippincott.

Copstead, L. C., & Banasik, J. L. (2000). *Pathophysiology: Biological and behavioral perspectives* (2nd ed.). Philadephia: Saunders.

Day, S. W., & Wynn, L. W. (2000). Sickle cell pain & hydroxyurea. *American Journal of Nursing, 100*(11), 34–38.

Druker, B. J., Sawyers, C. L., Capdeville, R., Ford, J. M., Baccarani, M., & Goldman, J. M. (2001). Chronic myelogenous leukemia. *Hematology (American Society of Hematology Education Program),* 87–113. Abstract from National Cancer Institute. Available: www. nci.nih.gov/cancerinformation/doc_ cit.aspx?args= 22; 11722980

Fontaine, K. L. (2000). *Healing practices: Alternative therapies for nursing.* Upper Saddle River, NJ: Prentice Hall Health.

Gorman, K. (1999). Sickle cell disease. *American Journal of Nursing, 99*(3), 38–43.

Gutaj, D. (2000). Oncology today: Lymphoma. *RN, 63*(8), 32–37.

Johnson, M., Bulechek, G., Dochterman, J. M., Maas, M., & Moorhead, S. (2001). *Nursing diagnoses, outcomes, & interventions.* St. Louis: Mosby.

Johnson, M., Maas, M., & Moorhead, S. (Eds.). (2000). *Nursing outcomes classification (NOC)* (2nd ed.). St. Louis: Mosby.

Kuhn, M. A. (1999). *Complementary therapies for health care providers.* Philadelphia: Lippincott.

Lea, D. H., & Williams, J. K. (2002). Genetic testing and screening. *American Journal of Nursing, 102*(7), 36–43.

Lehne, R. A. (2001). *Pharmacology for nursing care* (4th ed.). Philadelphia: Saunders.

Malarkey, L. M., & McMorrow, M. E. (2000). *Nurse's manual of laboratory tests and diagnostic procedures* (2nd ed.). Philadelphia: Saunders.

McCance, K. L., & Huether, S. E. (2002). Pathophysiology: *The biologic basis for disease in adults & children* (4th ed.). St. Louis: Mosby.

McCloskey, J. C., & Bulechek, G. M. (Eds.) (2000). *Nursing interventions classification (NIC)* (3rd ed.). St. Louis: Mosby.

Medoff, E. (2000). Oncology today: Leukemia. *RN, 63*(9), 42–49.

Mitchell, R. (1999). AJN Clinical Snapshot. Sickle cell anemia. *American Journal of Nursing, 99*(5), 36.

National Heart, Lung, and Blood Institute, National Institutes of Health. (2002). *Morbidity & mortality: 2002 chart book of cardiovascular, lung, and blood diseases.* Bethesda, MD: Author.

Navuluri, R. (2001). Understanding hemostasis. *American Journal of Nursing, 101*(9), Hospital extra: 24B, 24C.

North American Nursing Diagnosis Association. (2001). *NANDA nursing diagnoses: Definitions & classification 2001–2002.* Philadelphia: NANDA.

Persson, L., Hallberg, I. R., & Ohlsson, O. (1997). Survivors of acute leukemia and highly malignant lymphoma—retrospective views of daily life problems during treatment and when in remission. *Journal of Advanced Nursing, 25*(1), 68–78.

Porth, C. M. (2002). *Pathophysiology: Concepts of altered health states* (6th ed.). Philadelphia: Lippincott.

Spahis, J. (2002). Human genetics: Constructing a family pedigree. *American Journal of Nursing, 102*(7), 44–49.

Spatto, G. R., & Woods, A. L. (2003). *2003 edition PDR® nurse's drug handbook.* Clifton Park, NY: Delmar.

Springhouse. (1999). *Nurse's handbook of alternative & complementary therapies.* Springhouse, PA: Author.

Thompson, K. A. (1999). Adolescent health: Detecting Hodgkin's disease. *American Journal of Nursing, 99*(5), 61–64.

Tierney, L. M., McPhee, S. J., & Papadakis, M. A. (2001). *Current medical diagnosis & treatment* (40th ed.). New York: Lange Medical Books/McGraw-Hill.

U. S. Food and Drug Administration, Center for Drug Evaluation and Research. (2001). *Drug information. Gleevec (imatinib mesylate) questions and answers.* Available: www.fda.gov/cder/drug/infopage/gleevec/qa.htm

Wilkinson, J. M. (2000). *Nursing diagnosis handbook with NIC interventions and NOC outcomes* (7th ed.). Upper Saddle River, NJ: Prentice Hall Health.

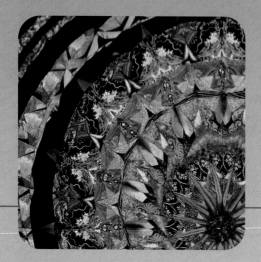

# Nursing Care of Clients with Peripheral Vascular and Lymphatic Disorders

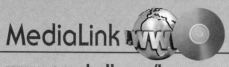

## www.prenhall.com/lemone

Additional resources for this chapter
can be found on the Student
CD-ROM accompanying this textbook,
and on the Companion Website
at www.prenhall.com/lemone. Click on
Chapter 33 to select the activities for
this chapter.

**CD-ROM**
• Audio Glossary
• NCLEX Review

*Animations*
• Lisinopril
• Warfarin

**Companion Website**
• More NCLEX Review
• Case Study
   Abdominal Aortic Aneurysm
• Care Plan Activity
   Lymphedema
• MediaLink Application
   Peripheral Vascular Disease

## LEARNING OUTCOMES

After completing this chapter, you will be able to:

▪ Relate the anatomy, physiology, and assessment of the peripheral vascular and lymphatic systems discussed in Chapter 31 to common disorders of these systems.

▪ Describe the pathophysiology of common peripheral vascular and lymphatic disorders.

▪ Identify tests used to diagnose and assess peripheral vascular and lymphatic disorders.

▪ Explain the nursing implications for medications used to treat clients with peripheral vascular and lymphatic disorders.

▪ Describe preoperative and postoperative nursing care of clients having vascular surgery.

▪ Provide client and family teaching to promote, maintain, and restore health in clients with common peripheral vascular and lymphatic disorders.

▪ Use the nursing process to plan and provide individualized care for clients with peripheral vascular and lymphatic disorders.

The major processes that interfere with peripheral blood flow and that of lymphatic fluid include constriction, obstruction, inflammation, and vasospasm. These conditions lead to disorders of blood pressure regulation, peripheral artery function, aortic structure, venous circulation, and lymphatic circulation.

A holistic approach is important when caring for clients with disorders of the peripheral vascular and lymphatic systems.

The focus of care is on teaching long-term care measures, pain relief, improving peripheral blood and lymphatic circulation, preventing tissue damage, and promoting healing. The prescribed treatment may have emotional, social, and economic effects on the client and family.

# DISORDERS OF BLOOD PRESSURE REGULATION

Blood flows through the circulatory system from areas of higher pressure to areas of lower pressure. The amount of pressure in any portion of the vascular system is affected by a number of factors, including blood volume, vascular resistance, and cardiac output. The **blood pressure** is the tension or pressure exerted by blood against arterial walls. A certain amount of pressure within the system is necessary to maintain open vessels, capillary perfusion, and oxygenation of all body tissues. Excess pressure, however, has harmful effects, increasing the workload of the heart, altering the structure of the vessels, and affecting sensitive body tissues such as the kidneys, eyes, and central nervous system.

This section focuses on **hypertension,** or excess pressure in the arterial portion of systemic circulation. Excessively low blood pressure, *hypotension,* is discussed in the shock section of Chapter 6. Altered pulmonary vascular pressures are discussed in Chapter 36. ⊕⊙

## PHYSIOLOGY REVIEW

Blood flow through the circulatory system requires *sufficient blood volume* to fill the blood vessels and *pressure differences* within the system that allow blood to move forward. The arterial, or supply side, of the circulation has relatively high pressures created by the thick elastic walls of the arteries and arterioles. The venous, or return side of the system, on the other hand, is a low pressure system of thin-walled, distensible veins. Blood flows through the capillaries linking these two systems from the higher pressure arterial side to the lower pressure venous side.

The arterial blood pressure is created by the ejection of blood from the heart during systole (*cardiac output* or *CO*) and the tension, or resistance to blood flow, created by the elastic arterial walls (*systemic vascular resistance* or *SVR*). The blood pressure rises as the heart contracts during systole, ejecting its blood. This pressure wave, or the **systolic blood pressure,** is felt as the peripheral pulse and heard as the Korotkoff's sounds during blood pressure measurement. In healthy adults the average systolic pressure is 120 mmHg. During diastole, or cardiac relaxation and filling, elastic arterial walls maintain a minimum pressure, the **diastolic blood pressure,** to maintain blood flow through the capillary beds. The average diastolic pressure in a healthy adult is 80 mmHg. The difference between the systolic and diastolic pressure, normally about 40 mmHg, is known as the **pulse pressure.** The **mean arterial pressure**

**(MAP)** is the average pressure in the arterial circulation throughout the cardiac cycle. The formula MAP = CO × SVR often is used to show the relationships between factors determining the blood pressure.

Cardiac output is determined by the blood volume and the ability of the ventricles to fill and effectively pump that blood. A number of factors contribute to systemic vascular resistance, including vessel length, blood viscosity, and vessel diameter and distensibility (compliance). While vessel length and blood viscosity remain relatively constant, vessel diameter and compliance are subject to normal regulatory activities and disease.

The arterioles normally determine the SVR as their diameter changes in response to a variety of stimuli:

- *Sympathetic nervous system (SNS)* stimulation. Baroreceptors in the aortic arch and carotid sinus signal the SNS via the cardiovascular control center in the medulla when the MAP changes. A drop in MAP stimulates the SNS, increasing the heart rate, cardiac output, and constricting arterioles (except in skeletal muscle). As a result, BP rises. A rise in MAP has the opposite effect, decreasing the heart rate and cardiac output, and causing arteriolar vasodilation.

- *Circulating epinephrine and norepinephrine* from the adrenal cortex (e.g., the fight-or-flight response) have the same effect as SNS stimulation.

- *Renin-angiotensin-aldosterone system* responds to renal perfusion. A drop in renal perfusion stimulates renin release. Renin converts angiotensinogen to angiotensin I, which is subsequently converted to angiotensin II in the lungs by angiotensin-converting enzyme (ACE). Angiotensin II is a potent vasoconstrictor. It also promotes sodium and water retention both directly and by stimulating the adrenal medulla to release aldosterone. Both SVR and CO increase, raising BP.

- *Atrial natriuretic peptide* is released from atrial cells in response to stretching by excess blood volume. It promotes vasodilation and sodium and water excretion, lowering BP.

- *Adrenomedullin* is a peptide synthesized and released by endothelial and smooth muscle cells in blood vessels. It is a potent vasodilator.

- *Vasopressin* or *antidiuretic hormone* (from the posterior pituitary gland) promotes water retention and vasoconstriction, raising BP.

- *Local factors* such as inflammatory mediators and various metabolites can promote vasodilation, affecting BP.

**Figure 33–1** ■ Factors affecting blood pressure.

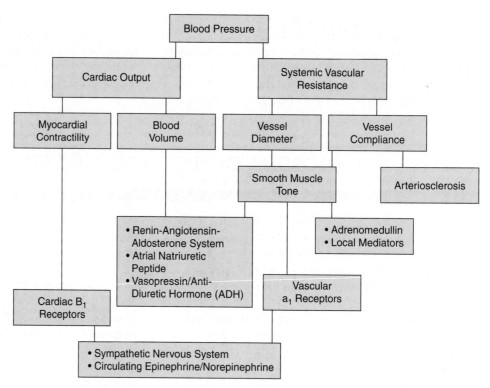

In addition to the above, the primary factor affecting vessel compliance is the extent of arteriosclerosis (hardening of the arteries) and atherosclerosis (plaque accumulation). Figure 33–1 ■ summarizes the interrelationships of major factors regulating blood pressure.

## THE CLIENT WITH PRIMARY HYPERTENSION

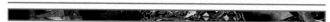

**Primary hypertension,** also known as *essential hypertension,* is a persistently elevated systemic blood pressure. About 50 million people in the United States have hypertension. More than 90% of these have primary hypertension, which has no identified cause.

Hypertension primarily affects middle-aged and older adults: 38% of people age 50 to 59 and 71% of people age 80 and older are hypertensive (National Heart, Lung, and Blood Institute [NHLBI], 2002). Hypertension is often called a "silent killer," because affected people often have no symptoms of the disease. Awareness and effective treatment of hypertension have significantly improved. Thirty years ago, only 51% of people with hypertension were aware of their condition and only 16% were effectively treated and controlled. In 1994, 88% of people with hypertension were aware of the disease, and 65% were effectively treated and controlled (NHLBI, 2002).

The prevalence of hypertension is significantly higher in blacks than in whites and Hispanics. More than 35% of black adults are hypertensive, whereas less than 25% of adult white and Hispanic people are affected. In whites and Hispanics, more males than females are hypertensive; in blacks the prevalence in men and women is nearly equal (NHLBI, 2002). Es-

sential hypertension affects people of all income groups, having great financial effects because of its effects on other body systems: cerebrovascular accident (stroke), coronary artery disease, and chronic renal failure.

Hypertension is defined as systolic blood pressure of 140 mmHg or higher, or diastolic pressure of 90 mmHg or higher, based on the average of three or more readings taken on separate occasions (NHLBI, 2002). Exceptions include clients being treated for hypertension and an initial reading of a systolic pressure of 210 mmHg or higher and/or a diastolic blood pressure of 120 mmHg or higher. Table 33–1 identifies classifications of blood pressure for adults age 18 and older as defined by the Joint National Committee.

A number of risk factors have been identified for primary hypertension (Box 33–1). Genetics play a role, as do environmental factors.

- *Family history.* Studies show a genetic link in 30% to 40% of primary hypertension (Porth, 2002). Genes involved in the renin-angiotensin-aldosterone system and others that affect vascular tone, salt and water transportation in the kidney, obesity, and insulin resistance are likely involved in the development of hypertension.
- *Age.* The incidence of hypertension rises with increasing age. Aging affects baroreceptors involved in blood pressure regulation as well as arterial compliance. As the arteries become less compliant, pressure within the vessels increases. This is often most apparent as a gradual increase in the systolic pressure with aging. Systolic hypertension increases the risk for cerebrovascular accident (stroke). See the Nursing Care of the Older Adult box on page 983.
- *Race.* Essential hypertension is more common and more severe in blacks than in people of other ethnic backgrounds.

TABLE 33–1  Classification of Blood Pressure for Adults Age 18 and Older*

| Category | Systolic (mmHg) | | Diastolic (mmHg) |
|----------|-----------------|------|-------------------|
| Optimal | <120 | and | <80 |
| Normal | <130 | and | <85 |
| High-normal | 130–139 | or | 85–89 |
| Hypertension‡ | | | |
|    Stage 1 | 140–159 | or | 90–99 |
|    Stage 2 | 160–179 | or | 100–109 |
|    Stage 3 | ≥180 | or | ≥110 |

*When systolic and diastolic blood pressures fall into different categories, the higher category is used to classify blood pressure status.
‡Based on the average of two or more readings taken at each of two or more visits after an initial screening.

Note. Adapted from The Sixth Report of the Joint National Committee on Prevention, Detection, Education, and Treatment of High Blood Pressure, NIH Publication No. 98-4080 by NHLBI, 1997, Bethesda, MD: National Institutes of Health. Available: http://www.nhlbi.nih.gov/guidelines/hypertension

---

## BOX 33–1 ■ Factors Contributing to Hypertension

### MODIFIABLE FACTORS

- High sodium intake
- Low potassium, calcium, and magnesium intake
- Obesity
- Excess alcohol consumption
- Smoking
- Glucose intolerance

### NONMODIFIABLE FACTORS

- Family history
- Age
- Race

---

This may relate to the genes controlling the renin-angiotensin-aldosterone system, although the exact mechanism for this increased risk is not yet understood.

- *Mineral intake.* High sodium intake often is associated with fluid retention. Although salt and water retention increase blood volume and cardiac output, it is not clear how salt intake contributes to the onset of hypertension or why some people are affected but others are not. Increased sodium intake does not cause hypertension, nor does the blood pressure fall with salt restriction in all hypertensive clients. Low potassium, calcium, and magnesium intakes also contribute to hypertension by unknown mechanisms. The ratio of sodium to potassium intake appears to play a role; possibly through the effects of increased potassium intake on sodium excretion. Potassium also may reduce vasoconstriction related to norepinephrine and other vasoactive substances (Porth, 2002). The link between low calcium and magnesium intakes and hypertension is unclear.
- *Obesity.* Central obesity (fat cell deposits in the abdomen), determined by an increased waist-to-hip ratio, has a stronger correlation with hypertension than body mass index or skinfold thickness. Although a clear correlation exists between obesity and hypertension, the relationship may be one of common cause: Genetic factors appear to play a role in the common triad of obesity, hypertension, and insulin resistance.
- *Insulin resistance.* Insulin resistance, with resulting hyperinsulinemia, is linked with hypertension by an unknown mechanism. Activation of the sympathetic nervous system, vascular smooth muscle growth due to excess insulin, the effect of insulin on renal regulation of sodium and water, and changes in cell membrane transport of sodium and calcium have been proposed as mechanisms in this relationship.
- *Excess alcohol consumption.* Regular consumption of three or more drinks a day increases the risk of hypertension.

---

## Nursing Care of the Older Adult

### HYPERTENSION

Controlling high blood pressure is as important in the older adult as in younger adults. In the United States, 60% of non-Hispanic whites, 61% of Mexican Americans, and 71% of African Americans age 60 and older have high blood pressure (NHLBI, 1997). Isolated systolic hypertension is common, as is an elevated pulse pressure (systolic BP minus diastolic BP), indicating decreased compliance of large arteries.

The Framingham Heart Study shows that cardiovascular deaths are 2 to 5 times more common in older adults with isolated systolic hypertension than in people with normal blood pressures. Stroke also is more common in older adults with systolic hypertension. These findings appear to relate to changes in blood vessels associated with aging: decreased compliance and decreased baroreceptor sensitivity. Decreased compliance impairs the ability of the vessels to expand and contract with varying amounts of blood, increasing peripheral vascular resistance and decreasing renal blood flow.

To obtain accurate blood pressure readings for older clients, slightly different procedures may be required. Palpation of the artery during cuff inflation is recommended to prevent inaccurate systolic readings due to an auscultatory gap, present in many older adults. The reflexes that maintain blood pressure during position changes diminish with aging. Allow the older client to sit upright or stand for 2 to 5 minutes before evaluating the blood pressure for true orthostatic readings.

Decreasing or discontinuing alcohol consumption reduces the blood pressure, particularly systolic readings. Lifestyle factors associated with excessive alcohol intake (obesity and lack of exercise) may contribute to hypertension as well.

- *Smoking.* In recent years, a relationship between serum norepinephrine levels (elevated by smoking) and hypertension has been documented. The goal of ongoing research is to clarify the long-term effects of smoking on blood pressure.
- *Stress.* Physical and emotional stress cause transient elevations of blood pressure, but the role of stress in primary hypertension is less clear. Blood pressure normally fluctuates throughout the day, increasing with activity, discomfort, or emotional responses such as anger. Frequent or continued stress may cause vascular smooth muscle hypertrophy or affect central integrative pathways of the brain (Porth, 2002).

## PATHOPHYSIOLOGY

Primary hypertension is thought to develop from a complex interaction of factors that regulate cardiac output and systemic vascular resistance. These interactions may include:

- Sympathetic nervous system overactivity with overstimulation of α- and β-adrenergic receptors, resulting in vasoconstriction and increased cardiac output.
- Renin-angiotensin-aldosterone system overactivity affects vasomotor tone and salt and water excretion. In addition, angiotensin II mediates arteriolar remodeling which permanently increases SVR.
- Other chemical mediators of vasomotor tone and blood volume such as atrial natriuretic peptide (factor) also play a role by affecting vasomotor tone and sodium and water excretion.
- The interaction between insulin resistance and endothelial function may be a primary cause of hypertension. Insulin resistance decreases the release of nitric oxide and other endogenous vasodilators, affects renal function, and increases sympathetic nervous system activity (McCance & Huether, 2002).

The result is sustained increases in blood volume and peripheral resistance. The cardiovascular system adapts to increased blood volume by increasing cardiac output. Autoregulatory mechanisms in the systemic arteries react to the increased volume, causing vasoconstriction. The increased systemic vascular resistance causes hypertension. Sustained hypertension, in turn, affects the cardiovascular system. The rate of atherosclerosis accelerates, increasing the risk for coronary heart disease and stroke. The workload of the left ventricle increases, leading to ventricular hypertrophy, which then increases the risk for coronary heart disease, dysrhythmias, and heart failure. Hypertension also can lead to nephrosclerosis and renal insufficiency (Porth, 2002).

## MANIFESTATIONS

The early stages of primary hypertension typically are asymptomatic, marked only by elevated blood pressure. Blood pressure elevations are initially transient but eventually become permanent. When symptoms do appear, they are usually vague. Headache, usually in the back of the head and neck, may be present on awakening, subsiding during the day. Other symptoms result from target organ damage, and may include nocturia, confusion, nausea and vomiting, and visual disturbances. Examination of the retina of the eye may reveal narrowed arterioles, hemorrhages, exudates, and papilledema (swelling of the optic nerve).

## COLLABORATIVE CARE

Hypertension management focuses on reducing the blood pressure to less than 140 mmHg systolic and 90 mmHg diastolic. The *Sixth Report of the Joint National Committee on Prevention, Detection, Evaluation, and Treatment of High Blood Pressure* (NHLBI, 1997) recommends a treatment plan based on cardiovascular disease risk factors, the presence or absence of target organ damage, and blood pressure levels (Table 33–2). Emphasis is placed on adherence to the treatment plan to prevent long-term consequences of hypertension (e.g., stroke, heart failure, and renal failure). Both pharmacologic and nonpharmacologic approaches are used. There is no cure for hypertension, but it can be controlled.

| TABLE 33–2 Recommended Hypertension Treatment | | | |
|---|---|---|---|
| **Stage** | **Risk Group A*** | **Risk Group B**** | **Risk Group C***** |
| High-normal (130–139/85–89) | Lifestyle modification | Lifestyle modification | Drug therapy plus lifestyle modification |
| Stage 1 (140–159/90–99) | Lifestyle modification for up to 12 months, then drug therapy | Lifestyle modification for up to 6 months, then drug therapy | Drug therapy plus lifestyle modification |
| Stages 2 and 3 (>160/>100) | Drug therapy plus lifestyle modification | Drug therapy plus lifestyle modification | Drug therapy plus lifestyle modification |

*Risk Group A: High normal blood pressure or stage 1, 2, or 3 hypertension; no clinical cardiovascular disease, target organ damage, or other risk factors

**Risk Group B: Hypertension; no clinical cardiovascular disease or target organ damage, one or more major risk factors such as smoking, hyperlipidemia, older age (>60 years), male gender or postmenopausal female, family history of cardiovascular disease

***Risk Group C: Hypertension; clinical cardiovascular disease or target organ damage; presence of diabetes with or without other risk factors

*Note. Adapted from The Sixth Report of the Joint National Committee on Prevention, Detection, Evaluation, and Treatment of High Blood Pressure NIH Publication No. 98-4080 by the NHLBI, 1997, Bethesda, MD: National Institutes of Health. Available: http://www.nhlbi.nih.gov/guidelines/hypertension*

| BOX 33–2 ■ Lifestyle Modifications for Hypertension |
| --- |
| ■ Lose weight if overweight. |
| ■ Dietary modifications. |
|   ■ Reduce sodium intake. |
|   ■ Maintain adequate dietary potassium intake. |
|   ■ Maintain adequate dietary calcium and magnesium intake. |
|   ■ Reduce intake of saturated fat and cholesterol. |
| ■ Limit alcohol intake to no more than 1 oz per day. |
| ■ Stop smoking. |
| ■ Engage in aerobic exercise for 30 to 45 minutes most days of the week. |
| ■ Use stress management techniques such as relaxation therapy. |

| BOX 33–3 ■ DASH Diet Recommendations |
| --- |
| ■ Grains—7 to 8 servings per day |
| ■ Vegetables—4 to 5 servings per day |
| ■ Fruits—4 to 5 servings per day |
| ■ Nonfat/lowfat milk—2 to 3 servings per day |
| ■ Lean meat (including fish and poultry)—2 or less servings per day |
| ■ Nuts, seeds, and dry beans—4 to 5 servings per week |
| ■ Calories—2000 per day |

## Diagnostic Tests

There are no specific diagnostic tests for essential hypertension. Diagnostic testing focuses on identifying possible causes of secondary hypertension (discussed later in this section) and determining target organ damage and other cardiovascular risk factors. Routine laboratory tests such as urinalysis, complete blood count, and blood chemistries (including electrolytes, glucose, and cholesterol levels) are done before treatment is started.

## Lifestyle Modifications

Lifestyle modifications generally are recommended for all clients with high normal blood pressure or intermittent or sustained hypertension. These modifications include weight loss, dietary changes, restricted alcohol use and cigarette smoking, increased physical activity, and stress reduction (Box 33–2).

### Diet

Dietary approaches to managing hypertension focus on reducing sodium intake, maintaining adequate potassium and calcium intakes, and reducing total and saturated fat intake. A mild to moderate sodium restriction (no added salt) lowers blood pressure and potentiates the effect of antihypertensive drugs for most hypertensive clients. The DASH (Dietary Approaches to Stop Hypertension) diet has proven beneficial effects in lowering blood pressure. This diet (Box 33–3) focuses on whole foods rather than individual nutrients. It is rich in fruits and vegetables (up to 10 servings per day), and low in total and saturated fats.

Weight loss is recommended for clients who are obese. A balanced diet such as the DASH diet is recommended for weight loss.

### Alcohol and Cigarette Use

The recommended alcohol intake for clients with hypertension is no more than 15 mL of ethanol per day. This translates to 12 oz of beer, 5 oz of wine, or 1 oz of whiskey. Women and lighter-weight people should reduce this limit by half. Although alcohol withdrawal may increase blood pressure, this is usually temporary and diminishes as abstinence or restricted intake continues.

Although nicotine is a vasoconstrictor, substantial data linking smoking to hypertension are lacking. A definitive link exists between smoking and heart disease, however. Clients who smoke are strongly urged to quit. Smoking also reduces the effect of some antihypertensive medications such as propranolol (Inderal). Smoking cessation aids such as nicotine patches and gum contain lower amounts of nicotine and usually do not raise blood pressure.

### Physical Activity

Regular exercise (such as walking, cycling, jogging, or swimming) reduces blood pressure and contributes to weight loss, stress reduction, and feelings of overall well-being. Previously sedentary clients are encouraged to engage in aerobic exercise for 30 to 45 minutes per day most days of the week. Isometric exercise (such as weight training) may not be appropriate, as it can raise the systolic blood pressure.

### Stress Reduction

Stress stimulates the sympathetic nervous system, increasing vasoconstriction, systemic vascular resistance, cardiac output, and the blood pressure. Regular, moderate exercise is the treatment of choice for reducing stress in hypertensive clients. Relaxation techniques such as biofeedback, therapeutic touch, yoga, and meditation to relax both mind and body may also lower blood pressure, although their effect has not been proven in hypertension management.

## Medications

Current pharmacologic treatment of hypertension involves using one or more of the following drug classes: diuretics, beta-adrenergic blockers, centrally acting sympatholytics, vasodilators, angiotensin-converting enzyme (ACE) inhibitors, and calcium channel blockers. These drug classes have different sites of action (Figure 33–2 ■)

Treatment usually is initiated using a single antihypertensive drug at a low dose. The dose is slowly increased until optimal blood pressure control is achieved. If the drug does not effectively lower the blood pressure or has troubling side effects, a different drug from another class of antihypertensive medications is substituted. If, on the other hand, the drug is tolerated well but has not lowered blood pressure to the desired level, a second drug from another class may be added to the treatment regimen.

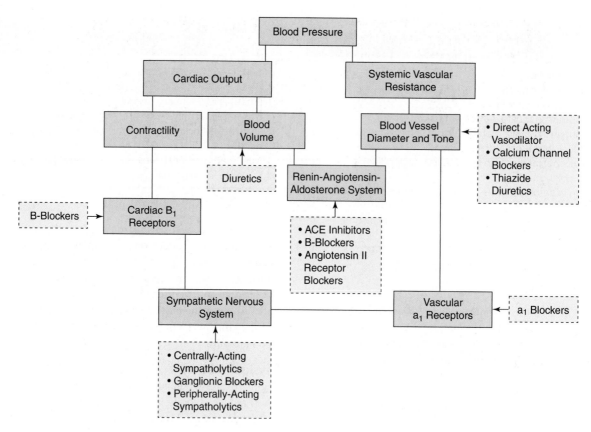

**Figure 33–2** ■ Sites of Antihypertensive Drug Action.

A diuretic or a beta blocker often is prescribed initially for uncomplicated hypertension. These drugs lower blood pressure and reduce the risk of complications such as heart failure and stroke. Diuretics are the preferred treatment for isolated systolic hypertension in older adults. ACE inhibitors also are commonly used in initial treatment of hypertension, particularly for clients who are diabetic or who have heart failure or a history of MI.

Other factors considered in selecting drugs for treating hypertension include demographic characteristics of the client, concurrent conditions, quality of life, cost, and possible interactions among prescribed drugs. In general, diuretics and calcium channel blockers are more effective for treating hypertension in blacks than beta blockers or ACE inhibitors. Beta blockers are preferred to treat hypertension with concurrent coronary heart disease and angina, but are contraindicated for clients who have asthma or depression. Beta blockers also reduce exercise tolerance and may adversely affect lifestyle for some clients. Nursing implications for administration of antihypertensive drugs (other than diuretics) are outlined on pages 987–988.

Thiazide diuretics, such as hydrochlorothiazide (Hydro-DIURIL), are widely used to control hypertension. In major clinical studies, single therapy with diuretics controlled blood pressure in about 50% of the clients and reduced hypertension-linked morbidity and mortality related to coronary heart disease. Diuretics control hypertension primarily by preventing tubular reabsorption of sodium, thus promoting sodium and water excretion and reducing blood volume. Thiazide diuretics

also reduce systemic vascular resistance through an unknown mechanism. Diuretics are particularly effective in blacks and in clients who are obese, older, or who have increased plasma volume or low renin activity. The adverse effects of diuretics generally are dose related. In addition to hypokalemia, diuretics may affect serum levels of glucose, triglycerides, uric acid, low-density lipoproteins, and insulin. More information about diuretics can be found in Chapters 5 and 27. ☜

Treatment of clients in risk group C generally is more aggressive to minimize the risk of MI, heart failure, or stroke. When the average blood pressure is greater than 200/120, immediate therapy, and possible hospitalization, is vital.

After a year of effective hypertension control, an effort may be made to reduce the dosage and number of drugs. This is known as step-down therapy. It is more successful in clients who have made lifestyle modifications. Careful blood pressure monitoring is necessary during and after step-down therapy, as the blood pressure often rises again to hypertensive levels.

## NURSING CARE

### Health Promotion

Health promotion teaching and activities focus on the modifiable risk factors for hypertension. Advise all clients (as well as children and adolescents) to stop or never start smoking. Discuss the risks of obesity, excess alcohol intake, and a sedentary

# Medication Administration

## Antihypertensive Drugs

### ALPHA-ADRENERGIC BLOCKERS

Doxazosin (Cardura)
Prazosin (Minipress)
Terazosin (Hytrin)

Alpha-adrenergic blocking agents block alpha receptors in vascular smooth muscle, decreasing vasomotor tone and vasoconstriction. They also reduce serum levels of low-density (LDL) and very low-density lipoproteins (VLDL). However, vasodilation may cause orthostatic hypotension and reflex stimulation of the heart, resulting in tachycardia and palpitations. A beta blocker may be ordered to minimize this effect.

#### Nursing Responsibilities
- Give the first dose at bedtime to minimize risk of fainting (called "first-dose syncope"). If the first dose is given in the daytime (or if the dose is increased), instruct to remain in bed for 3 to 4 hours.
- Assess blood pressure and apical pulse before each dose and as indicated thereafter.

#### Client and Family Teaching
- There is a risk of fainting after taking the first dose of this drug. Take the drug at bedtime to reduce this risk, and do not drive or engage in other hazardous activities for 12 to 24 hours after the first dose.
- This drug may cause dizziness or lightheadedness. Change positions slowly, and sit down if you become dizzy or lightheaded.
- Notify your primary care provider if you develop nasal congestion or impotence while taking this drug.
- Notify your primary care provider before discontinuing this medication.

### ANGIOTENSIN-CONVERTING ENZYME (ACE) INHIBITORS

Benazepril (Lotensin)
Captopril (Capoten)
Enalapril (Vasotec)
Fosinopril (Monopril)
Lisinopril (Zestril)

Moexipril (Univasc)
Perindopril (Aceon)
Quinapril (Accupril)
Ramipril (Altace)
Trandolapril (Mavik)

### Angiotensin II Receptor Blockers

Eprosartan (Teveten)
Irbersartan (Avapro)
Candesartan (Atacand)

Losartan (Cozaar)
Valsartan (Diovan)

The ACE inhibitors lower blood pressure by preventing conversion of angiotensin I to angiotensin II. This in turn prevents vasoconstriction and sodium and water retention. Angiotensin II receptor blockers (ARBs) have the same effect, but they act by blocking the effect of angiotensin II on receptors. Both ACE inhibitors and ARBs are less effective in black clients and are contraindicated in pregnancy (Lehne, 2001). Their primary adverse effects are persistent cough, first-dose hypotension, and hyperkalemia.

#### Nursing Responsibilities
- Assess blood pressure and WBC before giving the first dose. Monitor blood pressure for 2 hours after the first dose and regularly thereafter.
- Administer PO 1 hour before meals; tablets may be crushed.

- Report changes in WBC or differential, hyperkalemia, or changes in BUN or serum creatinine to the primary care provider.
- Do not administer to clients with renal artery stenosis or who are pregnant.
- Immediately report and treat manifestations of angioedema (giant wheals and edema of the tongue, glottis, and pharynx). Initiate resuscitation measures as needed. Discontinue drug immediately and do not use in the future.

#### Client and Family Teaching
- Report peripheral edema, signs of infection, or difficulty breathing to your primary care provider.
- Change position (lying to sitting and sitting to standing) slowly to prevent dizziness; sit down if dizziness or lightheadedness develops.
- Do not take a potassium supplement or use a potassium-based salt substitute while taking this drug unless prescribed by your physician.
- Notify your physician if you become pregnant while taking this drug. Although it is safe early in pregnancy, taking the drug during the second and third trimesters may harm the fetus.

### BETA-ADRENERGIC BLOCKING AGENTS

Acebutolol (Sectral)
Atenolol (Tenormin)
Betaxolol (Kerlone)
Bisoprolol (Zebeta)
Carteolol (Cartrol)
Metoprolol tartrate (Lopressor)

Nadolol (Corgard)
Penbutolol (Levatol)
Pindolol (Visken)
Propranolol (Inderal)
Timolol (Blocadren)

Beta-adrenergic blockers are commonly used to control hypertension. Beta blockers reduce blood pressure by preventing beta-receptor stimulation in the heart, thereby decreasing heart rate and cardiac output. Beta blockers also interfere with renin release by the kidneys, decreasing the effects of angiotensin and aldosterone. Potential adverse effects of beta blockers include bronchospasm, fatigue, sleep disturbances, nightmares, bradycardia, heart block, worsening of heart failure, gastrointestinal disturbances, impotence, and increased triglyceride levels.

#### Nursing Responsibilities
- Before giving initial dose, assess for contraindications to beta blockers such as asthma, chronic lung disease, bradycardia, or heart block.
- Assess blood pressure and apical pulse before giving; notify primary care provider if vital signs are outside established parameters.
- Report adverse effects such as bradycardia, decreased cardiac output (fatigue, dyspnea with exertion, hypotension, decreased level of consciousness), heart failure, heart block, bronchoconstriction (wheezing, dyspnea), or altered blood glucose levels (in diabetic clients).
- Carefully monitor responses of the older client.

#### Client and Family Teaching
- Monitor blood pressure and pulse daily as instructed.
- Change position (lying to sitting and sitting to standing) slowly to prevent dizziness and possible falls.
- Report effects such as fatigue, lethargy, and impotence to your primary care provider.

(continued on page 988)

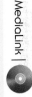

MediaLink | LISINOPRIL ANIMATION

# Medication Administration

## Antihypertensive Drugs (continued)

- Notify your physician if you become short of breath or develop a cough or swelling of your extremities.
- If you have diabetes, check blood glucose levels more frequently as hypoglycemia may develop with few symptoms.
- Talk to your primary care provider before taking any over-the-counter medications.
- Carry an adequate supply of the drug when traveling. Do not stop taking this drug without notifying your primary care provider.

### CALCIUM CHANNEL BLOCKERS

Amlodipine (Norvasc)
Diltiazem (Cardizem)
Felodipine (Plendil)
Isradipine (DynaCirc)
Nicardipine (Cardene)

Nifedipine (Procardia)
Nimodipine (Nimotop)
Nisoldipine (Sular)
Verapamil (Isoptin)

Calcium channel blockers inhibit the flow of calcium ions across the cell membrane of vascular tissue and cardiac cells. In doing so, they relax arterial smooth muscle, lowering peripheral resistance through vasodilation. Calcium channel blockers can cause reflex tachycardia, and some (e.g., verapamil and diltiazem) may impair cardiac function, worsening heart failure.

### Nursing Responsibilities

- Assess blood pressure, apical pulse, and liver and renal function tests prior to giving these drugs.
- Calcium channel blockers may be given orally or intravenously.
- Do not administer verapamil or diltiazem to clients with severe hypotension, sinus, or atrioventricular blocks. Administer with caution to clients also taking digoxin or a beta blocker.
- Periodically monitor blood pressure and apical pulse during therapy. Promptly report signs of bradycardia, AV block, or heart failure to the physician.

### Client and Family Teaching

- Take blood pressure and pulse daily as taught. Notify your physician if your pulse is less than 60 BPM or your blood pressure is not within the specified range.
- This drug may cause constipation. Drink six to eight glasses of water each day, and increase fiber in diet.
- Report shortness of breath, weight gain, or swelling in feet or ankles to your primary care provider.

### CENTRALLY ACTING SYMPATHOLYTICS

Clonidine (Catapres)
Guanabenz (Wytensin)

Guanfacine (Tenex)
Methyldopa (Aldomet)

The centrally acting sympatholytics stimulate the $\alpha_2$ receptors in the CNS to suppress sympathetic outflow to the heart and blood vessels. A fall in cardiac output and vasodilation result, reducing blood pressure. Dry mouth and sedation are common adverse effects. Severe reflex hypertension may occur if abruptly discontinued. Clonidine is contraindicated during pregnancy; methyldopa is contraindicated for clients with active liver disease.

### Nursing Responsibilities

- Assess for contraindications to therapy. Obtain baseline blood pressure, CBC, Coomb's test, and liver function studies.
- Administer oral doses at bedtime to minimize effects of sedation.

- Methyldopa may be given intravenously for hypertensive emergencies.
- Apply transdermal clonidine patch to dry, hairless area of intact skin on the chest or upper arm. Assess for rash, which indicates allergy, at area of application.
- Promptly report changes in laboratory values to the physician. Discontinue methyldopa if manifestations of liver dysfunction develop.

### Client and Family Teaching

- Relieve dry mouth by sipping water or chewing sugarless gum.
- Take with meals if gastric upset or nausea develop.
- Change position (lying to sitting and sitting to standing) slowly to prevent dizziness and possible falls.
- Do not suddenly discontinue medication or skip doses; this could cause serious hypertension.
- Report mental depression or decreased mental acuity to your health care provider.
- Side effects (such as dry mouth, nausea, and dizziness) tend to diminish over time.
- Do not drive a car if the medications cause drowsiness.

### VASODILATORS

Hydralazine (Apresoline)
Minoxidil (Loniten)

Vasodilators reduce blood pressure by relaxing vascular smooth muscle (especially in the arterioles), and decreasing peripheral vascular resistance. These drugs are often prescribed in combination with a diuretic or beta blocker, because they can cause reflex tachycardia and fluid retention. Because these drugs can have significant toxic effects, they are not routinely used to manage chronic hypertension.

### Nursing Responsibilities

- Hydralazine may be given orally or intravenously; minoxidil is given orally.
- Assess blood pressure and pulse before giving the drug and monitor during therapy as indicated. Report tachycardia or hypotension to the physician.
- Report peripheral edema and manifestations of volume overload and heart failure.
- Immediately report muffled heart sounds or paradoxical pulse as pericardial effusion and possible cardiac tamponade may develop during minoxidil therapy.
- Discontinue hydralazine and report manifestations of a SLE-like syndrome: muscle or joint pain, fever, or symptoms of nephritis or pericarditis.

### Client and Family Teaching

- Change position (lying to sitting and sitting to standing) slowly to prevent dizziness and possible falls.
- Report muscle, joint aches, and fever to your health care provider.
- Headache, palpitations, and rapid pulse may develop but should abate in about 10 days.
- Do not discontinue the medication without talking to your health care provider.
- Minoxidil may cause excessive hair growth. Contact your physician if this becomes troublesome.

## TABLE 33-3  Recommended Blood Pressure Follow-Up

| Category | Blood Pressure (mm Hg) | Recommended Follow-Up |
|---|---|---|
| Optimal | <120/80 | Recheck in 2 years |
| Normal | <130/85 | Recheck in 2 years |
| High-normal | 130–139/85–89 | Recheck in 1 year |
| Stage 1 hypertension | 140–159/90–99 | Confirm within 2 months |
| Stage 2 hypertension | 160–179/100–109 | Evaluate or refer to care provider within 1 month |
| Stage 3 hypertension | ≥180/≥110 | Evaluate or refer to care provider immediately or within 1 week as indicated |

*Note. Adapted from The Sixth Report of the Joint National Committee on Prevention, Detection, Education, and Treatment of High Blood Pressure, NIH Publication No. 98-4080, by NHLBI, 1997, Bethesda, MD: National Institutes of Health. Available: http://www.nhlbi.nih.gov/guidelines/hypertension*

lifestyle with clients. Encourage all clients to eat a diet rich in fruits and vegetables and low in total and saturated fat. Discuss the potential benefits of maintaining an adequate calcium and potassium intake and provide lists of foods containing these nutrients. Advise all clients to remain active and engage in aerobic exercise 4 or more days a week. Discuss the stress-reducing benefits of exercise.

Offer blood pressure screening, and refer clients for follow-up as indicated (Table 33–3).

## Assessment

Focused assessment of the client with hypertension includes:

- Health history: complaints of morning headache, cervical pain; cardiovascular or central nervous system manifestations; history of hypertension, renal disease, diabetes; family history of high blood pressure, heart failure, or kidney disease; current medications
- Physical examination: vital signs including blood pressure in both arms, apical and peripheral pulses; ophthalmologic exam of retinal fundus

## Nursing Diagnoses and Interventions

All clients with primary hypertension and their families need significant teaching to manage this chronic condition. Health maintenance is a high-priority problem. Depending on the stage of hypertension and concurrent illnesses, other appropriate nursing diagnoses may include imbalanced nutrition, fluid volume excess, and risk for noncompliance.

### Ineffective Health Maintenance

Unhealthy lifestyle and behaviors can lead to health problems such as hypertension. When hypertension has been identified, knowledge of the disease and its management is vital for the client. Willingness to take responsibility for hypertension management is central to effective blood pressure control. Adopting healthy lifestyle changes enhances drug therapy; in some cases, the need for medications may be eliminated or reduced. Because hypertension is often an asymptomatic disease and many antihypertensive drugs have unpleasant side effects, it is vital that the client understand the chronic progressive nature of the disease and its long-term consequences.

- Assist with identifying current behaviors that contribute to hypertension. *The client must first identify contributory behaviors before he or she can change them. Using knowledge of hypertension risk factors, the nurse can help identify behaviors and factors contributing to hypertension that can be changed. Including the family in this process is important to reduce potential sabotage of the client's efforts to adopt healthier behaviors.*
- Assist in developing a realistic health maintenance plan. *Preparing a health maintenance plan for the client does little to encourage personal responsibility for health. However, nurses can guide clients in developing realistic goals and expectations for the treatment plan and modifying risk factors such as smoking, exercise, diet, and stress.*
- Help the client and family identify strengths and weaknesses in maintaining health. *Discussing areas of the health maintenance plan that are working well and those that present difficulties can help to identify necessary changes in the plan and additional strategies for implementing it.*

### Risk for Noncompliance

Noncompliance, or failure to follow the identified treatment plan, is a continuing risk for any client with a chronic disease. Recommended lifestyle changes such as diet, exercise, restricted alcohol intake, stress reduction, and smoking cessation often are difficult to maintain on a continuing basis. In addition, prescribed medications may have undesirable effects whereas hypertension itself often has no symptoms or noticeable effects.

- Inquire about reasons for noncompliance with recommended treatment plan. Listen openly and without judging. *Nonthreatening discussion of factors contributing to noncompliance validates the client's self-esteem and partnership in the treatment plan.*

**PRACTICE ALERT** *Work with the client to develop mutual outcomes for the treatment plan. Discuss measures to improve compliance. The client has absolute control over compliance with the treatment plan. Demonstrating respect and involving the client in decision making and planning can improve compliance.* ∎

- Evaluate knowledge of hypertension, its long-term effects, and treatment. Provide additional information and reinforce teaching as needed. *Knowledge increases the sense of control, which also increases the likelihood of compliance with treatment.*

**PRACTICE ALERT** *Assess factors contributing to noncompliance, such as adverse drug effects. Suggest measures to manage adverse effects or, if indicated, contact the primary care provider about possible alternative drugs. Some adverse effects of antihypertensive drugs, such as gastric upset, lightheadedness, or nocturia may be easily managed by changing the timing of the drug dose. Others, such as fatigue, decreased exercise tolerance, or impotence may interfere with lifestyle and life roles to the extent that the client finds them intolerable.* ■

- Assist to develop realistic short-term goals for lifestyle changes. *Attempting to lose weight, exercise daily, stop smoking, and dramatically change the diet all at the same time may be overwhelming, leading to a sense of failure. Smaller, gradual changes are more easily incorporated into lifestyle and daily activities, improving compliance.*
- Help the client identify cues and develop reminders (e.g., written notes, a medication box filled weekly) to assist with maintaining a schedule for exercise and medications. *Cues and other devices provide helpful reminders of activities and schedules until they are incorporated into habits.*
- Reassure the client that relapse into old habits and behaviors is common. Encourage avoiding feelings of guilt associated with relapse, and use the circumstance to renew efforts to comply with treatment. *Guilt and feelings of failure can lead to further noncompliance unless the event is used to identify reasons for noncompliance and ways to prevent it from recurring in the future.*

## Imbalanced Nutrition:
## More Than Body Requirements

The relationship between obesity, excess alcohol intake, and hypertension is well documented. Hypertension is particularly associated with central obesity, identified by waist circumference greater than hip circumference. While weight loss is difficult and takes commitment to changing eating and exercise habits, it is possible for most clients to achieve.

- Assess usual daily food intake, and discuss possible contributing factors to excess weight, such as sedentary lifestyle, or using food as a reward or stress reliever. Inquire about diversional activities, exercise patterns, and previous weight reduction efforts (e.g., participation in weight reduction programs or using fad or crash diets). *Assessment data provides clues about contributing factors to obesity, the client's knowledge base about the relationship between eating and exercise habits and weight, and safe weight loss strategies. This provides direction for further teaching and for developing a realistic weight reduction plan.*
- Mutually determine with the client a realistic target weight (e.g., loss of 10% of current body weight over a 6-month period). Regularly monitor weight. Encourage a system of

nonfood rewards for achieving small, incremental goals. *Setting weight loss goals helps formalize the process and provides motivation for continued progress. Developing realistic goals may be difficult; unrealistic goals, however, set the client up for failure. Continuous incremental weight loss provides reassurance that it can be achieved and promotes permanent weight reduction.*

- Refer to a dietitian for information about low-fat, low-calorie foods and eating plans. Focus on changing eating habits as opposed to "following a diet." *Focusing on changing eating habits promotes the sense that low-fat, low-calorie eating patterns should become a part of lifestyle rather than a short-term measure to be endured until the weight loss goal is achieved.*
- Recommend participating in an approved weight loss program such as Weight Watchers, Overeaters Anonymous, or Take off Pounds Sensibly (TOPS). *Organized weight loss programs provide structure for a balanced weight reduction program, as well as mutual support from others trying to lose weight.*

## Excess Fluid Volume

Excess fluid volume often contributes to hypertension by increasing the cardiac output. A number of factors associated with hypertension can cause excess fluid volume, including sodium retention and disruption of the renin-angiotensin-aldosterone system. In addition, some antihypertensive drugs, such as calcium channel blockers and vasodilators, can contribute to excess fluid in the interstitial spaces and peripheral edema.

**PRACTICE ALERT** *Monitor blood pressure and other vital signs as indicated: every 1 to 2 hours or more frequently during acute hypertensive states; once a week or more frequently during initial treatment in the community. Vital signs are an indicator of fluid balance and the effectiveness of treatment. An elevated blood pressure, pulse, and respiratory rate may indicate fluid retention, whereas orthostatic hypotension and tachycardia may indicate fluid volume deficit.* ■

- Monitor intake and output, and weigh daily (if in an acute or long-term care facility) or weekly (in the community). *Rapid weight changes (over days) more accurately reflect fluid balance than intake and output records. One liter of fluid weighs 1 kg (2.2 lb). Weight changes and intake and output records help monitor the effects of therapy.*
- Monitor for peripheral edema (sacral edema in the bedridden client). *Drugs such as vasodilators can cause fluid accumulation in interstitial tissues, leading to peripheral or dependent edema. Adding a diuretic to the treatment plan may be necessary.*

**PRACTICE ALERT** *Monitor laboratory values, such as blood urea nitrogen (BUN), urine specific gravity, creatinine, electrolytes, and hematocrit and hemoglobin. Hypertension can alter renal perfusion and function, leading to fluid retention and altered laboratory values. Changes in BUN and creatinine indicate impaired renal function, whereas changes in hematocrit and hemoglobin often reflect changes in fluid volume.* ■

- Refer to a dietitian for teaching about a restricted sodium diet. Discuss the relationship between sodium intake and fluid retention. Provide opportunities to choose low-sodium foods from simulated menus. Support efforts, and reassure that lifestyle changes such as consuming less sodium take time. *Knowledge provides the power to take control of sodium intake. Patience and perseverance are needed to succeed; positive reinforcement of efforts to change long-standing dietary patterns is important.*

- Discuss the importance of adhering to treatment plans such as dietary restrictions and medication schedules. *Understanding the rationale for treatment measures promotes the client's sense of control and encourages compliance with the treatment regimen.*

## Using NANDA, NIC, and NOC

Chart 33–1 shows links between NANDA nursing diagnoses, NIC, and NOC for the client with hypertension.

## Home Care

Effective control of hypertension requires the client to not only participate in the plan of care, but also to take an active role in managing the disease. Treatment is managed in community settings, with regular visits to a clinic or office to monitor blood pressure and effects of treatment measures. Include the following topics when teaching the client and family about hypertension:

- Specific lifestyle changes recommended for the client and suggestions for implementing them. For example:
  - Increase activity gradually. Develop a realistic exercise program that is enjoyable and fits into lifestyle. Identify an exercise buddy for additional motivation. Activity and exercise, through a gradual conditioning of muscles and blood vessels, lower blood pressure by reducing peripheral vascular resistance. As the heart becomes conditioned and pumps more efficiently, kidney perfusion improves and intravascular volume falls, further reducing blood pressure.

Exercise also reduces stress and contributes to weight loss and maintenance. Aerobic exercise, such as walking, jogging, swimming, and cycling are appropriate; isometric activities (such as weight lifting) should be avoided without physician approval.

- Adopt healthy eating patterns, following a low-fat, low-cholesterol, moderate sodium diet that also is rich in fruits and vegetables and includes at least two servings of low-fat milk or milk products daily. Do not give up if you slip into old eating habits on occasion; use such occasions to identify ways to avoid future lapses.

- Stop smoking. Participating in organized smoking cessation programs or using aids such as nicotine patches can help.

- Use alcohol in moderation if at all, consuming no more than 1 oz of hard liquor, 5 oz of wine, or 12 oz of beer per day.

- Use stress-reducing techniques such as meditation, relaxation, deep breathing, and exercise to manage stress. Anger and hostility intensify vasoconstriction; channeling these emotions into more positive responses such as using a change process to modify factors that provoke these emotions can reduce their harmful effects on blood pressure.

- Prescribed medications, their intended effect, dose and timing, interactions, and possible adverse effects. Discuss effects that should be reported to the physician, and those that can be managed by the client or that will diminish over time.

- The importance of monitoring blood pressure and regular visits to the primary care provider or hypertension clinic to monitor treatment. During follow-up visits, assess the blood pressure and specific laboratory work (such as serum creatinine, BUN, and/or serum electrolytes) to evaluate the disease and the effects of antihypertensive medications.

Refer the client to community blood pressure clinics, and to home health services as needed for regular follow-up and reinforcement of teaching. Refer to a dietitian or to an organized weight loss program as indicated for further teaching and weight loss support.

## CHART 33–1  NANDA, NIC, AND NOC LINKAGES

### The Client with Hypertension

| NURSING DIAGNOSES | NURSING INTERVENTIONS | NURSING OUTCOMES |
|---|---|---|
| • Decisional Conflict | • Mutual Goal Setting<br>• Decision-Making Support | • Decision Making<br>• Information Processing |
| • Imbalanced Nutrition: More than Body Requirements | • Teaching: Prescribed Diet<br>• Weight Reduction Assistance | • Nutritional Status: Nutrient Intake<br>• Weight Control |
| • Ineffective Health Maintenance | • Self-Modification Assistance<br>• Self-Responsibility Facilitation | • Health-Promoting Behavior<br>• Treatment Behavior: Illness or Injury |
| • Noncompliance | • Health Education | • Adherence Behavior |

*Note. Data from Nursing Outcomes Classification (NOC) by M. Johnson & M. Maas (Eds.), 1997, St. Louis: Mosby; Nursing Diagnoses: Definitions & Classification 2001–2002 by North American Nursing Diagnosis Association, 2001, Philadelphia: NANDA; Nursing Interventions Classification (NIC) by J.C. McCloskey & G. M. Bulechek (Eds.), 2000, St. Louis: Mosby. Reprinted by permission.*

## Nursing Care Plan

# A Client with Hypertension

Margaret Spezia is a married, 49-year-old Italian American with eight children whose ages range from 3 to 18 years. For the past 2 months, Mrs. Spezia has had frequent morning headaches, and occasional dizziness and blurred vision. At her annual physical examination 1 month ago, her blood pressure was 168/104 and 156/94. She was instructed to reduce her fat and cholesterol intake, to avoid using salt at the table, and to start walking for 30 to 45 minutes daily. Mrs. Spezia returns to the clinic for follow-up.

### ASSESSMENT

While escorting Mrs. Spezia to the exam room and obtaining her weight, blood pressure, and history, Lisa Christos, RN, notices that Mrs. Spezia seems restless and upset. Ms. Christos says, "You look upset about something. Is everything OK?" Mrs. Spezia responds, "Well, my head is throbbing, and I'm sort of dizzy. I think I'm just overdoing it and not getting enough rest. You know, raising eight children is a lot of work and expense. I just started working part time so we wouldn't get behind in our bills. I thought the extra money might relieve some of my stress, but I'm not so sure that's really happening. I'm not getting any better and I'm worried that I'll lose my job or become disabled and that my husband won't be able to manage the children by himself. I really need to go home, but first, I want to get rid of this awful headache. Would you please get me a couple of aspirin or something?"

Mrs. Spezia's history shows a steady weight gain over the past 18 years. She has no known family history of hypertension. Physical findings include height 63 inches (160 cm), weight 225 lb (102 kg), T 99°F (37.2°C), P 100 regular, R 16, BP 180/115 (lying), 170/110 (sitting), 165/105 (standing), average 10-point difference in readings between right and left arm (lower on left). Skin cool and dry, capillary refill 4 seconds right hand, 3 seconds left hand. Mrs. Spezia's total serum cholesterol is 245 mg/dL (normal < 200 mg/dL). All other blood and urine studies are within normal limits. Based on analysis of the data, Mrs. Spezia is started on enalapril 5 mg and hydrochlorothiazide 12.5 mg in a combination drug (Vaseretic), and placed on a low-fat low-cholesterol, no-added-salt diet.

### DIAGNOSIS

- *Fatigue* related to effects of hypertension and stresses of daily life
- *Imbalanced nutrition: More than body requirements* related to excessive food intake
- *Ineffective health maintenance* related to inability to modify lifestyle
- *Deficient knowledge* related to effects of prescribed treatment

### EXPECTED OUTCOMES

- Reduce blood pressure readings to less than 150 systolic and 90 diastolic by return visit next week.

- Incorporate low-sodium and low-fat foods from a list provided into her diet.
- Develop a plan for regular exercise.
- Verbalize understanding of the effects of prescribed drug, dietary restrictions, exercise, and follow-up visits to help control hypertension.

### PLANNING AND IMPLEMENTATION

- Teach to take own blood pressure daily and record it, bringing the record to scheduled clinic visits.
- Teach name, dose, action, and side effects of her antihypertensive medication.
- Instruct to walk for 15 minutes each day this week, and to investigate swimming classes at the local pool.
- Discuss strategies for achieving a realistic weight loss goal.
- Refer for a dietary consultation for further teaching about fat and sodium restrictions.
- Discuss stress-reducing techniques, helping identify possible choices.

### EVALUATION

Mrs. Spezia returns to the clinic 1 week later. Her average blood pressure is now 148/88 mmHg. She has lost 1.5 lb, and states that her oldest daughter has suggested that they join a weight reduction program together. Mrs. Spezia is walking for an average of 20 minutes at a local mall each day. She verbalizes an understanding of her medication, and is taking it in the morning and before dinner each day. She met with the dietitian and discussed ways to reduce the sodium and fat in her diet. The dietitian provided a list of low-fat, low-sodium foods and recommended cookbooks to help Mrs. Spezia modify her cooking. Mrs. Spezia tells Ms. Christos, "I just can't believe how much better I feel already. My headaches are gone, and I've actually lost some weight—and I feel motivated to keep going. If I had only known how much better I could feel! I don't expect I'll ever go back to my old habits again; it's just not worth it!"

### Critical Thinking in the Nursing Process

1. Identify the factors that contributed to Mrs. Spezia's hypertension. Which were modifiable and which were not?
2. What is the rationale for reducing sodium and fat in Mrs. Spezia's diet?
3. Suppose your hypertensive client is homeless and has no source of income. How could you help ensure your client would follow the treatment plan? What would you do if the client did not follow it?
4. Discuss the role of stress in hypertension. What factors in Mrs. Spezia's life contribute to her stress level?
5. Develop a plan of care for the diagnosis, *Low self-esteem* related to obesity.

See Evaluating Your Response in Appendix C.

# THE CLIENT WITH SECONDARY HYPERTENSION

**Secondary hypertension** is elevated blood pressure resulting from an identifiable underlying process. It accounts for only 5% to 10% of identified cases of hypertension. Kidney disease and coarctation of the aorta are common causes of secondary hypertension. In older adults, renovascular disease is the most common cause of sudden hypertension. The pathophysiology of selected causes of secondary hypertension are summarized below.

- *Kidney disease.* Any disease that affects renal blood flow (e.g., renal artery stenosis) or renal function (e.g., glomerulonephritis, renal failure) can lead to hypertension. Disruption of the blood supply stimulates the renin-angiotensin-aldosterone system, with resulting vasoconstriction and sodium and water retention. Altered kidney function affects the elimination of water and electrolytes, leading to hypertension.
- *Coarctation of the aorta.* Coarctation of the aorta is narrowing of the aorta, usually just distal to the subclavian arteries. Reduced renal and peripheral blood flow stimulates the renin-angiotensin-aldosterone system and local vasocontrictive responses, raising the blood pressure. A marked difference between pressures in the upper and lower extremities is common, with weak pulses and poor capillary refill in the lower extremities.
- *Endocrine disorders.* Adrenal gland disorders such as Cushing's syndrome and primary aldosteronism can cause hypertension. A rare tumor of the adrenal medulla, *pheochromocytoma,* causes persistent or intermittent hypertension. Other endocrine disorders such as hyperthyroidism and pituitary disorders also can lead to hypertension.
- *Neurologic disorders.* Increased intracranial pressure causes an elevated blood pressure as the body attempts to maintain cerebral blood flow. Disorders that interfere with autonomic nervous system regulation (such as high spinal cord injury) may allow the sympathetic nervous system to predominate, increasing systemic vascular resistance and blood pressure.
- *Drug use.* Estrogen and oral contraceptive use may lead to hypertension, possibly by prompting sodium and water retention and affecting the renin-angiotensin-aldosterone system. Stimulant drugs, such as cocaine and methamphetamines, increase systemic vascular resistance and cardiac output, resulting in hypertension.
- *Pregnancy.* About 10% of all pregnant women are hypertensive. Hypertension may predate pregnancy or occur as a direct response to the pregnancy. The mechanism of pregnancy-induced hypertension (PIH) is unclear. It is a significant cause of maternal and fetal morbidity and mortality and requires careful perinatal management.

The pattern of secondary hypertension varies, depending on its cause. Pheochromocytoma may cause attacks of hypertension that last for minutes to hours, accompanied by anxiety, palpitations, diaphoresis, pallor, and nausea and vomiting. Primary aldosteronism may cause hypertension, weakness, paresthesias, polyuria, and nocturia (see Chapter 17). ⊂⊃ Symptoms of kidney disease accompany hypertension when a renal disorder is the cause.

The following diagnostic tests may be ordered to differentiate primary from secondary hypertension.

- *Renal function studies* and *urinalysis* to identify renal causes of hypertension. Elevated serum creatinine and BUN, reduced creatinine clearance, and hematuria, proteinuria, and casts often indicate kidney disease.
- *Serum potassium* is decreased in hyperaldosteronism.
- *Blood chemistries,* including serum electrolytes, glucose, and lipid studies are done to detect abnormalities indicative of endocrine or cardiovascular disease.
- *Intravenous pyelography (IVP), renal ultrasonography, renal arteriography,* and *CT* or *MRI* may be done when secondary hypertension is suspected.

Collaborative and nursing care for the client with secondary hypertension is the same as that for primary hypertension, discussed in the previous section. In addition, the underlying process is treated. See chapters covering specific disorders for more information about treatment measures.

# THE CLIENT WITH HYPERTENSIVE CRISIS

Some clients with hypertension may, for reasons not clearly understood, develop rapid, significant elevations in systolic and/or diastolic pressures. In a *hypertensive emergency,* the systolic pressure may be greater than 240 mmHg and the diastolic pressure higher than 130 mmHg. Immediate treatment (within 1 hour) is vital to prevent cardiac, renal, and vascular damage, and reduce morbidity and mortality. Most hypertensive emergencies occur when clients suddenly stop taking their medications or their hypertension is poorly controlled. Manifestations of hypertensive emergencies are listed in the box below.

**Malignant hypertension** is a hypertensive emergency, marked by a diastolic pressure greater than 120 mmHg. It most commonly affects younger clients (30 to 50 years old), African American men, pregnant women with toxemia, and people with collagen and/or renal disease (Porth, 2002). Malignant hypertension must be rapidly diagnosed and aggressively (yet carefully) treated to prevent encephalopathy and irreversible renal and cardiac failure (Tierney et al., 2001). Intense cerebral artery spasms help protect the brain from excess pressure; however, cerebral edema often develops. It may cause manifestations such as headache, confusion, swelling of the optic nerve

## Manifestations of Hypertensive Emergencies

- Rapid onset
- Blurred vision, papilledema
- Systolic pressure >240 mmHg
- Diastolic pressure >130 mmHg
- Headache
- Confusion
- Motor and sensory deficits

| TABLE 33–4 | Intravenous Drugs Used to Treat Hypertensive Emergencies | | | |
|---|---|---|---|---|
| Type | Name | Onset | Duration | Nursing Tips |
| Vasodilator | Nipride | seconds | 3 to 5 min | • Most effective drug<br>• Easy to titrate |
| Vasodilator | Nitroglycerin | 2 to 5 min | 3 to 5 min | • Tolerances may develop |
| Vasodilator | Diazoxide (Hyperstat) | 1 to 2 min | 4 to 24 hr | • Avoided in clients with coronary artery disease<br>• Used with beta-blockers and diuretics<br>• Painful if it enters tissues |
| Vasodilator | Fenoldopam (Corlopam) | <5 min | 30 min | • Do not use concurrently with beta blockers<br>• Monitor for heart failure, ischemic heart disease (angina, MI) |
| Vasodilator | Hydralazine (Apresoline) | 10 to 30 min | 2 to 6 hr | • Avoided in clients with coronary artery disease |
| Beta/alpha blocker | Labetalol (Trandate) | 5 to 10 min | 3 to 6 hr | • Avoided in clients with heart failure and asthma |
| Beta blocker | Esmolol (Brevibloc) | 1 to 2 min | 10 to 30 min | • Avoided in clients with heart failure and asthma |
| ACE inhibitor | Enalaprilat (Vasotec) | 15 min | 6 hr or more | • Watch for hypotension |
| Diuretic | Furosemide (Lasix) | 15 min | 4 hr | • Watch for hypotension<br>• Watch for hypokalemia |
| Calcium channel blocker | Nicardipene (Cardene) | 1 to 5 min | 3 to 6 hr | • Watch for signs of myocardial ischemia |

(papilledema), blurred vision, restlessness, and motor and sensory deficits (Porth, 2002). Prolonged malignant hypertension damages walls of the arterioles and renal blood vessels, and may lead to intravascular coagulation and acute renal failure.

The goal of care in hypertensive emergencies is to reduce the blood pressure by no more than 25% within minutes to 2 hours, then toward 160/100 within 2 to 6 hours. It is important to avoid rapid or excessive blood pressure decreases that may lead to renal, cerebral, or cardiac ischemia (NHLBI, 1997). Blood pressure is monitored frequently (every 5 to 30 minutes) during a hypertensive emergency. The BUN, serum creatinine, calcium, and total protein levels are carefully monitored to help determine the prognosis for recovery. Drug treatment for malignant hypertension includes parenteral administration of a rapidly acting antihypertensive, such as the potent vasodilator sodium nitroprusside (Nipride). Other medications that may be used are outlined in Table 33–4. Management also focuses on treating any underlying or coexisting heart, kidney, and CNS disorders.

Nursing care for the client with a hypertensive emergency focuses on continuous monitoring of the blood pressure and titrating drugs (administered by intravenous bolus or infusion) as ordered to achieve desired blood pressure. Avoiding excessive or very rapid blood pressure reductions is as important as achieving the desired blood pressure readings. Reassure the client and family of the rapid effect of prescribed drugs. Provide psychologic and emotional support as needed. Maintain an attitude of confidence that the treatment will achieve the desired effect. Following resolution of the hypertensive crisis, review causes of the crisis. Teach the client and family measures to effectively manage hypertension and prevent future hypertensive emergencies.

# DISORDERS OF THE AORTA AND ITS BRANCHES

The aorta and its branches may be affected by occlusions, aneurysms, and inflammations. These disorders may be chronic or acute and life threatening (e.g., a thoracic dissection). This section focuses on aneurysms of the aorta and its branches.

## THE CLIENT WITH AN ANEURYSM

An **aneurysm** is an abnormal dilation of a blood vessel, commonly at a site of a weakness or a tear in the vessel wall.

Aneurysms commonly affect the aorta and peripheral arteries, because of the high pressure in these vessels. An aneurysm also may develop in the ventricular wall, usually affecting the left ventricle. Most arterial aneurysms are caused by arteriosclerosis or atherosclerosis; trauma also may lead to aneurysm formation.

Arterial aneurysms are most common in men over age 50, most of whom are asymptomatic at the time of diagnosis. Hypertension is a major contributing factor in the development of some types of aortic aneurysms.

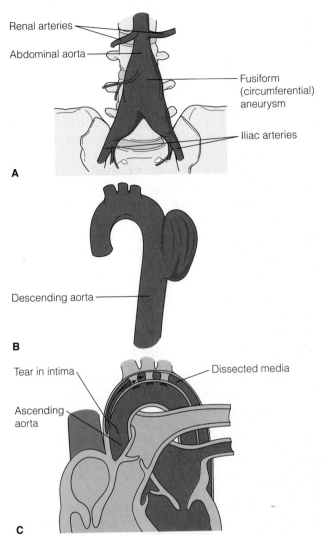

Renal arteries

Abdominal aorta

Fusiform
(circumferential)
aneurysm

Iliac arteries

**A**

Descending aorta

**B**

Tear in intima

Dissected media

Ascending
aorta

**C**

**Figure 33–3** ■ Aortic aneurysms. *A,* Fusiform aneurysm of the abdominal aorta and iliac arteries. *B,* Saccular aneurysm of the descending thoracic aorta. *C,* Dissection of the ascending thoracic aorta.

*Source: Bullock & Henze,* Focus on Pathology *(2000). Philadelphia: Lippincott, Williams & Wilkins. Reprinted with permission.*

# PATHOPHYSIOLOGY AND MANIFESTATIONS

Aneurysms form due to weakness of the arterial wall. *True aneurysms* are caused by slow weakening of the arterial wall due to the long-term, eroding effects of atherosclerosis and hypertension. True aneurysms affect all three layers of the vessel wall, and most are fusiform and circumferential. *Fusiform aneurysms* are spindle shaped and taper at both ends (Figure 33–3A■). *Circumferential* aneurysms involve the entire diameter of the vessel. They generally grow slowly but progressively. Their length and diameter vary considerably among clients. A large fusiform aneurysm may affect most of the ascending aorta as well as a large portion of the abdominal aorta.

*False aneurysms,* also known as traumatic aneurysms, are caused by a traumatic break in the vessel wall rather than weakening of the vessel. They often are *saccular,* shaped like small outpouchings (sacs) on a portion of the vessel wall (Figure 33–3B). A *berry aneurysm* is a type of saccular aneurysm. They are often small (less than 2 cm in diameter), caused by congenital weakness in the tunica media of the artery. Berry aneurysms are commonly found in the circle of Willis.

*Dissecting aneurysms* are unique, developing when a break or tear in the tunica intima and media allows blood to invade or *dissect* the layers of the vessel wall. The blood usually is contained by the adventitia, forming a saccular or longitudinal aneurysm (Figure 33–3C).

Aneurysms affect different segments of the aorta and its branches. Their manifestations generally are due to pressure of the aneurysm on adjacent structures. Table 33–5 summarizes the manifestations and complications of various types of aortic aneurysms.

## Thoracic Aortic Aneurysms

*Thoracic aortic aneurysms* account for about 10% of aortic aneurysms. They usually result from weakening of the aortic wall by arteriosclerosis and hypertension (Tierney et al., 2001). Other causes include trauma, coarctation of the aorta, tertiary

| TABLE 33–5 | Manifestations and Complications of Aortic Aneurysms | |
|---|---|---|
| **Type or Location** | **Manifestations** | **Complications** |
| Thoracic | • May be asymptomatic<br>• Back, neck, or substernal pain<br>• Dyspnea, stridor, or brassy cough if pressing on trachea<br>• Hoarseness and dysphagia if pressing on esophagus or laryngeal nerve<br>• Edema of the face and neck<br>• Distended neck veins | • Ruptured and hemorrhage |
| Abdominal | • Pulsating abdominal mass<br>• Aortic calcification noted on X-ray<br>• Mild to severe midabdominal or lumbar back pain<br>• Cool, cyanotic extremities if iliac arteries are involved<br>• Claudication (ischemic pain with exercise, relieved by rest) | • Peripheral emboli to lower extremities<br>• Rupture and hemorrage |
| Aortic dissection | • Abrupt, severe, ripping or tearing pain in area of aneurysm<br>• Mild or marked hypertension early<br>• Weak or absent pulses and blood pressure in upper extremities<br>• Syncope | • Hemorrhage<br>• Renal failure<br>• MI, heart failure, cardiac tamponade<br>• Sepsis<br>• Weakness or paralysis of lower extremities |

syphilis, fungal infections, and Marfan syndrome. The syphilis spirochete can invade and weaken aortic smooth muscle, causing an aneurysm to develop as long as 20 years after the primary infection. Marfan's syndrome fragments elastic fibers of the aortic media, weakening the vessel wall. (See the box on page 903 for more information about Marfan syndrome.)

Thoracic aneurysms frequently are asymptomatic. When present, symptoms vary by the location, size, and growth rate of the aneurysm. Substernal, neck, or back pain may occur. Pressure on the trachea, esophagus, laryngeal nerve, or superior vena cava may cause dyspnea, stridor, cough, difficult or painful swallowing, hoarseness, edema of the face and neck, and distended neck veins.

Aneurysms of the ascending aortic arch typically cause angina. Aneurysms of the aortic arch often cause dysphagia, dyspnea, hoarseness, confusion, and dizziness. Aneurysms of the thoracic aorta tend to enlarge progressively and may rupture, causing death.

## Abdominal Aortic Aneurysms

*Abdominal aortic aneurysms* are associated with arteriosclerosis and hypertension. Increasing age and smoking are believed to contribute as well. Most abdominal aortic aneurysms are found in adults over age 70. The vast majority (over 90%) develop below the renal arteries, usually where the abdominal aorta branches to form the iliac arteries.

Most abdominal aneurysms are asymptomatic, but a pulsating mass in the mid and upper abdomen and a bruit over the mass are found on exam. When pain is present, it may be constant or intermittent, usually felt in the midabdominal region or lower back. Its intensity may range from mild discomfort to severe pain. Pain intensity often correlates with the size and severity of the aneurysm. Severe pain may indicate impending rupture.

Sluggish blood flow within the aneurysm may cause thrombi (blood clots) to form. These can become emboli (circulating clots), traveling to the lower extremities and occluding peripheral arteries. The aneurysm may also rupture, with hemorrhage and hypovolemic shock. Rupture causes death before hospitalization in up to 50% of all clients; others die before surgery. Only about 10% to 20% of clients survive rupture of an abdominal aortic aneurysm.

## Popliteal and Femoral Aneurysms

Most popliteal and femoral aneurysms are due to arteriosclerosis. They are often bilateral and usually affect men.

*Popliteal aneurysms* may be asymptomatic. Manifestations, if any, are due to decreased blood flow to the lower extremity and include **intermittent claudication** (cramping or pain in the leg muscles brought on by exercise and relieved by rest), rest pain, and numbness. A pulsating mass may be palpable in the popliteal fossa (behind the knee). Thrombosis and embolism are complications; gangrene may result, often necessitating amputation.

A *femoral aneurysm* usually is detected as a pulsating mass in the femoral area. The manifestations are similar to those of popliteal aneurysms, resulting from impaired blood flow. Femoral aneurysms may rupture.

## Aortic Dissections

**Dissection** is a life-threatening emergency caused by a tear in the intima of the aorta with hemorrhage into the media. The hemorrhage dissects or splits the vessel wall, forming a blood-filled channel between its layers. Dissection can occur anywhere along the aorta. *Type A dissection* (also called *proximal dissection*) affects the ascending aorta; *type B dissection* (*distal dissection*) is limited to the descending aorta.

Hypertension is a major predisposing factor for aortic dissection. Other risk factors include male gender, advancing age, Marfan syndrome, pregnancy, congenital defects of the aortic valve, coarctation of the aorta, and inflammatory aortitis (Braunwald et al., 2001).

Dissection of the thoracic aortic walls progresses along the length of the vessel, moving both proximally and distally. As the aneurysm expands, pressure may prevent the aortic valve from closing or may occlude the branches of the aorta. Descending aortic dissection may extend into the renal, iliac, or femoral arteries.

The primary symptom of an aortic dissection is sudden, excruciating pain. The pain, often described as a ripping or tearing sensation, is usually over the area of dissection. Thoracic dissections cause chest or back pain. Other symptoms may include syncope, dyspnea, and weakness. The blood pressure may initially be increased, but rapidly falls and is often inaudible as the dissection occludes blood flow. Peripheral pulses are absent for the same reason.

Complications develop if major arteries are affected. Obstruction of the carotid artery causes neurologic symptoms such as weakness or paralysis. The myocardium, kidneys, or bowel may become ischemic or infarct. Acute aortic regurgitation may develop with dissection of the ascending aorta. With treatment, the long-term prognosis is generally good, although the in-hospital mortality rate following surgery is 15% to 20% (Braunwald et al., 2001).

## COLLABORATIVE CARE

Most aneurysms are asymptomatic, detected through a routine physical examination. Treatment depends on the size of the aneurysm. Small, asymptomatic aneurysms are often not treated; large aneurysms at risk for rupture require surgery.

## Diagnostic Tests

Diagnostic studies done to establish the diagnosis and determine the size and location of the aneurysm may include:

- *Chest X-ray* to visualize thoracic aortic aneurysms.
- *Abdominal ultrasonography* to diagnose abdominal aortic aneurysms.
- *Transesophageal echocardiography* to identify the specific location and extent of a thoracic aneurysm and to visualize a dissecting aneurysm.

- *Contrast-enhanced CT* or *MRI* allows precise measurements of aneurysm size.
- *Angiography* uses contrast solution injected into the aorta or involved vessel to visualize the precise size and location of the aneurysm.

## Medications

Thoracic aortic aneurysms are treated with long-term beta-blocker therapy and additional antihypertensive drugs as needed to control heart rate and blood pressure.

Clients with aortic dissection are initially treated with intravenous beta blockers such as propranolol (Inderal), metoprolol (Lopressor), labetalol (Normodyne), or esmolol (Brevibloc) to reduce the heart rate to about 60 BPM. Sodium nitroprusside (Nipride) infusion is started concurrently to reduce the systolic pressure to 120 mmHg or less. Calcium channel blockers also may be used. Direct vasodilators such as diazoxide (Hyperstat) and hydralazine (Apresoline) are avoided as they may actually worsen the dissection (Braunwald et al., 2001). Constant monitoring of vital signs, hemodynamic pressures (via Swan-Ganz catheter; see Chapter 30 ⊖⊖ for more information about hemodynamic hydrostatic pressure monitoring), and urine output are vital to ensure adequate perfusion of vital organs.

Following surgical correction of an aneurysm, anticoagulant therapy may be initiated. Heparin therapy is used initially, with conversion to oral anticoagulation prior to discharge. Many clients are maintained indefinitely on anticoagulant therapy; others may use lifelong, low-dose aspirin therapy to reduce the risk of clot formation.

## Surgery

Operative repair of aortic aneurysms is indicated when the aneurysm is symptomatic or expanding rapidly. Thoracic aneurysms more than 6 cm in diameter are surgically repaired; asymptomatic abdominal aneurysms greater than 5 cm in diameter may be repaired, depending on the client's operative risk factors. Type A dissections are repaired as soon as feasible; type B dissections may be surgically repaired, depending on the extent of involvement and risk for rupture (Braunwald et al., 2001).

An open surgical procedure in which the aneurysm is excised and replaced with a synthetic fabric graft is the standard treatment for expanding abdominal aortic aneurysms. Although the aneurysm walls may be excised, they usually are left intact and used to cover the graft (Figure 33–4 ■). Surgical repair of thoracic aneurysms is similar but more complex due to major vessels exiting at the aortic arch. Cardiopulmonary bypass is required if the ascending aorta is involved. The aortic valve also may be replaced during surgery. See the box on page 998 for nursing care of the client having surgery on the aorta.

Endovascular stent grafts are increasingly being used to treat abdominal aortic aneurysms. The stent, which consists of a metal sheath covered with polyester fabric, is placed percutaneously using fluoroscopy to guide its placement. Both straight and bifurcated grafts are available. This option may be pre-

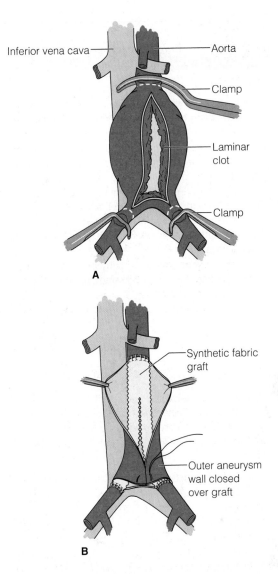

**Figure 33–4** ■ Repair of an abdominal aortic aneurysm. *A,* The aorta is exposed and clamped between the renal and iliac arteries. Atherosclerotic plaque and thrombotic material is removed. *B,* A synthetic graft is used to replace the aneurysm. The aneurysm walls are then sutured around the graft.

ferred in clients who have a high surgical risk (Meeker & Rothrock, 1999).

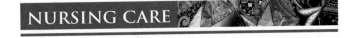

## NURSING CARE

### Assessment

Focused assessment for the client with a suspected aortic aneurysm includes:

- Health history: complaints of chest, back, or abdominal pain; extremity weakness; shortness of breath, cough, difficult or painful swallowing, hoarseness; history of hypertension, coronary heart disease, heart failure, or peripheral vascular disease

## NURSING CARE OF THE THE CLIENT HAVING SURGERY OF THE AORTA

### PREOPERATIVE CARE

- As time permits, provide routine preoperative care and teaching as outlined in Chapter 7. ⊝⊙ *Clients having vascular surgery have similar preoperative nursing care needs to other clients having major abdominal or thoracic surgery. If emergent surgery is required, time for preoperative care and teaching may be limited.*
- Implement measures to reduce fear and anxiety:
  a. Orient to the intensive care unit, if appropriate.
  b. Describe and explain the reason for all equipment and tubes, such as cardiac monitors, ventilators, nasogastric tubes, urinary catheters, intravenous lines and fluids, and intra-arterial lines.
  c. Explain what to expect following surgery (sights, sounds, frequency of taking vital signs, dressings, pain relief measures, communication strategies).
  d. Allow time for questions and expression of fears and concerns.
  *These explanations provide a sense of control for the client and family.*

### POSTOPERATIVE CARE

- Provide routine postoperative care and specific measures as ordered by the physician. *Clients undergoing aneurysm repair require nursing care similar to that provided to all clients with major thoracic or abdominal surgery, in addition to specific measures related to vascular surgery.*

**PRACTICE ALERT** *Monitor for and report manifestations of graft leakage:*
  a. *Ecchymoses of the scrotum, perineum, or penis; a new or expanding hematoma*
  b. *Increased abdominal girth*
  c. *Weak or absent peripheral pulses; tachycardia; hypotension*

  d. *Decreased motor function or sensation in the extremities*
  e. *Fall in hemoglobin and hematocrit*
  f. *Increasing abdominal, pelvic, back, or groin pain*
  g. *Decreasing urinary output (less than 30 mL/ hour)*
  h. *Decreasing CVP, pulmonary artery pressure, or pulmonary artery wedge pressure*
*These manifestations may signal graft leakage and possible hemorrhage. Pain may be due to pressure from an expanding hematoma or bowel ischemia. Decreased renal perfusion causes the glomerular filtration rate and urine output to fall.* ■

- Maintain fluid replacement and blood or volume expanders as ordered. Promptly report changes in vital signs, level of consciousness, and urine output. *Hypovolemic shock may develop due to blood loss during surgery, third spacing, inadequate fluid replacement, and/or hemorrhage if graft separation or leakage occurs.*
- Report manifestations of lower extremity embolism: pain and numbness in lower extremities, decreasing pulses, and pale, cool, or cyanotic skin. *Pulses may be absent for 4 to 12 hours postoperatively due to vasospasm; however, absent pulses with pain, changes in sensation, and a pale, cool extremity are indicative of arterial occulsion.*
- Report manifestations of bowel ischemia or gangrene: abdominal pain and distention, occult or fresh blood in stools, and diarrhea. *Bowel ischemia may result from an embolism or occur as a complication of surgery.*
- Report manifestations of impaired renal function: urine output less than 30 mL per hour, fixed specific gravity, increasing BUN and serum creatinine levels. *Hypovolemia or clamping of the aorta during surgery may impair renal perfusion, leading to acute renal failure.*
- Report manifestations of spinal cord ischemia: lower extremity weakness or paraplegia. *Impaired spinal cord perfusion may lead to ischemia and impaired function.*

---

- Physical examination: vital signs including blood pressure in upper and lower extremities; peripheral pulses; skin color and temperature; neck veins; abdominal exam including gentle palpation for masses and auscultation for bruits; neurologic exam including level of consciousness, sensation, and movement of extremities

### Nursing Diagnoses and Interventions

Nursing care for clients with an aneurysm of the aorta or its branches focuses on monitoring and maintaining tissue perfusion, relieving pain, and reducing anxiety. Nursing care usually is acute, precipitated by a complication or surgical repair of the aneurysm.

### Risk for Ineffective Tissue Perfusion

Clients with aortic aneurysms are at risk for impaired tissue perfusion due to aneurysm rupture with resulting hemorrhage and lack of blood flow to tissues distal to the rupture. In addition, thrombi often form within the aneurysm and may become emboli, obstructing distal arterial blood flow.

**PRACTICE ALERT** *Immediately report manifestations of impending rupture, expansion, or dissection of the aneurysm: increased pain; discrepancy between upper and lower extremity blood pressures and peripheral pulses; increased mass size; change in LOC or motor or sensory function; laboratory results. Rapid expansion may indicate increased risk for rupture, with resulting hemorrhage, shock, and possible death. Elective or planned surgery may rapidly become emergency surgery to prevent complications.* ■

- Implement interventions to reduce the risk of aneurysm rupture:
  a. Maintain bed rest with legs flat.
  b. Maintain a calm environment, implementing measures to reduce psychologic stress.
  c. Prevent straining during defecation and instruct to avoid holding the breath while moving.
  d. Administer beta blockers and antihypertensives as prescribed.

*Activity, stress, and the Valsalva maneuver increase blood pressure, increasing the risk of rupture. Elevating or crossing the legs restricts peripheral blood flow and increases pressure in the aorta or iliac arteries. Beta blockers and antihypertensives often are ordered to reduce pressure in the dilated vessel.*

**PRACTICE ALERT** *Report manifestations of arterial thrombosis or embolism: absent peripheral pulses; a pale or cyanotic, cool extremity; severe, diffuse abdominal pain with guarding; or increased groin, lumbar, or lower extremity pain. Sluggish blood flow within the aneurysm often causes thrombi to form. These thrombi can break loose, becoming emboli that can occlude peripheral arteries or arteries to the kidneys or mesentery. Arterial occlusion may necessitate emergency surgery to restore blood flow and prevent tissue infarct or gangrene.* ■

- Continuously monitor cardiac rhythm. Report complaints of chest pain or changes in ECG tracing. Administer oxygen as indicated. *Aortic dissection and repair place the client at significant risk for myocardial infarction (MI), a major cause of postoperative mortality and morbidity (Braunwald et al., 2001). Rapid identification and treatment of this complication can reduce the risk of death or long-term adverse effects of MI.*

**PRACTICE ALERT** *Immediately report changes in mental status or symptoms of peripheral neurologic impairment (weakness, paresthesias, paralysis). The expanding aneurysm or dissection can affect carotid and cerebral blood flow or spinal cord perfusion, leading to neurologic symptoms. Immediate restoration of blood flow is vital to prevent permanent neurologic deficits.* ■

### Risk for Injury

Potent antihypertensive drugs often are given intravenously to reduce the pressure on an expanding or dissecting aneurysm. Continuous monitoring of infusions and hemodynamic parameters such as arterial pressure, pulmonary pressures, and cardiac output is vital to ensure that adequate tissue perfusion is maintained during infusions of these potent drugs.

**PRACTICE ALERT** *Use an infusion control device for all drug infusions. These devices prevent accidental or inadvertent changes in the rate of the infusion and dose of the drug.* ■

- Continuously monitor arterial pressure and hemodynamic parameters as indicated. Promptly report results outside the specified parameters to the physician. *Many of the drugs used are effective within minutes. Responses vary among individuals, particularly in the older adult, necessitating continuous monitoring.*
- Monitor urine output hourly. Report output less than 30 mL/hr. *The kidneys are very sensitive to reduced perfusion pressure; inadequate renal blood flow can lead to acute renal failure.*

### Anxiety

Clients with aortic aneurysms often are highly anxious because of the urgent nature of the disorder. The nurse must manage the anxiety levels of both the client and family members to effectively address physiologic care needs. Stress reduction also is necessary to help maintain the blood pressure within desired limits.

- Explain all procedures and treatments, using simple and understandable terms. *Simplified explanations are necessary when anxiety levels interfere with learning and understanding.*
- Respond to all questions honestly, using a calm, empathetic, but matter-of-fact manner. *Honesty with the client and family promotes trust and provides reassurance that the true nature of the situation is not being "hidden" from them.*
- Provide care in a calm, efficient manner. *Using a calm manner even during preparations for emergency surgery reassures the client and family that although the situation is critical, the staff is prepared to handle things effectively.*
- Spend as much time as possible with the client. Allow supportive family members to remain with the client when possible. *The presence of a health professional and supportive family member reassures the client that he or she is not alone in facing this crisis.*

### Home Care

Topics to discuss when preparing clients and their families for home care depend on the treatment plan. Discuss the following topics when surgical repair is not immediately planned and the aneurysm will be monitored.

- Measures to control hypertension, including lifestyle and prescribed drugs
- The benefits of smoking cessation
- Manifestations of increasing aneurysm size or complications to report to the physician

Following surgery, discuss the following topics in preparing the client and family for home care.

- Wound care and preventing infection; manifestations of impaired healing or infection to be reported
- Prescribed antihypertensive and anticoagulant medications and their expected and unintended effects
- The importance of adequate rest and nutrition for healing
- Measures to prevent constipation and straining at stool (such as increasing fluid and fiber in the diet)
- The importance of avoiding prolonged sitting, lifting heavy objects, engaging in strenuous exercise, and having sexual intercourse until approved by the physician (usually 6 to 12 weeks)
- Signs and symptoms of complications to report to the physician

Provide referrals to a home health agency or community health service as necessary. Referrals are especially important for older adults and their caregivers, who may require additional assistance with the complex care needs.

# DISORDERS OF THE PERIPHERAL ARTERIES

Disorders that impair peripheral arterial blood flow may be *acute* (e.g., arterial thrombosis) or *chronic* (e.g., peripheral arteriosclerosis). Chronic occlusive disorders may be due to structural defects of the arterial walls or spasm of affected arteries. Impaired peripheral arterial circulation limits the availability of oxygen and nutrients to the tissues, and can have significant adverse effects. This section focuses on acute and chronic disorders affecting peripheral arteries.

## PHYSIOLOGY REVIEW

Peripheral arteries are the part of the systemic circulation that delivers oxygen and nutrients to the skin and the extremities. Arterial walls have three layers: the intima, which includes the endothelium and a layer of connective tissue and the basement membrane; the media, composed of smooth muscle and elastic fibers; and the adventitia, a thin layer of connective tissue that contains elastic and collagenous fibers. The muscular peripheral arteries control blood flow as their smooth muscle contracts and relaxes. Contraction narrows the vessel lumen (**vasoconstriction**), whereas smooth muscle relaxation expands the vessel (**vasodilation**). Peripheral arteries become progressively smaller; arterioles are less than 0.5 mm in diameter and are primarily smooth muscle. The arterioles control blood flow through the capillary beds where gas, nutrient, and waste product exchange occurs. Capillary walls are very thin, consisting of a single layer of endothelial cells surrounded by a thin basement membrane.

Blood flows from an area of higher pressure to an area of lower pressure. *Resistance* opposes blood flow. Resistance is created by friction of the blood itself, although the primary determinants of vascular resistance are the diameter and length of the blood vessel. See the physiology review section under "The Client with Hypertension" for more information about factors that determine vessel resistance.

## THE CLIENT WITH ACUTE ARTERIAL OCCLUSION

A peripheral artery may be acutely occluded by development of a thrombus (blood clot) or by an embolism. Blood flow to tissues supplied by the artery is impaired, resulting in acute tissue ischemia and a risk for necrosis and gangrene.

## PATHOPHYSIOLOGY

### Arterial Thrombosis

A **thrombus** is a blood clot that adheres to the vessel wall. Thrombi tend to develop in areas where intravascular factors stimulate coagulation (e.g., where a vessel lumen is partially obstructed and its wall is damaged and roughened by atherosclerosis). Other disorders, such as infection or inflammation of the vessel wall or pooling of blood (e.g., in an aneurysm) also can prompt coagulation and thrombus formation (McCance & Huether, 2002). A developing thrombus can occlude arterial blood flow through the vessel, leading to ischemia of tissues supplied by that artery. The extent of ischemia depends on the size of the affected artery and the degree of collateral circulation. In gradual processes of arterial occlusion such as atherosclerosis, collateral vessels often develop to compensate for impaired arterial flow. The extent of collateral circulation affects the degree of tissue ischemia distal to the thrombus.

### Arterial Embolism

An **embolism** is sudden obstruction of a blood vessel by debris. A thrombus can break loose from the arterial wall to become a **thromboembolus.** Other substances also can become emboli: atherosclerotic plaque, masses of bacteria, cancer cells, amniotic fluid, bone marrow fat, and foreign objects such as air bubbles or broken intravenous catheters. Regardless of cause, an embolus eventually lodges in a vessel that is too small to allow it to pass.

Arterial emboli often originate in the left side of the heart. They are associated with myocardial infarction, valvular heart disease, left-sided heart failure, atrial fibrillation, or infectious heart diseases. Emboli from the left heart often enter the carotid arteries and become trapped in the cerebral circulation, causing neurologic deficits (see Chapter 41). Thromboemboli that develop in the aorta or peripheral arterial circulation tend to lodge in areas where the arterial lumen is narrowed by atherosclerotic plaque and at arterial bifurcations.

### Manifestations

The manifestations of arterial thrombosis and embolism are those of tissue ischemia. Ischemic tissues are painful, pale, and cool or cold. Distal pulses are absent. Paresthesias (numbness and tingling) develop in the extremity. Cyanosis and mottling are common. Paralysis and muscle spasms may develop in the affected extremity. A line of demarcation between normal and ischemic tissue may be seen, particularly with embolism. Tissue below the line is cool or cold, and pale, cyanotic, or mottled. See the box below.

Arterial occlusion can result in permanent vessel and limb damage. Complete arterial occlusion leads to tissue necrosis and gangrene unless blood flow is promptly restored.

## Manifestations of Arterial Thrombosis and Embolus

- Pain
- Pallor or mottling
- Paresthesias (numbness and tingling)
- Cool or cold skin
- Pulselessness distal to the blockage
- Possible paralysis, weakness, or muscle spasms
- Possible line of demarcation; with pallor, cyanosis, and cooler skin distal to the blockage (especially with arterial embolism)

## COLLABORATIVE CARE

Acute arterial occlusions may require emergency treatment to preserve the limb if the obstructed vessel is large or collateral circulation is minimal. If the limb is not in jeopardy, more conservative management may be initiated.

### Diagnostic Tests

The diagnosis of acute arterial occlusion often is apparent by the signs and symptoms. *Arteriography* is used to confirm the diagnosis, locate the occlusion, and determine its extent.

### Medications

Anticoagulation with intravenous heparin is initiated to prevent further clot propagation and recurrent embolism. Anticoagulation is continued with oral anticoagulants after discharge. See the section on deep vein thrombosis later in this chapter for more information about anticoagulant therapy.

Arterial thrombosis may be treated with intra-arterial thrombolytic therapy using streptokinase, urokinase, or tissue plasminogen activator (t-PA) (see Chapter 29). Lysis of the thrombus or embolus is achieved in 50% to 80% of the cases (Tierney et al., 2001). Local intra-arterial injection of the thrombolytic drug allows use of lower doses and reduces the bleeding risk associated with thrombolytic drugs.

### Surgery

Immediate *embolectomy* (within 4 to 6 hours) is the treatment of choice for acute arterial occlusion by an embolus to prevent tissue necrosis and gangrene. When the involved vessel is in an extremity, local anesthesia and a special balloon-tipped catheter known as a Fogarty catheter may be used for high surgical risk clients (Tierney et al., 2001). An embolus in the mesenteric circulation necessitates emergency laparotomy. The risk of complications and limb loss increases significantly if surgery is delayed by 12 or more hours. Potential major complications include compartment syndrome (see Chapter 38), acute respiratory distress syndrome (Chapter 36), or acute renal failure (Chapter 27).

Arterial thrombosis also may be treated surgically, although the required surgery may be more extensive due to the length of the vessel involved. *Thromboendarterectomy* is done to remove the thrombus and plaque in the artery. An arterial graft may be required. Nursing care for clients who have undergone embolectomy or thrombus removal is discussed in the nursing care section that follows.

## NURSING CARE

### Assessment

Nursing assessment for the client with an acute arterial occlusion is highly focused due to the emergency nature of the problem.

- Health history: complaints of pain, numbness, tingling, or weakness in the involved extremity; history of atherosclerotic vessel disease, heart disease, or recent invasive procedure (e.g., angiography, percutaneous revascularization procedure)
- Physical examination: vital signs; peripheral pulses in both extremities; color, temperature, sensation, and movement of involved extremity; skin condition; presence of a line of demarcation

### Nursing Diagnoses and Interventions

Nursing care related to acute arterial occlusion focuses on protecting the affected extremity, managing anxiety, and reducing the risk of complications related to anticoagulant therapy.

#### Ineffective Tissue Perfusion: Peripheral

Protecting ischemic tissue from injury prior to surgery or medical thrombolysis is vital. Following surgery, there is a risk for thrombosis at the graft site or impaired perfusion due to edema of the surgical site.

**PRACTICE ALERT** *Monitor extremity perfusion, comparing affected and unaffected extremities. Assess peripheral pulses (using the Doppler stethoscope as needed), skin temperature and color, capillary refill, movement, and sensation every 1 to 4 hours. Promptly report changes or complaints of increased or unrelieved pain. Propagation of a thrombus can further obstruct arterial flow, increasing tissue ischemia. Following surgery, arterial spasms may cause a cyanotic, pulseless extremity; normal color and pulses should return within 12 hours. A thrombus may form at the surgical site or within a graft, causing tissue ischemia with pain and other manifestations of arterial occlusion. Further measures to restore circulation may be necessary.* ■

- Maintain intravenous fluids as ordered. *Adequate circulating blood volume is necessary to maintain cardiac output and tissue perfusion.*
- Protect the extremity, keeping it horizontal or lower than the heart. Use a cradle to keep bedclothes off the extremity and sheepskin or foam pad to protect it from hard or abrasive surfaces. Do not apply heat or cold. *Keeping the extremity lower than the heart promotes collateral blood flow. Ischemic tissue is easily damaged by minimal trauma such as shearing by bed linens, or heat or cold application.*
- Following surgery, avoid raising the knee gatch, placing pillows under the knees, or sitting with 90-degree hip flexion. *These activities may impair blood flow through the affected vessel.*

#### Anxiety

Clients with an acute arterial occlusion often are very anxious. The rapid and intense nature of preoperative activities can be overwhelming, increasing anxiety about the disorder and its outcome. Manifestations of anxiety may include trembling, palpitations, restlessness, dry mouth, helplessness, inability to relax, irritability, forgetfulness, and lack of awareness of surroundings. Nursing measures focus on establishing trust and minimizing the effects of anxiety to decrease surgical risk and improve recovery.

- Spend as much time as possible with the client. Provide opportunities to verbalize anxiety; offer reassurance and support. Support adaptive coping mechanisms. *The presence of a caring nurse provides a safe environment for expressing fears and anxieties. Coping mechanisms reduce the immediate perceived threat and increase the ability to deal with the situational crisis.*
- Perform required measures in an expedient but calm manner. *Calm, confident performance of treatment measures reassures the client and family that appropriate care is being given to treat the problem at hand.*
- Assess anxiety level at least every 8 hours; more often as needed. Intervene as indicated to reduce anxiety. *Assessment helps determine the intensity of anxiety, the client's ability to control it, and directs interventions to reduce it.*
- Decrease sensory stimuli as much as possible. *Reducing environmental stimuli provides the client a degree of control over anxiety.*
- Speak slowly and clearly and avoid unnecessary interruptions when listening. Give concise directions, focusing on the present. Involve the client in simple tasks and decisions to the extent possible. *High levels of anxiety interfere with learning. Keeping interactions focused on the present situation directs the client's focus and provides reassurance that it is the most important focus of the nurse as well. Providing opportunities for self-care and decision making reinforces the client's importance and power to control the situation.*

### Altered Protection

Thombolytic and/or anticoagulant therapy used to dissolve existing clots and prevent further clot formation increase the risk for bleeding. Close monitoring of physical status and laboratory data is vital, as are measures to reduce the risk for injury and bleeding.

**PRACTICE ALERT** *Assess for and report manifestations of impaired clotting, including excessive incisional bleeding; prolonged oozing from injection sites; bleeding gums, nose bleed, or hematuria; petechiae, bruising, or purpura. Anticoagulants and thrombolytics interfere with the clotting cascade and may cause abnormal bleeding.* ∎

- Monitor activated partial thromboplastin time (APTT) during heparin therapy and prothrombin time (PT) or international normalized ratio (INR) during oral anticoagulant therapy. Report values outside desired range. *The APTT, PT, and INR are prolonged by anticoagulant therapy. Values higher than the desired range may indicate an increased risk for bleeding; values below the target may indicate inadequate anticoagulation.*
- Protect from injury: Use side rails or other measures as needed to prevent falls; avoid parenteral injections and other invasive procedures as much as possible; hold firm pressure over injection and intravenous sites for 5 minutes and over arterial punctures for 20 minutes; use a soft toothbrush or sponge for oral care; use an electric razor for shaving. *Minor trauma can lead to extensive bleeding, particularly in the client who has received a thrombolytic drug.*

## Home Care

When preparing the client and family for home care related to an acute arterial occlusion, discuss the following topics as indicated.

- Care of the incision
- Manifestations of complications to be reported, including symptoms of infection or occlusion of the graft or artery
- Long-term anticoagulant therapy, including the reason, prescribed dose, follow-up laboratory testing and appointments, interactions with other drugs, and manifestations of excessive bleeding
- Any activity restrictions or dietary modifications
- Lifestyle modifications to slow atherosclerosis and control hypertension
- Measures to promote peripheral circulation and maintain tissue integrity (see the discussion of peripheral atherosclerosis that follows)

Refer for home care services (nursing care, physical therapy, housekeeping services) as indicated.

## THE CLIENT WITH PERIPHERAL ATHEROSCLEROSIS

*Arteriosclerosis* is the most common chronic arterial disorder, characterized by thickening, loss of elasticity, and calcification of arterial walls. **Atherosclerosis** is a form of arteriosclerosis in which deposits of fat and fibrin obstruct and harden the arteries. In the peripheral circulation, these pathologic changes impair the blood supply to peripheral tissues, particularly the lower extremities. This is known as **peripheral vascular disease (PVD).**

PVD usually affects people in their 60s and 70s; men are more often affected than women. Deaths attributed to peripheral arterial disease are about the same for black and white males, but are higher among black women than white women (NHLBI, 2002).

Risk factors for PVD are similar to those for atherosclerosis and coronary heart disease (see Chapter 29). ⬡ Diabetes mellitus, hypercholesterolemia, hypertension, cigarette smoking, and high homocystine levels are clear risk factors for PVD (Brauwald et al., 2001).

## PATHOPHYSIOLOGY

The pathophysiology of atherosclerosis is detailed in Chapter 29. ⬡ Atherosclerotic lesions involve both the intima and the media of the involved arteries. Lesions typically develop in large and midsize arteries, particularly the abdominal aorta and iliac arteries (30% of symptomatic clients), the femoral and popliteal arteries (80% to 90% of clients), and more distal arteries (40% to 50% of clients) (Braunwald et al., 2001). Arteriosclerosis in the abdominal aorta leads to the development of aneurysms as plaque erodes the vessel wall.

Plaque tends to form at arterial bifurcations. The vessel lumen is progressively obstructed, decreasing blood flow to the

## Manifestations of Peripheral Atherosclerosis

- Intermittent claudication
- Rest pain
- Paresthesias (numbness, decreased sensation)
- Diminished or absent peripheral pulses
- Pallor with extremity elevation, dependent rubor when dependent
- Thin, shiny, hairless skin; thickened toenails
- Areas of discoloration or skin breakdown

lower extremities. Tissue hypoxia or anoxia results. With gradual obstruction of the vessel, collateral circulation often develops. However, it is usually not adequate to supply tissue needs, especially when metabolic demand increases (e.g., during exercise). Manifestations typically develop only when the vessel is occluded by 60% or more.

## MANIFESTATIONS AND COMPLICATIONS

Pain is the primary symptom of peripheral atherosclerosis. **Intermittent claudication,** a cramping or aching pain in the calves of the legs, the thighs, and the buttocks that occurs with a predictable level of activity, is characteristic of PVD. The pain is often accompanied by weakness and is relieved by rest.

*Rest pain,* in contrast, occurs during periods of inactivity. It is often described as a burning sensation in the lower legs. Rest pain increases when the legs are elevated and decreases when the legs are dependent (e.g., hanging over the side of the bed). The legs also may feel cold or numb along with the pain. Sensation is diminished and the muscles may atrophy.

Peripheral pulses may be decreased or absent. A bruit may be heard over large affected arteries, such as the femoral artery and the abdominal aorta. The legs are pale when elevated, but often are dark red (*dependent rubor*) when dependent. The skin often is thin, shiny, and hairless, with discolored areas. Toenails may be thickened. Areas of skin breakdown and ulceration may be evident. Edema may develop with severe PVD. See the box above for manifestations of peripheral atherosclerosis.

Complications of peripheral atherosclerosis include gangrene and extremity amputation, rupture of abdominal aortic aneurysms, and possible infection and sepsis.

## COLLABORATIVE CARE

Management of peripheral atherosclerosis focuses on slowing the atherosclerotic process and maintaining tissue perfusion.

### Diagnostic Tests

Although PVD often can be diagnosed by the history and physical examination, diagnostic tests may be ordered to evaluate its extent. Noninvasive studies often are sufficient.

- *Segmental pressure measurements* use sphygmomanometer cuffs and a Doppler device to compare blood pressures between the upper and lower extremities (normally similar)

and within different segments of the affected extremity. In PVD, the BP may be lower in the legs than in the arms.
- *Stress testing* using a treadmill provides functional assessment of limitations. In PVD, pressure at the ankle may decline even further with exercise, confirming the diagnosis. Evaluation for coronary heart disease may be done simultaneously during exercise testing (Braunwald et al., 2001).
- *Doppler ultrasound* uses sound waves reflected off moving red blood cells within a vessel to evaluate blood flow. The impulses may be translated into an audible signal or a graphic waveform. With significant PVD, the waveform becomes progressively flatter as the transducer is moved distally along the affected vessel. Segmental pressures may be used to locate the site of obstruction.
- *Duplex Doppler ultrasound* combines the audible or graphic Doppler ultrasound with ultrasound imaging to identify arterial or venous abnormalities. Ultrasonic imaging provides views of the affected vessel while Doppler ultrasound evaluates blood flow. *Color-flow Doppler ultrasound (CDU)* provides color images of the vessel and blood flow.
- *Transcutaneous oximetry* evaluates oxygenation of tissues.
- *Angiography* or *magnetic resonance angiography* is done before revascularization procedures to locate and evaluate the extent of arterial obstruction. For angiography, a contrast medium is injected and vessels are visualized using fluoroscopy and X-rays. Magnetic resonance angiography does not require injection of a contrast medium and may replace angiography.

### Medications

Drug treatment of peripheral atherosclerosis is less effective than with coronary heart disease. Medications to inhibit platelet aggregation, such as aspirin or clopidogrel (Plavix) are ordered to reduce the risk of arterial thrombosis. Cilostazol (Pletal), a platelet inhibitor with vasodilator properties, improves claudication. Pentoxifylliune (Trental) decreases blood viscosity and increases red blood cell flexibility, increasing blood flow to the microcirculation and tissues of the extremities. Parenteral vasodilator prostaglandins may be given on a long-term basis to decrease pain and facilitate healing in clients with severe limb ischemia (Braunwald et al., 2001).

### Treatments

Smoking cessation is vital. Nicotine not only promotes atherosclerosis, but also causes vasospasm, further reducing blood flow to the extremities.

Meticulous foot care is vital to prevent ulceration and infection (Box 33–4). Elastic support hose, which reduce circulation to the skin, are avoided. Elevating the head of the bed on blocks may help relieve rest pain. Regular, progressively strenuous exercise, such as 30 to 45 minutes of walking daily, is important. The client is taught to rest at the onset of claudication, resuming activity when the pain resolves.

Other measures to slow the process of atherosclerosis, such as controlling diabetes and hypertension, lowering cholesterol levels, and weight loss, also are recommended (see Chapter 29). See the box on page 1004 for care of the older adult.

## BOX 33-4 ■ Foot Care for the Client with Peripheral Atherosclerosis

1. Keep legs and feet clean, dry, and comfortable.
   - Wash legs and feet daily in warm water, using mild soap.
   - Pat dry using a soft towel; be sure to dry between the toes.
   - Apply moisturizing cream to prevent drying.
   - Use powder on the feet and between the toes.
   - Buy shoes in the afternoon (when feet are largest); never buy shoes that are uncomfortable. Be sure toes have adequate room.
   - Wear a clean pair of cotton socks each day.
2. Prevent accidents and injuries to the feet.
   - Always wear shoes or slippers when getting out of bed.
   - Walk on level ground and avoid crowds, if possible.
   - Do not go barefoot.
   - Inspect legs and feet daily; use a mirror to examine backs of legs and bottoms of feet.
   - Have a professional foot care provider trim toenails and care for corns, calluses, ingrown toenails, or athlete's foot.
   - Always check the temperature of the water before stepping into the tub.
   - Do not get the legs or tops of the feet sunburned.
   - Report leg or foot problems (increased pain, cuts, bruises, blistering, redness, or open areas) to your health care provider.
3. Improve blood supply to the legs and feet.
   - Do not cross legs.
   - Do not wear garters or knee stockings.
   - Do not swim or wade in cold water.

## Revascularization

Revascularization may be done if symptoms are progressive, severe, or disabling. Other indications for surgery include symptoms that significantly interfere with activities of daily living, rest pain, and pregangrenous or gangrenous lesions. Either nonsurgical revascularization procedures or surgery may be performed.

Nonsurgical procedures include percutaneous transluminal angioplasty (PTA), stent placement, or atherectomy. Techniques may include balloon angioplasty to dilate the narrowed lumen, mechanical atherectomy to remove plaque, or laser or thermal angioplasty to vaporize the occluding material. Iliac and femoral-popliteal PTA initially reestablish good blood flow and relieve symptoms in more than 80% of clients. While the 3-year success rate is lower, stent placement improves the duration of symptom relief (Braunwald et al., 2001). See Chapter 29 for more information about revascularization procedures.

Surgical options include endarterectomy to remove occlusive plaque from the artery and bypass grafts. Knitted Dacron bypass grafts are commonly used. Both immediate and long-term graft patency is better with bypass grafting than with nonsurgical revascularization procedures, but the risk for operative complications such as myocardial infarction, stoke, infection, and peripheral embolization is higher (Braunwald et al., 2001). Nursing care for the client having revascularization surgery is similar to that provided for clients having an aortic aneurysm repair (see the box on page 998).

## Complementary Therapies

Complementary therapies for peripheral vascular disease include interventions to improve circulation and to reduce stress. A number of complementary therapies may improve peripheral circulation, including aromatherapy with rosemary or vetiver; biofeedback; healing or therapeutic touch and massage; herbals such as ginko, garlic, cayenne, hawthorn, and bilberry; and exercise including yoga. Aromatherapy and yoga also may reduce stress, as can breathing exercises, meditation, and counseling. In addition, complementary therapies to reduce atherosclerosis and lower cholesterol levels may slow the progress of PVD. Measures such as a very low-fat or vegetarian diet, including antioxidant nutrients or using vitamin C, vitamin E, or garlic supplements, and traditional Chinese medicine may be useful.

## NURSING CARE

### Health Promotion

Discuss healthy lifestyle habits with community and religious groups, school children (grades K through 12), and through the print media to reduce the incidence and slow the progression of atherosclerosis.

Strongly encourage all clients to avoid smoking in the first place, and to stop all forms of tobacco use. Discuss the adverse effects of smoking and the benefits of quitting. Provide information about dietary recommendations to maintain a healthy

## Nursing Care of the Older Adult

### PERIPHERAL ATHEROSCLEROSIS

With aging, blood vessels thicken and become less compliant. These changes reduce oxygen delivery to the tissues and impair carbon dioxide and waste product removal from the tissues. When normal effects of aging combine with an increased risk of atherosclerosis, the risk of peripheral vascular disease is high.

The older adult with peripheral atherosclerosis requires the same care and teaching as other clients. However, visual deficits and osteoarthritis may make foot care more difficult. Long-standing smoking habits are difficult to break. Mobility may be impaired by arthritis or the effects of neurologic disorders. The client who lives alone may resist walking. Periodic visits by a community or home health nurse may be helpful, as may be encouraging the client to join a support group for stopping smoking, changing eating habits, and taking part in regular activity.

weight and optimal cholesterol levels. Discuss the benefits and importance of regular exercise. Finally, encourage clients with cardiovascular risk factors to undergo regular screening for hypertension, diabetes, and hyperlipidemia.

## Assessment

Focused assessment related to peripheral atherosclerosis includes the following:

- Health history: complaints of pain, its relationship to exercise or rest, timing, associated symptoms, and relief measures; history of coronary heart disease, peripheral vascular disease, hyperlipidemia, hypertension, or diabetes; current medications; smoking history; usual diet and activity patterns
- Physical examination: vital signs; strength and equality of peripheral pulses of all extremities; capillary refill; skin color, temperature, hair distribution, presence of any discolorations or lesions; movement and sensation of lower extremities

## Nursing Diagnoses and Interventions

Impaired tissue perfusion is an obvious problem in peripheral atherosclerosis. Acute and chronic pain may interfere with activities of daily living, and ambulation may be limited. The possibility of losing a lower extremity is frightening. For a summary of clients' concerns about peripheral atherosclerosis see the Nursing Research box below.

### Ineffective Tissue Perfusion: Peripheral

Impaired blood flow to the lower extremities affects gas, nutrient, and waste product exchange between the capillaries and cells. Oxygen and nutrient deprivation impairs cell function and tissue integrity, causing pain and impaired healing. Pain develops with exercise and when extremities are elevated.

- Assess peripheral pulses, pain, color, temperature, and capillary refill every 4 hours and as needed. Use a Doppler device if pulses are not palpable. Mark pulse locations with an indelible marker. *Assessment data provide a baseline for evaluating the effectiveness of interventions and identifies changes in arterial blood flow.*
- Position with extremities dependent. *Gravity promotes arterial flow to the dependent extremity, increasing tissue perfusion and relieving pain.*

**PRACTICE ALERT** *Instruct to avoid smoking. If necessary, obtain an order for a nicotine patch or gum from the physician. Nicotine is a potent vasoconstrictor that further impairs arterial blood flow. Smoking cessation is a vital component of care. Nicotine patches and gum contain less nicotine than cigarettes, and can help reduce the stress of smoking cessation.* ■

- Discuss the benefits of regular exercise. *Exercise promotes development of collateral circulation to ischemic tissues and slows the process of atherosclerosis.*
- Use a foot cradle and lightweight blankets, socks, and slippers to keep extremities warm. Avoid electric heating pads or hot water bottles. *Keeping extremities warm conserves heat, prevents vasospasm, and promotes arterial flow. External heating devices are avoided to reduce the risk of burns in the client with impaired sensation. The foot cradle protects tissues from compression by linens.*
- Encourage frequent position changes. Instruct to avoid crossing legs or using a pillow under the knees. *Position changes promote blood flow and reduce damage caused by pressure. Leg crossing and excessive flexion of the hip or knee joints can compress partially obstructed arteries and impair blood flow to distal tissues.*

## Nursing Research

### Evidence-Based Practice for the Client with Peripheral Atherosclerosis

Peripheral vascular disease (PVD) affects millions of people in the United States. Peripheral atherosclerosis, a common type of PVD, develops insidiously as the arteries of the legs are gradually occluded by atherosclerotic plaque, causing symptoms such as intermittent claudication, ulceration, and gangrene. This study explored the lived experience of PVD, identifying key themes and categories through one-to-one interviews with a group of clients who had vascular bypass surgery within the past 18 months (Gibson & Kenrick, 1998). Major and minor categories and their interrelationships were identified. Powerlessness related to the direct effects of PVD and its treatment was a common theme. Clients often had unrealistic expectations of treatment measures such as surgery. Unrealistic expectations, in turn, led to the sense of powerlessness.

#### IMPLICATIONS FOR NURSING

Nurses may assume that clients with PVD understand the chronicity of their condition and the need to continue strategies to slow the process of atherosclerosis following bypass surgery. Clients, in contrast, may see surgery as curative, and the need to continue following a low-fat diet, smoking abstinence, and skin care precautions as indicative of failure. Nursing interventions to promote independence, manage pain, and reduce anxiety are vital. Teaching self-management and providing psychologic support can reduce the sense of powerlessness and improve quality of life.

#### Critical Thinking in Client Care

1. Teaching about leg and foot care is an important intervention for clients with PVD. What normal changes of aging (such as decreased visual acuity) might necessitate adaptations of a teaching plan?
2. React to the statement: Decreased mobility means decreased independence. What aspects of independent living are threatened if this statement is true?
3. You are providing immediate postoperative care to a client who has had abdominal surgery and also has peripheral arterial occlusive disease. How will the latter affect your assessments and interventions for this client?
4. While making a home visit, your client tells you he is very worried that his leg might be amputated. How would you respond?

## Pain

Impaired blood flow results in tissue ischemia. Metabolism shifts from an efficient aerobic process to an anaerobic process. Lactic acid and metabolic waste products accumulate in tissues, causing pain. Severe and cramping pain generally occurs with exercise early in the disease. Rest initially produces relief, similar to the process of angina (see Chapter 29). ⊂⊃ As the disease progresses, pain develops with less exercise and often occurs even at rest. Rest pain disrupts sleep, the sense of well-being, and has significant disruptive effects on life roles.

- Assess pain at least every 4 hours; using a standard pain scale more often as needed. *Pain is a subjective experience. Using a standard pain scale allows evaluation of treatment measures in relieving pain and restoring blood flow.*
- Keep extremities warm. *Cooling leads to vasoconstriction, increasing pain. Warming the extremities promotes vasodilation and improves arterial flow, reducing pain.*
- Teach pain relief and stress reduction techniques such as relaxation, meditation, and guided imagery. *Pain increases stress. The stress response leads to vasoconstriction, increasing pain. Stress reduction techniques, when combined with other measures to promote blood flow, can help reduce pain.*

## Impaired Skin Integrity

Clients with PVD are at risk for impaired skin integrity as a result of oxygen and nutrient deprivation. Chronic tissue ischemia leads to dry, scaly, and atrophied skin. Pruritus can lead to scratching; minor injuries may go unnoticed due to impaired sensation. Impaired tissue healing can lead to ulceration, infection, and potential gangrene.

**PRACTICE ALERT** *Assess and document skin condition at least every 8 hours a with each home visit; more frequently as indicated. Tissue ischemia increases the risk for damage, even with minor trauma such as pressure from poorly fitting shoes or bed linens. Frequent inspection and documentation of skin condition is vital to identify early indicators of impaired skin integrity and reduce the risk of complications such as infection.* ■

- Provide meticulous daily skin care, keeping the skin clean and dry. Apply a moisturizing cream to dry or scaly areas. *Intact skin is the body's first defense against bacterial invasion. Ischemic tissues of the injured extremity provide an excellent medium for microorganism growth. Clean, dry, supple skin decreases the risk of breakdown.*
- Apply a bed cradle. *The bed cradle suspends bed linens over the legs, preventing them from placing pressure on extremities and injured tissues. Minimizing pressure on the tissues promotes capillary blood flow.*
- Provide an egg crate mattress, flotation pad, sheepskin, or heel protectors. *Ischemic tissues may be damaged by minor trauma such as that created by the shearing forces of skin against bed linens.*

## Activity Intolerance

Pain and impaired perfusion of peripheral tissues may limit the client's ability to engage in desired activities, even impairing self-care.

- Assist with care activities as needed. *Severe claudication or rest pain may limit activities. Muscle atrophy of affected extremities is common, leading to fatigue and weakness.*
- Unless contraindicated, encourage gradual increases in duration and intensity of exercise. Teach to rest with extremities dependent when claudication develops, resuming activity after pain has abated. *Gradual increases in the duration and intensity of exercise promote development of collateral circulation, improve exercise tolerance, provide a sense of well-being, and support self-esteem.*
- Provide diversional activities during periods of prescribed bed rest. Encourage relaxation techniques to reduce muscle tension. *Diversional activities help prevent boredom and stress associated with enforced rest. Relaxation techniques reduce vasoconstriction induced by stress, improving peripheral circulation.*
- Encourage frequent position changes and active range-of-motion exercises. Encourage self-care to the extent possible. *Position changes relieve pressure on tissues, improving capillary circulation and reducing tissue ischemia. Range-of-motion exercises help prevent muscle atrophy and joint contractures. Self-care supports self-esteem.*

## Using NANDA, NIC, and NOC

Chart 33-2 shows links between NANDA nursing diagnoses, NIC, and NOC for the client with peripheral atherosclerosis.

## Home Care

Discuss the following topics when preparing the client and family for home care.

- Smoking cessation strategies and ways to avoid secondhand smoke
- Prescribed medications and anticoagulants, their purpose, doses, desired and adverse effects
- Signs of excess bleeding to report to the physician
- Skin surveillance and foot care (see Box 33–4)
- Recommended diet and exercise
- Weight loss strategies if appropriate

If revascularization or surgery has been performed, include the following topics as appropriate.

- Incision care
- Manifestations of complications (e.g., infection, graft leakage, or thrombosis) to be reported to the physician
- Activity limitations

Provide referrals to home health services, physical or occupational therapy, and home maintenance assistance services as indicated. Consider resources such as Meals-on-Wheels for clients who are severely limited by their disease.

## CHART 33-2  NANDA, NIC, AND NOC LINKAGES

### The Client with Peripheral Atherosclerosis

| NURSING DIAGNOSES | NURSING INTERVENTIONS | NURSING OUTCOMES |
|---|---|---|
| • Activity Intolerance | • Exercise Promotion<br>• Self-Care Assistance<br>• Home Maintenance Assistance | • Activity Tolerance<br>• Self-Care: Instrumental Activities of Daily Living |
| • Chronic Pain | • Coping Enhancement<br>• Positioning<br>• Medication Management | • Comfort Level<br>• Pain: Disruptive Effects |
| • Ineffective Health Maintenance | • Behavior Modification<br>• Self-Responsibility Facilitation<br>• Teaching: Prescribed Activity/Exercise | • Health-Promoting Behavior<br>• Knowledge: Treatment Regimen<br>• Self-Direction of Care |
| • Ineffective Tissue Perfusion: Peripheral | • Circulatory Care: Arterial Insufficiency<br>• Positioning<br>• Neurologic Monitoring<br>• Skin Surveillance | • Tissue Integrity: Skin and Mucous Membranes<br>• Tissue Perfusion: Peripheral |

*Note. Data from Nursing Outcomes Classification (NOC) by M. Johnson & M. Maas (Eds.), 1997, St. Louis: Mosby; Nursing Diagnoses: Definitions & Classification 2001–2002 by North American Nursing Diagnosis Association, 2001, Philadelphia: NANDA; Nursing Interventions Classification (NIC) by J.C. McCloskey & G. M. Bulechek (Eds.), 2000, St. Louis: Mosby. Reprinted by permission.*

## Nursing Care Plan
## A Client with Peripheral Atherosclerosis

William Duffy, age 69, is retired. His wife convinces him to see his primary care provider for increasing leg pain with walking and other exercise.

### ASSESSMENT

Katie Kotson, RN, obtains Mr. Duffy's history before he sees his physician. He states that he can only walk about a block before the pain in his calves gets so bad that he has to stop and rest. As a result, he has been less and less active, spending most of his time the past few months watching sports on television. He denies rest pain. He was diagnosed with type 2 diabetes about 15 years ago, which he manages with daily glyburide (DiaBeta), an oral hypoglycemic. He also has stable angina, for which he takes atenolol (Tenormin) and an occasional nitroglycerin tablet. His alcohol intake is moderate, averaging 1 to 2 beers per day, and he smokes about a pack of cigarettes per day. He states he tried to quit smoking after developing angina, but "after nearly 50 years of smoking, I think that's impossible!"

Physical exam findings include: height 68 inches (173 cm), weight 235 lb (107 kg), BP 168/78, P 66, R 16, T 97.6°F (36.5°C); upper extremities warm and pink, normal hair distribution, pulses strong and equal; lower extremities below knees cool and ruddy when dependent, pale to pink when elevated, skin shiny, scant hair; posterior tibial pulses weak bilaterally; weak pedal pulse on R, unable to palpate on L; 1+ to 2+ edema both feet and ankles.

The physician finds that Mr. Duffy's systolic blood pressure in his legs is an average of 28 mmHg lower than in his arms. He makes the diagnosis of peripheral atherosclerosis, and schedules Mr. Duffy for an exercise stress test with ankle pressure measurements before and after exercise and a color-flow Doppler ultrasound. Mr. Duffy is to return in 3 weeks after these studies have been completed.

### DIAGNOSIS

- *Activity intolerance* related to poor blood flow to lower extremities
- *Ineffective health maintenance* related to smoking and lack of information about disease management
- *Risk for impaired skin integrity* related to ischemic tissues of legs and feet
- *Risk for peripheral neurovascular dysfunction* related to impaired peripheral blood flow to lower extremities

### EXPECTED OUTCOMES

- Walk for at least 15 minutes three to four times per day, gradually increasing his pace and duration of exercise.
- Relate the benefits of smoking cessation.
- Identify strategies to improve chances for success in stopping smoking.
- Meet with dietitian before next visit to discuss dietary measures to promote weight loss and slow atherosclerosis.
- Verbalize an understanding of appropriate foot care measures.
- Identify measures to prevent inadvertent injury of feet and legs.

*(continued on page 1008)*

## Nursing Care Plan
## A Client with Peripheral Atherosclerosis (continued)

### PLANNING AND IMPLEMENTATION

- Teach about peripheral atherosclerosis and its relationship to Mr. Duffy's symptoms.
- With Mr. and Mrs. Duffy, plan strategies to start and maintain a program of regular exercise.
- Instruct to warm up slowly, and to stop exercise and rest for 3 minutes (or until pain is relieved) when claudication develops, then resume exercising.
- Discuss the effects of smoking on blood vessels.
- Help Mr. Duffy identify smoking cessation strategies such as support groups, clinics, and nicotine patches.
- Schedule an appointment with the dietitian to develop a low-calorie, low-fat, and low-cholesterol ADA diet that includes preferred foods and considers usual eating patterns.
- Reinforce and supplement previous foot care teaching.
- Discuss effects of impaired circulation on sensation in feet and legs and measures to prevent injury.

### EVALUATION

When Mr. Duffy returns to the office 3 weeks later, his diagnosis has been confirmed by the diagnostic studies. The physician decides to continue conservative therapy, now prescribing atorvastatin (Lipitor) to lower Mr. Duffy's serum cholesterol level, and cilostazol (Pletal) to reduce the risk of thrombosis and improve symptoms of claudication. Mr. Duffy also asks his physician for a prescription for nicotine patches, saying he is ready to quit smoking, but thinks he needs help to be successful. Mr. and Mrs. Duffy tell Miss Kotson that they are walking before every meal and really enjoying being outside more. They plan to walk in the local shopping mall when the weather gets worse. Mrs. Duffy has bought an American Heart Association cookbook, and is carefully planning their meals. Both Mr. and Mrs. Duffy have lost 5 lb since the previous visit. Mr. Duffy's skin on his legs and feet remains intact, and he identifies the measures he is using to protect his lower extremities from injury.

### Critical Thinking in the Nursing Process

1. What additional lifestyle changes related to peripheral atherosclerosis might be appropriate to suggest to Mr. Duffy at this time? Why?
2. Explain the relationship between physical exercise and pain in the client with peripheral atherosclerosis. Compare this relationship to that between exercise and angina.
3. Mr. Duffy uses a beta blocker, atenolol, to prevent angina. Why is this drug not effective in preventing claudication?
4. Develop a nursing care plan for the diagnosis, *Imbalanced nutrition: More than body requirements*.

See Evaluating Your Response in Appendix C.

## THE CLIENT WITH THROMBOANGIITIS OBLITERANS

**Thromboangiitis obliterans** (also called *Buerger's disease*) is an occlusive vascular disease in which small and midsize peripheral arteries become inflamed and spastic, causing clots to form. This disease may affect either the upper or lower extremities; it often affects a leg or foot. Its exact etiology is unknown.

Thromboangiitis obliterans primarily affects men under age 40 who smoke. Cigarette smoking is the single most significant cause of Buerger's disease. The disease is more prevalent in Asians and people of Eastern European descent. The incidence of HLA-B5 and 2A9 antigens is higher in people with Buerger's disease, suggesting a genetic link.

The course of the disease is intermittent with dramatic exacerbations and marked remissions. The disease may remain dormant for periods of weeks, months, or years. As the disease progresses, collateral vessels are more extensively involved. Consequently, subsequent episodes are more intense and prolonged. Prolonged periods of tissue hypoxia increase the risk for tissue ulceration and gangrene.

### PATHOPHYSIOLOGY AND MANIFESTATIONS

Inflammatory cells infiltrate the wall of small and midsize arteries in the feet and possibly the hands. This inflammatory process is accompanied by thrombus formation and vasospasms of arterial segments that impair blood flow. Adjacent veins and nerves also may be affected. As the disease progresses, affected vessels become scarred and fibrotic.

Pain in the affected extremities is the primary manifestation of thromboangiitis obliterans. Both claudication, cramping pain in calves and feet or the forearms and hands, and rest pain in the fingers and toes may occur. Sensation is diminished. Eventually, the skin becomes thin and shiny and the nails are thickened and malformed. On examination, the involved digits and/or extremities are pale, cyanotic, or ruddy, and cool or cold to touch. Distal pulses (e.g., the dorsalis pedis, posterior tibial, ulnar, or radial) are either difficult to locate or absent, even with a Doppler device.

Painful ulcers and gangrene may develop in the fingers and toes, as a result of severely impaired blood flow. Amputation may be necessary to remove necrotic tissue.

## COLLABORATIVE CARE

Thromboangiitis obliterans usually is diagnosed by the history and physical examination. Doppler studies may be used to locate and determine the extent of the disease. Angiography and magnetic resonance imaging may also be used to evaluate the extent of the disease, but usually are unnecessary.

The one most important component in managing this disease is smoking cessation. While stopping smoking does not cure the disease, it may slow its extension to other vessels. With continued smoking, attacks become increasingly intense and last much longer, significantly increasing the risk for ulcerations and gangrene.

Additional conservative measures are used to prevent vasoconstriction, improve peripheral blood flow, and prevent complications of chronic ischemia. These measures include keeping extremities warm, managing stress, keeping affected extremities in a dependent position, preventing injury to affected tissues, and regular exercise. Walking for 20 or more minutes several times a day is recommended.

There are no specific drugs for thromboangiitis obliterans. A calcium channel blocker such as diltiazem (Cardizem) or verapamil (Isoptin), or pentoxifylline (Trental), which decreases blood viscosity and increases red blood cell flexibility to improve peripheral blood flow, may provide some symptom relief.

Surgical approaches for thromboangiitis obliterans include sympathectomy or arterial bypass graft. Sympathectomy interrupts sympathetic nervous system input to affected vessels, reducing vasoconstriction and spasm. Arterial bypass grafts may be useful when larger vessels are affected by the disease. Amputation of an affected digit or extremity may be necessary if gangrene develops (see Chapter 38 for more information about amputation). Only portions of digits or of limbs (e.g., below the knee) may be amputated, to preserve as much healthy tissue as possible.

The prognosis for thromboangiitis obliterans depends significantly on the client's ability and willingness to stop smoking. With smoking cessation and good foot care, the prognosis for saving the extremities is good, even though no cure is available.

## NURSING CARE

Health promotion activities to prevent thromboangiitis obliterans focus on preventing smoking, especially in high-risk populations. Nursing assessment and care for clients with this disease is similar to that provided for clients with other arterial occlusive diseases. Nursing care focuses on promoting arterial circulation and preventing prolonged tissue hypoxia. Because inflammatory, spastic episodes may be unpredictable, care focuses on smoking cessation and relieving acute manifestations. In addition, postsurgical care is necessary if surgery has been performed. See the nursing care section for peripheral atherosclerosis as well as nursing care of the postsurgical client (Chapter 7) and following amputation (Chapter 38).

### Home Care

Discuss the following topics when preparing clients with thromboangiitis obliterans and their families for home care.

- Absolute necessity of smoking cessation
- Foot care
- Protecting affected extremities from injury
- Purpose, dose, desired and adverse effects, interactions, and any precautions associated with prescribed medications
- Signs and symptoms to report to the physician

## THE CLIENT WITH RAYNAUD'S DISEASE

**Raynaud's disease** and **phenomenon** are characterized by episodes of intense vasospasm in the small arteries and arterioles of the fingers and sometimes the toes (Porth, 2002). Raynaud's disease and phenomenon differ only in terms of cause. Raynaud's disease has no identifiable cause; Raynaud's phenomenon occurs secondarily to another disease (such as collagen vascular diseases like scleroderma and rheumatoid arthritis), other known causes of vasospasm, or long-term exposure to cold or machinery (McCance & Huether, 2002; Porth, 2002).

Raynaud's disease primarily affects young women between the ages of 20 and 40. Genetic predisposition may play a role in its development, although the actual cause is unknown. Table 33–6 compares thromboangiitis obliterans and Raynaud's disease.

## PATHOPHYSIOLOGY AND MANIFESTATIONS

Raynaud's disease and phenomenon are characterized by spasms of the small arteries in the digits. The arterial spasms limit arterial blood flow to the fingers and possibly the toes. Initial attacks may involve only the tips of one or two fingers; with disease progression, the entire finger and all fingers may be affected.

The manifestations of Raynaud's occur intermittently when spasms develop. Raynaud's disease has been called "the blue-white-red disease," because affected digits initially turn blue as blood flow is reduced due to vasospasm, then white as circulation is more severely limited, and finally very red as the fingers are warmed and the spasm resolves. Sensory changes may occur during attacks, including numbness, stiffness, decreased sensation, and aching pain.

The attacks tend to become more frequent and prolonged over time. With repeated attacks (and resultant decrease in oxygenation), the fingertips thicken and the nails become brittle. Ulceration and gangrene are serious complications that rarely occur.

## COLLABORATIVE CARE

Raynaud's disease and phenomenon are primarily diagnosed by the history and physical examination. There are no specific diagnostic tests for these disorders.

Vasodilators may be prescribed to provide symptomatic relief. Low doses of a sustained release calcium channel blocker such as nifedipine (Procardia) or diltiazem (Cardizem) may be prescribed. The α-adrenergic blocker prazosin (Minipress) also may reduce the frequency and severity of attacks. Transdermal nitroglycerine (or longer-acting oral nitrates) helps some clients by decreasing the amount of time necessary for the hands to return to normal following an attack (Tierney et al., 2001).

Conservative measures are a mainstay of treatment. Clients are instructed to keep their hands warm, wearing gloves when outside in cold weather and kitchen gloves when handling cold items (for instance, when preparing and serving cold foods and cleaning the refrigerator). Measures to avoid injury to the hands are taught. Sometimes attacks can be stopped by

| TABLE 33–6 | Comparison of Raynaud's Disease and Thromboangiitis Obliterans | |
| --- | --- | --- |
| **Topic** | **Raynaud's Disease** | **Thromboangiitis Obliterans** |
| Etiology | • Unknown<br>• Possible genetic predisposition | • Cigarette smoking most probable single cause<br>• Possible autoimmune response |
| Incidence/course of the disease | • Onset commonly between 15 and 45 years of age<br>• Usually affects young women<br>• Becomes progressively worse over time | • Occurs predominantly in men under 40<br>• More common in Asians and people of European heritage<br>• Intermittent course with exacerbations and remissions<br>• Increase severity and duration of attacks over time |
| Triggering stimuli | • Emotional stress<br>• Exposure to cold | • Cigarette smoking |
| Assessment findings | • Usually affects hands, sometimes toes<br>• Pain becomes more severe and prolonged as disease progresses<br>• "Blue-white-red" changes in color of hands with accompanying changes in skin temperature | • Claudication and pain<br>• Numbness or diminished sensation<br>• Cool, pale or cyanotic skin<br>• Shiny, thin skin and white, malformed nails in affected extremities<br>• Distal pulses difficult to find or absent<br>• Trophic changes to nail beds<br>• Ulceration and gangrene in later stages<br>• Small, red, tender vascular cords in affected extremities |
| Management | • Avoid unnecessary cold exposure<br>• Emphasize smoking cessation<br>• Medications such as calcium channel or alpha adrenergic blockers as indicated<br>• Teach stress management | • Stop smoking (crucial)<br>• Regular exercise<br>• Protect extremities from cold injury<br>• Teach stress management |

swinging the arms back and forth, increasing perfusion pressure in the small arteries by centrifugal force.

Smoking cessation is important. Stress reduction measures such as exercise, relaxation techniques, massage therapy, hobbies, aroma therapy, and counseling are taught or suggested. Additional lifestyle habits that contribute to vascular health are encouraged, such as reducing dietary fat, increasing activity level, and maintaining normal body weight.

## NURSING CARE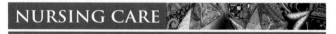

Nursing care for the client with Raynaud's disease or phenomenon is primarily educative and supportive. Protecting the hands and feet from exposure to cold and trauma is the major teaching topic. Nursing diagnoses and interventions previously outlined for peripheral atherosclerosis also are appropriate for clients with Raynaud's.

### Home Care

Reassure clients with Raynaud's phenomenon that most people with the disorder experience only mild, infrequent episodes. Discuss the following topics in preparing the client for managing the disorder.

• Dress warmly, keeping the trunk and hands warm.
• Avoid unnecessary exposure to cold.
• Stop smoking or do not start.
• The use, purpose, desired and potential adverse effects of prescribed medications, if any.

# DISORDERS OF VENOUS CIRCULATION

The two primary categories of venous system disorders are occlusive disorders and those related to ineffective venous blood flow. Impaired venous blood flow can lead to stasis and clotting, as well as tissue changes associated with venous congestion.

## PHYSIOLOGY REVIEW

The venous system is a low-pressure system in comparison with the arterial circulation. Veins and venules are thin-walled, distensible vessels. While they contain smooth muscle that allows them to contract or expand, the media (muscle layer) of veins is significantly thinner than that of arteries. The low pressures in the venous system allow it to serve as a reservoir for blood. Stimulation by the sympathetic nervous system causes veins to contract, helping maintain vascular volume. The low pressure venous system relies on skeletal muscle contractions and pressure changes in the abdomen and thorax to facilitate blood return to the heart. Unlike arteries, veins of the extremities contain valves to prevent retrograde blood flow.

## THE CLIENT WITH VENOUS THROMBOSIS

**Venous thrombosis** (also known as *thrombophlebitis*) is a condition in which a blood clot (thrombus) forms on the wall of a vein, accompanied by inflammation of the vein wall and some degree of obstructed venous blood flow.

Venous thrombi are more common than arterial thrombi because of lower pressures and flow within the venous system (McCance & Huether, 2002). Thrombi can form in either superficial or deep veins. **Deep venous thrombosis (DVT)** is a common complication of hospitalization, surgery, and immobilization. Obstetric and orthopedic procedures carry a higher risk for venous thrombosis; it may develop in more than 50% of clients having orthopedic surgery, particularly surgeries involving hip or knee (Braunwald et al., 2001). Other significant risk factors for venous thrombosis include abdominal or thoracic surgery, certain cancers, trauma, pregnancy, and use of oral contraceptives or hormone replacement therapy. See Box 33–5.

## PATHOPHYSIOLOGY AND MANIFESTATIONS

Three pathologic factors, called *Virchow's triad,* are associated with thrombophlebitis: stasis of blood, vessel damage, and increased blood coagulability. Vessel trauma stimulates the clotting cascade. Platelets aggregate at the site, particularly when venous stasis is present. Platelets and fibrin form the initial clot. Red blood cells are trapped in the fibrin meshwork, and the thrombus propagates (grows) in the direction of blood flow. The inflammatory response is triggered, causing tenderness,

| BOX 33–5 | ■ Factors Associated with Thrombophlebitis |
|---|---|

- ■ Immobilization: myocardial infarction, heart failure, stroke, postoperative
- ■ Surgery: orthopedic, thoracic, abdominal, genitourinary
- ■ Cancer: pancreatic, lung, ovary, testes, urinary tract, breast, stomach
- ■ Trauma: fractures of the spine, pelvis, femur, tibia; spinal cord injury
- ■ Pregnancy and delivery
- ■ Hormone therapy: oral contraceptives, hormone replacement therapy
- ■ Coagulation disorders

swelling, and erythema in the area of the thrombus. Initially the thrombus floats within the vein. Pieces of the thrombus may break loose and travel through the circulation as emboli. Fibroblasts eventually invade the thrombus, scarring the vein wall and destroying venous valves. Although patency of the vein may be restored, valve damage is permanent, affecting directional flow (Tierney et al., 2001).

### Deep Vein Thrombosis

The deep veins of the legs, primarily in the calf, and the pelvis provide the most hospitable environment for venous thrombosis. Approximately 80% of deep vein thromboses begin in the deep veins of the calf, often propagating into the popliteal and femoral veins (Figure 33–5 ■) (Tierney et al., 2001). DVT

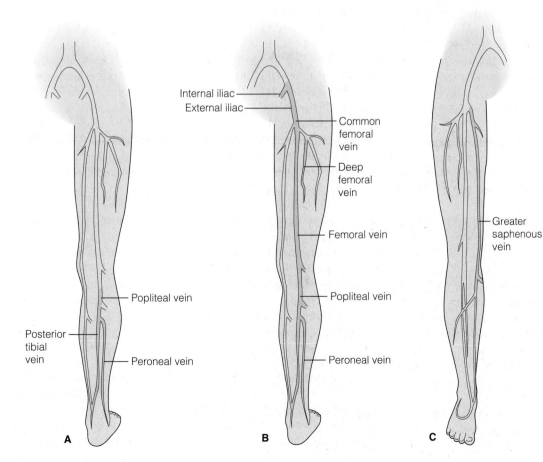

**Figure 33–5 ■** Common locations of venous thrombosis. *A,* The most common sites of deep vein thrombosis. *B,* DVT extending from the calf to the iliac veins. *C,* superficial venous thrombosis.

Internal iliac
External iliac
Common femoral vein
Deep femoral vein
Femoral vein
Popliteal vein
Peroneal vein

Posterior tibial vein
Popliteal vein
Peroneal vein

Greater saphenous vein

A    B    C

usually is asymptomatic; in some clients, a pulmonary embolism may be the first indication.

When present, the manifestations of DVT are primarily due to the inflammatory process accompanying the thrombus. Calf pain, which may be described as tightness or a dull, aching pain in the affected extremity, particularly upon walking, is the most common symptom. Tenderness, swelling, warmth, and erythema may be noted along the course of involved veins. The affected extremity may be cyanotic and often is edematous. Rarely, a cord may be palpated over the affected vein. A positive Homan's sign (pain in the calf when the foot is dorsiflexed) is an unreliable indicator of DVT. See the box below for a summary of the manifestations of deep and superficial venous thrombosis.

## Complications

The major complications of deep vein thrombosis are chronic venous insufficiency (see the next section of this chapter) and pulmonary embolism. Pulmonary embolism occurs when the clot fragments or breaks loose from the vein wall. As the clot travels, it moves through progressively larger veins and into the right side of the heart. From there it enters the pulmonary circulation, where it eventually occludes arterial flow to a portion of the lungs. The result is a mismatch between ventilation (air flow) and perfusion (blood flow) in a portion of the lungs. The effect on gas exchange depends on the size of the embolism and the vessel it occludes. See Chapter 36 ⊙ for more information about pulmonary emboli.

## Superficial Vein Thrombosis

Venous catheters and infusions are the primary risk factors for superficial venous thrombosis. Superficial vein thrombosis also may develop in conjunction with thromboangitis obliterans, varicose veins, or deep vein thrombosis. It may develop spontaneously in pregnant women or following delivery. In some cases, superficial venous thrombosis of the long saphenous vein is the earliest sign of an abdominal cancer such as pancreatic cancer (Tierney et al., 2001).

Superficial vein thrombosis is marked by pain and tenderness at the site of the thrombus. A reddened, warm, tender cord extending along the affected vein can be palpated. The area surrounding the vein may be swollen and red (see the box below).

## Manifestations of Venous Thrombosis

### DEEP VEIN THROMBOSIS
- Usually asymptomatic
- Dull, aching pain in affected extremity, especially when walking
- Possible tenderness, warmth, erythema along affected vein
- Cyanosis of affected extremity
- Edema of affected extremity

### SUPERFICIAL VEIN THROMBOSIS
- Localized pain and tenderness over the affected vein
- Redness and warmth along the course of the vein
- Palpable cordlike structure along the affected vein
- Swelling and redness of surrounding tissue

## COLLABORATIVE CARE

It is important to differentiate venous thrombosis from other causes of extremity pain, such as cellulitis, muscle strain, contusion, and lymphedema. The history, physical examination, and diagnostic tests are used to establish the diagnosis. Treatment focuses on preventing further clotting or extension of the clot and addressing underlying causes.

### Diagnostic Tests

- *Duplex venous ultrasonography* is a noninvasive test used to visualize the vein and measure the velocity of blood flow in the veins. Although the clot often cannot be visualized directly, its presence can be inferred by an inability to compress the vein during the examination.
- *Plethysmography* is a noninvasive test that measures changes in blood flow through the veins. It is often used in conjunction with Doppler ultrasonography. Plethysmography is most valuable in diagnosing thromboses of larger or more superficial veins.
- *Magnetic resonance imaging (MRI)* is another noninvasive means of detecting deep vein thrombosis. It is particularly useful when thrombosis of the vena cavae or pelvic veins is suspected.
- *Ascending contrast venography* uses an injected contrast medium to assess the location and extent of venous thrombosis. Although invasive, expensive, and uncomfortable, contrast venography is the most accurate diagnostic tool for venous thrombosis. It is used when the results of less invasive tests leave the diagnosis unclear (Tierney et al., 2001).

### Prophylaxis

Medications and other measures are used to prevent venous thrombosis when the risk is high. Low-molecular-weight heparins (see below) prevent deep vein thrombosis in clients who are undergoing general or orthopedic surgery, experiencing acute medical illness, or on prolonged bed rest. Oral anticoagulation also may be used as a prophylactic measure in clients with fractures or who are undergoing orthopedic surgery.

Elevating the foot of the bed with the knees slightly flexed promotes venous return. Early mobilization and leg exercises such as ankle flexion and extension assist venous flow by muscle compression. Intermittent pneumatic compression devices applied to the legs are effective to prevent DVT. They also are used when anticoagulation is contraindicated due to the increased risk for bleeding (Braunwald et al., 2001). Elastic stockings are used to prevent venous thrombosis as well in clients at risk.

### Medications

Anticoagulants to prevent clot propagation and enable the body's own lytic system to dissolve the clot are the mainstay of treatment for venous thrombosis. Thrombolytic drugs such as streptokinase or tissue plasminogen activator (t-PA) may accelerate the process of clot lysis and prevent damage to venous valves. There is, however, no evidence that thrombolytic therapy is more effective in preventing pulmonary embolism than anticoagulants (Braunwald et al., 2001). It also significantly increases the risk for bleeding and hemorrhage.

Nonsteroidal anti-inflammatory agents such as indomethacin (Indocin) or naproxen (Naprosyn) may be ordered to reduce inflammation in the veins and provide symptomatic relief, particularly for clients with superficial vein thrombosis.

### Anticoagulants

Anticoagulants are given to prevent clot extension and reduce the risk of subsequent pulmonary embolism. Anticoagulation is initiated with unfractionated heparin or low-molecular-weight (LMW) heparin. Following an initial intravenous bolus of 7,500 to 10,000 units of unfractionated heparin, a continuous heparin infusion of 1000 to 1500 IU per hour is started. The dosage is calculated to maintain the activated partial thromboplastin time (aPTT) at approximately twice the control or normal value. An infusion pump is used to deliver the prescribed dosage. Frequent monitoring of the infusion is an important nursing responsibility. Subcutanous heparin injections may be used as an alternate to intravenous infusion in some instances.

LMW heparins are increasingly used to prevent and treat venous thrombosis. They do not require the close laboratory monitoring of unfractionated heparins. LMW heparin is administered subcutaneously in fixed doses once or twice daily, allowing the option of outpatient treatment. LMW heparins have additional advantages, in that they are more effective and carry lower risks for bleeding and thrombocytopenia than conventional, unfractionated heparins.

Oral anticoagulation with warfarin may be initiated concurrently with heparin therapy. Overlapping heparin and warfarin therapy for 4 to 5 days is important because the full anticoagulant effect of warfarin is delayed, and it may actually promote clotting during the first few days of therapy (Tierney et al., 2001). Warfarin doses are adjusted to maintain the international normalized ratio (INR) at 2.0 to 3.0 (Braunwald et al., 2001).

Once this level is achieved, the heparin is discontinued and a maintenance dose of warfarin is prescribed to prevent recurrent thrombosis. Anticoagulation generally is continued for at least 3 months. When DVT is recurrent or risk factors such as altered coagulability or cancer are present, anticoagulant therapy may be prolonged. Regular follow-up is necessary to be sure prothrombin times (INR) remain within the desirable range for anticoagulation. See the Medication Administration box below for the nursing implications for anticoagulant therapy.

## Medication Administration

### Anticoagulant Therapy

#### HEPARIN

Heparin interferes with the clotting cascade by inhibiting the effects of thrombin and preventing the conversion of fibrinogen to fibrin. This prevents the formation of a stable fibrin clot. At therapeutic levels, heparin prolongs the thrombin time, clotting time, and activated partial thromboplastin time. When given intravenously, its effect is immediate. Given subcutaneously, its onset of action is within 1 hour. When heparin is discontinued, clotting times return to normal within 2 to 6 hours (Spratto & Woods, 2003).

#### Nursing Responsibilities

- Assess for history of unexplained or active bleeding. Assess laboratory results for abnormal clotting profile or evidence of active bleeding.
- Give a test dose as indicated to clients with a history of multiple allergies or a history of asthma.
- Administer by deep subcutaneous injection; abdominal sites are preferred. Avoid injecting within 2 inches of the umbilicus. Rotate sites. Do not aspirate prior to injecting or massage after the injection.
- Intravenous solutions may be diluted with dextrose, normal saline, or Ringer's solution. Use an infusion pump.
- Keep protamine sulfate, a heparin antagonist, available to treat excessive bleeding.
- Monitor and report abnormal laboratory results and aPTT values outside the desired range.
- Promptly report evidence of bleeding such as hematemesis, hematuria, bleeding gums, or unexplained abdominal or back pain.

#### Client and Family Teaching

- Report unusual bleeding or excessive menstrual flow.
- Use an electric razor and a soft-bristle toothbrush; prevent injury by clearing pathways, using a night light, and other measures. Do not consume alcohol.
- Avoid contact sports while on anticoagulant therapy.
- Do not consume large amounts of food rich in vitamin K (yellow and dark green vegetables).
- Do not use aspirin or NSAIDs while on heparin therapy unless advised to do so by your physician.
- Wear a MedicAlert tag and advise all health care providers (including dentists and podiatrists) of therapy.

#### LOW-MOLECULAR-WEIGHT HEPARINS

| | |
|---|---|
| Ardeparin (Normiflo) | Enoxaparin (Lovenox) |
| Dalteparin (Fragmin) | Tinzaparin (Innohep) |

LMW heparins are the most bioavailable fraction of heparin. They provide a more precise and predictable anticoagulant effect than unfractionated heparins. Like unfractionated heparin, LMW heparin prevents conversion of prothrombin to thrombin, liberation of thromboplastin from platelets, and formation of a stable clot. LMW heparins cannot be used interchangeably with each other or with unfractionated heparin.

#### Nursing Responsibilities

- Assess for evidence of active bleeding, a history of bleeding disorders or thrombocytopenia, or sensitivity to heparin, sulfites, or pork products.

*(continued on page 1014)*

## Medication Administration

### Anticoagulant Therapy (continued)

- Monitor for unusual or masked bleeding. PT and aPTT levels may be within normal levels even in the presence of hemorrhage.
- Administer by deep subcutaneous injection into abdominal wall, thigh, or buttocks. Rotate sites. Do not aspirate or massage.

#### Client and Family Teaching

- Subcutaneous self-administration technique, timing of doses, and site rotation. Do not rub site after administering to minimize bruising.
- Do not take aspirin, NSAIDs, or other over-the-counter drugs unless recommended by your physician.
- Promptly report excessive bruising or bleeding, chest pain, difficulty breathing, itching, rash, or swelling to your health care provider.
- Keep follow-up appointments as scheduled.

#### ORAL ANTICOAGULANT

Warfarin (Coumadin)

Warfarin interferes with synthesis of vitamin K–dependent clotting factors by the liver, leading to depletion of these factors. It has no effect on already circulating clotting factors or on existing clots. Warfarin inhibits extension of existing thrombi and the formation of new clots. Its action is cumulative and more prolonged than that of heparin.

#### Nursing Responsibilities

- Assess laboratory results and history for evidence of abnormal bleeding.
- Multiple drugs affect the metabolism and protein binding of warfarin; note all medications and assess for interactions with warfarin.

- Do not give during pregnancy as warfarin may cause congenital malformations.
- Oral tablets may be crushed and given without regard to meals.
- Dilute intravenous warfarin with supplied diluent; administer within 4 hours by direct intravenous injection at a rate of 25 mg/min.
- Keep vitamin K available to reverse effects of warfarin in the event of excessive bleeding or hemorrhage.
- Monitor PT or INR; report values outside the desired range.

#### Client and Family Teaching

- Do not take your prescribed dose and notify your physician immediately if bleeding occurs (hematemesis, bright red or black tarry feces, hematuria, bleeding gums, excessive bruising, etc.). Report rash or manifestations of hepatitis (dark urine, malaise, yellow skin or sclera).
- Take your warfarin at the same time every day; do not change brands as their effects may differ.
- Menstrual bleeding may be slightly increased; contact your health care provider if it increases significantly. Use reliable birth control to prevent pregnancy while taking warfarin. Immediately contact your health care provider if you think you may be pregnant.
- Take precautions to prevent injury and bleeding: use a soft toothbrush and electric razor, wear shoes, and use a night light. Avoid participating in contact sports.
- Do not smoke, use alcohol, or take any over-the-counter drugs unless specifically recommended by your health care provider. Notify all health care providers, including dentists and podiatrists, of therapy. Wear a MedicAlert tag.
- Obtain lab tests as scheduled and keep all scheduled follow-up appointments.

MediaLink | WARFARIN ANIMAITON

## Treatments

Treatment of venous thrombosis also includes measures to relieve symptoms and reduce inflammation. With superficial vein thrombosis, applying warm, moist compresses over the affected vein, extremity rest, and anti-inflammatory agents usually provide relief of symptoms.

Bed rest may be ordered for deep vein thrombosis. The duration of bed rest typically is determined by the extent of leg edema. The legs are elevated 15 to 20 degrees, with the knees slightly flexed, above the level of the heart to promote venous return and discourage venous pooling. Elastic antiembolism stockings (TEDS) or pneumatic compression devices are also frequently ordered to stimulate the muscle-pumping mechanism that promotes the return of blood to the heart. When permitted, walking is encouraged while avoiding prolonged standing or sitting. Crossing the legs also is avoided, as are tight-fitting garments or stockings that bind.

## Surgery

Venous thrombosis usually is effectively treated with conservative measures and anticoagulation. In some cases, however,

surgery is required to remove the thrombus, prevent its extension into deep veins, or prevent the effects of embolization.

*Venous thrombectomy* is done when thrombi lodge in the femoral vein and their removal is necessary to prevent pulmonary embolism or gangrene. Successful thrombus removal rapidly improves venous circulation. The duration of this effect varies.

When venous thrombosis is recurrent and anticoagulant therapy is contraindicated, a filter may be inserted into the vena cava to capture emboli from the pelvis and lower extremities, preventing pulmonary embolism. Several different filters are available (Figure 33–6 ■). The Greenfield filter is widely used for its ability to trap emboli within its apex while maintaining patency of the vena cava. The filter can be inserted under fluoroscopy with local anesthesia. Mortality and morbidity associated with the filter are very low (Meeker & Rothrock, 1999).

Extensive thrombosis of the saphenous vein may necessitate ligation and division of the saphenous vein where it joins the femoral vein to prevent clot extension into the deep venous system. A vein affected by septic venous thrombosis is excised to control the infection. Antibiotic therapy also is initiated.

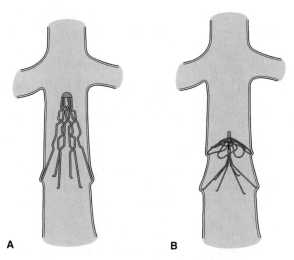

**Figure 33–6** ■ Venal caval filters. *A*, Greenfield filter. *B*, Nitinol filter.

## NURSING CARE

### Health Promotion

Prevention of venous thrombosis is an important component of nursing care for all at-risk clients. Position clients to promote venous blood flow from the lower extremities, with the feet elevated and the knees slightly bent. Avoid placing pillows under the knees and positions in which the hips and knees are sharply flexed. Use a recliner chair or foot stool when sitting. Ambulate clients as soon as possible, and maintain a regular schedule of ambulation throughout the day. Teach ankle flexion and extension exercises, and frequently remind clients to perform them. Apply elastic hose and pneumatic compression devices when appropriate. Instruct clients to avoid crossing legs when in bed or sitting. Inquire about possible prophylactic heparin or warfarin therapy for clients undergoing orthopedic surgery or other high-risk procedures. Frequently assess intravenous sites. Change the site and catheter as dictated by agency protocol and if evidence of local inflammation is noted.

### Assessment

Assess clients at risk for venous thrombosis for manifestations and risk factors.

- Health history: complaints of leg or calf pain, its duration and characteristics, and the effect of walking on the pain; history of venous thrombosis or other clotting disorders; current medications
- Physical examination: inspect affected extremity for redness, edema; palpate for tenderness, warmth, cordlike structures; body temperature

### Nursing Diagnoses and Interventions

In addition to the preventive measures identified earlier, priority nursing diagnoses for the client with venous thrombosis relate to pain, maintenance of tissue perfusion and integrity, and the potential adverse effects of prescribed treatments.

### Pain

The pain associated with venous thrombosis results from inflammation of the involved vein. It may be aggravated by use of the involved extremity. Associated edema and swelling may contribute to discomfort. Measures to reduce the inflammation often help relieve the pain.

- Regularly assess pain location, characteristics, and level using a standardized pain scale. Report increasing pain or changes in its location or characteristics. *Tissue substances released during the inflammatory process can stimulate pain receptors. In addition, localized swelling presses on pain-sensitive structures in the area of the inflammation, contributing to discomfort. As inflammation and swelling are reduced, pain should abate. Continued or increasing pain may indicate extension of the thrombosis. Sudden chest pain may indicate a pulmonary embolism, necessitating immediate intervention.*
- Measure calf and thigh diameter of the affected extremity on admission and daily thereafter. Report increases promptly. *The inflammatory process causes vasodilation and increases vessel permeability, causing edema of the affected extremity. Baseline and subsequent measurements provide a measure of treatment effectiveness.*
- Apply warm, moist heat to affected extremity at least four times daily, using warm, moist compresses or an aqua-K pad. *Moist heat penetrates tissues to a greater depth. Warmth promotes vasodilation, allowing reabsorption of excess fluid into the circulation. Vasodilation also reduces resistance within the affected vessel, reducing pain. As edema subsides, pressure on surrounding tissues is relieved, thereby reducing pain.*
- Maintain bed rest as ordered. *Using leg muscles during walking exacerbates the inflammatory process and increases edema. This, in turn, increases venous compression and pain.*

### Ineffective Tissue Perfusion: Peripheral

As thrombi develop, they occlude the lumen of the vein and obstruct blood flow. In addition, the accompanying inflammatory response may precipitate vessel spasms, further impairing arterial and venous blood flow and tissue perfusion. Impaired tissue perfusion, in turn, deprives tissues of nutrients and oxygen. As a result, distal tissues of the affected extremity are at risk for ulceration and infection.

**PRACTICE ALERT** *Assess peripheral pulses, skin integrity, capillary refill times, and color of extremities at least every 8 hours. Report changes promptly. Assessment of both extremities allows comparison of the affected and unaffected limbs. Weak or absent pulses, impaired capillary refill, or significant color changes in the affected extremity may indicate extension of the thrombus or a possible complication.* ■

- Assess skin of the affected lower leg and foot at least every 8 hours; more often as indicated. *Frequent assessment is important to rapidly detect early signs of tissue breakdown and implementation of measures to protect vulnerable tissues. Early intervention allows healing and restoration of tissue integrity; allowed to continue, the process can lead to necrosis and potential gangrene.*
- Elevate extremities at all times, keeping knees slightly flexed and legs above the level of the heart. *Elevation of the extremities promotes venous return and reduces peripheral edema. Knee flexion promotes muscle relaxation.*

**PRACTICE ALERT** *Remove antiembolic stockings or pneumatic compression device for 30 to 60 minutes during daily hygiene. Antiembolic stockings (e.g., TED hose) and pneumatic compression devices exert pressure on the extremity and promote venous return. They can, however, impair perfusion of the dermis. Removing them periodically allows assessment of the underlying tissue and restores perfusion of the dermis, reducing the risk for skin breakdown. Their use may be continued following discharge to reduce the risk of recurrent venous thrombosis.* ■

- Use mild soaps, solutions, and lotions to clean the affected leg and foot daily. Pat dry after washing, and apply a nonalcohol-based lotion or moisturizing cream. *Daily hygiene with nondrying soaps and solutions removes potential pathogens from the skin surface, and maintains skin integrity and the first line of defense against infection. Caustic or harsh soaps or solutions can dry and crack the skin. Dry, cracked skin permits bacteria and other microorganisms to enter and infect the tissue, potentially leading to ulceration and venous gangrene.*
- Use egg crate mattress or sheepskin on the bed as needed. *Egg crate mattresses and sheepskins distribute weight more evenly, preventing excess pressure on affected tissues.*
- Encourage frequent position changes, at least every 2 hours while awake. *Frequent position changes reduce pressure on bony prominences and edematous tissue, reducing the risk of tissue breakdown.*

### Ineffective Protection

Anticoagulant therapy interferes with the body's normal clotting mechanisms, increasing the risk for bleeding and hemorrhage.

**PRACTICE ALERT** *Assess for and promptly report evidence of bleeding, such as petechiae, bruising, bleeding gums, obvious or occult blood in vomitus, stool, or urine, unexplained back or abdominal pain. Anticoagulants interfere with the ability to form a stable clot and prevent excessive bleeding. Even minor trauma such as toothbrushing or bumping into furniture can result in bleeding.* ■

- Monitor laboratory results, including the INR (prothrombin time), aPTT, hemoglobin, and hematocrit as indicated. Report values outside the normal or desired range. *Coagulation studies are used to monitor the effect of anticoagulant medications. Values within the desired range prevent further clot*

*development while carrying a low risk for bleeding and hemorrhage. A fall in the hemoglobin and hematocrit may indicate undetected bleeding.*

### Impaired Physical Mobility

Although prolonged bed rest rarely is required, it is associated with many problems, including constipation, joint contractures, muscle atrophy, and boredom. Nursing care goals include maintaining joint range of motion, minimizing muscle atrophy, and reducing boredom.

- Encourage active range-of-motion exercises at least every 8 hours. Provide passive range of motion as needed. *Range-of-motion exercises maintain joint mobility and prevent contractures. Active range of motion (performed by the client) also helps prevent muscle atrophy and preserve function. While passive range-of-motion exercises do not prevent muscle atrophy, they do maintain joint mobility.*
- Encourage frequent position changes, deep breathing, and coughing. *Prolonged immobility can lead to impaired airway clearance and respiratory complications, such as atelectasis or pneumonia. Turning, coughing, and deep breathing facilitate expulsion of secretions from the respiratory tract, airway clearance, and alveolar ventilation.*
- Encourage increased fluid and dietary fiber intake. *Constipation is a frequent complication of immobility due to decreased gastrointestinal motility and loss of abdominal muscle strength. Increasing fluid and fiber intake helps maintain soft, easily expelled stools.*
- Assist with and encourage ambulation as allowed. *Ambulation promotes venous blood flow, helps maintain muscle tone and joint mobility, and increases the sense of well-being.*
- Encourage diversional activities such as reading, handiwork or other hobbies, television or video games, and socializing. *Boredom may lead to dozing and inertia, with little physical movement or mental stimulation, increasing the risk for complications of immobility.*

### Risk for Ineffective Tissue Perfusion: Cardiopulmonary

A thrombus that forms in the deep veins of the legs or pelvis may break loose or fragment, becoming an embolism. Emboli that originate in the venous system usually become trapped in the pulmonary circulation (pulmonary embolism). Gas exchange in the affected area is impaired as blood flow ceases or is reduced to an area of the lungs that is well ventilated (see Chapter 36). ∞

- Frequently assess respiratory status, including rate, depth, ease, and oxygen saturation levels. *A mismatch of ventilation and perfusion can significantly affect gas exchange, leading to rapid, shallow respirations, dyspnea and air hunger, and a fall in oxygen saturation levels.*

**PRACTICE ALERT** *Immediately report complaints of chest pain and shortness of breath, anxiety, or a sense of impending doom. The manifestations of pulmonary embolism are similar to those of myocardial infarction. Prompt intervention to restore pulmonary blood flow can reduce the risk of significant adverse effects.* ■

## CHART 33-3 NANDA, NIC, AND NOC LINKAGES

### The Client with Venous Thrombosis

| NURSING DIAGNOSES | NURSING INTERVENTIONS | NURSING OUTCOMES |
|---|---|---|
| • Impaired Physical Mobility | • Exercise Therapy: Joint Mobility<br>• Environmental Management: Safety | • Joint Movement: Active<br>• Ambulation: Walking |
| • Ineffective Health Maintenance | • Teaching: Prescribed Activity/Exercise<br>• Teaching: Prescribed Medication | • Knowledge: Health Behaviors<br>• Knowledge: Treatment Regimen |
| • Ineffective Protection | • Bleeding Precautions | • Coagulation Status |
| • Ineffective Tissue Perfusion: Peripheral | • Circulatory Care: Venous Insufficiency<br>• Positioning | • Tissue Integrity: Skin and Mucous Membranes<br>• Tissue Perfusion: Peripheral |
| • Pain | • Heat/Cold Application<br>• Coping Enhancement | • Comfort Level<br>• Pain: Disruptive Effects |

*Note. Data from Nursing Outcomes Classification (NOC) by M. Johnson & M. Maas (Eds.), 1997, St. Louis: Mosby; Nursing Diagnoses: Definitions & Classification 2001–2002 by North American Nursing Diagnosis Association, 2001, Philadelphia: NANDA; Nursing Interventions Classification (NIC) by J.C. McCloskey & G. M. Bulechek (Eds.), 2000, St. Louis: Mosby. Reprinted by permission.*

- Initiate oxygen therapy, elevate the head of the bed, and reassure the client who is experiencing manifestations of pulmonary embolism. *Oxygen therapy and elevating the head of the bed promote ventilation and gas exchange in those alveoli that are well perfused, helping maintain tissue oxygenation. Reassurance helps reduce anxiety and slow the respiratory rate, promoting greater respiratory depth and alveolar ventilation.*

## Using NANDA, NIC, and NOC

Chart 33–3 shows links between NANDA nursing diagnoses, NIC, and NOC for the client with venous thrombosis.

## Home Care

Treatment measures for venous thrombosis may be initiated and carried out on an outpatient basis or continued for an ex-

tended period of time following hospital discharge. Include the following topics when teaching for home care.

- Explanation of the disease process
- Treatment measures, including laboratory tests and their purposes, medications and adverse effects that should be reported
- Appropriate methods of heat application
- Prescribed activity restrictions
- Measures to prevent future episodes of venous thrombosis
- The importance of follow-up visits and laboratory tests as scheduled

Refer clients for community nursing services for continued assessment and reinforcement of teaching. Provide referrals for assistance with ADLs and home maintenance services as indicated. Consider referral for physical therapy if needed.

## Nursing Care Plan
## A Client with Deep Vein Thrombosis

Mrs. Opal Hipps, age 75, lives alone with her dog, Chester, in her family home in the suburbs. She retired from her job as a postal clerk 10 years ago and now spends a lot of time reading and watching television. Over the past week she has developed a vague aching pain in her right leg. She ignored the pain until last night when it developed into a much more severe pain in her right calf. She noticed that her right lower leg seemed larger than the left, and it was very tender to the touch. After seeing her physician and undergoing Doppler ultrasound studies, Mrs. Hipps is admitted to the hospital with the diagnosis of deep vein thrombosis in the right leg. She is placed on bed rest, and intravenous heparin. Michael Cookson, RN, is assigned to admit and care for Mrs. Hipps.

### ASSESSMENT

Mr. Cookson notices that Mrs. Hipps was admitted 14 months ago for repair of a fractured femur. Mrs. Hipps says, "This business about a blood clot really has me worried." She also tells Mr. Cookson that she is worried about who will care for her dog while she is in the hospital. Physical findings include: height 62 inches (157 cm), weight 149 lb (68 kg), T 99.2 F (37.3°C); vital signs within normal limits otherwise. Her left leg is warm and pink, with strong peripheral pulses and good capillary refill. Her right calf is dark red, very warm, and dry to touch. It is tender to palpation. The right femoral and popliteal pulses are strong, but the pedal and posterior tibial pulses are difficult to locate. The right calf diameter is 0.5 inch (1.27 cm) larger than the left.

(continued on page 1018)

## Nursing Care Plan
## A Client with Deep Vein Thrombosis *(continued)*

### DIAGNOSIS
- *Pain* related to inflammatory response in affected vein
- *Anxiety* related to unexpected hospitalization and uncertainty about the seriousness of her illness
- *Ineffective tissue perfusion: Peripheral* related to decreased venous circulation in the right leg
- *Risk for impaired skin integrity* related to pooling of venous blood in the right leg

### EXPECTED OUTCOMES
- Verbalize relief of right leg pain by day of discharge.
- Verbalize reduced anxiety by the second day of her hospitalization.
- Demonstrate reduced right leg diameter by 0.25 inch (0.64 cm) by the fifth day of hospitalization.
- Maintain intact skin in the right foot throughout the hospital stay.

### PLANNING AND IMPLEMENTATION
- Elevate legs, maintaining slight knee flexion, while in bed.
- Apply warm, moist compresses to right leg using a 2-hour-on, 2-hour-off schedule around the clock.
- Administer prescribed analgesics and evaluate effectiveness.
- Spend time with Mrs. Hipps to explain venous thrombosis and its treatment.
- Arrange for a friend or neighbor to care for Mrs. Hipps's dog.
- Apply antiembolism stockings as ordered; remove for 30 minutes every 8 hours.
- Monitor laboratory values to assess effect of anticoagulant therapy; report values outside desired range.
- Assist with progressive ambulation when allowed.
- Inspect legs and feet and record findings every 8 hours.

### EVALUATION
Seven days after admission, the pain in Mrs. Hipps's right leg has subsided and the diameter of her right calf is equal to her left calf. Mrs. Hipps admits to Mr. Cookson that her fears really relate to a cousin who was hospitalized for a similar problem and had his leg amputated. After talking about her condition and the steps she can take to prevent its recurrence, she is much less anxious. Before discharge, Mr. Cookson reviews instructions for antiembolism stockings, daily walking, warfarin schedule, and scheduled follow-up appointment. Her neighbor, Kate, came to pick her up. As Mr. Cookson was helping Mrs. Hipps into the car, Kate handed her a small brown dog and said, "I took good care of Chester for you, but he's missed you." Mrs. Hipps smiled, and assured Mr. Cookson that she would call the number he provided if she had any questions.

### Critical Thinking in the Nursing Process
1. Describe the pathophysiologic reasons for the pain in Mrs. Hipps's right leg.
2. How would you respond if Mrs. Hipps tells you she does not have the money to buy the prescribed anticoagulant when she goes home?
3. How would you change your teaching and discharge planning if Mrs. Hipps had difficulty caring for herself?
4. Design a plan of care for Mrs. Hipps for the diagnosis, *Activity intolerance.*

See Evaluating Your Response in Appendix C.

## THE CLIENT WITH CHRONIC VENOUS INSUFFICIENCY

**Chronic venous insufficiency** is a disorder of inadequate venous return over a prolonged period. Deep vein thrombosis is the most frequent cause of chronic venous insufficiency. Other conditions, such as varicose veins or leg trauma, may contribute; in some instances, it develops without an identified precipitating cause (Braunwald et al., 2001; Tierney et al., 2001).

## PATHOPHYSIOLOGY

Following DVT, large veins may remain occluded, increasing the pressure in other veins of the extremity. This increased pressure distends the veins, separating valve leaflets and impairing their ability to close. DVT also damages valve leaflets, causing them to thicken and contract. The result is impaired unidirectional blood flow and deep vein emptying (Porth, 2002).

When venous valves are incompetent, the muscle-pumping action produced during activity cannot propel blood back to the heart. Venous blood collects and stagnates in the lower leg (*venous stasis*). Venous pressures in the calf and lower leg increase, particularly during ambulation. This increased pressure impairs arterial circulation to the lower extremities as well. The body's ability to provide sufficient oxygen and nutrients to the cells and remove metabolic waste products diminishes. Eventually, there is so little oxygen and nutrients that cells begin to die. The skin atrophies, and subcutaneous fat deposits necrose. Breakdown of red blood cells in the congested tissues causes brown skin pigmentation (Porth, 2002). Venous stasis ulcers develop. Congested tissues impair the body's ability to increase the supply of oxygen, nutrients, and metabolic energy to heal the ulcer. As a result, the condition worsens and, over time, the ulcers enlarge. The congested venous circulation also prevents the blood from mounting effective inflammatory and immune responses, significantly increasing the risk for infection in the ulcerated tissue (McCance & Huether, 2002).

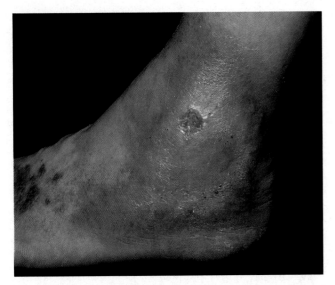

**Figure 33–7** ■ Chronic venous insufficiency. Note the discoloration of the ankle and the stasis ulcer.

*Source: Camera M. D. Studios. Carroll H. Weiss, Director. 8290 N. W. 26th Place. Sunrise, FL 33322.*

## MANIFESTATIONS

Manifestations of chronic venous insufficiency include lower leg edema, itching, and discomfort of the affected extremity that increase with prolonged standing. The extremity is cyanotic. Recurrent stasis ulcers develop (Figure 33–7 ■), usually forming just above the ankle, on the medial or anterior aspect of the leg. They heal poorly, forming scar tissue that breaks down easily. Tissue surrounding the ulcer is shiny, atrophic, and cyanotic, and there is a brownish pigmentation to the skin. Other skin changes may develop as well, such as eczema or stasis dermatitis. Necrosis and fibrosis of subcutaneous tissue causes the affected area of the leg to feel hard and somewhat leathery to the touch, but even the slightest trauma to the area can produce serious tissue breakdown. See the box on this page for the manifestations of chronic venous insufficiency. Table 33–7 compares venous and arterial ulcers.

### Manifestations of Chronic Venous Insufficiency

- Lower extremity edema that worsens with standing
- Itching, dull leg discomfort or pain that increases with standing
- Thin, shiny, atrophic skin
- Cyanosis and brown skin pigmentation of lower leg and foot
- Possible weeping dermatitis
- Thick, fibrous (hard) subcutaneous tissue
- Recurrent ulcerations of medial or anterior ankle

## COLLABORATIVE CARE

Collaborative care for the client with venous insufficiency focuses on relieving symptoms, promoting adequate circulation, and healing and preventing tissue damage.

The history and physical examination often establish the diagnosis of chronic venous insufficiency. Because a history of deep vein thrombosis is a major risk factor, careful evaluation of the past medical history and questioning of the client is important. There are no specific diagnostic tests to confirm the diagnosis of chronic venous insufficiency.

Conservative management of venous insufficiency focuses on reducing edema and treating ulcerations. Prolonged standing or sitting is discouraged. Graduated compression hosiery is ordered for daytime use, and frequent elevation of the legs and feet during the day is recommended. At night, the legs and feet should be elevated above the level of the heart by raising the foot of the mattress.

Treatment of associated stasis dermatitis varies, based on the duration of the condition. Wet compresses of boric acid, buffered aluminum actetate (Burrow's solution), or isotonic saline solution are applied to acute weeping dermatitis four times a day for 1-hour periods. Following the compress, a topical corticosteroid (such as 0.5% hydrocortisone cream) is applied. Bed rest is prescribed during the acute period. Stasis dermatitis that is subsiding or chronic may be treated with a topical

| TABLE 33–7 | Comparison of Arterial and Venous Leg Ulcers | |
| --- | --- | --- |
| **Factor** | **Arterial Ulcers** | **Venous Ulcers** |
| Location | Toes, feet, shin | Over medial or anterior ankle |
| Ulcer appearance | Deep, pale | Superficial, pink |
| Skin appearance | Normal to atrophic<br>Pallor on elevation<br>Rubor on dependency | Brown discoloration<br>Stasis dermatitis<br>Cyanosis on dependency |
| Skin temperature | Cool | Normal |
| Edema | Absent or mild | May be significant |
| Pain | Usually severe<br>Intermittent claudication<br>Rest pain | Usually mild<br>Aching pain |
| Gangrene | May occur | Does not occur |
| Pulses | Decreased or absent | Normal |

corticosteroid, zinc oxide ointment, or a topical broad-spectrum antifungal cream such as clotrimazole (Lotrimin) cream or miconazole (Monistat) cream (Tierney et al., 2001).

Isotonic saline compresses or wet-to-dry dressings are applied to stasis ulcers to promote healing. A dilute topical antibiotic solution also may be used (Braunwald et al., 2001). The ulcer may be treated by using a semirigid boot applied to the foot and lower leg. This device may be made of Unna's paste or Gauzetex bandage. Bony prominences must be well padded. The boot must be changed every 1 to 2 weeks, depending on the amount of drainage from the ulcer. This device often allows ambulatory treatment.

A very large, chronic ulcer may require surgery. In this case, the incompetent veins are ligated, the ulcer is excised, and the area is covered with a skin graft (see Chapter 14).

## NURSING CARE

Nursing care for the client with chronic venous insufficiency is primarily educative and supportive. Client teaching includes the following recommendations.

- Elevate the legs while resting and during sleep. See the box below for a nursing research study that suggests the supine position for resting.
- Walk as much as possible, but avoid sitting or standing for long periods of time.
- When sitting, do not cross your legs or allow pressure on the back of the knees (such as sitting on the side of the bed).
- Do not wear anything that pinches your legs (such as knee-high hose, garters, or girdles).

- Wear elastic hose as prescribed. The elastic hose should be tighter over the feet than at the top of the leg. Be sure the tops of the elastic hose do not cut into your legs. Put on the hose after you have had your legs elevated.
- Keep the skin on your feet and legs clean, soft, and dry.
- Follow guidelines in Box 33–4 for care of the legs and feet.

The following nursing diagnoses may apply to the client with chronic venous insufficiency.

- *Disturbed body image* related to edema and stasis ulcers on lower leg
- *Ineffective health maintenance* related to lack of knowledge about disorder and prescribed treatments
- *Risk for infection* related to ulcerations
- *Impaired physical mobility* related to pain and edema in lower legs
- *Impaired skin integrity* related to presence of stasis ulcers
- *Ineffective tissue perfusion: Peripheral* related to incompetent venous valves

See other sections of this chapter for specific nursing interventions related to many of these diagnoses. See the box on page 1021 for nursing care for the older adult with chronic venous stasis.

## THE CLIENT WITH VARICOSE VEINS

**Varicose veins** are irregular, tortuous veins with incompetent valves. Varicosities may develop in any veins, and may be called by other names, such as hemorrhoids in the rectum and varices in the esophagus. Varicosities usually affect the veins of the lower extremities; the long saphenous vein is often affected, and they also may develop in the short saphenous vein (Figure 33–8 ■).

## Nursing Research

### Evidence-Based Practice for the Client with Venous Leg Ulcers

Chronic leg ulcers due to venous insufficiency are a challenge to treat and heal. Oxygen is necessary for tissue repair and to prevent infection; however, peripheral perfusion to deliver oxygen to the tissues is impaired in clients with chronic venous insufficiency. Using measurements of transcutaneous tissue oxygen ($TcPo_2$), a group of nurse researchers evaluated the effects of four different positions and supplemental oxygen on a small group of subjects with venous ulcers (Wipke-Tevis, Stotts, Williams, Froelicher, & Hunt, 2001). Not surprisingly, these researchers found lower extremity resting $TcPo_2$ levels in clients with venous ulcers than in healthy adults. Changes in position resulted in minimal $TcPo_2$ changes in tissue surrounding the ulcer. When supplemental oxygen was given, $TcPo_2$ levels were higher in the supine position than with the legs elevated, sitting, or standing. These results suggest that control of peripheral circulation and tissue oxygenation may be impaired in clients with venous ulcers.

#### IMPLICATIONS FOR NURSING
The results of this study support advising clients with chronic venous ulcers to stay off their feet and rest in bed as much as possi-

ble to promote healing of venous ulcers. Remove compression stockings and devices while the client is in bed to promote perfusion of subcutaneous tissues and of the region surrounding the ulcer itself. Discuss the effects of position on peripheral tissue perfusion with clients, and encourage frequent rest periods during the day. Consider discussing the option of supplemental oxygen therapy for a client with delayed ulcer healing with the primary care provider.

#### Critical Thinking in Client Care
1. What is the usual response of blood vessels to changing positions from supine or sitting to standing? How does this compare with the results found here?
2. What is required for tissue healing? What measures can the nurse take to promote tissue healing in a client with impaired peripheral tissue perfusion?
3. How do the measures used to treat arterial and venous ulcers compare? Explain the rationale for differing treatment measures.

## Nursing Care of the Older Adult

### CHRONIC VENOUS STASIS

Disorders of venous stasis are common after the fifth decade of life. Aging affects vessels and tissues, increasing the risk for venous insufficiency and varicose veins. In addition, mobility frequently declines with aging, reducing the effect of the muscle pump in promoting venous return.

Regular exercise, walking in particular, is an important part of the treatment plan. Safety when walking is an important issue for older clients. Assess the client's mobility and stability during ambulation. If appropriate, suggest using a walker and quad-cane as needed. Assist older clients holding jobs that require prolonged standing to identify strategies to minimize standing and incorporate periods of activity into their work.

Following surgery or during treatment for stasis ulcers, older clients may need additional assistance with home care and maintenance. Initiate referral to social services as needed to arrange for home nursing care, meals, assistance with ADLs, and home maintenance services as indicated. In some instances, temporary placement in an extended care facility is necessary until the client and family can assume care.

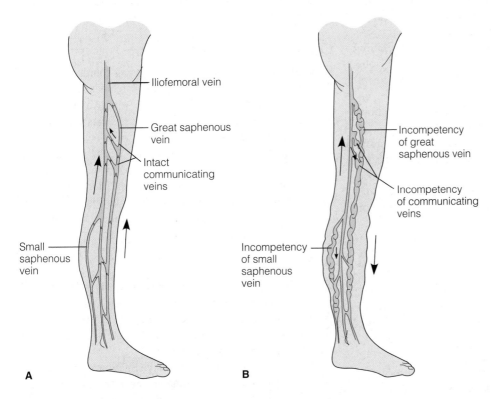

**Figure 33–8** ■ *A*, The normal venous structure of the leg. *B*, Varicose veins resulting from incompetent valves.

Varicose veins affect about 2% of people in industrialized nations. They are more common in women over age 35. Studies also suggest that the increased risk for varicose veins in women may relate to venous stasis during pregnancy. Aging is a risk factor, possibly related to decreased exercise and other factors that contribute to venous stasis. People in occupations that involve prolonged standing (such as beauticians, salespeople, and nurses) also have an increased incidence of varicose veins. Race is a risk factor: Whites are more frequently affected than blacks.

Most varicosities occur in the deep veins of the legs. Contributing causes include obesity, venous thrombosis, congenital arteriovenous malformations, or sustained pressure on abdominal veins (as in pregnancy and/or the presence of abdominal tumors). The effects of gravity, produced by long periods of standing, are a major causative factor.

## PATHOPHYSIOLOGY AND MANIFESTATIONS

Varicose veins are classified as primary (with no involvement of deep veins) or secondary (caused by the obstruction of deep veins). In both cases, long-standing increased venous pressure stretches the vessel wall. This sustained stretching impairs the ability of the venous valves to close, causing them to become incompetent.

The erect position produces a twofold negative effect on the veins. When standing, the leg veins resemble vertical columns and must withstand the full force of venous blood pressure. Prolonged standing, the force of gravity, lack of leg exercise, and incompetent venous valves all weaken the muscle-pumping mechanism, reducing venous blood return to the heart. As standing continues, the amount of blood pooled in the veins increases, further stretching the vessel wall. The venous valves become increasingly incompetent.

## Manifestations of Varicose Veins

- Severe, aching pain in the leg
- Leg fatigue, heaviness
- Itching of the affected leg (stasis dermatitis)
- Feelings of warmth in the leg
- Visibly dilated veins
- Thin, discolored skin above the ankles
- Stasis ulcers

Although varicose veins may be asymptomatic, most cause manifestations such as severe aching leg pain, leg fatigue, leg heaviness, itching, or feelings of heat in the legs. The degree of valvular incompetence does not seem to correlate well with the extent of symptoms. The menstrual cycle tends to worsen symptoms, suggesting a possible correlation with hormonal factors in women. Assessment reveals obvious dilated, tortuous veins beneath the skin of the upper and lower leg. If varicose veins are long-standing, the skin above the ankles may be thin and discolored, with a brown pigmentation. See the box above.

Complications of varicose veins include venous insufficiency and stasis ulcers. Chronic stasis dermatitis may also develop. Superficial venous thrombosis may develop in varicose veins, especially during and after pregnancy, following surgery, and in clients on estrogen therapy (oral contraceptives or hormone replacement therapy).

## COLLABORATIVE CARE

Varicose veins usually can be managed using conservative measures, although surgery may be required if symptoms are severe, when complications develop, or for cosmetic reasons.

### Diagnostic Tests

While varicose veins often are diagnosed by the history and physical examination, diagnostic tests may be ordered.

- *Doppler ultrasonography* or *duplex Doppler ultrasound* may be performed to identify specific locations of incompetent valves. This test is particularly useful before surgery to identify valves that allow reflux of blood from the femoral, popliteal, or peripheral deep veins into the superficial veins (Tierney et al., 2001).
- *Trendelenburg test* may be performed to determine the underlying cause of superficial venous insufficiency. The leg is elevated, then an elastic tourniquet is placed around the distal thigh. The varicosities then are observed as the client stands. When valves of the deep veins are incompetent, the veins remain flat on standing; they rapidly distend when the superficial venous valves are the underlying cause.

### Treatments

Although there is no real cure for varicose veins, conservative measures are the core of treatment for most clients with un-complicated varicose veins. These measures often relieve symptoms and prevent complications by improving venous circulation and relieving pressure on venous tissues. Properly fitted graduated compression stockings are commonly prescribed. They compress the veins, propelling blood back to the heart. Compression stockings augment the muscle pumping action of the legs. When worn during times of prolonged standing and in combination with frequent leg elevation, compression stockings often prevent progression of the condition and development of complications.

Regular, daily walking also is important. Prolonged sitting and standing are discouraged, although elevating the legs for specified periods during the day is beneficial. Leg elevation promotes venous return, prevents venous stasis, and decreases leg heaviness and fatigue.

### Compression Sclerotherapy

In compression sclerotherapy, a sclerosing solution is injected into the varicose vein and a compression bandage is applied for a period of time. This obliterates the vein. Venous blood is rerouted through healthy vessels whose valves are not compromised. Compression sclerotherapy may be used to treat small, symptomatic varicosities. It may be the primary treatment, or it may be used in conjunction with varicose vein surgery. While compression sclerotherapy may be done for cosmetic reasons, complications such as phlebitis, tissue necrosis, or infection may occur and need to be considered prior to the procedures.

### Surgery

Surgical treatment of varicose veins generally is reserved for clients who are very symptomatic, experience recurrent superficial venous thrombosis, and/or develop stasis ulcers. The objective of surgery is to remove the diseased veins. It may be considered for cosmetic reasons.

Surgery usually involves extensive ligation and stripping of the greater and lesser saphenous veins (Braunwald et al., 2001). The evening before surgery, the surgeon marks all incompetent superficial and perforating varicose veins with a permanent ink marker. Under either regional or general anesthesia, the greater saphenous vein is removed and the connected smaller tributaries that have not naturally clotted off are tied off. Multiple small incisions may be made over the varicosities, allowing removal of the affected segments of the vein. Incompetent tributaries that communicate with larger vessels also are ligated. For clients with less extensive disease or clients seeking cosmetic improvement, surgery may involve only the removal of the lesser saphenous vein through an incision in the popliteal fossa.

Postoperative care includes applying pressure bandages for a minimum of 6 weeks, elevating the extremities to minimize postoperative edema, and gradually increasing amounts of ambulation. Sitting and standing are prohibited during the initial recovery period, and are gradually reintroduced as deemed appropriate by the surgeon.

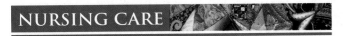

## NURSING CARE

### Health Promotion

Health promotion activities to reduce the incidence of varicose veins include teaching all clients, particularly young women, the benefits of regular exercise continued over the lifetime. Discuss the effect of prolonged sitting or standing on the legs, and encourage the client whose occupation involves these activities to periodically get up and move or to sit with the legs elevated. Encourage all clients to maintain normal weight for their height.

### Assessment

Focused assessment of the client with varicose veins includes the following:

- Health history: complaints of leg pain, aching, heaviness, or fatigue; ankle swelling; history of venous thrombosis
- Physical examination: visible, dilated, tortuous superficial veins in lower extremities

### Nursing Diagnoses and Interventions

In planning and providing nursing care for clients with varicose veins, emphasis is placed on the importance of health teaching to manage the symptoms of varicose veins, particularly because there is no cure for the disease. Nursing care for clients who have undergone surgical treatment for varicose veins focuses on assessing and promoting wound healing and preventing infection. Nursing diagnoses may include those related to pain, impaired tissue perfusion and skin integrity, and a risk for impaired neurovascular function.

### Chronic Pain

Varicose veins can lead to pooling of venous blood in the lower extremities. Venous congestion can cause a dull ache or feeling of pressure in the legs, particularly after prolonged standing. As venous pressure rises, arterial circulation and delivery of oxygen and nutrients to tissues is impaired. Tissue ischemia contributes to the pain. The pain associated with varicose veins tends to be chronic, developing and progressing gradually over a long period of time.

- Assess pain, including its intensity, duration, and aggravating and relieving factors. *Pain assessment allows collaborative planning with the client to identify appropriate interventions.*
- Inquire about current measures being used by the client to manage pain and its effects. Ask about the effectiveness of current management strategies and the desire to change. *Chronic pain management ultimately falls to the client. Strategies to address the pain must meet the client's needs.*

**PRACTICE ALERT** *Suggest keeping a diary of pain intensity, timing, precipitating events, and effectiveness of relief measures. Systematic tracking of pain is an important measure in improving its management.* ■

- Teach and reinforce nonpharmacologic pain management strategies such as progressive relaxation, imagery, deep breathing, distraction, and meditation. *The effectiveness of such strategies is well documented. Nonpharmacologic measures provide a variety of options for controlling pain while maintaining independence. These measures also can reduce reliance on analgesics.*
- Collaborate with the client to establish a pain control plan. *Collaborative planning for pain management increases the client's sense of control and reduces powerlessness. This, in turn, enhances the ability to cope with pain and its effects.*
- Regularly evaluate the effectiveness of planned interventions and pain management strategies. *Regular evaluation allows modification of the care plan as needed, as well as providing a measure of disease progression. Increasing or poorly controlled pain may necessitate additional collaborative interventions to manage the disorder.*

### Ineffective Tissue Perfusion: Peripheral

Varicose veins and venous stasis impair delivery of nutrients and oxygen to peripheral tissues as elevated venous pressures interfere with blood flow through the capillary beds. Improving venous blood flow reduces venous pressures and promotes arterial flow to peripheral tissues.

- Assess peripheral pulses, capillary refill, skin color and temperature, and extent of edema. *Assessment of arterial flow and tissue perfusion provide baseline and continuing data for evaluating the effectiveness of interventions.*
- Teach application and use of properly fitted elastic graduated compression stockings. *Elastic compression stockings compress the veins, promoting venous return from the lower extremities. During ambulation, the stockings enhance the blood-pumping action of the muscles. Because elastic stockings inhibit blood flow through small superficial vessels, they should be removed at least once each day for at least 30 minutes.*

**PRACTICE ALERT** *Instruct to maintain a program of regular exercise, such as walking for 20 to 30 minutes several times a day. Exercise stimulates circulation and promotes blood flow through the vascular system. When ambulation is restricted, active range-of-motion exercises help maintain muscle tone, joint mobility, and venous return.* ■

- Advise to elevate the legs for 15 to 20 minutes several times a day and to sleep with the legs elevated above the level of the heart. *Elevating the legs promotes venous return, reducing tissue congestion and improving arterial circulation. Improved venous return also increases the cardiac output and renal perfusion, promoting elimination of excess fluid and decreasing peripheral edema.*

### Risk for Impaired Skin Integrity

Ineffective venous valve function impairs venous return and increases venous pressures. These increased pressures oppose arterial blood flow and the delivery of oxygen and nutrients to the cells. As a result, tissues are vulnerable to any additional insult, and may break down.

- Assess lower extremity color, temperature, moisture, and for evidence of pressure or breakdown on admission and at each visit. *Initial and continuing assessment allows timely detection of early signs of skin and tissue breakdown. This, in turn, allows early institution of measures to prevent further tissue damage and promote healing.*
- Teach foot and skin care measures such as daily cleansing with nondrying soap, gentle drying, and lotions to prevent skin dryness and cracking. *Cleansing removes potentially harmful microorganisms and stimulates circulation. Care is taken to keep the skin moist and supple, promoting its function as the first line of defense against infection.*
- Discuss the importance of adequate nutrition and fluid intake. *Adequate nutrients are necessary to maintain tissue integrity and promote healing. A diet high in protein, carbohydrates, and vitamins and minerals promotes growth and maintenance of skin cells, provides energy, and helps prevent skin breakdown. Adequate hydration helps maintain the moisture and turgor of skin, reducing the risk of drying and breakdown.*

### Risk for Peripheral Neurovascular Dysfunction

Severe varicose veins can lead to chronic venous insufficiency, impaired arterial circulation, and ultimately, disrupted sensation in the affected extremity. Impaired neurologic function increases the client's risk for injury and infection of the extremity, as minor trauma may go unnoticed.

- Assess circulation, sensation, and movement of the lower extremities. *Disrupted circulation and venous congestion may interfere with sensory and motor function of the affected extremity. The potential for nerve and muscle involvement is especially high in clients with venous stasis ulcers.*

**PRACTICE ALERT** *Instruct to report signs of neurovascular dysfunction, such as numbness, coldness, pain, or tingling of an extremity. Early recognition of neurovascular dysfunction facilitates institution of interventions to prevent complications. Because the postoperative hospital stay following varicose vein surgery or venous stasis ulcer repair is brief, manifestations of neurovascular dysfunction may initially be detected by the client. Careful assessment and prompt reporting helps prevent potential complications such as skin breakdown, infection, and nerve damage.* ■

- Teach measures to protect the extremities from injury, such as always wearing shoes or firm slippers, cotton socks to absorb moisture, and testing the temperature of bath water with a thermometer or the upper extremities before stepping in. *Sensation in the lower extremities may be affected by poor circulation, necessitating additional measures to protect the legs and feet from injury.*

### Home Care

Most clients with varicose veins provide self-care at home. Include the following topics when preparing the client and family for home care.

- Leg elevation and exercise program
- Application and use of graduated elastic compression stockings
- Foot and leg care (see Box 33–4)
- Measures to avoid injury and skin breakdown
- Symptoms or potential complications to report to the physician

Provide information about suppliers for elastic stockings and any other required supplies. If venous stasis ulcers have developed, consider referral to home health services for regular assessment of healing and additional teaching.

## DISORDERS OF THE LYMPHATIC SYSTEM

The lymphatic system, which includes the lymphatic vessels and the lymph nodes, is a unique part of the circulatory system. The lymphatic system returns plasma and plasma proteins filtered out of the capillaries from interstitial tissues to the bloodstream. This fluid is called *lymph*. The lymphatic system consists of closed capillaries leading to larger lymphatic venules and lymphatic veins. These vessels contain smooth muscle and one-way valves that help move fluid toward the heart. Lymphatic vessels share the same sheath as arteries and veins; arterial pulsations and skeletal muscle contractions compress the lymphatic vessels to assist in maintaining lymph flow. As lymph moves through the lymphatic system, it is filtered through thousands of bean-shaped lymph nodes clustered along the vessels. Within these nodes, phagocytes remove foreign material from the lymph, preventing it from entering the bloodstream.

### THE CLIENT WITH LYMPHADENOPATHY

*Lymphadenopathy,* enlarged lymph nodes, may be localized or generalized. Localized lymphadenopathy usually results from an inflammatory process (e.g., streptococcal pharyngitis or an infected wound). The node enlarges as lymphocytes and monocytes proliferate within the node to destroy infectious material. Palpable lymph nodes often develop in response to minor trauma or a localized infection. Generalized lymphadenopathy usually is associated with malignancy or disease. Malignant cells or other abnormal cells invade the node, causing it to enlarge.

*Lymphangitis,* inflammation of the lymph vessels draining an infected area of the body, is characterized by a red streak along the inflamed vessels, pain, heat, and swelling. Fever and chills also may be present. Local lymph nodes are swollen and tender.

Treatment for lymphadenopathy and lymphangitis focuses on identifying and treating the underlying condition. Elevating the body part and applying heat to inflamed lymphatic vessels help reduce swelling and promote blood flow to the affected area.

## THE CLIENT WITH LYMPHEDEMA

**Lymphedema** may be a primary or a secondary disorder, resulting from inflammation, obstruction, or removal of lymphatic vessels. It is characterized by extremity edema due to accumulation of lymph. *Primary lymphedema* is uncommon, affecting about 1 in 10,000 people. It affects females more frequently than males, and may be associated with a genetic disorder (Braunwald et al., 2001).

*Secondary lymphedema* is an acquired condition, resulting from damage, obstruction, or removal of lymphatic vessels. The most common worldwide cause of secondary lymphedema is *filariasis,* infestation of the lymphatic vessels by filaria, a nematode worm. Other important causes of secondary lymphedema include recurrent episodes of bacterial lymphangitis, obstruction of lymph vessels by tumors, and surgical or radiation treatment for breast cancer (Braunwald et al., 2001).

## PATHOPHYSIOLOGY AND MANIFESTATIONS

Obstruction of lymph drainage prevents fluid and protein molecules from interstitial tissues from returning to the circulation. The protein molecules increase the osmotic pressure in interstitial tissues, drawing in additional fluid that causes edema in the soft tissues. One or both extremities may be affected.

The edema begins distally, progressing up the limb to involve the entire extremity (Figure 33–9 ■). Initial edema is soft and pitting; with chronic congestion, subcutaneous tissues become fibrotic, causing thick, rough skin and a woody texture of the limb (*brawny edema*). In contrast, the edema associated with venous disorders is softer, and the skin often is hyperpigmented with evidence of stasis dermatitis. Lymphedema generally is painless, although the limb may feel heavy.

## COLLABORATIVE CARE

Collaborative care for the client with lymphedema focuses on relieving edema and preventing or treating infection. The disorder may be difficult to treat effectively, and can lead to progressive disability due to the weight and awkwardness of the affected extremity.

### Diagnostic Tests

Abdominal or pelvic ultrasound and computed tomography (CT) scans are used to detect obstructing lesions. Magnetic resonance imaging (MRI) can show edema and identify lymph nodes and enlarged lymphatic vessels. More invasive procedures such as lymphangiography and radioactive isotope studies may occasionally be necessary to identify the lymphatic defect causing lymphedema.

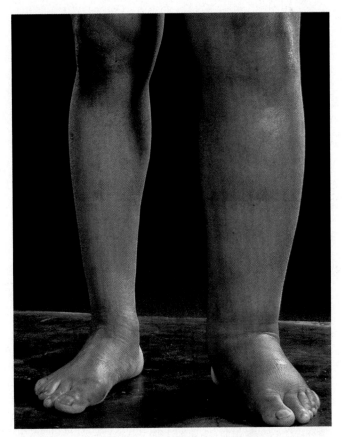

**Figure 33–9 ■** Severe lymphedema of the lower extremity.

*Source: MSNB/Custom Medical Stock Photo, Inc.*

- *Lymphangiography* uses injected contrast media to illustrate lymphatic vessels on X-rays. Organic dyes are used to identify a distal lymphatic vessel, and then a contrast medium is injected into the vessel for visualization of the lymphatic system of the limb. In primary lymphedema, lymph vessels are absent or hypoplastic (underdeveloped). In secondary lymphedema, lymph channels often are dilated; it may be possible to determine the level of obstruction (Braunwald et al., 2001).
- *Lymphoscintigraphy* involves injecting a radioactively tagged substance into distal subcutaneous tissues of the extremity, then mapping its flow through the lymphatic system. The pattern of lymph fluid distribution and transport is abnormal in clients with lymphedema.

### Treatments

Meticulous skin and foot care is vital to prevent infection in the affected extremity. Shoes should always be worn to reduce the risk of injury. Careful cleansing and use of emollient lotions are recommended to prevent drying of the skin. Exercise is encouraged, as are frequent periods of leg elevation. The foot of the bed is raised by 15 to 20 degrees at night to promote lymph flow. Elastic graduated compression stockings may be ordered for use during the day. In some cases, an intermittent pneumatic compression device to reduce edema may be prescribed for home use.

Antibiotics are given to prevent and treat infection, which can be recurrent and difficult to eradicate. Diuretic therapy may be used intermittently, particularly when primary lymphedema is exacerbated by the menstrual cycle or seasonal variability (Tierney et al., 2001).

Clients who do not respond to conservative treatment measures or who experience recurrent episodes of cellulitis and lymphangitis may require surgical treatment. Microvascular techniques may be used to create anatomoses between obstructed lymphatic vessels and adjacent veins, providing channels to redirect lymph into the venous system. Successful surgery may improve both extremity function and its cosmetic appearance (Tierney et al., 2001).

## NURSING CARE

Nursing care for clients with lymphatic disorders focuses on reducing edema, preventing tissue damage related to the edema, and promoting effective coping with the effect of the disorder on body image and function.

## Nursing Diagnoses and Interventions

Nursing diagnoses for the client with lymphedema may include *Impaired tissue integrity, Excess fluid volume,* and *Disturbed body image.*

### Impaired Tissue Integrity

Obstructed lymphatic flow leads to fluid congestion of the interstitial spaces of subcutaneous tissue. The resulting edema compresses and damages tissues of the affected extremity. Subcutaneous tissues become fibrotic, reducing their protective functions of shock absorption and insulation. In addition, obstructed lymphatic flow reduces the effectiveness of lymph nodes in filtering and removing foreign material and pathogens from the body. This increases the risk for local tissue infection such as *cellulitis,* a diffuse bacterial infection of the skin. Cellulitis increases the risk for skin and tissue breakdown and, if not effectively treated, can lead to sepsis.

> **PRACTICE ALERT** *Frequently inspect the skin of the affected extremity, documenting condition with each assessment. Promptly report areas of pallor, redness, or apparent inflammation. Breaks in the skin surface allow microbial invasion, and increase the risk for infection. Prompt identification and treatment of any lesions is vital to prevent further tissue breakdown and infection.* ∎

- Apply well-fitting elastic graduated compression stockings or intermittent pneumatic pressure devices as ordered. *Elastic stockings and/or pneumatic pressure devices oppose the movement of fluid out of capillaries and improve its reabsorption into vascular spaces for transportation back to the heart.*

> **PRACTICE ALERT** *Remove elastic stockings and intermittent pressure devices every 8 hours or at each home visit to inspect the underlying skin for evidence of redness, irritation, dryness, or breakdown. Elastic graduated compression stockings, antiembolic stockings, and pneumatic compression devices compress small vessels nourishing the skin and subcutaneous tissue. Periodic removal not only allows inspection of the underlying skin, but also allows restoration of blood flow to these small vessels and the tissues.* ∎

- Instruct to elevate the extremities while seated and during sleep. *Elevation of the extremities diminishes venous congestion, promotes venous return, facilitates arterial circulation and tissue perfusion, and helps reduce the accumulation of excess fluids in interstitial spaces of the affected extremity.*

> **PRACTICE ALERT** *Use preventive skin care devices as indicated. Collected fluid in the affected extremity increases its weight and interferes with regular movement. The increased weight places greater pressure on surfaces of the limb that come in contact with furniture. Protective devices such as egg crate foam, sheepskin, pillows, or padding help prevent tissue compression, promoting circulation and reducing the risk of skin and tissue breakdown.* ∎

- Keep skin clean and dry, especially in interdigital spaces. Teach skin and foot care to the client and family. *Clean, dry skin provides the first line of defense against infection. Significant limb edema can interfere with reaching the distal extremity and cleaning interdigital spaces. The dark, moist spaces between the toes are an excellent environment for bacterial growth. Teaching fosters self-care and independence, as well as preparing the client and family to manage this often chronic condition.*
- Discuss the importance of adhering to the therapeutic regimen. *Lymphedema generally is a chronic condition; effective management requires active client participation in planning and implementing care to reduce edema and maintain tissue integrity.*

### Excess Fluid Volume

In lymphedema, obstruction, destruction, or congenital malformation of lymphatic vessels interferes with the normal circulation of lymphatic fluid. As a result, lymph collects in the subcutaneous tissues of the affected extremity, causing excess fluid volume of that extremity. Some clients may benefit from intermittent diuretic therapy and dietary sodium restriction.

- Discuss the rationale for restricted sodium intake if ordered. Teach ways to maintain the recommended sodium restriction, and assist to choose foods that are low in sodium. *Sodium causes retention of extracellular water; restricting dietary sodium may help prevent additional fluid accumulation in interstitial spaces.*

> **PRACTICE ALERT** *Monitor intake and output and/or weight (daily or weekly). Use consistent scales, timing, and clothing for accurate weight measurements. Intake and output records and short-term changes in weight reflect fluid balance. Measures of fluid balance permit evaluation of the effectiveness of interventions such as restricted sodium intake and diuretic therapy.* ∎

• During acute periods, assess the affected extremity daily for increased edema; measure girth of the extremity using consistent technique. *The size of the affected extremity provides a measure of the effectiveness of ordered interventions and progression of the disorder.*

### Disturbed Body Image

The disproportionate size of an extremity or extremities due to lymphedema can profoundly affect body image. During early stages of the disease, conservative measures may effectively reduce the edema and size of the affected limb. However, as the disease progresses, conservative measures may become less effective, leading to more permanent disfigurement. Mobility may be impaired, and the client may develop an increasingly negative self-perception.

• Encourage discussions about usual coping patterns and perception of self. *Knowledge of existing coping patterns and behaviors helps the nurse assess the client's ability to cope with the current situation. This knowledge is then used to reinforce effective coping mechanisms and help develop more effective coping strategies. This exchange also allows the client to voice feelings related to actual or perceived changes in body image.*
• Accept the client's perception of self and of the impact of the changes in appearance. *Nonjudgmental acceptance of the client's view of self and of the effects of changes in appearance builds trust and promotes rapport. A trusting relationship promotes the client's ability to take an active role in managing the disorder, participate in health care decisions, and adhere to the plan of care. Nonjudgmental listening also promotes mutual respect and demonstrates caring and compassion.*
• Encourage active participation in self-care. Assist with identifying alternative self-care strategies when the extent of edema interferes with performing some aspects of self-care such as trimming toenails or washing feet. *The client initially may have difficulty viewing or touching the affected body part. Gentle encouragement and support from the nurse helps the client assume self-care and accept the affected body part. Brainstorming to identify alternative care strategies promotes the client's independence even when total self-care is not feasible.*

### Home Care

When preparing the client with chronic lymphedema and family to manage the disorder, include the following teaching topics.

• Recommended program of exercise and elevation of the extremity
• Foot and skin care
• Use of elastic graduated compression stockings and/or intermittent pressure devices
• Importance of wearing elastic stockings during the majority of waking hours, removing them once during the daytime and while sleeping
• Measures to prevent infection in the affected extremity, such as wearing gloves while gardening
• Signs and symptoms to report to the health care provider (e.g., manifestations of tissue breakdown or infection, increasing edema, or evidence of compromised circulation)
• Use and precautions associated with any prescribed medications
• Sodium-restricted diet if ordered

Provide information about contacts for questions, and make referrals as needed. Evaluate the need for home health, home maintenance assistance, and other services such as physical or occupational therapy.

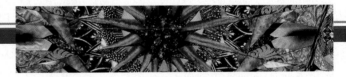

## EXPLORE MediaLink

NCLEX review questions, case studies, care plan activities, MediaLink applications, and other interactive resources for this chapter can be found on the Companion Website at www.prenhall.com/lemone.

Click on Chapter 33 to select the activities for this chapter. For animations, video clips, more NCLEX review questions, and an audio glossary, access the Student CD-ROM accompanying this textbook.

## TEST YOURSELF

1. A potential blood donor whose blood pressure is found to average 180/106 on two different readings tells the nurse, "I don't understand how it could be so high—I feel just fine." The appropriate response by the nurse is:

   a. "This is probably just a false reading due to 'white coat syndrome.' Don't worry about it."

   b. "It is unusual that you are not having some symptoms such as severe headaches and nosebleeds."

   c. "High blood pressure often has few or no symptoms; that's why it is called the 'silent killer.'"

   d. "You probably should have your blood pressure rechecked in 3 months or so and then follow up with your primary care provider if it is still high."

2. A client is complaining of new onset calf and foot pain. The nurse notes that the leg below the knee is cool, pale, and dorsalis pedis and posterior tibial pulses are absent. The nurse should:

   a. Immediately notify the physician
   b. Elevate the leg and apply a warm blanket
   c. Provide the ordered analgesic
   d. Apply antiembolism (TED) stockings

3. An expected assessment finding in a client with peripheral atherosclerosis would be:

   a. Pallor of the legs and feet when dependent
   b. Increased hair growth on the affected extremity
   c. Higher blood pressure readings in the affected extremity
   d. Impaired sensation in the affected extremity

4. The nurse evaluates her teaching of a client admitted with deep vein thrombosis as effective when the client states:

   a. "I'll use a hard-backed, upright chair when sitting instead of my recliner."
   b. "I'll get my blood drawn as scheduled and notify the doctor if I have any unusual bleeding or bruising."
   c. "I understand why I am not allowed to exercise for the next 6 weeks and will take it easy."
   d. "I'll have my wife buy a low-cholesterol cookbook and we'll make an appointment with the dietician to learn about a low-fat, low-cholesterol diet."

5. A client with visible varicose veins tells the nurse that she wants to have surgery to remove them, because "my legs ache every evening and they are really ugly!" The most appropriate response would be:

   a. "Often measures such as elevating your legs and elastic stockings can relieve the discomfort associated with varicose veins."
   b. "Surgery will have a good cosmetic effect, but will not relieve the discomfort associated with varicose veins."
   c. "All varicose veins should be surgically removed to restore adequate blood flow to your legs and prevent gangrene."
   d. "Surgery is never indicated unless the varicose veins are interfering with circulation. Have you tried cosmetic measures to cover them up?"

See Test Yourself answers in Appendix C.

# BIBLIOGRAPHY

Ackley, B. J., & Ladwig, G. B. (2002). *Nursing diagnosis handbook: A guide to planning care* (5th ed.). St. Louis: Mosby.

Braunwald, E., Fauci, A. S., Kasper, D. L., Hauser, S. L., Longo, D. L., & Jameson, J. L. (2001). *Harrison's principles of internal medicine* (15th ed.). New York: McGraw-Hill.

Breen, P. (2000). DVT: What every nurse should know. *RN, 63*(4), 58–62.

Chase, S. L. (2000). Hypertensive crisis. *RN, 63*(6), 62–67.

Church, V. (2000). Staying on guard for DVT & PE. *Nursing, 30*(2), 34–42.

Deglin, J. H., & Vallerand, A. H. (2003). *Davis's drug guide for nurses* (8th ed.). Philadelphia: F.A. Davis.

Ferguson, M., Cook, A., Rimmasch, H., Bender, S., & Voss, A. (2000). Pressure ulcer management: The importance of nutrition. *MEDSURG Nursing, 9*(4), 163–175.

Fontaine, K. L. (2000). *Healing practices: Alternative therapies for nursing.* Upper Saddle River, NJ: Prentice Hall Health.

Gallo, J. J., Busby-Whitehead, J., Rabins, P. V., Silliman, R. A., & Murphy, J. B. (Eds.). (1999). *Reichel's care of the elderly: Clinical aspects of aging* (5th ed.). Philadelphia: Lippincott Williams & Wilkins.

Gibson, J. M., & Kenrick, M. (1998). Pain and powerlessness: The experience of living with peripheral vascular disease. *Journal of Advanced Nursing, 27*(4), 737–745.

Hess, C. T. (2001). Putting the squeeze on venous ulcers. *Nursing, 31*(9), 58–63.

Johnson, M., Bulechek, G., Dochterman, J. M., Maas, M., & Moorhead, S. (2001). *Nursing diagnoses, outcomes, & interventions.* St. Louis: Mosby.

Johnson, M., Maas, M., & Moorhead, S. (Eds.). (2000). *Nursing outcomes classification (NOC)* (2nd ed.). St. Louis: Mosby.

Kuhn, M. A. (1999). *Complementary therapies for health care providers.* Philadelphia: Lippincott.

Lehne, R. A. (2001). *Pharmacology for nursing care* (4th ed.). Philadelphia: Saunders.

Malarkey, L. M., & McMorrow, M. E. (2000). *Nurse's manual of laboratory tests and diagnostic procedures* (2nd ed.). Philadelphia: Saunders.

McCance, K. L., & Huether, S. E. (2002). *Pathophysiology: The biologic basis for disease in adults and children* (4th ed.). St. Louis: Mosby.

McCloskey, J. C., & Bulechek, G. M. (Eds.) (2000). *Nursing interventions classification (NIC)* (3rd ed.). St. Louis: Mosby.

McConnell, E. A. (2002). Clinical do's & don'ts. Applying antiembolism stockings. *Nursing, 32*(4), 17.

Meeker, M. H., & Rothrock, J. C. (1999). *Alexander's care of the patient in surgery* (11th ed.). St. Louis: Mosby.

Miracle, V. A. (2001). Act fast during a hypertensive crisis. *Nursing, 31*(9), 50–51.

National Heart, Lung, and Blood Institute: National High Blood Pressure Education Program. (1997). *The sixth report of the Joint National Committee on Prevention, Detection, Evaluation, and Treatment of High Blood Pressure.* Bethesda, MD: National Institutes of Health.

National Heart, Lung, and Blood Institute, National Institutes of Health. (2002). *Morbidity & mortality: 2002 chart book of cardiovascular, lung, and blood diseases.* Bethesda, MD: Author.

Navuluri, R. (2001a). Anticoagulant therapy. *American Journal of Nursing, 101*(11), 24A–24D.

Navuluri, R. (2001b). Nursing implications of anticoagulant therapy. *American Journal of Nursing, 101*(12), 24A–B.

North American Nursing Diagnosis Association. (2001). *NANDA nursing diagnoses: Definitions & classification 2001–2002.* Philadelphia: NANDA.

Patel, C. T. C., Kinsey, G. C., Koperski-Moen, K. J., & Bungum, L. D. (2000). Vacuum-assisted wound closure. *American Journal of Nursing, 100*(12), 45–48.

Porth, C. M. (2002). *Pathophysiology: Concepts of altered health states* (6th ed.). Philadelphia: Lippincott.

Spratto, G. R., & Woods, A. L. (2003). *2003 edition PDR® nurse's drug handbook™.* Clifton Park, NY: Delmar Learning.

Tierney, L. M., McPhee, S. J., & Papadakis, M. A. (2001). *Current medical diagnosis & treatment* (40th ed.). New York: Lange Medical Books/McGraw-Hill.

Wipke-Tevis, D. D., Stotts, N. A., Williams, D. A., Froelicher, E. S., & Hunt, T. K. (2001). Tissue oxygenation, perfusion, and position in patients with venous leg ulcers. *Nursing Research, 50*(1), 24–32.

Woods, S. L., Froelicher, E. S. S., & Motzer, S. U. (2000). *Cardiac nursing* (4th ed.). Philadelphia: Lippincott.

Woods, A. (2002). Patient education series. High blood pressure (hypertension). *Nursing, 32*(4), 54–55.

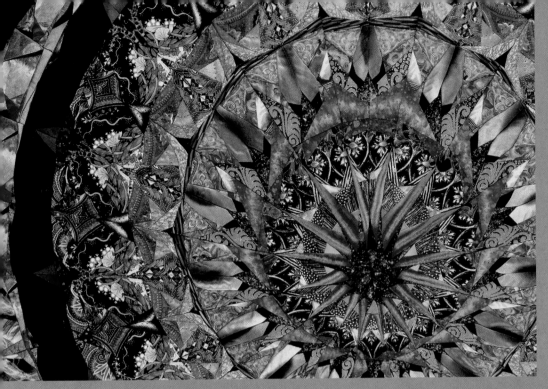

# RESPONSES TO ALTERED RESPIRATORY FUNCTION

CHAPTER | 34

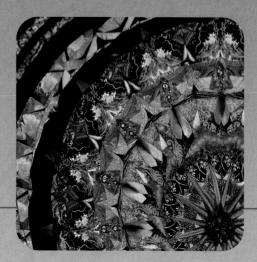

# Assessing Clients with Respiratory Disorders

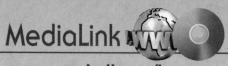

## MediaLink

### www.prenhall.com/lemone

Additional resources for this chapter can be found on the Student CD-ROM accompanying this textbook, and on the Companion Website at www.prenhall.com/lemone. Click on Chapter 34 to select the activities for this chapter.

**CD-ROM**
- Audio Glossary
- NCLEX Review

*Animations*
- Respiratory System
- Carbon Dioxide Transport
- Gas Exchange
- Oxygen Transport

**Companion Website**
- More NCLEX Review
- Functional Health Pattern Assessment
- Case Study
    Respiratory Assessment

## LEARNING OUTCOMES

After completing this chapter, you will be able to:

- Review the anatomy and physiology of the respiratory system.

- Explain the mechanics of ventilation.

- Describe factors affecting respiration.

- Identify specific topics for consideration during a health history interview of the client with health problems involving the respiratory system.

- Describe physical assessment techniques for respiratory function.

- Identify abnormal findings that may indicate impairment in the function of the respiratory system.

The respiratory system provides the cells of the body with oxygen and eliminates carbon dioxide, formed as a waste product of cellular metabolism. The events in this process, called respiration, are:

- *Pulmonary ventilation:* Air is moved into and out of the lungs.
- *External respiration:* Exchange of oxygen and carbon dioxide occurs between the alveoli and the blood.
- *Gas transport:* Oxygen and carbon dioxide are transported to and from the lungs and the cells of the body via the blood.
- *Internal respiration:* Exchange of oxygen and carbon dioxide is made between the blood and the cells.

## REVIEW OF ANATOMY AND PHYSIOLOGY

Although the system functions as a whole, this unit contains separate chapters dealing with the upper respiratory system (the nose, pharynx, larynx, and trachea) and the lower respiratory system (the lungs).

### The Upper Respiratory System

The upper respiratory system serves as a passageway for air moving into the lungs and carbon dioxide moving out to the external environment (Figure 34–1 ■). As air moves through these structures, it is cleaned, humidified, and warmed.

#### The Nose

The nose is the external opening of the respiratory system. The external nose is given structure by the nasal, frontal, and maxillary bones as well as plates of hyaline cartilage. The nostrils (also called the external nares) are two cavities within the nose, separated by the nasal septum. These cavities open into the nasal portion of the pharynx through the internal nares. The nasal cavities just behind the nasal openings are lined with skin

that contains hair follicles, sweat glands, and sebaceous glands. The nasal hairs filter the air as it enters the nares. The rest of the cavity is lined with mucous membranes that contain olfactory neurons and goblet cells that secrete thick mucus. The mucus not only traps dust and bacteria but also contains lysozyme, an enzyme that destroys bacteria as they enter the nose. As mucus and debris accumulate, mucosal ciliated cells move it toward the pharynx, where it is swallowed. The mucosa is highly vascular, warming air that moves across its surface.

Three structures project outward from the lateral wall of each nasal cavity: the superior, middle, and inferior turbinates. The turbinates cause air entering the nose to become turbulent and also increase the surface area of mucosa exposed to the air. As air moves through this area, heavier particles of debris drop out and are trapped in the mucosa of the turbinates.

#### The Sinuses

The nasal cavity is surrounded by paranasal sinuses (Figure 34–2 ■). These openings are located in the frontal, sphenoid, ethmoid, and maxillary bones. Sinuses lighten the skull, assist in speech, and produce mucus that drains into the nasal cavities to help trap debris.

#### The Pharynx

The pharynx, a funnel-shaped passageway about 5 inches (13 cm) long, extends from the base of the skull to the level of the C6 vertebra. The pharynx serves as a passageway for both air and food. It is divided into three regions: the nasopharynx, the oropharynx, and the laryngopharynx.

The nasopharynx serves only as a passageway for air. Located beneath the sphenoid bone and above the level of the soft palate, the nasopharynx is continuous with the nasal cavities. This segment is lined with ciliated epithelium, which continues

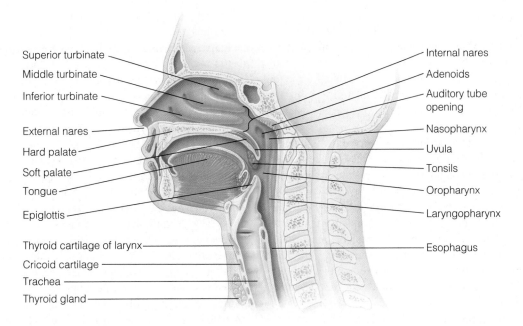

**Figure 34–1** ■ The upper respiratory system.

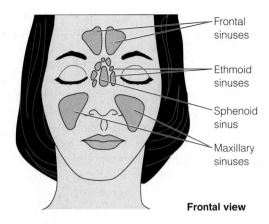

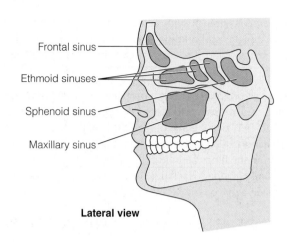

**Frontal view**

**Lateral view**

**Figure 34–2** ■ Sinuses, frontal and lateral views.

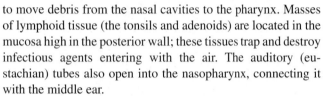

to move debris from the nasal cavities to the pharynx. Masses of lymphoid tissue (the tonsils and adenoids) are located in the mucosa high in the posterior wall; these tissues trap and destroy infectious agents entering with the air. The auditory (eustachian) tubes also open into the nasopharynx, connecting it with the middle ear.

The oropharynx lies behind the oral cavity and extends from the soft palate to the level of the hyoid bone. It serves as a passageway for both air and food. An upward rise of the soft palate prevents food from entering the nasopharynx during swallowing. The oropharynx is lined with stratified squamous epithelium that protects it from the friction of food and damage from the chemicals found in food and fluids.

The laryngopharynx extends from the hyoid bone to the larynx. It is also lined with stratified squamous epithelium, and serves as a passageway for both food and air. Air does not move into the lungs while food is being swallowed and moved into the esophagus.

### The Larynx

The larynx is about 2 inches (5 cm) long. It opens superiorly at the laryngopharynx and is continuous inferiorly with the trachea. The larynx provides an airway and routes air and food into the proper passageway. As long as air is moving through the larynx, its inlet is open; however, the inlet closes during swallowing. The larynx also contains the vocal cords, necessary for voice production.

The larynx is framed by cartilages, connected by ligaments and membranes. The thyroid cartilage is formed by the fusion of two cartilages; the fusion point is visible as the Adam's apple. The cricoid cartilage lies below the thyroid cartilage; other pairs of cartilages form the walls of the larynx. The epiglottis, also a cartilage, is covered with mucosa that contains taste buds. This structure normally projects upward to the base of the tongue; however, during swallowing, the larynx moves upward and the epiglottis tips to cover the opening to the larynx. If anything other than air enters the larynx, a cough reflex expels the foreign substance before it can enter the lungs. This protective reflex does not work if the person is unconscious.

### The Trachea

The trachea begins at the inferior larynx and descends anteriorly to the esophagus to enter the mediastinum, where it divides to become the right and left primary bronchi of the lungs. The trachea is about 4 to 5 inches (12 to 15 cm) long and 1 inch (2.5 cm) in diameter. It contains 16 to 20 C-shaped rings of cartilage joined by connective tissue. The mucosa lining the trachea consists of pseudostratified ciliated columnar epithelium containing seromucous glands that produce thick mucus. Dust and debris in the inspired air are trapped in this mucus, moved toward the throat by the cilia, and then either swallowed or coughed out through the mouth.

## The Lower Respiratory System

The lower respiratory system includes the lungs and the bronchi (Figures 34–3 ■ and 34–4 ■).

### The Lungs

The center of the thoracic cavity is filled by the *mediastinum,* which contains the heart, great blood vessels, bronchi, trachea, and esophagus. The mediastinum is flanked on either side by the lungs (see Figure 34–3). Each lung is suspended in its own pleural cavity, with the anterior, lateral, and posterior lung surfaces lying close to the ribs. The hilus, on the mediastinal surface of each lung, is where blood vessels of the pulmonary and circulatory systems enter and exit the lungs. The primary bronchus also enters in this area. The apex of each lung lies just below the clavicle, whereas the base of each lung rests on the diaphragm. The lungs are elastic connective tissue, called stroma, and are soft and spongy.

The two lungs differ in size and shape. The left lung is smaller and has two lobes, whereas the right lung has three lobes. Each of the lung lobes contains a different number of bronchopulmonary segments. These segments are separated by connective tissue. There are eight segments in the two lobes of the left lung and ten segments in the three lobes of the right lung.

The vascular system of the lungs consists of the pulmonary arteries, which deliver blood to the lungs for oxygenation, and the pulmonary veins, which deliver oxygenated blood to the heart. Within the lungs, the pulmonary arteries branch into a

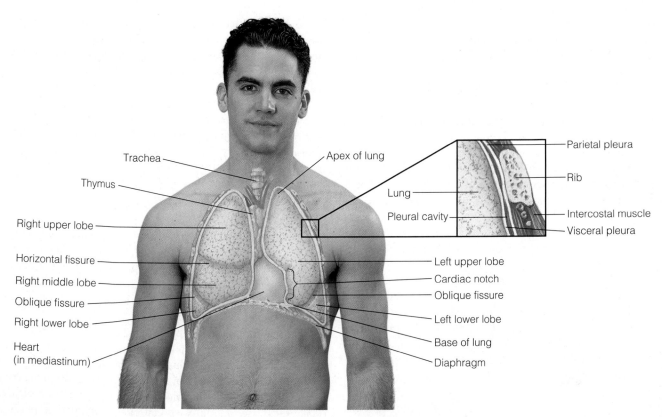

**Figure 34–3** ■ The lower respiratory system, showing the location of the lungs, the mediastinum, and layers of visceral and parietal pleura.

pulmonary capillary network that surrounds the avleoli. Lung tissue receives its blood supply from the bronchial arteries and drains by the bronchial and pulmonary veins.

### The Pleura

The pleura is a double-layered membrane that covers the lungs and the inside of the thoracic cavities (see Figure 34–3). The *parietal pleura* lines the thoracic wall and mediastinum. It is continuous with the *visceral pleura*, which covers the external lung surfaces. The pleura produces pleural fluid, a lubricating, serous fluid that allows the lungs to move easily over the thoracic wall during breathing. The pleura's two layers also cling tightly together and hold the lungs to the thoracic wall. The structure of the pleura creates a slightly negative pressure in the pleural space (which is actually a potential rather than an actual space), necessary for lung function.

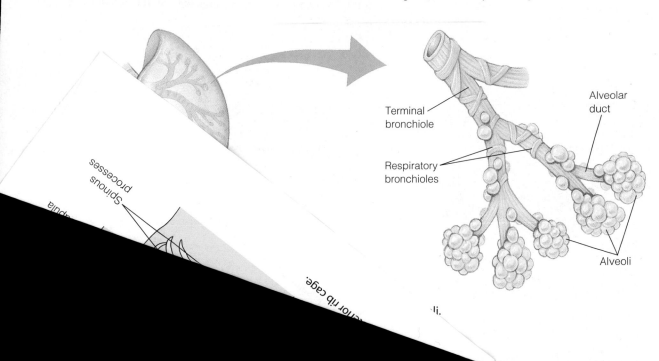

## The Bronchi and Alveoli

The trachea divides into right and left primary bronchi. These main bronchi subdivide into the secondary (lobar) bronchi, then branch into the tertiary (segmental) bronchi, and then into smaller and smaller bronchioles, ending in the terminal bronchioles, which are extremely small (see Figure 34–4). These branching passageways collectively are called the bronchial or respiratory tree. From the terminal bronchioles, air moves into air sacs (called respiratory bronchioles), which further branch into alveolar ducts that lead to alveolar sacs and then to the tiny alveoli. During inspiration, air enters the lungs through the primary bronchus and then moves through the increasingly smaller passageways of the lungs to the alveoli, where oxygen and carbon dioxide exchange occurs in the process of external respiration. During expiration, the carbon dioxide is expelled.

Alveoli cluster around the alveolar sacs, which open into a common chamber called the atrium. There are millions of alveoli in each lung, providing an enormous surface for gas exchange. Alveoli have extremely thin walls of a single layer of squamous epithelial cells over a very thin basement membrane. The external surface of the alveoli are covered with pulmonary capillaries. The alveolar and capillary walls form the respiratory membrane. Gas exchange across the respiratory membrane occurs by simple diffusion. The alveolar walls also contain cells that secrete a surfactant-containing fluid, necessary for maintaining a moist surface and reducing the surface tension of the alveolar fluid to help prevent collapse of the lungs.

## The Rib Cage and Intercostal Muscles

The lungs are protected by the bones of the rib cage and the intercostal muscles. There are 12 pairs of ribs, which all articulate with the thoracic vertebrae (Figure 34–5 ■). Anteriorly, the first 7 ribs articulate with the body of the sternum. The eighth, ninth, and tenth ribs articulate with the cartilage immediately above the ribs. The eleventh and twelfth ribs are called floating ribs, because they are unattached.

The sternum has three parts: the manubrium, the body, and the xiphoid process. The junction between the manubrium and the body of the sternum is called the manubriosternal junction or the angle of Louis. The depression above the manubrium is called the suprasternal notch.

The spaces between the ribs are called the intercostal spaces. Each intercostal space is named for the rib immediately above it (e.g., the space between the third and fourth ribs is designated as the third intercostal space). The intercostal muscles between the ribs, along with the diaphragm, are called the inspiratory muscles.

## Mechanics of Ventilation

Pulmonary ventilation depends on volume changes within the thoracic cavity. A change in the volume of air in the thoracic cavity leads to a change in the air pressure within the cavity. Because gases always flow along their pressure gradients, a change in pressure results in gases flowing into or out of the lungs to equalize the pressure.

The pressures normally present in the thoracic cavity are the intrapulmonary pressure and the intrapleural pressure. The intrapulmonary pressure, within the alveoli of the lungs, rises and falls constantly as a result of the acts of ventilation (inhalation and exhalation). The intrapleural pressure, within the pleural space, also rises and falls with the acts of ventilation, but it is always less than (or negative to) the intrapulmonary pressure. Intrapulmonary and intrapleural pressures are necessary not only to expand and contract the lungs, but also to prevent their collapse.

Pulmonary ventilation has two phases: inspiration, during which air flows into the lungs; and expiration, during which gases flow out of the lungs. The two phases make up a single breath, and normally occur from 12 to 20 times each minute. A single inspiration lasts for about 1 to 1.5 seconds, whereas an expiration lasts for about 2 to 3 seconds.

During inspiration, the diaphragm contracts and flattens out to increase the vertical diameter of the thoracic cavity

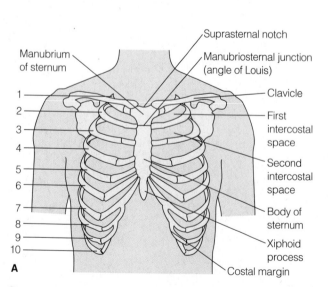

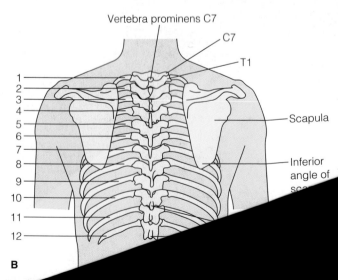

**Figure 34–5** ■ *A*, Anterior rib cage, showing intercostal spaces. *B*, Poste

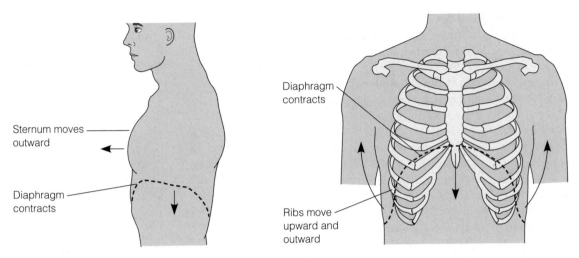

**Figure 34–6** ■ Respiratory inspiration: lateral and anterior views. Note the volume expansion of the thorax as the diaphragm flattens.

(Figure 34–6 ■). The external intercostal muscles contract, elevating the rib cage and moving the sternum forward to expand the lateral and anteroposterior diameter of the thoracic cavity, decreasing intrapleural pressure. The lungs stretch and the intrapulmonary volume increases, decreasing intrapulmonary pressure slightly below atmospheric pressure. Air rushes into the lungs as a result of this pressure gradient until the intrapulmonary and atmospheric pressures equalize.

Expiration is primarily a passive process that occurs as a result of the elasticity of the lungs (Figure 34–7 ■). The inspiratory muscles relax, the diaphragm rises, the ribs descend, and the lungs recoil. Both the thoracic and intrapulmonary pressures increase, compressing the alveoli. The intrapulmonary pressure rises to a level greater than atmospheric pressure, and gases flow out of the lungs.

## FACTORS AFFECTING RESPIRATION

The rate and depth of respirations are controlled by respiratory centers in the medulla oblongata and pons of the brain and by chemoreceptors located in the medulla and in the carotid and aortic bodies. The centers and chemoreceptors respond to changes in the concentration of oxygen, carbon dioxide, and hydrogen ions in arterial blood. For example, when carbon dioxide concentration increases or the pH decreases, the respiratory rate increases.

In addition, respiratory passageway resistance, lung compliance, lung elasticity, and alveolar surface tension forces affect respiration.

- Respiratory passageway resistance is created by the friction encountered as gases move along the respiratory passageways, by constriction of the passageways (especially the larger bronchioles), by accumulations of mucus or infectious material, and by tumors. As resistance increases, gas flow decreases.
- Lung compliance is the distensibility of the lungs. It depends on the elasticity of the lung tissue and the flexibility of the rib cage. Compliance is decreased by factors that decrease the elasticity of the lungs, block the respiratory passageways, or interfere with movement of the rib cage.
- Lung elasticity is essential for lung distention during inspiration and lung recoil during expiration. Decreased elasticity from disease such as emphysema impairs respiration.

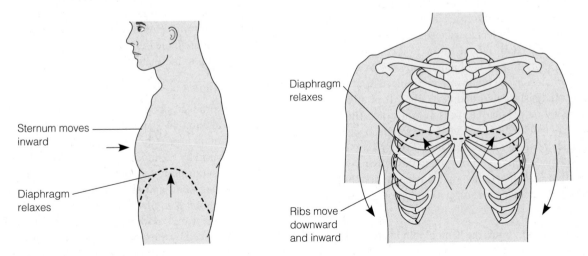

**Figure 34–7** ■ Respiratory expiration: lateral and anterior views.

- A liquid film of mostly water covers the alveolar walls. At any gas-liquid boundary, the molecules of liquid are more strongly attracted to each other than to gas molecules. This produces a state of tension, called surface tension, that draws the liquid molecules even more closely together. The water content of the alveolar film compacts the alveoli and aids in the lungs' recoil during expiration. In fact, if the alveolar film were pure water, the alveoli would collapse between breaths. Surfactant, a lipoprotein produced by the alveolar cells, interferes with this adhesiveness of the water molecules, reducing surface tension, and helping expand the lungs. With insufficient surfactant, the surface tension forces can become great enough to collapse the alveoli between breaths, requiring tremendous energy to reinflate the lungs for inspiration.

## Respiratory Volume and Capacity

Respiratory volume and capacity are affected by gender, age, weight, and health status.

- Tidal volume (TV) is the amount of air (approximately 500 mL) moved in and out of the lungs with each normal, quiet breath.
- Inspiratory reserve volume (IRV) is the amount of air (approximately 2100 to 3100 mL) that can be inhaled forcibly over the tidal volume.
- Expiratory reserve volume (ERV) is the approximately 1000 mL of air that can be forced out over the tidal volume.
- The residual volume is the volume of air (approximately 1100 mL) that remains in the lungs after a forced expiration.
- Vital capacity refers to the sum of TV + IRV + ERV and is approximately 4500 mL in the healthy client.
- About 150 mL of air never reaches the alveoli (the amount remaining in the passageways) and is called anatomical dead space volume.

## Oxygen Transport and Unloading

Oxygen is carried in the blood either bound to hemoglobin or dissolved in the plasma. Oxygen is not very soluble in water, so almost all oxygen that enters the blood from the respiratory system is carried to the cells of the body by hemoglobin. This combination of hemoglobin and oxygen is called *oxyhemoglobin*.

Each hemoglobin molecule is made of four polypeptide chains, with each chain bound to an iron-containing heme group. The iron groups are the binding sites for oxygen; each hemoglobin molecule can bind with four molecules of oxygen.

Oxygen binding is rapid and reversible. It is affected by temperature, blood pH, partial pressure of oxygen ($PO_2$), partial pressure of carbon dioxide ($PCO_2$), and serum concentration of an organic chemical called 2,3-DPG. These factors interact to ensure adequate delivery of oxygen to the cells.

The relative saturation of hemoglobin depends on the $PO_2$ of the blood, as illustrated in the oxygen-hemoglobin dissociation curve (Figure 34–8 ■).

- Under normal conditions, the hemoglobin in arterial blood is 97.4% saturated with oxygen. Hemoglobin is almost fully saturated at a $PO_2$ of 70 mmHg. As arterial blood flows

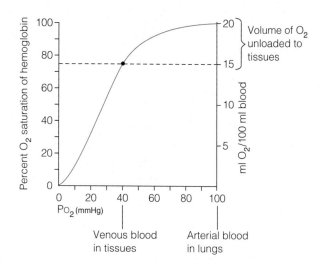

**Figure 34–8** ■ Oxygen-hemoglobin dissociation curve. The percent $O_2$ saturation of hemoglobin and total blood oxygen volume are shown for different oxygen partial pressures ($PO_2$). Arterial blood in the lungs is almost completely saturated. During one pass through the body, about 25% of hemoglobin-bound oxygen is unloaded to the tissues. Thus, venous blood is still about 75% saturated with oxygen. The steep portion of the curve shows that hemoglobin readily off-loads or on-loads oxygen at $PO_2$ levels below about 50 mmHg.

through the capillaries, oxygen is unloaded, so that the oxygen saturation of hemoglobin in venous blood is 75%.

- The affinity of oxygen and hemoglobin decreases as the temperature of body tissues increases above normal. As a result, less oxygen binds with hemoglobin, and oxygen unloading is enhanced. Conversely, as the body is chilled, oxygen unloading is inhibited.
- The oxygen-hemoglobin bond is weakened by increased hydrogen ion concentrations. As blood becomes more acidotic, oxygen unloading to the tissues is enhanced. The same process occurs when the partial pressure of carbon dioxide increases because this decreases the pH.
- The organic chemical 2,3-DPG is formed in red blood cells and enhances the release of oxygen from hemoglobin by binding to it during times of increased metabolism (as when body temperature increases). This binding alters the structure of hemoglobin to facilitate oxygen unloading.

## Carbon Dioxide Transport

Active cells produce about 200 mL of carbon dioxide each minute; this amount is exactly the same as that excreted by the lungs each minute. Excretion of carbon dioxide from the body requires transport by the blood from the cells to the lungs. Carbon dioxide is transported in three forms: dissolved in plasma, bound to hemoglobin, and as bicarbonate ions in the plasma (the largest amount is in this form).

The amount of carbon dioxide transported in the blood is strongly influenced by the oxygenation of the blood. When the $PO_2$ decreases, with a corresponding decrease in oxygen saturation, increased amounts of carbon dioxide can be carried in the blood. Carbon dioxide entering the systemic circulation from the cells causes more oxygen to dissociate from hemoglobin, in turn allowing more carbon dioxide to combine with hemoglobin and more bicarbonate ions to be generated. This situation is reversed in the pulmonary circulation, where the uptake of oxygen facilitates the release of carbon dioxide.

## ASSESSING RESPIRATORY FUNCTION

The nurse assesses the respiratory system both during a health assessment interview to collect subjective data and a physical assessment to collect objective data.

### The Health Assessment Interview

This section provides guidelines for collecting subjective data through a health assessment interview specific to the function of the respiratory system. A health assessment interview to determine problems of the respiratory system may be done as part of a health screening or as part of a total health assessment. Alternatively, the interview may focus on a chief complaint (such as difficulty breathing). If the client has a problem of any part of the respiratory system, analyze its onset, characteristics and course, severity, precipitating and relieving factors, and any associated symptoms, noting the timing and circumstances. For example, you may ask the client the following:

- What problems are you having with your breathing? Is your breathing more difficult if you lie flat? Is it painful to breathe in or out?
- When did you first notice that your cough was becoming a problem? Do you cough up mucus? What color is the mucus?
- Have you had nosebleeds in the past?

During the interview, carefully observe the client for difficulty in breathing, pausing to breathe in the middle of a sentence, hoarseness, changes in voice quality, and cough. Ask about present health status, medical history, family health history, and risk factors for illness. These areas of the client's health status include information about the nose, throat, and lungs.

To determine present health status, ask about pain in the nose, throat, or chest. Information about cough includes what type of cough, when it occurs, and how it is relieved. The client should describe any sputum associated with the cough. Is the client experiencing any dyspnea (difficult or labored breathing)? How is the dyspnea associated with activity levels and time of day? Is the client having chest pain? How is this related to activity and time of day? Note the severity, type, and location of the pain. Explore problems with swallowing, smelling, or taste. Also ask about nosebleeds and nasal or sinus stuffiness or pain, and about current medication use, aerosols or inhalants, and oxygen use.

Document past medical history by asking questions about a history of allergies, asthma, bronchitis, emphysema, pneumonia, tuberculosis, or congestive heart failure. Other questions include a history of surgery or trauma to the respiratory structures and a history of other chronic illnesses such as cancer, kidney disease, and heart disease. If the client has a health problem involving the respiratory system, ask about medica-

tions used to relieve nasal congestion, cough, dyspnea, or chest pain. Document a family history of allergies, tuberculosis, emphysema, and cancer.

The client's personal lifestyle, environment, and occupation may provide clues to risk factors for actual or potential health problems. Question the client about a history of smoking and/or exposure to environmental chemicals (including smog), dust, vapors, animals, coal dust, asbestos, fumes, or pollens. Other risk factors include a sedentary lifestyle and obesity. Also ask the client about use of alcohol and substances that are injected (such as heroin) or inhaled (such as cocaine or marijuana).

Other questions and leading statements, categorized by functional health patterns, can be found on the Companion Website.

### Physical Assessment

Physical assessment of the respiratory system may be performed as part of a total assessment, or alone for a client with known or suspected problems. Assess the respiratory system through inspection, palpation, percussion, and auscultation of the nose, throat, thorax, and lungs. In addition, note the client's level of consciousness and assess the color of the lips, nail beds, nose, ears, and tongue for signs of respiratory distress.

The equipment needed to assess the respiratory system includes a tongue blade, penlight, nasal speculum, metric ruler, marking pen, and stethoscope with diaphragm. The room should be warm and well lighted. Ask the client to remove all clothing above the waist; give female clients a gown to wear during the examination. Conduct the examination with the client in the sitting position. Prior to the examination, collect all necessary equipment and explain the techniques to the client to decrease anxiety.

The three different types of normal breath sounds are vesicular, bronchovesicular, and bronchial. Assessment of these sounds is discussed in Table 34–1.

### Nasal Assessment with Abnormal Findings (✓)

- Inspect the nose for changes in size, shape, or color.
  - ✓ The nose may be asymmetrical as a result of previous surgery or trauma.
  - ✓ The skin around the nostrils may be red and swollen in allergies.
- Inspect the nasal cavity. Use an otoscope with a broad, short speculum. Gently insert the speculum into each of the nares and assess the condition of the mucous membranes and the turbinates.
  - ✓ The septum may be deviated.
  - ✓ Perforation of the septum may occur with chronic cocaine abuse.
  - ✓ Red mucosa indicates infection.
  - ✓ Purulent drainage indicates nasal or sinus infection.
  - ✓ Allergies may be indicated by watery nasal drainage, pale turbinates, and polyps on the turbinates.
- Assess ability to smell. Ask the client to breathe through one nostril while pressing the other one closed. Ask the client to close his or her eyes. Place a substance with an aromatic odor

MediaLink | FUNCTIONAL HEALTH PATTERN ASSESSMENT

| TABLE 34–1   Normal Breath Sounds | |
| --- | --- |
| **Type of Breath Sound** | **Characteristics** |
| Vesicular | • Soft, low-pitched, gentle sounds<br>• Heard over all areas of the lungs except the major bronchi<br>• Have a 3:1 ratio for inspiration and expiration, with inspiration lasting longer than expiration |
| Bronchovesicular | • Medium pitch and intensity of sounds<br>• Have a 1:1 ratio, with inspiration and expiration being equal in duration<br>• Heard anteriorly over the primary bronchus on each side of the sternum, and posteriorly between the scapulae |
| Bronchial | • Loud, high-pitched sounds<br>• Gap between inspiration and expiration<br>• Have a 2:3 ratio for inspiration and expiration, with expiration longer than inspiration<br>• Heard over the manubrium |

under the client's nose (use ground coffee or alcohol) and ask the client to identify the odor. Test each nostril separately. This test is usually done only if the client has problems with the sense of smell.

✓ Changes in the ability to smell may be the result of damage to the olfactory nerve or to chronic inflammation of the nose.

✓ Zinc deficiency may also cause a loss of the sense of smell.

## Thoracic Assessment with Abnormal Findings (✓)

• Assess respiratory rate.

✓ **Tachypnea** (rapid respiratory rate) is seen in **atelectasis** (collapse of lung tissue following obstruction of the bronchus or bronchioles), pneumonia, asthma, pleural effusion, pneumothorax, and congestive heart failure.

✓ Damage to the brainstem from a stroke or head injury may result in either tachypnea or **bradypnea** (low respiratory rate).

✓ Bradypnea is seen with some circulatory disorders, lung disorders, as a side effect of some medications, and as a response to pain.

✓ **Apnea,** cessation of breathing lasting from a few seconds to a few minutes, may occur following a stroke or head trauma, as a side effect of some medications, or following airway obstruction.

• Inspect the anteroposterior diameter of the chest. The anteroposterior diameter of the chest should be less than the transverse diameter. Normal ratios vary from 1:2 to 5:7.

✓ The anteroposterior diameter is equal to the transverse diameter in barrel chest, which typically occurs with emphysema.

• Inspect for intercostal retraction.

✓ Retraction of intercostal spaces may be seen in asthma.

✓ Bulging of intercostal spaces may be seen in pneumothorax.

• Inspect and palpate for chest expansion. Place your hands with the fingers spread apart palm down on the client's posterolateral chest. Gently press the skin between your thumbs (Figure 34–9 ■). Ask the client to breathe deeply. As the client inhales, watch your hands for symmetry of movement.

✓ Thoracic expansion is decreased on the affected side in atelectasis, pneumonia, pneumothorax, and pleural effusion.

✓ Bilateral chest expansion is decreased in emphysema.

• Gently palpate the location and position of the trachea.

✓ The trachea shifts to the unaffected side in pleural effusion and pneumothorax and shifts to the affected side in atelectasis.

• Palpate for tactile fremitus. Ask the client to say "ninety-nine" as you palpate at three different levels for a vibratory sensation called tactile fremitus, which occurs as sound waves from the larynx travel through patent bronchi and lungs to the chest wall.

✓ Tactile fremitus is decreased in atelectasis, emphysema, asthma, pleural effusion, and pneumothorax. It is increased in pneumonia if the bronchus is patent.

• Percuss the lungs for dullness over shoulder apices and over anterior, posterior, and lateral intercostal spaces (Figure 34–10 ■).

✓ Dullness is heard in clients with atelectasis, lobar pneumonia, and pleural effusion.

✓ Hyperresonance is heard in those with chronic asthma and pneumothorax.

• Percuss the posterior chest for diaphragmatic excursion. Systematic percussion of the posterior chest from a level of lung resonance to the level of diaphragmatic dullness reveals

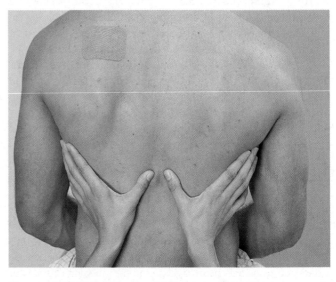

**Figure 34–9 ■** Palpating for chest expansion.

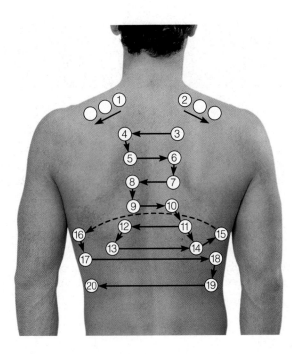

**Figure 34–10** ■ Sequence for lung percussion.

diaphragmatic excursion, a measurement of the level of the diaphragm. First percuss downward over the posterior thorax while the client exhales fully and holds the breath. Mark the spot at which the sound changes from resonant to dull. Then ask the client to inhale and hold the breath while you percuss downward again to note the descent of the diaphragm. Again mark the spot where the sound changes. Measure the difference, which normally varies from about 3 to 5 cm (Figure 34–11 ■).

✓ Diaphragmatic excursion is decreased in emphysema, on the affected side in pleural effusion, and in pneumothorax.

✓ A high level of dullness or a lack of excursion may indicate atelectasis or pleural effusion.

## Breath Sound Assessment with Abnormal Findings (✓)

- Auscultate the lungs for breath sounds with the diaphragm of the stethoscope by having the client take slow deep breaths through the mouth. Listen over anterior, posterior, and lateral intercostal spaces (Figure 34–12 ■).
  - ✓ Bronchial breath sounds (expiration > inspiration) and bronchovesicular breath sounds (inspiration = expiration) are heard over lungs filled with fluid or solid tissue.
  - ✓ Breath sounds are decreased over atelectasis, emphysema, asthma, pleural effusion, and pneumothorax.
  - ✓ Breath sounds are increased over lobar pneumonia.
  - ✓ Breath sounds are absent over collapsed lung, pleural effusion, and primary bronchus obstruction.
- Auscultate for crackles, wheezes, and friction rubs. If crackles or wheezes are heard, ask the client to cough and note if adventitious sound is cleared.
  - ✓ Crackles (short, discrete, crackling or bubbling sounds) may be noted in pneumonia, bronchitis, and congestive heart failure.
  - ✓ Wheezes (continuous, musical sounds) may be heard in clients with bronchitis, emphysema, and asthma.
  - ✓ A friction rub is a loud, dry, creaking sound that indicates pleural inflammation.
- Auscultate voice sounds where any abnormal breath sound is noted by having client say "ninety-nine" (bronchophony); whisper "one, two, three" (whispered pectoriloquy); and say "ee" (egophony). Normally, these sounds are heard by the examiner, but are muffled.
  - ✓ Voice sounds are decreased or absent over areas of atelectasis, asthma, pleural effusion, and pneumothorax.
  - ✓ Voice sounds are increased and clearer over lobar pneumonia.

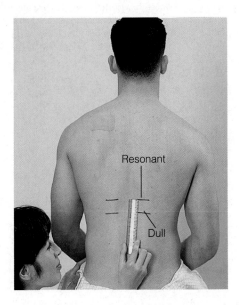

**Figure 34–11** ■ Measuring diaphragmatic excursion.

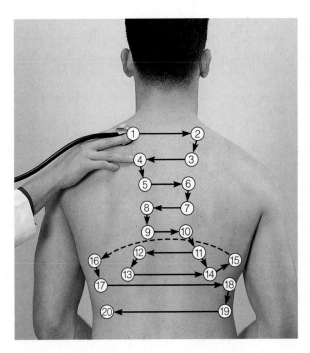

**Figure 34–12** ■ Sequence for lung auscultation.

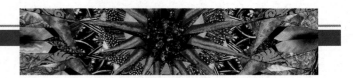

 EXPLORE MediaLink

NCLEX review questions, case studies, care plan activities, MediaLink applications, and other interactive resources for this chapter can be found on the Companion Website at www.prenhall.com/lemone.

Click on Chapter 34 to select the activities for this chapter. For animations, video clips, more NCLEX review questions, and an audio glossary, access the Student CD-ROM accompanying this textbook.

## TEST YOURSELF

1. Where is the apex of each lung located?

    a. In the mediastinum
    b. Resting on the diaphragm
    c. Within the parietal pleura
    d. Just below the clavicle

2. What physiologic process is involved in gas exchange at the respiratory membrane?

    a. Facilitates transport
    b. Active transport
    c. Simple diffusion
    d. Hydrostatic pressure

2. While auscultating your client's breath sounds, you note continuous musical sounds. You document these sounds as:

    a. Murmurs
    b. Wheezes
    c. Crackles
    d. Rales

3. Your client has had a lung removed. What type of breath sound would you expect to assess over this area?

    a. Hyperresonance
    b. Crackles
    c. Bronchovesicular
    d. Absent

4. What would you ask the client to do as you auscultate the lungs?

    a. "Hold your breath."
    b. "Repeat the numbers 99 several times."
    c. "Take slow deep breaths through your mouth."
    d. " Breathe in and out through your nose."

See Test Yourself answers in Appendix C.

## BIBLIOGRAPHY

Andresen, G. (1998). Assessing the older patient. *RN, 61*(3), 46–56.

Basfield-Holland, E. (1997). Assessing pulmonary status: It's more than listening to breath sounds. *Nursing, 27*(8), 1–2, 4–9.

Connolly, M. (2001). Chest x-rays: Completing the picture. *RN, 64*(6), 56–62, 64.

Jevon, P., & Ewens, B. (2001). Assessment of a breathless patient. *Nursing Standard, 15*(16), 48–53.

Kirton, C. (1996). Assessing breath sounds. *Nursing, 26*(6), 50–51.

Lyneham, J. (2001). Physical examination (abdomen, thorax and lungs): A review. *Australian Journal of Advanced Nursing, 18*(3), 31.

O'Hanlon-Nichols, T. (1998). Basic assessment series: The adult pulmonary system. *American Journal of Nursing, 98*(2), 39–45.

Walton, J., & Miller, J. (1998). Evaluating physical and behavioral changes in older adults. *MEDSURG Nursing, 7*(2), 85–90.

Watson, R. (2000). Assessing pulmonary function in older people. *Nursing Older People, 12*(8), 27–28.

Weber, J., & Kelley, J. (2002). *Health assessment in nursing* (2nd ed). Philadelphia: Lippincott.

Wilson, S., & Giddens, J. (2001). *Health assessment for nursing practice.* St. Louis: Mosby.

### CHAPTER 35

# Nursing Care of Clients with Upper Respiratory Disorders

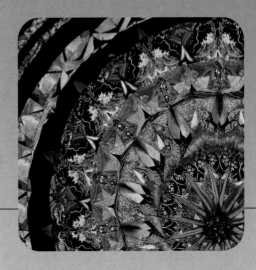

**MediaLink**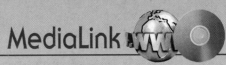

**www.prenhall.com/lemone**

Additional resources for this chapter can be found on the Student CD-ROM accompanying this textbook, and on the Companion Website at www.prenhall.com/lemone. Click on Chapter 35 to select the activities for this chapter.

**CD-ROM**
- Audio Glossary
- NCLEX Review

**Companion Website**
- More NCLEX Review
- Case Study
    Sleep Apnea
- Care Plan Activity
    Epistaxis
- MediaLink Application
    Laryngectomy

## LEARNING OUTCOMES

After completing this chapter, you will be able to:

- Relate anatomy, physiology, and assessment of the upper respiratory tract to commonly occurring disorders.

- Describe the pathophysiology of common upper respiratory tract disorders, relating their manifestations to the pathophysiologic process.

- Discuss nursing implications for diagnostic tests, medications, and other collaborative care measures to treat upper respiratory disorders.

- Provide care for clients having surgery involving the upper respiratory system.

- Identify nursing care needs for the client with a tracheostomy.

- Use the nursing process to assess needs, plan and implement individualized care, and evaluate responses for clients with upper respiratory disorders.

Upper respiratory disorders may affect the nose, paranasal sinuses, tonsils, adenoids, larynx, and pharynx. See Chapter 34 to review the anatomy and physiology of these structures as well as their assessment. ⟴ Upper respiratory disorders may be very minor, such as the common cold. However, a patent upper airway is necessary for effective breathing. Acute and even life-threatening problems develop when upper airway patency is affected (e.g., by laryngeal edema). Upper respiratory disorders can affect breathing, communication, and body image. When breathing is compromised because of swelling, bleeding, or accumulation of secretions, fear and anxiety develop.

Nursing care focuses on maintaining the airway, managing pain and symptoms, promoting effective communication, and providing psychologic support for the client and family.

# INFECTIOUS OR INFLAMMATORY DISORDERS

Constant exposure of the upper respiratory tract to the environment makes it vulnerable to a variety of infectious and inflammatory conditions. Although most upper respiratory infections and inflammations are minor, complications may result. In the frail older adult, the risk of serious problems following an upper respiratory infection can be significant.

**Rhinitis,** inflammation of the nasal cavities, is the most common upper respiratory disorder. Rhinitis may be either acute or chronic. *Acute viral rhinitis,* or the common cold, is discussed below. Chronic rhinitis includes allergic, vasomotor, and atrophic rhinitis. *Allergic rhinitis,* or hay fever, results from a sensitivity reaction to allergens such as plant pollens. It tends to occur seasonally. The etiology of *vasomotor rhinitis* is unknown. Although its manifestations are similar to those of allergic rhinitis, it is not linked to allergens. *Atrophic rhinitis* is characterized by changes in the mucous membrane of the nasal cavities.

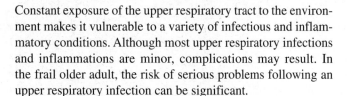

## THE CLIENT WITH VIRAL UPPER RESPIRATORY INFECTION

Viral upper respiratory infections (URIs or the common cold) are the most common respiratory tract infections and are among the most common human diseases. URIs are highly contagious and are prevalent in schools and work environments. The incidence of acute URI peaks during September and late January, coinciding with the opening of schools, as well as toward the end of April. Most adults experience two to four colds each year (Porth, 2002).

### PATHOPHYSIOLOGY

More than 200 strains of virus cause URI, including rhinoviruses, adenoviruses, parainfluenza viruses, coronaviruses, and respiratory syncytial virus. Occasionally, more than one virus may be present. Viruses causing acute URI spread by aerosolized droplet nuclei during sneezing or coughing or by direct contact. The virus usually spreads when the hands and fingers pick it up from contaminated surfaces and carry it to the eyes and mucous membranes of the susceptible host. Infected clients are highly contagious, shedding virus for a few days prior to and after the appearance of symptoms. Although immunity is produced to the individual virus strain, the number of viruses causing URI ensures that most people continue to experience colds throughout their lifetime.

Viscous mucus secretions in the upper respiratory tract trap invading organisms, preventing contamination of more vulnerable areas. Cells of the upper respiratory tract are infected when the virus attaches to receptors on the cell. Local immunologic defenses, such as secretory IgA antibodies in respiratory secretions, then attempt to inactivate the antigen, producing a local inflammatory response. The mucous membranes of the nasal passages swell and become hyperemic and engorged. Mucus-secreting glands become hyperactive. These responses to the virus produce the typical manifestations of viral URI.

### MANIFESTATIONS

Acute viral upper respiratory infection often presents as the common cold. Nasal mucous membranes appear red (*erythematous*) and *boggy* (swollen). Swollen mucous membranes, local vasodilation, and secretions cause nasal congestion. Clear, watery secretions lead to **coryza** or *rhinorrhea*, profuse nasal discharge. Sneezing and coughing are common. Sore throat is common, and may be the initial symptom. Systemic manifestations of acute viral URI may include low-grade fever, headache, malaise, and muscle aches. Symptoms generally last for a few days up to 2 weeks. Although acute viral URI is typically mild and self-limited, its effects on the immune defenses of the upper respiratory tract can increase the risk for more serious bacterial infections, such as sinusitis or otitis media.

## COLLABORATIVE CARE

Because most acute viral upper respiratory infections are self-limiting, self-care is appropriate and encouraged. Medical treatment is usually required only when complications such as sinusitis or otitis media develop.

Diagnosis of acute viral URI is usually based on the history and physical examination. Diagnostic testing may be indicated if a complication such as bacterial infection is suspected. A white blood count (WBC) may be ordered to assess for leukocytosis (an elevated WBC). Cultures of purulent discharge may also be obtained.

Treatment is symptomatic. Adequate rest, maintaining fluid intake, and avoiding chilling help relieve systemic symptoms such as fever, malaise, and muscle ache. Instruct clients to cover the mouth and nose with tissue when coughing or sneezing, and to dispose of soiled tissues properly. Additionally, avoiding crowds helps prevent spread of the infection to others.

## Medications

Medications may be recommended to shorten the duration of the illness and relieve symptoms. Mild decongestants or over-the-counter antihistamines may help relieve coryza and nasal congestion. Warm saltwater gargles, throat lozenges, or mild analgesics may be used for sore throat. Although no specific antiviral therapy has been shown to be effective, experimental vaccines to prevent acute viral URI are in developmental stages. For the nursing implications of decongestants and common antihistamines see the box below.

## Complementary Therapies

Complementary therapies are appropriate for treating most acute viral URI. Herbal remedies such as Echinacea and garlic have antiviral and antibiotic effects. Taken at the first sign of infection, Echinacea may reduce the duration and symptoms. The recommended dose of Echinacea varies, depending on the part of the plant used in the preparation. It should not be used for longer than 2 weeks. It is contraindicated for use during pregnancy and lactation, and in people who have an autoimmune disease such as rheumatoid arthritis.

Aromatherapy with essential oils such as basil, cedarwood, eucalyptus, frankincense, lavender, marjoram, peppermint, or rosemary can reduce congestion, and promote comfort and recovery. Teach clients that these essential oils are to be used only for inhalation, not for internal consumption.

## Medication Administration

### Decongestants and Antihistamines

#### DECONGESTANTS

Phenylephrine (Neo-Synephrine, others)
Phenylpropanolamine (Comtrex, Ornade, Triaminic, others)
Pseudoephedrine (Sudafed, Actifed, others)

Decongestants promote vasoconstriction, reducing the inflammation and edema of nasal mucosa and relieving nasal congestion. They are very effective when applied topically (by nasal spray) because of their rapid onset of action. However, the duration of effect is short, followed by vasodilation and rebound congestion. Because of their rapid effect and short duration, these preparations are habit-forming. Chronic use may lead to *rhinitis medicamentosa,* a rebound phenomenon of drug-induced nasal irritation and inflammation.

#### Nursing Responsibilities

- Assess for contraindications, such as hypertension or chronic heart disease. These drugs stimulate the sympathetic nervous system, increasing peripheral vascular resistance, blood pressure, and heart rate.
- Evaluate medication regimen for potential interactions such as antihypertensive medications and monoamine oxidase (MAO) inhibitors.

#### Client and Family Teaching

- Do not use more than the recommended dose.
- Check with the physician before taking decongestants if you are taking any prescription medications or are being treated for high blood pressure or heart disease.
- Use nasal sprays for no more than 3 to 5 days.
- Increase fluid intake to relieve mouth dryness.
- These drugs may cause nervousness, shakiness, or difficulty sleeping. Stop the drug if these effects occur.

#### ANTIHISTAMINES

Brompheniramine (Dimetane, others)
Chlorpheniramine (Chlor-Trimeton, others)
Clesmastine (Tavist)
Dexchlorpheniramine (Dexchlor, others)
Triprolidine (Actidil, Myidil)

*Nonsedating*

Cetirizine (Zyrtec)
Fexofenadine (Allegra)
Loratadine (Claritin)

Antihistamines are widely available with and without a prescription. They are frequently combined with decongestants in over-the-counter cold and allergy preparations. Antihistamines relieve the systemic effects of histamine and dry respiratory secretions through an anticholinergic effect. Most antihistamines cause drowsiness; nonsedating forms are less likely to interfere with alertness.

#### Nursing Responsibilities

- Before administering or recommending these drugs, assess for possible contraindications, including the following:
  - Acute asthma or lower respiratory disease that may be aggravated by drying of secretions
  - Hypersensitivity to antihistamines
  - Glaucoma (increased intraocular pressure)
  - Impaired gastrointestinal motility or obstruction
  - Prostatic hypertrophy or other urinary tract obstruction
  - Heart disease
- For clients who must remain alert while on antihistamine therapy, recommend nonsedating forms.

#### Client and Family Teaching

- Do not drive or operate machinery while taking over-the-counter or prescription forms of antihistamines known to be sedating.
- Stop the drug and notify your doctor immediately if you develop confusion, excessive sedation, chest tightness, wheezing, bleeding, or easy bruising while taking antihistamines.
- Do not use alcohol or other CNS depressants while taking antihistamines.
- Hard candy, gum, ice chips, and liquids help relieve mouth dryness caused by antihistamines.

## NURSING CARE

### Health Promotion

Clients can limit their incidence of acute viral URI by frequent handwashing and avoiding exposure to crowds. Maintaining good general health and stress-reducing activities support the immune system and help prevent acute viral URI (see the box below). Teach the client that chilling or going out in the rain do not cause colds, and that URI are more likely to occur during periods of physical or psychologic stress.

### Home Care

The primary nursing role in caring for clients with acute viral URI is educational. Self-care is appropriate for most clients unless the problem is recurrent or a complication occurs. Acute viral URI may interfere with work and recreational activities. Unless limited by symptoms, normal daily activities and roles usually can be maintained. Additional rest during the acute phase of illness is recommended. Additional fluid intake and a well-balanced diet help support the immune response, hastening recovery.

## Nursing Research

### Evidence-Based Practice for the Older Adult

A volunteer population of healthy older adults participated in a 3-year study to determine the effects of moderate exercise on the incidence of respiratory tract infections. Participants walked for 30 to 35 minutes at least three times a week, with 10-minute warmup and cooldown sessions. Stress levels as perceived by the study participants were considered an additional variable, because previous studies have shown an increased incidence of upper respiratory infections in people who have high levels of stress. After just 1 year of the study, 79% of the subjects reported reduced stress and fewer symptoms of respiratory infections. Preliminary data also indicated that the majority of volunteers maintained a low incidence of upper and lower respiratory infections.

#### IMPLICATIONS FOR NURSING

Nurses can play an important role in educating older adults about the beneficial effects of regular moderate exercise such as walking. The client is likely not only to reduce the incidence of respiratory infections but also to realize other benefits, such as improved cardiac and respiratory function, and improved musculoskeletal strength, endurance, and flexibility.

#### Critical Thinking in Client Care Level

1. How does stress level affect susceptibility to infection of the upper respiratory tract?
2. Why is regular exercise beneficial in reducing the perceived level of stress?
3. Plan an exercise program to meet the needs of a mixed group of older adults living in a rural area of the Pacific Northwest. Consider probable access to facilities, weather (usually cool and rainy), age range, and possible gender differences.

Include the following topics in teaching for home care:

- Using disposable tissues to cover the mouth and nose while coughing or sneezing to reduce airborne spread of the virus.
- Blowing the nose with both nostrils open to prevent infected matter from being forced into the eustachian tubes.
- Washing hands frequently, especially after coughing or sneezing, to limit viral transmission.
- Using over-the-counter preparations for symptomatic relief; precautions related to the sedating effects of antihistamines.
- Limiting use of nasal decongestants to every 4 hours for only a few days at a time to prevent rebound effect.

## THE CLIENT WITH INFLUENZA

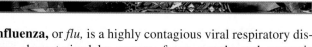

**Influenza,** or *flu,* is a highly contagious viral respiratory disease characterized by coryza, fever, cough, and systemic symptoms such as headache and malaise. Influenza usually occurs in epidemics or pandemics, although sporadic cases do occur. Localized outbreaks of influenza usually occur about every 1 to 3 years. Global epidemics (pandemics) are less frequent, developing every 10 to 15 years until the past two decades. Although influenza tends to be mild and self-limited in healthy adults, older adults and people with chronic heart or pulmonary disease have a high incidence of complications (such as pneumonia) and a higher risk for mortality related to the disease and its complications (Braunwald et al., 2001).

### PATHOPHYSIOLOGY

Influenza virus is transmitted by airborne droplet and direct contact. Three major strains of the virus have been identified as influenza A virus, influenza B virus, and influenza C virus. Influenza A is responsible for most infections and the most severe outbreaks of influenza. This is primarily due to its ability to alter its surface antigens, bypassing previously developed immune defenses to the virus. New strains of influenza virus are named according to the strain, geographic origin, and year (e.g., A/Taiwan/89). Outbreaks of influenza B virus are generally less extensive and less severe than those caused by influenza A virus. Illness associated with influenza C virus is mild and often goes unrecognized.

The incubation period for influenza is short, only 18 to 72 hours. The virus infects the respiratory epithelium. It rapidly replicates in infected cells and is released to infect neighboring cells. Inflammation leads to necrosis and shedding of serous and ciliated cells of the respiratory tract. This allows extracellular fluid to escape, producing rhinorrhea. With recovery, serous cells are replaced more rapidly than ciliated cells, leading to continued cough and coryza. Systemic manifestations of influenza likely are caused by release of inflammatory mediators such as tumor necrosis factor α and interleukin 6 (Braunwald et al., 2001).

The respiratory epithelial necrosis caused by influenza increases the risk for secondary bacterial infections. Sinusitis and otitis media are frequent complications of influenza. Tracheobronchitis, inflammation of the trachea and bronchi, may develop. While tracheobronchitis is not a serious health risk, its manifestations may persist for up to 3 weeks.

Influenza is clearly linked to an increased risk for pneumonia, particularly in older adults. Changes in respiratory function associated with aging, including decreased effectiveness of cough and increased residual lung volume, pose little risk in the healthy older adult but greatly increase the risk for pneumonia associated with influenza. Viral pneumonia is a serious complication that may be fatal. It typically develops within 48 hours of the onset of influenza, often in clients with preexisting heart valve or pulmonary disease. Influenza pneumonia progresses rapidly and can cause hypoxemia and death within a few days. Bacterial pneumonia is more likely to occur in older at-risk adults but also may affect otherwise healthy adults. It usually presents as a relapse of influenza, with a productive cough and evidence of pneumonia on the chest X-ray. See Chapter 36 for more information about pneumonia. 

*Reye's syndrome* is a rare but potentially fatal complication of influenza. Although it is more likely to affect children, it also has been identified in older adults. It is most often associated with influenza B virus. Reye's syndrome develops within 2 to 3 weeks after the onset of influenza. It has a 30% mortality rate. Hepatic failure and encephalopathy develop rapidly in clients with Reye's syndrome.

## MANIFESTATIONS

Infection with influenza virus produces one of three syndromes: uncomplicated nasopharyngeal inflammation, viral upper respiratory infection followed by bacterial infection, or viral pneumonia. The onset is rapid; profound malaise may develop in a matter of minutes.

Manifestations of influenza include abrupt onset of chills and fever, malaise, muscle aches, and headache. Respiratory manifestations include dry, nonproductive cough, sore throat, substernal burning, and coryza (see the box below). Acute symptoms subside within 2 to 3 days, although fever may last as long as a week. The cough may be severe and productive. Along with fatigue and weakness, the cough can persist for days or several weeks.

---

## Manifestations of Influenza

### RESPIRATORY MANIFESTATIONS

- Coryza
- Cough, initially dry becoming productive
- Substernal burning
- Sore throat

### SYSTEMIC MANIFESTATIONS

- Fever and chills
- Malaise
- Muscle aches
- Fatigue

---

## COLLABORATIVE CARE

Preventing influenza by immunizing at-risk populations is an important aspect of care. Immunization with polyvalent (containing antigens of several viral strains) influenza virus vaccine is about 85% effective in preventing influenza infection for several months to a year (Tierney et al., 2001). Annual immunization is recommended for at-risk clients, including people over the age of 65, residents of nursing homes, adults and children with chronic cardiopulmonary disorders (e.g., asthma) or chronic metabolic diseases such as diabetes, and health care workers who have frequent contact with high-risk clients. Additionally, family members of at-risk clients should be vaccinated to reduce the client's risk of exposure. The vaccine is given in the fall, prior to the annual winter outbreak. (See the box below.) Medical treatment of influenza focuses on establishing the diagnosis, providing symptomatic relief, and preventing complications.

---

## Nursing Research
### Evidence-Based Practice to Prevent Influenza

Older adults are disproportionately affected by influenza and related disorders: approximately 80% to 90% of all influenza-related deaths in the United States occur in people who are 65 or older (Hughes & Tartasky, 1996). Additionally, costs associated with influenza-related hospitalizations during epidemics are staggering. Previous studies have found that older adults are most likely to use strategies such as dressing warmly, ensuring adequate nutrition and taking vitamins to prevent influenza, with only 38% of participants getting influenza immunization. Few identify pneumonia as a possible consequence of influenza and upper respiratory infection. Hughes & Tartasky (1996) describe developing and implementing an immunization program for home-bound elders using the Health Belief Model as a theoretical framework.

### IMPLICATIONS FOR NURSING

The population at highest risk for serious sequelae from colds or influenza is older adults. Nurses can have a positive influence on client outcomes by teaching appropriate prevention strategies and symptom management. It is important to include information about possible adverse consequences and indicators for medical attention when teaching self-care. Nurses in community-based settings and those providing home care should plan immunization clinics to reach older adults in accessible settings such as homes, senior centers, assisted living facilities, and grocery stores.

### Critical Thinking in Client Care

1. Identify five common reasons given for not getting an influenza immunization.
2. For each reason given, identify at least one nursing strategy to encourage at-risk clients to seek immunization.
3. What additional measures can nurses take to reduce the risk of an influenza epidemic in their communities?

## Diagnostic Tests

The diagnosis of influenza is based on history, clinical findings, and knowledge of an influenza outbreak in the community. A chest X-ray and white blood cell (WBC) count may be done to rule out complications such as pneumonia. The WBC is commonly decreased in influenza; bacterial infections usually cause increased WBCs.

## Medications

Yearly immunization with influenza vaccine is the single most important measure to prevent or minimize symptoms of influenza. Although the vaccine is readily available and inexpensive, only about 30% of at-risk clients are vaccinated each year. Many may fear a reaction from the vaccine, although the vaccines are highly purified and reactions are rare. About 5% of people experience mild symptoms of low-grade fever, malaise, or myalgia for up to 24 hours after vaccination. Because the vaccine is produced in eggs, it should not be given to people who are allergic to egg protein. Serious adverse reactions to influenza vaccine are rare. *Guillain-Barré syndrome,* an acute neurologic disorder characterized by muscle weakness and distal sensory loss, has been associated with certain batches of vaccine.

Amantadine (Symmetrel) or rimantadine (Flumadine) may be used for prophylaxis in unvaccinated people who are exposed to the virus. If the drug is given before or within 48 hours of exposure, it inhibits viral shedding and prevents or decreases the symptoms of influenza. If possible, unvaccinated people should receive the vaccine along with the antiviral drug. The drug is continued for several weeks or for the duration of the influenza outbreak.

Amantadine, rimantadine, and the antiviral drugs zanamivir (Relenza), oseltamivir (Tamiflu), and ribavirin (Virazole) also may be used to reduce the duration and severity of flu symptoms. Both zanamivir and ribavirin are administered by inhalation; the other drugs are given orally. See Chapter 8 ⊖⊃ for nursing implications for antiviral drugs.

Over-the-counter analgesics such as aspirin, acetaminophen, or NSAIDs provide symptomatic relief of fever and muscle ache. Antitussives may decrease cough, promoting rest. Antibiotics are not indicated unless secondary bacterial infection occurs.

## NURSING CARE

### Health Promotion

Stress the importance of yearly influenza vaccination for clients in high-risk groups and their families. Teach about spread of the disease, including measures to reduce the risk of contracting influenza, such as avoiding crowds and people who are ill.

### Assessment

Unless there is a known outbreak of influenza in the community, it can be difficult to differentiate the manifestations of influenza from those of other URI.

- Health history: known exposure to virus; current symptoms, their onset and duration; presence of dyspnea, chest pain, productive cough, facial pain or pressure in sinus areas; current medications, history of influenza vaccine; chronic diseases such as heart disease, chronic obstructive pulmonary disease (COPD), or diabetes; known medication allergies.
- Physical examination: general appearance; vital signs including temperature; skin color; lung sounds; abdominal exam

## Nursing Diagnoses and Interventions

Although the symptoms of influenza are distressing, most people with the illness provide self-care and do not contact a health care provider. Recommendations to rest in bed during the acute phase of the illness and limit activities until recovery are appropriate for influenza.

Severe disease or complications of influenza may necessitate hospitalization for respiratory support and management. For these clients, nursing care focuses on maintaining airway clearance, breathing patterns, and adequate rest.

### Ineffective Breathing Pattern

Muscle aches, malaise, and elevated temperature may increase the respiratory rate and alter the depth of respirations, decreasing effective alveolar ventilation. Shallow respirations also increase the risk of *atelectasis,* lack of ventilation in an area of lung.

> **PRACTICE ALERT** *Monitor respiratory rate and pattern. Tachypnea and/or rapid, shallow respirations may impair effective alveolar ventilation and gas exchange.* ■

- Pace activities to provide for periods of rest. *Tachypnea increases the work of breathing, causing fatigue; fatigue, in turn, can further impair ventilation and reduce the effectiveness of coughing.*
- Elevate the head of the bed. *The upright position improves lung excursion and reduces the work of breathing by lowering the diaphragm, moving abdominal contents downward, creating less resistance to diaphragmatic excursion, and slightly decreasing venous return.*

### Ineffective Airway Clearance

Swelling and congestion of mucous membranes, extracellular fluid exudate, and impaired ciliary action due to cell damage increase the risk of impaired airway clearance in influenza. The older adult is at particular risk because of normally reduced ciliary activity and increased lung compliance.

> **PRACTICE ALERT** *Monitor the effectiveness of cough and ability to remove airway secretions. Fatigue and general malaise may impair the ability to cough effectively and mobilize secretions.* ■

## CHART 35–1 NANDA, NIC, AND NOC LINKAGES

### The Client with Influenza

| NURSING DIAGNOSES | NURSING INTERVENTIONS | NURSING OUTCOMES |
|---|---|---|
| • Ineffective Breathing Pattern | • Cough Enhancement<br>• Respiratory Monitoring | • Respiratory Status: Ventilation |
| • Deficient Fluid Volume | • Fluid Management | • Hydration |
| • Hyperthermia | • Fever Treatment | • Thermoregulation |
| • Health-Seeking Behaviors | • Health Education<br>• Immunization/Vaccination Management | • Health-Promoting Behavior<br>• Immunization Behavior |

*Note. Data from* Nursing Outcomes Classification (NOC) *by M. Johnson & M. Maas (Eds.), 1997, St. Louis: Mosby;* Nursing Diagnoses: Definitions & Classification 2001–2002 *by North American Nursing Diagnosis Association, 2001, Philadelphia: NANDA;* Nursing Interventions Classification (NIC) *by J.C. McCloskey & G. M. Bulechek (Eds.), 2000, St. Louis: Mosby. Reprinted by permission.*

• Maintain adequate hydration. Assess mucous membranes and skin turgor for evidence of dehydration. *Fever and decreased oral fluid intake may lead to dehydration and increased viscosity of secretions. Thick, viscous secretions are more difficult to expectorate.*

• Increase the humidity of inspired air with a bedside humidifier. *Increasing the water content of inhaled air helps loosen thick secretions and soothe mucous membranes.*

• Teach effective cough techniques. Administer analgesics as ordered. *The huff cough is effective to maintain open airways and spares energy (see Chapter 36 ⊂⊃ for client teaching of this technique). Relieving muscle ache increases the ability to cough effectively.*

### Disturbed Sleep Pattern

Airway congestion, malaise, muscle aches, and persistent cough may interfere with the ability to rest, increasing fatigue and prolonging recovery.

• Assess sleep patterns using subjective and objective information. *The client may appear to be sleeping but not achieving normal sleep patterns because of influenza symptoms. Both subjective and objective data are important to accurately assess sleep.*

• Provide antipyretic and analgesic medications at or shortly before bedtime. *These drugs promote comfort by reducing fever and relieving muscle aches.*

**PRACTICE ALERT** *If necessary, request a cough suppressant for nighttime use. Cough suppressants are not recommended during the day because coughing promotes airway clearance. They may, however, be necessary at night to allow rest.* ∎

### Using NANDA, NIC, and NOC

Chart 35–1 shows links between NANDA nursing diagnoses, NIC, and NOC for the client with influenza.

### Home Care

Encourage appropriate self-care for clients with influenza. Discuss the following topics related to home care:

• Increase rest during the acute, febrile phase of the illness.
• Maintain a liberal fluid intake even if anorexic.
• Appropriately use over-the-counter medications for symptom relief.
• Employ hygiene measures such as using disposable tissues and frequent handwashing to reduce spread of the disease.
• Know manifestations of potential complications of influenza to report to the primary care provider.

## THE CLIENT WITH SINUSITIS

**Sinusitis** is inflammation of the mucous membranes of one or more of the sinuses (see Figure 34–2). Sinusitis is a common condition that usually follows an upper respiratory infection such as acute viral upper respiratory infection or influenza. Common causative organisms include streptococci, *S. pneumoniae, Haemophilus influenzae,* and staphylococci. The risk of sinusitis is higher when the immune system is suppressed by immunosuppressive drugs or HIV infection. Sinusitis is common and difficult to treat in people who have AIDS.

### PHYSIOLOGY REVIEW

The sinuses (or *paranasal sinuses*) are air-filled cavities in the facial bones that open into the turbinates of the nasal cavity. They are lined with ciliated mucous membranes that help move fluid and microorganisms out of the sinuses into the nasal cavity. The sinuses normally are sterile. Air within the sinuses has a lower oxygen content than inspired air.

### PATHOPHYSIOLOGY

Sinusitis develops when nasal mucous membranes swell or other disorders obstruct sinus openings, impairing drainage. Mucus secretions collect in the sinus cavity, serving as a medium for bacterial growth. The nasal and sinus mucous membranes are continuous; therefore, bacteria generally spread to the sinuses via the opening into the nasal turbinates. The inflammatory response provoked by bacterial invasion draws serum and leukocytes to the area to combat the infection, increasing swelling and pressure.

Any process that impairs drainage from the sinuses may precipitate sinusitis. These include nasal polyps, deviated septum, rhinitis, tooth abscess, or swimming or diving trauma. In hospitalized clients, sinusitis may develop following prolonged nasotracheal intubation. Usually more than one sinus is infected. The frontal and maxillary sinuses are usually involved in adults.

Sinusitis may be acute or chronic. Chronic sinusitis results when acute sinusitis is untreated or inadequately treated. With continued infection, bacteria can become isolated, producing chronic inflammation. Over time, mucous membranes become thickened. Fungal infections may cause chronic infections, especially in immunosuppressed clients. Other factors that may contribute to chronic sinusitis are smoking, a history of allergy, and habitual use of nasal sprays or inhalants.

Complications develop when the infection spreads to surrounding structures (Box 35–1). These include periorbital abscess, or cellulitis, cavernous sinus thrombosis, meningitis, brain abscess, or sepsis. Eustachian tube edema may lead to hearing loss.

## MANIFESTATIONS

The client with acute sinusitis often looks sick. Manifestations of sinusitis include pain and tenderness across the infected sinuses, headache, fever, and malaise. The pain usually increases with leaning forward. When the maxillary sinuses are involved, pain and pressure are felt over the cheek. The pain may be referred to the upper teeth. Frontal sinusitis causes pain and tenderness across the lower forehead. Infection of the ethmoid sinus produces retro-orbital pain and pain over the high lateral aspect of the nose. Sphenoid sinusitis, the rarest form, may cause pain in the occiput, vertex, or middle of the head. Symptoms often worsen for 3 to 4 hours after awakening and then become less severe in the afternoon and evening as secretions drain. The intensity and location of headache pain may change as sinuses drain. In acute sinusitis, the pain is usually constant and severe. In chronic sinusitis, the pain is described as dull and may be constant or intermittent.

| BOX 35–1 | ■ Potential Complications of Sinusitis |
|---|---|

### LOCAL COMPLICATIONS
| | |
|---|---|
| ■ Orbital cellulitis | ■ Cavernous sinus thrombosis |
| ■ Subperiosteal abscess | ■ Mucocele |
| ■ Orbital abscess | ■ Osteomyelitis |

### INTRACRANIAL COMPLICATIONS
| | |
|---|---|
| ■ Meningitis | ■ Brain abscess |
| ■ Epidural abscess | ■ Venous sinus thrombosis |
| ■ Subdural abscess | |

Other symptoms include nasal congestion, purulent nasal discharge, and bad breath. The nasal mucous membrane is red and swollen. Purulent drainage may be noted at the opening to the middle turbinate. This may be the only sign of chronic sinusitis. Swallowed secretions irritate and inflame the throat, and may cause nausea or vomiting.

## COLLABORATIVE CARE

Treatment of sinusitis focuses on restoring drainage of obstructed sinuses, controlling infection, relieving pain, and preventing complications.

### Diagnostic Tests

The diagnosis of acute sinusitis usually can be made using the history and physical exam.

* *Sinus X-rays* are evaluated. Sinuses are normally translucent because they are filled with air; affected sinuses appear cloudy or opaque. A visible air-fluid level or thickening of the sinus mucosa may be seen in infected sinuses.
* *CT scan* is a more sensitive indicator of acute and chronic sinusitis and often is performed without preceding X-rays.
* *Magnetic resonance imaging (MRI)* may be ordered if malignancy of the sinus is suspected.

### Medications

Antibiotic therapy directed at the usual organisms causing sinusitis typically is prescribed. Amoxicillin (possibly combined with clavulanate [Augmentin]), trimethoprim-sulfamethoxazole (Bactrim, Septra), cefuroxime (Ceftin), cefaclor (Ceclor), ciprofloxacin (Cipro), or clarithromycin (Biaxin) are commonly used antibiotics for sinusitis. Antibiotic therapy is continued for a full 2-week course; occasionally a longer course is prescribed to prevent relapse. If the sinusitis does not respond to treatment with oral antibiotics, hospitalization and intravenous antibiotic therapy may be required. See Chapter 8 for nursing care related to antibiotic therapy. ⚭

Oral or topical (in the form of nasal sprays) decongestants such as pseudoephedrine or phenylephrine are also prescribed to reduce mucosal edema and promote sinus drainage. Antihistamines may decrease nasal congestion and facilitate sinus drainage, but they also tend to increase the viscosity of secretions and hinder drainage. For this reason, they may not be as effective as decongestants. Saline nose drops or sprays promote sinus drainage, as does inhalation of warm steam. To administer topical drugs, the client's head is tilted backward and to the side on which the drops are to be instilled. The client may need to remain in position for 5 minutes to allow the drops to reach the posterior nares. Systemic mucolytic agents such as guaifenesin may be useful to liquefy secretions, promoting sinus drainage. Aerobic exercise also promotes mucous flow and may be recommended.

### Surgery

Clients who do not respond to pharmacologic measures and who experience persistent facial pain, headache, or nasal congestion may require *endoscopic sinus surgery*. Detailed evaluation of the sinuses by CT scan is done prior to surgery. Under local or general anesthesia, a fiberoptic nasal endoscope is inserted to visualize the sinus opening. If obstruction is present, it can be removed, restoring patency and drainage. This surgery is most effective for local disease, recurrent acute sinusitis, and for removing anatomic obstructions (Way & Doherty, 2003). Clients who have endoscopic sinus surgery usually do not require nasal packing postoperatively. Instead, frequent nasal cleaning and irrigation with normal saline are performed. The client is instructed to sneeze with the mouth open and avoid blowing the nose, lifting, or straining for a week following surgery.

*Antral irrigation* can be done in the physician's office under local anesthesia. A 16-gauge needle is inserted under the inferior turbinate of the nose into the maxillary sinus on the affected side. Saline solution is instilled to irrigate the area and wash out the sinus of purulent exudate. The client is seated with the head forward and mouth open to allow drainage of the solution through the nose and mouth. A culture of the exudate may be obtained to determine appropriate antibiotic therapy.

The *Caldwell-Luc procedure* may be necessary if endoscopic sinus surgery is unsuccessful. It is performed under local or general anesthesia. An incision is made under the upper lip into the maxillary sinus, and diseased mucous membrane and periosteum are removed. An opening between the maxillary sinus and lateral nasal wall, a "nasal antral window," is created to increase aeration of the sinus and promote drainage into the nasal cavity. The area is packed with gauze for 24 to 48 hours postoperatively. The gauze packing obstructs nasal breathing while it is in place. As the maxillary sinus heals, exposed bone is covered by mucosa. The upper lip and teeth may be numb for several months after the procedure because of nerve trauma. Chewing may be impaired on the affected side. Only liquids are given for the first 24 hours, followed by a soft diet. The client is instructed to avoid wearing dentures and the Valsalva maneuver (no blowing the nose, coughing, or straining at stool) for about 2 weeks after the packing has been removed to prevent bleeding.

In *external sphenoethmoidectomy,* an incision along the side of the nose from the middle of the eyebrow is used to open and remove diseased tissue from the sphenoid or ethmoid sinuses (Figure 35–1 ■). Nasal polyps may also be removed using this

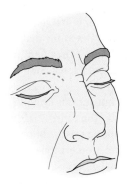

**Figure 35–1** ■ Incision to access ethmoid and frontal sinuses. Resulting scar is nearly invisible in folds of the eye.

approach. Nasal packing is inserted, and an eye pressure patch is applied to decrease periorbital edema. Care is similar to that following the Caldwell-Luc procedure.

## NURSING CARE

### Assessment

Focused assessment of the client with suspected sinusitis includes the following:

- Health history: complaints of frontal or periorbital headache, cheek, teeth, or ear pain; timing of pain and changes in intensity over course of the day; nasal discharge or postnasal drip; other symptoms; previous sinus problems; current medications, known medication allergies
- Physical examination: general appearance, vital signs including temperature; inspect nasal and pharyngeal mucous membranes; percuss sinuses for tenderness

### Nursing Diagnoses and Interventions

The client with sinusitis is often acutely uncomfortable. Obstructed and congested sinuses cause pain and pressure that increase with position changes and leaning forward. Treatment usually is community based, making education the key nursing role. When the client is hospitalized for intravenous antibiotic therapy or sinus surgery, *Pain* and *Imbalanced nutrition* are priority nursing diagnoses.

#### Pain

Although sinus surgery is relatively minor, both the incision and postoperative swelling can cause discomfort. Nasal packing, if used, contributes to the discomfort.

- Assess pain using a standardized pain scale. Administer analgesics as ordered. *Relief of pain promotes a feeling of well-being and enhances recovery.*
- Apply ice packs to the nose. *Cold compresses reduce swelling, control bleeding, and provide local analgesia.*
- Elevate the head of the bed to Fowler's or high-Fowler's position for 24 to 48 hours after surgery. *Elevating the operative site minimizes tissue swelling and promotes comfort.*

#### Imbalanced Nutrition: Less Than Body Requirements

Postoperatively, the sense of smell, an appetite stimulus, is diminished by nasal packing. Mouth discomfort from the incision and numbness of the upper teeth also may impact appetite and eating.

- Provide clear liquid diet progressing to soft foods as tolerated. High-calorie dietary supplements may be used. *A progressive diet is used to assess the ability to swallow without choking and allay fears. Foods high in calories and nutritional value provide for metabolic and healing requirements.*
- Monitor intake, output, and weight. *This information allows assessment of overall fluid balance and the adequacy of dietary intake.*
- Elevate the head of the bed during meals. *The upright position facilitates swallowing and minimizes risk of aspiration.*

## Home Care

Teaching for clients with sinusitis and their families focuses on following through with appropriate treatment and promoting comfort. Discuss the following topics when preparing for home care:

- The importance of completing the entire course of prescribed antibiotics to achieve cure and prevent the development of antibiotic-resistant bacteria. Assist in developing a schedule that helps ensure all doses are taken.
- Measures to prevent superinfections (such as vaginitis or oral thrush) during the prolonged course of treatment (e.g., consume 8 oz of yogurt containing live bacterial cultures daily while on antibiotics).
- Use systemic or topical decongestants to promote sinus drainage.
- Maintain a liberal fluid intake to reduce the viscosity of mucous drainage.
- Use a humidifier or steam inhalation to promote sinus drainage.
- Sleep with the head of the bed elevated to a 45-degree angle and on the unaffected side to promote drainage of affected sinuses.
- Application of a warm, moist pack to the area of pain and tenderness to promote comfort.
- Notify the physician if symptoms do not improve with treatment or if signs of a complication develop, such as increased pain, and redness and swelling on the side of the nose or around the eyes.
- Postoperative instructions to prevent bleeding, such as avoiding blowing the nose for 7 to 10 days and avoiding strenuous activity such as heavy lifting for about 2 weeks.
- Use saline nasal sprays postoperatively to keep the nasal mucosa moist.

## THE CLIENT WITH PHARYNGITIS OR TONSILLITIS

**Pharyngitis,** acute inflammation of the pharynx, is one of the most commonly identified clinical problems. Although it is usually viral in origin, pharyngitis may also be caused by bacterial infection. *Group A beta-hemolytic streptococcus* (strep throat) is the most common cause of bacterial pharyngitis. Other bacteria that may cause pharyngitis include *Neisseria gonorrheae,* a gram-negative diplococcus that is sexually transmitted, *Mycoplasma,* and *Chlamydia trachomatis.*

**Tonsillitis** is acute inflammation of the palatine tonsils. Although it is sometimes viral in origin, tonsillitis is usually due to streptococcal infection. The incidence of streptococcal infections is greatest between late fall and spring, especially in cold climates. Viral tonsillitis may occur in epidemics in people living in crowded conditions, such as military recruits.

## PATHOPHYSIOLOGY AND MANIFESTATIONS

Pharyngitis and tonsillitis are contagious and spread by droplet nuclei. Incubation varies from a few hours to several days, depending on the organism. Viral infections are communicable for 2 to 3 days. Symptoms usually resolve within 3 to 10 days after onset.

Viral pharyngitis may be attributed to the same viruses causing the common cold, rhinovirus, coronavirus, or parainfluenza virus. Pharyngitis caused by adenovirus, influenza virus, or Epstein-Barr virus (associated with infectious mononucleosis) may be particularly severe.

Although bacterial pharyngitis may be mild and indistinguishable from viral pharyngitis by its signs and symptoms, it can lead to significant complications such as abscess, scarlet fever, toxic shock syndrome, rheumatic fever, or acute post-streptococcal glomerulonephritis.

Acute pharyngitis causes pain and fever. The pain may vary from a scratchy sore throat to one so painful that swallowing is difficult. Streptococcal pharyngitis is usually marked by an abrupt onset, with fever of 101° F (38.3° C) or higher, severe sore throat with dysphagia, malaise, and often arthralgias and myalgias. Anterior lymph nodes are often enlarged and tender. Exudate (pus) may be seen on the pharynx and tonsils. In contrast, the onset of viral pharyngitis is often gradual, with manifestations of low-grade fever, sore throat, mild hoarseness, headache, and rhinorrhea. The pharyngeal membranes appear mildly red with vascular congestion. Infectious mononucleosis, caused by the Epstein-Barr virus, often presents as acute pharyngitis, with visible patches of exudate on the pharynx or tonsils (Braunwald et al., 2001). The cervical lymph nodes are enlarged and tender as well.

In tonsillitis, the tonsils appear bright red and edematous. White exudate is present on the tonsils; pressing on a tonsil may produce purulent drainage. The uvula may also be reddened and swollen. Cervical lymph nodes are usually tender and enlarged.

The client with tonsillitis complains of a sore throat, difficulty swallowing, general malaise, fever, and otalgia (pain referred to the ear). Manifestations are often more severe in adolescents and adults than in children. Infection may extend via the eustachian tubes to cause acute otitis media. This may lead to further damage such as spontaneous rupture of the eardrums and mastoiditis. See Chapter 45 ⌘ for more information about otitis media.

*Peritonsillar abscess,* or *quinsy,* is a potential complication of tonsillitis. It usually results from group A beta-hemolytic streptococcus infection extending from the tonsils to the surrounding tissue. The abscess causes pus formation behind the tonsil with marked swelling and asymmetric deviation of the uvula. The degree of swelling may make it difficult to swallow anything other than liquids. The client may exhibit thickening of the voice, drooling, and a tonic contraction of the muscles of mastication, called trismus.

Rare (1% to 3%) but serious complications of streptococcal pharyngitis and tonsillitis include acute glomerulonephritis and rheumatic fever, abnormal immune responses to the infection. Acute glomerulonephritis generally presents with sudden onset of hematuria, proteinuria, and less commonly, hypertension and edema within 7 to 10 days after the acute infection. Rheumatic fever typically presents 3 to 5 weeks after acute infection with fever, painful or swollen joints, rash, and heart murmur. Other complications of bacterial infection include sinusitis, otitis media, mastoiditis, and cervical adenitis.

## COLLABORATIVE CARE

Both viral and bacterial pharyngitis are usually self-limited diseases. However, because of the risk for serious complications associated with streptococcal sore throat, an effort is usually made to establish an accurate diagnosis and treat bacterial pharyngitis.

- *Throat swab* is obtained and examined for streptococcus antigen using the latex agglutination (LA) antigen test or enzyme immunoassay (ELISA) testing. These tests allow rapid identification of the antigen (in as little as 10 minutes for the LA test) but are not highly sensitive. When the test is positive, treatment for strep throat is initiated. If the test is negative, the swab is cultured to ensure that streptococcus organisms are not present. Even throat cultures are not always accurate, with approximately 10% false negative and 20% false positive results.
- *Complete blood count (CBC)* may be done on severely ill clients or to rule out other causes of pharyngitis. The WBC count is usually normal or low in viral infections and elevated in bacterial infections.

Antipyretics and mild analgesics such as aspirin or acetaminophen provide symptomatic relief for throat pain and associated myalgias. Penicillin is the drug of choice for group A streptococci. Erythromycin, amoxicillin, or cefuroxime (Ceftin, Kefurox) may be used if the client is allergic to penicillin. Antibiotic therapy is continued for at least 10 days. The client is no longer contagious after 24 hours of antibiotic therapy.

A peritonsillar abscess is drained by needle aspiration or by incision and drainage. The area is first sprayed with a topical anesthetic such as cetacaine and then injected with a local anesthetic. The sitting position is preferred for the procedure, because it enables expectoration of blood and pus. Tonsillectomy is done either immediately or 6 weeks after incision and drainage of peritonsillar abscess.

*Tonsillectomy* (surgical removal of the tonsils) is indicated for recurrent or chronic infections that have not responded to antibiotic therapy, hypertrophy of the tonsils with risk of airway obstruction, peritonsillar abscess, repeated attacks of purulent otitis media, and tonsil malignancy. Adenoid tissue usually is removed at the same time. Bleeding is the most significant postoperative complication of tonsillectomy.

## NURSING CARE

Because of the risk of significant complications associated with streptococcal pharyngitis, encourage all clients with symptoms that persist for several days or that include fever, lymphadenopathy, and myalgias to seek evaluation and treatment.

Home care is appropriate for acute uncomplicated pharyngitis. Treatment focuses on adequate rest and relief of symptoms. A liquid or soft diet is useful when swallowing is difficult. Increased fluid intake is encouraged, especially when febrile. Warm saline gargles, moist inhalations, and application of an ice collar are soothing to the sore throat.

Following tonsillectomy, ensure a patent airway by placing the client in semi-Fowler's position with the head turned to the side to allow secretions to drain from the mouth and pharynx. Keep the airway in place until the gag and swallowing reflexes have returned. Apply an ice collar to reduce swelling and pain. Notify the surgeon immediately if excessive bleeding or hemorrhage occurs. If there is no bleeding, allow water and cracked ice as desired. Warm saline mouthwashes are helpful in managing thick oral secretions following tonsillectomy. A liquid or semiliquid diet is recommended for several days.

### Home Care

Discuss the following topics when preparing the client for home care.

- The importance of completing the full 10 days of antibiotic therapy if prescribed
- Using warm saline gargles or throat lozenges for symptomatic relief
- Signs and symptoms of possible complications of streptococcal infection such as glomerulonephritis or rheumatic fever
- Monitoring temperature in the morning and evening until well to ensure that the infection has not spread to deeper tissues
- Proper use and disposal of tissues and frequent handwashing to prevent spreading the infection to others

For the client who has had a peritonsillar abscess drainage or tonsillectomy, provide the following instructions.

- Postoperative mouth and throat care
- Avoiding use of aspirin for 2 weeks to reduce the risk of postoperative bleeding
- Manifestations of bleeding to report to the physician (delayed hemorrhage may occur for up to 1 week post surgery)

## THE CLIENT WITH A LARYNGEAL INFECTION

The larynx, located between the upper airways and the lungs, protects the lower respiratory tract from inhaled substances other than air, and allows speech. The larynx includes the epiglottis, which covers the larynx during swallowing, and the glottis, or vocal cords. Either portion of the larynx may become inflamed.

### EPIGLOTTITIS

*Epiglottitis,* inflammation of the epiglottis, is an uncommon disorder that presents as a medical emergency. *H. influenzae* infection is the most common cause of epiglottitis. Epiglottitis is

## Nursing Care Plan

## A Client with Peritonsillar Abscess

Monica Wunderman, age 27, was recently treated for tonsillitis caused by infection by group A streptococcus. She presents to the emergency department 10 days later appearing acutely ill. She states that her throat is so sore that she has difficulty swallowing even liquids. Barbara Ironhorse, the ED nurse, completes an assessment of Ms. Wunderman.

### ASSESSMENT

Findings include T 102°F (38.8°C). An acutely swollen and reddened area of the soft palate is noted in her mouth, half occluding the orifice from the mouth into the pharynx. Yellow exudate is present. CBC reveals an elevated WBC of 16,000/mm³. A diagnosis of peritonsillar abscess is made. Needle aspiration of the abscess is performed.

### DIAGNOSIS

• *Acute pain* related to swelling
• *Risk for ineffective airway clearance* related to pain and swelling
• *Deficient fluid volume* related to fever and difficulty in swallowing fluids

### EXPECTED OUTCOMES

• Have minimal or no pain.
• Maintain a patent airway as demonstrated by normal respiratory rate and rhythm.
• Maintain optimal fluid intake as evidenced by consumption of fluids and semiliquid foods, moist mucous membranes, normal skin turgor, and normal temperature.

### PLANNING AND IMPLEMENTATION

• Teach that ice-cold fluids may be easier to swallow than hot or room-temperature beverages and may provide a local analgesic effect.
• Advise to avoid citrus juices, hot or spicy foods, and rough-textured foods for 1 week.
• Teach pain management strategies such as applying an ice collar as desired and gargling with warm saline or mouthwash solution every 1 to 2 hours for the first 24 to 48 hours after aspiration of the abscess.
• Instruct to take medications as prescribed.

### EVALUATION

When Ms. Ironhorse contacts Ms. Wunderman by telephone 2 days after her visit to the emergency department, she reports complete relief of symptoms. She is afebrile, taking fluids without difficulty, and has had no difficulty breathing. She has not experienced any pain.

### Critical Thinking in the Nursing Process

1. Describe common symptoms of infectious or inflammatory diseases of the upper airway and discuss methods of symptom relief.
2. Describe common pharmacologic interventions for these disorders.
3. What themes of nursing diagnoses emerge for these clients?

See Evaluating Your Response in Appendix C.

---

a rapidly progressive cellulitis that begins between the base of the tongue and the epiglottis. The epiglottis itself becomes swollen and inflamed; swelling of adjacent tissues pushes the epiglottis posteriorly. This swelling and edema threatens the airway. Adults usually present with a 1 to 2 day history of sore throat, *odynophagia* (painful swallowing), dyspnea, and possibly drooling and stridor.

Using a tongue blade to view the oropharynx is avoided; this may precipitate laryngospasm and airway obstruction. The epiglottis is visualized using a flexible fiberoptic laryngoscope to establish the diagnosis. The epiglottis appears red, swollen, and edematous. Nasotracheal intubation may be required to ensure airway patency. The client is admitted to a critical care unit and intravenous antibiotic therapy is initiated. Ceftriaxone (Rocephin), cefuroxime (Ceftin), or ampicillin/sulbactam (Unasyn) may be prescribed. If allergic to penicillin, a combination of clindamycin (Cleocin) and either trimethoprim-sulfamthoxazole (TMP-SMZ) or ciprofloxacin (Cipro) may be used. Dexamethasone, a systemic corticosteroid, is also given to suppress the inflammatory response and rapidly reduce swelling of the epiglottis.

Nursing care for the client with acute epiglottitis focuses on monitoring and maintaining airway patency. Monitor oxygen saturation continuously. Observe closely for signs of airway obstruction, including nasal flaring, restlessness, stridor, use of accessory muscles, and decreased oxygen saturation measurements. If the client is not intubated, supplies for emergency intubation should be kept in the unit. Epiglottitis is frightening for both the client and the nurse. Maintaining a calm, reassuring manner is an essential nursing role.

## LARYNGITIS

**Laryngitis,** inflammation of the larynx, is a common disorder that may occur alone or in conjunction with other upper respiratory infections. It is commonly associated with viral URI such as influenza. It may also occur with bronchitis, pneumonia, or other respiratory infections. Excessive use of the voice, sudden changes in temperature or exposure to dust, irritating fumes, smoke, or other pollutants can also cause acute or chronic laryngitis. It is more common in the winter and in colder climates.

In laryngitis, the mucous membrane lining the larynx becomes inflamed; the vocal cords also may become edematous.

The primary symptom of laryngitis is a change in the voice. Hoarseness or *aphonia,* complete loss of the voice, may occur. The throat is often sore and scratchy, and a dry, harsh cough may be present.

There is no specific treatment for viral laryngitis. Any identified precipitating factors such as overuse of the voice and exposure to irritants should be eliminated. Voice rest is advised, as is abstinence from tobacco and alcohol, which are chemical irritants. Treatment may also include inhaling steam or spraying the throat with antiseptic solutions. Identifying and eliminating irritants is helpful to prevent future attacks.

Impaired verbal communication is the priority nursing problem for clients with laryngitis. The meaning of messages is conveyed not only by the words used, but also by the tone and loudness of voice. Instruct to rest the voice as much as possible. Encourage speaking in short sentences or using alternate methods of communication, such as writing. Resting the voice hastens recovery and decreases throat discomfort. Advise to use soothing throat lozenges, sprays, or other comfort measures such as gargling with a warm antiseptic solution. Help identify potential irritants, such as fumes, chemicals, or cold temperature, to prevent future bouts of laryngitis.

## THE CLIENT WITH DIPHTHERIA

*Diphtheria* is an acute, contagious disease caused by *Corynebacterium diphtheriae,* a small aerobic pathogen. This disease, which primarily affects adults, is uncommon in the United States. Waning immunity due to lack of periodic booster immunizations is the primary risk factor for diphtheria in the United States.

The disease is spread through droplet nuclei and by contamination of articles such as eating utensils. Asymptomatic carriers can be a factor in spreading this infection. People who have recovered from diphtheria can harbor bacteria in their throats for up to 4 weeks. Diphtheria is easily spread in areas where sanitation is poor, living conditions are crowded, and access to health care is limited. Immunization is readily available, and infants and children are usually immunized against diphtheria, pertussis, and tetanus concurrently.

## PATHOPHYSIOLOGY AND MANIFESTATIONS

*C. diphtheriae* infects the mucous membranes of the respiratory tract and can invade skin lesions. The tonsils and pharynx are common sites of infection. Toxins released by the organism inflame mucosal surfaces of the pharynx. Exudate from inflamed tissues forms a thick, grayish, rubbery pseudomembrane over the posterior pharynx and sometimes into the trachea. This pseudomembrane adheres to inflamed, eroded surfaces and interferes with eating, drinking, and breathing. The airway may be obstructed, necessitating tracheostomy to maintain respirations. The toxins damage the heart and central

nervous system and may cause myocarditis and paralysis of cranial or peripheral nerves.

Clients with diphtheria develop fever, malaise, sore throat, and malodorous breath. In severe cases, the neck may be warm and swollen because of lymphadenopathy. Isolated patches of gray or white exudate grow and extend to form a gray membrane that becomes progressively thicker. Dislodging the membrane often causes bleeding. Symptoms of airway obstruction, such as stridor and cyanosis, can develop quickly.

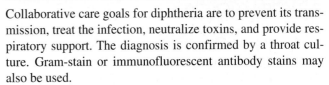

## COLLABORATIVE CARE

Collaborative care goals for diphtheria are to prevent its transmission, treat the infection, neutralize toxins, and provide respiratory support. The diagnosis is confirmed by a throat culture. Gram-stain or immunofluorescent antibody stains may also be used.

Strict isolation procedures are instituted, and all contacts are screened and immunized. Booster shots are given to people who were immunized 5 or more years previously. Unimmunized contacts are treated with immunization and antibiotics.

Diphtheria antitoxin is given to neutralize free toxin and prevent further toxin production. Diphtheria antitoxin is produced in horses; a skin test for sensitivity to horse serum should precede immunization. Anaphylaxis is a risk during antitoxin therapy; epinephrine must be readily available. Antibiotics such as penicillin or erythromycin are administered to eliminate the organism.

## NURSING CARE

Clients with diphtheria require intensive nursing care. The client is placed on bed rest and monitored closely for airway obstruction, cardiac manifestations, and CNS complications. Nutrition and fluid balance may be affected by difficulty swallowing. Upright positioning can promote fluid intake during the acute phase of the disease. Equipment for suction, emergency intubation, and tracheostomy are kept at the bedside.

**PRACTICE ALERT** *Diphtheria is a reportable disease. Immediately contact the local health department and the Centers for Disease Control and Prevention of all suspected and confirmed cases.* ■

Preventing further cases of diphtheria is a nursing responsibility. Symptomatic clients are isolated and treated until two negative throat cultures are obtained. Nasopharyngeal and throat cultures are also obtained from all close contacts. Asymptomatic disease carriers are confined to home until at least 3 days of antibiotic therapy have been completed. All contacts, including hospital personnel, receive tetanus and diphtheria toxoids (Td).

## THE CLIENT WITH PERTUSSIS

**Pertussis,** or *whooping cough,* is a highly contagious acute upper respiratory infection caused by the bacterium *Bordetella pertussis.* Although it is thought to be a childhood disease that has been virtually eliminated by aggressive immunization of infants, pertussis still occurs in North America. Up to 45% of people affected by pertussis are adolescents and adults. Adults are thought to be an important reservoir for this disease (Braunwald et al., 2001).

## PATHOPHYSIOLOGY

*B. pertussis* is a gram-negative rod that is spread by respiratory droplets. The bacteria attach to ciliated epithelial cells of the nasopharynx, multiplying and invading respiratory tissues. The damage and effects of pertussis are not due to the infection itself, but to toxins produced by the bacteria. These toxins damage the mucosa and paralyze the cilia. As a result, clearance of respiratory secretions is impaired, increasing the risk for pneumonia. The toxins also prompt an inflammatory response and inhibit immune defenses.

Although immunization does not appear to confer lifetime immunity, the disease tends to be milder in adolescents, adults, and people who have been immunized. These infected individuals can, however, transmit the disease to other susceptible people, including unimmunized or underimmunized infants (Atkinson, Wolfe, Humiston, & Nelson, 2000).

Young infants have the highest risk for complications of the disease, such as pneumonia and neurologic complications. Neurologic complications are thought to result from hypoxia due to prolonged paroxysms of coughing. Complications in adolescents and adults may occur as a result of increased intrathoracic pressure during prolonged coughing spells. These may include pneumothorax, weight loss, inguinal hernia, rib fracture, and *cough syncope* (fainting due to hypoxia) (Braunwald et al., 2001).

## MANIFESTATIONS

Classic pertussis follows a predictable pattern, with typical upper respiratory infection symptoms (coryza, sneezing, low-grade fever, and mild cough) beginning 7 to 10 days after exposure. After 1 to 2 weeks, the cough becomes more frequent, occurring in paroxysms or bursts of rapid coughs, often ending with an audible whoop caused by rapid inspiration. This whoop is less common in adolescents and adults, often delaying diagnosis. Vomiting commonly follows an episode of coughing. Coughing paroxysms vary in frequency from several per hour to 5 to 10 per day, interfering with eating and sleep. This stage of the disease, called the *paroxysmal stage,* usually lasts no more than 6 weeks, after which coughing becomes less severe and gradually resolves over a period of up to 3 months.

In adolescents and adults, pertussis is suspected when an upper respiratory infection produces a cough that persists longer than 7 days, is accompanied by vomiting, and is worse at night. See the box in next column.

### Manifestations of Pertussis

**CLASSIC**
- Catarrhal phase: coryza, malaise, low-grade fever, sneezing, cough
- Paroxysmal phase: frequent spasms of sometimes violent coughing, worse at night; characteristic whoop on inspiration following cough paroxysm; vomiting, fatigue, weight loss resulting from severe cough
- Convalescent phase: gradually decreasing frequency and severity of coughing episodes

**ATYPICAL (often seen in adolescents and adults)**
- Severe, prolonged cough that may not be paroxysmal; whoop uncommon
- Vomiting with cough
- Cough at night

## COLLABORATIVE CARE

Active immunization with pertussis vaccine is the primary preventive strategy for pertussis. Acellular pertussis vaccines that are effective but produce fewer adverse reactions than traditional whole-cell vaccines are available and preferred for immunization.

The diagnosis of pertussis is established by culture of nasopharyngeal secretions. However, nasopharyngeal secretions may remain positive for the organism for only about 3 weeks after the onset of symptoms, so blood tests for antibodies to the organism may be necessary to confirm the diagnosis. Lymphocytosis (elevated lymphocyte count) may be present.

Erythromycin is the antibiotic of choice to eradicate *B. pertussis* infection. Trimethoprim-sulfamethoxazole (TMP-SMZ) may be used as an alternate to erythromycin. Hospitalization rarely is required for adults, although children and infants with severe disease often are hospitalized to prevent complications such as neurologic effects of hypoxia and malnutrition. Respiratory isolation is instituted for 5 days after antibiotic therapy is started. Prophylactic erythromycin or TMP-SMZ is prescribed for all household and close contacts of the infected client.

## NURSING CARE

Nurses are instrumental in promoting effective immunization of all infants and young children against pertussis. Education is a key nursing role related to immunization, as significant controversy currently exists about potential long-term adverse consequences of the vaccine. Recommend that all parents request acellular vaccine due to its lower risk of adverse effects.

Recommend nasopharyngeal culture for clients complaining of persistent cough, especially when the cough is accompanied by vomiting or significantly worse at night, or if other members of the household or close contacts have a similar illness.

Education is a primary nursing role related to pertussis. Adult clients usually remain in the community for treatment. Teach respiratory isolation measures to be used until the disease is no longer communicable to others. Discuss ways to control respiratory secretions, and the importance of disposing of tissues and secretions personally to prevent exposure of others. Stress the importance of prophylactic treatment for all household and close contacts. Discuss measures to maintain fluid and nutrient intake, and use of a cough suppressant at night to promote rest. Encourage increased fluid intake to promote expectoration of respiratory secretions. Teach about the prescribed antibiotic, including its potential adverse effects and measures to reduce them, such as taking erythromycin with meals to prevent gastric upset. Contact the local county health department for follow-up of contacts and compliance with prescribed treatment.

# UPPER RESPIRATORY TRAUMA OR OBSTRUCTION

## THE CLIENT WITH EPISTAXIS

The nose has a rich blood supply, receiving major arterial vessels from both the internal and external carotid artery systems. **Epistaxis,** or nosebleed, may be precipitated by a number of factors. Trauma (picking the nose or blunt trauma) can cause epistaxis, as can drying of nasal mucous membranes, infection, substance abuse (e.g., cocaine), arteriosclerosis, or hypertension. Epistaxis may also indicate a bleeding disorder related to acute leukemia, thrombocytopenia, aplastic anemia, or severe liver disease. Additionally, treatment with an anticoagulant or antiplatelet drug may cause nosebleed. In adults, men more frequently have nosebleeds than women.

## PATHOPHYSIOLOGY

Ninety percent of all nosebleeds arise in the anterior nasal septum from Kiesselbach's area, a rich vascular plexus. Because of their location, these vessels are susceptible to trauma from nose picking, drying, and infection. Posterior epistaxis more often develops secondarily to systemic disorders such as blood dyscrasias, hypertension, or diabetes. In posterior epistaxis, bleeding is from the terminal branches of the sphenopalatine and internal maxillary arteries. Posterior epistaxis tends to be more severe and occurs more frequently in the older adult.

## COLLABORATIVE CARE

The goal of treatment for epistaxis is to identify and control the source of bleeding.

Anterior bleeding can usually be managed by simple first-aid measures, such as applying pressure (pinching the nose toward the septum) for 5 to 10 minutes and applying ice packs to the nose and forehead to cause vasoconstriction. The client is placed in a sitting position to decrease blood flow to the head and reduce venous pressure. Leaning forward reduces drainage of blood backward into the nasopharynx and decreases swallowing of blood. The client is instructed to spit out the blood to help estimate the amount of bleeding and to prevent nausea and vomiting as a result of swallowed blood.

If applying pressure does not control the bleeding, medications, nasal packing, or surgery may be necessary.

### Medications

Topical vasoconstrictors such as cocaine (0.5%), phenylephrine (Neo-Synephrine) (1:1000), or adrenaline (1:1000) may be used to control anterior bleeding. These medications may be applied by nasal spray or on a cotton swab held against the bleeding site. Chemical cauterization of the bleeding vessel may be done using agents such as silver nitrate or Gelfoam. A topical anesthetic such as tetracaine, lidocaine, or cocaine may be used prior to nasal packing. If posterior nasal packing is required, prophylactic antibiotic therapy is initiated to prevent sinusitis or possible toxic shock syndrome.

### Nasal Packing

If bleeding cannot be controlled with pressure and local medications, the nasal cavity may be packed with 0.25-inch petroleum gauze. For an anterior pack, several feet of packing are placed carefully and systematically along the floor of the nasal cavity and then into the vault of the nose. Anterior nasal packs are usually left in place for 24 to 72 hours. If epistaxis is caused by a bleeding disorder, the packing may be left in place for 4 to 5 days while the disorder is treated.

Posterior nosebleeds are more difficult to control, requiring both anterior and posterior packing (Figure 35–2 ■). Posterior packs are usually left in place for 2 to 5 days. A loose anterior nasal pack may also be inserted. Posterior nasal packing is very uncomfortable, and can cause respiratory and cardiovascular complications. Hypoxemia is common; supplementary oxygen is administered. Narcotic analgesics are prescribed to manage the discomfort. Hypertension, dysrhythmias, and even acute myocardial infarction may occur in clients with severe cardiovascular disease. Toxic shock syndrome is another potential complication of posterior nasal packing. The pack may occlude

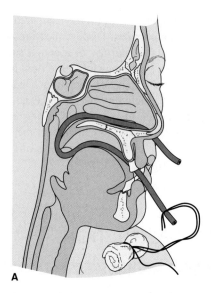 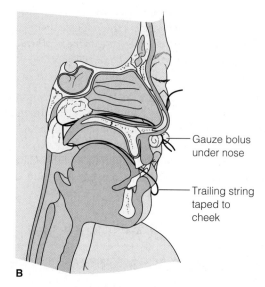

Gauze bolus
under nose

Trailing string
taped to
cheek

A                                                    B

**Figure 35–2** ■ Posterior nasal packing. *A,* A rubber catheter is inserted through the nose and out the mouth and attached to the packing. *B,* The catheter is withdrawn through the nose to position the packing in the posterior nasopharynx. Ties exiting through the nose and mouth are used to stabilize the packing in position and remove it when it is no longer needed.

the eustachian tube and sinus openings, resulting in ear discomfort, possible otitis media, or sinusitis. Oral and nasal dryness can be minimized by use of a high-humidity face tent. Nursing care of the client with nasal packing is outlined in the box below.

A Foley catheter or inflatable nasal balloons may be used as an alternative to posterior nasal packing for effective tamponade. The catheter or nasal balloon is inserted through the nose into the nasopharynx, inflated, and left in place for 2 to 3 days.

## Surgery

Chemical or surgical cautery procedures may be used to sclerose involved vessels in the anterior aspect of the nose. The resulting scab must be left undisturbed until the mucosa has healed, or further bleeding may occur.

Surgical procedures to control bleeding are often preferred to posterior nasal packing for posterior bleeding. The bleeding vessel may be cauterized using an endoscopic approach. In some cases, surgery is required to occlude the internal maxil-

## NURSING CARE OF THE CLIENT WITH NASAL PACKING

- Continuously monitor oxygen saturation. Administer supplementary oxygen as ordered. *Posterior nasal packing causes hypoxemia. Supplemental oxygen is given to maintain tissue oxygenation.*
- Frequently monitor vital signs and respiratory rate or pattern. *Posterior nasal packing increases the risk for respiratory and cardiovascular complications. Tachycardia and tachypnea may be early signs of cardiac or respiratory compromise.*
- Inspect the mouth and oropharynx. Notify the physician if the packing is seen in the oropharynx. *Misplacement of nasal packing can obstruct the upper airway.*
- Elevate the head of the bed. *Elevating the head of the bed facilitates ventilation.*
- Encourage deep, slow breathing through the mouth. Provide psychologic support, reassurance, and teaching. *Inability to breathe through the nose causes anxiety and fear.*

- Check for blood at the back of the throat and frequent swallowing. *Visible blood or frequent swallowing could indicate posterior bleeding.*
- Report hematemesis. *Bleeding from the posterior portion of the nose often drains down the nasopharynx and is swallowed. Hematemesis may indicate continued bleeding.*
- Apply cold compresses to nose. *An ice or cold compress decreases pain and promotes vasoconstriction, decreasing bleeding and swelling.*
- Provide for rest. *Rest reduces the metabolic demands and oxygen consumption.*
- Ensure adequate oral fluid intake. *Fluid intake helps maintain fluid balance and decreases dryness of oral mucous membranes because of mouth breathing.*
- Provide frequent oral hygiene. Use a bedside humidifier. *These measures reduce drying of oral mucous membranes and promote comfort.*

lary artery by ligation (tying off) or embolization. These procedures may be done under either conscious sedation and local anesthesia or general anesthesia. Facial paralysis, paresthesias, facial pain, and dental injury are potential complications (Way & Doherty, 2003).

## NURSING CARE

### Assessment

Nursing assessment of the client with a nosebleed focuses on the immediate problem and possible underlying conditions.

- Health history: duration of current bleed; any identified precipitating factors such as trauma; history of prior nosebleeds; current medications; chronic conditions such as hypertension, bleeding disorders, etc.
- Physical examination: estimated amount of bleeding; presence of blood in oropharynx; vital signs; evidence of facial or nasal trauma

### Nursing Diagnoses and Interventions

Nosebleeds can be frightening, particularly when they occur without preceding trauma. Nurses provide care for clients with epistaxis in outpatient and emergency settings, and may care for hospitalized clients with nasal packing. Support, reassurance, and education are important nursing roles related to epistaxis. Priority nursing diagnoses include *Anxiety* and *Risk for aspiration*.

#### Anxiety

The amount of blood lost in a nosebleed can be frightening. The sensation of blood draining down the throat and inability to breathe through the nose contribute to anxiety. Spontaneous epistaxis may lead to fear of a major health problem such as high blood pressure.

**PRACTICE ALERT** *Maintain an attitude of calm reassurance. By remaining calm and confident, the nurse reassures the client that the nosebleed is not a life-threatening event.* ■

- Instruct the client to pinch the nares together at the bridge of the nose. *Most nosebleeds are anterior in origin; direct pressure usually stops the bleeding. Having the client place pressure on the nose provides a focus and helps restore a sense of control, reducing anxiety.*
- Encourage slow, deep breathing through the mouth. *Controlled mouth breathing maintains lung ventilation and reduces anxiety.*
- Provide a basin and tissues; encourage the client to expectorate blood, not swallow it. *These measures give the client greater control and reduce the fear of choking on blood.*

**PRACTICE ALERT** *Assess the client with nasal packing frequently for adequate oxygenation. Maintain supplemental oxygen as ordered. Cerebral hypoxia produces a sense of apprehension and fear.* ■

#### Risk for Aspiration

Anxiety and blood draining into the nasopharynx increase the risk for aspiration of blood into the trachea. When nasal packing is in place, the client is unable to breathe through the nose, increasing the risk of aspiration when food or fluids are consumed.

**PRACTICE ALERT** *Position upright with the head forward. Provide a basin for expectorating blood. These measures minimize the amount of blood draining down the nasopharynx and swallowed, reducing the risk of aspiration and minimizing nausea from swallowed blood. Vomiting of swallowed blood increases the risk of aspiration.* ■

- Apply ice or a cold compress to the nose. *Cold causes vasoconstriction, reducing bleeding.*

**PRACTICE ALERT** *Position the client with nasal packing with the head elevated and on the side when asleep. This position reduces the risk of aspiration of oral secretions.* ■

### Home Care

Following an episode of epistaxis, teaching for home care focuses on measures to prevent further bleeding. Include the following teaching topics.

- Avoid strenuous exercise for several days or weeks, depending on the severity of the nosebleed and its treatment.
- Do not blow the nose or engage in activities such as heavy lifting or bending that could increase pressure and dislodge the crust; sneeze with the mouth open to avoid increasing pressure in nasal vessels.
- For an anterior nose bleed, use petroleum jelly, a water-soluble lubricant, or bacitracin ointment to lubricate nasal mucosa and reduce the risk of spontaneous bleeding.
- Use a humidifier or vaporizer to minimize dryness of the mucous membranes.
- Do not forcefully blow the nose or pick the nose.
- For spontaneous nose bleed, seek medical evaluation for any possible underlying problem, such as hypertension or a bleeding disorder.

## THE CLIENT WITH NASAL TRAUMA OR SURGERY

The nose is the most commonly broken bone of the face. A nasal fracture (broken nose) usually is caused by a sports injury or trauma related to violence or motor vehicle crashes. The nasal septum normally divides the nose into two equal parts. Deviation of the septum can result from nasal trauma. Soft tissue trauma commonly accompanies nasal fracture.

MediaLink | EPISTAXIS CARE PLAN

## Manifestations of Nasal Fracture

- Epistaxis
- Deformity or displacement to one side
- Crepitus
- Periorbital edema and ecchymosis
- Nasal bridge instability

## PATHOPHYSIOLOGY AND MANIFESTATIONS

One or both sides of the nose may be broken. A *unilateral fracture* involves only one side of the nose. It causes little displacement or cosmetic deformity. It is usually not serious, but septal deviation and swelling can obstruct the airway. *Bilateral fractures* are more common, with depression or displacement of both nasal bones to one side. The nose appears flattened or deviated with an S or C configuration. *Complex fractures* may also involve the septum, ascending processes of the maxilla, and frontal bones of the face.

Soft-tissue trauma commonly accompanies nasal fracture. Mucous membrane tears cause epistaxis. Soft-tissue hematomas (black eye) are also frequent. Swelling develops rapidly following the injury and may obscure the fracture. Boney crepitus may be felt on gentle palpation. Septal hematoma may develop, increasing the risk for infection. The manifestations of nasal fracture are listed in the box above.

Potential complications of nasal fracture include septal hematoma and abscess formation, septal perforation or deviation, and cerebrospinal fluid (CSF) leakage. Septal hematoma can lead to complete and bilateral nasal obstruction. If undrained, hematoma increases the risk of staphylococcal abscess, which can lead to necrosis of septal cartilage and *saddle nose deformity.*

Septal deviation causes varying degrees of nasal obstruction. The septal cartilage bulges or deviates to one side, partially or totally obstructing the nares. Mild deviation is generally asymptomatic. Partial obstruction of air flow through one side may cause noisy breathing while awake and snoring during sleep. Major deviations can cause pain because of sinus obstruction or infection. They may also cause nosebleeds due to dryness of the nasal mucosa. Occasionally, the defect is severe enough to cause cosmetic deformity. Perforations are usually not serious and do not usually require repair unless obstruction or external deformity occur.

Fractures of other facial bones may accompany a broken nose, particularly when facial trauma is severe. Fractures in the nasoethmoidal or frontal region can disrupt the dura, causing CSF leakage or rhinorrhea. CSF rhinorrhea is suspected by watery nasal drainage tests positive for glucose.

## COLLABORATIVE CARE

The major treatment goals for nasal fractures are to maintain a patent airway and prevent deformity. Respirations are closely monitored.

## Diagnostic Tests

Head and facial X-rays are done to identify the fracture and assess for other facial fractures. The intranasal cavity is examined using a nasal speculum to rule out septal hematoma. If a CSF leak is suspected, a CT scan is done. A radiopaque substance or fluorescein dye may be instilled into the intrathecal or lumbar subarachnoid space to identify the site of leakage.

## Treatments

Ideally, the fracture is reduced early, before significant edema develops. Nasal fractures heal rapidly. Simple reduction may be done in the emergency department with local anesthesia. An external splint may be applied for 7 to 10 days to maintain proper alignment until healing occurs. The splint is padded to prevent skin breakdown. Ice may be gently applied to the face and nose to control edema and bleeding. Nasal packing may be used to control epistaxis.

## Surgery

Complex nasal fractures, nasal septal deviation, or persistent CSF leakage may require surgical repair or realignment of nasal bones. Rhinoplasty with concurrent septoplasty is the most common procedure used to repair nasal fracture or a deviated nasal septum.

**Rhinoplasty** is surgical reconstruction of the nose. It is done to relieve airway obstruction and repair visible deformity of the nose following fracture. If edema is excessive after nasal fracture, surgery is delayed for 7 to 10 days to allow swelling to subside. Using an intranasal incision, the nasal skin is lifted and the framework of the nose reshaped by removing, rearranging, or augmenting bone or cartilage. The skin is then repositioned over the reconstructed frame. Prosthetic implants may help reshape the nose. Either local or general anesthesia may be used; hospitalization is often unnecessary. Following surgery, nasal packing is left in place for up to 72 hours to minimize bleeding and provide tissue support. A temporary plastic splint molded to the shape of the nose is removed in 3 to 5 days. The splint protects the reshaped nose and helps to control swelling. Most swelling and bruising subside within 10 to 14 days; normal sensation returns within several months following surgery. Rhinoplasty generally has few complications.

Either a septoplasty or a submucous resection (SMR) may be done under local anesthesia to correct a deviated septum. *Septoplasty* involves incising one side of the septum, elevating the mucous membrane, and removing or straightening the deviated portion of septal cartilage. In a *submucous resection,* bone and cartilage are removed. In both procedures, packing is applied to both sides of the nose to prevent bleeding and to keep the septal mucosa in midline position.

Small defects in the cribriform plate, fovea ethmoidalis, or sphenoid sinus associated with persistent CSF leakage may require endoscopic repair. Either a tissue graft or fibrin glue may be used to repair the defect. The graft or glue is held in place with an absorbable packing. Large defects may require craniotomy for repair (Way & Doherty, 2003).

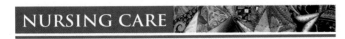

## NURSING CARE

### Health Promotion

Teach all people, children and adolescents in particular, about the importance of wearing helmets and facial protectors when participating in high-risk sports such as football, hockey, and baseball catching. Promote the use of seatbelts with shoulder harness and airbags in vehicles to reduce the risk of facial injury in motor vehicle crashes.

### Assessment

Focused nursing assessment for the client with a suspected nasal fracture includes:

- Health history: nature and circumstances of the injury; pain; ability to breathe through the nose
- Physical examination: evident trauma, swelling, ecchymosis, or deformity of the nose; vital signs, respiratory rate and ease; gently palpate nose and facial bones for crepitus; inspect oropharynx for drainage; test nasal discharge for glucose

### Nursing Diagnoses and Interventions

Nursing care for clients with nasal fracture focuses on controlling pain, bleeding, and swelling. Airway management is a priority. Most nasal fractures are managed on an outpatient basis, and education is a vital nursing function.

### Ineffective Airway Clearance

Immediately following nasal trauma and fracture, the airway is at risk for obstruction by bleeding and edema. Deformity resulting from inappropriate fracture position during healing also can impair nasal airway clearance. This is a consideration when inserting nasogastric tubes or suctioning clients with septal deviation.

**PRACTICE ALERT** *Monitor airway patency. Edema and bleeding may obstruct the airway, causing signs of respiratory distress such as tachypnea, dyspnea, shortness of breath, tachycardia, and use of accessory muscles.* ■

- Monitor cough effectiveness and ability to clear airway secretions. *Pain, edema, and nasal bleeding may impair the ability to cough effectively.*

**PRACTICE ALERT** *Have suction equipment available. Airway patency is a priority; oropharyngeal suctioning may be necessary to remove secretions and maintain a clear airway. Suctioning of the nasopharynx is avoided to prevent additional tissue trauma.* ■

- Maintain adequate hydration. Assess mucous membranes and skin turgor for evidence of dehydration. *Decreased oral fluid intake may lead to dehydration and thick, viscous secretions that are more difficult to expectorate.*

- Assess patency of both nares before inserting a nasogastric tube or feeding tube. If airflow is obstructed through one side, insert the tube through the unobstructed nare. Carefully monitor respiratory status following tube insertion. *The nasogastric tube is inserted through the unobstructed nare to avoid mucosal trauma; however, a large gastric tube may interfere with nasal breathing, necessitating close monitoring.*

### Risk for Infection

The client with a nasal fracture is at increased risk for infection. The nasal mucosa is a natural barrier to infection, and trauma increases the risk for invasion by pathogens. Septal hematoma can lead to abscess formation and staphylococcal infection. A CSF leak indicates disruption of the dura, increasing the risk of ascending infection and meningitis.

**PRACTICE ALERT** *Test watery, clear fluid dripping from the ear or nose for glucose. CSF will test positive for glucose on a Dextrostrip.* ■

- Avoid suctioning if possible. *Suctioning catheters could introduce microorganisms and cause additional trauma to tissues.*
- Monitor vital signs every 4 hours. *A rise in temperature may indicate infection.*
- Administer antibiotics as ordered. *Antibiotics may be prescribed to prevent abscess formation, and, if CSF leakage is present, to prevent meningitis.*

### Home Care

Provide the following teaching when preparing the client with a nasal fracture for home care.

- Elevate the head of the bed with blocks and apply ice or cold packs to the nose for 20 minutes four times a day to reduce swelling.
- Swelling usually subsides in several days; bruising may persist for several weeks.
- It is difficult to determine the final cosmetic outcome until swelling has subsided.
- If indicated by delayed fracture reduction or malformation, discuss rhinoplasty and its potential benefits.

If CSF leakage is present, also include the following instructions.

- Rest in bed with the head of the bed elevated to 30 to 45 degrees.
- Restrict fluid intake as ordered and take the prescribed diuretic to reduce intracranial pressure and CSF leakage.
- Distribute allowed fluids throughout the day.
- List name, purpose, effects, and precautions for any prescribed medication.
- Avoid straining, blowing the nose, sneezing, or vigorous coughing until allowed by the physician.
- Immediately report manifestations of infection, including stiff neck, headache, and fever to the physician.

Following rhinoplasty or septoplasty, provide the following instructions.

- Apply ice packs to the nose to relieve discomfort and reduce swelling.
- Elevate the head of the bed on blocks to decrease local edema.

- Do not blow the nose for 48 hours after the packing is removed to prevent bleeding.
- Vigorous coughing or straining at stool may cause bleeding and should be avoided.
- Clean teeth and mouth frequently and increase fluid intake to decrease oral dryness due to mouth breathing.
- Bruising around the eyes and nose will last for several days.

## Nursing Care Plan
## A Client with Nasal Trauma

Clifton Kavanaugh is a 36-year-old mailman who broke his nose when he was hit in the face by a baseball. He is admitted to the emergency department accompanied by a friend.

### ASSESSMENT
Mr. Kavanaugh presents with obvious deformity of the nose. It is swollen, bloody, and deviated to one side. The nose is bleeding slightly. Mr. Kavanaugh rates the pain as a 6 on a scale of 1 to 10. Vital signs are BP 132/70, P 120 and regular, R 22, T 98.6°F (37°C) axillary.

Mr. Kavanaugh is breathing through his mouth and holding an ice compress to his nose. Boney crepitus and edema are felt on palpation. There is no evidence of CSF leak from either nose or ears. X-ray confirms a nasal fracture.

### DIAGNOSES
- *Acute pain* related to nasal fracture
- *Ineffective breathing pattern* related to nasal swelling and bleeding
- *Anxiety* related to pain and need for emergency care
- *Disturbed body image* related to nasal deformity

### EXPECTED OUTCOMES
- Verbalize relief of pain.
- Maintain a patent airway and normalize his breathing pattern.
- Demonstrate reduced anxiety.
- Express concerns about potential body image change.

### PLANNING AND IMPLEMENTATION
- Administer analgesics as ordered.
- Apply ice compress to nose.
- Inspect oropharynx for evidence of bleeding.
- Encourage deep, slow breathing through the mouth.
- Provide oral hygiene.
- Discuss concerns regarding injury.
- Assist with nasal splint application.

### EVALUATION
Following treatment, Mr. Kavanaugh reports his pain has decreased to a level of 2 on a scale of 1 to 10. He appears more relaxed, no longer grimacing and with a relaxed posture. His respirations are easy at 18. The nasal splint is intact. Mr. Kavanaugh is able to look in a mirror and state with a laugh, "I look like a raccoon." He is admitted to the hospital for rhinoplasty.

### Critical Thinking in the Nursing Process
1. A client in the emergency department with nasal trauma becomes extremely panicky because of blood draining down his throat. How would you intervene to reduce this client's anxiety without using nasal suction? Why is it important to avoid suctioning the nasopharynx in the client with nasal trauma?
2. Develop a plan of care for the client with a leak of CSF from a nasal fracture.
3. Compare immediate versus delayed rhinoplasty for the client with nasal fracture.

See Evaluating Your Response in Appendix C.

## THE CLIENT WITH LARYNGEAL OBSTRUCTION OR TRAUMA

The larynx is the narrowest portion of the upper airway. As such, it is at risk for obstruction. Laryngeal obstruction is a life-threatening emergency. Blows to the neck or other traumatic injuries may damage the larynx, interfering with its patency and function.

## PATHOPHYSIOLOGY AND MANIFESTATIONS
### Laryngeal Obstruction

The larynx may be partially or fully obstructed by aspirated food or foreign objects, or by laryngospasm or edema due to inflammation, injury, or anaphylaxis. Anything that occludes the larynx can obstruct the airway. The most common cause of

obstruction in adults is ingested meat that lodges in the airway (the so-called *café coronary*). Risk factors for food aspiration include ingesting large boluses of food and chewing them insufficiently, consuming excess alcohol, and wearing dentures. A foreign body in the larynx causes pain, laryngospasm, dyspnea, and inspiratory stridor. Aspirated foreign bodies may pass through the larynx into the trachea and lungs, causing pneumonitis.

Laryngospasm occurs due to repeated or traumatic intubation attempts, chemical irritation, or hypocalcemia. An acute type I hypersensitivity response may cause anaphylaxis with release of inflammatory mediators leading to angioedema of upper airways and severe laryngeal edema.

The most common manifestations of laryngeal obstruction are coughing, choking, gagging, obvious difficulty breathing with use of accessory muscles, and inspiratory stridor. As the airway is obstructed, signs of asphyxia become apparent. Respirations are labored and noisy with wheezing and stridor. Cyanosis may develop. Respiratory arrest and death may result without prompt treatment.

## Laryngeal Trauma

Trauma to the larynx can occur in motor vehicle crashes or assaults (e.g., blows to the neck or attempted strangulation). The larynx also may be traumatized during endotracheal intubation or tracheotomy. Trauma may fracture thyroid and/or cricoid cartilage, resulting in loss of airway patency. Soft-tissue injuries can cause swelling that further impairs the airway. Manifestations of laryngeal trauma may include subcutaneous emphysema or crepitus, voice change, dysphagia and pain with swallowing, inspiratory stridor, hemoptysis, and cough.

## COLLABORATIVE CARE

The treatment goal is to maintain an open airway. If airway obstruction is partial and the client is able to cough and move air in and out of the lungs, radiologic and laryngoscopic examination may be done to locate the foreign body. An endotracheal tube may be inserted to maintain airflow through the larynx in spasm or an edematous larynx. For anaphylaxis, epinephrine may be administered to reduce laryngeal edema and relieve obstruction.

When airway obstruction is complete, the Heimlich maneuver is performed immediately to clear the obstruction. For the conscious person, the rescuer wraps his or her arms around the victim from behind, places one fist between the umbilicus and xiphoid process, covers the fist with the other hand and forcefully thrusts the hands upward (Figure 35–3A■). For the unconscious victim, the rescuer straddles the victim's thighs and delivers thrusts upward and inward on the upper abdomen

(Figure 35–3B). These moves are continued until the obstruction is relieved or more definitive care can be given. Endotracheal intubation may be attempted. If intubation is unsuccessful, an immediate cricothyrotomy or tracheotomy must be performed to open the airway.

CT scan is used to identify laryngeal fractures; however, emergency treatment may be required prior to diagnosis to ensure airway patency and preserve life. Soft-tissue injuries may be managed conservatively with bedside humidifier, intravenous fluids, antibiotics, and corticosteroids to reduce edema. More severe injuries require endotracheal intubation or immediate tracheostomy.

## NURSING CARE

**PRACTICE ALERT** *The priority of nursing care in laryngeal obstruction or trauma is restoring a patent airway to prevent cerebral anoxia and death. Laryngeal obstruction and trauma are medical emergencies requiring immediate intervention.* ■

Closely monitor clients at risk for laryngeal obstruction (e.g., following neck trauma, newly extubated clients, and people receiving medications with a high risk of anaphylaxis, such as intravenous antibiotics or radiologic dyes) for manifestations of obstruction, including dyspnea, nasal flaring, tachypnea, anxiety, wheezing, and stridor. Suction the airway as needed; small aspirated foreign bodies might possibly be removed by suctioning. If obstruction is complete, initiate a cardiopulmonary arrest procedure and perform the Heimlich maneuver until the obstruction is relieved or the emergency response team arrives. Prepare to assist with emergency intubation or tracheotomy as needed. Provide emotional support, reassurance, and teaching for the client and family to reduce anxiety.

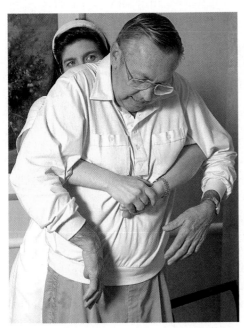

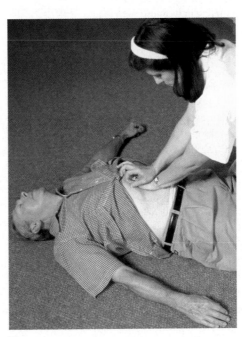

**Figure 35–3** ■ Administering abdominal thrusts (the Heimlich maneuver) to *A*, a conscious victim, and *B*, an unconscious victim.

**A**　　　　　　**B**

Health promotion and teaching for home care focus on preventing laryngeal obstruction and early intervention techniques. Everyone should be aware of the risk factors for adult aspiration. Caution clients who wear dentures to take small bites, chewing each bite carefully before swallowing. Discuss the relationship between excess alcohol intake and food aspiration. Participate in promoting training of the general public in CPR and the Heimlich maneuver. The more people who are adequately trained in emergency procedures, the more likely it is that emergency procedures will be initiated in a timely manner. Clients with a known risk for anaphylaxis, such as people with a previous anaphylactic response and those allergic to bee venom, should wear a MedicAlert tag and carry a bee-sting kit to allow early intervention to prevent severe laryngeal edema and spasm.

# THE CLIENT WITH OBSTRUCTIVE SLEEP APNEA

**Sleep apnea,** intermittent absence of airflow through the mouth and nose during sleep, is a serious and potentially life-threatening disorder. It affects at least 2% of middle-aged women and 4% of middle-aged men. Sleep apnea is a leading cause of excessive daytime sleepiness, and may contribute to other problems such as poor work performance and motor vehicle crashes (Braunwald et al., 2001; McCance & Huether, 2002).

Types of sleep apnea include obstructive and central. In *obstructive sleep apnea,* the more common type, the respiratory drive remains intact, but airflow ceases due to occlusion of the oropharyngeal airway. *Central sleep apnea* is a neurologic disorder that involves transient impairment of the neurologic drive to respiratory muscles.

In addition to male gender, risk factors for obstructive sleep apnea include increasing age and obesity. Large neck circumference (>17 inches in men and >16 inches in women) also is a known risk factor for obstructive sleep apnea (Porth, 2002). Use of alcohol and other central nervous system depressants may contribute to sleep apnea.

## PATHOPHYSIOLOGY

During sleep, skeletal muscle tone decreases (except the diaphragm). The most significant decrease occurs during rapid eye movement (REM) sleep (Porth, 2002). Loss of normal pharyngeal muscle tone permits the pharynx to collapse during inspiration as pressure within the airways becomes negative in relation to atmospheric pressure. The tongue is also pulled against the posterior pharyngeal wall by gravity during sleep, causing further obstruction. Obesity or skeletal or soft-tissue changes that decrease inspiratory tone, such as a relatively large tongue in a relatively small oropharynx, contribute to the problem. Airflow obstruction causes the oxygen saturation, $Po_2$, and pH to fall, and the $Pco_2$ to rise. This progressive asphyxia causes brief arousal from sleep, which restores airway patency and airflow. Sleep can be severely fragmented as these episodes may occur hundreds of times each night.

## Manifestations of Obstructive Sleep Apnea

- Loud, cyclic snoring
- Periods of apnea lasting 15 to 120 seconds during sleep
- Gasping or choking during sleep
- Restlessness, thrashing during sleep
- Daytime fatigue and sleepiness
- Morning headache
- Personality changes, depression
- Intellectual impairment
- Impotence
- Hypertension

Recurrent episodes of apnea and arousal during sleep have secondary physiologic effects. Sleep fragmentation and loss of slow-wave sleep are thought to contribute to neurologic and behavior problems such as excessive daytime sleepiness, impaired intellect, memory loss, and personality changes. Recurrent nocturnal asphyxia and negative intrathoracic pressure due to airway obstruction increase the workload of the heart. People with coronary heart disease may develop myocardial ischemia and angina. Dysrhythmias such as significant bradycardia and dangerous tachydysrhythmias may develop. Left ventricular function may be impaired and heart failure may occur. Systemic blood pressure remains high during sleep and may contribute to systemic hypertension that affects more than 50% of people with obstructive sleep apnea (Braunwald et al., 2001). Pulmonary hypertension also may develop. Sudden cardiac death is believed to be a potential fatal complication of obstructive sleep apnea.

## MANIFESTATIONS

Narrowed upper airways produce loud snoring during sleep, often years before obstructive sleep apnea occurs. Excessive daytime sleepiness, headache, irritability, and restless sleep also are common manifestations. See the box above.

## COLLABORATIVE CARE

The goal of care for obstructive sleep apnea is to restore airflow and prevent the adverse effects of the disorder. Sustained weight loss may cure obstructive sleep apnea.

### Diagnostic Tests

The diagnosis of obstructive sleep apnea is based on *polysomnography,* an overnight sleep study. Several variables are recorded during the study, including:

- Electroencephalogram and measurements of ocular activity and muscle tone
- Recordings of ventilatory activity and airflow
- Continuous arterial oxygen saturation readings
- Heart rate

Transcutaneous arterial $Pco_2$ readings also may be monitored during the study. Because sleep studies are time consuming and expensive, overnight monitoring of oxygen saturation by pulse

SLEEP APNEA CASE STUDY   MediaLink

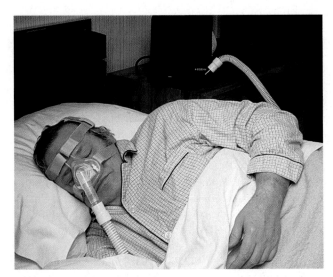

**Figure 35–4** ■ A client using a nasal mask and CPAP to treat sleep apnea.

*Courtesy of Respironics, Inc.*

oximetry may be used to confirm the diagnosis of sleep apnea when symptoms indicate a high probability of the disorder (Braunwald et al., 2001).

## Treatments

Mild to moderate obstructive sleep apnea may be treated by weight reduction, alcohol abstinence, improving nasal patency, and avoiding the supine position for sleep. Although weight reduction often cures the disorder, maintaining optimal weight is difficult. Oral appliances designed to keep the mandible and tongue forward also may be prescribed.

Nasal continuous positive airway pressure (CPAP) is the treatment of choice for obstructive sleep apnea. Positive pressure generated by an air compressor and administered through a tight-fitting nasal mask (Figure 35–4 ■) splints the pharyngeal airway, preventing collapse and obstruction. With proper training, this device is well tolerated by the client. Nasal airways can become dry and irritated with CPAP, so in-line humidifier or a room humidifier is recommended. A newer device, the BiPaP ventilator, delivers higher pressures during inhalation and lower pressures during expiration, providing less resistance to exhaling.

## Surgery

Tonsillectomy and adenoidectomy may relieve upper airway obstruction in some clients. Excision of obstructive tissue from the soft palate, uvula, and posterior lateral pharyngeal wall may be accomplished by *uvulopalatopharyngoplasty* (*UPPP*). Although only about 50% of these surgeries are successful in treating sleep apnea, UPPP is useful in selected cases. In severe cases, tracheostomy may also be performed to bypass the area of obstruction.

## NURSING CARE

Obstructive sleep apnea usually is treated in the home. Nursing care focuses on teaching the client and family about equipment use and strategies to decrease contributing factors such as obesity and alcohol intake. The following nursing diagnoses are appropriate for clients with sleep apnea.

- *Disturbed sleep pattern* related to repeated apneic episodes
- *Fatigue* related to interrupted sleep patterns
- *Ineffective breathing pattern* related to obstruction of upper airway during sleep
- *Impaired gas exchange* related to altered lung ventilation during obstructive episodes
- *Risk for injury* related to daytime somnolence and altered judgment
- *Risk for sexual dysfunction* related to impotence resulting from sleep apnea

## Home Care

Effective sleep apnea management depends on the client's willingness to participate in care. Provide teaching about the following topics.

- Relationship between obesity and sleep apnea
- Plans, resources, and referrals as needed for weight loss (e.g., programs such as Weight Watchers to provide additional support)
- Relationship of alcohol and sedatives to sleep apnea; referral to an alcohol treatment program or Alcoholics Anonymous as indicated
- How to use CPAP if ordered
- The importance of using CPAP continuously at night
- Measures to reduce airway dryness, including supplemental humidity and an adequate fluid intake to maintain moist mucous membranes

If a support group for people with sleep apnea syndrome is available in the local area, refer the client and family to the group.

# UPPER RESPIRATORY TUMORS

Although tumors of the upper respiratory tract are relatively uncommon, they have the potential to impair the upper airways and interfere with breathing and ventilation of the lungs. Of the upper respiratory tract structures, the larynx is affected by abnormal growths most often.

## THE CLIENT WITH NASAL POLYPS

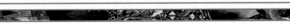

*Nasal polyps* are benign grapelike growths of the mucous membrane lining the nose. These benign tumors can interfere with air movement through nasal passages or obstruct sinus openings, leading to sinusitis. They usually affect people who have chronic allergic rhinitis or asthma.

## PATHOPHYSIOLOGY AND MANIFESTATIONS

Chronic irritation and swelling of the mucous membranes from allergic rhinitis may cause slow polyp formation. Polyps form in areas of dependent mucous membrane, presenting as pale, edematous masses covered with mucous membrane. They are usually bilateral and have a stemlike base, making them fairly moveable. Polyps can continue to enlarge, eventually becoming larger than a grape. Polyps may be asymptomatic, although large polyps may cause nasal obstruction, rhinorrhea, and loss of sense of smell. Manifestations of sinusitis may develop. The voice may have a nasal tone. Asthmatics who have nasal polyps may have an associated aspirin allergy of which they are not aware.

## COLLABORATIVE CARE

When polyps occur in conjunction with an acute upper respiratory infection, they may regress spontaneously with resolution of the infection. When symptomatic, polyps may be managed with topical corticosteroid nasal sprays or low-dose oral corticosteroids to shrink the edematous polyps and manage allergic symptoms. However, polyps continue to enlarge when corticosteroid therapy is discontinued.

Surgery may be required to restore normal breathing. Surgical removal of polyps (*polypectomy*) often is done in the physician's office under local anesthesia. A wire snare is used to clip the polyps from their stemlike base. Nasal packing is inserted to control bleeding after removal. Alternatively, laser surgery may be used to remove polyps. Healing is more rapid following laser intervention, and the risk of bleeding is reduced. Because polyps tend to recur, repeated surgeries may be necessary.

## NURSING CARE

Teaching about home care following polypectomy is the primary nursing responsibility for the client with nasal polyps. Provide postoperative care instructions, and discuss measures to reduce the risk of bleeding.

  a. Apply ice or cold compresses to the nose to decrease swelling, promote comfort, and prevent bleeding.
  b. Avoid blowing the nose for 24 to 48 hours after nasal packing is removed.
  c. Avoid straining at stool, vigorous coughing, and strenuous exercise.

Discuss manifestations of possible bleeding, such as frequent swallowing or visible blood at the back of the throat. Swallowed blood may cause nausea and vomiting. Encourage the client to rest for 2 to 3 days after surgery to reduce the risk of bleeding. Instruct to increase fluid intake and clean mouth frequently to reduce oral dryness associated with mouth breathing while nasal packing is in place.

# THE CLIENT WITH A LARYNGEAL TUMOR

Laryngeal tumors may be either benign or malignant. Benign tumors of the larynx include papillomas, nodules, and polyps. People who chronically shout, project, or vocalize in an abnormally high or low tone, abusing the voice, are at risk for developing benign laryngeal tumors. In adults, vocal cord nodules are often referred to as "singer's nodules"; cheerleaders and public speakers may also develop them. Voice abuse also contributes to the development of vocal cord polyps, as does cigarette smoking and chronic irritation from industrial pollutants.

Malignancy, or cancer of the larynx is uncommon and is often curable if detected early. However, an estimated 3700 people died from laryngeal cancer in 2002; and 8900 new cases were diagnosed (ACS, 2002a). Men are affected more than 3 times as often as women. Cancer of the larynx usually develops between age 50 and 70. Cigarette smoking is the major risk factor for laryngeal cancer: The risk of developing laryngeal cancer is 5 to 35 times greater in smokers than in nonsmokers. Alcohol consumption is a significant cofactor in increasing the risk. When combined with smoking, the risk increases significantly, perhaps as much as 100 times (ACS, 2002b). Other risk factors include poor nutrition, human papillomavirus infection, exposure to asbestos and other occupational pollutants, and race (laryngeal cancer is more common in African Americans than among whites).

## PATHOPHYSIOLOGY AND MANIFESTATIONS
### Benign Tumors

Papillomas are small, wartlike growths believed to be viral in origin. Polyps and nodules may develop on the vocal cords of the larynx as a result of voice abuse. Nodules occur as paired lesions on the free edges of the vocal cords. Hoarseness and a breathy voice quality are manifestations of benign vocal cord tumors.

### Laryngeal Cancer

Squamous cell carcinoma is the most common malignancy of the larynx. Changes in the laryngeal mucosa occur over time as it is subjected to noxious irritants such as cigarette smoke. White, patchy, precancerous lesions known as *leukoplakia* appear. Red, velvety patches, called *erythroplakia,* are thought to represent a later stage of carcinoma development. The initial cancerous lesion, carcinoma in situ (CIS), is superficial. Malignant cells replace the lining layer, but do not invade into deeper tissues. Untreated, about 30% of CIS lesions develop into squamous cell cancer (ACS, 2002b). Laryngeal cancer spreads by both direct invasion of surrounding tissues and metastasis. It may metastasize to the lungs; however, metastases of other cancers to the larynx are rare.

Laryngeal cancer may develop in any of the three areas of the larynx—the glottis, the supraglottis, and the subglottis. Manifestations vary according to site of the lesion.

Lesions of the true vocal cords or glottis account for nearly 65% of all laryngeal cancers (Figure 35–5 ■). Fortunately, these cancers tend to be well differentiated and slow growing. Metastasis occurs late in the course of the disease because of a

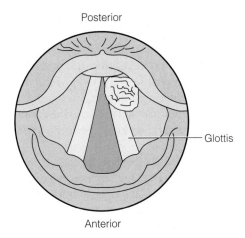

Posterior

Glottis

Anterior

**Figure 35–5** ■ Cancer of the larynx. Most lesions form along the edges of the glottis.

limited lymphatic supply. The usual symptom of glottic cancer is hoarseness, or a change in the voice because the tumor prevents complete closure of the vocal cords during speech.

Approximately 35% of laryngeal cancers develop in the supraglottic area, which includes the epiglottis, aryepiglottic folds, arytenoid muscles and cartilage, and false vocal cords. Lymphatic supply to this region of the larynx is rich; tumors often invade locally and metastasize early. Symptoms often do not develop until the tumor is relatively large, delaying diagnosis. Manifestations of supraglottic cancer include painful swallowing, sore throat, or a feeling of a lump in the throat. Later manifestations include dyspnea, foul breath, and pain that radiates to the ear.

Subglottic tumors (below the vocal cords) are the least common. They often are asymptomatic until the enlarging tumor obstructs the airway.

Common manifestations of laryngeal cancer are listed in the box on this page.

## COLLABORATIVE CARE

Benign laryngeal tumors may resolve with correction of the underlying problem, such as voice training with a speech thera-

---

### Manifestations of Laryngeal Cancer

- Hoarseness
- Change in the voice
- Painful swallowing
- Dyspnea
- Foul breath
- Palpable lump in neck
- Earache

---

pist or smoking cessation. Treatment of laryngeal malignancy varies with the extent of the cancer. Early diagnosis and treatment are important: 80% to 95% of early stage tumors can be cured, whereas 50% to 80% of people with advanced laryngeal cancer die of the disease.

### Diagnostic Tests

- *Direct* or *indirect laryngoscopy* is used for initial evaluation when laryngeal cancer is suspected. A fiberoptic laryngoscope is used for direct laryngoscopy; mirrors are used to visualize the larynx in indirect laryngoscopy.
- *Biopsy* is obtained from suspicious lesions to examine the cells. Biopsy is usually obtained under general anesthesia. Tissue may be obtained via endoscopy or by fine needle aspiration of the mass.
- *Imaging studies* such as CT scan, MRI, and chest X-ray are obtained to evaluate the size of the mass, possible extension into deeper tissues, involvement of lymph nodes, and possible metastasis to the lungs. A barium swallow may be done to evaluate the effects of the tumor on swallowing.

### Treatments

An inhaled steroid spray may be used for vocal cord polyps. In some cases, surgical excision of benign nodules or polyps is required. This usually is performed via laryngoscopy, using microforceps or a laser. A biopsy of the tumor is done to rule out malignancy.

Laryngeal cancer treatment is determined by *staging* the cancer. Information such as tumor size and location (T), number of involved lymph nodes (N), and presence or absence of metastases (M) is combined to assign a stage, designated by Roman numerals I to IV. Table 35–1 outlines laryngeal cancer stages.

---

| TABLE 35–1 | Staging of Laryngeal Tumors |
|---|---|
| Stage 0 | • Carcinoma in situ<br>• No lymph node involvement or metastasis |
| Stage I | • Tumor confined to site of origin with normal vocal cord mobility<br>• No lymph node involvement or metastasis |
| Stage II | • Tumor involves adjacent tissues<br>• No lymph node involvement or metastasis |
| Stage III | • Tumor confined to larynx with fixation of vocal cords; immediately surrounding supraglottic tissues may be involved<br>• No lymph node involvement or a single positive node on the side of the tumor<br>• No metastasis |
| Stage IV | • Massive tumor that extends beyond boundaries of larynx to involve surrounding tissues<br>• Single or multiple lymph nodes may be involved<br>• Distant metastasis may be present |

## Radiation Therapy

Radiation therapy is often the treatment of choice for early laryngeal cancer. Radiation disrupts the DNA of the cell, causing it to die. External radiation may be used, or implants of iridium seeds can be placed into hollow plastic needles that are inserted directly into or near the tumor site during surgery to deliver radiation. Radiation therapy is extremely effective for treating glottic cancer, with cure rates equal to those achieved by surgery. Radiation therapy preserves the voice, although the tone or timber of the voice may be affected.

Radiation therapy may be used in combination with chemotherapy to treat more advanced laryngeal cancers. Nearly two-thirds of clients with locally invasive cancers can avoid total laryngectomy when treated with combination radiation and chemotherapy. Survival rates are equal to those achieved with total laryngectomy (Way & Doherty, 2003).

Radiation therapy also may be used in conjunction with surgery to destroy any remaining cancerous cells, or as a palliative treatment for advanced tumors. See Chapter 10 for more information about radiation therapy and its nursing implications.

## Chemotherapy

Chemotherapy is used in combination with radiation therapy as the primary treatment for some laryngeal cancers. It also is used to treat distant metastasis and for palliation when the tumor is unresectable. The most commonly used chemotherapy drugs to treat laryngeal cancer are cisplatin (Platinol) and 5-fluorouracil (5-FU). Other drugs that may be used include methotrexate (Mexate), bleomycin sulfate (Blenoxane), and carboplatin (Paraplatin). A multiple-drug treatment regimen may be employed to maximize therapeutic effects. See Chapter 10 ⊙⊃ for the nursing implications for chemotherapy.

## Surgery

The type of surgery used to treat laryngeal cancer is based on site, size, and invasiveness of the tumor into the larynx. The goals of surgery are to remove the malignancy, maintain airway patency, and achieve optimal cosmetic appearance.

Carcinoma in situ, vocal cord polyps, and early vocal cord cancers may be removed by laser during a laryngoscopy procedure. The cure rate for early tumors using this method is excellent. This surgery may be performed on an outpatient basis. The degree of trauma to the vocal cords varies, depending on the size of the lesion. The voice is preserved, but total voice rest with whispering only may be ordered for a week or more following surgery. In some cases, a temporary tracheostomy may be done at the time of surgery to ensure that swelling does not interfere with airway patency. Once the tracheostomy tube is removed and the opening is closed, the client can eat, speak, and breathe normally.

**Laryngectomy,** removal of the larynx, may be necessary. A *partial laryngectomy* (hemilaryngectomy, vertical partial laryngectomy) may be used for tumors localized to a portion of the larynx with limited extension beyond the larynx. In a partial laryngectomy, 50% or more of the larynx is removed. The voice generally is well preserved, although it may be

changed by the surgery. A tracheostomy tube may be inserted for early postoperative airway management. It is usually removed in 5 to 7 days as postoperative swelling subsides, and the stoma is allowed to close. Normal speaking, breathing, and swallowing are restored. If the epiglottis has been removed, careful monitoring for aspiration is necessary. Enteral tube feedings or parenteral nutrition may be required for several weeks after surgery. Swallowing techniques to prevent aspiration are taught.

A *total laryngectomy* is required for cancers that extend beyond the vocal cords. The entire larynx is removed, along with the epiglottis, thyroid cartilage, several tracheal rings, and the hyoid bone. Because the trachea and the esophagus are permanently separated by this surgery (Figure 35–6 ■), there is no risk of aspiration during swallowing. Normal speech is lost, and a permanent tracheostomy is created in a total laryngectomy. The tracheostomy tube inserted during surgery may be left in place for several weeks and then removed, leaving a natural stoma, or it may be left in place permanently. See page 1067 for nursing care of the client undergoing a total laryngectomy. Procedure 35–1 on page 1068 outlines tracheostomy care.

If cervical lymph nodes are involved but there is no evidence of distal metastasis, *radical* or *modified neck dissection* may be performed along with total laryngectomy. In a radical neck dissection, all soft tissue from the lower edge of the mandible down

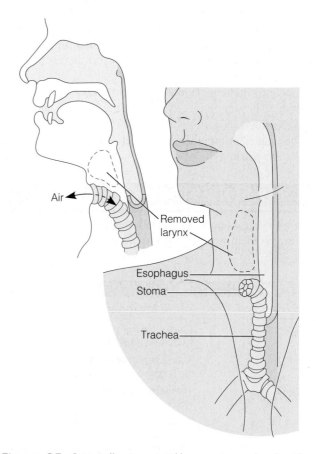

**Figure 35–6** ■ Following a total laryngectomy, the client has a permanent tracheostomy. No connection between the trachea and esophagus remains.

# NURSING CARE OF THE CLIENT HAVING A TOTAL LARYNGECTOMY

## PREOPERATIVE CARE

- Assess knowledge and understanding of the diagnosis and proposed surgery. Clarify information and reinforce previous teaching as needed. *A clear understanding by the client and family of the purpose, anticipated benefits, and consequences of total laryngectomy prior to surgery is vital to promote postoperative recovery.*
- Provide routine preoperative care and teaching as explained in Chapter 7. ⊖⊙
- Assess anxiety levels of the client and family related to the diagnosis and proposed surgery. *High levels of anxiety interfere with learning and the ability to cooperate in care. Interventions to reduce anxiety may be required prior to teaching and providing preoperative instructions.*
- Without increasing fear, emphasize that total laryngectomy results in a loss of speech and that the client will breathe through a permanent stoma in the neck. *Although clients and family members may verbalize an understanding of the loss of speech following surgery, they may believe that verbal communication will still be possible through the stoma.*
- Establish a means of communicating postoperatively, using a magic slate, alphabet board, eye or hand signals, or other strategies. *Learning techniques for communicating preoperatively decreases the client's and family's postoperative anxiety. Long-term speech rehabilitation measures, such as the tracheoesophageal puncture are not appropriate for use in the immediate postoperative period.*
- Point out that surgery will affect the sense of taste and smell, and eating in the initial postoperative period. Reassure that nutritional and fluid needs will be met with intravenous or enteral feedings until eating can be resumed. *The client may not be prepared for the effect of surgery on taste and smell, and therefore the enjoyment of food.*
- If possible and desired by the client and family, arrange a visit by a postlaryngectomy client who effectively uses an alternate form of verbal communication. *The client and family may feel more comfortable expressing their fears and asking questions of someone who has gone through the same experience they are facing.*

## POSTOPERATIVE CARE

- Provide routine postoperative nursing care and monitoring as explained in Chapter 7.

- Frequently monitor airway patency and respiratory status, including respiratory rate and pattern; lung sounds; oxygen saturation. *Excessive or retained respiratory secretions can impair gas exchange, increase the work of breathing, and lead to complications such as pneumonia.*
- Encourage deep breathing and coughing. *Deep breathing helps ensure adequate ventilation of lower airways; coughing helps to move secretions out of airways.*
- Elevate the head of the bed. *The upright position promotes effective ventilation of the lungs, and reduces edema and swelling of the neck.*
- Maintain humidification of inspired gases. *With a tracheostomy, humidification of inspired air in the upper airways is lost. Humidified air helps maintain moist mucous membranes and secretions, promoting secretion removal by coughing or suctioning.*
- Maintain an adequate fluid intake (intravenously, enteral, and oral when allowed). *Adequate hydration keeps secretions liquid and mucous membranes moist.*
- Suction via tracheostomy using sterile technique as needed. *Surgery, impaired nutrition, and the effects of radiation therapy may cause fatigue and a weak cough effort. Suctioning may be necessary to clear secretions and maintain airway patency.*
- Provide tracheostomy care as needed. See Procedure 35–1. *Periodic cleaning of the tracheostomy tube is necessary to remove accumulated secretions and maintain airway patency.*
- Teach to protect the stoma from particulate matter in the air with a gauze square or other stoma protector. *Permanent tracheostomy results in loss of the protective mechanisms of the upper airway that prevent foreign material from entering the lungs.*
- Instruct to support the head when moving in bed. *Additional head support reduces the strain on tissues in the operative area.*
- Place the call light within easy reach at all times; answer the call light promptly. *The client who is unable to speak needs reassurance that help is within reach at all times.*
- Encourage family members to remain present when possible. *Supportive family presence helps reassure the client that he or she will not be left alone or helpless.*
- Spend as much time as possible with the client. When leaving the room, specify the time when you will return. *These measures help establish trust and relieve anxiety.*

---

to the clavicle is removed, including cervical lymph nodes, the sternocleidomastoid muscle, internal jugular vein, cranial nerve XI (spinal accessory), and submaxillary salivary gland. Extensive tissue dissection can result in significant deformity. Skin grafts or flaps may be used to close the wound. Hemovac drains are placed in the wound to prevent hematoma and extensive edema formation. After surgery, the client may have difficulty lifting and turning the head because of muscle loss. Resection of the spinal accessory nerve causes shoulder drop on the affected side. In a modified neck dissection, neck contents are removed, with the exception of the sternocleidomastoid muscle, internal jugular vein, and spinal accessory nerve.

## Speech Rehabilitation

Various techniques may be used to restore speech after total laryngectomy. *Tracheoesophageal puncture (TEP)* is the usual method used to restore speech. A small fistula is created between the posterior tracheal wall and the anterior esophagus. A small, one-way shunt valve is fitted into the fistula (Figure 35–7 ■). Occluding the tracheostomy stoma with a finger forces exhaled air through the valve into the esophagus and hypopharynx, creating vibration and sound. The muscles of speech are used to form words. The one-way valve prevents aspiration from the esophagus into the trachea. An external tracheostoma valve may be used to avoid using the hand to

- Health history: current symptoms, including voice change, difficulty swallowing, throat pain; risk factors such as voice abuse, family history of cancer, occupational exposures; smoking history, use of alcohol and amount.
- Physical examination: voice character; general appearance and apparent state of health; swallowing ability; visible or palpable mass in neck.

## Nursing Diagnoses and Interventions

Nursing care for the client with a benign tumor of the larynx focuses on maintaining a patent airway and teaching about the disorder and strategies to prevent its recurrence. The client with laryngeal cancer has multiple nursing care needs. The risk for impaired verbal communication is significant. Dysphagia may interfere with swallowing and nutrition. Nutrition also may be impaired by radiation, chemotherapy, and surgery. The diagnosis of cancer is frightening for most clients, no matter what the potential for cure is with treatment.

### Risk for Impaired Airway Clearance

Following resection of a benign or malignant vocal cord nodule, local tissue edema may interfere with airway patency.

**PRACTICE ALERT** *During the immediate postoperative period, closely monitor for signs of airway obstruction, such as labored breathing or inspiratory stridor. The larynx is the narrowest portion of the upper airways. Tissue edema following surgery can further restrict the airway, interfering with lung ventilation and gas exchange.* ■

- Apply cold packs to the neck as ordered or indicated. *Cold application constricts local blood vessels and reduces edema development.*
- Withhold food and fluids until the cough and gag reflexes have returned. *Local anesthesia used during removal of benign tumors and nodules impairs the cough and gag reflexes, increasing the risk for aspiration.*

### Impaired Verbal Communication

Treatment of laryngeal cancer often alters the quality of the voice, results in short-term restriction on speaking, or, in the case of total laryngectomy, causes loss of the voice. The client ultimately determines treatment choices for laryngeal cancer; some choose to forgo laryngectomy to avoid voice loss when the chance for long-term success and cancer cure is minimal.

- Prior to surgery, assess for additional obstacles to communication. *Communication may be impaired by hearing loss, illiteracy, or weakness associated with the disease process, altering the ability to use alternative communication strategies.*
- Assess the importance of verbal communication to self-concept, occupation, and lifestyle. *Many factors influence adaptation to the loss of normal verbal communication. If the ability to speak is central to an occupation (e.g., elementary school teacher, singer) or self-concept (e.g., a politician or attorney), adapting to a total laryngectomy may be difficult. For these clients, laryngectomy may mean a loss of employment or career.*

**PRACTICE ALERT** *Prior to surgery, introduce nonverbal communication strategies such as pencil and paper, magic slate, or an alphabet board. Encourage the client to practice using each method and to choose the most acceptable one. Having the client determine a means of communication prior to surgery helps to alleviate anxiety and increases the sense of control.* ■

- Arrange consultation with a speech therapist about alternate forms of oral communication prior to surgery if possible. *Determining a means of communicating on a continuing basis prior to surgery helps to relieve fear of inability to communicate and may guide the choice of a surgical procedure.*

**PRACTICE ALERT** *After surgery, assess frequently. Place the call bell at hand. The presence of a caring nurse helps to decrease anxiety and promotes communication. Knowing that help is readily available enhances feelings of security and decreases anxiety.* ■

- Reinforce teaching about alternative communication strategies. *Anxiety or information overload may impair the ability to retain information; reinforcement facilitates learning.*
- Maintain a positive attitude about postoperative communication, but do not promote unrealistic expectations. *Not all clients are able to use all alternative methods of verbal communication after the laryngectomy. Some clients remain nonverbal.*
- If desired, arrange a visit by a rehabilitated laryngectomy client who has mastered an alternative form of verbal communication and has a positive attitude about rehabilitation. *Many clients and their families find that they are better able to communicate their fears with someone who has gone through the same experience they are facing.*

### Impaired Swallowing

Disruption of laryngeal structures by the tumor itself or due to radiation or surgery can impair the swallowing mechanism. Additionally, even when a total laryngectomy has been performed and a connection between the oropharynx and trachea no longer exists, swallowing may cause fear of choking.

- Maintain intravenous fluids and enteral feedings or parenteral nutrition until adequate food and fluids can be ingested orally. *It is important to maintain nutritional and fluid balance until normal eating can be resumed.*
- Postoperatively, initiate oral intake with soft foods, not liquids. *Soft foods are easier to handle and swallow initially. As recovery progresses, thickened liquids can be swallowed and, eventually, a normal diet.*
- Following total laryngectomy, reassure that choking is not possible, because there is no connection between the esophagus and trachea. *Clients often fear that swallowing will result in choking and they will be unable to cough effectively.*
- Instruct to initiate a swallow by placing a small amount of food on the back of the tongue, flex the head forward, and then think "swallow." *Swallowing is no longer an automatic function and needs to be relearned.*

*Provide for privacy during initial attempts at eating. Eating in the presence of others may cause embarrassment until confidence in eating is regained. Privacy also reduces distractions, allowing concentration on swallowing.* ■

## Imbalanced Nutrition: Less Than Body Requirements

Large laryngeal tumors often place pressure on the esophagus and may cause dysphagia (difficulty swallowing) or odynophagia (painful swallowing). In either case, difficulty eating may ultimately impair nutrition. Additionally, cancer often produces a hypermetabolic state, increasing calorie requirements. If surgery is performed, difficulty swallowing and a fear of aspiration in the early postoperative period also interfere with eating. Enteral or parenteral feedings are usually needed initially to meet nutritional status. After a total laryngectomy, the senses of taste and smell are disrupted. Although the sense of taste may be partially recovered, clients may complain that eating no longer is pleasurable.

- Assess nutritional status using height and weight charts, reported weight loss, and anthropometric measurements such as skinfolds. *Thorough assessment of nutritional status is important in planning to meet current and anticipated calorie needs.*

*Monitor food and fluid intake and urinary output. Pain or fatigue, rather than a sensation of fullness, may prompt the decision to stop eating, resulting in inadequate intake.* ■

- Evaluate current and preferred eating habits and foods, as well as understanding of nutrition. *This evaluation provides additional information about nutrition as well as a basis for future planning.*

*Weigh daily. Daily weight is an accurate measure of both fluid balance and nutritional status.* ■

- Refer to a dietitian for further evaluation, planning, and education. *A professional can identify nutritional needs and help plan a diet that will meet them.*
- Encourage experimentation with foods of different textures and temperatures. *Very cold foods or foods of a soft texture may be easier to swallow.*
- Encourage frequent, small meals rather than three large meals per day. *Frequent, small quantities of food improve overall intake when dysphagia, odynophagia, or fatigue interfere with nutrition.*
- Recommend liquid supplements such as Ensure when calorie needs are not being met. Provide information about where to obtain nutritional supplements. *Liquid dietary supplements provide balanced nutrition as well as additional calories and are an effective way of increasing intake. They are available without prescription in major supermarkets.*

- Provide mouth care before meals and supplemental feedings. Provide a topical anesthetic such as viscous lidocaine before eating for stomatitis or esophagitis related to radiation or chemotherapy. *The tumor or its treatment may cause bad breath or a foul taste in the mouth, which suppresses appetite. Inflamed mucosa may make eating uncomfortable. A topical anesthetic may relieve this discomfort and thus promote food intake.*
- Provide an antiemetic 30 minutes before eating as needed to relieve nausea. *Nausea interferes with food intake. An antiemetic can relieve nausea and make eating possible.*
- Suggest enteral (tube) feedings via nasogastric or gastrostomy tube if the client is unable to consume enough food to maintain weight and nutritional status. *Both cancer and surgery increase calorie needs. Supplemental enteral feedings may be necessary to prevent catabolism and to promote healing and recovery.*

*Following laryngectomy, place in semi-Fowler's or Fowler's position. Elevating the head of the bed facilitates swallowing of oral secretions and helps prevent regurgitation of tube feedings.* ■

- Instruct to perform mouth rinses before initiating feeding postoperatively. *Rinsing helps clean the mouth and also provides practice in using tongue and cheek muscles to control fluid in the mouth.*
- Refer to a physical or speech therapist for swallowing rehabilitation following laryngectomy. *Because surgery changes the relationship of the trachea, esophagus, and oropharynx, swallowing needs to be relearned before eating.*
- Reinforce swallowing instructions. *Reinforcement promotes learning.*

## Anticipatory Grieving

The client with laryngeal cancer faces not only the diagnosis of cancer, which is often perceived as a death sentence, but also the prospect of mutilating surgery. If laryngectomy is necessary, the client grieves the loss of both a body part and an important function, speech, a vital aspect of social interaction and often necessary for one's career. It also enables people to express their needs when they cannot meet them alone. The loss of speech, therefore, is a major loss. In addition, the tracheal stoma changes the manner in which the client breathes. If radical neck dissection is required, loss of neck musculature and function also alters body image and self-concept.

- Provide opportunities for expressing feelings of grief, anger, or fear about the diagnosis of cancer, the impending surgery, and the anticipated loss of speech. *The client with laryngeal cancer needs the opportunity (and may need permission) to grieve anticipated losses. A cancer diagnosis may precipitate grieving for unfulfilled plans and expectations, even though a cure may be anticipated. Laryngectomy causes a major change in body image, with loss of a vital body part and creation of a stoma. The client also grieves the loss of speech. This loss can have a significant impact on occupation and social interaction.*

**PRACTICE ALERT** *Provide a calm, supportive environment with adequate privacy and emotional support for the client and family members as they work through the grieving process. It is important for the client and family to know that their feelings of loss are real and accepted by caregivers.* ■

- Help the client and family discuss the potential impact of the loss on family structure and function. *Discussion helps family members understand each other's feelings and support one another.*
- Refer for psychologic or spiritual counseling as appropriate. *Counseling and spiritual guidance can help the client and family deal with the diagnosis and proposed treatment, and help prevent a sense of defeat and hopelessness.*
- Help identify additional resources, such as coping strategies that have been successfully used in the past to deal with crises. *This exercise helps the client and family identify strengths they can use to deal with the present situation.*

## Using NANDA, NIC, and NOC

Chart 35–2 shows links between NANDA nursing diagnoses, NIC, and NOC for the client with laryngeal cancer.

## Home Care

Teaching for the client with a benign laryngeal tumor emphasizes management of contributing factors. Stress the importance of not yelling or screaming. Refer clients, particularly singers, to a speech therapist for voice training. Emphasize the need to keep the voice within its normal range to reduce vocal cord stress. Encourage smoking cessation, particularly if the

client is also a singer. Discuss the relationship of industrial pollutants to laryngeal tumors and help explore ways of reducing pollutant exposure.

Teaching the client and family about laryngeal cancer, treatment options, and home care related to those treatments is an important nursing responsibility. Include the following topics when teaching.

- Clarification of treatment options, including risks and benefits
- Importance of early intervention to reduce the risk of local spread and metastasis
- If a total laryngectomy is proposed, options for communication after surgery, including the pros and cons of each:
  a. The tracheoesophageal puncture device requires some manual dexterity to manipulate.
  b. Only about 30% of clients are able to master esophageal speech.
  c. A trial of the speech generator prior to surgery may reduce frustration in learning to use it postoperatively.
- Care related to radiation therapy, including skin and mouth care, management of secretions (see Chapter 10 ⊕ for more information about radiation therapy and its effects)
- Strategies and resources for smoking cessation and alcohol abstinence
- Ways to achieve and maintain optimal nutrition.
- Tracheostomy stoma care and preventing respiratory infection. Provide opportunities to practice and redemonstrate techniques. Clean technique (rather than sterile) is used; the tracheostomy tube may not be needed once the stoma is fully healed. Discuss these additional measures.
  a. Using a humidifier or vaporizer to add humidity to inspired air.

---

## CHART 35–2 NANDA, NIC, AND NOC LINKAGES

### The Client with Laryngeal Cancer

| NURSING DIAGNOSES | NURSING INTERVENTIONS | NURSING OUTCOMES |
|---|---|---|
| • Impaired Verbal Communication | • Communication Enhancement: Speech Deficit<br>• Anxiety Reduction<br>• Support System Enhancement | • Communication Ability<br>• Communication: Expressive Ability<br>• Coping |
| • Ineffective Airway Clearance | • Airway Management<br>• Airway Suctioning<br>• Artificial Airway Management | • Respiratory Status: Ventilation<br>• Knowledge: Treatment Regimen |
| • Impaired Swallowing | • Aspiration Precautions<br>• Swallowing Therapy<br>• Enteral Tube Feeding<br>• Positioning | • Aspiration Control<br>• Swallowing Status<br>• Nutritional Status: Food and Fluid Intake |

*Note. Data from Nursing Outcomes Classification (NOC) by M. Johnson & M. Maas (Eds.), 1997, St. Louis: Mosby; Nursing Diagnoses: Definitions & Classification 2001–2002 by North American Nursing Diagnosis Association, 2001, Philadelphia: NANDA; Nursing Interventions Classification (NIC) by J.C. McCloskey & G. M. Bulechek (Eds.), 2000, St. Louis: Mosby. Reprinted by permission.*

b. Increasing fluid intake to maintain mucosal moisture and loosen secretions.

c. Shielding the stoma with a stoma guard, such as a gauze square on a tie around the neck, to prevent particulate matter from entering the lower respiratory tract.

d. Promptly removing secretions from skin surrounding the stoma to prevent irritation and skin breakdown.

e. Water sports are contraindicated with a permanent tracheostomy; there is no restriction on other activities although lifting may be more difficult because of inability to hold the breath (the Valsalva maneuver).

f. Showering and bathing (without submerging the neck or head) are allowed; protect the stoma with a cupped hand or washcloth.

• Manifestations of potential complications of laryngectomy to be reported to the physician, including loss of hearing or facial expression due to auditory or facial nerve injury, or shoulder drop due to damage to the spinal accessory nerve.

The client and family need emotional and motivational support through this trying time. Refer to local support groups such as a laryngectomy club or lost cord club. If the client and family are having difficulty adjusting to the diagnosis of cancer and the effects of treatment, provide referral to counseling.

---

## Nursing Care Plan
## A Client with Total Laryngectomy

David Tom is a 61-year-old accountant who is divorced and has two adult children. He has smoked two packs of cigarettes daily since high school, and usually has three or four cocktails each evening. After several months of persistent sore throat and hoarseness, Mr. Tom was diagnosed with cancer of the larynx. He has been admitted to the surgical care unit from the ICU 2 days post total laryngectomy.

### ASSESSMENT

Mr. Tom's vital signs are stable: BP 146/84, P 92 and regular, R 18, T 98°F (36.7°C) axillary. A tracheostomy tube is sutured in place, and he is receiving humidified oxygen at 28% per tracheostomy collar. Pulse oximetry is 94%. He is receiving continuous tube feeding per nasogastric feeding tube. Two Hemovac wound drains are present in the right neck area. A moderate amount of edema is noted in the right facial and submandibular area. Mr. Tom is ambulatory within the room.

### DIAGNOSIS

• *Risk for ineffective airway clearance* related to postoperative edema
• *Risk for ineffective breathing pattern* related to pain and anxiety
• *Disturbed body image* related to total laryngectomy and presence of tracheostomy stoma
• *Impaired verbal communication* related to total laryngectomy
• *Pain* related to surgical procedure
• *Risk for imbalanced nutrition: Less than body requirements* related to difficulty eating after surgery

### EXPECTED OUTCOMES

• Maintain clear airways and lung sounds.
• Maintain oxygen saturation level greater than 92%.
• Demonstrate interest in providing incision and stoma care.
• Accept information about potential communication strategies.
• Communicate effective pain management.
• Maintain appropriate body weight, intake, and output.

### PLANNING AND IMPLEMENTATION

• Assess respiratory status including rate, pattern, lung sounds, and cough effectiveness at least every 4 hours.
• Monitor quantity, color, and odor of secretions.
• Assess vital signs and pain at least every 4 hours. Administer analgesics as ordered.
• Schedule time to sit with Mr. Tom and discuss his concerns and feelings at least three times per day.
• Provide written information as requested.
• Monitor intake, output, and daily weight.
• Arrange dietary consultation to determine caloric requirements.

### EVALUATION

Mr. Tom reports in writing that his pain is adequately controlled. His respiratory status is stable with clear breath sounds throughout and an oxygen saturation of 94%. He is afebrile. Mr. Tom is tolerating tube feedings well and expresses a desire to begin eating. The dietitian has visited and assisted in planning to begin oral feedings. Intake and output are stable, as is his weight. Mr. Tom has been receptive to receiving information about follow-up care and exploration of various modalities of speech.

### Critical Thinking in the Nursing Process

1. Compare and contrast advantages and disadvantages of various methods to allow speech following total laryngectomy.
2. Develop a plan of care for Mr. Tom for the nursing diagnosis, *Disturbed body image*.
3. Discuss nursing interventions to provide wound care for the client with laryngectomy and radical neck dissection.
4. List strategies to optimize ventilation.

See Evaluating Your Response in Appendix C.

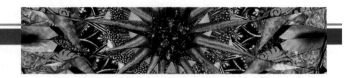

 **EXPLORE MediaLink**

NCLEX review questions, case studies, care plan activities, MediaLink applications, and other interactive resources for this chapter can be found on the Companion Website at www.prenhall.com/lemone.

Click on Chapter 35 to select the activities for this chapter. For animations, video clips, more NCLEX review questions, and an audio glossary, access the Student CD-ROM accompanying this textbook.

# TEST YOURSELF

1. Which of the following health promotion activities planned by a nurse working with a group of community-dwelling senior citizens would be most likely to prevent influenza and pneumonia?

   a. Indoor exercise programs during winter months
   b. Influenza vaccine clinics at the senior center
   c. Teaching effective handwashing
   d. Advising seniors to avoid crowds

2. A client in the emergency department following facial trauma complains that his nose "just keeps dripping." The drainage appears like watery blood. The most appropriate nursing action would be to:

   a. Provide a box of tissues
   b. Reassure the client that this is expected with a nasal fracture
   c. Suction the nasopharynx
   d. Obtain a specimen for glucose testing

3. An expected finding in a client with obstructive sleep apnea would be:

   a. Confusion and signs of dementia
   b. Enlarged tongue
   c. Complaints of daytime sleepiness
   d. Decreased oxygen saturation levels while awake

4. The nurse in a physician's office notes that a regular client's voice is hoarse, a change from previous visits. The most appropriate question to ask the client would be:

   a. "How long has your voice been hoarse?"
   b. "Do you smoke?"
   c. "Do you have a sore throat?"
   d. "Would you like a prescription for throat lozenges?"

5. The nurse evaluates his teaching as effective when a client with stage 1 laryngeal cancer states:

   a. "I'm glad I don't have to worry about treating this cancer now because it is so early."
   b. "I hate to think about eventually losing the ability to speak, but I'd rather treat it aggressively than lose my life to cancer."
   c. "I'm glad this was diagnosed early, when it can be treated with radiation so I won't lose my voice."
   d. "Thank goodness this type of cancer usually doesn't spread anywhere else."

See Test Yourself answers in Appendix C.

# BIBLIOGRAPHY

Ackley, B. J., & Ladwig, G. B. (2002). *Nursing diagnosis handbook: A guide to planning care* (5th ed.). St. Louis: Mosby.

American Cancer Society. (2002a). *Cancer facts and figures 2002*. Atlanta: Author.
_____.(2002b). *Laryngeal and hypopharyngeal cancer.* Available: www.cancer.org

Atkinson, W., Wolfe, C., Humiston, S., & Nelson, R. (Eds.). (2000). *Epidemiology and prevention of vaccine-preventable diseases* (6th ed.) Atlanta: Centers for Disease Control and Prevention.

Braunwald, E., Fauci, A. S., Kasper, D. L., Hauser, S. L., Longo, D. L., & Jameson, J. L. (2001). *Harrison's principles of internal medicine* (15th ed.). New York: McGraw-Hill.

Bullock, B. A., & Henze, R. L. (2000). *Focus on pathophysiology.* Philadelphia: Lippincott.

Conn, V. (1991). Self-care actions taken by older adults for influenza and colds. *Nursing Research, 40*(3), 176–181.

Deglin, J. H., & Vallerand, A. H. (2001). *Davis's drug guide for nurses* (7th ed.). Philadelphia: F.A. Davis.

Fontaine, K. L. (2000). *Healing practices: Alternative therapies for nursing.* Upper Saddle River, NJ: Prentice Hall Health.

Hakemi, A. (2001). Diagnosing and managing rhinosinusitis. *Physician Assistant, 25*(11), 16–25.

Hughes, D. L., & Tartasky, D. (1996). Implementation of a flu immunization program for homebound elders: A graduate student practicum. *Geriatric Nursing, 17*(5), 217–221.

Johnson, M., Bulechek, G., Dochterman, J. M., Maas, M., & Moorhead, S. (2001). *Nursing diagnoses, outcomes, & interventions.* St. Louis: Mosby.

Johnson, M., Maas, M., & Moorhead, S. (Eds.). (2000). *Nursing outcomes classification (NOC)* (2nd ed.). St. Louis: Mosby.

Kearney, K. (2001). Emergency. Epiglottitis. *American Journal of Nursing, 101*(8), 37–38.

Kirchner, J. T. (1999). Manifestations of pertussis in immunized children and adults. *American Family Physician, 60*(7), 2148–2149.

Klein, L. (2001). Sinusitis: When to treat and how. *RN, 64*(1), 42–44, 46, 48.

Kuhn, M. A. (1999). *Complementary therapies for health care providers.* Philadelphia: Lippincott.

Lehne, R. A. (2001). *Pharmacology for nursing care* (4th ed.). Philadelphia: Saunders.

Loud, B. (2001). A water pick to clear sinuses? *RN, 64*(1), 48–49.

Malarkey, L. M., & McMorrow, M. E. (2000). *Nurse's manual of laboratory tests and diagnostic procedures* (2nd ed.). Philadelphia: Saunders.

Marchiondo, K. (2000). Pickwickian syndrome: The challenge of severe sleep apnea. *MEDSURG Nursing, 9*(4), 183–188.

McCloskey, J. C., & Bulechek, G. M. (Eds.). (2000). *Nursing interventions classification (NIC)* (3rd ed.). St. Louis: Mosby.

Meeker, M. H., & Rothrock, J. C. (1999). *Alexander's care of the patient in surgery* (11th ed.). St. Louis: Mosby.

Merritt, S. L. (2000). Putting sleep disorders to rest. *RN, 63*(7), 26–30.

North American Nursing Diagnosis Association. (2001). *NANDA nursing diagnoses: Definitions & classification 2001–2002*. Philadelphia: NANDA.

Porth, C. M. (2002). *Pathophysiology: Concepts of altered health states* (6th ed.). Philadelphia: Lippincott.

Seay, S. J., Gay, S. L., & Strauss, M. (2002). Emergency. Tracheostomy emergencies. *American Journal of Nursing, 102*(3), 59, 61, 63.

Shellenbarger, T., & Wolfe, S. (2000). Nosebleeds: Not just kids' stuff. *RN, 63*(2), 50–55.

Springhouse. (1999). *Nurse's handbook of alternative & complementary therapies*. Springhouse, PA: Author.

Tierney, L. M., McPhee, S. J., & Papadakis, M. A. (2001). *Current medical diagnosis & treatment* (40th ed.). New York: Lange Medical Books/McGraw-Hill.

Urden, L. D., Stacy, K. M., & Lough, M. E. (2002). *Thelan's critical care nursing: Diagnosis and management* (4th ed.). St. Louis: Mosby.

The Voice Center. (2002). Speech after a total laryngectomy. Available: www.voice-center.com/alaryngeal_speech.htm

Way, L. W., & Doherty, G. M. (2003). *Current surgical diagnosis and treatment* (11th ed.). New York: McGraw-Hill.

Whitney, E. N., & Rolfes, S. R. (2002). *Understanding nutrition* (9th ed.). Belmont, CA: Wadsworth.

Wilkinson, J. M. (2000). *Nursing diagnosis handbook with NIC interventions and NOC outcomes* (7th ed.). Upper Saddle River, NJ: Prentice Hall Health.

Yantis, M. A. (2002). Pain control. Obstructive sleep apnea syndrome. *American Journal of Nursing, 102*(6), 83, 85.

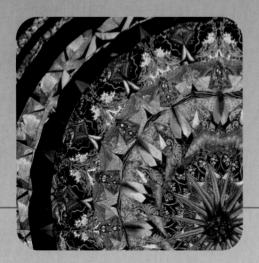

# CHAPTER 36

# Nursing Care of Clients with Lower Respiratory Disorders

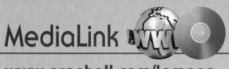

## MediaLink

**www.prenhall.com/lemone**

Additional resources for this chapter can be found on the Student CD-ROM accompanying this textbook, and on the Companion Website at www.prenhall.com/lemone. Click on Chapter 36 to select the activities for this chapter.

**CD-ROM**
- Audio Glossary
- NCLEX Review

**Animation**
- ARDS
- Asthma
- Salmeterol

**Companion Website**
- More NCLEX Review
- Case Study
  Acute Asthma Attack
- Care Plan Activity
  Pneumonia
- MediaLink Application
  Respiratory Disorders

## LEARNING OUTCOMES

After completing this chapter, you will be able to:

- Relate anatomy, physiology, and assessment of the lower respiratory tract and its function to common disorders affecting the lower respiratory system.

- Describe the pathophysiology and manifestations of common lower respiratory disorders.

- Identify tests used to diagnose disorders of the lower respiratory system.

- Discuss nursing implications for medications and treatments prescribed for lower respiratory disorders.

- Provide appropriate care for the client having thoracic surgery.

- Effectively teach clients with lower respiratory disorders and their families.

- Use the nursing process to assess, plan and implement individualized care, and evaluate responses for a client with a lower respiratory disorder.

Many clients in acute care, long-term care, and the community experience acute or chronic disorders affecting the lower respiratory system. These disorders often lead to lost work time and account for a significant portion of health care costs.

Normal function of the lower respiratory system depends on several organ systems: the central nervous system, which stimulates and controls breathing; chemoreceptors in the brain, aortic arch, and carotid bodies, which monitor the pH and oxygen content of blood; the heart and circulatory system, which provide for blood supply and gas exchange; the musculoskeletal system, which provides an intact thoracic cavity capable of expanding and contracting; and the lungs and bronchial tree, which allow air movement and gas exchange. Impaired function of any of these systems affects ventilation and respiration. As a result, tissues may become *hypoxic*, with inadequate oxygen to support metabolic activity.

Disorders of the lower respiratory tract have both local and systemic effects. Local effects include cough, excess mucus production, shortness of breath or **dyspnea** (difficult or labored breathing), **hemoptysis** (bloody sputum), and chest pain. Systemic effects may include fever, anorexia and malaise, **cyanosis** (gray to blue or purple skin color caused by deoxygenated hemoglobin), **clubbing** of fingers and toes (enlargement and blunting of terminal digits), and other manifestations of impaired gas exchange.

Disorders of the lower respiratory system discussed in this chapter include infectious or inflammatory conditions, obstructive and restrictive lung diseases, pulmonary vascular disorders, lung cancer, chest and respiratory trauma, and respiratory failure. Before continuing, review the anatomy, physiology, and assessment of the lower respiratory system in Chapter 34.

# INFECTIONS AND INFLAMMATORY DISORDERS

Infections and inflammation of the lower respiratory system are common. The respiratory tree is constantly exposed to the environment as air moves into and out of the lower respiratory tract. In addition, the oropharynx is colonized by huge numbers of microorganisms that may be aspirated into the bronchial tree. Both anatomic and physiologic defenses help maintain the sterility of the lower respiratory tract. When these defenses are impaired, the risk for infection increases. For example, drugs, alcohol, or neuromuscular disease may suppress the cough reflex, and the influenza virus can leave the respiratory epithelium vulnerable to bacterial infection. Even in healthy people, microorganisms and other foreign material occasionally enter the bronchial tree and lung parenchyma.

## THE CLIENT WITH ACUTE BRONCHITIS

**Bronchitis,** inflammation of the bronchi, may be either an acute or a chronic condition. Acute bronchitis is relatively common in adults. Impaired immune defenses and cigarette smoking increase the risk for acute bronchitis. In otherwise healthy adults, it typically follows a viral upper respiratory infection. Chronic bronchitis is a component of chronic obstructive pulmonary disease (COPD) and is discussed later in this chapter.

## PATHOPHYSIOLOGY AND MANIFESTATIONS

Infectious bronchitis can be caused by either viruses or bacteria that damage the respiratory mucosa. Inhalation of toxic gases or chemicals can lead to inflammatory bronchitis. In either case, the inflammatory response causes vasodilation and edema of the mucosal lining of the bronchi. Mucosal irritation increases mucus production and initiates the cough reflex.

Acute bronchitis is typically heralded by a nonproductive cough that later becomes productive. The cough often occurs in paroxysms, and may be aggravated by cold, dry, or dusty air. Chest pain, often substernal, is common. Other manifestations include moderate fever and general malaise.

## COLLABORATIVE CARE

The diagnosis of acute bronchitis typically is based on the history and clinical presentation. A chest X-ray may be ordered to rule out pneumonia, because the presenting manifestations can be similar. Other diagnostic testing is rarely indicated. Treatment is symptomatic and includes rest, increased fluid intake, and the use of aspirin or acetaminophen to relieve fever and malaise. Many physicians prescribe a broad-spectrum antibiotic such as erythromycin or penicillin, because approximately 50% of acute bronchitis is bacterial in origin. An expectorant cough medication is recommended for use during the day and a cough suppressant for night to facilitate rest.

## NURSING CARE

Nursing interventions for clients with acute bronchitis are primarily educational. Include the following teaching topics.

- Increase fluid intake to keep mucus thin and meet increased needs related to fever.
- Use over-the-counter analgesics and cough preparations containing dextromethorphan for symptom relief.
- Use and effects of any prescribed medications.
- The importance of smoking cessation (as appropriate).

## THE CLIENT WITH PNEUMONIA

Inflammation of the lung parenchyma (the respiratory bronchioles and alveoli) is known as **pneumonia.** Despite significant advances in antibiotic therapy, pneumonia remains the sixth leading cause of death in the United States, and the leading cause of death from infectious disease (Porth, 2002). In 1999, nearly 64,000 deaths in the United States were attributed to pneumonia (NHLBI, 2002). Its incidence and mortality are highest in older adults and people with debilitating diseases. Pneumonia currently accounts for about 10% of adult hospital admissions in the United States.

Pneumonia may be either infectious or noninfectious. Bacteria, viruses, fungi, protozoa, and other microbes can lead to infectious pneumonia. Noninfectious causes include aspiration of gastric contents and inhalation of toxic or irritating gases. Pneumonias often are classified as community acquired, nosocomial (hospital acquired), or opportunistic. Different organisms are implicated in each of these classifications (Table 36–1). The most common causative organism for community-acquired pneumonia is *Streptococcus pneumoniae* (also called pneumococcus), a gram-positive bacterium. This organism causes 70% to 75% of all diagnosed cases of pneumonia. *Mycoplasma pneumoniae, Haemophilus influenzae,* and the influenza virus are also leading causes of community-acquired pneumonia. *Staphylococcus aureus* and gram-negative bacteria such as *Klebsiella pneumoniae, Pseudomonas aeruginosa,* and enteric bacilli, including *Escherichia coli,* are often implicated as nosocomial causes of pneumonia. Organisms such as *Pneumonocystis carinii* generally cause infections only in immunocompromised people (opportunistic infections).

### PHYSIOLOGY REVIEW

The lower respiratory tract normally is sterile. A number of defense mechanisms help maintain this sterile environment. Infectious particles trapped by the mucous membranes of the nose are removed by sneezing, while those deposited in the nasopharynx usually are swallowed or expectorated. Reflex closure of the epiglottis and the branching bronchial tree present anatomic barriers to entry of microorganisms and other possible contaminants. The cilia and mucus that line the respiratory tract, and the cough reflex, serve to trap and eliminate foreign matter that enters the lower respiratory tract. Organisms that make it past these barriers usually are rapidly phagocytized in the alveolus by resident macrophages, then attacked by the in-

### Nursing Care of the Older Adult

#### PNEUMONIA

Several changes associated with aging and disease affect respiratory function and airway clearance. The number of cilia decreases, and the cough weakens. Gag and cough reflexes diminish. The older adult is at greater risk for dehydration, leading to thick, viscous mucus that is difficult to expectorate. Immune function declines with aging. These factors increase the risk of pulmonary infection and reduce the older adult's ability to respond effectively to infectious processes.

Other factors also may increase the risk for and severity of lower respiratory infections in the older adult: immobility, smoking history, surgical procedures, use of multiple medications, malnutrition, and such diseases as chronic obstructive pulmonary disease (COPD) and heart disease.

flammatory and immune defenses of the body. Aging impairs these immune responses, increasing the risk for pneumonia (see the box above).

### PATHOPHYSIOLOGY

The most common means of entry of pathogens into the lung is aspiration of oropharyngeal secretions containing microbes. Microorganisms also may be inhaled after having been released when an infected person coughs, sneezes, or talks. Contaminated aerosolized water also may be inhaled, an important means of spread for viral and some other types of pneumonia. Finally, bacteria may spread to the lungs through the bloodstream from infection elsewhere in the body.

When the invading microorganisms colonize the alveoli, an inflammatory and immune response is initiated. The antigen-antibody response and endotoxins released by some organisms damage bronchial and alveolar mucous membranes, causing inflammation and edema. Infectious debris and exudate can fill alveoli, interfering with ventilation and gas exchange.

The pathologic process, anatomic location, and manifestations of pneumonias vary according to the infective organism.

### Acute Bacterial Pneumonia

Of the bacterial pneumonias, the pathogenesis of pneumococcal (*Streptococcus pneumoniae*) pneumonia is best understood (Figure 36–1 ■). These bacteria reside in the upper respiratory tract of up to 70% of adults. They may be spread by direct person-to-person contact via droplets. In many cases, infection results from aspiration of resident bacteria. In the lower respi-

| TABLE 36–1 Common Organisms Causing Pneumonia in Adults |||
|---|---|---|
| **Community Acquired** | **Hospital Acquired** | **Opportunistic** |
| • *Streptococcus pneumoniae*<br>• *Mycoplasma pneumoniae*<br>• *Haemophilus influenzae*<br>• Influenza virus<br>• *Chlamydia pneumoniae*<br>• *Legionella pneumophila* | • *Staphylococcus aureus*<br>• *Pseudomonas aeruginosa*<br>• *Klebsiella pneumoniae*<br>• *Escherichia coli* | • *Pneumocystis carinii*<br>• *Mycobacterium tuberculosis*<br>• Cytomegalovirus (CMV)<br>• Atypical mycobacteria<br>• Fungi |

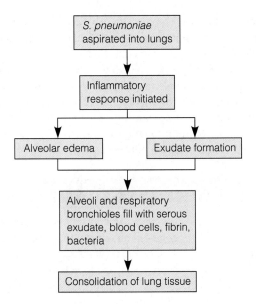

**Figure 36–1** ■ The pathogenesis of pneumococcal pneumonia.

ratory tract, the inflammatory response initiated by these organisms causes alveolar edema and the formation of exudate. As alveoli and respiratory bronchioles fill with serous exudate, blood cells, fibrin, and bacteria, *consolidation* (solidification) of lung tissue occurs. The lower lobes of the lungs are usually affected because of gravity. Consolidation of a large portion of an entire lung lobe is known as *lobar pneumonia*. This is the typical pattern for pneumococcal pneumonia. *Bronchopneumonia* is patchy consolidation involving several lobules. Other bacterial pneumonias often present with the patchy involvement of bronchopneumonia; pneumococcal pneumonia may also follow this pattern. The process resolves when macrophages predominate, digesting and removing inflammatory exudate from the infected lung.

## MANIFESTATIONS AND COMPLICATIONS

The presentation of bacterial pneumonia is usually acute, with rapid onset of shaking chills, fever, and cough productive of rust-colored or purulent sputum. Chest aching or *pleuritic pain* (sharp localized chest pain that increases with breathing and coughing) is common. Limited breath sounds and fine crackles or rales are heard over the affected area of lung. A pleural friction rub may be audible. If the involved area is large and gas exchange is impaired, dyspnea and cyanosis may be noted.

A more insidious onset with low-grade fever, cough, and scattered crackles is more typical of bronchopneumonia. Dyspnea is less commonly seen. The older adult or debilitated client may have atypical manifestations of pneumonia, with little cough, scant sputum, and minimal evidence of respiratory distress. Fever, tachypnea, and altered mentation or agitation may be the primary presenting symptoms.

Pneumococcal pneumonia typically resolves uneventfully; normal lung structure is restored on completion of the process. Local extension of the infection to involve the pleura (*pleuritis*) is the most common complication. Bacteremia can spread the infection to other tissues, leading to meningitis, endocarditis, or peritonitis, and increasing the risk of mortality.

Pneumonias caused by *Staphylococcus aureus* and gram-negative bacteria often cause extensive parenchymal damage with necrosis, lung abscess, and empyema. **Empyema** is accumulation of purulent exudate in the pleural cavity. Progressive destruction of lung tissue and functional impairment is a possible consequence of *Klebsiella* pneumonia.

### Legionnaires' Disease

Legionnaires' disease is a form of bronchopneumonia caused by *Legionella pneumophila*, a gram-negative bacterium widely found in water, particularly warm standing water. Legionnaires' disease occurs sporadically and in outbreaks, such as that which occurred at an American Legion convention in 1976, when the disease was first recognized. Contaminated water-cooled air-conditioning systems and other water sources have been implicated in its spread.

Smokers, older adults, and people with chronic diseases or impaired immune defenses are most susceptible to Legionnaires' disease. Symptoms develop gradually, beginning 2 to 10 days after exposure. Dry cough, dyspnea, general malaise, chills and fever, headache, confusion, anorexia and diarrhea, myalgias and arthralgias are common manifestations. Consolidation of lung tissue is patchy or lobar. The mortality rate in Legionnaires' disease is up to 31% without treatment in otherwise healthy people and up to 80% in people who are immunocompromised (Braunwald et al., 2001).

### Primary Atypical Pneumonia

Pneumonia caused by *Mycoplasma pneumoniae* is generally classified as *primary atypical pneumonia,* because its presentation and course significantly differ from other bacterial pneumonias. Mycoplasma infection often causes pharyngitis or bronchitis. When pneumonia develops, patchy inflammatory changes in the alveolar septum and interstitial tissue of the lung occur. Alveolar exudate and consolidation of lung tissue are not features of atypical pneumonia.

Young adults—college students and military recruits in particular—are the primary affected population. Primary atypical pneumonia is highly contagious. Its manifestations resemble those of viral pneumonia; systemic manifestations of fever, headache, myalgias, and arthralgias often predominate. The cough associated with atypical pneumonia is dry, hacking, and nonproductive. Because of the typically mild nature and predominant systemic manifestations, mycoplasmal and viral pneumonia are often referred to as "walking pneumonias."

### Viral Pneumonia

Approximately 10% of pneumonias in adults are viral. Influenza and adenovirus are the most common organisms; however, the incidence of cytomegalovirus (CMV) pneumonia is increasing in immunocompromised people. Other viruses such as herpesviruses and measles virus also may cause viral pneumonia. As in primary atypical pneumonia, lung involvement in viral pneumonia is limited to the alveolar septum and interstitial spaces.

Viral pneumonia is typically a mild disease that often affects older adults and people with chronic conditions. It usually occurs in community epidemics. Flulike symptoms of headache, fever, fatigue, malaise, and muscle aching are common, along with a dry cough.

## Pneumocystis carinii Pneumonia

As many as 75% to 80% of people with acquired immune deficiency syndrome (AIDS) develop an opportunistic pneumonia caused by *Pneumocystis carinii*, a common parasite found worldwide. Immunity to *P. carinii* is nearly universal, except in immunocompromised people. Opportunistic infection may develop in people treated with immunosuppressive or cytotoxic drugs for cancer or organ transplant and in people with genetic or acquired immunodeficiency.

Infection with *P. carinii* produces patchy involvement throughout the lungs, causing affected alveoli to thicken, become edematous, and fill with foamy, protein-rich fluid. Gas exchange is severely impaired as the disease progresses.

*P. carinii* pneumonia (PCP) has an abrupt onset with fever, tachypnea and shortness of breath, and a dry, nonproductive cough. Respiratory distress can be significant, with intercostal retractions and cyanosis.

Table 36–2 compares the manifestations of infectious pneumonias.

## Aspiration Pneumonia

Aspiration of gastric contents into the lungs results in a chemical and bacterial pneumonia known as *aspiration pneumonia.* Major risk factors for aspiration pneumonia include emergency surgery or obstetric procedures, depressed cough and gag reflexes, and impaired swallowing. Older surgical clients are at significant risk. Enteral nutrition by either nasogastric or gastric tube also increases the risk for aspiration pneumonia. Vomiting is not always apparent; silent regurgitation of gastric contents may occur when the level of consciousness is decreased. Measures to reduce the risk for aspiration pneumonia include

minimizing the use of preoperative medications, promoting anesthetic elimination from the body, and preventing nausea and gastric distention.

The low pH of gastric contents causes a severe inflammatory response when aspirated into the respiratory tract. Pulmonary edema and respiratory failure may result. Common complications of aspiration pneumonia include abscesses, bronchiectasis (chronic dilation of the bronchi and bronchioles), and gangrene of pulmonary tissue.

## COLLABORATIVE CARE

Prevention is a key component in managing pneumonia. Identifying vulnerable populations and instituting preventive strategies are measures to reduce the mortality and morbidity associated with pneumonia. With early identification of the infecting organism, appropriate treatment, and support of respiratory function, most clients recover uneventfully. However, pneumonia remains a serious disease with significant mortality, especially in aged and debilitated populations.

## Diagnostic Tests

Diagnostic testing for pneumonia focuses on establishing a diagnosis, determining the extent of lung involvement, and identifying the causative organism.

- *Sputum gram stain* rapidly identifies the infecting organisms as gram-positive or gram-negative bacteria. Antibiotic therapy can then be directed at the predominant type of organism until culture and sensitivity results are obtained.
- *Sputum culture and sensitivity* is ordered to identify the infecting organism and determine the most effective antibiotic therapy. When obtaining sputum for culture, it is important to obtain secretions from the lower respiratory tract, not the mouth and nasal passages. See Procedure 36–1.
- *Complete blood count (CBC) with white blood cell (WBC) differential* shows an elevated WBC (11,000/mm$^3$ or higher)

## TABLE 36–2   Manifestations of Infectious Pneumonias

| Type | Onset | Respiratory Manifestations | Systemic Manifestations |
|---|---|---|---|
| Pneumococcal or lobar pneumonia | Abrupt | Cough productive of purulent or rust-colored sputum; pleuritic or aching chest pain; decreased breath sounds and crackles over affected area; possible dyspnea and cyanosis | Chills and fever |
| Bronchopneumonia | Gradual | Cough, scattered crackles; minimal dyspnea and respiratory distress | Low-grade fever |
| Legionnaires' disease | Gradual | Dry cough; dyspnea | Chills and fever; general malaise; headache; confusion; anorexia and diarrhea; myalgias and arthralgias |
| Primary atypical pneumonia | Gradual | Dry, hacking, nonproductive cough | Fever, headache, myalgias, and arthralgias predominate |
| Viral pneumonia | Sudden or gradual | Dry cough | Flulike symptoms |
| *Pneumocystis carinii* pneumonia | Abrupt | Dry cough; tachypnea and shortness of breath; significant respiratory distress | Fever |

## Procedure 36–1 — Obtaining a Sputum Specimen

### SUPPLIES

- Sterile sputum container, specimen cup, or mucus trap
- Mouth care supplies
- Sterile suction kit, if necessary
- Gloves

### BEFORE THE PROCEDURE

If the sputum specimen is to establish the initial diagnosis, obtain the specimen before starting oxygen and/or antibiotic therapy. Antibiotics reduce the bacterial count, making it difficult to identify the infecting organism. Oxygen therapy dries mucous membranes, making it more difficult to obtain a specimen. Unless otherwise instructed, obtain the specimen early in the morning, just after awakening. Respiratory secretions tend to pool during sleep; it is easier to obtain a specimen before normal coughing and daily activity has cleared them.

Provide for privacy, and explain the procedure. Emphasize the importance of coughing deeply to obtain sputum from the lower respiratory tract, avoiding expectoration of saliva. Increasing fluid intake prior to obtaining the specimen can help liquefy secretions, making them easier to expectorate.

### DURING THE PROCEDURE

1. Use standard precautions.
2. Provide for mouth care prior to obtaining the specimen to reduce contamination by oral flora.
3. Instruct to cough deeply several times, expectorating mucus into the container.
4. Close the container securely using aseptic technique.
5. Label the container with name and other identifying data, time and date, and any special conditions, such as antibiotic or oxygen therapy. Enclose specimen container in a clean plastic bag, and take to the laboratory or refrigerate as ordered to preserve the specimen.
6. To obtain a specimen by suctioning:
   - Provide mouth care as indicated above.
   - Obtain a sterile mucus trap. Using aseptic technique, attach the trap to the suction apparatus between the suction catheter and tubing.
   - Preoxygenate for suctioning as needed.
   - Perform tracheal suctioning using aseptic technique via either the nasotracheal route, endotracheal tube, or tracheostomy. Lubricate the catheter with sterile normal saline. Apply no suction as the catheter is being inserted into the trachea; apply suction for no longer than 10 seconds while withdrawing the catheter.
   - Detach the mucus trap; close and label. Clear the suction catheter and tubing with normal saline after removing the mucus trap. Dispose of equipment appropriately.
7. A sputum specimen also may be obtained during bronchoscopy procedure.

### AFTER THE PROCEDURE

Provide mouth care as needed. Teach the importance of completing all ordered antibiotic prescriptions to ensure complete eradication of microorganisms. Document the time and date that the specimen was obtained; and note color, consistency, and odor of sputum.

---

with increased circulating immature leukocytes (a left shift) in response to the infectious process. White blood cell changes are minimal in viral and other pneumonias.

- *Arterial blood gases (ABGs)* may be ordered to evaluate gas exchange. Alveolar inflammation can interfere with gas exchange across the alveolar-capillary membrane, especially if exudate or consolidation is present. Respiratory secretions or pleuritic pain also can interfere with alveolar ventilation. An arterial oxygen tension ($Po_2$) of less than 75 to 80 mmHg indicates impaired gas exchange or alveolar ventilation.
- *Pulse oximetry,* a noninvasive method of measuring arterial oxygen saturation, is ordered to continuously monitor gas exchange. The $Sao_2$ is the percentage of arterial hemoglobin that is saturated or combined with oxygen; it normally is 95% or higher. An $Sao_2$ of less than 95% may indicate impaired alveolar gas exchange.
- *Chest X-ray* is obtained to determine the extent and pattern of lung involvement. Fluid, infiltrates, consolidated lung tissue, and atelectasis (areas of alveolar collapse) appear as densities on the film.
- *Fiberoptic bronchoscopy* may be done to obtain a sputum specimen or remove secretions from the bronchial tree (Figure 36–2 ■). In this procedure, a flexible bronchoscope

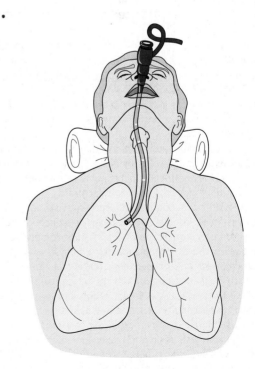

**Figure 36–2** ■ Fiberoptic bronchoscopy.

is inserted through the mouth and larynx into the tracheo-bronchial tree, allowing direct visualization of tissues and collection of specimens for analysis. Nursing responsibilities related to bronchoscopy are summarized in the box below.

## Immunization

Vaccines offer some degree of protection against the most common bacterial and viral pneumonias.

Pneumococcal vaccine, made of antigens from 23 types of pneumococcus, usually imparts lifetime immunity with a single dose. The vaccine is recommended for people who have a high risk of adverse outcome from bacterial pneumonias: people over age 65; those with chronic cardiac or respiratory conditions, diabetes mellitus, alcoholism, or other chronic diseases; and immunocompromised people.

Influenza vaccine is also recommended for high-risk populations. The predominant strain of influenza virus varies from year to year. A new vaccine formulation is prepared yearly, incorporating antigens of the influenza strains predicted to be the most prevalent for the upcoming flu season (typically the winter months). Vulnerable populations for whom yearly vaccine is recommended include those listed above as well as health care workers and residents of long-term care facilities. The vaccine contains egg protein, and is not recommended for people who have a severe allergy to eggs or who have previously experienced a severe hypersensitivity response to the vaccine.

## Medications

Medications used to treat pneumonia may include antibiotics to eradicate the infection and bronchodilators to reduce bronchospasm and improve ventilation.

Initial antibiotic therapy is based on the results of sputum Gram stain and the pattern of lung involvement shown on the chest X-ray. Typically, a broad-spectrum antibiotic such as a penicillin, cephalosporin, erythromycin, or aminoglycoside is ordered until the results of sputum culture and sensitivity tests are available. Table 36–3 lists commonly prescribed antibiotics for selected pneumonias; nursing implications for selected antibiotics are summarized on pages 224–226.

When an inflammatory response to the infection causes bronchospasm and constriction, bronchodilators may be ordered to improve ventilation and reduce hypoxia. Bronchodilators generally belong to one of two major groups: the sympathomimetic drugs, such as albuterol sulfate (Proventil) and metaproterenol (Alupent); or the methylxanthines, such as theophylline and aminophylline. Use of these drugs and related nursing implications are discussed in detail in the section on asthma.

An agent to "break up" mucus or reduce its viscosity may be prescribed. Acetylcysteine (Mucomyst), potassium iodide, and guaifenesin (a common ingredient in expectorant cough syrups), help to liquefy mucus, making it easier to expectorate. For many clients, however, increasing fluid intake is an effective means of liquefying mucus.

## Nursing Implications for Diagnostic Tests

### Bronchoscopy

#### Nursing Responsibilities

- Provide routine preoperative care as ordered. *Bronchoscopy is an invasive procedure requiring conscious sedation or anesthesia. Care provided prior to the procedure is similar to that provided before many minor surgical procedures.*
- Provide mouth care just prior to bronchoscopy. *Mouth care reduces oral microorganisms and the risk of introducing them into the lungs.*
- Bring resuscitation and suction equipment to the bedside. *Laryngospasm and respiratory distress may occur following the procedure. The anesthetic suppresses the cough and gag reflexes, and secretions may be difficult to expectorate.*
- Following the procedure, closely monitor vital signs and respiratory status. *Possible complications of bronchoscopy include laryngospasm, bronchospasm, bronchial perforation with possible pneumothorax or subcutaneous emphysema, hemorrhage, hypoxia, pneumonia or bacteremia, and cardiac stress.*
- Instruct to avoid eating or drinking for approximately 2 hours or until fully awake with intact cough and gag reflexes. *Suppression of the cough and gag reflexes by systemic and local anesthesia used during the procedure increase the risk for aspiration.*
- Provide an emesis basin and tissues for expectorating sputum and saliva. *Until reflexes have returned, the client may be unable to swallow sputum and saliva safely.*

- Monitor color and character of respiratory secretions. Secretions normally are blood tinged for several hours following bronchoscopy, especially if biopsy has been obtained. Notify the physician if sputum is grossly bloody. *Grossly bloody sputum may indicate a complication such as perforation.*
- Collect postbronchoscopy sputum specimens for cytologic examination as ordered. *Cells in the sputum may be examined if a tumor is suspected.*

#### Client and Family Teaching

- Fiberoptic bronchoscopy requires 30 to 45 minutes to complete. It may be done at the bedside, in a special procedure room, or in the surgical suite.
- The procedure usually causes little pain or discomfort, because an anesthetic is given. You will be able to breathe during the bronchoscopy.
- Some voice hoarseness and a sore throat are common following the procedure. Throat lozenges or warm saline gargles may help relieve discomfort.
- You may develop a mild fever within the first 24 hours following the procedure. This is a normal response.
- Persistent cough, bloody or purulent sputum, wheezing, shortness of breath, difficulty breathing, or chest pain may indicate a complication. Notify your physician if they develop.

TABLE 36-3  Antibiotic Therapy for Selected Pneumonias

| Causative Organism | Antibiotic of Choice | Alternative Antibiotics |
| --- | --- | --- |
| Streptococcus pneumoniae | Penicillin G or V; doxycycline; amoxicillin | Erythromycin, cephalosporins, fluoroquinolone, vancomycin |
| Staphylococcus aureus | Penicillinase-resistant penicillin (e.g., nafcillin); vancomycin for methicillin-resistant organisms | Cephalosporins, vancomycin, clindamycin; ciprofloxacin, fluoroquinlones, TMP-SMZ* |
| Mycoplasma pneumoniae | Erythromycin | Doxycycline, clarithromycin, azithromycin, fluoroquinolone |
| Klebsiella pneumoniae | Third-generation cephalosporin (with aminoglycoside if severe); methronidazole | Aztreonam, imipenem-cilastatin, fluoroquinolone |
| Legionella pneumophila | Erythromycin + rifampin; fluoroquinolone | TMP-SMZ*, azithromycin, clarithromycin, ciprofloxacin |
| Pneumocystis carinii | TMP-SMZ*, pentamidine | Dapsone + trimethoprim, clindamycin + primaquine, trimetrexate + folinic acid |

*Trimethoprim-sulfamethoxazole

## Treatments

When mucous secretions are thick and viscous, increasing fluid intake to 2500 to 3000 mL per day helps liquefy secretions, making them easier to cough up and expectorate. If the client is unable to maintain an adequate oral intake, intravenous fluids and nutrition may be required.

Incentive spirometry may be used to promote deep breathing, coughing, and clearance of respiratory secretions. Endotracheal suctioning may be required if the cough is ineffective. This invasive technique is discussed in the section describing nursing care for the client with acute respiratory failure. On occasion, bronchoscopy is used to perform pulmonary toilet and remove secretions.

### Oxygen Therapy

Oxygen therapy may be indicated for the client who is tachypneic or hypoxemic.

Inflammation of the alveolar-capillary membrane interferes with diffusion of gases across the membrane. Diffusion is affected by several other factors, including the partial pressure of gases on each side of the membrane. Increasing the percentage of inspired oxygen above that of room air (21%) increases the partial pressure of oxygen in the alveoli and enhances its diffusion into the capillaries. Supplemental oxygen therefore improves oxygenation of the blood and tissues in clients with pneumonia.

Depending on the degree of hypoxia, oxygen may be administered by either a low-flow or high-flow system. Low-flow systems include the nasal cannula, simple face mask, partial rebreathing mask, and nonrebreathing mask (Figure 36–3 ■). A nasal cannula can deliver 24% to 45% oxygen concentrations with flow rates of 2 to 6 L/min. The nasal cannula is comfortable and does not interfere with eating or talking. A simple face mask delivers 40% to 60% oxygen concentrations with flow rates of 5 to 8 L/min. Up to 100% oxygen can be delivered by the nonrebreather mask, the highest concentration possible without mechanical ventilation. When the amount of oxygen delivered must be precisely regulated, a high-flow

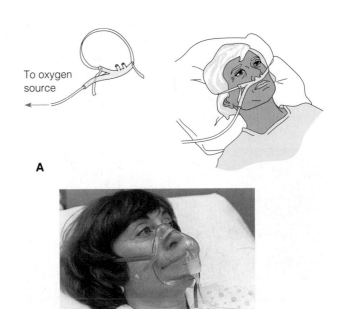

To oxygen source

A

B

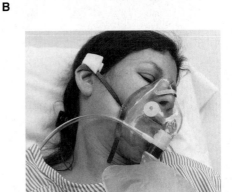

C

**Figure 36–3** ■ Low-flow oxygen delivery devices: *A*, nasal cannula; *B*, simple face mask; *C*, nonrebreather mask.

*Source: NMSB, Custom Medical Stock Photos, Inc.*

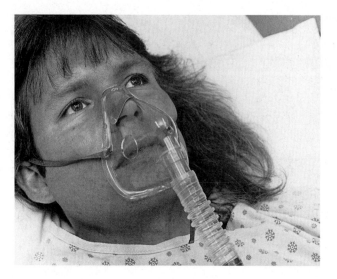

**Figure 36–4** ■ Venturi mask, a high-flow oxygen delivery system.

system such as a Venturi mask is used (Figure 36–4 ■). The Venturi mask regulates the ratio of oxygen to room air, allowing precise regulation of the oxygen percentage delivered, from 24% to 50%. Severe hypoxia may necessitate intubation and mechanical ventilation. Endotracheal intubation and methods of mechanical ventilation are discussed in the section on respiratory failure.

## Chest Physiotherapy

Chest physiotherapy, including percussion, vibration, and postural drainage, may be prescribed to reduce lung consolidation and prevent atelectasis. *Percussion* is performed by rhythmically striking or clapping the chest wall with cupped hands (Figure 36–5A ■), using rapid wrist flexion and extension. Cupping traps air between the palm and the client's skin, setting up vibrations through the chest wall that loosen respiratory secretions. The trapped air also provides a cushion, preventing injury. When performed correctly, percussion produces a hollow, popping sound. Percussion may also be done using a mechanical percussion cup. The breasts, sternum, spinal column, and kidney regions are avoided during percussion.

*Vibration* facilitates secretion movement into larger airways. It usually is combined with percussion, although it may be used when percussion is contraindicated or poorly tolerated. Vibration is performed by repeatedly tensing the arm and hand muscles while maintaining firm but gentle pressure over the affected area with the flat of the hand (Figure 36–5B).

Percussion and vibration are done in conjunction with *postural drainage,* which uses gravity to facilitate removal of secretions from a particular lung segment. The client is positioned with the segment to be drained superior to or above the trachea or mainstem bronchus. Drainage of all lung segments requires a variety of positions (Figure 36–6 ■); rarely do all segments require drainage. Bronchodilators or nebulizer treat-

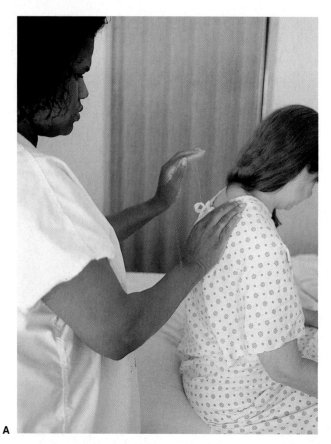

**A**

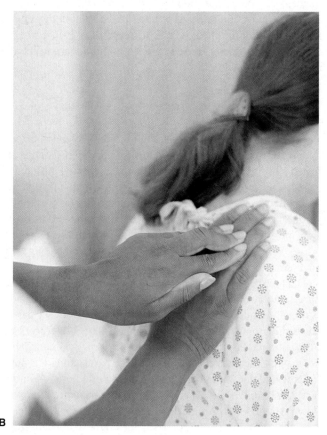

**B**

**Figure 36–5** ■ *A,* Percussing (clapping) the upper posterior chest. Notice the cupped position of the nurse's hands. *B,* Vibrating the upper posterior chest.

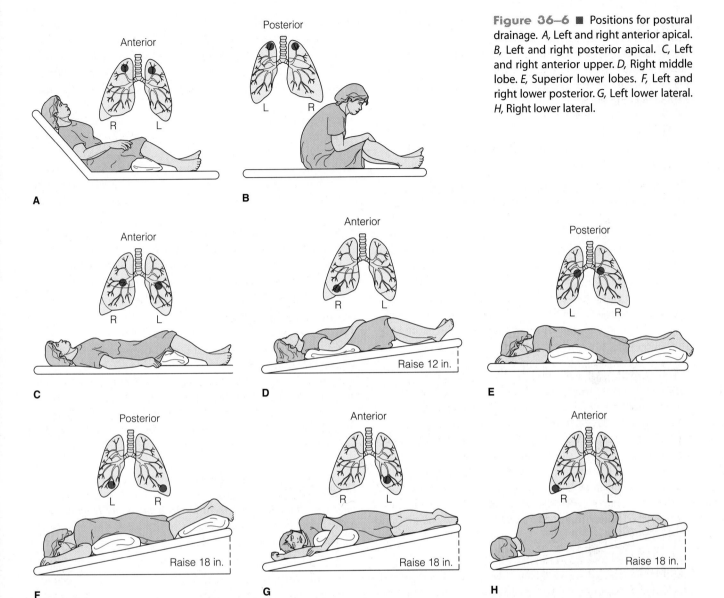

**Figure 36–6** ■ Positions for postural drainage. *A,* Left and right anterior apical. *B,* Left and right posterior apical. *C,* Left and right anterior upper. *D,* Right middle lobe. *E,* Superior lower lobes. *F,* Left and right lower posterior. *G,* Left lower lateral. *H,* Right lower lateral.

ments are administered as ordered prior to postural drainage. It is best to perform postural drainage before meals to avoid nausea and vomiting.

## Complementary Therapies

Although complementary therapies do not replace conventional treatment for pneumonia, they often promote comfort and speed recovery. The herb Echinacea is widely used to stimulate immune function and treat upper respiratory infections (URIs). Because viral URIs often precede pneumonia, it may be helpful in preventing pneumonia. Goldenseal, which often is sold in combination with Echinaciea, is used to treat bacterial, fungal, and protozoal infections of the mucous membranes of the respiratory tract (Lehne, 2001). Ma huang contains the active ingredient ephedra, which may help relieve bronchospasm and ease breathing. Because the pharmacology of ephedra is identical to ephedrine, this herb should not be used by clients with heart disease, hypertension, diabetes, or prostatic hypertrophy (Lehne, 2001).

## NURSING CARE

### Health Promotion

Health promotion activities focus on pneumonia prevention. Make clients in high-risk groups aware of the benefits of immunizations against influenza and pneumococcal pneumonia. A single dose of pneumococcus vaccine usually produces immunity to most strains of pneumococcal pneumonia, although repeat doses may be needed for older adults and people who are immunosuppressed. (Pneumococcus vaccine is contraindicated for people receiving immunosuppressive therapy.) Annual influenza vaccine helps prevent pneumonia, because pneumonia often occurs as a sequella to influenza.

**PRACTICE ALERT** *Inquire about allergic responses to eggs or previous influenza vaccinations prior to administering influenza vaccine. A significant hypersensitivity response may occur in clients who are allergic to egg protein.* ■

Additional measures to screen for and detect pneumonia in older adults are appropriate. Frequent pulmonary assessment and aggressive interventions help prevent problems. Restoring and maintaining mobility improves ventilation and helps mobilize secretions. Promoting adequate fluid intake liquefies secretions, making them easier to expectorate.

## Assessment

Focused assessment of the client with pneumonia includes the following:

- Health history: current symptoms and their duration; presence of shortness of breath or difficulty breathing, chest pain and its relationship to breathing; cough, productive or nonproductive, color, consistency of sputum; other symptoms; recent upper respiratory or other acute illness; chronic diseases such as diabetes, chronic lung disease, or heart disease; current medications; medication allergies
- Physical examination: presentation, apparent distress, level of consciousness; vital signs including temperature; skin color, temperature; respiratory excursion, use of accessory muscles of respiration; lung sounds

## Nursing Diagnoses and Interventions

Clients with lower respiratory disorders such as pneumonia may have multiple nursing care needs, depending on the severity of the illness. Alveolar ventilation and the process of alveolar respiration can be affected by inflammation and secretions. **Hypoxemia,** low levels of oxygen in the blood, and tissue hypoxia may result. Nursing care focuses on supporting optimal respiratory function and promoting rest to reduce metabolic and oxygen needs. Priority nursing diagnoses include *Ineffective airway clearance, Ineffective breathing pattern,* and *Activity intolerance.*

### Ineffective Airway Clearance

The inflammatory response to infection causes tissue edema and exudate formation. In the lungs, the inflammatory response can narrow and potentially obstruct bronchial passages and alveoli. Assessment findings supporting this nursing diagnosis include adventitious breath sounds such as crackles (rales), rhonchi, and wheezes; dyspnea and tachypnea; coughing; and indicators of hypoxia such as cyanosis, reduced $SaO_2$ levels, anxiety, and apprehension.

- Assess respiratory status, including vital signs, breath sounds, $SaO_2$, and skin color at least every 4 hours. *Early identification of respiratory compromise allows intervention before tissue hypoxia is significant.*
- Assess cough and sputum (amount, color, consistency, and possible odor). *Assessment of the cough and nature of sputum produced allow evaluation of the effectiveness of respiratory clearance and the response to therapy.*
- Monitor arterial blood gas results; report increasing hypoxemia and other abnormal results to the physician. *Blood gas changes may be an early indicator of impaired gas exchange due to airway narrowing or obstruction.*
- Place in Fowler's or high-Fowler's position. Encourage frequent position changes and ambulation as allowed. *The up-*

*right position promotes lung expansion; position changes and ambulation facilitate the movement of secretions.*
- Assist to cough, deep breathe, and use assistive devices. Provide endotracheal suctioning using aseptic technique as ordered. *Coughing, deep breathing, and suctioning help clear airways.*
- Provide a fluid intake of at least 2500 to 3000 mL per day. *A liberal fluid intake helps liquefy secretions, facilitating their clearance.*
- Work with the physician and respiratory therapist to provide pulmonary hygiene measures, such as postural drainage, percussion, and vibration. *These techniques help mobilize and clear secretions.*
- Administer prescribed medications as ordered, and monitor their effects. *If the infecting organism is resistant to the prescribed antibiotic, little improvement may be seen with treatment. Bronchodilators help maintain open airways but may have adverse effects such as anxiety and restlessness.*

### Ineffective Breathing Pattern

Pleural inflammation often accompanies pneumonia, causing sharp localized pain that increases with deep breathing, coughing, and movement, which can lead to rapid and shallow breathing. Distal airways and alveoli may not expand optimally with each breath, increasing the risk for atelectasis and decreasing gas exchange. Fatigue from the increased work of breathing is an additional problem in pneumonia. This, too, can lead to decreased lung inflation and an ineffective breathing pattern.

---

**PRACTICE ALERT** *Assess respiratory rate, depth, and lung sounds at least every 4 hours. Tachypnea and diminished or adventitious breath sounds may be early indicators of respiratory compromise.* ■

---

- Provide for rest periods. *Rest reduces metabolic demands, fatigue, and the work of breathing, promoting a more effective breathing pattern.*
- Assess for pleuritic discomfort. Provide analgesics as ordered. *Adequate pain relief minimizes splinting and promotes adequate ventilation.*
- Provide reassurance during periods of respiratory distress. *Hypoxia and respiratory distress produce high levels of anxiety, which tends to further increase tachypnea and fatigue and decrease ventilation.*
- Administer oxygen as ordered. *Oxygen therapy increases the alveolar oxygen concentration and facilitates its diffusion across the alveolar-capillary membrane, reducing hypoxia and anxiety.*
- Teach slow abdominal breathing. *This breathing pattern promotes lung expansion.*
- Teach use of relaxation techniques, such as visualization and meditation. *These techniques help reduce anxiety and slow the breathing pattern.*

### Activity Intolerance

Impaired airway clearance and gas exchange interfere with oxygen delivery to body cells and tissues. At the same time, the infectious process and the body's response to it increase metabolic demands on the cells. The net result of this imbalance between oxygen delivery and oxygen demand is a lack of physiologic energy to maintain normal daily activities.

- Assess activity tolerance, noting any increase in pulse, respirations, dyspnea, diaphoresis, or cyanosis. *These assessment findings may indicate limited or impaired activity tolerance.*
- Assist with self-care activities, such as bathing. *Assistance with ADLs reduces energy demands.*
- Schedule activities, planning for rest periods. *Rest periods minimize fatigue and improve activity tolerance.*
- Provide assistive devices, such as an overhead trapeze. *These assistive devices facilitate movement and reduce energy demands.*
- Enlist the family's help to minimize stress and anxiety levels. *Stress and anxiety increase metabolic demands and can decrease activity tolerance.*
- Perform active or passive ROM exercises. *Exercises help maintain muscle tone and joint mobility, and prevent contractures if bed rest is prolonged.*
- Provide emotional support and reassurance that strength and energy will return to normal when the infectious process has resolved and the balance of oxygen supply and demand is restored. *The client may be concerned that activity intolerance will continue to be a problem after the acute infection is resolved.*

## Using NANDA, NIC, and NOC

Chart 36–1 shows links between NANDA nursing diagnoses, NIC, and NOC for the client with pneumonia.

## Home Care

Clients with pneumonia usually are treated in the community, unless their respiratory status is significantly compromised. Discuss the following topics when preparing the client and family for home care.

- The importance of completing the prescribed medication regimen as ordered; potential drug side effects and their management, including manifestations that necessitate stopping the drug and notifying the physician
- Recommendations for limiting activities and increasing rest
- Maintaining adequate fluid intake to keep mucus thin for easier expectoration
- Ways to maintain adequate nutritional intake, such as small, frequent, well-balanced meals
- The importance of avoiding smoking or exposure to secondhand smoke to prevent further irritation of the lungs
- Manifestations to report to the physician, such as increasing shortness of breath, difficulty breathing, increased fever, fatigue, headache, sleepiness, or confusion
- The importance of keeping all follow-up appointments to ensure disease cure

Clients with severe respiratory compromise or who are elderly or debilitated may require home care assistance to remain at home. Provide referrals to home intravenous services, home health nursing services, and home maintenance services as indicated. Community services such as Meals-on-Wheels can provide support to reduce the energy demands of meal preparation.

## CHART 36–1 NANDA, NIC, AND NOC LINKAGES

### The Client with Pneumonia

| NURSING DIAGNOSES | NURSING INTERVENTIONS | NURSING OUTCOMES |
|---|---|---|
| • Activity Intolerance | • Energy Management<br>• Environmental Management<br>• Self-Care Assistance | • Activity Tolerance<br>• Energy Conservation<br>• Self-Care: Activities of Daily Living (ADLs) |
| • Deficient Knowledge | • Infection Protection<br>• Teaching: Disease Process<br>• Teaching: Prescribed Medication | • Knowledge: Health Behaviors<br>• Knowledge: Energy Conservation<br>• Knowledge: Illness Care |
| • Impaired Gas Exchange | • Anxiety Reduction<br>• Oxygen Therapy<br>• Respiratory Monitoring | • Respiratory Status: Gas Exchange |
| • Ineffective Airway Clearance | • Cough Enhancement<br>• Chest Physiotherapy<br>• Positioning | • Respiratory Status: Airway Patency<br>• Respiratory Status: Ventilation |

*Note. Data from Nursing Outcomes Classification (NOC) by M. Johnson & M. Maas (Eds.), 1997, St. Louis: Mosby; Nursing Diagnoses: Definitions & Classification 2001–2002 by North American Nursing Diagnosis Association, 2001, Philadelphia: NANDA; Nursing Interventions Classification (NIC) by J.C. McCloskey & G. M. Bulechek (Eds.), 2000, St. Louis: Mosby. Reprinted by permission.*

# Nursing Care Plan
## A Client with Pneumonia

Mary O'Neal is a 35-year-old executive assistant and a part-time college student. On returning home from class one evening, she begins to chill. She alternates between chills and sweats all night. Staying home from work, she remains in bed most of the next day. Her fever continues, and she develops a cough and dull aching chest pain. When the cough becomes productive of rust-colored sputum the following day, she seeks medical treatment from her family doctor.

### ASSESSMENT

Debby Kowalski, RN, the family practice clinic nurse, admits Mrs. O'Neal to the clinic and obtains the nursing assessment. Mrs. O'Neal denies any previous history of respiratory diseases "other than the usual colds, flu, and such." She also denies any history of smoking or medication allergies. She says her symptoms began abruptly with the onset of the chills. She describes her chest pain as a dull ache that was initially substernal but now is localized in her lower lateral right chest. The pain increases with deep breathing, coughing, and moving. Her cough is increasing in frequency and severity, and her sputum appears rusty brown. Her vital signs are BP 116/74, P 104 and regular, R 26, T 101.8°F (38.7°C). Skin warm and flushed, with no evidence of cyanosis. Respirations shallow, unlabored; respiratory excursion equal. Diminished breath sounds in bases bilaterally, crackles noted in right posterior and lateral base. Faint pleural rub heard at right midaxillary line.

A STAT CBC shows a WBC of 18,900/mm³; differential shows increased numbers of neutrophils and immature WBCs (bands). Ms. Kowalski has Mrs. O'Neal rinse with an antiseptic mouthwash and collect a sputum specimen for culture and Gram stain prior to seeing the physician.

The physician orders a chest X-ray after examining Mrs. O'Neal. Based on her history, examination, and the chest X-ray, he makes the diagnosis of acute bacterial pneumonia, probably pneumococcal. He prescribes oral penicillin V, 500 mg every 6 hours for 10 days. He asks Mrs. O'Neal to return for a follow-up appointment in 10 days and refers her back to Ms. Kowalski for appropriate teaching.

### DIAGNOSIS

- *Ineffective breathing pattern* related to pleuritic chest pain
- *Hyperthermia* related to inflammatory process
- *Deficient knowledge* about pneumonia and its treatment

### EXPECTED OUTCOMES

- Maintain normal pulmonary function.
- Describe measures to minimize elevations in body temperature.
- Identify a schedule for taking her medication that will facilitate compliance with the regimen.
- Describe manifestations that should be reported to the physician.

### PLANNING AND IMPLEMENTATION

- Assess knowledge and understanding of pneumonia and its effects.
- Assist to develop a medication schedule that coordinates with normal daily routine.
- Teach about the following:
  a. Importance of avoiding use of a cough suppressant except at night to facilitate rest
  b. Ways to increase fluid intake to reduce fever and maintain thin mucus for easy expectoration
  c. Beneficial effects of rest, especially during the acute phase of her illness
  d. Safe use of aspirin and acetaminophen to reduce fever
  e. Importance of taking all prescribed medication doses as scheduled
  f. Common side effects of penicillin V and their management
  g. Early manifestations of penicillin allergy that necessitate stopping the medication and notifying the physician
  h. Signs of complications of pneumonia or worsening pneumonia to report

### EVALUATION

The sputum culture confirms *S. pneumoniae* as the cause of Mrs. O'Neal's pneumonia. When she returns for her follow-up appointment, she reports that she began to feel better after 2 days on the penicillin and returned to work the following Monday. Her examination reveals good breath sounds throughout with no adventitious sounds. The follow-up sputum culture is free of pathogens.

### Critical Thinking in the Nursing Process

1. Do any of the factors identified in the case study increase Mrs. O'Neal's risk for acute bacterial pneumonia?
2. Mrs. O'Neal's WBC differential showed increased neutrophil and band counts. Describe the reason for and effect of this change.
3. Even though Mrs. O'Neal has no history of medication allergies, anaphylactic shock remains a potential risk. Describe the sequence of events leading to anaphylactic shock, its initial symptoms, and immediate nursing interventions.
4. Had Mrs. O'Neal required hospitalization to treat her acute pneumonia, interruption of her usual activities and responsibilities could lead to anxiety. Develop a care plan for this situation, using the nursing diagnosis, *Altered role performance* related to hospitalization.

See Evaluating Your Response in Appendix C.

## THE CLIENT WITH SEVERE ACUTE RESPIRATORY SYNDROME

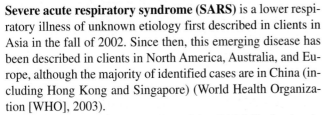

**Severe acute respiratory syndrome (SARS)** is a lower respiratory illness of unknown etiology first described in clients in Asia in the fall of 2002. Since then, this emerging disease has been described in clients in North America, Australia, and Europe, although the majority of identified cases are in China (including Hong Kong and Singapore) (World Health Organization [WHO], 2003).

The primary population affected by SARS is previously healthy adults age 25 to 70 years. Recent travel (within 10 days of the onset of symptoms) to an area with documented or suspected community transmission of SARS or close contact with a person known or suspected to have SARS are the primary risk factors for this disease.

## PATHOPHYSIOLOGY AND MANIFESTATIONS

Although not yet proven, the infective agent responsible for SARS is thought to be a newly identified coronavirus. This virus appears to spread by close person-to-person contact. Other potential sources of the infection are through direct contact with an infected person or contaminated object, and exposure of the eyes or mucous membranes to respiratory secretions (Centers for Disease Control and Prevention [CDC], 2003c).

The incubation period for SARS is generally 2 to 7 days, although it may be as long as 10 days in some people. Fever higher than 100.4°F (38°C) is typically the initial manifestation of the disease. The high fever may be accompanied by chills, headache, malaise, and muscle aches. After 3 to 7 days, respiratory manifestations of SARS develop, including nonproductive cough, shortness of breath, dyspnea, and possible hypoxemia.

While the majority of people with SARS recover, up to 20% of affected clients require intubation and mechanical ventilation (see the section on respiratory failure). About 3 in 100 clients with SARS die.

## COLLABORATIVE CARE

Prompt identification of SARS, infection control measures, and reporting of the disease are vital to control this potentially deadly disease. Health care providers and public health personnel should report cases of SARS to state and local health departments.

### Diagnostic Tests

At this time, no laboratory test is available to diagnose SARS. Initial diagnostic testing for a client with suspected SARS may include the following:

- *Serology tests* for antibodies to the new coronavirus may be available in some research centers.
- *Chest X-ray* may be normal or show interstitial infiltrates in a focal or generalized patchy pattern. In late stages of SARS, consolidation may be evident.

- *Pulse oximetry (oxygen saturation)* often shows hypoxemia in the respiratory phase of the illness.
- *Complete blood count (CBC)* often demonstrates a low lymphocyte count early in the disease. Leukopenia and thrombocytopenia may develop at the peak of the respiratory illness.
- *Creatinine phosphokinase (CPK or CK), ALT,* and *AST* levels may be markedly increased in SARS.
- *Sputum specimen* is obtained. Gram stain and culture are performed on the specimen to rule out other causes of pneumonia.
- *Blood culture* may be done to identify possible bacteremia.

### Medications

At this time, no medications have been shown to be consistently effective in treating SARS. Antibiotic and/or antiviral therapy targeted at community-acquired forms of pneumonia may be administered.

### Infection Control

Because health care workers are at risk for developing SARS after caring for infected clients, infection control precautions should be immediately instituted when SARS is suspected. Standard precautions (see Appendix A ⊕ ) are implemented along with contact and airborne precautions. The Centers for Disease Control and Prevention (2003b) recommends hand hygiene, gown, gloves, eye protection, and an N95 respirator to prevent transmission of SARS in healthcare settings.

When clients with SARS are managed in the community, they are advised to remain home for 10 days after the fever has resolved and until respiratory symptoms are absent or minimal. Members of the household are advised to wash hands frequently or use alcohol-based hand rubs. The client is advised to cover the mouth and nose with tissue when coughing or sneezing and to wear a surgical mask during close contact with uninfected people. Sharing of utensils, towels, and bedding should be avoided. Routine cleaning (e.g., washing with soap and hot water) is adequate to disinfect objects and no special precautions are necessary for disposing of waste.

### Treatments

Care of the client with SARS is supportive. Oxygen may be administered to treat hypoxemia. Intubation and mechanical ventilation may be required if respiratory failure or acute respiratory distress syndrome (ARDS) develops.

## NURSING CARE

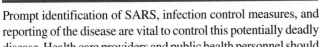

Nursing care of the client with SARS focuses on preventing spread of the disease to others and providing respiratory support.

### Health Promotion

Advise clients planning elective or nonessential travel to mainland China and Hong Kong, Singapore, and Hanoi, Vietnam, that they may wish to postpone their trips. Use respiratory and contact infection control precautions in addition to standard precautions when caring for all clients with suspected SARS to prevent spread of the disease to health care workers or other clients.

## Assessment

Focused assessment data for the client with suspected SARS include the following. For more complete respiratory assessment, see Chapter 34.

- Health history: current symptoms, including fever, malaise, shortness of breath, and cough; onset of symptoms; recent international travel or exposure to a person known to have SARS
- Physical assessment: vital signs including temperature; respiratory status, including respiratory rate, depth, and effort; presence of cough; adventitious lung sounds

## Nursing Diagnoses and Interventions

The client with SARS poses a risk for spread of the infection to health care workers and others. In addition, while many people with this disease experience only mild symptoms and recover fully and uneventfully, others develop severe respiratory distress and may require significant respiratory support. Gas exchange may be impaired, leading to significant hypoxemia. In addition to the nursing diagnoses discussed in the previous section on pneumonia, *Impaired gas exchange* and *Risk for infection* are priority nursing diagnoses.

## Impaired Gas Exchange

Although the pathophysiology of SARS is not fully understood, this disorder is known to cause hypoxemia of varying degrees in some clients. Significant hypoxemia may necessitate intubation and mechanical ventilation to support cellular function until recovery occurs.

- Monitor vital signs, color, oxygen saturation, and arterial blood gases. Assess for manifestations such as anxiety or apprehension, restlessness, confusion or lethargy, or complaints of headache. *These assessment data alert the nurse and care providers to potential hypoxemia or hypercapnia due to impaired gas exchange.*

**PRACTICE ALERT**   *Promptly report signs of respiratory distress, including tachypnea, tachycardia, nasal flaring, use of accessory muscles, intercostal retractions, cyanosis, increasing restlessness, anxiety, or decreased level of consciousness. These may be early manifestations of respiratory failure and inability to maintain ventilatory effort.* ■

- Promptly report worsening arterial blood gases and oxygen saturation levels. *Close assessment of these values allows timely intervention as needed.*
- Maintain oxygen therapy and mechanical ventilation as ordered. Hyperoxygenate prior to suctioning. *Oxygen and mechanical ventilation support alveolar gas exchange. Hyperoxygenation prior to suctioning reduces the degree of hypoxemia that occurs during suctioning.*

- Place in Fowler's or high Fowler's position. *Sitting positions decrease pressure on the diaphragm and chest, improving lung ventilation and decreasing the work of breathing.*
- Minimize activities and energy expenditures by assisting with ADLs, spacing procedures and activities, and allowing uninterrupted rest periods. *Rest is vital to reduce oxygen and energy demands.*

**PRACTICE ALERT**   *Avoid sedatives and respiratory depressant drugs unless mechanically ventilated. These medications can further depress the respiratory drive, worsening respiratory failure.* ■

- If intubation and mechanical ventilation is necessary, explain the procedure and its purpose to the client and family, providing reassurance that this *temporary* measure improves oxygenation and reduces the work of breathing. Alert that talking is not possible while the endotracheal tube is in place, and establish a means of communication. *Thorough explanation is important to relieve anxiety.*

See the section on respiratory failure later in this chapter for more information about caring for a client who is intubated and mechanically ventilated.

### Risk for Infection

The spread of SARS is a risk both in the health care facility and the community in which the client resides. Respiratory and contract precautions are recommended to prevent the spread of SARS via respiratory secretions or contact with the virus.

- Place the client in a private room with airflow control that prevents air within the room from circulating into the hallway or other rooms. A negative flow room in which air is diluted by at least six fresh-air exchanges per hour is recommended. *A negative flow room and multiple fresh-air exchanges dilute the concentration of virus within the room and prevent its spread to adjacent areas.*
- Use standard precautions and respiratory and contact isolation techniques as recommended by the CDC, including wearing respirators, gowns, and eye protection when caring for clients with SARS. *These measures are important to prevent the spread of SARS to others.*
- Discuss the reasons for and importance of respiratory and contact isolation procedures during treatment. *Maintenance of infection control precautions during and immediately following the febrile and respiratory phases of SARS is vital to prevent its spread to health care workers and the community.*
- Place a mask on the client when transporting to other parts of the facility for diagnostic or treatment procedures. *Covering the client's nose and mouth during transport minimizes air contamination and the risk to visitors and personnel.*
- Inform all personnel having contact with the client of the diagnosis. *This allows personnel to take appropriate precautions.*
- Assist visitors to mask prior to entering the room. *Providing visitors with appropriate masks or respirators reduces their risk of infection.*

- Teach the client how to limit transmitting the disease to others:
  a. Always cough and expectorate into tissues.
  b. Dispose of tissues properly, placing them in a closed bag.
  c. Wear a mask if sneezing or unable to control respiratory secretions.
  d. Do not share eating utensils, towels, bedding, or other objects with others, as this disease may also be spread by contact with contaminated objects.

*Teaching appropriate precautions helps prevent the spread of SARS to others while allowing as much freedom from restraints as possible.*

## Home Care

Many clients with SARS experience only mild symptoms and are appropriately cared for in the community. Teaching about home care and infection control precautions is vital to prevent spread of this disease to the community. Include the following topics when teaching for home care.

- The disease, its origin, and how it is spread
- Manifestations of impaired respiratory status to report to the physician
- Preventing spread of the disease to others:
  1. Cover the mouth and nose with tissues when coughing or sneezing. Personally dispose of tissues in a paper bag or the garbage. Wear a surgical mask during close contact with other members of the household.
  2. Limit interactions outside the home; do not go to work, school, or other public areas until you have been free of fever for 10 days and your respiratory symptoms are resolving.
  3. Remind all members of the household to wash hands (or use an alcohol-based hand sanitizer) frequently, particularly after direct contact with body fluids.
  4. Do not share eating utensils, towels, or bedding with others. These items can be cleaned with soap and hot water between uses. Clean contaminated surfaces with a household disinfectant.
- Monitoring uninfected members of the household for signs of the illness (Instruct to report fever or respiratory symptoms to the physician.)

## THE CLIENT WITH LUNG ABSCESS

A **lung abscess** is a localized area of lung destruction or necrosis and pus formation. The most common cause of lung abscess is aspiration and resulting pneumonia. Risk factors, therefore, are those for aspiration: decreased level of consciousness due to anesthesia, injury or disease of the central nervous system, seizure, excessive sedation, or alcohol abuse; swallowing disorders; dental caries; and debilitation secondary to cancer or chronic disease. Lung abscess also may occur as a complication of some types of pneumonia, including those due to *Staphylococcus aureus, Klebsiella,* and *Legionella.*

## PATHOPHYSIOLOGY AND MANIFESTATIONS

A lung abscess forms after lung tissue becomes consolidated (i.e., after alveoli become filled with fluid, pus, and microorganisms). Consolidated tissue becomes necrotic. This necrotic process can spread to involve the entire bronchopulmonary segment and progress proximally until it ruptures into a bronchus. With rupture, the contents of the abscess empty into the bronchus, leaving a cavity filled with air and fluid, a process known as *cavitation.* If purulent material from the abscess is not expectorated, the infection may spread, leading to diffuse pneumonia or a syndrome similar to acute respiratory distress syndrome (ARDS, discussed later in this chapter).

Manifestations of lung abscess typically develop about 2 weeks after the precipitating event (aspiration, pneumonia, and so on). Their onset may be either acute or insidious. Early symptoms are those of pneumonia: productive cough, chills and fever, pleuritic chest pain, malaise, and anorexia. The temperature may be significantly elevated, 103°F (39.4°C) or higher. When the abscess ruptures, the client may expectorate large amounts of foul-smelling, purulent, and possibly blood-streaked sputum. Breath sounds are diminished, and crackles may be noted in the region of the abscess. A dull percussion tone is also present.

## COLLABORATIVE CARE

The diagnosis of lung abscess usually is based on the history and presentation. The CBC may indicate leukocytosis. Sputum culture may not show the organism involved unless rupture occurs. Chest X-ray shows a thick-walled, solitary cavity with surrounding consolidation, although differentiating lung abscess from consolidation can be difficult until cavitation occurs.

Lung abscess is treated with antibiotic therapy, usually intravenous clindamycin (Cleocin), amoxicillin-clavulanate (Augmentin), or penicillin (Tierney et al., 2001). Postural drainage may be ordered to relieve obstruction and promote drainage. In some cases, bronchoscopy is used to drain the abscess. If the pleural space becomes involved, a chest tube (tube thoracostomy) may be used to drain the abscess. See the section on pneumothorax for further discussion of chest tubes.

## NURSING CARE

Although most clients with lung abscess recover fully with appropriate antibiotic treatment, rupture and drainage of the abscess into a bronchus is a frightening experience. Nursing care needs of the client relate primarily to maintaining a patent airway and adequate gas exchange. The following nursing diagnoses may be appropriate for the client with lung abscess.

- *Risk for ineffective airway clearance* related to large amounts of purulent drainage in bronchi
- *Impaired gas exchange* related to necrotic and consolidated lung tissue

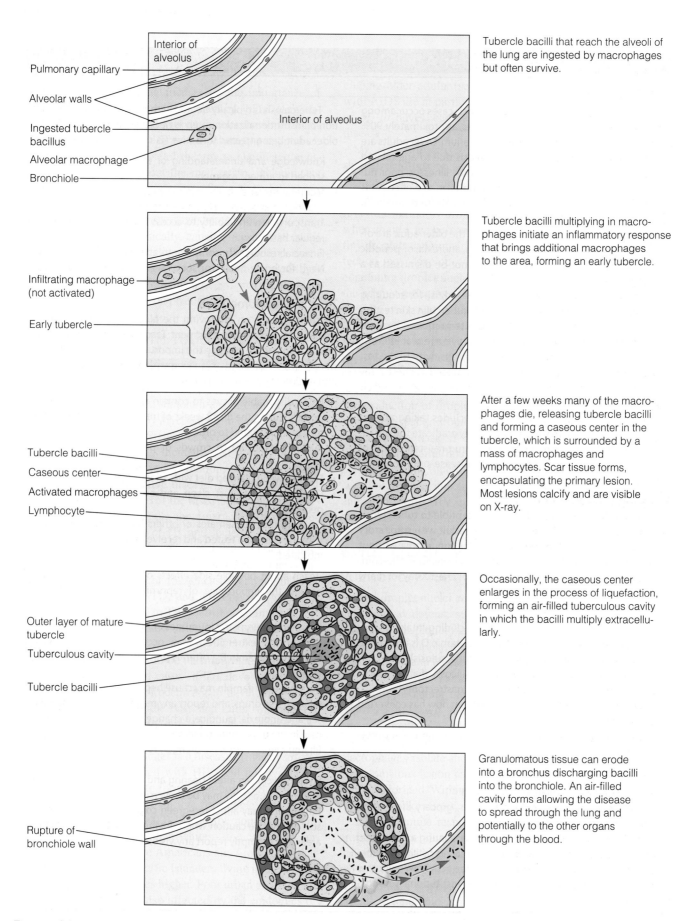

Interior of
alveolus

Pulmonary capillary

Alveolar walls

Ingested tubercle
bacillus

Alveolar macrophage

Bronchiole

Interior of alveolus

Tubercle bacilli that reach the alveoli of
the lung are ingested by macrophages
but often survive.

Infiltrating macrophage
(not activated)

Early tubercle

Tubercle bacilli multiplying in macrophages initiate an inflammatory response
that brings additional macrophages
to the area, forming an early tubercle.

Tubercle bacilli

Caseous center

Activated macrophages

Lymphocyte

After a few weeks many of the macrophages die, releasing tubercle bacilli
and forming a caseous center in the
tubercle, which is surrounded by a
mass of macrophages and
lymphocytes. Scar tissue forms,
encapsulating the primary lesion.
Most lesions calcify and are visible
on X-ray.

Outer layer of mature
tubercle

Tuberculous cavity

Tubercle bacilli

Occasionally, the caseous center
enlarges in the process of liquefaction,
forming an air-filled tuberculous cavity
in which the bacilli multiply extracellu-
larly.

Rupture of
bronchiole wall

Granulomatous tissue can erode
into a bronchus discharging bacilli
into the bronchiole. An air-filled
cavity forms allowing the disease
to spread through the lung and
potentially to the other organs
through the blood.

**Figure 36–7** ■ The pathogenesis of tuberculosis.

throughout the lung or other organs. This severe form of tuberculosis is uncommon in adults (Braunwald et al., 2001).

A previously healed tuberculosis lesion may be reactivated. *Reactivation tuberculosis* occurs when the immune system is suppressed due to age, disease, or use of immunosuppressive drugs. The extent of lung disease can vary from small lesions to extensive cavitation of lung tissue. Tubercles rupture, spreading bacilli into the airways to form satellite lesions and produce tuberculosis pneumonia. Without treatment, massive lung involvement can lead to death, or a more chronic process of tubercle formation and cavitation may result. People with chronic disease continue to spread *M. tb* into the environment, potentially infecting others. Figure 36–7 ■ illustrates the pathogenesis of tuberculosis.

Clients with HIV disease are at high risk for developing active tuberculosis, due to primary infection or reactivation. HIV infection suppresses cellular immunity, which is vital to limiting the replication and spread of *M. tb*.

## MANIFESTATIONS AND COMPLICATIONS

The initial infection causes few symptoms and typically goes unnoticed until the tuberculin test becomes positive or calcified lesions are seen on chest X-ray. Manifestations of primary progressive or reactivation tuberculosis often develop insidiously and are initially nonspecific (see the box below). Fatigue, weight loss, anorexia, low-grade afternoon fever, and night sweats are common. A dry cough develops, which later becomes productive of purulent and/or blood-tinged sputum. It is often at this stage that the client seeks medical attention.

Tuberculosis empyema and bronchopleural fistula are the most serious complications of pulmonary tuberculosis. When a tuberculosis lesion ruptures, bacilli may contaminate the pleural space. Rupture also may allow air to enter the pleural space from the lung, causing pneumothorax.

## Extrapulmonary Tuberculosis

When primary disease or reactivation allows live bacilli to enter the bronchi, the disease may spread through the blood and lymph system to other organs. These distant disease metastases may produce an active lesion, or they may become dormant and reactivate at a later time. Extrapulmonary tuberculosis is especially prevalent in people with HIV disease.

### Miliary Tuberculosis
*Miliary tuberculosis* results from hematogenous spread (through the blood) of the bacilli throughout the body. Miliary tuberculosis causes chills and fever, weakness, malaise, and progressive dyspnea. Multiple lesions evenly distributed throughout the lungs are noted on X-ray. The sputum rarely contains organisms. The bone marrow is usually involved, causing anemia, thrombocytopenia, and leukocytosis. Without appropriate treatment, the prognosis is poor.

### Genitourinary Tuberculosis
The kidney and genitourinary tract are common extrapulmonary sites for tuberculosis. The organism spreads to the kidney through the blood, initiating an inflammatory process similar to that which occurs in the lungs. Reactivation can occur years after the original infection. As the lesion then enlarges and caseates, a large portion of the renal parenchyma is destroyed. The infection then can spread to rest of the urinary tract, including the ureters and bladder. Scarring and strictures commonly result. In men, the prostate, seminal vesicles, and epididymis may be involved. In women, tuberculosis may affect the fallopian tubes and ovaries.

Manifestations of genitourinary tuberculosis develop insidiously. Symptoms of a urinary tract infection, including malaise, dysuria, hematuria, and pyuria, develop. Flank pain may be present. Men may develop manifestations of epididymitis or prostatitis: perineal, sacral, or scrotal pain and tenderness; difficulty voiding; and fever. Women may have manifestations of pelvic inflammatory disease, impaired fertility, or ectopic pregnancy.

### Tuberculosis Meningitis
Tuberculosis meningitis results when tuberculosis spreads to the subarachnoid space. In the United States, this complication most often affects older adults, usually from reactivation of latent disease. Manifestations develop gradually, with listlessness, irritability, anorexia, and fever. Headache and behavior changes are common early symptoms in the older adult. As the disease progresses, the headache increases in intensity, vomiting develops, and the level of consciousness decreases. Convulsions and coma may follow. Without appropriate treatment, neurologic effects may become permanent.

### Skeletal Tuberculosis
Tuberculosis of the bones and joints is most likely to occur during childhood, when bone epiphyses are open and their blood supply is rich. The organisms spread via the blood to vertebrae, the ends of long bones, and joints. Immune and inflammatory processes isolate the bacilli, and the disease often becomes evident years or decades later.

Tuberculous spondylitis usually involves the thoracic vertebrae, eroding vertebral bodies and causing them to collapse. Significant kyphosis develops, and the spinal cord may be compressed. The large, weight-bearing joints (hips and knees) are most often affected by tuberculous arthritis, although other joints may be affected, particularly if they have been previously damaged. The involved joint is painful, warm, and tender.

## COLLABORATIVE CARE

Tuberculosis was a major public health concern earlier in this century, before the development of effective sanitation measures and drug treatment. Developing drug-resistant strains,

---

### Manifestations of Pulmonary Tuberculosis

- Fatigue
- Weight loss
- Anorexia
- Low-grade afternoon fever and night sweats
- Cough: initially dry, later productive of purulent and/or blood-tinged sputum

susceptibility of people with HIV disease, and inadequate access to health care for high-risk populations contribute to the continuing significance of tuberculosis as a significant public health threat. Collaborative care, therefore, focuses on the following:

- Early detection
- Accurate diagnosis
- Effective disease treatment
- Preventing tuberculosis spread to others

Hospitalization is rarely required to treat tuberculosis. With appropriate treatment, clients become noninfective to others fairly rapidly. However, a client with active tuberculosis may be admitted for a concurrent problem or a complication of the disease. Nurses and other health care workers are at risk for exposure if the disease has not yet been diagnosed. When a client with tuberculosis is institutionalized, maintain respiratory isolation to minimize the risk of infection to other clients and to the health care workers.

Noncompliance with prescribed treatment is a major problem in treating active tuberculosis: The client can continue transmitting the disease to others, and drug-resistant strains of bacteria can develop when treatment is incomplete. Tuberculosis must be reported to local and state public health departments; contacts are identified and examined. People who share living or work environments with the client are tested and receive prophylactic treatment. Continuing contact with clients who have active TB is vital to ensure effective cure.

## Screening

The tuberculin test is used to screen for tuberculosis infection. A cellular, or delayed hypersensitivity, response to *M. tuberculosis* develops within 3 to 10 weeks after the infection. Injecting a small amount of *purified protein derivative (PPD)* of tuberculin any time thereafter activates this response, attracting macrophages to the area and causing a pronounced local inflammatory response. The amount of induration surrounding the injection site is used to determine infection (see Table 36–4 and Figure 36–8 ■). It is important to remember that a positive response indicates that infection and a cellular (T-cell) response have developed; however, it does not mean that active disease is present or that the client is infectious to others.

Several methods are currently available for tuberculin testing:

- *Intradermal PPD (Mantoux) test:* 0.1 mL of PPD (5 tuberculin units, or TU) is injected intradermally into the dorsal aspect of the forearm. This test is read within 48 to 72 hours, the peak reaction period, and recorded as the diameter of induration (raised area, not erythema) in millimeters.
- *Multiple-puncture (tine) test:* A multiple-puncture device is used to introduce tuberculin into the skin. This test is less accurate than other testing methods. A vesicular reaction is considered positive; any other reaction must be confirmed using a Mantoux test.

Although it is impractical and unnecessary to screen the entire population, the Centers for Disease Control and Preven-

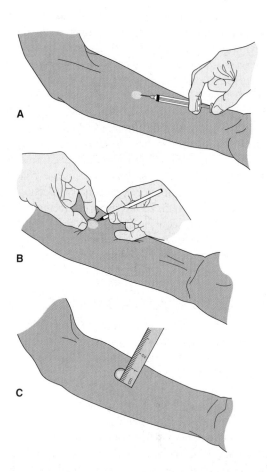

**Figure 36–8** ■ *A,* Intradermal injection for tuberculin testing. *B,* The injection causes a local inflammatory response (wheal). *C,* Measurement of induration following tuberculin testing.

| TABLE 36–4 | Interpreting Tuberculin Test Results |
|---|---|
| **Area of Induration** | **Significance** |
| Less than 5 mm | Negative response; does not rule out infection. |
| 5 to 9 mm | Positive for people who:<br>• Are in close contact with a client with infective TB.<br>• Have an abnormal chest X-ray.<br>• Have HIV infection.<br>Negative for all others. |
| 10 to 15 mm | Positive for people who have other risk factors:<br>• Birth in a high-incidence country<br>• Low socioeconomic status<br>• African American, Hispanic, Asian American in poverty areas<br>• Injection drug use<br>• Residence in a long-term care facility<br>• Identified local risk factors |
| Greater than 15 mm | Positive for all people |

tion (CDC) recommends screening people in the following risk groups.

- People with or at high risk for HIV infection
- Close contacts of people who have or are suspected of having infectious TB
- People with medical risk factors, such as silicosis, chronic malabsorption, end-stage renal failure, diabetes mellitus, immunosuppression, and hematologic and other malignancies
- People born in countries with a high prevalence of TB
- Medically underserved low-income populations, including racial and ethnic minorities
- Alcoholics and injection drug users
- Residents and staff of long-term residential facilities, such as long-term care facilities, correctional institutions, and mental health facilities

False-negative responses are common in people who are immunosuppressed. A two-step procedure may be necessary to elicit a positive response. If the first test elicits a negative response, a second PPD test is given 1 week later. If the second test also is negative, the client either is free of infection or is *anergic* (unable to react to common antigens). This two-step procedure is recommended for long-term care residents and workers.

## Diagnostic Tests

A positive tuberculin test alone does not indicate active disease. Sputum tests for the bacillus and chest X-rays are routinely used to diagnose and evaluate active disease. A series of three consecutive early-morning sputum specimens is typically examined for bacilli (see Procedure 36–1). Use special procedures or personal protective devices when obtaining sputum specimens. If possible, collect specimens in a room equipped with airflow control devices, ultraviolet light, or both. Alternatively, have the client step outside to collect the specimen. Wear a mask capable of filtering droplet nuclei when collecting sputum specimens. Aerosol therapy, percussion, and postural drainage may help the client produce sputum. Occasionally, endotracheal suctioning, bronchoscopy, or gastric lavage may be necessary to obtain a specimen. See the box on page 1082 for nursing care related to bronchoscopy.

- *Sputum smear* is microscopically examined for *acid-fast bacilli*. *M. tuberculosis* resists decolorizing chemicals after staining. This property is called "acid-fast." The acid-fast smear provides a rapid indicator of the tubercle bacillus.
- *Sputum culture* positive for *M. tuberculosis* provides the definitive diagnosis. However, *M. tuberculosis* is slow growing, requiring 4 to 8 weeks before it can be detected using traditional culture techniques. Automated radiometric culture systems (such as Bactec) allow detection of *M. tuberculosis* in several days.
- Once the organism is detected, *sensitivity testing* is performed to identify appropriate drug therapy.
- *Polymerase chain reaction (PCR)* permits rapid detection of DNA from *M. tuberculosis.*

- *Chest X-ray* is ordered to diagnose and evaluate TB. Typical findings in pulmonary TB include dense lesions in the apical and posterior segments of the upper lobe and possible cavity formation.

Prior to initiating antituberculosis drug therapy, several additional diagnostic tests may be done to establish baseline data for monitoring potential adverse effects of the drugs.

- *Liver function tests* are obtained prior to treatment with isoniazid (INH) as this drug is hepatotoxic.
- A thorough *vision examination* is done prior to treatment with ethambutol, a commonly used antituberculosis medication. Optic neuritis is a potential adverse effect of this drug. Periodic eye examinations are scheduled during the course of therapy.
- *Audiometric testing* is performed before streptomycin therapy is initiated. Ototoxicity is a significant adverse effect of streptomycin and other aminoglycoside antibiotics. Hearing also is evaluated periodically during the course of therapy to detect any hearing loss.

## Medications

Chemotherapeutic medications are used both to prevent and treat tuberculosis infection. Goals of the pharmacologic treatment of TB are to:

- Make the disease noncommunicable to others.
- Reduce symptoms of the disease.
- Effect a cure in the shortest possible time.

Prophylactic treatment is used to prevent active tuberculosis. Clients with a recent skin test conversion from negative to positive are often started on prophylactic therapy, especially when other risk factors are present. Prophylactic therapy also is used for people in close household contact with a person whose sputum is positive for bacilli. Single-drug therapy is effective for prophylactic treatment, whereas treatment of active disease always involves two or more chemotherapeutic medications. For adults, isoniazid (INH), 300 mg per day for a period of 6 to 12 months, is commonly used to prevent active TB.

When isoniazid prophylaxis is contraindicted, bacilli Calmette-Guérin (BCG) vaccine may be prescribed. This vaccine is widely used in developing countries. BCG is made from an attenuated strain of *M. bovis,* a closely related bacillus that causes tuberculosis in cattle. In the United States, BCG vaccine is recommended only for infants, children, and health care workers with a negative tuberculin test who are repeatedly exposed to untreated or ineffectively treated people with active disease. After vaccination with BCG, a positive reaction to tuberculin testing is common. Periodic chest X-rays may be required for screening purposes.

The tuberculosis bacillus mutates readily to drug-resistant forms when only one anti-infective agent is used. Active disease is always treated with concurrent use of at least two antibacterial medications to which the organism is sensitive. The primary antituberculosis drugs can prevent development of resistance because all act by different mechanisms. However, the

more information about anthrax and the section of this chapter on respiratory failure for nursing care measures for the client with inhalation anthrax.

## THE CLIENT WITH A FUNGAL INFECTION

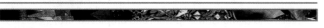

Fungal spores are endemic, present in the air everyone breathes. Normal respiratory defense mechanisms allow few of these spores to reach the lungs. If they reach the lungs, pulmonary macrophages and neutrophils efficiently remove them in most people. When they do cause infection, it is typically mild and self-limiting. Most fungi are opportunistic, able to cause infection only in people who are immunocompromised. For this reason, clients with AIDS, renal failure, leukemia, burns, or chronic diseases, as well as people receiving corticosteroids or immunosuppressants, are particularly susceptible to fungal diseases.

Many fungal lung diseases have a geographic distribution pattern. Histoplasmosis and blastomycosis are more common in the southeastern, mid-Atlantic, and central states. California, Arizona, and western Texas are the primary sites for coccidioidomycosis, also known as San Joaquin valley fever (Braunwald et al., 2001).

The course and manifestations of fungal lung diseases resemble those of tuberculosis. Lung lesions are slow to develop, and symptoms are mild. The fungus can disseminate from the lung to other organs.

## PATHOPHYSIOLOGY

### Histoplasmosis

Histoplasmosis, an infectious disease caused by *Histoplasma capsulatum,* is the most common fungal lung infection in the United States. The organism is found in the soil and is linked to exposure to bird droppings and bats. Infection occurs when the spores are inhaled and reach the alveoli. Most infections develop into *latent asymptomatic disease,* much like tuberculosis, or *primary acute histoplasmosis,* a mild, self-limiting influenzalike illness. Initial chest X-rays are nonspecific; later ones show areas of calcification. *Chronic progressive disease,* usually seen in older adults, typically is limited to the lung but may involve any organ. Progressive lung changes and cavitation occur, with increasing dyspnea and eventual disabling pulmonary disease.

Regional lymph vessels spread the organism from the lungs to other parts of the body, much like the process that occurs in tuberculosis. In the healthy host, normal immune responses inactivate and remove the organism. In the immunocompromised host, however, macrophages remove the fungi but are unable to destroy them, resulting in *disseminated histoplasmosis.* This type of histoplasmosis is often fatal. Manifestations of fever, dyspnea, cough, weight loss, and muscle wasting are usual. Ulcerations of the mouth and oropharynx may be present, and the liver and spleen are enlarged.

## Coccidioidomycosis

Coccidioidomycosis is an infectious disease caused by the fungus *Coccidioides immitis.* This mold grows in the soil of the arid Southwest, Mexico, and Central and South America. When inhaled, the fungus typically causes an acute, self-limiting pulmonary infection that often is asymptomatic and goes unrecognized. If manifestations do occur, they resemble those of influenza, with malaise, fever, body aches, and cough. Pleuritic pain, skin rash, and arthritis of the knees and ankles also may develop. Disseminated disease, which may affect the lymph nodes, meninges, spleen, liver, kidney, skin, and adrenal glands, is rare in immunocompetent people. When it does occur, the mortality rate is high. Meningitis is the usual cause of death.

## Blastomycosis

The fungus *Blastomyces dermatitidis* causes the infectious disease blastomycosis. It occurs primarily in the south central and midwestern regions of the United States and in Canada. Men are affected more frequently than women. The lungs are the primary site for the disease, although it may spread to involve the skin, bones, genitourinary system, and, rarely, the central nervous system. Pulmonary symptoms include fever, dyspnea, pleuritic chest pain, and cough, which may become productive of bloody or purulent sputum. If untreated, the disseminated disease is slowly progressive and ultimately fatal.

## Aspergillosis

*Aspergillus* spores are common in the environment, but rarely cause disease except in the immunocompromised. When they do cause infection, *Aspergillus* species invade blood vessels and produce hyphae that branch at acute angles, frequently causing venous or arterial thrombosis. In the lungs, aspergillosis can cause an acute, diffuse, self-limited pneumonitis. The manifestations of pulmonary aspergillosis include dyspnea, nonproductive cough, pleuritic chest pain, chills, and fever. If the organism invades a pulmonary blood vessel, hemoptysis or massive pulmonary hemorrhage can occur. In clients with underlying lung disease, balls of *Aspergillus* hyphae may form within cysts or cavities, usually in the upper lobes of the lung. Symptoms often are milder and more insidious in onset, with fever, weight loss, night sweats, and cough (Braunwald et al., 2001; Morrison & Lew, 2001).

## COLLABORATIVE CARE

Most fungal lung infections can be diagnosed by microscopic examination of a sputum specimen for the fungus. Blood cultures also may be done, as well as cultures of cerebrospinal fluid if indicated. Chest X-ray may show typical changes in lung tissue or widening of the mediastinum, depending on the infecting organism.

Acute pulmonary histoplasmosis and acute pulmonary coccidioidomycosis usually resolve without treatment, although antifungal drugs may be given to shorten the disease course. Oral itraconazole (Sporanox), a broad-spectrum antifungal agent, is commonly prescribed to treat histoplasmosis. Other fungal lung diseases and clients who are immunocompromised are often treated with intravenous amphotericin B. Surgery (lobectomy) may be indicated for clients with severe hemoptysis associated with aspergillosis.

## NURSING CARE

Clients with fungal lung infections have different nursing care needs, depending on the disease and their immune status. For most clients, nursing care focuses on education. People living in high-prevalence areas or who have specific risk factors such as exposure to bird droppings (for example, by cleaning chicken coops, pigeon lofts, or barns where birds roost), decomposed vegetation, rotting wood, or stored grain need to be aware of the risk, common symptoms, and measures to reduce

the risk. Clients with latent histoplasmosis may need education to maintain good general health to prevent reactivation. Teach clients receiving antifungal drugs about the specific drug, its intended and adverse effects, the duration of therapy, and symptoms to report to the physician. Include teaching about any specific precautions such as drug or food interactions. Itraconazole interacts with many medications; verify the safety of concurrent usage with all other prescribed drugs. Its use is contraindicated during pregnancy and lactation; emphasize the importance of effective birth control and of notifying the physician immediately if pregnancy occurs. Amphotericin B is a toxic drug. Administer the intial intravenous dose slowly after premedicating with an antihistamine and antiemetic as ordered to manage its adverse effects. Monitor carefully during infusion and therapy for changes in vital signs, hydration, nutrition, weight, or urine output.

# OBSTRUCTIVE DISORDERS OF THE AIRWAYS

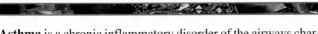

Many pulmonary disorders and diseases can affect the airways. Although their pathophysiology differs, these diseases are characterized by limited airflow. Airflow is limited when:

- Elastic recoil of the lungs is reduced, decreasing the force to push air out.
- Airway lumen are obstructed by secretions, increasing resistance.
- Airway walls are thickened.
- Smooth muscle of the airways is activated, causing bronchoconstriction.
- Interstitial support necessary to maintain airway distention and patency is lost.

Aging contributes to airflow limitation. The number of alveoli decrease, and emphysematous changes (senile emphysema) reduce the surface area for gas exchange. Alveoli become less elastic, causing increased air trapping and dead space.

Limited airflow increases the work of breathing and the residual volume of the lungs as air is trapped behind narrowed or collapsed airways. Inspired air mixes with an abnormally large volume of residual air, effectively reducing the amount of oxygen available in the alveoli. Decreased alveolar ventilation further reduces oxygen available for exchange.

## THE CLIENT WITH ASTHMA

**Asthma** is a chronic inflammatory disorder of the airways characterized by recurrent episodes of wheezing, breathlessness, chest tightness, and coughing. Inflammation causes increased responsiveness of the airways to multiple stimuli. The widespread airflow obstruction that occurs during acute episodes usually reverses either spontaneously or with treatment.

In the United States, approximately 11 million people experienced at least one asthma attack in the year 2000. Although it is more common in children than adults, about 4% of the adult population is affected. After several years of increase, the prevalence of asthma currently is relatively stable. Asthma is a serious disease, causing more than 4000 deaths in the United States in 1999. Mortality due to asthma is higher in blacks than in whites and higher in females than in males (NHLBI, 2002).

A number of risk factors can be identified for asthma, although many clients develop the disease in the absence of known risk factors. Allergies play a strong role in childhood asthma, although less so in adults. There is a strong genetic component to the disease, although a specific pattern of inheritance has not been identified. Environmental factors, including air pollution and occupational exposure to industrial compounds, may contribute. Respiratory viruses such as rhinovirus and influenza can precipitate asthma attacks. Other contributory factors include exercise (particularly in cold air) and emotional stress.

## PHYSIOLOGY REVIEW

Airways within the lungs contain crisscrossing strips of smooth muscle that control their diameter. This muscle is innervated by the autonomic nervous system. Parasympathetic (cholinergic) stimulation leads to bronchoconstriction, or narrowing of the airways. Sympathetic stimulation through $\beta_2$-adrenergic receptors causes bronchodilation, or expansion of the airways. Slight bronchoconstriction normally predominates. However, when increased airflow is necessary (e.g., during exercise), the parasympathetic system is inhibited, and stimulation of the sympathetic system causes bronchodilation. Inflammatory mediators (such as histamine) released during an antigen-antibody response act directly on bronchial smooth muscle to produce bronchoconstriction.

# PATHOPHYSIOLOGY

During symptom-free periods, airway inflammation in asthma is subacute or quiet. An acute inflammatory response may be triggered by a variety of factors. Common triggers for an acute asthma attack include exposure to allergens, respiratory tract infection, exercise, inhaled irritants, and emotional upsets.

Childhood asthma (which may continue into adulthood) is most often linked to inhalation of allergens such as pollen, animal dander, or household dust. Clients with allergic asthma often have a history of other allergies. Environmental pollutants, such as tobacco smoke and irritant gases (e.g., sulfur dioxide, nitrogen dioxide, and ozone) can provoke asthma. Exposure to secondhand smoke as a child is associated with a higher risk for and increased severity of asthma. Agents found in the workplace, such as noxious fumes and gases, chemicals, and dusts, may cause occupational asthma.

Respiratory infections, viral in particular, are a common internal stimulus for an asthmatic attack. Exercise-induced asthma attacks also are common, affecting 40% to 90% of people with bronchial asthma (Porth, 2002). Loss of heat or water from the bronchial surface may contribute to exercise-induced asthma. Exercising in cold, dry air increases the risk of an asthma attack in susceptible people.

Emotional stress is a significant etiologic factor for attacks in as many as half of clients with asthma. Common pharmacologic triggers include aspirin and other NSAIDs, sulfites (which are used as preservatives in wine, beer, fresh fruits, and salad), and beta blockers.

When a trigger such as inhalation of an allergen or irritant occurs, an *acute* or *early response* develops in the hyperreactive airways predisposed to bronchospasm. Sensitized mast cells in the bronchial mucosa release inflammatory mediators such as histamine, prostaglandins, and leukotrienes. These mediators stimulate parasympathetic receptors and bronchial smooth muscle to produce bronchoconstriction. They also increase capillary permeability, leading to mucosal edema, and stimulate mucus production.

The attack is prolonged by the *late phase response,* which develops 4 to 12 hours after exposure to the trigger. Inflammatory cells such as basophils and eosinophils are activated, which damage airway epithelium, produce mucosal edema, impair mucociliary clearance, and produce or prolong bronchoconstriction. The degree of hyperreactivity depends on the extent of inflammation. Together, bronchoconstriction, edema and inflammation, and mucous secretion narrow the airway. Airway resistance increases, limiting airflow, and increasing the work of breathing (Figure 36–9 ■).

Limited expiratory airflow traps air distal to the spastic airways. Trapped air mixes with inspired air in the alveoli, reducing its oxygen tension and gas exchange across the alveolar-capillary membrane. Blood flow is reduced to distended alveoli, further affecting gas exchange. As a result, hypoxemia develops. Hypoxemia and increased lung volume due to trapping stimulate the respiratory rate. As a result, the $Paco_2$ falls, leading to respiratory alkalosis. (See Chapter 5 ⊙⊙ for more information about acid-base imbalances.)

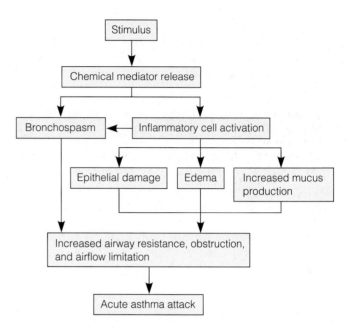

**Figure 36–9** ■ The pathogenesis of an acute episode of asthma.

## Manifestations of Acute Asthma

- Chest tightness
- Dyspnea
- Wheezing
- Cough
- Tachypnea and tachycardia
- Anxiety and apprehension

## MANIFESTATIONS AND COMPLICATIONS

An asthma attack is characterized by a subjective sensation of chest tightness, dyspnea, wheezing, and cough (see the box above). The onset of symptoms may be either abrupt or insidious, and an attack may subside rapidly or persist for hours or days. During an attack, tachycardia, tachypnea, and prolonged expiration are common. Diffuse wheezing is heard on auscultation. With more severe attacks, use of accessory muscles of respiration, intercostal retractions, loud wheezing, and distant breath sounds may be noted. Fatigue, anxiety, apprehension, and severe dyspnea that allows speaking only one or two words between breaths, may occur with persistent severe episodes. The onset of respiratory failure is marked by inaudible breath sounds with reduced wheezing and an ineffective cough. Without careful assessment, this apparent relief of symptoms can be misinterpreted as an improvement.

The frequency of attacks and severity of symptoms vary greatly from person to person. Although some people have infrequent, mild episodes, others have nearly continuous manifestations of cough and wheezing with periodic severe exacerbations (Table 36–6).

**Status asthmaticus** is severe, prolonged asthma that does not respond to routine treatment. Without aggressive therapy, status asthmaticus can lead to respiratory failure with hypox-

TABLE 36-6  Classification of Asthma Severity

| Classification | Symptom Frequency | Nighttime Symptoms |
|---|---|---|
| Mild intermittent | • No more than twice a week<br>• Brief attacks (hours to days) of varied intensity<br>• Asymptomatic and normal peak expiratory flow (PEF) rate between attacks | No more than twice a month |
| Mild persistent | • More than twice a week but less than once a day<br>• Exacerbations may affect activity | More than twice a month |
| Moderate persistent | • Daily symptoms<br>• Daily short-acting bronchodilator use<br>• Exacerbations affect activity<br>• Exacerbations more than twice a week, may last for days | More than once a week |
| Severe persistent | • Continual symptoms<br>• Limited physical activity<br>• Frequent exacerbations | Frequent |

*Note. Adapted from* Expert Panel Report 2: Guidelines for the Diagnosis and Management of Asthma, *Publication No. 97-4051 by National Education and Prevention Program, 1997, Bethesda, MD: National Institutes of Health.*

emia, hypercapnia, and acidosis. Endotracheal intubation, mechanical ventilation, and aggressive drug treatment may be necessary to sustain life.

In addition to acute respiratory failure, other complications associated with acute asthma include dehydration, respiratory infection, atelectasis, pneumothorax, and cor pulmonale.

## COLLABORATIVE CARE

The diagnosis of asthma is based primarily on the history and manifestations. Treatment goals are twofold. Daily management focuses on controlling symptoms and preventing acute attacks. During an acute attack, therapy is directed toward restoring airway patency and alveolar ventilation.

### Diagnostic Tests

Diagnostic tests are used to determine the degree of airway involvement during and between acute episodes and identify causative factors such as allergens.

- *Pulmonary function tests (PFTs)* are used to evaluate the degree of airway obstruction. Pulmonary function testing done before and after use of an aerosolized bronchodilator helps determine the reversibility of airway obstruction. The residual volume (RV) of the lungs may be increased and vital capacity decreased or normal even during periods of remission. The forced expiratory volume ($FEV_1$) and peak expiratory flow rate (PEFR) are the most valuable pulmonary function studies to evaluate the severity of an asthma attack and the effectiveness of treatment measures. See Box 36–1.
- *Challenge or bronchial provocation testing* uses an inhaled substance such as methacholine or histamine with PFTs to confirm the diagnosis of asthma by detecting airway hyper-responsiveness.

- *ABGs* are drawn during an acute attack to evaluate oxygenation, carbon dioxide elimination, and acid-base status. ABGs initially show hypoxemia with a low $PO_2$, and mild respiratory alkalosis with an elevated pH and low $PCO_2$ due to tachypnea. Severe airflow obstruction causes significant hypoxemia and respiratory acidosis (pH less than 7.35 and $PCO_2$ greater than 42 mmHg), indicative of respiratory failure and the need for mechanical ventilation.
- *Skin testing* may be done to identify specific allergens if an allergic trigger is suspected for asthma attacks.

### Disease Monitoring

*Peak expiratory flow rate (PEFR)* is used on a day-to-day basis to evaluate the severity of bronchial hyperresponsiveness. Small, inexpensive meters to measure PEFR are available. Readings taken at varying times of day over several weeks are used to establish the client's personal best or normal PEFR. This value is then used to evaluate the severity of airway obstruction. Traffic signal colors are used for simplicity: *green* (80% to 100% of personal best) indicates asthma that is under control; *yellow* (50% to 80%) is caution, indicating a need for further medication or treatment; and *red* (50% or less) signals an immediate need for a bronchodilator and medical treatment if the level does not immediately return to the yellow range (Porth, 2002).

### Preventive Measures

Asthma attacks often can be prevented by avoiding allergens and environmental triggers. Modifying the home environment by controlling dust, removing carpets, covering mattresses and pillows to reduce dust mite populations, and installing air filtering systems may be useful. Pets may need to be removed from the household. Eliminating all tobacco smoke in the home is vital. Wearing a mask that retains humidity and warm air while exercising in cold weather may help prevent attacks of exercise-induced asthma. Early treatment of respiratory infections is vital to prevent asthma exacerbations.

## BOX 36–1 ■ Pulmonary Function Tests

Pulmonary function tests (PFTs) are performed in a pulmonary function laboratory. After preparing the client, a nose clip is applied and the unsedated client breathes into a spirometer or body plethysmograph, a device for measuring and recording lung volume in liters versus time in seconds. The client is instruced how to breathe for specific tests: for example, to inhale as deeply as possible and then exhale to the maximal extent possible. Using measured lung volumes, respiratory capacities are calculated to assess pulmonary status. The specific values determined by PFT and illustrated in the figure include the following:

■ *Total lung capacity (TLC)* is the total volume of the lungs at their maximum inflation. Four values are used to calculate TLC:
  a. *Tidal volume ($V_T$),* the volume inhaled and exhaled with normal quiet breathing.
  b. *Inspiratory reserve volume (IRV),* the maximum amount that can be inhaled over and above a normal inspiration.
  c. *Expiratory reserve volume (ERV),* the maximum amount that can be exhaled following a normal exhalation.
  d. *Residual volume (RV),* the amount of air remaining in the lungs after maximal exhalation.
■ *Vital capacity (VC)* is the total amount of air that can be exhaled after a maximal inspiration. It is calculated by adding together the IRV, $V_T$, and the ERV.

■ *Inspiratory capacity* is the total amount of air that can be inhaled following a normal quiet exhalation. It is calculated by adding the $V_T$ and IRV.
■ *Functional residual capacity (FRC)* is the volume of air left in the lungs after a normal exhalation. The ERV and RV are added to determine the FRC.
■ *Forced expiratory volume ($FEV_1$)* is the amount of air that can be exhaled in 1 second.
■ *Forced vital capacity (FVC)* is the amount of air that can be exhaled forcefully and rapidly after maximum air intake.
■ *Minute volume (MV)* is the total amount or volume of air breathed in 1 minute.

In older clients, residual capacity is increased, and vital capacity is decreased. These age-related changes result from the following:

■ Calcification of the costal cartilage and weakening of the intercostal muscles, which reduce movement of the chest wall.
■ Vertebral osteoporosis, which decreases spinal flexibility and increases the degree of kyphosis, further increasing the anterior-posterior diameter of the chest.
■ Diaphragmatic flattening and loss of elasticity.

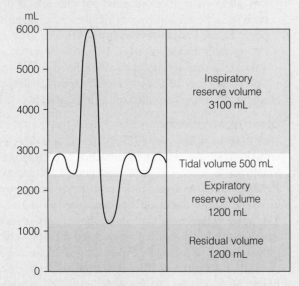
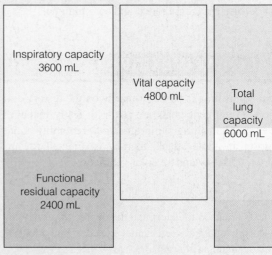

The relationship of lung volumes and capacities. Volumes (mL) shown are for an average adult male.

## Medications

Medications are used to prevent and control asthma symptoms, reduce the frequency and severity of exacerbations, and reverse airway obstruction. Drugs used for long-term control of asthma are taken daily to maintain control of the disease. The primary drugs in this group are anti-inflammatory agents, long-acting bronchodilators, and leukotriene modifiers. Quick-relief medications provide prompt relief of bronchoconstriction and airflow obstruction with associated wheezing, cough, and chest tightness. Short-acting adrenergic stimulants (rapid-acting bronchodilators), anticholinergic drugs, and methylxanthines fall into this category.

## Bronchodilators

Most asthmatics need bronchodilator therapy to control their symptoms. Inhalation of nebulized medication is the preferred means of administration. The primary bronchodilators used include adrenergic stimulants, methylxanthines, and anticholinergic agents.

Adrenergic stimulants affect receptors on smooth muscle cells of the respiratory tract, causing smooth muscle relaxation and bronchodilation. Long-acting adrenergic stimulants such as inhaled salmeterol and oral sustained-release albuterol are used in conjunction with anti-inflammatory drugs to control symptoms, but are not appropriate to treat an acute episode of

## BOX 36–2 ■ Client Teaching: Using a Metered-Dose Inhaler

- Firmly insert a charged metered-dose inhaler (MDI) canister into the mouthpiece unit.
- Remove mouthpiece cap. Shake canister vigorously for 3 to 5 seconds.
- Exhale slowly and completely.
- Holding the canister upside down, place the mouthpiece in the mouth, closing lips around it, or directly in front of the mouth.
- Press and hold the canister down while inhaling deeply and slowly for 3 to 5 seconds (see figure).
- Hold breath for 10 seconds, release pressure on the container, remove from mouth, and exhale. Wait 20 to 30 seconds before repeating the procedure for a second puff.
- Rinse the mouth after using the inhaler to minimize systemic absorption and drying the mucous membranes.
- Rinse the inhaler mouthpiece at least once a day.

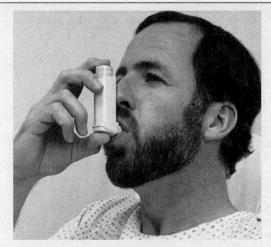

Use of a metered-dose inhaler.

asthma. Inhaled short-acting beta-adrenergic agonists such as albuterol, bitolterol, pirbuterol, and terbutaline, administered by metered-dose inhalers (MDIs), are the treatment of choice for quick relief (Box 36–2). They act within minutes, but their duration generally is short, lasting only 4 to 6 hours. Tachycardia and muscle tremors, common side effects of adrenergic agonists, are minimal with inhalation therapy.

Anticholinergic medications prevent bronchoconstriction by blocking parasympathetic input to bronchial smooth muscle. Ipratropium bromide, an anticholinergic drug administered by metered-dose inhaler, is useful when asthma symptoms are poorly controlled by adrenergic stimulants alone. Anticholinergic drugs act more slowly than adrenergic stimulants, requiring up to 60 to 90 minutes to achieve maximal effect.

Theophylline is a methylxanthine used as adjunctive treatment for asthma. It relaxes bronchial smooth muscle and may also inhibit the release of chemical mediators of the inflammatory response. Monitoring of serum theophylline levels is necessary because of wide individual variations in metabolism and elimination of the drug and its toxic effects. Serum levels of 10 to 20 µg/mL or lower are recommended. Theophylline may be used as a long-term bronchodilator, given once or twice daily. A related drug, aminophylline, may be administered intravenously to treat an acute, severe exacerbation of the disease.

### Anti-Inflammatory Agents

Corticosteroids and two nonsteroidal anti-inflammatory agents, cromolyn sodium and nedocromil, are used to suppress airway inflammation and reduce asthma symptoms.

Corticosteroids block the late response to inhaled allergens and reduce bronchial hyperresponsiveness. The preferred route of administration is by metered-dose inhaler to minimize systemic absorption and reduce the adverse effects of prolonged steroid use (cushingoid effects). For a severe acute attack, corticosteroids may be given systemically to alleviate symptoms and induce remission.

Cromolyn sodium and nedocromil are used to prevent acute episodes of asthma. They reduce airway hyperreactivity and inhibit the release of mediator substances. These drugs are used for long-term control of asthma, not quick relief. They have a wide margin of safety and few side effects.

### Leukotriene Modifiers

Leukotriene modifiers, zafirlukast (Accolate) and zileuton (Zyflo Filmtab), are new oral medications that reduce the inflammatory response in asthma. They appear to improve lung function, diminish symptoms, and reduce the need for short-acting bronchodilators. These drugs affect the metabolism and excretion of other medications such as warfarin and theophylline and may cause liver toxicity.

Nursing implications for medications used to treat asthma are outlined on pages 1110–1111.

### Complementary Therapies

A number of herbal preparations and other complementary therapies have been shown to be helpful in treating asthma. Herbal preparations may include atopa belladonna (the natural form of atropine) or ephedra (also called ma huang), an herb that contains ephedrine. These herbals have effects similar to those of drugs used to treat asthma, and should not be used in combination with sympathetic stimulants or anticholinergic preparations. The safety of ephedra is currently in question; advise clients to always check with a physician before using preparations containing ephedra. Capsaicin also may relieve acute asthma symptoms. Other herbal preparations include quercetin and grape seed extract. Refer clients interested in using natural preparations to a qualified herbalist, and emphasize the importance of talking to the physician before using these preparations along with conventional treatment.

In addition to herbals, other complementary therapies such as biofeedback, yoga, breathing techniques, acupuncture, homeopathy, and massage have been found to alleviate or help control asthma symptoms.

# Medication Administration

## Asthma

### ADRENERGIC STIMULANTS

Epinephrine
Isoproterenol (Isuprel)
Metaproterenol (Alupent, Metaprel)
Terbutaline (Brethaire, Brethine)
Isoetharine (Bronkosol, Bronkometer)
Albuterol (Proventil, Ventolin)
Bitolterol (Tornalate)
Pirbuterol (Maxair)
Salmeterol (Serevent)

Adrenergic stimulants affect sympathetic receptors in the respiratory tract, resulting in smooth muscle relaxation and bronchodilation. Administered by metered-dose inhalers, these drugs are the treatment of choice for acute bronchial asthma. Oral forms may be used for prophylaxis but are not effective in treating an acute attack because of their slow onset. When administered orally or parenterally, their effect on the sympathetic nervous system can produce undesirable side effects such as nervousness, irritability, tachycardia, and cardiac dysrhythmias.

### Nursing Responsibilities

- Use with caution in clients with hypertension, cardiovascular disease or dysrhythmias, hyperthyroidism, or diabetes.
- When given to a client who is hypoxemic and acidotic, these drugs may cause potentially dangerous cardiac stimulation.
- When given by MDI wait 1 to 2 minutes between puffs to allow airways to dilate, permitting the second dose to reach distal airways.
- Observe for desired effect of reduced dyspnea and wheezing. Central nervous system stimulation (anxiety, irritability, and insomnia) and tremor are common side effects.

### Client and Family Teaching

- Use the prescribed inhaler or nebulizer as directed.
- If you are taking a bronchodilator along with another medication by inhalation, use the bronchodilator first to open airways and enhance the effectiveness of the second medication.
- Rinse the mouth after using inhalers to reduce systemic absorption of the medication.
- Keep a log to track your bronchodilator use. If the drug becomes less effective, or if you need a higher dosage or more frequent doses than prescribed, contact your physician.
- Report palpitations, irregular pulse, and other side effects to the physician.

### METHYLXANTHINES

Theophylline (Bronkotabs, Quibron, Slo-Phyllin Theolair, Theo-Dur, others)
Aminophylline (Somophyllin)

The methylxanthines are chemically related to caffeine. Once the drugs of choice for preventing and treating asthma attacks, they are now are used primarily to prevent nocturnal asthma in affected adult clients. Theophylline has a narrow margin of safety and high potential for toxicity. Because the metabolism and excretion of theophylline vary significantly from person to person—affected by such factors as age, smoking, genetic factors, alcoholism, and other chronic diseases—monitoring of serum levels is vital.

### Nursing Responsibilities

- The therapeutic blood level for theophylline is 10 to 20 µg/mL.
- Monitor for manifestations of toxicity. Anorexia, nausea, vomiting, restlessness, insomnia, cardiac dysrhythmias, and seizures are early manifestations. Other manifestations include epigastric pain, hematemesis, diarrhea, headache, irritability, muscle twitching, palpitations, tachycardia, flushing, and circulatory failure.
- Administer with meals or a full glass of water or milk to minimize gastric irritation.
- Monitor effect closely when administering concurrently with other medications such as barbiturates, anticonvulsants, thyroid hormone, beta blockers, bronchodilators, and others.
- Aminophylline is incompatible with many other intravenous drugs. Use a separate line or flush the line with normal saline before and after administering any other preparation.

### Client and Family Teaching

- Oral methylxanthines are ineffective to treat an acute asthma attack; do not delay other treatment by using these drugs.
- Check with the physician before taking any over-the-counter medications or other prescription drugs while on theophylline.
- Do not smoke while using this drug.
- Report adverse effects to the physician.

### ANTICHOLINERGICS

Atropine
Ipratropium bromide (Atrovent)

Anticholinergics are potent bronchodilators, blocking input from the parasympathetic nervous system. Atropine is used infrequently because of its tendency to dry secretions of the mucous membranes and other side effects. Ipratropium bromide is available as an inhaler and has fewer side effects than atropine.

### Nursing Responsibilities

- Assess for possible contraindications to the drug, including hypersensitivity, glaucoma, prostatic hypertrophy, or bladder-neck obstruction.
- Assess for desired and/or adverse effects: improving or worsening symptoms; nausea, vomiting, abdominal cramping, anxiety, dizziness; headache.
- Provide ice chips, fluids, or hard candy to relieve dry mouth.

### Client and Family Teaching

- To prevent overdose, take no more than the prescribed number of doses per day.
- If the drug becomes less effective over time, notify the physician; an adjustment in dosage may be needed.

### CORTICOSTEROIDS

Beclomethasone dipropionate (Vanceril, Beclovent)
Triamcinalone acetonide (Azmacort)
Flunisolide (AeroBid)
Dexamethasone sodium phosphate (Decadron Phosphate Respihaler)

The anti-inflammatory effect of corticosteroids helps both prevent and treat acute episodes. Corticosteroids are used to reduce

## Medication Administration

### Asthma (continued)

the frequency and severity of asthma attacks and allow reduced dosages of other drugs. The cushingoid side effects of corticosteroids, always a major concern with their use, are minimized when they are inhaled.

#### Nursing Responsibilities
- Administer inhaler doses after bronchodilators to facilitate transit of the medication to distal airways.
- Assess for common side effects: sore throat; hoarseness; and oropharyngeal or laryngeal *Candida albicans* infection.
- Administer antifungal medications or gargles as ordered.

#### Client and Family Teaching
- Rinse the mouth after using the inhaler and maintain good oral hygiene to reduce the risk of fungal infections.
- These medications should not be used to alleviate the symptoms of an acute attack.
- Several weeks of continued therapy may be required before a beneficial effect is noticed.
- Notify the physician if you develop weight gain, fluid retention, muscle weakness, redistribution of fat, or mood changes.

### MAST CELL STABILIZERS

Cromolyn sodium (Intal, Nasalcrom)
Nedocromil (Tilade)

Cromolyn sodium and nedocromil inhibit inflammatory cells in the airway, blocking early and late responses to inhaled antigens. Both also prevent bronchoconstriction in response to inhaling cold air. They are administered by metered-dose inhaler, and have a wide margin of safety. Clients using nedocromil may complain of an unpleasant taste.

#### Nursing Responsibilities
- Evaluate for potential adverse effects of wheezing and bronchoconstriction.

#### Client and Family Teaching
- Gargling or sipping water can decrease the throat irritation associated with nebulizer treatment.
- Use appropriate technique. Inhale deeply with head tipped back to open airways, hold breath, and then exhale. Repeat until all of the drug has been inhaled.
- These drugs are used only to prevent asthma attacks; they are not effective in treating an acute attack.
- Several weeks may be required before a beneficial effect is noted.

### LEUKOTRIENE MODIFIERS

Zafirlukast (Accolate)
Zileuton (Zyflo)

Leukotriene modifiers interfere with the inflammatory process in the airways, improving airflow, decreasing symptoms, and reducing the need for short-acting bronchodilators. They are used for maintenance therapy in adults and children over the age of 12 as an alternative to inhaled corticosteroid therapy. They are not used to treat an acute attack.

#### Nursing Responsibilities
- Administer at least 1 hour before or 2 hours after meals.
- These drugs inhibit some liver enzymes, affecting the metabolism of warfarin and possibly terfenadine and theophylline. Monitor prothrombin times and theophylline blood levels.
- Monitor liver enzymes, as these drugs may be toxic to the liver.

#### Client and Family Teaching
- Take the drugs as prescribed on an empty stomach.
- Notify the physician if a change in color of stools or urine is noted or if jaundice develops.

## NURSING CARE

Nurses encounter clients with asthma both in the acute care setting during an acute exacerbation and as outpatients or in homes. The priority nursing care needs differ with each setting.

### Health Promotion

Although specific measures to prevent asthma have not yet been identified, the link between parental smoking and childhood asthma is strong. Discuss this link with young people and families with children. Encourage all clients to not start smoking, and if they do smoke, to quit. Provide referrals to smoking cessation clinics, help groups, or a care provider for nicotine patches as needed to facilitate quitting.

### Assessment

Assessment of the client experiencing an acute asthma attack must be very focused and timely.

- Health history: current symptoms, including chest tightness, shortness of breath, dyspnea; duration of current attack; measures used to relieve symptoms and their effect; identified precipitating factors for the attack; frequency of attacks; current medications; known allergies
- Physical examination: apparent level of distress; color; vital signs; respiratory rate and excursion, breath sounds throughout lung fields; apical pulse

### Nursing Diagnoses and Interventions

An acute asthma attack causes fear as breathing becomes increasingly difficult and hypoxemia develops. Anxiety in turn tends to increase the severity and manifestations of the attack. Priority nursing care needs during an acute attack focus on improving airway clearance and reducing fear and anxiety. Teaching about prevention of future attacks and home management must be postponed until adequate ventilation is restored.

#### Ineffective Airway Clearance

Bronchospasm and bronchoconstriction, increased mucus secretion, and airway edema narrow the airways and impair airflow during an acute attack of asthma. Both inspiratory and expiratory volume are affected, decreasing the oxygen available at the alveolus for the process of respiration. Narrowed air passages increase the work of breathing, increasing the metabolic rate and tissue demand for oxygen.

**PRACTICE ALERT** *Frequently assess respiratory status (at least every 1 to 2 hours): respiratory rate and depth, chest movement or excursion, breath sounds, and peak expiratory flow rate. Respiratory status can change rapidly during an acute asthma attack and its treatment. Decreasing PEFRs indicate worsening airflow restriction. Slowed, shallow respirations with significantly diminished breath sounds and decreased wheezing may indicate exhaustion and impending respiratory failure. Immediate intervention is necessary.* ■

- Monitor skin color and temperature and level of consciousness. *Cyanosis, cool clammy skin, and changes in level of consciousness (agitation, lethargy, or confusion) indicate worsening hypoxia.*
- Assess arterial blood gas results and pulse oximetry readings; notify the physician of abnormal values or changes in status. *These values provide information about gas exchange and the adequacy of alveolar ventilation. A fall in oxygen saturation levels is an early indicator of impaired gas exchange.*

**PRACTICE ALERT** *Assess cough effort and sputum for color, consistency, and amount. Ineffective cough may also signal impending respiratory failure.* ■

- Place in Fowler's, high-Fowler's, or orthopneic (with head and arms supported on the overbed table) position to facilitate breathing and lung expansion. *These positions reduce the work of breathing and increase lung expansion, especially of basilar areas.*
- Administer oxygen as ordered. If a mask is used, monitor closely for feelings of claustrophobia or suffocation. *Supplemental oxygen reduces hypoxemia. Although the mask is a very effective oxygen delivery system, it may increase anxiety.*
- Administer nebulizer treatments and provide humidification as ordered. *Nebulizer treatments are used to administer bronchodilators and other medications; humidity helps loosen secretions.*
- Initiate or assist with chest physiotherapy, including percussion and postural drainage. *Percussion and postural drainage facilitate the movement of secretions and airway clearance.*
- Increase fluid intake. *Increasing fluids helps keep secretions thin.*
- Provide endotracheal suctioning as needed. *Endotracheal suctioning may be necessary to remove secretions and improve ventilation if the client is unable to clear secretions by coughing.*

## Ineffective Breathing Pattern

The physiologic changes in lung ventilation that occur during an acute asthma attack impair both lung expansion and emptying. Anxiety caused by hypoxia and dyspnea compounds the problem by increasing the respiratory rate. Collaborative and nursing interventions can help restore a more normal breathing pattern and adequate lung ventilation.

**PRACTICE ALERT** *Frequently assess respiratory rate, pattern, and breath sounds. Note manifestations of ineffective breathing, including rapid rate, shallow respirations, nasal flaring, use of accessory muscles, intercostal retractions, and diminished or absent breath sounds. Early identification of ineffective respirations allows timely initiation of interventions.* ■

- Monitor vital signs and laboratory results. *Tachypnea, tachycardia, an elevated blood pressure, and increasing hypoxemia and hypercapnia are signs of compromised respiratory status.*
- Assist with ADLs as needed. *This conserves energy and reduces fatigue.*
- Provide rest periods between scheduled activities and treatments. *Scheduled rest is important to prevent fatigue and reduce oxygen demands.*
- Teach and assist to use techniques to control breathing pattern:
  a. Pursed-lip breathing
  b. Abdominal breathing
  c. Relaxation techniques including visualization, meditation, and others
  *Pursed-lip breathing helps keep airways open by maintaining positive pressure, and abdominal breathing improves lung expansion. Relaxation techniques reduce anxiety and its effect on the respiratory rate.*
- Administer medications, including bronchodilators and anti-inflammatory drugs, as ordered. Monitor for desired and possible adverse effects. *Medications are used to improve airway status and facilitate breathing.*

### Anxiety

Acute exacerbations of asthma can produce significant anxiety. Fear of being unable to breathe and feelings of suffocation associated with acute asthma are significant. Financial or other concerns may cause the client to want to avoid hospitalization. Increasingly frequent and severe episodes may cause fear for the future. Hypoxia contributes to anxiety as well, stimulating the sympathetic nervous system and the fight-or-flight response.

- Assess level of anxiety. *Interventions for severe anxiety or panic differ from those for mild or moderate anxiety.*
- Assist to identify coping skills that have been successful in the past. *Successful coping helps the client regain control of the situation, reducing anxiety.*

**PRACTICE ALERT** *Provide physical and emotional support. Remain with the client during episodes of severe anxiety; schedule time every 1 to 2 hours to be with the mildly or moderately anxious client. Answer call lights promptly. The severely anxious client may fear being alone or believe that he or she will die if someone is not on hand. Knowing that the nurse is readily available and will return regardless if help is needed reduces anxiety.* ■

- Listen actively to concerns; do not deny or negate the fear of dying or of being unable to breathe. *Active listening promotes trust and helps the client express concerns.*

**PRACTICE ALERT** *Provide clear, concise directions and explanations about procedures. Avoid presenting more information than the client is able to assimilate. Anxiety interferes with the ability to learn. Explanations may need to be repeated frequently.* ■

- Include the client in care planning and decisions as appropriate, without making excessive demands. *Participating in decision making increases the client's sense of control. Because high levels of anxiety interfere with the ability to make decisions, it is important to avoid placing demands on the client that may further increase the level of anxiety.*
- Reduce excessive environmental stimuli, and maintain a calm demeanor. *This promotes rest.*
- Allow supportive family members to remain with the client. *Significant others provide additional support and can help reduce anxiety.*
- Assist to use relaxation techniques, such as guided imagery, muscle relaxation, and meditation. *These techniques help restore psychologic balance and reduce sympathetic stimulation and responses.*

### Ineffective Therapeutic Regimen Management

Once acute asthma is under control and effective respirations have been reestablished, it is important to help the client identify contributing factors to the attack. This helps the client prevent future episodes.

- Assess level of understanding about asthma and the prescribed treatment regimen. Provide additional information and teaching as indicated. *Assessment helps to identify and clarify misperceptions and difficulties with disease management.*
- Discuss the client's perception of the illness and its effect on his or her lifestyle. *Open discussion can help identify conflicts between lifestyle and the treatment regimen.*

**PRACTICE ALERT** *Assist to identify factors that contributed to the acute episode. Identifying contributing factors increases the client's awareness of the disease and strategies to prevent future exacerbations.* ■

- Assist the client and significant others to identify problems or difficulties integrating the treatment regimen into their lifestyle. *Asthma and its management may necessitate lifestyle modifications to prevent acute exacerbations. This can significantly impact family members, for example, eliminating cigarette smoking or pets from the household, removing carpets, or daily damp-dusting to remove dust mites.*
- Assess knowledge and understanding of prescribed medications and use of over-the-counter preparations. *This is important to determine misperceptions or possible misuse of medications.*

- Provide verbal and written instructions. *Written instructions reinforce teaching and allow future reference.*
- Refer to counseling, support groups, or self-help organizations. *Counseling, support groups, and self-help organizations can help the client and family adapt to living with asthma and the treatment regimen.*

### Home Care

Asthma is a chronic disease that is best managed by the client with assistance from medical personnel. Teaching for home care focuses on promoting the highest level of wellness and preventing and managing acute episodes and exacerbations of the disease. Topics to include in teaching are as follows:

- Suggestions for lifestyle changes to avoid specific triggers for asthma attacks, for example:
  - Warm up slowly before exercising in cold weather; wear a special mask or scarf to retain air warmth and humidity while exercising.
  - Substitute indoor exercises during cold, dry weather.
  - Reduce the risk for respiratory infections (e.g., adequate rest, good nutrition, and stress management to maintain immune function, yearly influenza vaccines and immunization against pneumococcal pneumonia).
  - Use techniques to reduce or manage physical and psychologic stress.
- Using PEFR meter to monitor airway status; how to manage the disease based on results
- Using prescribed medications, including:
  - Name, frequency, dose, and desired effect.
  - Potential adverse effects and their management, including effects to report to the physician.
  - Potential interactions with other drugs (including over-the-counter herbal preparations) or foods.
  - If tolerance is a potential risk, how to identify it and steps to take.

Provide referrals to local or regional resources for further teaching and support as needed. Consider the need for home health services, home respiratory care services, and others as needed. See Box 36–3 for selected national resource agencies.

| BOX 36–3 ■ **Home Care Resources for Clients with Asthma** |
| --- |

American Lung Association
800-LUNG-USA (800-586-4872)
www.lungusa.org

Asthma and Allergy Foundation of America
800-7-ASTHMA (800-727-8462)

Asthma Information Center
www.mdnet.de/asthma

National Asthma Education and Prevention Program
National Heart, Lung, and Blood Institute Information Center
301-251-1222
www.nhlbi.nih.gov

MediaLink | ASTHMA RESOURCES

# THE CLIENT WITH CHRONIC OBSTRUCTIVE PULMONARY DISEASE

Clients with chronic airflow obstruction due to chronic bronchitis and/or emphysema are said to have **chronic obstructive pulmonary disease (COPD).**

In 2000, approximately 11.4 million Americans were affected by COPD. It is more common in whites than in blacks and affects men more frequently than women. It is the fourth leading cause of death in the United States. The death rate from COPD continues to rise, particularly among black males and females of all ethnic groups. In the year 2000, COPD and other chronic obstructive lung diseases accounted for over 123,500 deaths (NHLBI, 2002). In addition, COPD morbidity is significant. In people under age 65, COPD is second only to heart disease as a cause of disability, resulting in an estimated 250 million lost work hours yearly.

Obstructive lung disease typically affects middle-aged and older adults. Cigarette smoking is clearly implicated as the primary cause of COPD, even though it develops in only 10% to 15% of smokers. Cigarette smoke and the irritants it contains impair ciliary movement, inhibit the function of alveolar macrophages, and cause mucus-secreting glands to hypertrophy. It also produces emphysema or airway destruction and constricts smooth muscle, increasing airway resistance. Other contributing factors include air pollution, occupational exposure to noxious dusts and gases, airway infection, and familial and genetic factors.

## PATHOPHYSIOLOGY AND MANIFESTATIONS

COPD is characterized by slowly progressive obstruction of the airways. The disease is one of periodic exacerbations, often related to respiratory infection, with increased symptoms of dyspnea and sputum production. Unlike acute processes in which lung tissues recover, airways and lung parenchyma do not return to normal following an exacerbation; instead, they demonstrate progressive destructive changes.

Although one or the other may predominate, COPD typically includes components of both chronic bronchitis and emphysema, two distinctly different processes. Chronic asthma is also often present. Through different mechanisms, these processes cause airways to narrow, resistance to airflow to increase, and expiration to become slow or difficult (Figure 36–10 ■). The result is a mismatch between alveolar ventilation and blood flow or perfusion, leading to impaired gas exchange.

The clinical presentation of COPD varies from simple chronic bronchitis without disability to chronic respiratory failure and severe disability. Manifestations are typically absent or minor early in the disease. When the client finally seeks care, productive cough, dyspnea, and exercise intolerance often have been present for as long as 10 years. The cough typically occurs in the mornings and often is attributed to "smoker's cough." Initially, dyspnea occurs only on extreme exertion; as the disease progresses, dyspnea becomes more severe and accompanies mild activity. Manifestations characteristic of chronic bronchi-

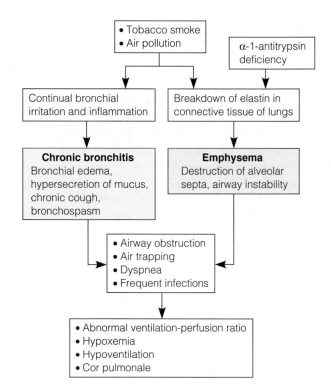

**Figure 36–10 ■** The pathogenesis of chronic obstructive pulmonary disease.

tis and emphysema develop. The clinical features and manifestations of COPD are summarized in Table 36–7.

## Chronic Bronchitis

**Chronic bronchitis** is a disorder of excessive bronchial mucus secretion. It is characterized by a productive cough lasting 3 or more months in 2 consecutive years (Porth, 2002). Cigarette smoke is the major factor implicated in the development of chronic bronchitis.

Inhaled irritants lead to a chronic inflammatory process with vasodilation, congestion, and edema of the bronchial mucosa. Thick, tenacious mucus is produced in increased amounts. Narrowed airways and excess secretions obstruct airflow; expiration is affected first, then inspiration. Because ciliary function is impaired, normal defense mechanisms are unable to clear the mucus and any inhaled pathogens. Recurrent infection is common in chronic bronchitis. An imbalance between ventilation and perfusion leads to hypoxemia, hypercapnia, and pulmonary hypertension. Pulmonary hypertension often leads to right-sided heart failure.

Manifestations of chronic bronchitis are a cough productive of copious amounts of thick, tenacious sputum, cyanosis, and evidence of right-sided heart failure, including distended neck veins, edema, liver engorgement, and an enlarged heart. Adventitious sounds, including loud rhonchi and possible wheezes, are prominent on auscultation.

## Emphysema

**Emphysema** is characterized by destruction of the walls of the alveoli, with resulting enlargement of abnormal air spaces. As

**TABLE 36–7   Clinical Features and Manifestations of COPD**

| | Feature | Chronic Bronchitis | Emphysema |
|---|---|---|---|
| History | Onset<br>Smoking<br>Cough | After age 35; recurrent respiratory infections<br>Usual<br>Persistent, productive of copious mucopurulent sputum | After age 50; insidious progressive dyspnea<br>Usual<br>Absent or mild with scant clear sputum, if any |
| Physical Examination | Appearance<br><br><br>Chest | Often obese; edematous and cyanotic; distended neck veins and other symptoms of right-sided heart failure<br>Adventitious sounds with wheezing and rhonchi; normal percussion note | Usually thin and cachectic; barrel chest; prominent accessory muscles of respiration<br>Distant or diminished breath sounds; hyperresonant percussion note |
| Other Features | Blood gases<br><br>Pulmonary function studies<br>Pulmonary hypertension | Hypercapnia and hypoxemia; respiratory acidosis<br>Normal or decreased total lung capacity; moderately increased residual volume<br>May be severe | Normal or mild hypoxemia; normal pH<br><br>Increased total lung capacity; markedly increased residual volume<br>Only when advanced |

in chronic bronchitis, cigarette smoking is strongly implicated as a causative factor in most cases of emphysema. Deficiency of alpha₁-antitrypsin, an enzyme that normally inhibits the activity of proteolytic enzymes and tissue destruction in the lungs, leads to an early onset of emphysema, often before age 40 (Braunwald et al., 2001).

Alveolar wall destruction causes alveoli and air spaces to enlarge with loss of corresponding portions of the pulmonary capillary bed. As a result, the surface area for alveolar-capillary diffusion is reduced, affecting gas exchange. Elastic recoil is lost, reducing the volume of air that is passively expired. The loss of support tissue also affects airways, increasing the risk of expiratory collapse and further air trapping. Anatomically, either respiratory bronchioles or alveoli may be the primary tissue involved.

Emphysema is insidious in onset. Dyspnea is the initial symptom. Initially occurring only with exertion, dyspnea may progress to become severe even at rest. Cough is minimal or absent. Air trapping and hyperinflation increase the anterior-posterior chest diameter, causing *barrel chest.* The client often is thin, tachypneic, uses accessory muscles of respiration and often assumes a position of sitting and leaning forward (Figure 36–11 ■). The expiratory phase of the respiratory cycle is prolonged. On auscultation, breath sounds are diminished, and the percussion tone is hyperresonant.

## COLLABORATIVE CARE

Although COPD can be prevented in most people, it cannot be cured. Smoking abstinence is the only certain way to prevent COPD and to slow its progression. To a certain extent, airway obstruction can be reversed and disability minimized early in the disease. Treatment generally focuses on relieving symptoms, minimizing obstruction, and slowing disability.

## Diagnostic Tests

Diagnostic tests are used to help establish the diagnosis of chronic obstructive pulmonary disease and identify the predominant component, emphysema or chronic bronchitis. These procedures also are used to assess respiratory status and monitor treatment effectiveness.

* *Pulmonary function testing* is performed to establish the diagnosis and evaluate the extent and progress of COPD (see Box 36–1). Fasting is not required for this noninvasive test; however, tobacco products, bronchodilators, and eating a heavy meal should be avoided for 4 to 6 hours prior to testing. Results are based on calculated norms for each person

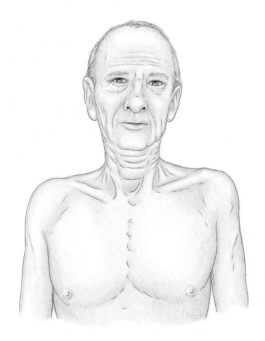

**Figure 36–11** ■ Typical appearance of a client with emphysema.

by age, height, sex, and weight; note these as well as all current medications on the requisition. In COPD, the total lung capacity and residual volume typically are increased. The forced expiratory volume ($FEV_1$) and forced vital capacity (FVC) are decreased due to narrowed airways and resistance to airflow.

- *Ventilation-perfusion scanning* may be performed to determine the extent of ventilation/perfusion mismatch—that is, the extent to which lung tissue is ventilated but not perfused (dead space), or perfused but inadequately ventilated (physiologic shunting). A radioisotope is injected or inhaled to illustrate areas of shunting and absent capillaries (Figure 36–12 ■).
- *Serum alpha₁-antitrypsin levels* may be drawn to screen for deficiency, particularly in clients with a family history of obstructive airway disease, those with an early onset, women, and nonsmokers. Normal adult serum alpha₁-antitrypsin levels range from 80 to 260 mg/dL. Fasting is not required prior to this test.
- *Arterial blood gases (ABGs)* are drawn to evaluate gas exchange, particularly during acute exacerbations of COPD. Clients with predominant emphysema often have mild hypoxemia and normal or low carbon dioxide tension. Respiratory alkalosis may be present due to an increased respiratory rate. Predominant chronic bronchitis and airway obstruction may cause marked hypoxemia and hypercapnia with respiratory acidosis. Oxygen saturation levels are low due to marked hypoxemia. See page 122 for steps to interpret ABGs.

**PRACTICE ALERT** *Hypercapnia (elevated $Paco_2$ levels) often is chronic in clients with COPD. This reduces the stimulatory effect of the $Paco_2$ and pH on the respiratory center; instead, breathing is driven by a fall in arterial oxygen levels. Administering oxygen can lead to respiratory arrest because the drive to breathe is suppressed.* ■

- *Pulse oximetry* is used to monitor oxygen saturation of the blood. Marked airway obstruction and hypoxemia often causes oxygen saturation levels less than 95%. Pulse oximetry may be continuously monitored to assess the need for supplemental oxygen.
- *Exhaled carbon dioxide (capnogram or $ETco_2$)* may be measured to evaluate alveolar ventilation. The normal $ETco_2$ reading is 35 to 45 mmHg; it is elevated when ventilation is inadequate, and decreased when pulmonary perfusion is impaired. $ETco_2$ monitoring can reduce the frequency of ABG determinations.
- *CBC with WBC differential* often shows increased RBCs and hematocrit (erythrocytosis) as chronic hypoxia stimulates increased erythropoiesis to increase the oxygen-carrying capacity of the blood. *Polycythemia,* increased numbers of all blood cells, may be evident. Increased WBC count and a higher percentage of immature WBCs (bands) are often indicative of bacterial infection.
- *Chest X-ray* may show flattening of the diaphragm due to hyperinflation and evidence of pulmonary infection if present.

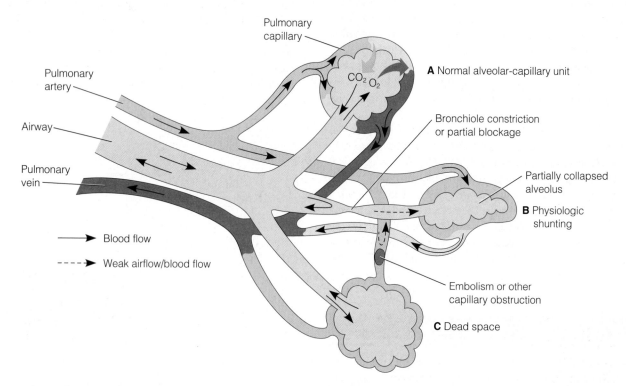

**Figure 36–12** ■ Ventilation-perfusion relationships. *A,* Normal alveolar-capillary unit with an ideal match of ventilation and blood flow. Maximum gas exchange occurs between alveolus and blood. *B,* Physiologic shunting: A unit with adequate perfusion but inadequate ventilation. *C,* Dead space: A unit with adequate ventilation but inadequate perfusion. In the latter two cases, gas exchange is impaired.

## Smoking Cessation

Smoking cessation can not only prevent COPD from developing, but also can improve lung function once the disease has been diagnosed. Forced expiratory volume ($FEV_1$) improves, and survival is prolonged, largely due to lower rates of lung cancer and heart disease. Sustained quitting is difficult; only 6% of smokers succeed in long-term abstinence from smoking (Braunwald et al., 2001). Use of nicotine patches or gum and an antidepressant such as bupropion (Wellbutrin, Zyban) improve the chances of success.

## Medications

Immunization against pneumococcal pneumonia and yearly influenza vaccine are recommended to reduce the risk of respiratory infections. A broad-spectrum antibiotic is prescribed if infection is suspected. Recent studies indicate that clients with purulent sputum and increased dyspnea will likely benefit from antibiotic therapy, even if no other signs of infection are present. Prophylactic antibiotics may be ordered for clients who experience four or more disease exacerbations per year (Braunwald et al., 2001).

Bronchodilators improve airflow and reduce air trapping in COPD, resulting in improved dyspnea and exercise tolerance. Bronchodilators may be given by metered-dose inhaler (MDI), by nebulizer, or orally. Oral administration may promote adherence, but is associated with much higher rates of adverse effects. A spacer or holding chamber may facilitate effective use of an MDI. Ipratropium bromide, an anticholinergic agent administered by MDI, is frequently prescribed. It has a longer duration of action than the short-acting $\beta_2$-adrenergic stimulant bronchodilators and few side effects. Salmeterol, a longer-acting $\beta_2$ agonist, may be used in combination therapy. Oral theophylline, a methylxanthine, is a weak bronchodilator and has a narrow therapeutic range, but often is prescribed for its other effects. Theophylline stimulates the respiratory drive, strengthens diaphragmatic contractions, and improves cardiac output. As a result, dyspnea, exercise tolerance, and quality of life improve for the client with COPD. Bronchodilators are discussed in further detail in the section on asthma, and their nursing implications are outlined in the box on page 1110.

Corticosteroid therapy may be used when asthma is a major component of COPD. It also improves symptoms and exercise tolerance, and may reduce the severity of exacerbations and the need for hospitalization. Oral corticosteroids, such as prednisone, are used initially. If a beneficial response occurs, the amount is reduced to the lowest effective dose. Every-other-day dosing or administration by inhaler is preferred to minimize steroid side effects, such as cushingoid effects and an increased risk for osteoporosis and vertebral fractures.

Alpha$_1$-antitrypsin ($\alpha_1$AT) replacement therapy is available for clients with emphysema due to a genetic deficiency of the enzyme. Although expensive and inconvenient ($\alpha_1$AT is administered weekly by intravenous infusion), it has been shown to reduce the rate of airflow decline and mortality.

## Treatments

In addition to refraining from smoking, exposure to other airway irritants and allergens should be avoided. The client should remain indoors during periods of significant air pollution to prevent exacerbations of the disease. Air filtering systems or air conditioning may be useful.

Pulmonary hygiene measures, including hydration, effective cough, percussion, and postural drainage, are used to improve clearance of airway secretions. Maintaining adequate systemic hydration is essential to keep secretions thin. Forceful coughing is often less effective than leaning forward and repeatedly "huffing," with relaxed breathing between huffs. Percussion and postural drainage may be necessary if the client is unable to clear secretions by usual means. Cough suppressants and sedatives generally are avoided as they may cause retention of secretions.

Unless disabling cardiac disease is present, a regular exercise program is beneficial in:

- Improving exercise tolerance.
- Enhancing ability to perform activities of daily living.
- Preventing deterioration of physical condition.

A program of regular aerobic exercise (e.g., walking for 20 minutes at least three times weekly) designed to gradually increase exercise tolerance is recommended. Activities that strengthen the muscles used for breathing and ADLs, such as swimming and golf, also are beneficial. See the Nursing Research box on page 1118.

Breathing exercises are used to slow the respiratory rate and relieve accessory muscle fatigue. Pursed-lip breathing slows the respiratory rate and helps maintain open airways during exhalation by keeping positive pressure in the airways. Abdominal breathing relieves the work of accessory muscles of respiration.

### Oxygen

Long-term oxygen therapy is used for severe and progressive hypoxemia. Oxygen therapy improves exercise tolerance, mental functioning, and quality of life in advanced COPD. It also reduces the rate of hospitalization and increases length of survival. Oxygen may be used intermittently, at night, or continuously. For severely hypoxemic clients, the greatest benefit is seen with continuous oxygen. Home oxygen may be supplied as liquid oxygen, compressed gas cylinders, or oxygen concentrators.

An acute exacerbation of COPD may necessitate oxygenation and inspiratory positive-pressure assistance with a face mask or intubation and mechanical ventilation. Oxygen administered without intubation and mechanical ventilation requires caution: Chronic elevated carbon dioxide levels in the blood inhibit this normal stimulus to breathe, leaving only the stimulus of low blood oxygen tension. Oxygen administered at high flow rates or a high percentage can reduce this stimulus, leading to respiratory insufficiency or arrest.

### Surgery

When medical therapy is no longer effective, lung transplantation may be an option. Both single and bilateral transplants

## Nursing Research

### Evidence-Based Practice for the Client with COPD

The correlation between physical activity and performance of essential activities of daily living, quality of life, and higher level functioning is well established. This is particularly true for the elderly and people with disease-related impairment in physical abilities. Physical inactivity is both a cause and an effect of declining physical function in the elderly. A study by Belza, Steele, Hunziker, Lakshminaryan, Holt, and Buchner (2001) sought to describe the relationships between functional performance measured as physical activity, functional capacity, symptoms, and health-related quality of life in a group of clients with chronic obstructive pulmonary disease.

A number of variables were used to evaluate physical activity and functional capacity (degree of airways obstruction, exercise capacity, and self-sufficiency in walking). Physical activity was not found to correlate well with self-reported functional status. A 6-minute walk test was, however, identified as a good predictor of physical activity and symptom severity.

### IMPLICATIONS FOR NURSING

Although this study is preliminary and replication of the results is necessary to generalize its findings, it supports a program of regular physical activity as a measure to maintain functional status and reduce symptom progression. Encourage COPD clients to enroll in a pulmonary rehabilitation program if one is available. If there is no organized program in the area, work with a pulmonologist, respiratory therapist, and physical therapist to develop an exercise program for clients with COPD.

### Critical Thinking in Nursing

1. Why do you think the 6-minute walk test was found to be a better measure of physical activity than the clients' self-reports?
2. Use the physiologic and psychologic effects of regular exercise to explain the correlation between the 6-minute walk test and improved symptoms in the client with COPD.
3. Consider the age of most clients with COPD. What other physical or psychosocial factors commonly limit physical activity in this population? How can you use this information in designing an appropriate exercise program?

---

have been performed successfully, with a 2-year survival rate of 75%. Lung reduction surgery is an experimental surgical intervention for advanced diffuse emphysema and lung hyperinflation. The procedure reduces the overall volume of the lung, reshapes it, and improves elastic recoil. As a result, pulmonary function and exercise tolerance improve and dyspnea is reduced. See the box on page 1140 for nursing care of the client undergoing lung surgery.

## Complementary Therapies

Complementary therapies may be useful to help manage symptoms of COPD. Dietary measures such as minimizing intake of dairy products and salt may help reduce mucous production and to keep mucus more liquefied. Be sure to recommend measures to replace the protein and calcium in dairy products to help maintain nutritional balance.

Herbal teas made with peppermint and yarrow, coltsfoot, or comfrey may act as expectorants to help relieve chest congestion. Licorice root, which may be taken in several forms, also has expectorant and anti-inflammatory effects that may be beneficial. Licorice root can, however, cause toxicity when used for extended periods of time. Refer clients to a qualified herbalist for treatment.

Acupuncture may help the client with smoking cessation, and also has been used to treat asthma and other respiratory conditions. Hypnotherapy and guided imagery are used to assist with smoking cessation. These techniques also can help the client control anxiety and breathing patterns. Refer clients to a trained professional. Nurses, physicians, psychologists, counselors, social workers and others can take professional training in hypnotherapy and guided imagery (Fontaine, 2000).

## NURSING CARE

### Health Promotion

Not smoking—never start, or quit—is the best preventive measure for chronic obstructive pulmonary disease. Even in clients with COPD, smoking cessation improves lung function and increases survival. Educate all clients, including preschool and school-age children, about the risks of smoking. See Box 36–4.

### Assessment

Focused assessment for the client with chronic obstructive pulmonary disease includes:

- Health history: current symptoms, including cough, sputum production, shortness of breath or dyspnea, activity tolerance; frequency of respiratory infections and most recent episode; previous diagnosis of emphysema, chronic bronchitis, or asthma; current medications; smoking history (in pack years—packs per day times number of years smoked), history of exposure to secondhand smoke, occupational or other pollutants
- Physical examination: general appearance, weight for height, mental status; vital signs including temperature; skin color and temperature; anterior-posterior:lateral chest diameter, use of accessory muscles, nasal flaring or pursed-lip breathing; respiratory excursion and diaphragmatic excursion; percussion tone; breath sounds throughout; neck veins, apical pulse and heart sounds, peripheral pulses, edema

## BOX 36–4    ■ Cigarette Smoking and Tobacco Use

The use of tobacco reaches back to early civilizations, when it was used in religious ceremonies and as an offering of friendship. At one time, tobacco was thought to have medicinal qualities effective against all common diseases. Widespread use of tobacco among the male population of the industrialized world began during World War I.

Tobacco is now recognized as the leading cause of preventable illness in the world. In spite of this knowledge, aggressive marketing of the product continues, and its worldwide use is increasing, especially in underdeveloped countries.

The link between tobacco use and lung cancer was reported as early as 1912. In 1987, lung cancer became the leading cause of cancer-related death in the United States among both men and women.

Cigarette smoke contains approximately 4000 chemicals, including nicotine. Nicotine is a highly addictive psychoactive substance that is relatively cheap and readily available. It produces euphoria, which acts as a positive reinforcer for continued use. In North American society, tobacco is more acceptable than many other dependency-producing drugs.

Tar is the particulate matter in cigarette smoke that is responsible for most of its carcinogenic and pathologic effects on the lungs. Smoke also paralyzes the cilia, reducing their ability to remove tars from contact with the respiratory epithelium. The risk for cancer and other lung diseases is dose related, affected by the age at which smoking began, the number of cigarettes smoked per day, and the number of years smoked. Smoking cessation reduces the risks associated with tobacco use. For some, such as the risk of coronary heart disease, quitting smoking yields rapid benefits. For others, the degree of risk reduction is less immediate, but still significant.

Nurses need to do more than simply advise clients to quit smoking and talk about the risks of smoking. Nurses can take an active role in smoking cessation. Identify smoking habits, smoking-related illnesses, and previous efforts to quit. Work with the client to identify barriers and obstacles to quitting. Educate about the addictive nature of nicotine, and explain the manifestations of nicotine withdrawal (anxiety, irritability, headache, and disturbed sleep). Develop a plan with the client that specifies a target date to quit and includes ways to deal with obstacles to quitting, withdrawal symptoms, and the temptation to resume smoking. Offer self-help material at an appropriate reading level. Refer to a counselor, physician, self-help group, or smoking cessation clinic. If a relapse occurs, accept it as a normal part of rehabilitation from any addictive substance. Continue to provide support and encouragement, helping the client avoid further relapses.

Nurses can be especially effective in primary prevention of cigarette smoking and the diseases associated with it. Just as tobacco companies direct advertising at women and teens, nurses can target these populations and younger children for programs to prevent smoking. In addition, nurses need to become active in reducing minors' access to tobacco products, especially cigarettes and chewing tobacco (often the first product used by teens).

Nursing diagnoses that may be appropriate related to smoking include the following:

- *Ineffective health maintenance* related to tobacco use
- *Decisional conflict* related to tobacco use
- *Ineffective denial* related to acknowledgment of substance abuse and dependence

## Nursing Diagnoses and Interventions

Clients with chronic obstructive pulmonary disease, whether hospitalized or in the community, have multiple nursing care needs. Because of the obstructive nature of the disease, airway clearance is a high priority. Nutritional deficit is common, particularly when emphysema is predominant. Because this chronic disease affects all functional health patterns, psychosocial issues are also of concern in planning nursing care.

### Ineffective Airway Clearance

Both chronic bronchitis and emphysema affect the ability to maintain open airways. In chronic bronchitis, copious amounts of thick, tenacious mucus are produced. Ciliary action is impaired, making it difficult to clear mucus from the airways. The loss of supporting tissue caused by emphysema increases the the risk for airway collapse. In both cases, air is trapped distally, and less oxygen is available to the alveoli for diffusion. Normal respiratory defense mechanisms are impaired, and mucus-plugged airways provide an ideal environment for bacterial growth. Respiratory infection further impairs airway clearance and is often the cause of an acute exacerbation.

- Assess respiratory status every 1 to 2 hours or as indicated. Assess rate and pattern; cough and secretions (color, amount,

consistency, and odor); and breath sounds, both normal and adventitious. *Frequent assessment is vital to monitor current status and response to treatment. Adventitious sounds should decrease with effective intervention. Diminished or absent breath sounds may indicate increasing airway obstruction and possible atelectasis.*

**PRACTICE ALERT** *Promptly report changes in oxygen saturation, skin color, or mental status. A drop in oxygen saturation levels, increasing cyanosis, or altered level of consciousness indicate hypoxemia, possibly related to airway obstruction.* ■

- Monitor arterial blood gas results. *Increasing hypoxemia, hypercapnia, and respiratory acidosis may indicate increasing airway obstruction.*
- Weigh daily, monitor intake and output, and assess mucous membranes and skin turgor. *Dehydration causes respiratory secretions to become thicker, more tenacious, and difficult to expectorate; fluid overload can further compromise respiratory status.*
- Encourage a fluid intake of at least 2000 to 2500 mL per day unless contraindicated. *Adequate fluid intake helps keep mucous secretions thin.*

- Place in Fowler's, high-Fowler's, or orthopneic position; encourage movement and activity to tolerance. *Upright positions improve ventilation and reduce the work of breathing. Activity helps mobilize secretions and prevent them from pooling.*
- Assist with coughing and deep breathing at least every 2 hours while awake. Position seated upright, leaning forward during coughing. *The upright position promotes chest expansion, increasing the effectiveness of coughing and reducing the work involved.*
- Provide tissues and a paper bag to dispose of expectorated sputum. *This important infection control measure reduces the spread of respiratory organisms to other people.*
- Refer to a respiratory therapist, and assist with or perform percussion and postural drainage as needed. *Percussion helps loosen secretions in airways; postural drainage facilitates movement of these secretions out of the respiratory tract.*

**PRACTICE ALERT** *Provide endotracheal, oral, or nasopharyngeal suctioning as necessary. Suctioning may be necessary to stimulate cough and help clear secretions.* ■

- Provide rest periods between treatments and procedures. *The client with COPD fatigues easily; adequate rest is important to conserve energy and reduce fatigue.*
- Administer expectorant and bronchodilator medications as ordered. Correlate timing with respiratory treatments. *Using expectorants and bronchodilators prior to coughing, percussion, and postural drainage increases their effectiveness in clearing airways.*
- Provide supplemental oxygen as ordered. *Supplemental oxygen helps maintain adequate blood and tissue oxygenation.*

**PRACTICE ALERT** *Prepare for intubation and mechanical ventilation if respiratory status deteriorates (increasing hypoxemia and hypercapnia, decreased level of consciousness, cyanosis, or worsening airway obstruction). Respiratory failure is a possible complication of an acute exacerbation of COPD and requires immediate intervention to preserve life.* ■

## Imbalanced Nutrition: Less Than Body Requirements

With advanced COPD, minimal activity, including eating, can cause fatigue and dyspnea. The client may be unable to consume a full meal without resting. At the same time, the increased work of breathing increases metabolic demands, and more calories are required. The client may appear cachectic (thin and wasted). Poor nutritional status further impairs immune function and increases the risk of a complicating infection.

- Assess nutritional status, including diet history, weight for height (use reference tables of desired weights), and anthropometric (skinfold) measurements. *It is important to differentiate nutritional status from body type rather than assume a nutritional impairment.*
- Observe and document food intake, including types, amounts, and caloric intake. *This information can provide direction for supplementation, if needed.*

- Monitor laboratory values, including serum albumin and electrolyte levels. *These values provide information about the adequacy of nutritional intake, including protein.*
- Consult with a dietitian to plan meals and nutritional supplements that meet caloric needs. *More concentrated sources of high-energy foods may be required to maintain caloric intake without excess fatigue. A diet high in proteins and fats without excess carbohydrates is recommended to minimize carbon dioxide production during metabolism (carbohydrates are metabolized to form $CO_2$ and water).*
- Provide frequent, small feedings with between-meal supplements. *Frequent, small meals help maintain intake and reduce fatigue associated with eating.*
- Place seated or in high-Fowler's position for meals. *An upright position promotes lung expansion and reduces dyspnea.*
- Assist to choose preferred foods from the menu; encourage family members to bring food from home if allowed. *Providing preferred foods encourages eating.*
- Keep snacks at the bedside. *Snacks provide additional caloric intake.*
- Provide mouth care prior to meals. *This helps enhance the appetite.*
- If unable to maintain oral intake, consult with the physician about enteral or parenteral feedings. *Maintenance of caloric and nutrient intake is vital to prevent catabolism.*

## Compromised Family Coping

Chronic illness affects the entire family structure. Roles and relationships change; additional demands are placed on the family. Family members may blame the client for causing the illness or have distorted perceptions about it, even denying its existence. They may refuse to assist or participate in care. The client may develop an attitude of helplessness or dependence or may demonstrate anger, hostility, or aggression.

- Assess interactions between client and family. *Assessment helps identify desired and potential destructive behaviors.*
- Assess the effect of the illness on the family. *Assessment of family interactions, roles, and relationships assists in planning appropriate interventions.*
- Help the client and family identify strengths for coping with the situation. *Identifying personal and family strengths helps the family regain a sense of control.*
- Provide information and teaching about COPD. *Education helps the family gain an understanding of the client's condition and needs.*
- Encourage expression of feelings. Avoid judging feelings expressed or family members as "good" or "bad," "right" or "wrong." *It is important that the nurse remain objective to maintain the therapeutic relationship.*
- Help family members recognize behaviors and attitudes that may hinder effective treatment, such as continuing to smoke in the house. *Family members may be unaware of the effect of their behavior on the client's ability to change habits and cope with a disabling disease.*
- Encourage family members to participate in care. *This helps develop skills for use at home.*

- Initiate a care conference involving the client, family, and health care team members from a variety of disciplines. *A wide range of perspectives and areas of expertise aids in problem solving and facilitates communication.*
- If dysfunctional family relationships interfere with measures to enhance coping, advocate for the client, reaffirming his or her right to make decisions. *Dysfunctional family relationships are not likely to change simply because of illness. The nurse can better meet the client's needs by accepting his or her limitations in dealing with family members.*
- Refer the client and family to support groups and pulmonary rehabilitation programs, as available. *Support groups and structured rehabilitation programs enhance coping abilities.*
- Arrange a social services consultation. *This can help the client and family identify care and support service needs.*
- Refer community agencies or services such as home health, homemaker services, or Meals-on-Wheels as appropriate. *Agencies or community services can provide additional support beyond the family's means or capability.*

### Decisional Conflict: Smoking

Smoking is more than a habit; it is an addiction. The client who must quit is facing a significant loss, not only of nicotine but also of a lifestyle. Although the client may fully comprehend the consequences of continuing to smoke, the decision to give up a part of his or her life is not easy. This fear may be expressed in such concerns as "I'll gain weight," or "What will I do with my hands?" In addition to providing practical information, a plan, and assistance with nicotine withdrawal, the nurse must support the client's decision-making process to comply with an order to stop smoking.

- Assess knowledge and understanding of the choices involved and possible consequences of each. *The decision to quit smoking ultimately belongs to the client. He or she needs a full understanding of the consequences of quitting or continuing to smoke.*
- Acknowledge concerns, values, and beliefs; listen nonjudgmentally. *The nurse needs to avoid imposing his or her values and beliefs about smoking on the client.*
- Spend time with the client, encouraging expression of feelings. *This demonstrates acceptance of the client and his or her right to make the decision.*
- Help plan a course of action for quitting smoking and adapt it as necessary. *When the client develops the plan, he or she has more ownership in it and interest in making it work.*
- Demonstrate respect for decisions and the right to choose. *Respect supports self-esteem and the ability to cope.*
- Provide referral to a counselor or other professional as needed. *Counselors or other people trained to assist with smoking cessation can help with decision making.*

## Using NANDA, NIC, and NOC

Chart 36–3 shows links between NANDA nursing diagnoses, NIC, and NOC for the client with COPD.

## Home Care

As with any chronic disease, the client and family will have primary responsibility for disease management. Teaching is vital to promote optimal health and slow disease progression. Teaching for home care focuses on effective coughing and breathing techniques, preventing exacerbations, and managing prescribed therapies.

### CHART 36–3 NANDA, NIC, AND NOC LINKAGES

#### The Client with COPD

| NURSING DIAGNOSES | NURSING INTERVENTIONS | NURSING OUTCOMES |
| --- | --- | --- |
| • Anxiety | • Anxiety Reduction<br>• Coping Enhancement | • Anxiety Control<br>• Coping |
| • Decisional Conflict | • Decision-Making Support<br>• Health System Guidance | • Decision Making<br>• Participation: Health Care Decisions |
| • Imbalanced Nutrition: Less than Body Requirements | • Nutrition Management<br>• Weight Gain Assistance | • Nutritional Status: Food and Fluid Intake |
| • Ineffective Airway Clearance | • Airway Management<br>• Cough Enhancement<br>• Oxygen Therapy<br>• Respiratory Monitoring | • Respiratory Status: Airway Patency<br>• Respiratory Status: Gas Exchange |
| • Ineffective Breathing Pattern | • Energy Management<br>• Positioning | • Respiratory Status: Ventilation<br>• Vital Signs Status |
| • Ineffective Health Maintenance | • Self-Responsibility Facilitation<br>• Teaching: Disease Process | • Self-Direction of Care<br>• Treatment Behavior: Illness or Injury |

*Note. Data from Nursing Outcomes Classification (NOC) by M. Johnson & M. Maas (Eds.), 1997, St. Louis: Mosby; Nursing Diagnoses: Definitions & Classification 2001–2002 by North American Nursing Diagnosis Association, 2001, Philadelphia: NANDA; Nursing Interventions Classification (NIC) by J.C. McCloskey & G. M. Bulechek (Eds.), 2000, St. Louis: Mosby. Reprinted by permission.*

## THE CLIENT WITH ATELECTASIS

**Atelectasis** is not a disease but a condition associated with many respiratory disorders. It is a state of partial or total lung collapse and airlessness. It may be acute or chronic. The most common cause of atelectasis is obstruction of the bronchus ventilating a segment of lung tissue. The affected segment may be small or an entire lobe. Other causes include compression of the lung by pneumothorax, pleural effusion, or tumor; or loss of pulmonary surfactant and inability to maintain open alveoli.

The manifestations of atelectasis depend on its size. Diminished breath sounds over the affected area may be the only sign of a small atelectasis. If a large lung segment is affected, manifestations may include tachycardia, tachypnea, dyspnea, cyanosis, and other signs of hypoxemia. Chest expansion may be reduced and breath sounds absent on the affected side. Fever and other manifestations of infection may be present.

Chest X-ray shows an area of airless lung. CT scan may help determine the cause of atelectasis.

The primary therapy for atelectasis is prevention. High risk clients, such as those with COPD, smokers undergoing surgery, and people on prolonged bed rest or mechanical ventilation, should have vigorous chest physiotherapy to maintain open airways. Frequently assess respiratory status, including rate, breath sounds, and spirometry readings for early detection and treatment.

When atelectasis develops, treatment focuses on the underlying cause. Vigorous coughing and chest therapy may relieve obstruction by a mucus plug. Bronchoscopy may be necessary to remove the obstruction. Antibiotic therapy is ordered to treat infectious causes.

Nursing care to prevent and treat atelectasis is directed toward airway clearance. Position the client with atelectasis on the unaffected side to promote gravity drainage of affected segment. Encourage frequent position changes, ambulation, coughing, and deep breathing. Unless contraindicated, encourage fluids to help liquefy secretions. Teach the client at high risk for developing atelectasis about pulmonary care measures, fluid intake, and preventing pulmonary infections.

## THE CLIENT WITH BRONCHIECTASIS

**Bronchiectasis** is characterized by permanent abnormal dilation of one or more large bronchi and destruction of bronchial walls. Infection often is present. The destructive process of bronchiectasis is initiated by inflammation, usually due to recurrent airways infection. About half of all cases of bronchiectasis are related to cystic fibrosis. Other causes include infections, such as severe pneumonia, tuberculosis, or fungal infections; lung abscess; exposure to toxic gases; abnormal lung or immunologic defenses; and localized airway obstruction due to a foreign body or tumor. Inflammation and airway obstruction are common to all these processes. Bronchial walls become weakened and dilated as a result, leading to pooling of secretions and further infection and inflammation.

A chronic cough productive of large amounts of mucopurulent sputum is characteristic. Other manifestations of bronchiectasis include hemoptysis, recurrent pneumonia, wheezing and shortness of breath, malnutrition, right-sided heart failure, and cor pulmonale.

Collaborative care for bronchiectasis focuses on maintaining optimal pulmonary function and preventing progression of the disorder. The diagnosis is typically based on the history and physical examination. Chest X-ray and CT scan may be ordered to help confirm the diagnosis and determine the extent of lung damage.

Antibiotics are prescribed at the first indication of infection and may also be used prophylactically. Inhaled bronchodilators may be ordered. Chest physiotherapy is a vital component of continuing care for bronchiectasis. Percussion and postural drainage help mobilize secretions. Oxygen may be prescribed. Bronchoscopy may be used to clear retained secretions or obstruction or to evaluate hemoptysis. If lung destruction is localized and unresponsive to conservative management, surgical lung resection may be necessary.

Nursing care of the client with bronchiectasis is similar to that for clients with other obstructive lung diseases. Airway clearance is a primary problem, as is ineffective breathing pattern. Other applicable nursing diagnoses may include Impaired Gas Exchange, Imbalanced Nutrition: Less Than Body Requirements and Self-Care Deficit.

# INTERSTITIAL PULMONARY DISORDERS

Many lung diseases damage the interstitial or connective tissue of the lung. Occupational lung diseases and sarcoidosis are interstitial lung diseases. Toxic drugs and radiation also cause interstitial damage. Table 36–8 identifies common causes of interstitial lung disorders.

These disorders may be acute or insidious. Their rate of progression varies from person to person, as does the degree of disability they produce.

## THE CLIENT WITH AN OCCUPATIONAL LUNG DISEASE

Occupational lung diseases are a diverse group of disorders directly related to inhalation of noxious substances in the work environment. There are two major classifications of occupational lung diseases:

| TABLE 36–8 | Selected Causes of Interstitial Lung Disorders |
| --- | --- |
| **Cause** | **Examples** |
| Inorganic dusts | Silica (silicosis), asbestos (asbestosis), coal (coal workers' pneumoconioses), talc (talcosis) |
| Organic dusts | Cotton (byssinosis), sugar cane (bagassosis), moldy hay (farmer's lung) |
| Drugs | Antineoplastic agents, antibiotics, gold salts, phenytoin |
| Radiation | External radiation or inhaled radioactive materials |
| Infections | Widespread TB or fungal infections, viral or *Pneumocystis carinii* pneumonia |
| Poisons and noxious gases | Paraquat, nitrogen dioxide, chlorine, ammonia, sulfur dioxide |
| Systemic diseases | Uremia, pulmonary edema |
| Unknown causes | Sarcoidosis, idiopathic pulmonary fibrosis, connective tissue disorders |

- *Pneumoconioses,* chronic fibrotic lung diseases caused by inhalation of inorganic dusts and particulate matter
- *Hypersensitivity pneumonitis,* allergic pulmonary diseases caused by exposure to inhaled organic dusts

## PHYSIOLOGY REVIEW

Lung tissue contains elastin and collagen fibers. Elastin fibers are easily stretched, facilitating lung expansion. Collagen fibers, in contrast, resist stretching. This increases the work of breathing. Both elastin and collagen affect lung compliance, or the ease with which the lungs are inflated. Other factors affecting compliance include the water content of lung tissue and surface tension (Porth, 2002).

## PATHOPHYSIOLOGY

When a noxious substance is inhaled, the response to that substance depends on:

- The size of particulates;
- Its nature (organic or inorganic);
- Where it deposits in the respiratory tract; and
- The susceptibility of the individual.

Relatively large particles, larger than 6 microns, are too big to reach lower airways and often are deposited in the nose. Smaller particles can be carried with inspired air into the alveoli. Normal lung defenses, including alveolar macrophages, lymph channels, and the mucociliary escalator, attempt to remove particulate matter from the alveoli. Cigarette smoking, alcohol ingestion, or hypersensitivity reactions can impair these defenses.

The inhaled substance damages alveolar epithelium, leading to an inflammatory process of the alveoli and interstitial tissue of the lung. The inflammatory response produces further damage, and abnormal fibrotic (scar) tissue replaces the elastin fibers of normal lung tissue. As a result, the lungs become stiff and noncompliant. Lung volumes decrease, the work of breathing increases, and alveolar-capillary diffusion is impaired, leading to hypoxemia.

## Asbestosis

Inhalation of asbestos fibers is a common cause of occupational lung disease. *Asbestosis* is a diffuse interstitial fibrotic disease involving the terminal airways, alveoli, and pleurae. Exposure to asbestos fibers occurs during mining, milling, manufacturing, and application of asbestos products. Although symptoms may not become apparent until 20 years after exposure, they tend to progress, even when further exposure has been halted. Asbestosis is also associated with an increased risk of bronchogenic carcinoma, especially in cigarette smokers, malignant mesothelioma (an uncommon tumor of membranes such as the pleura and peritoneum), and pleural plaques (Tierney et al., 2001).

The manifestations of asbestosis include exertional dyspnea, exercise intolerance, and inspiratory crackles. Diffuse, small, irregular or linear opacities appear on chest X-ray, primarily in the lower lobes. As the disease progresses, respiratory failure and marked hypoxemia may develop.

## Silicosis

Inhalation of silica dust by hard-rock miners, foundry workers, sandblasters, pottery makers, and granite cutters can lead to *silicosis,* a nodular pulmonary fibrosis. Silicosis affects 1.2 to 3 million workers in the United States. Although generally associated with long-term exposure to silica, it can develop in as little as 10 months of intense exposure (Braunwald et al., 2001). In silicosis, macrophages are destroyed as they engulf silica particles, releasing substances that damage lung tissue and lead to fibrosis and scarring.

Simple silicosis is asymptomatic with no demonstrable respiratory impairment. Complicated silicosis, in contrast, is characterized by large conglomerate densities in the upper lungs. These clients may be severely dyspneic and have a productive cough. Pulmonary function testing shows both restrictive and obstructive changes. Increasing size of conglomerate masses can lead to severe disability, cor pulmonale, and death.

## Coal Worker's Pneumoconiosis

Ingestion of coal dust by alveolar macrophages causes "coal macules" to form, leading to *coal worker's pneumoconiosis,* or *"black lung disease."* This occupational lung disease affects 12% of all miners, with a higher incidence in the eastern United States than in the West (Braunwald et al., 2001). Coal macules appear on chest X-ray as diffuse, small opacities primarily affecting the upper lungs.

Simple coal worker's pneumoconiosis (CWP) generally is asymptomatic. A small percentage of clients (1% to 2%) develop progressive massive fibrosis which destroys the pulmonary vascular bed and airways of the upper lungs. This progressive form of the disease causes symptoms similar to those of complicated silicosis.

lining of the capillary, and a thin basement membrane between the alveolar and capillary cells. Oxygen and carbon dioxide readily diffuse across this very thin membrane. Diffusion is driven by a concentration gradient: The partial pressure of oxygen in the alveolus is greater than that in the capillary, therefore it diffuses into the blood. Carbon dioxide, in contrast, diffuses from the capillaries into the alveoli, driven by the higher pressure of dissolved carbon dioxide in venous blood.

A match between blood flow through the pulmonary vascular system (perfusion) and lung ventilation is necessary for effective *respiration* (the exchange of gases between the organism and the environment). Local factors regulate ventilation and perfusion to maintain this match. A low alveolar $PO_2$ causes alveolar capillary constriction, directing blood flow to areas of the lung where the alveolar $PO_2$ is higher. Likewise, high alveolar $PCO_2$ levels cause local bronchodilation, increasing airflow and eliminating excess carbon dioxide.

## PATHOPHYSIOLOGY

Thrombi affecting only the deep veins of the calf rarely embolize to the pulmonary circulation. However, thrombi often propogate proximally to the popliteal and ileofemoral veins. From there, they may break loose to become an embolus. As vessels of the venous system become progressively larger, the embolus rarely is trapped until it enters the pulmonary arterial system with its progressively smaller vessels leading to the pulmonary capillary beds.

The impact of a pulmonary embolus depends on the extent to which pulmonary blood flow is obstructed, the size of the embolus, its nature, and secondary effects of the obstruction. The effects can range widely:

- Occlusion of a large pulmonary artery with sudden death. Gas exchange is significantly reduced or prevented, and cardiac output falls dramatically as blood fails to move through the pulmonary vascular system and return to the left heart.
- Lung tissue infarction due to occlusion of a significant portion of pulmonary blood flow. Fewer than 10% of pulmonary emboli result in pulmonary infarction.
- Obstruction of a small segment of the pulmonary circulation with no permanent lung injury.
- Chronic or recurrent small emboli which may be multiple.

Obstruction of pulmonary blood flow by an embolus affects both perfusion and ventilation. Neurohumoral reflexes triggered by obstruction cause vasoconstriction, increasing pulmonary vascular resistance. In severe cases, this can lead to pulmonary hypertension and right ventricular heart failure. Systemically, hypotension and a drop in cardiac output may develop. Bronchoconstriction occurs in the affected area of lung. Dead space (areas of the lung that are ventilated but not perfused) increases. Alveolar surfactant decreases, increasing the risk for atelectasis.

If infarction does not occur, the fibrinolytic system (see Chapter 32) ultimately dissolves the clot, and pulmonary function returns to normal. Infarcted tissue becomes scarred and fibrotic.

Fat emboli are the most common nonthrombotic pulmonary emboli. A fat embolism usually occurs after fracture of long bone (typically the femur) releases bone marrow fat into the circulation. Adipose tissue or liver trauma may also lead to fat emboli.

## MANIFESTATIONS

The manifestations of pulmonary embolism depend on its size and location. Small emboli may be asymptomatic. Manifestations usually develop abruptly, over a period of minutes. The most common symptoms are dyspnea and pleuritic chest pain. Anxiety, a sense of impending doom, and cough are also common. See the box below. Diaphoresis and hemoptysis may develop. Massive pulmonary embolus can cause syncope and cyanosis. On examination, tachycardia and tachypnea are noted. Crackles may be heard on auscultation of the chest, and a cardiac gallop ($S_3$ and possibly $S_4$) may be noted. A low-grade fever may develop. It is difficult to differentiate pulmonary embolism from myocardial infarction or pneumonia by manifestations.

Characteristic manifestations of fat emboli include sudden onset of cardiopulmonary and neurologic symptoms: dyspnea, tachypnea, tachycardia, confusion, delirium, and decreased level of consciousness. Petechiae often develop on the chest and arms.

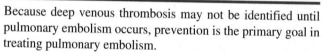

## COLLABORATIVE CARE

Because deep venous thrombosis may not be identified until pulmonary embolism occurs, prevention is the primary goal in treating pulmonary embolism.

Early ambulation of medical and surgical clients is an effective means of preventing venous stasis and reducing the incidence of pulmonary embolism. External pneumatic compression of the legs is also effective for clients undergoing neurosurgery, urologic surgery, or major surgery of the hip or knee, or when anticoagulant therapy is contraindicated. Other preventive measures include elevating the legs and active and passive leg exercises.

When pulmonary embolism occurs, treatment is supportive. Oxygen therapy is initiated, and analgesics may be ordered to relieve severe pleuritic pain and anxiety. Pulmonary artery and wedge pressures are monitored with a balloon (Swan-Ganz) catheter. Cardiac outputs also may be assessed. Cardiac rhythm is monitored to detect dysrhythmias.

| Manifestations of Pulmonary Embolism | |
|---|---|
| **COMMON** | |
| • Dyspnea and shortness of breath | • Cough |
| • Chest pain | • Tachycardia and tachypnea |
| • Anxiety and apprehension | • Crackles (rales) |
| | • Low-grade fever |
| **LESS COMMON** | |
| • Diaphoresis | • Cyanosis |
| • Hemoptysis | • $S_3$ and/or $S_4$ gallop |
| • Syncope | |

## Diagnostic Tests

The studies performed to identify DVT differ from those used to diagnose a pulmonary embolism. See Chapter 33 for diagnostic studies for venous thrombosis.

- *Plasma D-dimer levels* are highly specific to the presence of a thrombus. D-dimer is a fragment of fibrin formed during lysis of a blood clot; elevated blood levels indicate thrombus formation and lysis (e.g., DVT and pulmonary embolism).
- *Lung scans,* including perfusion and ventilation scans are performed, alone or in combination, to diagnose pulmonary embolism. In a perfusion lung scan, radiotagged albumin is injected intravenously and distributed in the lungs by the pulmonary blood flow. The lungs are then scanned for distribution of the isotope. An area of lung in which the isotope is undetectable is suggestive of occluded blood flow and pulmonary embolism (Figure 36–14 ■). For a ventilation scan, a radiotagged gas such as krypton or xenon-133 is inhaled. The lungs are scanned for gas distribution. Combined perfusion and ventilation scans allow identification of areas of the lungs that are ventilated but not perfused, a characteristic of pulmonary embolism.
- *Pulmonary angiography* is the definitive test for pulmonary embolism when other, less invasive tests are inconclusive. It is possible to detect very small emboli with angiography. A contrast medium injected into the pulmonary arteries illustrates the pulmonary vascular system on X-ray.
- *Chest X-ray* often shows pulmonary infiltration and occasionally pleural effusion.
- *Electrocardiogram (ECG)* is ordered to rule out acute myocardial infarction as the cause of symptoms. ECG findings commonly associated with pulmonary embolism include tachycardia and nonspecific T wave changes.
- *ABGs* usually show hypoxemia ($PO_2$ less than 80 mmHg), and often respiratory alkalosis (pH >7.45, $PCO_2$ <38 mmHg) due to tachypnea and hyperventilation.
- *Exhaled carbon dioxide ($ETCO_2$)* may be measured to evaluate alveolar perfusion. The normal $ETCO_2$ reading is 35 to 45 mmHg; it is decreased when pulmonary perfusion is impaired.
- *Coagulation studies* are ordered to monitor the response to therapy. The *activated partial thromboplastin time (aPTT or PTT)* is used to assess the intrinsic clotting pathway and the response to heparin therapy. Desired levels with anticoagulant therapy are 1.5 to 2 times the control value. The risk of recurrent thromboembolism is high at levels less than 1.5 times the control; the risk of bleeding increases at levels greater than 2 times the control. The *prothrombin time (PT or Pro-time)* or *International Normalized Ratio (INR)* is used to assess the extrinsic clotting system and oral anticoagulation with warfarin (Coumadin). The goal of anticoagulant therapy is to achieve a prothrombin time 1.25 to 1.5 times the control time. The therapeutic range for the INR is 2.0 to 3.0.

## Medications

Anticoagulant therapy is the standard treatment to prevent pulmonary emboli. It is often instituted in high-risk clients who have no evidence of pulmonary embolism, to prevent possible devastating effects. In the client with DVT or a pulmonary embolus, anticoagulants are administered to prevent further clotting and embolization. See Chapter 33 for more information about anticoagulant therapy to prevent and treat DVT. See the Medication Administration box on pages 1013 and 1014 for the nursing implications for anticoagulant therapy.

For pulmonary embolus, heparin therapy is initiated with an intravenous bolus of 5,000 to 10,000 units of heparin, followed by continuous infusion at the rate of 1000 to 1500 units per hour. The aPTT or PTT is monitored frequently until stabilized. Heparin therapy is typically continued for about 5 days or until oral anticoagulant therapy has become fully effective.

Oral anticoagulant therapy with warfarin sodium (Coumadin) is initiated at the same time as heparin. Warfarin alters the synthesis of vitamin K–dependent clotting factors and requires 5 to 7 days to be fully effective. Anticoagulant therapy is continued for 2 to 3 months when few risk factors for thromboemboli exist; long-term therapy is used when chronic disorders that increase the risk of thromboemboli are present.

Bleeding is a risk associated with anticoagulant therapy. Although major hemorrhage is uncommon, it occurs in approximately 5% of clients receiving intravenous heparin. Cardiac, hepatic, and renal disease increase the risk of significant bleeding, as does age over 60 years. Protamine, a protein that combines with heparin to inactivate it, is used to stop its anticoagulant effect if major bleeding occurs. Vitamin K is given to treat bleeding associated with Coumadin therapy.

Thrombolytic therapy may be used to treat massive pulmonary embolus and hypotension. Streptokinase, urokinase, or tissue plasminogen activator (t-PA) are used to *lyse* (disintegrate) the embolus, restore pulmonary blood flow, and reduce pulmonary artery and right heart pressures. Although thrombolytic therapy may not reduce mortality associated with pulmonary embolus, it may reduce the incidence of pulmonary hypertension, which develops 3 to 5 years after an embolism. Thrombolysis significantly increases the risk of bleeding, particularly cerebral bleeding. Contraindications to thrombolysis include intracranial disease, recent stroke, active bleeding or a bleeding disorder, pregnancy, severe hypertension, and recent

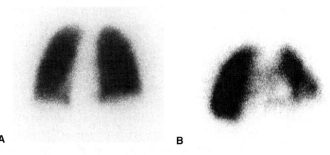

**A**        **B**

**Figure 36–14** ■ *A,* Normal perfusion lung scan showing smooth outlines and complete lung fields. *B,* Perfusion lung scan of a client with pulmonary embolus showing uneven densities in right lung, indicating impaired blood flow.

*Courtesy of University of California, Davis Medical Center.*

surgery or trauma. Because of the increased risk of hemorrhage, invasive procedures are avoided after thrombolysis. See Chapter 29 ⊖ for further discussion of thrombolytic therapy and its nursing implications.

## Surgery

When anticoagulant therapy fails to prevent recurrent emboli or is contraindicated, an umbrellalike filter may be inserted into the inferior vena cava to trap large emboli while allowing continued blood flow (see Figure 33-6). The filter usually is inserted percutaneously, via either the femoral or jugular vein.

## NURSING CARE

### Health Promotion

Nurses are key in preventing pulmonary embolism. Encouraging clients to ambulate after surgery or illness, applying compression stockings or pneumatic compression devices, teaching and encouraging leg exercises, discouraging the use of pillows under the knees—all these measures help prevent DVT and subsequent pulmonary emboli.

Teach clients to reduce the risks associated with long periods of immobility, stopping every 1 to 2 hours during long automobile trips for a brief stretch and walk, getting up every hour or so and doing leg exercises while seated during long flights, and avoiding crossing the legs to prevent venous stasis and pooling. Regular exercise such as walking also reduces the risk of DVT. Instruct clients who stand for long periods to use well-fitted elastic stockings, being careful to avoid hose that bind around the knee or thigh.

### Assessment

Because pulmonary embolus can be a medical emergency, assessment may be very focused. In other instances, when emboli are small and not life threatening, a more extensive nursing assessment may be done.

- Health history: chest pain, shortness of breath, other symptoms, including onset, severity, precipitating factors; history of recent surgery, venous thrombosis, or other risk factor such as childbirth or malignancy; current medications
- Physical examination: level of consciousness, presence of respirations and pulse; color, skin temperature and moisture; vital signs including apical pulse and temperature; breath sounds and heart sounds; oxygen saturation level; neck vein distention, peripheral edema

### Nursing Diagnoses and Interventions

A large pulmonary embolus can cause a significant mismatch between pulmonary ventilation and circulation. Impaired gas exchange is a priority problem and focus for interventions. Cardiac output may be significantly affected by obstructed pulmonary blood flow. Thrombolytic and anticoagulant therapy affect the clotting process, increasing the risk for bleeding. Anxiety accompanies pulmonary embolism almost universally.

### Impaired Gas Exchange

Pulmonary embolism results in areas of the lung that are ventilated but not perfused; they receive no capillary blood flow. If the embolus is large and a major segment of the lung is unperfused, gas exchange is significantly affected. Nursing interventions are directed toward compensating for impaired gas exchange.

- Frequently assess respiratory status, including rate, depth, effort, lung sounds, and oxygen saturation. *Impaired ventilation will further compromise gas exchange and worsen hypoxemia. Oxygen saturation can be monitored continuously and noninvasively to evaluate gas exchange.*

**PRACTICE ALERT** *Monitor and record level of consciousness, mental status, and skin color. Hypoxemia often causes confusion and agitation; hypercapnia may reduce level of consciousness. Cyanosis indicates significant hypoxemia.* ∎

- Place in Fowler's or high-Fowler's position, with the lower extremities dependent. *This position facilitates maximal lung expansion and reduces venous return to the right side of the heart, lowering pressures in the pulmonary vascular system.*

**PRACTICE ALERT** *Start oxygen per nasal cannula or mask. Obtain a physician's order if one has not been written. Supplemental oxygen increases alveolar and arterial oxygenation. Oxygen is a drug and must be prescribed by the physician. It may, however, be initiated by the nurse in an emergency to prevent tissue hypoxia.* ∎

- Monitor arterial blood gas results, reporting abnormal findings as indicated. *ABGs are used to assess gas exchange and tissue oxygenation. An arterial line may be inserted for monitoring arterial pressure and arterial blood sampling.*
- Maintain bed rest. *Bed rest reduces metabolic demands and tissue needs for oxygen.*

### Decreased Cardiac Output

The impact of a large pulmonary embolus on hemodynamic status can be significant. Pressures in the pulmonary vascular system and right heart increase; blood return to the left heart and cardiac output may significantly decrease. Nursing interventions focus on preserving an adequate blood pressure and organ function until cardiopulmonary status stabilizes.

**PRACTICE ALERT** *Assess and record vital signs and cardiopulmonary status every 15 to 30 minutes initially, then every 2 to 4 hours as condition stabilizes. Frequent assessment facilitates timely interventions to maintain cardiovascular status and preserve organ function.* ∎

- Auscultate heart sounds every 2 to 4 hours, reporting any abnormalities. *Sounds such as an S3 or S4 gallop may indicate cardiac compromise.*

*Record intake and output hourly. Decreased urinary output often is an early indicator of decreased cardiac output. Maintaining renal perfusion is vital to preserve renal function and prevent acute renal failure.* ■

- Assess skin color and temperature. *These assessments monitor tissue perfusion.*
- Monitor cardiac rhythm. *A drop in cardiac output and other hemodynamic alterations resulting from pulmonary embolism can precipitate dysrhythmias. Dysrhythmias, in turn, can further impair cardiac output.*
- Administer vasopressors and other medications as ordered. Carefully monitor the response to prescribed medications. *Drugs may be prescribed to maintain adequate arterial pressure and tissue perfusion. Potent drugs such as vasopressors require careful monitoring for desired and adverse effects.*
- ...pulmonary artery pressures, neck vein distension, and peripheral ...... Report findings as indicated. *Right-sided heart failure is a potential complication of pulmonary embolism because of increased pulmonary artery pressures.*
- Maintain intravenous and arterial access sites as well as central lines. *The client may be in unstable and critical condition, potentially needing immediate interventions to maintain life.*

PRACTICE ALERT *Provide frequent skin care. Impaired tissue perfusion and oxygenation increase the risk of skin and tissue breakdown.* ■

- Instruct to report chest pain or other symptoms. *Decreased cardiac output and an increased workload due to pulmonary hypertension may cause anginal pain.*

### Ineffective Protection

Thrombolytics and anticoagulant therapy impair normal clotting mechanisms, increasing the risk for bleeding and hemorrhage. This risk is particularly acute during the first 24 to 48 hours following thrombolytic drug administration.

- Assess frequently for overt and covert signs of bleeding: bleeding gums; hematuria; obvious or occult blood in stool or vomitus; incisional bleeding, bleeding or bruising of injection sites or with minor trauma; joint pain or immobility; abdominal or flank pain. *Careful monitoring is necessary to identify early signs of abnormal bleeding and prevent potential hemorrhage.*

PRACTICE ALERT *Promptly report changes in neurologic status. Although cerebral bleeding is not evident externally, changes in level of consciousness and other neurologic signs suggest it and should be reported immediately.* ■

- Report coagulation study results outside the desired range for anticoagulant therapy. *Levels less than the target range may indicate an increased risk for further clot development and pulmonary emboli; levels above the target range indicate an increased risk for bleeding.*

- Keep protamine sulfate available for heparin therapy and vitamin K available for warfarin (Coumadin) therapy. *Bleeding or hemorrhage due to excess anticoagulant may require antidote administration to rapidly reverse anticoagulant effects.*
- Assess medication regimen for possible drug interactions that could potentiate or inhibit anticoagulant effects. *Drug interactions can increase the risk for hemorrhage or further embolus formation.*
- Avoid invasive procedures, injections, and venous punctures when possible, particularly during and following thrombolytic therapy. *Invasive procedures increase the risk of tissue trauma and bleeding.*
- Maintain firm pressure on injection and venipuncture sites. Maintain pressure for 30 minutes following arterial puncture. *Firm pressure reduces the risk for bleeding into the tissues.*

PRACTICE ALERT *Use an infusion device to administer heparin infusion. Using an infusion pump or device helps prevent administration of excess medication.* ■

- Maintain adequate fluid intake. Administer stool softeners as ordered. *These measures help prevent constipation and straining, which may precipitate bleeding of hemorrhoids.*

### Anxiety

Pulmonary embolism is a physiologic and psychologic threat to safety and integrity. It is a major physiologic stressor, eliciting a strong neuroendocrine stress response. The feeling of suffocation and inability to catch one's breath that accompanies a pulmonary embolus is also a strong psychologic stressor. Fear, anxiety, and apprehension are common responses.

- Assess anxiety level. *Appropriate interventions are determined by the level of anxiety.*

PRACTICE ALERT *Provide reassurance and emotional support, listening to fears. Do not negate the fear of dying, but reassure that treatment usually restores effective respiratory function. The fear of death is very real and must not be discounted; however, it is important to provide reassurance to alleviate excess anxiety.* ■

- Remain with the client as much as possible. *The presence of a caring nurse helps reduce fear.*
- Explain procedures and treatments, using short, simple sentences. *Providing clearly understood, simple instructions reduces fear of the unknown.*
- Reduce environmental stimuli, and use a calm, reassuring manner. *These measures help reduce anxiety (for both the nurse and the client).*
- Allow supportive family members to remain with the client as much as possible. *Calm, supportive family members provide further reassurance.*
- Administer morphine sulfate as ordered. *Morphine is given to reduce pain and anxiety.*

## Home Care

Discuss the following topics when preparing the client with pulmonary embolism and family members for home care.

- Use of prescribed anticoagulant, including drug interactions, scheduled laboratory testing, and manifestations of bleeding to report to the primary care provider
- Using a soft toothbrush and electric razor to reduce the risk of bleeding
- Avoiding aspirin (unless prescribed) and other over-the-counter medications without approval by the physician
- Importance of wearing a MedicAlert tag for anticoagulant use
- Health promotion measures to reduce the risk of recurrent pulmonary embolism
- Symptoms of recurrent pulmonary embolism, such as sudden chest pain, shortness of breath, and possibly bloody sputum

# THE CLIENT WITH PULMONARY HYPERTENSION

The pulmonary vascular system is normally a high-flow, low-pressure, low-resistance system that can accommodate large increases in blood flow when necessary (e.g., during exercise). The normal mean arterial pressure in the pulmonary system is 12 to 15 mmHg (25 to 28 systolic/8 diastolic). **Pulmonary hypertension** is abnormal elevation of the pulmonary arterial pressure.

## PATHOPHYSIOLOGY AND MANIFESTATIONS

Pulmonary hypertension can develop as a primary disorder, but usually occurs secondarily to another condition.

### Primary Pulmonary Hypertension

*Primary pulmonary hypertension* is an uncommon disorder characterized by increased pulmonary vascular pressure and resistance with no apparent cause. Its etiology is unknown. It affects primarily women in their 30s or 40s. The manifestations of primary pulmonary hypertension are progressive dyspnea, fatigue, angina, and syncope with exertion. This progressive disorder generally causes a steady decline to death within 3 to 4 years.

### Secondary Pulmonary Hypertension

*Secondary pulmonary hypertension* is more common than primary. Its usual cause is reduced size of the pulmonary vascular bed, which may be due to vasoconstriction or widespread vessel destruction or obstruction. Hypoxemia is a potent pulsel vasoconstrictor and a common initiating factor in pulmonary vasoconstrictor and a common initiating factor in pulmonary hypertension. Chronic lung diseases, sleep apnea, and hypoventilation due to obesity or neuromuscular disease can lead to hypoxemia. Alveolar wall destruction associated with emphysema leads to loss of pulmonary capillaries. Large or multiple pulmonary emboli may cause significant vessel obstruction. Other factors such as left ventricular failure or mitral

stenosis also can lead to elevated pulmonary pressures. Once initiated, pulmonary hypertension becomes self-sustaining, because pulmonary vessels undergo changes that further narrow the pulmonary bed.

Manifestations of secondary pulmonary hypertension often are masked by those of the underlying disease. Dyspnea and dull, retrosternal chest pain are typical, as well as fatigue and syncope on exertion.

## Cor Pulmonale

**Cor pulmonale** is a condition of right ventricular hypertrophy and failure resulting from long-standing pulmonary hypertension. Chronic obstructive pulmonary disease is the most common cause of cor pulmonale.

The manifestations of cor pulmonale are those of the underlying pulmonary disorder and right-sided heart failure. Chronic productive cough, progressive dyspnea, and wheezing common. With right-sided heart failure, peripheral edema and distended neck veins are seen. Skin is warm, moist, and both ruddy and cyanotic because of increased numbers of RBCs and hypoxemia.

## COLLABORATIVE CARE

The CBC commonly shows *polycythemia,* increased numbers of red blood cells. ABGs and oxygen saturation measurements reveal hypoxemia. The chest X-ray shows right heart enlargement and dilation of central pulmonary arteries. Typical ECG changes are those of right ventricular hypertrophy. An echocardiogram may be done to identify cardiac changes occurring either as a cause or result of pulmonary hypertension. Doppler ultrasonography is a noninvasive means of estimating pulmonary artery pressure, but cardiac catheterization may be required for definitive diagnosis. See page 817 for nursing care of the client undergoing cardiac catheterization.

Treatment for primary pulmonary hypertension is not particularly effective to reverse or slow the course of the disease. The calcium channel blockers nifedipine (Procardia) or diltiazem (Cardizem) may be given to reduce pulmonary vascular resistance and improve cardiac output. Short-acting direct vasodilators such as intravenous adenosine, inhaled nitric oxide, or intravenous prostacyclin may be used for severe disability. Bilateral lung or heart-lung transplant is the most effective long-term treatment for primary pulmonary hypertension.

Treatment of secondary pulmonary hypertension is directed toward the underlying disease process. Pulmonary hypertension often is advanced at the time of diagnosis and resistant to treatment. Supplemental oxygen may be ordered to reduce hypoxemia. Long-term anticoagulation or calcium channel blockers may be prescribed. If polycythemia is present, phlebotomy is performed to reduce the viscosity of the blood.

When cor pulmonale is present, salt and water restrictions as well as diuretic therapy are added to the above regimen to manage the right-sided heart failure.

## NURSING CARE

Nursing care for the client with pulmonary hypertension or cor pulmonale is largely supportive. The focus is toward the underlying lung disease. Impaired gas exchange due to contraction of the pulmonary vascular system is a significant problem that causes many secondary problems, such as activity intolerance, anxiety, fatigue, and others. Nursing interventions for impaired gas exchange are directed toward maintaining adequate alveolar ventilation, oxygenation, and perfusion. The following measures may be included.

- Monitoring breath sounds, respiratory rate, skin color, and use of accessory muscles
- Positioning for optimal lung expansion
- Coughing, deep breathing, and chest physiotherapy
- Administering prescribed vasodilators

It is important to assess fatigue and dyspnea with activities and to plan frequent rest periods. Assist with self-care as needed to conserve energy.

With primary pulmonary hypertension, *Anticipatory grieving* and *Hopelessness* are additional potential nursing diagnoses. When cor pulmonale is present, *Decreased cardiac output, Excess fluid volume,* and *Ineffective individual coping* must be considered.

### Home Care

Most care for these chronic conditions is provided in the home and community settings. Teaching is directed both at the underlying lung disease, if present, and the resulting hypertensive process. Refer to the section on COPD for teaching related to this disease, the most frequent underlying cause of cor pulmonale.

In addition, provide teaching about the following topics for the client and family.

- Disease process, its management, and the prognosis
- Manifestations or changes in condition to report to the physician, such as a change in activity tolerance, increased edema, and signs of respiratory infection or exacerbation
- Importance of planned rest periods between activities and measures to conserve energy, such as using a shower chair
- Importance of not smoking due to its irritant and vasoconstrictive effects
- Prescribed medications, including their use and effects

# LUNG CANCER

## THE CLIENT WITH LUNG CANCER

Lung cancer is the leading cause of cancer deaths among all racial groups in the United States, accounting for 31% of all cancer deaths in men and 25% of all cancer deaths in women. In 2002, nearly 155,000 people died from lung cancer in the United States; an estimated 169,400 new cases were diagnosed in that same year (ACS, 2002). It is a major health problem with a grim prognosis: Most people with lung cancer die within 1 year of the initial diagnosis.

The incidence of lung cancer varies from state to state and among nations. It increases with age, occurring most commonly in clients over age 50. Cigarette smoke, which contains 43 known chemical carcinogens and cancer promoters, is clearly the most significant cause of lung cancer. More than 80% of lung cancer cases are related to smoking, and the disease is 10 times more common in smokers than nonsmokers. There is a dose-response relationship between smoking and lung cancer; the more the person smokes and the longer the person smokes, the greater the risk. Exposure to ionizing radiation and inhaled irritants, asbestos in particular, is also recognized as a risk factor for lung cancer (Porth, 2002).

At the time of diagnosis, cancer of the lung typically is well advanced, with distant metastasis present in 55% of clients and regional lymph node involvement in another 25%. The prognosis is generally poor: The overall 5-year survival rate is only 15% (ACS, 2002).

## PATHOPHYSIOLOGY

The vast majority of primary lung lesions are *bronchogenic carcinoma,* tumors of the airway epithelium. These tumors are further differentiated by cell type: small-cell carcinoma, adenocarcinoma, squamous cell carcinoma, and large-cell carcinoma. For clinical purposes, the latter three cell types frequently are classified together as non-small-cell carcinomas. *Small-cell carcinomas,* which account for approximately 25% of lung cancers, grow rapidly and spread early. These tumors have paraneoplastic properties; that is, they produce manifestations at sites that are not directly affected by the tumor. Small-cell lung carcinomas can synthesize bioactive products and hormones such as adrenocorticotropic hormones (ACTH), antidiuretic hormone (ADH), a parathormone-like hormone, and gastrin-releasing peptide. *Non-small-cell carcinoma* accounts for about 75% of lung cancers. Each cell type differs in its incidence, presentation, and manner of spread. Table 36–9 outlines the incidence and unique characteristics of each cell type.

Bronchogenic cancer, regardless of cell type, tends to be aggressive, locally invasive, and have widespread metastatic lesions. Tumors begin as mucosal lesions that grow to form masses which obstruct the bronchi or invade adjacent lung tissue. All types frequently spread via the lymph system to nodes and other organs such as the brain, bones, and liver. *Superior vena cava syndrome,* partial or complete obstruction of the superior vena cava, is a potential complication of lung cancer, particularly when the tumor involves the superior mediastinum or the mediastinal lymph nodes.

## COLLABORATIVE CARE

Because lung cancer typically is advanced when diagnosed and the prognosis generally is poor, prevention of the disease must be a primary goal for all health care providers. With 80% of lung cancer related to cigarette smoking, reducing tobacco use can have a significant impact on the death rate from lung cancer—a far greater impact than advances in treatment. Unfortunately, declines in adult tobacco use have slowed in recent years and its use among teenagers increased significantly during the 1990s (ACS, 2002).

Establishing an accurate diagnosis is the first step in treating lung cancer. Treatment decisions are based on the tumor location, type of cancer cell, staging of the tumor, and the client's ability to tolerate treatment. Lung cancer is staged by the tumor size, location, degree of invasion of the primary tumor, and the presence of metastatic disease. Lung cancer staging is summarized in Table 36–10. Surgery is the treatment of choice for most forms of lung cancer.

## Diagnostic Tests

- *Chest X-ray* usually provides the first evidence of lung cancer. It is particularly reliable as a diagnostic tool when compared with previous chest X-ray. In high-risk populations, the chest X-ray may be used as a screening tool for lung cancer.
- *Sputum specimen* is sent for *cytologic examination* to establish the diagnosis of lung cancer. The sputum sample is collected on arising in the morning. If malignant cells are found in the sputum, more expensive and invasive examinations may be unnecessary. However, a sputum sample negative for malignant cells does not rule out lung cancer; it may simply indicate that the tumor is not shedding cells into mucous secretions.
- *Bronchoscopy* is frequently done to visualize and obtain tissue for biopsy from the tumor. A flexible fiberoptic bronchoscope is inserted through the mouth into the bronchus. When a tumor mass or suspicious tissue is identified visually, a cable-activated instrument is used to obtain a biopsy specimen. If the tumor cannot be seen, the airways may be flushed with a saline solution (bronchial washing) to obtain cells for cytologic examination. Nursing care of the client undergoing a bronchoscopy is included in the box on page 1080.
- *CT scan* is used to evaluate and localize tumors, particularly tumors in the lung parenchyma and pleura. It also is done prior to needle biopsy to localize the tumor. CT scanning can also detect distant tumor metastasis and evaluate tumor response to treatment.
- Cells or tissue for *cytologic examination and biopsy* may be obtained by aspirating fluid from a pleural effusion, percutaneous needle biopsy, and lymph node biopsy. These procedures may be done in an outpatient or a surgical setting.
- *CBC, liver function studies,* and *serum electrolytes* including calcium are obtained to evaluate for evidence of metastatic disease or paraneoplastic syndromes.

## Medications

Combination chemotherapy is the treatment of choice for small-cell lung cancer because of its rapid growth, dissemination, and sensitivity to cytotoxic drugs. Used in combination, chemotherapeutic drugs allow tumor cells to be attacked at different parts of the cell cycle and in different ways, in-

### TABLE 36–10  Lung Cancer Staging

| | Primary Tumor (T-Stage) | Regional Lymph Nodes (N) | Distant Metastasis (M) |
|---|---|---|---|
| | $T_0$–No evidence of primary tumor | | $M_X$–Presence of distant metastasis cannot be assessed |
| Stage 0 | $T_X$–Malignant cells in bronchopulmonary secretions, but no tumor visualized | | |
| Stage I | $T_1$S–Carcinoma in situ | $N_0$–No regional lymph node metastasis | $M_0$–No distant metastasis |
| | $T_1$–Tumor that is 3 cm diameter or less, with no evidence of invasion | | |
| Stage II | $T_2$–Tumor that is greater than 3 cm diameter, or invades visceral pleura, or has associated atelectasis or pneumonitis | $N_1$–Metastasis or direct extension to peribronchial or ipsilateral hilar nodes | |
| Stage III | $T_3$–Tumor with direct extension into an adjacent structure, or any tumor with associated pleural effusion or atelectasis or pneumonitis of entire lung | $N_2$–Metastasis to ipsilateral mediastinal or subcarinal nodes | |
| Stage IV | $T_4$–Tumor that invades mediastinum or involves the heart, great vessels, trachea, esophagus, vertebral body, or carina; presence of malignant pleural effusion | $N_3$–Metastasis to contralateral mediastinal, scalene, or supraclavicular nodes | $M_1$–Distant metastasis present |

creasing the effectiveness of therapy. Fifty percent of clients with tumors at early stages achieve complete tumor remission with combination chemotherapy. When a complete tumor response is achieved in the first few cycles of chemotherapy, the chances for long-term survival are much greater.

Combination chemotherapy is used also as an adjunct to surgery or radiation therapy for lung cancer. It may be used to reduce the size of advanced local tumors prior to surgery, and to lengthen survival when distant metastases are present. See Chapter 10 ⊙⊙ for further discussion of chemotherapy.

Bronchodilators may be prescribed to reduce airway obstruction. Analgesics and pain management strategies are vital when the cancer is advanced. See Chapter 4 ⊙⊙ for more information about postoperative and cancer pain management.

## Surgery

Surgery offers the only real chance for a cure in non-small-cell lung cancer. Unfortunately, most tumors are inoperable or only partially resectable at the time of diagnosis. The 5-year survival rate for clients with resectable tumors is between 20% and 50%, depending on the size of the tumor and the extent of lymph node involvement (Braunwald et al., 2001). The type of surgery performed depends on the location and size of the tumor, as well as the client's pulmonary and general health. The goal of surgery is to remove all involved tissue while preserving as much functional lung as possible. Table 36–11 outlines various surgical procedures used to treat lung cancer. Nursing care for the client having lung surgery is outlined in the box on page 1140.

## Radiation Therapy

Radiation therapy is used alone or in combination with surgery or chemotherapy for lung cancer. The treatment goal may be either cure or symptom relief (palliative). Prior to surgery, radiation therapy is used to "debulk" tumors. When cancer has spread by direct extension to other thoracic structures and surgery is not feasible, radiation therapy may be the treatment of choice. It also may be used to relieve manifestations such as cough, hemoptysis, pain due to bone metastasis, and dyspnea from bronchial obstruction. Complications of lung cancer, such as superior vena cava syndrome, may be treated with radiation.

Radiation therapy may be delivered by external beam to the primary tumor site or by intraluminal radiation, or brachytherapy. Radiation therapy and related nursing care is discussed further in Chapter 10. Specific nursing measures for the client undergoing radiation therapy for lung cancer are outlined in the Nursing Care box on page 1141.

## NURSING CARE

### Health Promotion

The incidence of lung cancer is decreasing as the use of tobacco products declines. Teach people of all ages, particularly children and teenagers, about the link between cigarette smoking and lung cancer. Not smoking and avoiding exposure to secondhand smoke is the primary preventive measure for lung cancer. In addition, explain the risk of lung cancer to clients with occupational risk factors, exposure to asbestos products in particular.

### Assessment

Nursing assessment related to lung cancer focuses on identifying risk factors for the disease, early manifestations of lung cancer, and respiratory function in the client undergoing treatment.

- Health history: current symptoms, including chronic cough, shortness of breath, blood-tinged sputum; systemic manifestations such as recent weight loss, fatigue, anorexia, bone pain; smoking history; occupational exposure to carcinogens; chronic diseases such as COPD
- Physical examination: general appearance; skin color, evidence of clubbing; weight and height; vital signs; respiratory rate, depth, excursion; lung sounds to percussion and auscultation

| TABLE 36–11 | Types of Lung Surgery for Lung Cancer | |
|---|---|---|
| **Procedure** | **Description** | **Used for** |
| Laser bronchoscopy | Bronchoscopy-guided laser used to resect tumor | Tumors localized in a main bronchus |
| Mediastinoscopy | Visualization of the mediastinum using an endoscope passed through a suprasternal incision | Evaluation and biopsy of a mediastinal tumor and lymph nodes |
| Thoracotomy | Incision into the chest wall | Access the lung and thoracic cavity for surgery |
| Wedge resection | Removal of a small section (wedge) of peripheral lung tissue | Small, peripheral lung tumors |
| Segmental resection | Removal of an individual bronchovascular segment of a lobe | Peripheral lung tumor with no evidence of extension to the chest wall or metastasis |
| Sleeve resection (bronchoplastic reconstruction) | Resection of a section of a major bronchus with reconstruction of remaining normal bronchus | Small lesion of a major bronchus |
| Lobectomy | Removal of a single lung lobe | Tumors confined to a single lobe |
| Pneumonectomy | Removal of an entire lung | Tumor widespread throughout the lung, involving the main bronchus, or fixed to the hilum |

# NURSING CARE OF THE CLIENT HAVING LUNG SURGERY

## PREOPERATIVE CARE

- Provide routine preoperative nursing care as outlined in Chapter 7. ∞
- Note any history of smoking, respiratory and cardiac diseases, and other chronic conditions in the nursing history. *These factors may affect the response to surgery and the risk for postoperative complications.*
- Provide emotional and psychologic support for the client and family. *In addition to facing surgery, the client may be adjusting to a new diagnosis of cancer and the possibility that surgical intervention will be only partially successful.*
- Instruct about postoperative procedures, including respiratory therapy, breathing exercises, and coughing techniques. Allow practice time. *Learning will be easier in the preoperative period, when pain and analgesia are not affecting mental function.*
- If the client will return from surgery with an endotracheal tube and mechanical ventilation, establish a means of communication using hand or eye signals or a magic slate. *Establishing a means of communication prior to surgery reduces postoperative anxiety at being unable to speak.*
- If the client will return to ICU, introduce the client and family to the unit and any machines, such as ventilators and monitors, that will be used. *The knowledge that this is an expected part of surgical recovery reduces the client's and family's postoperative anxiety.*

## POSTOPERATIVE CARE

- Assess and provide routine postoperative care as outlined in Chapter 7.
- Assess for adequate pain control, and provide analgesics as needed. *Incisional pain commonly causes altered breathing patterns in the client who has undergone lung surgery.*
- Frequently assess respiratory status, including color, oxygen saturation, respiratory rate and depth, chest expansion, lung sounds, percussion tone, and arterial blood gases. *Maintaining adequate ventilation and gas exchange postoperatively is vital to*

reduce mortality and morbidity. Gas exchange may be impaired by complications of lung surgery, including pneumothorax, atelectasis, bronchospasm, pulmonary embolus, bronchopleural fistula, and acute respiratory distress syndrome (ARDS).

- Assist with effective coughing techniques, postural drainage, and incentive spirometry. Perform endotracheal suctioning as needed while intubated. *Surgical manipulation and anesthesia can increase the mucous production, leading to airway obstruction. Aggressive pulmonary hygiene is important to prevent this complication.*
- Monitor and maintain effective mechanical ventilation. *This is vital to ensure adequate ventilation and gas exchange in the early postoperative period.*
- Maintain patent chest tubes and a closed drainage system. Monitor chest tube output every hour initially, then every 2 to 4 or 8 hours as indicated. Notify the physician if chest tube output exceeds 70 mL per hour and/or is bright red, warm, and free flowing. *Maintaining a patent, intact chest drainage system is vital to reestablish negative pressure within the chest cavity and reexpansion of the lungs. Increased amounts of warm, free-flowing blood indicate intrathoracic hemorrhage that may necessitate surgical intervention.*
- Assess for signs of infection involving the incision or chest tube site(s). Use strict aseptic technique in caring for incisions and invasive monitoring devices. *The postoperative client is at risk for incisional infections, empyema in the chest cavity, and pneumonia.*
- Assist with turning and to ambulate as soon as possible. *Early mobility is important to prevent possible complications, such as pneumonia or pulmonary embolus.*
- Assess and maintain nutritional status. Initiate enteral or parenteral nutrition early if intubation and mechanical ventilation will be required for an extended period. Provide frequent small feedings once extubated. *Maintaining nutritional status promotes wound healing and prevents negative nitrogen balance. Frequent small feedings reduce the fatigue associated with eating.*

## Nursing Diagnoses and Interventions

The client with lung cancer is facing invasive treatments with undesirable side effects, possibly surgery, and typically a poor prognosis for long-term survival. Nursing care needs are diverse, related to respiratory status, the cancer itself and possible metastases, and the treatment plan. Priority nursing diagnoses related to respiratory function include ineffective breathing pattern and activity intolerance. Pain and anticipatory grieving also are likely to be high-priority problems.

### Ineffective Breathing Pattern

Breathing pattern and ventilation may be affected by the tumor itself or by treatment of the tumor. Thoracic surgery increases the risk due to the incision and disruption of the muscles of respiration. Maintaining effective lung ventilation is particularly important postoperatively to reexpand remaining lung tissue and prevent surgical complications.

- Assess and document respiratory rate, depth, and lung sounds at least every 4 hours; evaluate more frequently in the immediate postoperative period or as indicated by condition. *Early detection of signs of respiratory compromise or adventitious lung sounds is vital for effective intervention.*

**PRACTICE ALERT** *Monitor oxygen saturation, exhaled carbon dioxide, and/or blood gas results, reporting changes from normal. Changes in levels of blood oxygen or exhaled $CO_2$ may be early indications of respiratory compromise.* ■

- Frequently assess and document pain level (using a standard pain scale); provide analgesics as needed. *Pain and attempting to avoid chest movement to prevent additional pain can lead to rapid, shallow respirations and ineffective ventilation.*

# NURSING CARE OF THE CLIENT RECEIVING RADIATION THERAPY

Although radiation therapy is well controlled and specifically directed toward the tumor cells, some normal cells are also damaged in the process of treatment. Nursing care and client teaching help the client cope with uncomfortable side effects associated with radiation therapy.

## Nursing Responsibilities

- Monitor for potential complications:
  a. Radiation pneumonitis—dyspnea on exertion, dry cough, fever
  b. Pericarditis—chest pain, pericardial friction rub; muffled heart sounds, paradoxical pulse, ECG abnormalities (Notify the physician if symptoms develop.)
  c. Esophagitis—pain, sore throat, difficulty swallowing
- Encourage adequate fluid intake to liquefy respiratory secretions.
- Provide local analgesics and local anesthetics such as viscous lidocaine as ordered to relieve dysphagia and sore throat.
- Offer small frequent meals of soft, cool foods and liquids to maintain nutritional status.

## Client and Family Teaching

- If dyspnea or pneumonitis develop, teach positioning, pursed-lip techniques, and relaxation exercises to facilitate breathing.
- Reassure that pneumonitis is generally a self-limiting process and should resolve when the course of radiotherapy is completed.
- Teach the manifestations of pericarditis, which may develop during treatment or up to 1 year after its completion. Chest pain or pressure, rapid heartbeat, and fever may signal pericarditis; increasing fatigue, dyspnea, and lightheadedness can indicate a chronic process with pericardial effusion and possible cardiac tamponade.
- Instruct to eliminate hot, spicy, or acidic foods from the diet if esophagitis is a problem. Alcohol and tobacco should also be avoided.
- Adequate rest and nutrition are important to alleviate the symptoms of radiation fatigue, which is common in clients receiving radiation therapy for lung cancer. The fatigue is generally temporary.

---

- Elevate the head of the bed to 60 degrees. *Elevating the head of the bed reduces pressure on the diaphragm and permits optimal lung expansion.*
- Assist to turn, cough, and deep breathe and use incentive spirometry. Help splint the chest with a pillow or blanket when coughing. *These measures promote airway clearance.*
- Suction airway as needed. *Suctioning may be required to remove secretions that the client is unable to cough up and expectorate.*

**PRACTICE ALERT** *Maintain chest tube integrity and patency by ensuring uninterrupted gravity flow. Chest tubes help reestablish negative pressure in the thoracic cavity, allowing the lung to fully reexpand.* ■

- Provide chest physiotherapy with percussion and postural drainage as needed or ordered. *Percussion and postural drainage help maintain airway patency and effective respirations.*
- If mechanical ventilation is instituted, work with respiratory therapy and use analgesia or sedation as needed to synchronize respirations with the ventilator. *Coordination of the client's respiratory effort with ventilator-delivered breaths is important for fully effective mechanical ventilation.*
- Provide reassurance and emotional support. *These measures help relieve anxiety and promote an effective breathing pattern.*

## Activity Intolerance

Both resectional lung surgery and inoperable lung cancer reduce the amount of functional lung tissue and surface area for gas diffusion. This can lead to activity intolerance if the oxygen supply is insufficient to meet the body's oxygen demand.

**PRACTICE ALERT** *Assess and document physiologic responses to activity, including pulse, respiratory rate, dyspnea, and fatigue. These assessments are good indicators of activity tolerance.* ■

- Plan rest periods between activities and procedures. *Rest periods reduce oxygen demands and fatigue.*
- Assist the postoperative client to increase activities gradually. *Increasing activity levels gradually improves exercise tolerance.*
- Teach measures to conserve energy while performing ADLs, such as sitting while showering and dressing and wearing slip-on shoes. *These energy-conserving measures reduce oxygen demand and allow the client to remain independent as long as possible.*
- Keep frequently used objects within easy reach. *This helps conserve energy.*
- Administer oxygen as prescribed. Teach the client and family about home oxygen use if appropriate. *Supplemental oxygen can help improve activity and exercise tolerance.*
- Encourage maintenance of physical activity to tolerance. *Maintaining activity levels to the degree possible improves physical and emotional well-being.*
- Allow family members to provide assistance as needed. *This helps the client conserve energy and allows the family to retain a sense of usefulness.*

## Pain

Pain is a priority problem in both the postoperative period as well as in the terminal stages of cancer. Poorly managed pain prolongs recovery from surgery. In the terminal cancer client, chronic and acute pain must be managed effectively to allow a peaceful death.

- Assess and document pain using a standardized pain scale and objective data. *Pain is a subjective experience, best evaluated by the client. Changes in vital signs, guarded movement, or unwillingness to move may indicate unreported pain.*

- Provide analgesics as needed to maintain comfort. *Postoperative recovery and restoration of function is facilitated by adequate pain management.*
- For cancer pain, maintain an around-the-clock medication schedule using narcotic, nonsteroidal anti-inflammatory drugs, and other medications as ordered. *Addiction is not a concern in terminal cancer; providing adequate pain relief that does not allow "breakthrough" pain is important.*
- Provide or assist with comfort measures, such as massage, positioning, distraction, and relaxation techniques. *These techniques promote relaxation and enhance pain relief.*
- Assist the client and family to plan and engage in activities that distract from pain such as reading, watching television, and engaging in social interactions. *Distraction helps the client focus away from the pain.*
- Spend as much time with the client as possible; allow family members to remain with the client. *Physical presence of the nurse and family provides emotional support for the client.*

### Anticipatory Grieving

Because lung cancer often is advanced when diagnosed, the client faces the very real prospect of dying from the disease. Grieving for the anticipated loss of life is a normal response as the client and family begin to adapt to the diagnosis. Nursing care goals are to promote expression of feelings and thoughts about the loss, and to help the client and family initiate grief work, make decisions, and use appropriate resources and coping mechanisms to deal with the loss.

- Spend time with the client and family. *Time is necessary to develop a trusting, therapeutic relationship.*

- Answer questions honestly; do not deny the probable outcome of the disease. *Honesty reinforces reality and provides a sense of control over decisions to be made.*
- Encourage the client and family to express their feelings, fears, and concerns. *Open expression of feelings helps to promote understanding and acceptance.*
- Assist with understanding the grieving process and acceptance of feelings as normal. *Feelings of guilt, anger, or depression may cause the client to withdraw from others. Explanation of the grieving process enhances understanding and ability to cope.*
- Help identify strengths and coping measures that have been used effectively in the past. Provide positive reinforcement for effective coping behavior. *Past effective coping measures can help the client and family deal with the present situation and regain a sense of control.*
- Help the client and family make decisions regarding treatment and care. *This also is important to give them a sense of control.*
- Encourage use of other support systems, such as spiritual and social groups. Refer the client and family to support groups, social support services, and hospice care as indicated. Provide American Cancer Society literature and information as appropriate. *These support systems provide emotional support and help the client and family cope with the diagnosis.*
- Discuss advance directives (the living will) and power of attorney for health care with the client and family. *These documents give the client and family a sense of control over medical care provided if the client is no longer able to express his or her own wishes.*

### Using NANDA, NIC, and NOC

Chart 36–4 shows links between NANDA nursing diagnoses, NIC, and NOC for the client with lung cancer.

---

## CHART 36–4 NANDA, NIC, AND NOC LINKAGES

### The Client with Lung Cancer

| NURSING DIAGNOSES | NURSING INTERVENTIONS | NURSING OUTCOMES |
|---|---|---|
| • Activity Intolerance | • Energy Management<br>• Self-Care Assistance | • Activity Tolerance<br>• Energy Conservation |
| • Acute and/or Chronic Pain | • Pain Management<br>• Patient-Controlled Analgesia (PCA) Assistance | • Comfort Level<br>• Pain Control<br>• Pain: Disruptive Effects |
| • Anticipatory Grieving | • Grief Work Facilitation<br>• Family Support | • Coping<br>• Family Coping |
| • Ineffective Breathing Pattern | • Airway Management<br>• Respiratory Monitoring | • Respiratory Status: Ventilation |
| • Ineffective Coping | • Coping Enhancement<br>• Decision-Making Support<br>• Support System Enhancement | • Coping<br>• Decision Making<br>• Social Support |

*Note. Data from Nursing Outcomes Classification (NOC) by M. Johnson & M. Maas (Eds.), 1997, St. Louis: Mosby; Nursing Diagnoses: Definitions & Classification 2001–2002 by North American Nursing Diagnosis Association, 2001, Philadelphia: NANDA; Nursing Interventions Classification (NIC) by J.C. McCloskey & G. M. Bulechek (Eds.), 2000, St. Louis: Mosby. Reprinted by permission.*

## Home Care

A primary teaching need to prepare the client and family affected by lung cancer for home care is information about the disease itself, expected prognosis, and planned treatment strategies. Provide honest information; do not promote false hope. Include the following additional topics in teaching for home care.

- Importance of quitting smoking, especially if surgery has been performed (The client with lung cancer may have difficulty recognizing the need to stop smoking. Include information about the effects of nicotine and the tars in cigarette smoke on healing and already compromised lung tissue.)
- Planned treatments such as chemotherapy or radiation therapy, including expected effects and usual side effects of each
- Strategies to cope with noxious effects of radiation or chemotherapy

- Activities and exercises to improve strength and regain function for the postoperative client
- The need to continue coughing and deep-breathing exercises at home
- Symptoms to report to the physician: fever, increasing or continued shortness of breath, cough, increased or purulent sputum, redness, pain, swelling, or incisional drainage
- Use of prescribed medications, including desired and potential side effects and interactions with other drugs or foods
- Use of analgesics and other pain relief measures for postoperative or cancer pain
- Information about hospice services, home health, local cancer support groups for clients and caregivers, and American Cancer Society services

Refer the client and family for home health services including nursing care, assistance with ADLs, respiratory care, and respite care as needed.

## Nursing Care Plan
## A Client with Lung Cancer

After coughing up bloody sputum one morning, James Mueller, a 68-year-old retired millworker, sees his physician. A chest X-ray shows a suspicious density in the central portion of his right lung. Mr. Mueller is admitted to the hospital the following Monday for diagnostic tests.

### ASSESSMENT

Anita Sarros, RN, admits Mr. Mueller to the oncology unit and obtains a nursing history. Mr. Mueller is married and has three grown children. He worked in a local paper mill for 35 years before retiring at age 62. He describes himself as "pretty healthy," except for a chronic smoker's cough. He started smoking as a young man in the army. He has a 50 pack-year smoking history, having smoked a pack a day for 50 years, since age 18. Mr. Mueller says he briefly quit smoking following a small heart attack 3 years ago, but started again after 4 months. On further questioning, Mr. Mueller says his cough has been productive for the past few months, especially in the morning, and that he is shorter of breath than usual with activity.

Mr. Mueller's examination data includes BP 162/86, P 78 and regular, R 20, and T 98.4°F (36.9 C). Color good, skin warm and dry. Inspiratory and expiratory wheezes noted in right chest but good breath sounds throughout. No other abnormal findings are noted on examination. The physician orders early-morning sputum specimens times 3 days for cytologic examination and schedules a CT scan of the chest the morning after admission.

Mr. Mueller's CBC shows mild anemia, but remaining routine laboratory tests are essentially normal. Sputum cytology is positive for small-cell bronchogenic cancer. The CT scan shows a central mass approximately 4 cm in diameter with involved mediastinal and subclavicular lymph nodes. A small mass is also noted on the lumbar spine. After conferring with his physician and an oncologist, Mr. Mueller decides to undergo a trial course of chemotherapy.

### DIAGNOSIS

- *Ineffective airway clearance* related to tumor mass
- *Risk for imbalanced nutrition: Less than body requirements* related to effects of chemotherapy
- *Risk for compromised family coping* related to new diagnosis of lung cancer
- *Deficient knowledge* about lung cancer and aids to smoking cessation

### EXPECTED OUTCOMES

- Maintain a patent airway.
- Maintain current weight.
- Express feelings and concerns about the effect of cancer on the family unit.
- Participate in care.
- Contact appropriate support groups.
- Verbalize an understanding of the disease, its treatment, and prognosis.
- Develop a plan to stop smoking.

### PLANNING AND IMPLEMENTATION

- Teach coughing, deep breathing, and hydration measures to facilitate airway clearance.
- Discuss symptoms to report to the physician: increased dyspnea or hemoptysis, severe stridor or wheezing, chest pain.
- Discuss measures to relieve nausea associated with chemotherapy, including premedication with a prescribed antiemetic.
- Have dietitian consult with Mr. and Mrs. Mueller to develop a diet plan for maintaining ideal weight.
- Discuss possible effects of lung cancer with Mr. and Mrs. Mueller.
- Encourage Mr. and Mrs. Mueller to call a family conference to discuss the disease with their children and grandchildren.

*(continued on page 1144)*

## Nursing Care Plan
## A Client with Lung Cancer (continued)

- Evaluate family members' knowledge and understanding of lung cancer, correcting misinformation and teaching as needed.
- Have an American Cancer Society volunteer contact the family.
- Refer to local cancer support group.
- Refer to home health department for follow-up and further teaching.
- Work with Mr. Mueller to develop a plan to stop smoking.
- Ask the physician for a prescription for nicotine patches or gum for Mr. Mueller.

### EVALUATION

Mr. Mueller had his first chemotherapy treatment in the hospital and was discharged 4 days after admission. After 3 months of chemotherapy, his tumor shows little regression, and a liver scan reveals further metastasis. He and his wife decide to stop chemotherapy, a decision with which the children reluctantly agree. Mr. and Mrs. Mueller are referred to hospice services. With the help of hospice nurses and volunteers, Mr. Mueller is able to remain at home. His pain is managed initially with oral MS Contin, a sustained-release form of morphine sulfate, and later with an intravenous morphine infusion. Mr. Mueller dies at home with his family at his side 9 months after his diagnosis of lung cancer.

### Critical Thinking in the Nursing Process

1. The oncologist prescribed a chemotherapy regimen of cyclophosphamide, doxorubicin, and vincristine. Describe how each of these drugs works against cancer cells, and discuss the rationale for using this combination.
2. Develop a care plan to deal with the specific side effects for the above treatment regimen.
3. Mr. Mueller had small-cell (oat cell) cancer. How would his presentation and treatment differ if the diagnosis had been non-small-cell adenocarcinoma, stage $T_2N_2M_0$?

See Evaluating Your Response in Appendix C.

# DISORDERS OF THE PLEURA

The *pleura* is a thin membrane with two layers: the visceral pleura, which overlies the lung surface, and the parietal pleura, which lines the inner chest wall. Between the layers of pleura is a potential space, the *pleural cavity,* which contains a thin layer of serous fluid. As the thoracic cavity expands during inspiration, the pressure in this space becomes negative in relation to atmospheric and alveolar pressure. The expansible lung is drawn out, and air rushes into the alveoli. When the pleura is inflamed or affected by disease or injury, air or fluid can collect in the pleural cavity, restricting lung expansion and air movement.

## Pleuritis

**Pleuritis,** or inflammation of the pleura, irritates sensory fibers of the parietal pleura, causing characteristic pain. Pleural inflammation usually occurs secondarily to another process, such as a viral respiratory illness, pneumonia, or rib injury.

The onset of pleuritis is typically abrupt. The pain is unilateral and well localized; it is usually sharp or stabbing in nature. Pain may be referred to the neck or the shoulder. Deep breathing, coughing, and movement aggravate the pain. Respirations are rapid and shallow, and chest wall movement is limited on the affected side. Breath sounds are diminished, and a pleural friction rub may be heard over the site.

The diagnosis of pleuritis is based on its manifestations. Chest X-ray and ECG may be ordered to rule out other causes of chest pain. Treatment for pleuritis is symptomatic. Analgesics and NSAIDs, indomethacin (Indocin) in particular, help relieve the pain. Codeine may be ordered, both to relieve pain and to suppress the cough.

Nursing care for the client with pleuritis is directed toward promoting comfort, including administration of NSAIDs and analgesics. Positioning and splinting the chest while coughing also are helpful. Although wrapping the chest with 6-inch-wide elastic bandages may help relieve pain, this may excessively restrict chest motion, increasing the risk of impaired airway clearance.

Teach the client and family that pleuritis is generally self-limited and of short duration. Discuss symptoms to report to the physician: increased fever, productive cough, difficulty breathing, or shortness of breath. Provide information about prescription and nonprescription NSAIDs and analgesics, including the drug ordered, how to use it, and its desired and possible adverse effects.

## THE CLIENT WITH A PLEURAL EFFUSION

The pleural space normally contains only about 10 to 20 mL of serous fluid. **Pleural effusion** is collection of excess fluid in the pleural space. Pleural effusions result from either systemic or local disease. Systemic disorders that may lead to pleural effusion include heart failure, liver or renal disease, and connective tissue disorders, such as rheumatoid arthritis and systemic lupus erythematosus. Pneumonia, atelectasis, tuberculosis, lung cancer, and trauma are local conditions that may cause pleural effusion.

## PATHOPHYSIOLOGY AND MANIFESTATIONS

Excess pleural fluid may be either *transudate,* formed when capillary pressure is high or plasma proteins are low, or *exudate,* the result of increased capillary permeability. Other pleural fluid collections include *empyema,* pus in the pleural cavity; *hemothorax,* the presence of blood in the cavity; and *hemorrhagic pleural effusion,* a mixture of blood and pleural fluid.

A large pleural effusion compresses adjacent lung tissue. This causes the characteristic manifestation of dyspnea. Pain may develop, although with inflammatory processes pleuritic pain often is relieved by formation of an effusion. Breath sounds are diminished or absent, and a dull percussion tone is heard over the affected area. Chest wall movement may be limited.

## COLLABORATIVE CARE

Chest X-ray often provides the first evidence of a pleural effusion. Because fluid typically collects in dependent regions, it is seen at the base of the affected lung on an upright chest X-ray, and along the lateral wall when the client is positioned on the affected side. CT scans and ultrasonography also are used to localize and differentiate pleural effusions.

If the cause of pleural effusion is not apparent, a thoracentesis is done. **Thoracentesis** is an invasive procedure in which fluid (or occasionally air) is removed from the pleural space with a needle. Aspirated fluid is analyzed for appearance, cell counts, protein and glucose content, the presence of enzymes such as LDH and amylase, abnormal cells, and culture.

When pleural effusion is significant and interferes with respirations, thoracentesis is the treatment of choice to remove the fluid (Figure 36–15 ■). Thoracentesis may be performed at the bedside, in a procedure room, or in an outpatient setting. Local anesthesia is used, and the procedure requires less than 30 minutes to complete. Percussion, auscultation, radiography, or ultrasonography are used to locate the effusion and needle in-

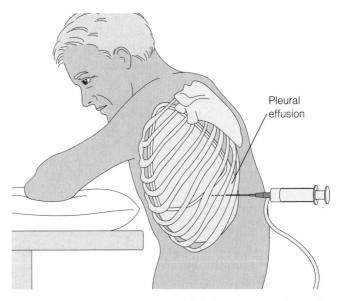

Pleural effusion

**Figure 36–15** ■ Thoracentesis. With the client seated, a needle is inserted between the ribs into the pleural space to withdraw accumulated fluid.

sertion site. The amount of fluid removed is limited to 1200 to 1500 mL at one time to reduce the risk of cardiovascular collapse from rapid removal of too much fluid. Pneumothorax is a possible complication of thoracentesis if the visceral pleura is punctured or a closed drainage system not maintained during the procedure. Nursing care for the client undergoing a thoracentesis is outlined in the box below.

## NURSING CARE OF THE CLIENT HAVING A THORACENTESIS

### PREPROCEDURE CARE

- Verify a signed informed consent for the procedure. *This invasive procedure requires informed consent.*
- Assess knowledge and understanding of the procedure and its purpose; provide additional information as needed. *An informed client will be less apprehensive and more able to cooperate during the thoracentesis.*
- Preprocedure fasting or sedation is not required. *Only local anesthesia is used in this procedure, and the gag and cough reflexes remain intact.*
- Administer a cough suppressant if indicated. *Movement and coughing during the procedure may cause inadvertent damage to the lung or pleura.*
- Obtain a thoracentesis tray, sterile gloves, injectable lidocaine, povidone-iodine, dressing supplies, and an extra overbed table or mayo stand. *These supplies are used by the physician performing the procedure.*
- Position the client upright, leaning forward with arms and head supported on an anchored overbed table. *This position spreads the ribs, enlarging the intercostal space for needle insertion.*
- Inform the client that although local anesthesia prevents pain as the needle is inserted, a sensation of pressure may be felt. *A pressure sensation occurs as the needle punctures the parietal pleura to enter the pleural space.*

### POSTPROCEDURE CARE

- Monitor pulse, color, oxygen saturation, and other signs during thoracentesis. *These are indicators of physiologic tolerance of the procedure.*
- Apply a dressing over the puncture site, and position on the unaffected side for 1 hour. *This allows the pleural puncture to heal.*
- Label obtained specimen with name, date, source, and diagnosis; send specimen to the laboratory for analysis. *Fluid obtained during thoracentesis may be examined for abnormal cells, bacteria, and other substances to determine the cause of the pleural effusion.*
- During the first several hours after thoracentesis, frequently assess and document vital signs; oxygen saturation; respiratory status, including, respiratory excursion, lung sounds, cough, or hemoptysis; and puncture site for bleeding or crepitus. *Frequent assessment is important to detect possible complications of thoracentesis, such as pneumothorax.*
- Obtain a chest X-ray. *Chest X-ray is ordered to detect possible pneumothorax.*
- Normal activities generally can be resumed after 1 hour if no evidence of pneumothorax or other complication is present. *The puncture wound of thoracentesis heals rapidly.*

Because pleural effusion usually occurs secondarily to another disease or disorder, medical management also focuses on treating the underlying condition to prevent further fluid accumulation. An empyema may require repeated drainage, as well as high doses of parenteral antibiotics. Occasionally, thoracotomy and surgical excision may be necessary. Recurrent pleural effusions, often due to cancer, may be prevented by instilling an irritant, such as doxycycline bleomycin, or talc, into the pleural space to cause adhesion of the parietal and visceral pleura (*pleurodesis*). Water-seal chest tube drainage is often employed for hemothorax.

## NURSING CARE

Nursing care for the client with a pleural effusion is directed toward supporting respiratory function and assisting with procedures to evacuate collected fluid. With a large pleural effusion and partial lung collapse, impaired gas exchange and activity intolerance are high-priority nursing problems. Risk for impaired gas exchange is also a priority problem during the initial period following thoracentesis.

Teaching for home care focuses on symptoms of recurrent effusion or complications following a thoracentesis to report to the physician: Increasing dyspnea or shortness of breath, cough, and hemoptysis. Pleuritic pain may be an early sign of effusion and also should be reported. Further teaching about an underlying condition also may be necessary; for example, the client with heart failure may need teaching about a salt-restricted diet.

## THE CLIENT WITH PNEUMOTHORAX

Accumulation of air in the pleural space is called **pneumothorax.** Pneumothorax can occur spontaneously, without apparent cause, as a complication of preexisting lung disease, as a result of blunt or penetrating trauma to the chest, or from an iatrogenic cause (e.g., following thoracentesis).

## PATHOPHYSIOLOGY AND MANIFESTATIONS

Pressure in the pleural space is normally negative in relation to atmospheric pressure. This negative pressure is vital to the process of breathing. Contraction of the diaphragm and the intercostal muscles enlarges the thoracic space. Negative intrapleural pressure draws the lung outward, increasing its volume so air rushes in to fill the expanded lung space.

When either the visceral or parietal pleura is breached, air enters the pleural space, equalizing this pressure. Lung expansion is impaired, and the natural recoil tendency of the lung causes it to collapse to a greater or lesser extent, depending on the size and rapidity of air accumulation. Table 36–12 illustrates the classifications of pneumothorax.

### Spontaneous Pneumothorax

*Spontaneous pneumothorax* develops when an air-filled bleb, or blister, on the lung surface ruptures. Rupture allows air from the airways to enter the pleural space. Air accumulates until pressures are equalized or until collapse of the involved lung section seals the leak. Spontaneous pneumothorax may be either *primary (simple)* or *secondary (complicated)*.

Primary pneumothorax affects previously healthy people, usually tall, slender men between ages 16 and 24 (Way & Doherty, 2003). The cause of primary pneumothorax is unknown. Risk factors include smoking and familial factors. Air-filled blebs tend to form in the apices of the lungs. This is considered to be a benign condition, although recurrences are common. Certain activities also increase the risk of spontaneous pneumothorax, such as high altitude flying and rapid decompression during scuba diving.

Secondary pneumothorax, generally caused by overdistention and rupture of an alveolus, is more serious and potentially life threatening. It develops in clients with underlying lung disease, usually COPD. Middle-age and older adults are primarily affected. Secondary pneumothorax also may be associated with asthma, cystic fibrosis, pulmonary fibrosis, tuberculosis, acute respiratory distress syndrome (ARDS), and other lung diseases. Rarely, a form of secondary pneumothorax called *catamenial pneumothorax* can develop in affected women within 24 to 48 hours of the onset of menstrual flow.

The manifestations of spontaneous pneumothorax depend on the size of pneumothorax, extent of lung collapse, and any underlying lung disease. Typically, pleuritic chest pain and shortness of breath begin abruptly, often while at rest. The respiratory and heart rates increase as gas exchange is affected. Chest wall movement may be asymmetrical, with less movement on the affected side than the unaffected side. The affected side is hyperresonant to percussion, and breath sounds may be diminished or absent. Hypoxemia may develop, although normal mechanisms that shunt blood flow to the unaffected lung often maintain normal oxygen saturation levels. Hypoxemia is more pronounced in secondary pneumothorax.

### Traumatic Pneumothorax

Blunt or penetrating trauma of the chest wall and pleura can cause pneumothorax. Blunt trauma, for example, due to a motor vehicle crash, fall, or during cardiopulmonary resuscitation (CPR), can lead to a *closed pneumothorax*. Fractured ribs penetrating the pleura are the leading cause of pneumothorax due to blunt trauma. Fracture of the trachea and a ruptured bronchus or esophagus also may result from blunt trauma, leading to closed pneumothorax.

*Open pneumothorax (sucking chest wound)* results from penetrating chest trauma such as a stab wound, gunshot wound, or impalement injury. With open pneumothorax, air moves freely between the pleural space and the atmosphere through the wound. Pressure on the affected side equalizes with the atmosphere, and the lung collapses rapidly. The result is significant hypoventilation.

*Iatrogenic pneumothorax* may result from puncture or laceration of the visceral pleura during central-line placement, thoracentesis, or lung biopsy. During bronchoscopy, bronchi or lung tissue can be disrupted. Alveoli can become overdistended and rupture during anesthesia, resuscitation procedures, or mechanical ventilation.

TABLE 36–12   Types of Pneumothorax

| Type | Pathophysiology | Manifestations |
|---|---|---|
| **Spontaneous**<br>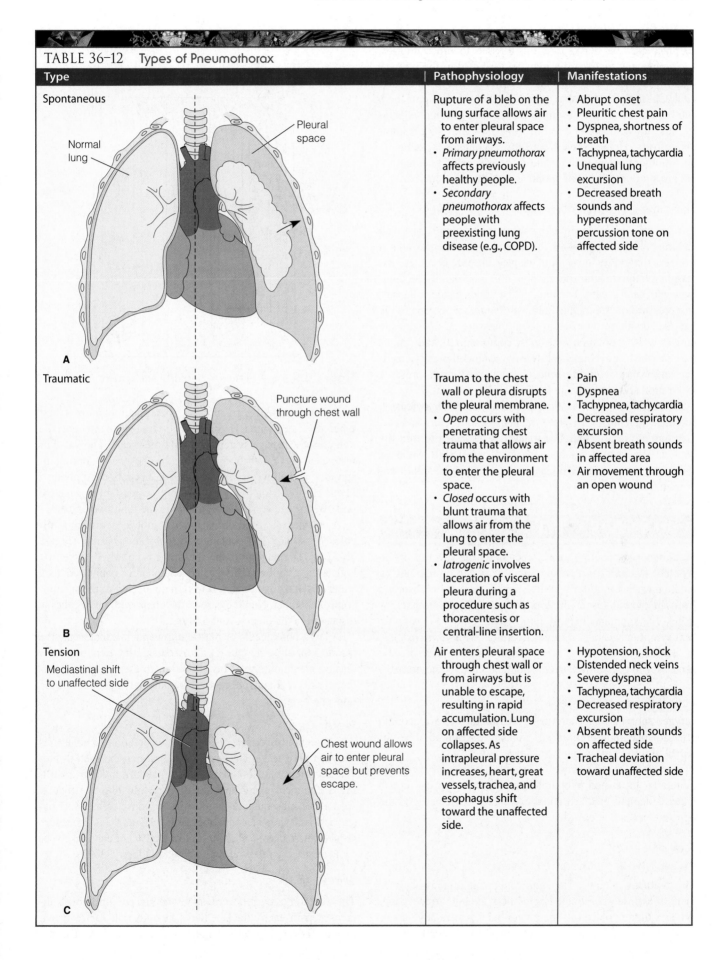 | Rupture of a bleb on the lung surface allows air to enter pleural space from airways.<br>• *Primary pneumothorax* affects previously healthy people.<br>• *Secondary pneumothorax* affects people with preexisting lung disease (e.g., COPD). | • Abrupt onset<br>• Pleuritic chest pain<br>• Dyspnea, shortness of breath<br>• Tachypnea, tachycardia<br>• Unequal lung excursion<br>• Decreased breath sounds and hyperresonant percussion tone on affected side |
| **Traumatic** | Trauma to the chest wall or pleura disrupts the pleural membrane.<br>• *Open* occurs with penetrating chest trauma that allows air from the environment to enter the pleural space.<br>• *Closed* occurs with blunt trauma that allows air from the lung to enter the pleural space.<br>• *Iatrogenic* involves laceration of visceral pleura during a procedure such as thoracentesis or central-line insertion. | • Pain<br>• Dyspnea<br>• Tachypnea, tachycardia<br>• Decreased respiratory excursion<br>• Absent breath sounds in affected area<br>• Air movement through an open wound |
| **Tension** | Air enters pleural space through chest wall or from airways but is unable to escape, resulting in rapid accumulation. Lung on affected side collapses. As intrapleural pressure increases, heart, great vessels, trachea, and esophagus shift toward the unaffected side. | • Hypotension, shock<br>• Distended neck veins<br>• Severe dyspnea<br>• Tachypnea, tachycardia<br>• Decreased respiratory excursion<br>• Absent breath sounds on affected side<br>• Tracheal deviation toward unaffected side |

Labels on figures:
Normal lung
Pleural space
A
Puncture wound through chest wall
B
Mediastinal shift to unaffected side
Chest wound allows air to enter pleural space but prevents escape.
C

With traumatic pneumothorax, manifestations of pain and dyspnea may be masked or missed due to other injuries. Tachypnea and tachycardia may be attributed to the primary injury. Focused assessment for evidence of pneumothorax is vital. Chest wall movement on the affected side is diminished, and breath sounds are absent. If a penetrating wound is present, air may be heard and felt moving through it with respiratory efforts. Hemothorax frequently accompanies traumatic pneumothorax. The manifestations of iatrogenic pneumothorax are similar to those of spontaneous pneumothorax.

## Tension Pneumothorax

*Tension pneumothorax* develops when injury to the chest wall or lungs allows air to enter the pleural space but prevents it from escaping. Pressure within the pleural space becomes positive in relation to atmospheric pressure as air rapidly accumulates with each breath. The lung on the affected side collapses, and pressure on the mediastinum shifts thoracic organs to the unaffected side of the chest, placing pressure on the opposite lung as well. Ventilation is severely compromised, and venous return to the heart is impaired. Tension pneumothorax is a medical emergency requiring immediate intervention to preserve respiration and cardiac output.

In addition to manifestations of pneumothorax, hypotension and distended neck veins are evident as venous return and cardiac output are affected. The trachea is displaced toward the unaffected side as a result of the mediastinal shift. Signs of shock may be present. See Chapter 6 ⊂⊃ for the manifestations and treatment of shock.

## COLLABORATIVE CARE

Treatment for pneumothorax depends on the severity of the problem. A small simple pneumothorax may require no treatment other than monitoring with serial X-rays. Air is absorbed from the pleural space, allowing most small pneumothoraces to resolve spontaneously. A large pneumothorax or significant symptoms usually requires treatment with *thoracostomy,* or the placement of chest tubes. Surgical intervention may be necessary to prevent recurrent spontaneous pneumothorax.

## Diagnostic Tests

Oxygen saturation measurements are obtained to evaluate the effect of pneumothorax on gas exchange. ABGs may be obtained to further assess gas exchange.

The chest X-ray is an effective diagnostic tool for pneumothorax. In tension pneumothorax, air is evident on the affected side, and mediastinal structures are shifted toward the opposite or unaffected side.

## Treatments

### Chest Tubes

The treatment of choice for significant pneumothorax is placement of a closed-chest catheter to allow the lung to reexpand. When a tube is placed in the pleural cavity to remove air or fluid, it must be sealed to prevent air from also entering the

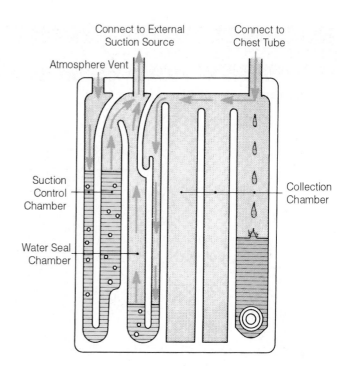

**Figure 36–16** ■ A closed-chest drainage system.

tube and, in essence, creating an open pneumothorax. Chest tubes are sealed with a Heimlich (one-way) valve or connected to a closed drainage system with a "water seal." The valve or water seal prevent air from entering the chest cavity during inspiration and allow air to escape during expiration. Applying a low level of suction to the system helps to reestablish negative pressure in the pleural space, allowing the lung to reexpand.

A number of closed-drainage chest tube systems are available. Most are self-contained disposable systems (Figure 36–16 ■). Drainage from the chest tube is collected in the first collection chamber. This sealed chamber is connected to a water-seal chamber, which is in turn connected to the suction-control chamber. Nursing care of the client with chest tubes is discussed in the box on page 1149.

A large-bore needle or plastic intravenous catheter may be inserted through the chest wall as emergency treatment of a tension pneumothorax. This allows air to escape from the affected side, relieving pressure on mediastinal structures and the opposite lung.

### Pleurodesis

Although controversial, *pleurodesis,* or creation of adhesions between the parietal and visceral pleura, may be used to prevent recurrent pneumothorax. This procedure involves instilling a chemical agent such as doxycycline into the pleural space. The subsequent inflammatory response creates scar tissue and adhesions between the pleural layers. This procedure reduces the recurrence rate to as low as 2% but can make subsequent surgery more difficult (Way & Doherty, 2003).

### Surgery

The risk for recurrence of spontaneous pneumothorax increases with each attack. Clients at high risk for recurrent pneumothorax may have surgery to reduce the risk of future

## NURSING CARE OF THE CLIENT WITH CHEST TUBES

### PREPROCEDURE CARE

- Ensure a signed informed consent for chest tube insertion. *This invasive procedure requires informed consent.*
- Provide additional information as indicated. Explain that local anesthesia will be used but that pressure may be felt as the trochar is inserted. Reassure that breathing will be easier once the chest tube is in place and the lung reexpands. *The client may be extremely dyspneic and anxious and may need reassurance that this invasive procedure will provide relief.*
- Gather all needed supplies, including thoracostomy tray, injectable lidocaine, sterile gloves, chest tube drainage system, sterile water, and a large sterile catheter-tipped syringe to use as a funnel for filling water-seal and suction chambers. *These supplies are used during the insertion procedure to establish a water-seal drainage system.*
- Position as indicated for the procedure. *Either an upright position (as for thoracentesis) or side-lying position may be used, depending on the site of the pneumothorax.*
- Assist with chest tube insertion as needed. The procedure may be performed in a procedure room, in the surgical suite, or at the bedside. *Although chest tube insertion is a relatively simple procedure, nursing assistance is necessary to support the client and rapidly establish a closed drainage system.*

### POSTPROCEDURE CARE

- Assess respiratory status at least every 4 hours. *Frequent assessment is necessary to monitor respiratory status and the effect of chest tube.*
- Maintain a closed system. Tape all connections, and secure the chest tube to the chest wall. *These measures are important to*

prevent inadvertent tube removal or disruption of the system integrity.
- Keep the collection apparatus below the level of the chest. *Pleural fluid drains into the collection apparatus by gravity flow.*
- Check tubes frequently for kinks or loops. *These could interfere with drainage.*
- Check the water seal frequently. The water level should fluctuate with respiratory effort. If it does not, the system may not be patent or intact. Periodic air bubbles in the water-seal chamber are normal and indicate that trapped air is being removed from the chest. *Frequent assessment of the system is important to ensure appropriate functioning.*
- Measure drainage every 8 hours, marking the level on the drainage chamber. Report drainage that is cloudy, in excess of 70 mL per hour, or red, warm, and free flowing. *Red, free-flowing drainage indicates hemorrhage; cloudiness may indicate an infection. Emptying the drainage would disrupt integrity of the closed system.*
- Periodically assess water level in the suction control chamber, adding water as necessary. *Adequate water in the suction control chamber prevents excess suction from being placed on delicate pleural tissue.*
- Assist with frequent position changes and sitting and ambulation as allowed. *Chest tubes should not prevent performance of allowed activities. Care is needed to prevent inadvertent disconnection or removal of the tubes.*
- When the chest tube is removed, immediately apply a sterile occlusive petroleum jelly dressing. *An occlusive dressing prevents air from reentering the pleural space through the chest wound.*

---

ruptures. A thoracotomy is done to excise or oversew blebs (usually at the apices of the lungs). The overlying pleura is then roughened or irritated to induce scarring and adhesion to the surface of the lung. In some cases, the parietal pleura may be partially excised. These procedures can be done using video-assisted thoracoscopic surgery (VATS), a minimally invasive surgical technique (Way & Doherty, 2003).

## NURSING CARE

### Health Promotion

Health promotion activities to prevent spontaneous and traumatic pneumothorax primarily involve health teaching. Initiate and participate in programs to prevent smoking among children and teenagers. Teach safe behaviors such as always wearing a seat beat in an automobile, driving safely, and using precautions to prevent falls when working or recreating in high places.

### Assessment

The client with pneumothorax may be in acute respiratory distress, necessitating rapid and focused assessment.

- Health history: current symptoms and their duration; precipitating factors or activities if known; previous episodes of pneumothorax; smoking history; chronic pulmonary diseases such as COPD
- Physical assessment: general appearance and degree of apparent respiratory distress; evidence of chest trauma; vital signs, oxygen saturation, skin color, level of consciousness; respiratory excursion, percussion tone, and breath sounds anterior and posterior chest; neck vein inspection, position of trachea; peripheral pulses

### Nursing Diagnoses and Interventions

Maintaining or restoring adequate alveolar ventilation and gas exchange is of highest priority for the client with a pneumothorax. Chest tubes may interfere with physical mobility, contributing to a high risk for injury.

### Impaired Gas Exchange

Loss of negative pressure in the pleural cavity and the resulting collapse of lung tissue can cause poor chest expansion and loss of alveolar ventilation. As the pneumothorax is removed or reabsorbed, ventilation and gas exchange improve.

- Assess and document vital signs and respiratory status, including rate, depth, lung sounds, and oxygen saturation at least every 4 hours. *Frequent assessment is important to monitor the adequacy of respirations and lung expansion.*

**PRACTICE ALERT** *Evaluate chest wall movement, position of the trachea, and neck veins frequently. Early identification of tension pneumothorax and appropriate interventions are vital to preserve cardiorespiratory function.* ■

- Place in Fowler's or high-Fowler's position. *This position facilitates lung expansion.*
- Administer oxygen as ordered. *Supplemental oxygen is given to improve oxygenation of the blood and tissues.*

**PRACTICE ALERT** *Provide emotional support, particularly in early stages and during chest tube insertion. Dyspnea and hypoxemia can cause extreme anxiety and apprehension, impairing the ability to cooperate with procedures.* ■

- Assess chest tube, system function, and drainage at least every 2 hours. *The system must remain patent and intact to function effectively.*
- Provide for rest. *Adequate rest is important to conserve energy and reduce oxygen demand.*

### Risk for Injury

Pain and the presence of chest tubes can reduce the perceived ability to ambulate and provide self-care. Moderate activity is encouraged unless respiratory function is significantly impaired. Caution is taken to maintain integrity of the chest tube system. If the tube is inadvertently pulled out or system integrity is disrupted, the pneumothorax may increase or infection may develop.

**PRACTICE ALERT** *Avoid placing tension on chest tubes during positioning, ambulation, and care activities. The chest tubes are minimally secured to the chest wall and can be dislodged if tension is placed on them.* ■

- Secure a loop of drainage tubing to the sheet or gown. *Looping the drainage tubing prevents direct pressure on the chest tube itself.*
- When turning to the affected side, ensure that neither the chest tube nor drainage tubing is kinked or occluded under the client. *This maintains patency of the system.*
- Teach the client how to ambulate with the drainage system, keeping the system lower than the chest. In most cases, suction can be discontinued during ambulation. *Ambulation facilitates lung ventilation and expansion. Drainage systems are portable to allow ambulation while chest tubes are in place. Keeping the drainage system lower than the chest promotes drainage and prevents reflux.*
- Observe insertion site for redness, swelling, pain, or drainage. Report any signs of infection, including fever, to the physician. *Interruption of skin integrity by chest tube insertion increases the risk for infection.*

- If a connection comes loose, reconnect it as soon as possible. *A closed, sealed system is vital to prevent air from entering the pleural space and an open pneumothorax.*

**PRACTICE ALERT** *Seal the wound of an open pneumothorax or from inadvertent tube removal as soon as possible with a sterile occlusive dressing, such as gauze impregnated with petroleum jelly. If a sterile dressing is not available, other occlusive material such as foil or plastic wrap can be used. Tape the dressing on three sides only. An occlusive dressing taped on three sides prevents the development of a tension pneumothorax by inhibiting air from entering the wound during inhalation but allowing it to escape during exhalation.* ■

### Home Care

Clients who have experienced spontaneous pneumothorax need education about their future risk. After a single episode of spontaneous pneumothorax, the risk of recurrence is 40% to 50%. This risk increases with subsequent episodes (Way & Doherty, 2003). Stress the importance of quitting smoking to reduce the risk. Other activities that can precipitate recurrent episodes include mountain climbing or those involving exposure to high altitudes, flying in unpressurized aircraft, and scuba diving (Tierney et al., 2001). The client may be advised to avoid contact sports.

Following a pneumothorax, instruct the client to gradually increase exercise and activity to previous levels. Stress the importance of follow-up care and monitoring. Discuss manifestations to report to the physician: upper respiratory infections; fever, cough, or difficulty breathing; sudden, sharp chest pain; or redness, pain, swelling, tenderness, or drainage from the chest tube puncture wound.

## THE CLIENT WITH HEMOTHORAX

**Hemothorax,** or blood in the pleural space, usually occurs as a result of chest trauma, surgery, or diagnostic procedures. Tumors, pulmonary infarction, and infections such as tuberculosis also can cause hemothorax. When blood collects in the pleural space, pressure on the affected lung impairs ventilation and gas exchange. With significant hemorrhage, a risk of shock exists.

Hemothorax causes symptoms similar to those of pneumothorax. Lung sounds are diminished, and a dull percussion tone is noted over the collected blood, typically at the base of the lung. Chest X-ray is used to confirm the diagnosis of hemothorax.

Thoracentesis or thoracostomy with chest tube drainage is used to remove blood from the pleural space. With significant hemorrhage (e.g., due to trauma or surgery), the blood may be collected for subsequent autotransfusion. Blood for autotransfusion should be collected and reinfused within 4 hours. Strict aseptic technique is used in collecting the blood. It is collected through a gross particulate filter into a container primed with anticoagulant and reinfused when the container is full or when transfusion is necessary. Air is removed from the blood container prior to reinfusion and a filter used to eliminate debris, such as degenerating blood cells, fat particles, and fibrin.

Priority nursing care for the client with hemothorax focuses on assessing and maintaining adequate respiratory function and cardiac output. The priority of care depends on the rate and extent of hemothorax. In a large, slow-developing hemothorax, ventilatory status may be affected significantly. In this instance, impaired gas exchange and ineffective breathing pattern are priority nursing diagnoses. When hemothorax develops rapidly and hemorrhage is significant, additional priority nursing diagnoses include *Decreased cardiac output* and *Risk for deficient fluid volume.*

When preparing the client for home care following a hemothorax, discuss the importance of avoiding smoking and preventing respiratory infection. Include symptoms to report to the physician. If trauma or infection caused the hemothorax, discuss measures to prevent future trauma and continuing treatment for the infection as indicated.

# TRAUMA OF THE CHEST OR LUNG

Chest injury is a leading cause of death from trauma. It is commonly associated with motor vehicle crashes, violent crime, and falls. Chest injuries can range from mild, such as a simple rib fracture, to severe and fatal. Traumatic injury to the chest may involve both the chest wall and underlying thoracic structures, including the lungs, heart, great vessels, and esophagus. Chest and lung injury can result from several different mechanisms: penetrating trauma, such as a stab or gunshot wound; blunt trauma, such as a fall, motor vehicle crash, vehicle-pedestrian impact, or crush injury; or inhalation injury, such as smoke inhalation or near drowning.

Rapid and continuing assessment of the airway, breathing, and circulation (ABCs) is vital in chest or lung injuries. Chest trauma can disrupt any or all of these functions. Chest injuries that may be life threatening include airway obstruction, tension pneumothorax, open pneumothorax, massive hemothorax, and flail chest with pulmonary contusion.

## THE CLIENT WITH A THORACIC INJURY

Thoracic injuries may be minor and have little effect on respiratory status, for example, simple rib fracture in a previously healthy client. When pain or chest wall instability impair breathing or the underlying lung tissue is damaged, the risk is more significant. Thoracic trauma usually is caused by motor vehicle crashes or falls.

## PATHOPHYSIOLOGY AND MANIFESTATIONS

Acceleration-deceleration injury and direct mechanisms of injury (e.g., crush injuries) are the most common mechanisms of thoracic injuries. Acceleration-deceleration injuries are caused by a rapid change in velocity as occurs in a motor vehicle crash or fall. The body stops suddenly, but the tissues and organs within the chest cavity continue to move forward until they impact with the chest wall. Injuries sustained can be significant, depending on the velocity (speed) of the vehicle or body at the point of impact, the surface with which the body impacts, and individual characteristics (e.g., size and bone structure).

## Rib Fracture

Simple rib fracture, usually involving a single rib, is the most common chest wall injury. Rib fracture generally is tolerated well and heals rapidly in a young, previously healthy person. In an older adult or person with preexisting lung disease, however, a fractured rib may lead to significant complications, such as pneumonia, atelectasis, and, potentially, respiratory failure. Displaced fractured ribs can penetrate the pleura, leading to pneumothorax and possible hemothorax. Fractures of certain ribs are more frequently associated with underlying tissue damage. Intrathoracic vessels may be damaged or torn with fractures of the first and second ribs. Fractures of the seventh through tenth ribs may cause liver or spleen injuries (Urden, Stacy, & Lough, 2002).

Rib fracture causes pain on inspiration and coughing. This leads to voluntary splinting, with rapid, shallow respirations and inhibited cough. Bruising may be seen over the fracture, and crepitus may be palpated with respiratory movement. Breath sounds are diminished, especially in the bases, due to splinting. If pneumothorax develops, chest wall movement on the affected side may be reduced, and breath sounds absent or significantly diminished. A hyperresonant percussion tone usually is noted. Hemothorax also causes diminished or absent breath sounds on the affected side, with a dull percussion note.

## Flail Chest

Multiple rib fractures may impair chest wall stability and normal chest wall function. When two or more consecutive ribs are fractured in multiple places, a free-floating segment of the chest wall, or **flail chest,** results. Physiologic function of the chest wall is impaired as the flail segment is sucked inward during inhalation and moves outward with exhalation. This is known as *paradoxic movement* (Figure 36–17 ■). Lung expansion is impaired and the work of breathing increases. Flail chest is frequently associated with underlying pulmonary contusion, which may lead to respiratory failure.

Flail chest causes dyspnea and pain, especially on inspiration. Paradoxic chest movement is evident with inspection. Chest expansion is unequal, and palpable crepitus is present. Breath sounds are diminished, and crackles may be heard on auscultation.

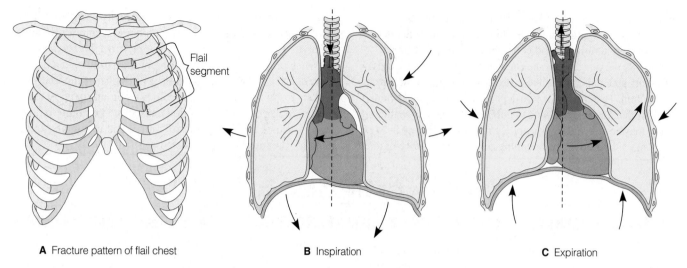

**A** Fracture pattern of flail chest    **B** Inspiration    **C** Expiration

**Figure 36–17** ■ Flail chest with paradoxic movement.

## Pulmonary Contusion

Pulmonary contusion, or lung tissue injury, is frequently associated with flail chest and other blunt chest trauma. It may occur unilaterally or bilaterally. Pulmonary contusion often results from abrupt chest compression followed by sudden decompression, as can occur with an MVC, significant fall, or crush injury. Alveoli and pulmonary arterioles rupture, causing intra-alveolar hemorrhage and interstitial and bronchial edema. The resulting inflammatory response increases capillary permeability, leading to edema which may be localized to the damaged lung tissue or more generalized. Inflammation and edema impair the production of surfactant within the alveoli, decreasing compliance. Pulmonary vascular resistance increases and blood flow decreases. Airway obstruction, atelectasis, and impaired gas diffusion result. Associated chest wall injury impairs the ability to clear secretions effectively, and the work of breathing is significantly increased.

Manifestations of pulmonary contusion may not be apparent until 12 to 24 hours after the injury. Increasing shortness of breath, restlessness, apprehension, and chest pain are early signs. Copious sputum, which may be blood tinged, is present. Later manifestations include tachycardia, tachypnea, dyspnea, and cyanosis. Even with appropriate treatment, pulmonary contusion can lead to acute respiratory distress and potential death.

## COLLABORATIVE CARE

Chest X-ray is used to identify most chest wall injuries. Rib fractures are evident on X-ray. Pulmonary contusion may show as initial patchy opacifications progressing to diffuse opacification, or "white-out." Changes in oxygen saturation and arterial blood gases depend on the degree to which ventilation and gas exchange are affected by the injury.

Simple rib fractures typically heal uneventfully. Providing adequate analgesia to promote breathing, coughing, and movement is the primary intervention. With multiple rib fractures, an intercostal nerve block may be used to ensure adequate ventilation. Rib belts, binders, and taping to stabilize the rib cage are not recommended, because they may interfere with ventilation and lead to atelectasis. Even with simple rib fracture, older clients and clients with preexisting lung disease require close monitoring to prevent and detect atelectasis, pneumonia, and other complications.

Intercostal nerve blocks or continuous epidural analgesia may be employed to manage the pain associated with flail chest. For a small flail chest, analgesia combined with supplemental oxygen therapy may be adequate. In some cases, internal or external fixation of the flail segment may be done.

The preferred treatment for flail chest is intubation and mechanical ventilation. Positive-pressure ventilation provides support and stabilization of the flail segment and improves ventilation and gas exchange. The work of breathing is decreased and healing improved.

Clients with pulmonary contusion often are critically ill, requiring intensive care management. Treatment is supportive, directed at maintaining adequate ventilation and alveolar gas exchange. Endotracheal intubation and mechanical ventilation are necessary in most cases. Repeated bronchoscopy may be done to remove secretions and cellular debris, preventing atelectasis. Although adequate hydration is necessary to prevent shock, overhydration can increase pulmonary edema. Pulmonary arterial pressure monitoring with a Swan-Ganz catheter and frequent arterial blood gas measurement is required for optimal fluid replacement and management of ventilatory support. See Chapter 30 ⬡ for more information about pulmonary artery pressure monitoring.

Unilateral pulmonary contusion may present a unique management problem. Mechanical ventilation with positive end-expiratory pressure (PEEP) to maintain open alveoli and adequate gas exchange can damage the unaffected lung. Intubation with a double-lumen endotracheal tube which permits independent ventilation of each lung may be used.

# NURSING CARE

Chest wall trauma can interfere with adequate chest expansion and alveolar ventilation. When a pulmonary contusion is also present, gas exchange is affected as well. Priorities for nursing management include controlling pain, ensuring adequate ventilation, and promoting gas exchange.

## Acute Pain

With many thoracic injuries, pain interferes with lung expansion and coughing, leading to such complications as pneumonia and atelectasis. Adequate pain management is a key component of medical and nursing management for these clients.

- Frequently assess pain, using a standard pain scale and objective data. *Increased respiratory rate, shallow respirations, diminished breath sounds, and reluctance to move and cough may indicate inadequate pain control in a thoracic injury.*
- Administer analgesics by patient-controlled analgesia or on a schedule to maintain pain control. *Analgesics are more effective when pain is not allowed to become intense.*

**PRACTICE ALERT** *Assess for possible respiratory depression due to narcotic analgesia. Respiratory depression can further compromise ventilation in the client with thoracic injury.* ■

- Notify the physician if pain relief is inadequate or excess sedation and respiratory depression occur. *An intercostal nerve block may be done to reduce the need for narcotic analgesia. Assess for bleeding and adequate ventilation following a nerve block.*

## Ineffective Airway Clearance

Aggressive respiratory hygiene may be necessary to maintain open airways and adequate ventilation.

- Assess lung sounds and respiratory rate, depth, and effort frequently. Encourage to cough, deep breathe, and change position every 1 to 2 hours, and use the incentive spirometer. *Frequent assessment and measures to maintain airway patency are vital to prevent complications in the client with thoracic injury.*
- Teach how to splint the affected area with a blanket or pillow when coughing. *Splinting reduces movement and discomfort of the affected area.*
- Suction airway as indicated. Work with respiratory therapy to maintain optimal mechanical ventilation. Secure the endotracheal tube to maintain appropriate position and lung ventilation. *Endotracheal tube security is particularly important when a double-lumen endotracheal tube is in place, because malposition can occlude one main bronchus and prevent ventilation of the affected lung.*

- Elevate the head of the bed. *Elevating the head of the bed facilitates lung expansion and reduces the work of breathing.*

**PRACTICE ALERT** *Promptly report to the physician signs of complications, such as diminished breath sounds, increasing crackles (rales) or rhonchi, dull or hyperresonant percussion tones, unequal chest movement, hemoptysis, chills or fever, or changes in vital signs. Prompt intervention for complications is vital to promote healing and recovery.* ■

## Impaired Gas Exchange

Impaired gas exchange is of particular concern in pulmonary contusion. Alveolar damage and pulmonary edema can significantly impair oxygenation of the blood and removal of carbon dioxide.

- Monitor vital signs, color, oxygen saturation, and arterial blood gases. Assess for manifestations such as anxiety or apprehension, restlessness, confusion or lethargy, or complaints of headache. *These assessment data alert the nurse and care providers to potential hypoxemia or hypercapnia due to impaired gas exchange.*
- Maintain oxygen therapy and mechanical ventilation as ordered. Hyperoxygenate prior to suctioning. *Oxygen and mechanical ventilation support alveolar gas exchange. Hyperoxygenation prior to suctioning reduces the degree of hypoxemia that occurs during suctioning.*
- Monitor intake and output, weigh daily, and monitor central venous pressure and pulmonary artery pressure as ordered. Maintain any ordered fluid restriction. *Fluid volume status is monitored to reduce the effects of pulmonary edema on lung tissues.*
- Maintain bed rest or activity restriction as ordered. Space activities to allow periods of uninterrupted rest. *Rest reduces the metabolic rate and oxygen consumption.*

## Home Care

Simple rib fracture and minor chest wall injuries often are managed on an outpatient basis. Include the following topics when teaching for home care.

- Pain management and its importance in preventing respiratory complications
- Importance of coughing and deep breathing; how to splint the rib cage during coughing
- Reasons for not taping or wrapping the chest continuously
- Symptoms to report to the physician: chills and fever, productive cough, purulent or bloody sputum, shortness of breath or difficulty breathing, and increasing chest pain
- Importance of avoiding respiratory irritants, such as cigarette smoke and occupational or environmental pollutants

Significant pulmonary contusion can result in long-term respiratory insufficiency. Discuss activity modifications and occupational changes with the client and family as indicated. Refer to home care services such as respiratory therapy and home health if needed.

## THE CLIENT WITH INHALATION INJURY

The internal environment of the lungs normally is protected from noxious substances by respiratory defense mechanisms. If these defenses are breached, inhaled agents, such as gases, fumes, toxins, and water, can cause internal trauma to the lungs.

## PATHOPHYSIOLOGY AND MANIFESTATIONS

### Smoke Inhalation

Pulmonary injury due to inhalation of hot air, toxic gases, or particulate matter is the leading cause of death in burn injury (Braunwald et al., 2001). Smoke inhalation affects up to one-third of clients admitted to burn units. Smoke inhalation can significantly affect normal respiratory function through three different mechanisms:

- Thermal damage to the airways, leading to impaired ventilation
- Carbon monoxide or cyanide poisoning, resulting in tissue hypoxia
- Chemical damage to the lung from noxious gases, which can impair gas exchange

Smoke inhalation is suspected whenever a burn occurs in a closed space; if there are burns to the face or upper torso or singed nasal hairs; if sputum contains ashlike material; and when manifestations such as dyspnea, wheezing, rales, or rhonchi develop.

The lower airways of the lungs typically are protected from thermal damage by cooling of the inhaled gases in the upper airway and laryngeal spasm. Upper airway obstruction due to tissue edema and laryngeal spasm can occur quickly, however, resulting in **asphyxiation,** or oxygen deprivation, without lung damage. Steam inhalation can cause thermal damage to tissues of the lower respiratory tract.

Inhalation of carbon monoxide or cyanide gas poses an immediate threat to life. Carbon monoxide is a colorless, odorless gas produced in a fire. It binds readily with hemoglobin. The affinity of carbon monoxide for hemoglobin is 200 to 250 times stronger than that of oxygen. Hemoglobin bound to carbon monoxide reduces the oxygen-carrying capacity of blood and oxygen delivery to cells of the body. Carbon monoxide poisoning is suspected if the burn occurred in a closed space, if there is evidence of inhalation injury, or if dyspnea develops.

The manifestations of carbon monoxide poisoning depend on the level of carboxyhemoglobin saturation. When hemoglobin is 10% to 20% saturated with carbon monoxide, symptoms include headache, dizziness, dyspnea, and nausea. A characteristic "cherry-red" color of the skin and mucous membranes may be seen. With increasing levels, confusion, visual disturbances, irritability, hallucinations, hypotension, seizures, and coma develop. Permanent neurologic deficit can occur in survivors of severe acute carbon monoxide poisoning.

Many other toxic chemicals may be present in smoke, especially in a house fire or industrial plant fire. Hydrogen cyanide can be lethal when inhaled. Inhalation of toxic chemicals causes bronchospasm and edema of the airways and alveoli. Acute respiratory distress syndrome may develop within 1 to 2 days. Sloughing of damaged mucosa leads to airway obstruction and atelectasis. Pneumonia is common following smoke inhalation.

### Near-Drowning

Drowning is a leading preventable cause of accidental death in the United States. Approximately 5500 people die of drowning every year in the United States. Alcohol ingestion is a factor in 25% to 33% of adult drowning deaths (Tierney et al., 2001). Asphyxiation and aspiration are the primary problems associated with drowning and near-drowning. About 10% of victims do not aspirate water; instead, laryngeal spasm causes asphyxia. This is known as "dry drowning." In most cases, however, asphyxia and hypoxemia are the result of fluid aspiration. The effects of hypoxemia occur rapidly; loss of consciousness can occur within 3 to 5 minutes after total immersion. Circulatory impairment, brain injury, and brain death can occur within 5 to 10 minutes. Immersion in very cold water and the *dive reflex*, a protective mechanism that slows the heartbeat, constricts peripheral vessels, and shunts blood to the brain and heart, may prolong survival.

Water aspiration can cause delayed death from near-drowning. Respiratory and systemic effects differ, depending on whether freshwater or saltwater has been aspirated. Freshwater is hypotonic; when aspirated, it is rapidly absorbed from the alveoli, leading to hypervolemia and hemodilution. Hemolysis occurs as blood cells are subjected to a hypotonic environment, and serum electrolytes are diluted. Electrolyte imbalances can cause cardiac dysrhythmias and death. Hemolysis can lead to acute tubular necrosis and acute renal failure. Aspiration of freshwater impairs pulmonary surfactant and damages the alveolar-capillary membrane. Respiratory failure can result.

Nearly the opposite effects occur with saltwater aspiration. As a hypertonic fluid, saltwater draws fluid into the alveoli, resulting in hypovolemia and hemoconcentration. Hemolysis is insignificant, and small elevations in serum sodium and chloride levels rarely cause life-threatening effects. With either type of near-drowning episode, inhaled microorganisms and debris can lead to pneumonia. The pathophysiologic changes associated with freshwater and saltwater near-drowning are illustrated in Figure 36–18 ■.

Manifestations of near-drowning may include altered level of consciousness, restlessness, and apprehension. The client may complain of headache or chest pain. Other signs include vomiting, possible cyanosis, apnea, tachypnea, and wheezing. If pulmonary edema is present, pink froth may be visible in the mouth and nose. Other manifestations include tachycardia, dysrhythmias, hypotension, shock, and cardiac arrest. Hypothermia may be present.

The near-drowning victim who never loses consciousness or is conscious on admission to the emergency department has a good prognosis for recovery. The prognosis is less optimistic when neurologic damage has occurred.

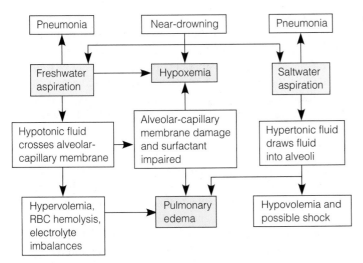

**Figure 36–18** ■ The pathogenesis of near-drowning, freshwater and saltwater.

## COLLABORATIVE CARE

With inhalation injuries, the most effective treatment is prevention. A working smoke detector (with functioning batteries) could prevent the majority of deaths from smoke inhalation occurring in the home. The line, "A smoke detector was found, but the batteries had been removed," is all too familiar in news reports of fire-related deaths.

To prevent drowning, life preservers and flotation vests or jackets should be worn on the body, not stored in the hold of the boat. These devices are designed to keep the head above water. Even accomplished swimmers should never enter the water alone in unguarded areas. Just as alcohol and driving do not mix, neither do alcohol and boating or other water sports.

The second most important line of defense against death or permanent injury from inhalation injuries is removing the victim from the area of the fire or water and administering effective cardiopulmonary resuscitation. In many cases, immediate restoration of effective breathing and circulation is key to preserving life. Hypoxemia progresses rapidly until breathing is restored; reversal of tissue hypoxia depends on adequate circulation. In both smoke inhalation and near drowning, intubation may be necessary to establish an airway. Oxygen is administered as soon as possible. Attempts to drain water from the lungs of the near-drowning victim waste time and are generally ineffective in restoring alveolar ventilation. External cardiac defibrillation may be necessary to reestablish an effective cardiac rhythm and circulation. When the victim is hypothermic, resuscitation measures are continued until the core body temperature reaches approximately 90°F (32°C). The basic rule in hypothermia is that the client is not declared dead until the body has been rewarmed and life signs remain absent.

### Diagnostic Tests

When inhalation injury is known or suspected, the following diagnostic tests may be done.

- *ABGs* are drawn to evaluate gas exchange and the degree of hypoxemia. Combined respiratory and metabolic acidosis may be apparent. With effective ventilation and supplemental oxygen, acidosis may reverse quickly. With carbon monoxide poisoning, arterial $PO_2$ may be normal, but oxyhemoglobin saturation is less than normal.
- *Carboxyhemoglobin levels* are drawn in suspected carbon monoxide poisoning. Normal levels are less than 5% in nonsmokers and less than 10% in smokers. Higher levels indicate carbon monoxide poisoning. Levels less than 20% are considered mild poisoning; between 20% and 40% is moderate poisoning; and 40% to 60% is severe poisoning. Levels higher than 60% are generally fatal.
- *Serum electrolytes* and *osmolality levels* vary in near-drowning, depending on the type of water aspirated. In freshwater drowning, serum electrolyte levels and osmolality may be significantly reduced. With saltwater drowning, serum sodium and chloride may be somewhat high, and osmolality is increased because of hypovolemia.
- *Chest X-ray* is done, but may not show changes until 12 or more hours after the insult. Evidence of acute respiratory distress syndrome may be seen 24 to 48 hours after inhalation injury.
- *Bronchoscopy* may be ordered to inspect damaged lung tissue, particularly with smoke inhalation and possible thermal injury.

### Treatments

Treatment of inhalation injury is generally supportive. Endotracheal intubation and mechanical ventilation often are required to maintain the airway and provide adequate alveolar ventilation and oxygenation. All clients with inhalation injury require supplemental oxygen, even when intubation and ventilation are not required. *Hyperbaric oxygen therapy,* the delivery of 100% oxygen at increased atmospheric pressure, may be used to treat carbon monoxide poisoning. This treatment carries some risks, such as oxygen toxicity and potential trauma to lung tissues, sinuses, and ears due to the increased pressures (Leifer, 2001).

Other treatment measures may include bronchodilator therapy to manage bronchospasm. Bronchodilators can be administered by aerosol inhalation or intravenous infusion. Coughing and suctioning is important to remove secretions and debris. Chest physiotherapy with percussion and postural drainage may be performed.

Intravenous fluids may be ordered; if significant hemolysis has occurred, packed red blood cells may be given to improve the oxygen-carrying capacity of the blood. Fluid therapy is monitored carefully, using pulmonary artery or central venous pressures to reduce the risk of pulmonary edema.

With near-drowning victims, measures such as inducing hypothermia or barbiturate-induced coma and administering corticosteroids and osmotic diuretics may be employed to help prevent neurologic damage.

Careful monitoring for complications such as pneumonia and acute respiratory distress syndrome is vital throughout the course of treatment. Respiratory status, vital signs, and other data are frequently assessed to identify complications and allow early intervention.

# NURSING CARE

## Health Promotion

Prevention of inhalation injuries is an important nursing responsibility. Teach everyone the value of a working smoke detector, especially in the sleeping areas of the house. Encourage families to develop an escape plan in case of fire and to use fire drills to rehearse getting out of the house. Smoldering cigarettes are a leading cause of house fires; help clients develop a plan to stop smoking. Teach people to drop and roll should clothing catch fire. (Flames rise, increasing the risk of respiratory injury when upright.)

Learning to swim safely is important to prevent drowning. Teach clients never to swim alone, when fatigued, or immediately following a meal. Remind clients that knowing how to swim will not prevent drowning in very cold water or in large bodies of water, such as lakes, rivers, or the ocean. Instruct to always wear flotation devices while boating, water-skiing, surfing, or wind-surfing. Wet suits help prevent hypothermia during activities in very cold water. Advise covering or fencing swimming pools, hot tubs, and ponds to prevent inadvertent entry and drowning.

A population well trained in effective, safe cardiopulmonary resuscitation (CPR) provides the best second line of defense against inhalation injury. Rapid restoration of breathing is essential to prevent hypoxia and brain damage. Encourage all people to be trained and regularly update CPR skills. Work with communities to increase the number of trained people. Refer clients to local chapters of the American Red Cross or American Heart Association for classes.

## Assessment

Inhalation injuries may be a medical emergency, necessitating focused and timely nursing assessment.

- Health history: circumstances of the injury, including duration of exposure to smoke or time under water, explosion or fire in a closed area, type and temperature of water immersed in; resuscitation measures used; allergies, and current medical problems
- Physical examination: airway, breathing, circulation; level of consciousness; color; vital signs; heart and lung sounds; urine output; evidence of burns or soot around nares or mouth

## Nursing Diagnoses and Interventions

Nursing care priorities for the client with an inhalation injury are determined by the type of injury or tissue damage. Airway clearance is a major concern in all inhalation injuries, as is impaired gas exchange. Tissue hypoxia also can be a significant problem.

### Ineffective Airway Clearance

Nursing measures to maintain an adequate airway begin with careful and frequent assessment of respiratory status, including rate, depth, and effort as well as breath sounds. Note amount, color, and consistency of sputum. Assist to cough frequently; suction the intubated client as needed to remove secretions. Elevate the head of the bed to facilitate alveolar ventilation unless otherwise ordered. Stabilize endotracheal tube with tape and ties to prevent displacement into a mainstem bronchus, which could lead to ventilation of only one lung. Report changes in the character of secretions that may indicate complications: pink, frothy sputum suggesting pulmonary edema, or purulent sputum suggestive of pneumonia. Administer bronchodilators as ordered. Perform percussion and postural drainage as ordered.

### Impaired Gas Exchange

Support gas exchange by administering supplemental oxygen, with or without mechanical ventilation. Frequently assess oxygen saturation, skin color, and mental status. Decreasing level of consciousness may be an early sign of hypoxemia. Monitor exhaled carbon dioxide, arterial blood gases, and pulmonary artery pressures as ordered and indicated. Report changes to the physician. Maintain oxygen flow rates as ordered. Provide frequent mouth care to reduce the discomfort of dry mucous membranes and prevent tissue breakdown. Work with respiratory therapy to maintain effective oxygen delivery with mechanical ventilation. Administer sedation as required. Maintain fluid restriction if ordered.

### Ineffective Tissue Perfusion: Cerebral

Impaired cerebral tissue perfusion is a priority problem, especially with near-drowning. Hypoxia and possible hypervolemia can lead to cerebral edema and increased intracranial pressure (IICP), further impairing blood flow. Monitor vital signs and neurologic status frequently. A change in level of consciousness or behavior is typically the earliest sign of IICP. Changes noted on an intracranial pressure monitor also provide early evidence of IICP. Increasing systolic blood pressure and pulse pressure and slowed heart rate are late signs. Other manifestations may include pupillary changes and decreasing muscle strength. Report changes promptly to the physician. Elevate the head of the bed and keep the head in neutral position to promote drainage from the cranial vault. Maintain effective ventilation and oxygenation; hypercapnia and hypoxemia increase cerebral edema. Administer sedation, osmotic diuretics, or corticosteroids as ordered to reduce cerebral edema. Maintain fluid restriction. Space activities and promote rest to reduce metabolic demands.

## Home Care

Teach clients who do not require hospitalization for inhalation injury about symptoms that may indicate a complication and should be reported to the physician: increasing dyspnea, cough productive of purulent or pink frothy mucus, confusion, or other changes. Manifestations of respiratory damage may not be apparent for 24 to 48 hours following the injury.

Significant hypoxia due to near-drowning or carbon monoxide poisoning may cause permanent neurologic effects. Work with the family to develop communication techniques and identify remaining strengths. Help the family identify future care needs and means for meeting them, such as home health, personal care aides, or long-term care facilities. Provide social services and support group referrals.

# RESPIRATORY FAILURE

Many of the conditions discussed in this chapter, from pneumonia to acute respiratory distress syndrome (ARDS), can lead to respiratory failure. In **respiratory failure,** the lungs are unable to oxygenate the blood and remove carbon dioxide adequately to meet the body's needs, even at rest.

## THE CLIENT WITH ACUTE RESPIRATORY FAILURE

Respiratory failure is not a disease but a consequence of severe respiratory dysfunction. It is often defined by arterial blood gas values. An arterial oxygen level ($Po_2$) of less than 50 to 60 mmHg and an arterial carbon dioxide level ($Pco_2$) of greater than 50 mmHg are generally accepted as indicators of respiratory failure. However, clients with advanced COPD may be alert and functional with blood gas values that would indicate respiratory failure in someone whose respiratory function was previously normal. In clients with COPD, respiratory failure is indicated by an acute drop in blood oxygen levels along with increased carbon dioxide levels.

Respiratory failure can result from inadequate alveolar ventilation (hypoventilation), impaired gas exchange, or a significant ventilation-perfusion mismatch. COPD is the most common cause of respiratory failure. Other lung diseases, chest injury, inhalation trauma, neuromuscular disorders, and cardiac conditions can also lead to respiratory failure. Selected causes of acute respiratory failure are identified in Table 36–13.

## PATHOPHYSIOLOGY

Respiratory failure may be characterized by primary hypoxemia or a combination of hypoxemia and hypercapnia (Figure 36–19 ■). In hypoxemic respiratory failure, $Po_2$ is significantly

| TABLE 36–13 | Selected Causes of Respiratory Failure |
|---|---|
| **Type of Dysfunction** | **Examples** |
| **Impaired ventilation:** | |
| • Airway obstruction | Laryngospasm, foreign body aspiration, airway edema |
| • Respiratory disease | Asthma, COPD |
| • Neurologic causes | Spinal cord injury, poliomyelitis, Guillain-Barré syndrome, drug overdose, stroke |
| • Chest wall injury | Flail chest, pneumothorax |
| **Impaired diffusion:** | |
| • Alveolar disorders | Pneumonia, pneumonitis, COPD |
| • Pulmonary edema | Heart failure, acute respiratory distress syndrome (ARDS), near-drowning |
| **Ventilation-perfusion mismatch** | Pulmonary embolism |

reduced, whereas $Pco_2$ remains normal or is low due to stimulation of the respiratory center and tachypnea. Impaired diffusion across the alveolar-capillary membrane, and a ventilation-perfusion mismatch can cause a drop in arterial oxygen levels that is more rapid than the rise in carbon dioxide. Metabolic acidosis results from tissue hypoxia. The increased work of breathing can eventually lead to respiratory muscle fatigue and hypoventilation.

Hypoventilation, or reduced movement of air into and out of the lung, causes carbon dioxide retention. With significant hypoventilation, the carbon dioxide level in the blood rises rapidly, leading to respiratory acidosis. Hypoxemia develops more slowly, and responds readily to administration of oxygen unless gas exchange also is impaired.

**Figure 36–19 ■** Respiratory failure, its causes and manifestations.

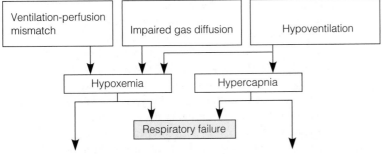

Manifestations:
• Dyspnea, tachypnea
• Cyanosis
• Restlessness, apprehension
• Confusion, impaired judgment
• Tachycardia, dysrhythmias
• Hypertension
• Metabolic acidosis

Manifestations:
• Dyspnea → respiratory depression
• Headache
• Papilledema
• Tachycardia, hypertension
• Drowsiness, coma
• Systemic vasodilation, heart failure
• Respiratory acidosis

In summary, hypoxemia without a corresponding rise in carbon dioxide levels indicates a failure of oxygenation; hypoxemia with hypercapnia is the result of lung hypoventilation.

The prognosis for acute respiratory failure varies, depending on the underlying disease process. Respiratory failure resulting from uncomplicated drug overdose generally resolves quickly without long-term effects. When respiratory failure results from underlying lung disease, the course may be prolonged and the outcome less favorable. Among adults requiring mechanical ventilation for acute respiratory failure, it is estimated that 62% survive to be weaned from the ventilator, but only 43% survive to be discharged from the hospital, and 30% remain alive at 1 year after discharge (Tierney et al., 2001).

## MANIFESTATIONS

The manifestations of respiratory failure are caused by hypoxemia and hypercapnia, as well as the underlying disease process. Hypoxemia causes dyspnea and neurologic symptoms such as restlessness, apprehension, impaired judgment, and motor impairment. Tachycardia and hypertension develop as the cardiac output increases in an effort to bring more oxygen to the tissues. Cyanosis is present. As hypoxemia progresses, dysrhythmias, hypotension, and decreased cardiac output may develop.

Increased carbon dioxide levels depress CNS function and cause vasodilation. Dyspnea and headache are early signs. Other manifestations include peripheral and conjunctival vasodilation, papilledema, neuromuscular irritability, and decreased level of consciousness. As hypercapnia worsens, the respiratory center may be depressed, reducing dyspnea and slowing respirations. Increased carbon dioxide and hydrogen ion concentrations not longer stimulate the respiratory center; hypoxemia provides the only active breathing stimulus. Administering oxygen without ventilatory support may eliminate any drive to breathe, leading to respiratory arrest.

## COLLABORATIVE CARE

Treatment of respiratory failure focuses on correcting the underlying cause or disease, supporting ventilation, and correcting hypoxemia and hypercapnia. Care related to disorders that can precipitate respiratory failure is discussed in the sections specific to each disorder.

### Diagnostic Tests

Exhaled carbon dioxide and arterial blood gases are used to diagnose and monitor treatment of respiratory failure.

- *Exhaled carbon dioxide (ETCO₂)* is used to evaluate alveolar ventilation. The normal ETCO₂ is 35 to 45 mmHg; it is elevated when ventilation is inadequate, and decreased when pulmonary perfusion is impaired.
- *Arterial blood gases* also are used to evaluate alveolar ventilation and gas exchange. With hypoxemic respiratory failure, the $P_{CO_2}$ may be normal, 38 to 42 mmHg, or even low due to tachypnea. A pH of less than 7.35 and low bicarbonate levels indicate metabolic acidosis, typical of hypoxemic respiratory failure.

In respiratory failure due to hypoventilation, the $P_{CO_2}$ is elevated, usually greater than 50 mmHg. The pH is low due to respiratory acidosis. Acidosis develops rapidly in hypoxemia and hypercapnia because of increased acid production (metabolic) and decreased acid elimination (respiratory).

### Medications

Drugs used in treating respiratory failure depend on the underlying cause of the failure and the need for intubation and mechanical ventilation.

Beta-adrenergic (sympathomimetic) or anticholinergic medications may be administered by inhalation to promote bronchodilation. If mechanical ventilation is required, the drugs may be given by nebulizer attached to the ventilator. Methyxanthine bronchodilators (theophylline derivatives) may be given intravenously. See the box on page 1110 and the asthma section of this chapter for more information about bronchodilators and their nursing implications. Corticosteriods, administered by inhalation or intravenously, may be ordered to reduce airway edema. Antibiotics are given to treat any underlying infection.

Sedation and analgesia often are required during mechanical ventilation to decrease pain and anxiety. Benzodiazepines such as diazepam (Valium), lorazepam (Ativan), or midazolam (Versed) may be used for sedation and to inhibit the respiratory drive. Intravenous morphine or fentanyl provide analgesia and also inhibit the respiratory drive, allowing more effective mechanical ventilation. Occasionally, the client's respiratory drive competes with the ventilator despite sedation, decreasing its effectiveness and increasing the work of breathing. A neuromuscular blocking agent may be necessary to induce paralysis and suppress the ability to breathe. Nursing implications of neuromuscular blockers are described in the Medication Administration box on page 1159.

### Oxygen Therapy

Oxygen is administered to reverse hypoxemia in acute respiratory failure. In general, the goal is to achieve an oxygen saturation of 90% or greater without oxygen toxicity. A $P_{O_2}$ of about 60 mmHg usually is adequate to meet the oxygen needs of body tissues. Higher levels do not significantly increase oxygen saturation and may lead to hypoventilation in clients with chronic hypercapnia. As little as 1 to 3 L of oxygen per nasal cannula or 28% oxygen per Venturi mask may correct hypoxemia in advanced COPD. Oxygen concentrations of 40% to 60% may be required when diffusion is impaired (e.g., in pneumonia or acute respiratory distress syndrome). High concentrations are used only for short periods to avoid oxygen toxicity. Both the oxygen concentration and duration of therapy contribute to oxygen toxicity. Continued high oxygen concentrations impair the synthesis of surfactant, reducing lung compliance (ease of inflation). Acute respiratory distress syndrome or absorption atelectasis may develop.

When respiratory failure is caused by hypoventilation or usual oxygen delivery systems do not correct hypoxemia, a tight-fitting mask to maintain *continuous positive airway pressure (CPAP)* may be used. CPAP increases lung volume,

## Medication Administration

### Neuromuscular Blockers

#### NONDEPOLARIZING NEUROMUSCULAR BLOCKERS
Rocuronium (Zemuron)
Pancuronium bromide (Pavulon)
Atracurium besylate (Tracrium)
Cisatracurium (Nimbex)

Nondepolarizing neuromuscular blockers competitively block the action of acetylcholine (ACh) at skeletal muscle receptors, preventing muscle depolarization and contraction. Complete muscle paralysis is achieved within minutes. Facial muscles are affected first, followed by muscles of the limbs, neck, and trunk. The muscles of respiration (the diaphragm and intercostal muscles) are least sensitive to the effects of neuromuscular blockers and are paralyzed last. When the drug is discontinued or an antagonist is given, muscles recover in reverse order, respiratory function is recovered first.

#### Nursing Responsibilities
- Prior to administering, assess endotracheal tube placement and ensure effective mechanical ventilator function. The risk of hypoxemia and organ damage is significant if respiratory muscles are paralyzed without adequate ventilatory support in place.
- Administer the drug by slow intravenous injection and/or intravenous infusion as prescribed.

- Keep an acetylcholinesterase (AChE) inhibitor such as neostigmine (Prostigmin) available at the bedside to rapidly reverse neuromuscular effects if needed.
- Administer morphine sulfate, diazepam (Valium), or other antianxiety agent or sedative as ordered. Neuromuscular blockers provide no sedation or pain relief; muscle paralysis produces extreme anxiety.
- Instill artificial tears every 2 to 4 hours.
- Suction oral cavity as needed to remove saliva.
- *Never* turn off ventilator alarms when administering neuromuscular blockers. Should the tubing become disconnected or plugged, the client is unable to breathe independently or call for help.
- Treat the client as though awake and alert. Although unable to respond, mental function is unaffected.

#### Client and Family Teaching
- Reassure that the ability to move and communicate will return when the drug is discontinued.
- Teach the family about the effects of the drug and the reason for its use. Explain that the client can hear and understand what is going on.

---

opening previously closed alveoli, improving ventilation of underventilated alveoli, and improving ventilation-perfusion relationships.

## Airway Management

If the upper airway is obstructed or positive pressure mechanical ventilation is necessary to correct hypoxemia and hypercapnia, an endotracheal tube that extends from the mouth or nose into the trachea is inserted (Figure 36–20 ■). To maintain positive pressure ventilation, the tube is cuffed with an air-filled or foam sac just above the end of the tube. When the cuff is inflated, it obstructs the upper airway, preventing air from escaping back into the nose or mouth. Excess pressure of the cuff can cause tissue ischemia and necrosis of the trachea. To minimize this risk, high-volume, low-pressure ("floppy") cuffs are used. Tubes with low-pressure cuffs may be left in place for 3 to 4 weeks.

A tracheostomy may be performed if long-term ventilatory support is required. Although a tracheostomy is more comfortable and easier to secure in place, complications such as cuff necrosis and increased risk of infection are associated with tracheostomy as well as endotracheal intubation. Table 36–14 compares the advantages, disadvantages, and possible complications of endotracheal tubes and tracheostomy.

When the client is able to maintain effective respirations and ventilatory support is no longer required, the endotracheal tube is removed (*extubation*). Gag, cough, and swallow reflexes must be intact to prevent aspiration. After oxygenation and suctioning, the cuff is deflated and the tube removed. Humidified oxygen is provided immediately following removal. Close observation for respiratory distress is vital following extubation. Inspiratory stridor within the first 24 hours indicates laryngeal edema, which may necessitate reintubation. Sore throat and a hoarse voice are common after extubation. Oral intake is reinitiated slowly, with careful assessment of swallowing.

## Mechanical Ventilation

Mechanical ventilation is indicated when alveolar ventilation is inadequate to maintain blood oxygen and carbon dioxide levels. Specific indications for mechanical ventilation include:

- Apnea or acute ventilatory failure.
- Hypoxemia unresponsive to oxygen therapy alone.
- Increased work of breathing with progressive client fatigue.

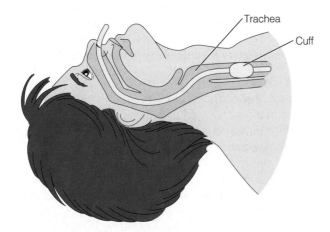

**Figure 36–20** ■ Nasal endotracheal (nasotracheal) intubation.

TABLE 36–14  A Comparison of Endotracheal Tubes and Tracheostomy

| | Advantages | Disadvantages | Potential Complications |
|---|---|---|---|
| Oral endotracheal tube | • More easily inserted<br>• Larger tube can be used, facilitating work of breathing, suctioning | • More difficult to secure<br>• Can be obstructed by biting<br>• Communication and mouth care more difficult<br>• Increased risk of lower respiratory infection | • Obstruction or displacement<br>• Pressure necrosis of lip<br>• Tracheoesophageal fistula |
| Nasal endotracheal tube | • More easily secured and stabilized<br>• Well tolerated by client<br>• Facilitate communication and oral hygiene | • Necessitate smaller tube which may impede removal of secretions<br>• Increased risk of lower respiratory infection | • Obstruction or displacement<br>• Pressure necrosis of nares<br>• Obstruction of sinus drainage, possible sinusitis<br>• Tracheoesphageal fistula |
| Tracheostomy | • Easily secured and stabilized<br>• Enable swallowing, speech, and oral hygiene<br>• Avoid upper airway complications | • Require surgical incision<br>• Increased risk of lower respiratory infection | • Hemorrhage due to incision or vessel erosion by tube<br>• Wound infection<br>• Subcutaneous emphysema |

Drug overdose, neural disorders, chest wall injury, and airway problems such as severe asthma or COPD can lead to acute ventilatory failure. Disorders that affect alveolar-capillary diffusion, such as pulmonary contusion, pneumonia, and ARDS, may necessitate mechanical ventilation to attain adequate oxygenation. Positive pressure ventilation increases lung volume, helps redistribute fluid from the alveolar to the interstitial space, and helps reduce the oxygen demand caused by increased work of breathing in many conditions leading to respiratory failure.

## Types of Ventilators

Two broad general classifications of mechanical ventilators are available. Negative-pressure ventilators create subatmospheric pressure externally to draw the chest outward and air into the lungs, mimicking spontaneous breathing. The iron lung, Curiass ventilator, and PulmoWrap are examples of negative-pressure ventilators (Figure 36–21 ■).

Positive-pressure ventilators are more commonly used, especially in treating acute respiratory failure (Figure 36–22 ■). These ventilators push air into the lungs, rather than drawing it in like negative-pressure ventilators. An endotracheal tube or tracheostomy is necessary for positive-pressure ventilation.

Several variables are used to trigger, cycle, and limit airflow with positive-pressure ventilators. The *trigger* prompts the ventilator to deliver a breath. The client's inspiratory effort triggers *ventilator-assisted breaths. Ventilator-controlled breaths* usually are triggered by a preset time interval (e.g., a breath is delivered every 5 seconds for a rate of 12 breaths per minute). The ventilator *cycle,* or duration of inspiration, can be limited by volume, pressure, flow, or time. *Volume-cycled ventilators* deliver air until a preset volume is delivered. *Pressure-cycled ventilators* cycle off when a preset pressure is achieved within the airways. *Flow-cycled ventilators* are cycled by a preset inspiratory flow rate, and *time-cycled ventila-*

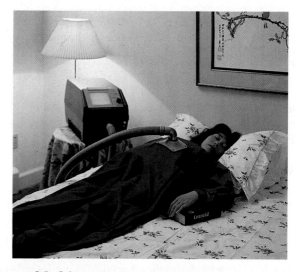

**Figure 36–21** ■ A negative-pressure ventilator.

*Courtesy of Life Care Corporation.*

*tors* deliver air for a set time interval. Airflow delivered by the ventilator also can be limited by factors such as airway pressure (e.g., a volume-cycled ventilator can be set to immediately stop inspiratory flow if airway pressure exceeds a preset value).

## Modes of Ventilation

A number of different *modes* or patterns of ventilation may be used with positive-pressure ventilators. Assist-control mode ventilation, synchronized intermittent mandatory ventilation, continuous positive airway pressure, positive end-expiratory pressure, pressure support ventilation, and pressure-control ventilation are common modes of ventilation in use today (Table 36–15).

*Assist-control mode ventilation (ACMV)* is frequently used to initiate mechanical ventilation and when the client is at risk

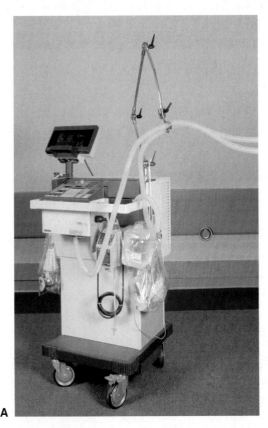

**A**

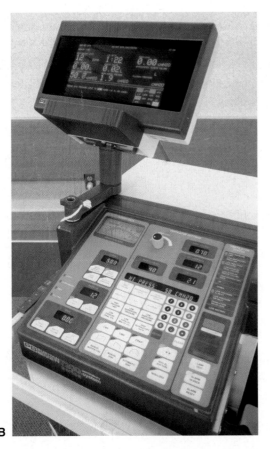

**B**

**Figure 36–22** ■ A positive-pressure ventilator and the control panel used to set the mode, rate, limits, and percentage of oxygen delivered.

for respiratory arrest (e.g., overdose or head injury). Assisted breaths are triggered by inspiratory effort; however, if the respiratory rate falls below a preset number (e.g., 14 per minute), ventilator-controlled breaths are delivered. All breaths, assisted and controlled, are delivered at a specific tidal volume or pressure and inspiratory flow rate.

*Synchronized intermittent mandatory ventilation (SIMV)* allows the client to breathe spontaneously, without ventilator assistance, between delivered ventilator breaths. Mandatory or ventilator-controlled breaths are delivered at a preset rate, volume, and/or pressure, coordinated with the client's inspiratory efforts. This mode of ventilation is used to support ventilation, to exercise respiratory muscles between ventilator-assisted breaths and during the weaning process (Braunwald et al., 2001).

*Continuous positive airway pressure (CPAP)* applies positive pressure to the airways of a spontaneously breathing client. CPAP may be used with either endotracheal intubation or a tight-fitting face mask. All breathing is spontaneous (client triggered) and pressure controlled. CPAP is used to help maintain open airways and alveoli, decreasing the work of breathing.

*Positive end-expiratory pressure (PEEP)* requires intubation and can be applied to any of the previously described ventilator modes. With PEEP, a positive pressure is maintained in the airways during exhalation and between breaths. Keeping alveoli

open between breaths improves ventilation-perfusion relationships and diffusion across the alveolar-capillary membrane. This reduces hypoxemia and allows use of lower percentages of inspired oxygen. PEEP is particularly useful for treating ARDS.

In *pressure support ventilation (PSV)*, ventilator-assisted breaths are delivered when the client initiates an inspiratory effort. The cycle is flow limited; inspiration is terminated when inspiratory airflow falls below a preset rate. This mode decreases the work of breathing. It can be used in combination with SIMV when the respiratory drive is depressed. Ventilatory support can be gradually withdrawn during weaning.

*Pressure-control ventilation (PCV)*, in contrast, controls pressure within the airways to reduce the risk of airway trauma (e.g., following thoracic surgery). Ventilation is time triggered and time cycled, but pressure is limited. The ventilator maintains a preset airway pressure throughout inspiration. Because all breaths are controlled by the ventilator, heavy sedation may be required to prevent competition between inspiratory effort and ventilator control.

*Noninvasive ventilation (NIV)* provides ventilator support using a tight-fitting facemask, thus avoiding intubation. Its primary use is to support clients with impending respiratory failure (e.g., advanced COPD). The degree of success varies, primarily limited to client intolerance due to the physical and psychologic discomfort of wearing a mask when dyspneic (Braunwald et al., 2001).

## TABLE 36-15  Modes of Positive-Pressure Ventilator Operation

| Mode | Description | Pattern |
|---|---|---|
| Spontaneous breathing | Client has full control of rate, tidal volume, pressures. | |
| Assist-control mode ventilation (ACMV) | Client can trigger ventilator to deliver breaths at preset volume or pressure and inspiratory flow rate; breaths will be delivered at preset rate if client does not initiate. | |
| Synchronized intermittent mandatory ventilation (SIMV) | Mandatory breaths delivered by ventilator are synchronized with client's inspiratory effort. | |
| Continuous positive airway pressure (CPAP) | Positive pressure is maintained in airways; all breaths are spontaneous. | |
| Positive end-expiratory pressure (PEEP) | Used in conjunction with other ventilator modes; positive airway pressure is maintained throughout respiratory cycle. | |
| Pressure support ventilation (PSV) | Pressurized inspiratory flow supports the client's inspiratory effort, decreasing the work of breathing. | |

TABLE 36–16   Ventilator Settings

| Parameter | Description |
|---|---|
| Rate (f) | Number of ventilator-delivered breaths per minute: usually 12 to 15 in adults using ACMV, may be lower in SIMV |
| Tidal volume ($V_t$) | Amount of gas delivered with each ventilator breath: usually 8 to 10 mL/kg of body weight |
| Oxygen concentration ($FIO_2$) | Percentage of oxygen delivered with ventilator breaths: can be set between 21% (room air) and 100% |
| I:E ratio | Duration of inspiration to expiration: usually 1:2 to 1:1.5 |
| Flow rate | Speed at which air is delivered |
| Sensitivity | Effort required by client to initiate a ventilator-assisted breath |
| Pressure limit | Maximal pressure within airways that will terminate a ventilator breath |

## Ventilator Settings

In addition to choosing the mode of ventilation, other parameters are set to meet individual client needs when positive-pressure ventilation is used (Table 36–16).

For most adult clients, the rate is initially set between 12 and 15 breaths per minute. With ACMV or SIMV, the client's respiratory rate often is higher than the ventilator setting due to spontaneous breathing. Exhaled carbon dioxide ($ETCO_2$) or the $PCO_2$ may be used to determine the rate. A $PCO_2$ less than 38 mmHg indicates hyperventilation and respiratory alkalosis; the set rate is reduced. A $PCO_2$ above 42 mmHg or an $ETCO_2$ greater than 45 mmHg indicates hypoventilation and a need to increase the rate.

The tidal volume setting controls the amount of gas delivered with each ventilator breath. The normal adult tidal volume at rest is about 7 mL/kg of body weight, or 400 to 550 mL. The tidal volume delivered by mechanical ventilation is slightly higher (500 to 750 mL) to compensate for tubing dead space. Higher tidal volumes can cause lung tissue trauma.

The percentage of oxygen delivered with ventilator breaths is adjusted to maintain the oxygen saturation and $PO_2$ within acceptable ranges. Because prolonged delivery of high oxygen concentrations increases the risk of oxygen toxicity and pulmonary fibrosis, the $FIO_2$ is set at the lowest possible level for adequate tissue oxygenation. For most clients, the goal is to maintain an oxygen saturation greater than 90%. Lower levels may be appropriate for clients with long-standing COPD.

## Complications

Although endotracheal intubation and mechanical ventilation can be life-saving in respiratory failure, they are not without risk. Improper endotracheal tube placement or advancement of the tube into a mainstem bronchus can result in ventilation of one lung only. The inflated lung becomes overdistended and traumatized, and the uninflated lung develops atelectasis.

**NOSOCOMIAL PNEUMONIA.**   Infection is a significant risk associated with intubation and mechanical ventilation. Normal upper respiratory tract defense mechanisms are bypassed, with loss of air humidification and trapping of pathogens. Oral secretions and gastric contents can enter the respiratory tree through the open epiglottis. Often the cough reflex is inhibited or impaired by the underlying disease process and the contin-

ued presence of the endotracheal tube. Even when strict asepsis is used for suctioning and other respiratory procedures, the lower airways are contaminated within 24 hours of intubation (Urden et al., 2002). Secretions often become thick and tenacious, increasing the risk of atelectasis.

**BAROTRAUMA.**   *Barotrauma* (also called *volutrauma*) is lung injury due to alveolar overdistention. Both the volume of delivered gas and the pressures under which it is delivered can contribute to barotraumas. As a result, overdistended alveoli rupture, allowing air to escape into the pulmonary interstitial spaces and the mediastinum, pleural space, and other tissues. Subcutaneous emphysema, pneumothorax, and pneumomediastinum are possible results of barotrauma. *Subcutaneous emphysema,* or air in the subcutaneous tissue, causes tissue swelling of the chest, neck, and face. A "crackling" or air-bubble-popping sensation is felt on palpation of subcutaneous emphysema. Swelling may be massive. Once the cause is corrected, the air is gradually reabsorbed.

*Pneumothorax* is identified by signs of unequal chest expansion, a sudden loss or significant decrease in breath sounds on the affected side, and a hyperresonant percussion tone. Rapid chest tube insertion is necessary to prevent tension pneumothorax and cardiovascular compromise. *Pneumomediastinum* is the presence of air in the mediastinum, the space between the lungs that contains the heart, great vessels, trachea, and esophagus. Air in the mediastinal space can interfere with the function of all these organs and lead to such complications as pneumopericardium (air in the pericardial sac). Pneumomediastinum may have few manifestations, but the chest X-ray shows widening of the mediastinal space.

**CARDIOVASCULAR EFFECTS.**   Positive-pressure ventilation increases intrathoracic pressure, which can interfere with venous return to the heart and ventricular filling. As a result, cardiac output falls. Use of PEEP increases the effects of mechanical ventilation on cardiac output. The decreased cardiac output can affect liver and kidney function secondarily.

**GASTROINTESTINAL EFFECTS.**   Gastrointestinal complications are commonly associated with prolonged mechanical ventilation. Stress ulcers (erosive gastritis) may develop, leading to painless gastrointestinal hemorrhage. Histamine $H_2$-receptor blockers or sucralfate are often used to prevent stress ulcers. Air leaks around the endotracheal tube can cause gastric distention; a nasogastric tube often is inserted to prevent vomiting. Sedation and other medications used during mechanical ventilation can slow intestinal motility, leading to constipation.

## Weaning

The process of removing ventilator support and reestablishing spontaneous, independent respirations is called **weaning.** Weaning begins only after the underlying process causing respiratory failure has been corrected or stabilized. The process and time required for weaning depend on factors such as preexisting lung condition, duration of mechanical ventilation, and the client's general condition, both physical and psychologic. In all cases, the vital signs, respiratory rate, extent of dyspnea, blood gases, and clinical status are used to evaluate weaning and its progress.

Following a brief period of mechanical ventilation, T-piece or CPAP may be used for weaning. In T-piece weaning, the ventilator is removed for brief periods during which oxygen is delivered using a T-piece (Figure 36–23 ■). The duration of periods off the ventilator is gradually increased until the client can maintain adequate independent respirations for several hours. Vital signs, oxygen saturation, $ETCO_2$, and $PO_2$ are carefully monitored during the process. When mechanical ventilation is no longer needed, the endotracheal tube is removed. CPAP weaning follows a similar process, with trials of spontaneous breathing supported by the ventilator in CPAP mode.

SIMV and PSV are used for weaning when the duration of mechanical ventilation has been longer and reconditioning of respiratory muscles is needed. When SIMV is used, the number of mandatory ventilator-assisted breaths is gradually decreased as ABGs, $ETCO_2$, and the respiratory rate are monitored. When the client is able to tolerate SIMV at 4 breaths per minute without rest periods of greater ventilatory support, CPAP or T-piece weaning is attempted prior to extubation (Braunwald et al., 2001).

Weaning is the primary use for pressure-support ventilation (PSV). Initially, PSV is set slightly below peak inspiratory pressures required during volume-cycled ventilation. Pressure support levels are gradually decreased, often in a cyclic pattern of periods of minimal support alternating with higher support to recondition respiratory muscles. When the

PSV level is just enough to overcome endotracheal tube resistance, support is discontinued and the client is extubated (Braunwald et al., 2001).

***TERMINAL WEANING.*** When an illness is terminal or irreversible with a poor prognosis, terminal weaning may be requested by the client or family. *Terminal weaning* is the gradual withdrawal of mechanical ventilation when survival without assisted ventilation is not expected. Unlike weaning when recovery is expected which usually occurs in an intensive care unit (ICU), the client is moved to a quiet medical-surgical or hospice room or even home prior to initiating terminal weaning. Family members are encouraged to remain with the client throughout the process. If possible, decisions about sedation and analgesia prior to and during weaning are made with the client, as are decisions about hydration and nutritional support following weaning. Ventilator support is gradually withdrawn using the same modes described earlier (SIMV, PSV). Analgesia and sedation are given to promote comfort during weaning.

## Other Treatments

Attention also must be paid to fluid and electrolyte status and adequate nutrition. Mechanical ventilation promotes sodium and water retention due to its effects on cardiac output. Renal perfusion is decreased, stimulating the renin-angiotensin-aldosterone system to retain sodium and water. A Swan-Ganz catheter is often inserted to monitor pulmonary artery pressures and cardiac output. An arterial line allows repeated blood gas analysis and continuous arterial pressure monitoring. Serum electrolytes are drawn frequently, and intake, output, and daily weight are carefully monitored.

Enteral or pareteral nutrition are provided during mechanical ventilation, because the endotracheal tube prohibits eating. A nasogastric, gastrostomy, or jejunostomy feeding tube is placed for enteral nutrition. A jejunostomy tube may be used to reduce the risk of regurgitation and aspiration.

## NURSING CARE

### Health Promotion

Education is a primary strategy to prevent respiratory failure. Teach all clients and the public about the risks of smoking, water safety, the value of a working smoke detector, and measures to prevent smoke inhalation in a fire. Discuss the importance of pneumococcal vaccine and annual influenza immunizations for people who are at high risk, including those over age 65 and people with chronic diseases. Teach clients with COPD about measures to reduce their risk of respiratory infection and symptoms to report to the physician.

### Assessment

Focused assessment data related to respiratory failure includes the following:

- Health history: current manifestations, their duration, and identified precipitating factors (may need to be obtained from family members if mental status is affected); history of

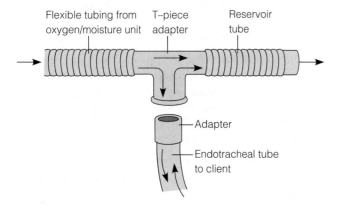

**Figure 36–23 ■** A T-piece, or "blow-by" unit, for weaning from mechanical ventilation.

Labels in figure: Flexible tubing from oxygen/moisture unit; T-piece adapter; Reservoir tube; Adapter; Endotracheal tube to client

previous episodes; chronic diseases such as COPD, occupational lung disease; current medications
- Physical examination: level of consciousness, mental status; vital signs; color and oxygen saturation; respiratory assessment including rate and depth, use of accessory muscles, respiratory excursion, auscultation; cardiovascular assessment including heart rate and sounds, neck vein distention, peripheral pulses, evidence of clubbing

## Nursing Diagnoses and Interventions

Clients in respiratory failure are often unstable and critically ill. They require both intensive medical care and intensive nursing care. Priority nursing needs relate to maintaining ventilation and a patent airway. Perhaps less obvious, but no less critical, nursing care needs relate to preventing injury and managing anxiety.

### Impaired Spontaneous Ventilation

In acute respiratory failure, fatigue from the work of breathing may impair the ability to maintain adequate ventilation. This is a concern both prior to initiation of mechanical ventilation and during the weaning process. See the box below.

- Assess and document respiratory rate, vital signs, and oxygen saturation every 15 to 30 minutes. *Close monitoring is vital to detect early signs of increasing respiratory distress and inability to sustain adequate breathing.*

**PRACTICE ALERT** *Promptly report signs of respiratory distress, including tachypnea, tachycardia, nasal flaring, use of accessory muscles, intercostal retractions, cyanosis, increasing restlessness, anxiety, or decreased level of consciousness. These may be early manifestations of respiratory failure and inability to maintain ventilatory effort.* ■

- Promptly report worsening arterial blood gases and oxygen saturation levels. *Close assessment of these values allows timely intervention as needed.*
- Administer oxygen as ordered, monitoring response. Observe closely for respiratory depression, especially in the client with COPD. *Oxygen administration reduces the hypoxemic respiratory drive. Chronically high $PCO_2$ levels depress the respiratory center; hypoxemia may provide the only respiratory drive.*
- Place in Fowler's or high-Fowler's position. *Sitting positions decrease pressure on the diaphragm and chest, improving lung ventilation and decreasing the work of breathing.*
- Minimize activities and energy expenditures by assisting with ADLs, spacing procedures and activities, and allowing uninterrupted rest periods. *Rest is vital to reduce oxygen and energy demands.*

**PRACTICE ALERT** *Avoid sedatives and respiratory depressant drugs unless mechanically ventilated. These medications can further depress the respiratory drive, worsening respiratory failure.* ■

## Nursing Research

### Evidence-Based Practice for the Client on Long-Term Mechanical Ventilation

Problems associated with long-term mechanical ventilation can further impair the client's ability to be weaned from ventilator support. These problems include symptom control, nutrition, psychologic and emotional problems, and sleep-rest deprivation. Fatigue, a psychologic and physiologic response to physical, situational, and psychologic stress, often is overlooked as a factor during weaning procedures. The client has had to relinquish control of his or her body and environment. Exposure to environmental, drug-related, mental, and emotional stressors is constant, and nutritional, sleep-rest, and activity patterns are altered for days or weeks. Technology impairs human interactions and increases vulnerability to energy depletion.

Higgins (1998) studied fatigue, nutrition, depression, and sleep-rest in a group of clients who were mechanically ventilated for at least 7 days. None of the clients had been ventilator dependent before hospital admission. They ranged in age from 24 to 79 years; 65% of the subjects had a primary diagnosis of acute respiratory failure on admission to critical care. Interestingly, five subjects declined to participate in the study because of fatigue. Descriptive and laboratory data obtained from the medical record and a questionnaire were used to measure the perception of fatigue, depression, and sleep-rest. All study participants perceived themselves as fatigued, with 45% reporting severe fatigue. Although all subjects were followed by a dietitian and received enteral nutrition, serum albumin levels fell during hospitalization. Moderate depression was noted on a standardized depression tool.

### IMPLICATIONS FOR NURSING

The data obtained in this study suggest that clients on long-term ventilator support are malnourished, and experience fatigue, depression, and disturbed sleep-rest. Nurses need to monitor nutritional status, and actively collaborate with the physician and dietitian to maintain adequate nutrition. Fatigue and related manifestations indicate a need for energy-conserving nursing interventions. Sleep is fragmented. Consideration should be given to moving clients on long-term ventilation to an intermediate care or step-down unit as soon as possible to provide for privacy and social interaction with family and to reduce noxious environmental stimuli.

### Critical Thinking in Client Care

1. Serum albumin and hemoglobin levels were used to evaluate the subjects' nutritional status. What other measures could be used to assess client nutrition?
2. Identify possible behavioral indicators of depression in the client who is intubated and on mechanical ventilation. What nursing measures would be appropriate related to depression in the critically ill client?
3. Develop a nursing care plan to improve the quality and duration of sleep for a client who is intubated and on mechanical ventilation.

- Prepare for endotracheal intubation and mechanical ventilation:
  a. Obtain an intubation tray with a selection of sterile endotracheal tubes and laryngoscope with a variety of adult blades.
  b. Check laryngoscope lamp; replace battery pack or bulb as needed.
  c. Set up for endotracheal suction, bringing continuous suction head, container, tubing, sterile catheter and glove kits, and sterile normal saline to the bedside.
  d. Notify respiratory therapy to set up the ventilator.
  e. Notify radiology that a portable chest X-ray will be needed on completion of intubation to verify correct placement of the endotracheal tube.
  *Intubation and mechanical ventilation may be required to maintain ventilation and gas exchange.*
- Explain the procedure and its purpose to the client and family, providing reassurance that this is a temporary measure to reduce the work of breathing and allow rest. Alert that talking is not possible while the endotracheal tube is in place, and establish a means of communication. *Thorough explanation is important to relieve anxiety.*

### Ineffective Airway Clearance

Ineffective airway clearance may either cause respiratory failure or occur as a result of interventions. Impaired ventilation frequently leads to acute respiratory failure, particularly in clients with COPD or asthma. Chest trauma also can impair airway patency as a result of pulmonary contusion and ineffective cough. Although intubation and mechanical ventilation can be life-saving measures, they also increase the risk of respiratory infection and ineffective secretion management.

**PRACTICE ALERT** *Frequently assess respiratory rate, chest movement, lung sounds, oxygen saturation, $ET_{CO_2}$, and ABGs. Intubation and mechanical ventilation do not ensure adequate oxygenation and ventilation. Displacement of the endotracheal tube or obstruction by respiratory secretions impair ventilation.* ■

- Suction as needed to maintain a patent airway. Indicators for suctioning include crackles and rhonchi on auscultation, frequent coughing or setting off the high-pressure alarm, and increasing restlessness or anxiety. Procedure 36–2 outlines endotracheal suctioning. *Although clients with a tracheostomy can usually cough up secretions, the length and diameter of endotracheal tubes makes this extremely difficult. Even with humidification, secretions often become thick and tenacious, further inhibiting their removal.*
- Obtain sputum for culture if it appears purulent or is odorous. *Culture is necessary to identify pathogens and guide antibiotic therapy.*
- Perform percussion, vibration, and postural drainage as ordered. *These techniques help loosen secretions and move them into larger airways for removal by coughing or suctioning.*

**PRACTICE ALERT** *Evaluate endotracheal tube cuff pressure by measurement (should have no more than 20 to 25 mmHg of pressure) or by auscultating the suprasternal notch for a hissing sound at the end of inspiration. The minimum effective cuff pressure to maintain alveolar ventilation is used to reduce the risk of tracheal ischemia and necrosis.* ■

- Firmly secure endotracheal or tracheostomy tube. Provide adequate slack on ventilator tubing to prevent tension on the tube when turning, positioning, or transferring to chair or stretcher. If necessary, loosely restrain hands. *These measures are important to ensure proper airway placement and prevent its inadvertent removal.*
- Assess fluid balance and maintain adequate hydration. *Adequate hydration helps liquefy secretions.*

### Risk for Injury

Many factors increase the risk for injury in acute respiratory failure. Hypoxemia and hypercapnia affect the level of consciousness and may impair mental status. Endotracheal intubation and mechanical ventilation carry risks of tracheal damage and trauma to the lungs. Neuromuscular blockade, if used, presents a significant risk for injury as the client is unable to breathe spontaneously, communicate, and move.

- Assess frequently, noting the following:
  a. Level of consciousness, orientation, and awareness
  b. Condition of mucosa of mouth and nose
  c. Respiratory: lung sounds, chest excursion, and ventilator pressures
  d. Cardiovascular: vital signs, skin color, capillary refill, and peripheral pulses
  e. Gastrointestinal: bowel sounds; test gastric secretions and feces for occult blood
  f. Genitourinary: urine output, daily weight
  g. Skin and extremities
  *Complications associated with respiratory failure and mechanical ventilation can affect many body systems. Frequent assessment allows early detection and intervention.*

**PRACTICE ALERT** *Do not bypass or turn off any ventilator alarms. The intubated client is unable to communicate verbally and cannot call for help. If neuromuscular blockers are used, the client is also unable to breathe without ventilator support.* ■

- Report condition changes such as increasing air leak around the cuff and decreased breath sounds or chest movement. *These may be manifestations of a complication of intubation and ventilation, such as tracheal necrosis, displacement of the endotracheal tube into the right mainstem bronchus, pneumothorax, or atelectasis.*
- Turn and reposition frequently, taking care to stabilize endotracheal tube during movement. *Repositioning helps maintain tissue perfusion and prevent skin and tissue breakdown.*
- Keep skin and linens clean, dry, and wrinkle-free. Protect pressure areas with padding, eggcrate, or heal and elbow protectors. *The client may not be able to perceive and report*

## Procedure 36–2 — Endotracheal Suctioning

### SUPPLIES

- Suction unit with connecting tubing and connector at the bedside
- If an in-line suction catheter is not present
  a. Sterile suction catheter (size 12 to 16 Fr) and glove-kit or suction catheter and sleeve
  b. Sterile normal saline
- Personal protective devices as indicated: goggles, mask, gown

### PREPROCEDURE

Explain the procedure and why it is being done. Tell the client that although suctioning is not painful, it is uncomfortable. While suction is being applied, breathing is difficult but these periods last only 10 seconds. Stress that suctioning allows removal of secretions and stimulates coughing, which helps clear secretions from smaller airways. Establish a means of communicating; for example, tell the client to raise a finger or rapidly blink if unable to tolerate suctioning.

### PROCEDURE

1. Use standard precautions.
2. Prepare the suction unit by turning it on and regulating it to no more than −80 to −120 mmHg.
3. Open sterile saline bottle, leaving the cap loosely in place.

**WITH AN IN-LINE CATHETER**

- Wearing exam gloves, attach the catheter to suction tubing.
- Adjust the oxygen ($FIO_2$) to 100%; allow three breaths.

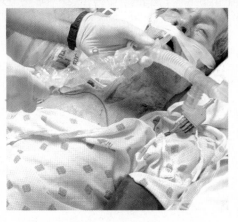

- Manipulating the catheter through the plastic shield (to maintain its sterility), insert the catheter without applying suction until resistance is met; apply suction while slowly withdrawing the catheter with a twirling motion (see figure)
- Suction for no longer than 10 seconds (count the seconds or watch the clock—the time passes more quickly than you think), then allow to rest for three to five breaths. Repeat the procedure as needed for a total of no more than three times.
- Remove suction tubing from the catheter, clear the tubing, turn off suction, and remove and discard gloves.

**WITH A SEPARATE CATHETER-AND-GLOVE KIT**

- Open suction catheter/glove kit. Remove saline cup, and fill with sterile normal saline.
- Put on sterile gloves, and attach catheter to suction tubing, keeping dominant hand sterile; lubricate catheter tip with sterile saline.

- Use the nondominant hand to adjust oxygen ($FIO_2$) to 100%; allow three breaths.
- Using the nondominant hand, disconnect ventilator tubing from the endotracheal tube. Manipulating the suction catheter with the dominant (sterile) hand and the suction control valve with the non-dominant (nonsterile) hand, insert the catheter, without applying suction until resistance is met. Then, apply suction while slowly withdrawing the catheter, using a twirling motion.
- Suction for no longer than 10 seconds. Reconnect the ventilator, and allow to rest for three to five breaths; clear suction tubing with sterile saline.
- Repeat the above two steps as needed for a total of three times.
- Reconnect ventilator tubing to the endotracheal tube.
- Clear suction tubing, turn off suction, and remove the catheter, discarding it with the gloves.
4. Provide three additional breaths at 100% oxygen, then readjust to the previous ordered level.
5. Note color, quantity, consistency, and odor of sputum.
6. Assess lung sounds and tolerance of the procedure.
7. Wash hands.

### POSTPROCEDURE

Document assessment before and after suctioning, along with the character of the sputum and the client's tolerance of the procedure. Report changes in sputum character, such as purulence or an odor that may indicate infection.

---

*pain, and move voluntarily to reduce pressure, necessitating excellent skin care.*

- Perform passive ROM exercises every 4 to 8 hours. *These exercises maintain joint flexibility and help prevent contractures associated with long-term immobility.*
- Keep side rails up and use soft restraints as needed. *These safety measures are important to prevent falls, inadvertent disconnection of the ventilator, or dislodging of the endotracheal tube.*
- Administer histamine $H_2$-blockers and sucralfate as ordered. *Stress gastritis and possible gastrointestinal hemorrhage are common, preventable complications of mechanical ventilation.*

### Anxiety

Critical illness creates anxiety for any client. In acute respiratory failure, this anxiety is compounded by the presence of an endotracheal tube or tracheostomy, mechanical ventilator, numerous monitors and equipment, and, potentially, neuromuscular blockade and paralysis of voluntary muscles. Fear of continued dependence on the mechanical ventilator and inability to return to a normal life may compound this anxiety.

**PRACTICE ALERT** *Frequently monitor anxiety level. High levels of anxiety increase oxygen use and often interfere with the ability to work with the respirator. This can increase hypoxemia and further increase anxiety; intervention is necessary to break this cycle.* ■

- Remain with the client as much as possible. *The frequent and continuing presence of a caregiver provides reassurance that help is readily available.*
- Explain all monitors, procedures, unusual sounds, and machinery. *Understanding of the environment and various sounds and alarms reduces anxiety.*
- Provide a simple means of communication, such as a slate, picture board, or alphabet board. If neuromuscular blockade is used, use methods such as looking to the right for "yes" and left for "no." Reassure that endotracheal tube removal restores the ability to speak. *The inability to speak and call out for help is frightening for the client. Providing an alternate means of communication helps reduce anxiety.*
- Encourage frequent family visits, especially if the time of visitations is being limited. Encourage family participation in care. *Family visits help reduce anxiety and feelings of abandonment. Allowing family members to participate in care helps reduce their anxiety as well.*
- Explain to the family that the client can hear and understand. Emphasize the importance of talking to the client, not over or about the client. *The family may not understand that the client may be mentally alert although unable to respond. Talking to the client about everyday things reduces the client's sense of isolation and fear.*
- Provide distraction with radio or television if allowed. *Distraction helps reduce the focus on machines and unusual sounds of monitors and alarms.*
- Attend to physical needs promptly and completely. *This provides reassurance that needs will be met even though the client is unable to ask for assistance.*
- Reassure that intubation and mechanical ventilation is a temporary measure to allow the lungs to rest and heal. Reinforce that the client will be able to breathe independently again. *The client may fear continued dependence on mechanical ventilation.*

**PRACTICE ALERT** *Provide sedation and antianxiety medications as needed, especially when neuromuscular blockade is used. Although neuromuscular blockade paralyzes voluntary muscles, the level of consciousness is unimpaired.* ■

## Using NANDA, NIC, and NOC

Chart 36–5 shows links between NANDA nursing diagnoses, NIC, and NOC for the client with respiratory failure.

## Home Care

Prior to hospital discharge, teach the client and family about the following topics.

- Factors that precipitated respiratory failure and measures to prevent it in the future (e.g., the impact of respiratory irritants on compromised lungs)
- Measures to prevent future episodes such as remaining indoors with an air filter or air conditioning when pollution levels are high, obtaining influenza and pneumonia immunizations, and avoiding exposure to cigarette smoke
- Effective coughing and pulmonary hygiene measures such as percussion, vibration, and postural drainage

Acute respiratory failure resulting from an acute insult such as pneumonia or near-drowning often resolves with few long-term sequelae. When respiratory failure results from an underlying disease such as COPD, the prognosis is less optimistic. Clients with end-stage COPD may have repeated episodes of respiratory failure, with a gradual loss of respiratory function and reserve. These clients may choose terminal weaning rather than a future of increasing disability. Discuss what to expect during the terminal weaning process with the client and family. Discuss use of sedation prior to and during the weaning process. Explain that medications are used to reduce respiratory distress and dyspnea during weaning. Assure

## CHART 36–5 NANDA, NIC, AND NOC LINKAGES

### The Client with Respiratory Failure

| NURSING DIAGNOSES | NURSING INTERVENTIONS | NURSING OUTCOMES |
|---|---|---|
| • Impaired Spontaneous Ventilation | • Respiratory Monitoring<br>• Artificial Airway Management<br>• Mechanical Ventilation | • Respiratory Status: Gas Exchange<br>• Respiratory Status: Ventilation |
| • Dysfunctional Ventilatory Weaning Response | • Anxiety Reduction<br>• Mechanical Ventilatory Weaning<br>• Energy Management | • Anxiety Control<br>• Respiratory Status: Ventilation<br>• Energy Conservation |
| • Ineffective Airway Clearance | • Airway Suctioning<br>• Airway Insertion and Stabilization | • Respiratory Status: Airway Patency |
| • Impaired Gas Exchange | • Oxygen Therapy | • Respiratory Status: Gas Exchange |

*Note. Data from Nursing Outcomes Classification (NOC) by M. Johnson & M. Maas (Eds.), 1997, St. Louis: Mosby; Nursing Diagnoses: Definitions & Classification 2001–2002 by North American Nursing Diagnosis Association, 2001, Philadelphia: NANDA; Nursing Interventions Classification (NIC) by J.C. McCloskey & G. M. Bulechek (Eds.), 2000, St. Louis: Mosby. Reprinted by permission.*

the client and family that nursing support is continuously available during the weaning process and that family and other supporters such as clergy are allowed to remain with the client.

## THE CLIENT WITH ACUTE RESPIRATORY DISTRESS SYNDROME

**Acute respiratory distress syndrome (ARDS)** is characterized by noncardiac pulmonary edema and progressive refractory hypoxemia. First identified in 1967, ARDS has been known by various names, such as shock lung, wet lung, Vietnam lung, and adult hyaline membrane disease. It is widely recognized as a severe form of acute respiratory failure. The mortality rate associated with acute respiratory distress syndrome, while declining, remains around 50%.

Although the exact cause of ARDS is unclear, it is known that ARDS does not occur as a primary process but may follow a number of diverse conditions producing direct or indirect lung injury (see Table 36–17).

## PATHOPHYSIOLOGY

The underlying pathology in ARDS is acute lung injury resulting from an unregulated systemic inflammatory response to acute injury or inflammation. Inflammatory cellular responses and biochemical mediators damage the alveolar-capillary membrane. This damage develops rapidly, often within 90 minutes of the systemic inflammatory response and within 24 hours of the initial insult (Figure 36–24 ■). Damaged capillary membranes allow plasma and blood cells to escape into the interstitial space. Increased interstitial pressure and damage to the alveolar membrane allow fluid to enter the alveoli. Within the alveolus, the fluid dilutes and inactivates

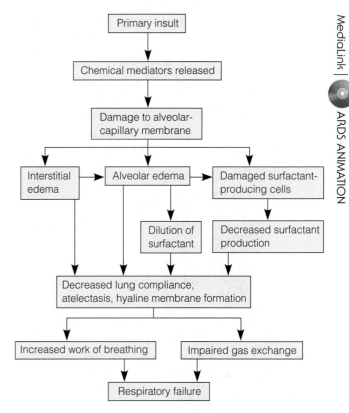

**Figure 36–24** ■ The pathogenesis of ARDS.

surfactant. Surfactant-producing cells are damaged by the inflammatory process, leading to a deficit of surfactant, increased alveolar surface tension, and alveolar collapse with atelectasis. The lungs become less compliant, and gas exchange is impaired. As the syndrome progresses, hyaline membranes form, further reducing gas exchange and compliance. Finally, fibrotic changes occur in the lungs. Intra-alveolar septa thicken, and alveolar surface area for gas exchange is reduced. Hypoxemia becomes refractory or resistant to improvement with supplemental oxygen, and the $P_{CO_2}$ rises as diffusion is further impaired. Figure 36–24 and the *Pathophysiology Illustrated* figure on pages 1170 and 1171 illustrate the pathophysiology of ARDS.

As ARDS progresses, tissue hypoxia becomes significant, and metabolic acidosis develops. Carbon dioxide exchange is impaired as well as oxygen exchange, leading to combined respiratory and metabolic acidosis. Sepsis and multiple organ system dysfunction of the kidneys, liver, gastrointestinal tract, central nervous system, and cardiovascular system are the leading causes of death in ARDS. If the process is halted before this occurs, the long-term prognosis for recovery is good.

## MANIFESTATIONS

Initial manifestations of ARDS typically develop 24 to 48 hours after the initial insult. Dyspnea, tachypnea, and anxiety are early manifestations. Progressive respiratory distress develops, with increasing respiratory rate, intercostal retractions, and use of accessory muscles of respiration. Cyanosis develops that may not improve with oxygen administration.

| TABLE 36–17 | Conditions Associated with the Development of ARDS |
| --- | --- |
| **Conditions** | **Examples** |
| Shock | Hemorrhagic shock, septic shock |
| Inhalation injuries | Aspiration of gastric contents, smoke and toxic gases, near-drowning, oxygen toxicity |
| Infections | Gram-negative sepsis, viral pneumonias, *Pneumocystis cariniii* pneumonia, miliary tuberculosis |
| Drug overdose | Heroin, methadone, propoxyphene, aspirin |
| Trauma | Burns, head injury, lung contusion, fat emboli |
| Other | Disseminated intravascular coagulation (DIC), pancreatitis, uremia, amniotic fluid and air emboli, multiple transfusions, open heart surgery with cardiopulmonary bypass |

Acute respiratory distress syndrome (ARDS) is a severe form of acute respiratory failure that occurs in response to pulmonary or systemic insults. ARDS is characterized by noncardiogenic pulmonary edema caused by inflammatory damage to alveolar and capillary walls. Many disorders may precipitate ARDS, although sepsis is the most common.

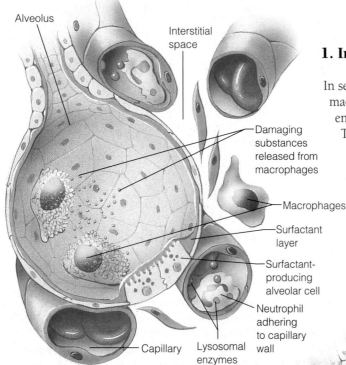

### 1. Initiation of ARDS

In sepsis-induced ARDS, bacterial toxins cause macrophages and neutrophils to adhere to endothelial surfaces of the alveoli and capillaries. The macrophages release oxidants, inflammatory mediators, enzymes, and peptides that damage the capillary and alveolar walls. In response, neutrophils release lysosomal enzymes causing further damage.

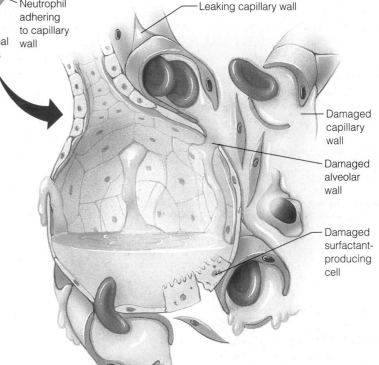

### 2. Onset of Pulmonary Edema

The damaged capillary and alveolar walls become more permeable, allowing plasma, proteins, and erythrocytes to enter the interstitial space. As interstitial edema increases, pressure in the interstitial space rises and fluid leaks into alveoli. Plasma proteins accumulating in the interstitial space lower the osmotic gradient between the capillary and interstitial compartment. As a result, the balance is disrupted between the osmotic force that pulls fluid from the interstitial space into the capillaries and the normal hydrostatic pressure that pushes fluid out of the capillaries. This imbalance causes even more fluid to enter alveoli.

## 4. End-Stage ARDS

Fibrin and cell debris from necrotic cells combine to form hyaline membranes, which line the interior of the alveoli and further reduce alveolar compliance and gas exchange. Because $CO_2$ cannot diffuse across hyaline membranes, $PCO_2$ levels now begin to rise while $PO_2$ levels continue to fall. Rising $PCO_2$ levels can lead to respiratory acidosis. Without respiratory support, respiratory failure will develop. Even with aggressive treatment, almost 50% of clients with ARDS die.

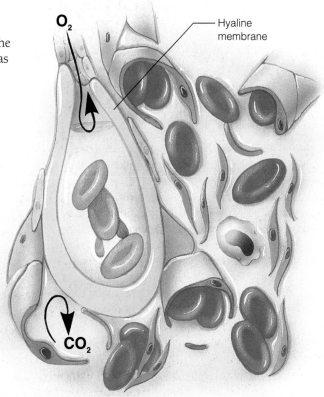

## 3. Alveolar Collapse

Protein-rich fluid accumulates in the alveoli, inactivating surfactant and damaging type II alveolar cells that produce surfactant. (Surfactant is important in maintaining alveolar compliance—the ability of tissue to stretch or distend.) As active surfactant is lost, the alveoli stiffen and collapse, leading to atelectasis, which increases breathing effort.

Decreased alveolar compliance, atelectasis, and fluid-filled alveoli interfere with gas exchange across the alveolar-capillary membrane. Blood oxygen ($PO_2$) levels fall. Because carbon dioxide diffuses more readily than oxygen, however, blood carbon dioxide ($PCO_2$) levels also fall initially as tachypnea causes more $CO_2$ to be expired.

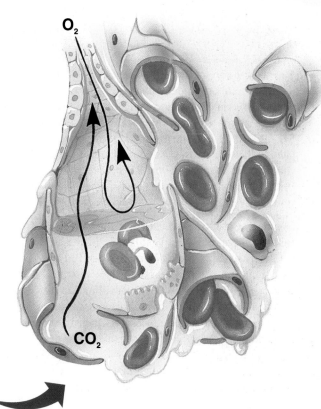

Breath sounds are initially clear, but crackles (rales) and rhonchi develop later. As respiratory failure progresses, mental status changes such as agitation, confusion, and lethargy occur.

## COLLABORATIVE CARE

ARDS management is directed toward identifying and treating its underlying cause and providing aggressive respiratory support.

### Diagnostic Tests

*Refractory hypoxemia* (hypoxemia that does not improve with oxygen administration) is the hallmark of ARDS.

- *Arterial blood gases* initially show hypoxemia with a $Po_2$ of less than 60 mmHg and respiratory alkalosis due to tachypnea.
- *Chest X-ray* changes may not be evident for as long as 24 hours after the onset of ARDS. Diffuse infiltrates are seen initially, progressing to a "white out" pattern.
- *Pulmonary function testing* shows decreased lung compliance with reduced vital capacity, minute volume, and functional vital capacity (see Box 36–1).
- *Pulmonary artery pressure monitoring* shows normal pressures in ARDS, helping distinguish ARDS from cardiogenic pulmonary edema.

### Medications

Although there is no definitive drug therapy for ARDS, a number of medications may be used. Inhaled nitric oxide reduces intrapulmonary shunting and improves oxygenation by dilating blood vessels in better-ventilated areas of the lungs. Surfactant therapy may be prescribed. Surfactant is a complex mixture of phospholipids, neutral lipids, and proteins that forms a thin layer atop a thin layer of water on the inner surface of the alveolus, reducing the surface tension within the alveoli. Surface tension tends to pull the walls of the alveoli together, increasing the likelihood of collapse during exhalation. Surfactant, by reducing surface tension, helps maintain open alveoli, decreasing the work of breathing, improving compliance and gas exchange, and preventing atelectasis.

Interventions to block the inflammatory response are under investigation, such as using nonsteroidal anti-inflammatory agents and corticosteroids. Corticosteroids may be used late in the course of ARDS to improve oxygenation and lung mechanics when fibrotic changes occur.

### Mechanical Ventilation

The mainstay of ARDS management is endotracheal intubation and mechanical ventilation. With ARDS, it is rarely possible to maintain adequate tissue oxygenation with oxygen therapy alone.

With mechanical ventilation, the $Fio_2$ is set at the lowest possible level to maintain a $Po_2$ higher than 60 mmHg and oxygen saturation of approximately 90%. When the $Po_2$ cannot be maintained with less than 50% inspired oxygen, there is a risk that oxygen toxicity will accentuate ARDS. Often it is necessary to add continuous positive airway pressure (CPAP) or positive end-expiratory pressure (PEEP) to mechanical ventilation settings to maintain blood and tissue oxygenation. Maintaining open airways and alveoli enhances gas diffusion and reduces ventilation-perfusion mismatch. PEEP decreases cardiac output and increases the risk of barotrauma, necessitating close monitoring. Either assist-control or SIMV may be used along with PEEP or CPAP in treating ARDS.

It is important to remember that mechanical ventilation does not cure ARDS; it simply supports respiratory function while the underlying problem is being identified and treated.

### Treatments

Atelectasis frequently occurs in dependent lung regions in ARDS. Prone positioning in conjunction with mechanical ventilation reduces the pressure of surrounding tissue on dependent regions and improves oxygenation.

Other management strategies include careful fluid replacement, attention to nutrition, treatment of any infection, and correction of the underlying condition. A Swan-Ganz line is placed to monitor pulmonary artery pressures and cardiac output. Fluid replacement is carefully tailored to these measurements to avoid fluid imbalances, which may worsen hypoxia and ARDS. Enteral or parenteral feeding is necessary to maintain nutritional status and prevent tissue catabolism. Infections are treated with intravenous antibiotic therapy tailored to the causative organism. Low-molecular-weight heparin may be ordered to prevent thrombophlebitis and possible pulmonary embolus or disseminated intravascular coagulation (DIC), a possible complication of ARDS.

## NURSING CARE

The nursing care needs of the client with ARDS are very similar to those of any client with acute respiratory failure. Maintaining adequate ventilation and respirations are of highest priority, along with preventing injury and managing anxiety. See the section on acute respiratory failure for nursing care related to these diagnoses. Additional high-priority nursing care concerns for the client with ARDS are related to the effects of PEEP on cardiac output and potential problems of weaning ventilatory support.

### Decreased Cardiac Output

With positive pressure ventilation, increased intrathoracic pressure decreases cardiac output. When PEEP is applied, intrathoracic pressure increases further; this can significantly decrease venous return, ventricular filling, stroke volume, and cardiac output. Manifestations of decreased cardiac output include hypotension and compensatory tachycardia as the heart attempts to maintain cardiac output despite decreased stoke volume. In the client who is already hypoxic because of ARDS, this drop in cardiac output can increase tissue damage. Urine output falls, and dysrhythmias may develop.

- Monitor and record vital signs, including apical pulse, at least every 2 hours; more frequently immediately following initiation of mechanical ventilation or addition of PEEP. *Frequent assessment is vital to detect early signs of decreased cardiac output.*

**PRACTICE ALERT** *Record urine output hourly. Because a significant portion of the cardiac output goes directly to the kidneys, a fall in urine output to less than 30 mL per hour is often the first sign of decreased cardiac output.* ■

- Assess level of consciousness at least every 4 hours. *Altered level of consciousness, confusion, and restlessness are early signs of cerebral hypoxia due to decreased cardiac output.*
- Monitor pulmonary artery pressures, central venous pressure, and cardiac output readings every 1 to 4 hours. *Changes in these measurements may indicate worsening cardiac status.*
- Assess heart and lung sounds frequently. *Increasing crackles or abnormal heart sounds may indicate heart failure.*
- Weigh daily at the same time. *Accurate daily weights are the best indicator of fluid volume status.*
- Frequently provide good skin care, keeping skin clean and dry and protecting pressure points. *Tissue hypoxia increases the risk of skin breakdown, which in turn increases the risk of infection and sepsis.*
- Maintain intravenous fluids as ordered. *Intravenous fluids are given to maintain vascular volume and prevent dehydration.*
- Administer analgesics, sedatives, and neuromuscular blockers as needed. *These medications may be prescribed to decrease cardiac workload.*

### Dysfunctional Ventilatory Weaning Response

The client with dysfunctional ventilatory weaning response has difficulty adjusting to reduced mechanical ventilator support, prolonging the weaning process. Airway congestion, inadequate rest or nutrition, pain, anxiety, and a nonsupportive environment are factors that can contribute to difficulty weaning. With ARDS, the pathologic processes of the disease and its effects on gas exchange may be responsible for a prolonged or ineffective weaning process.

Assessment findings indicative of dysfunctional weaning include:

- Dyspnea, apprehension, or agitation.
- Decreasing oxygen saturation level.
- Cyanosis or pallor, diaphoresis.
- Increased blood pressure, pulse, and respiratory rate.
- Diminished or adventitious breath sounds, use of accessory muscles.
- Decreased level of consciousness.
- Deteriorating arterial blood gas values.
- Shallow, gasping breaths or paradoxic abdominal breathing.

Nursing interventions for dysfunctional weaning include the following:

- Assess vital signs every 15 to 30 minutes following changes in ventilator settings and during T-piece trials. *Vital signs, heart and respiratory rates in particular, can provide early signs of hypoxemia and poor tolerance of the weaning process.*

**PRACTICE ALERT** *Frequently monitor oxygen saturation, ETco₂, and arterial blood gases following changes in ventilator settings. These values are used to assess the adequacy of ventilation and gas exchange during the weaning process.* ■

- Place in Fowler's or high-Fowler's position. *Fowler's position facilitates lung expansion and reduces the work of breathing.*
- Fully explain all weaning procedures, along with expected changes in breathing. *Adequate explanations help reduce anxiety and improve the ability to cooperate.*
- Remain with the client during initial periods following changes of ventilator settings or T-piece trials. *This provides reassurance and allows close monitoring of the response.*
- Limit procedures and activities during weaning periods. *Reducing energy expenditures and cardiac work facilitates the weaning process.*
- Provide diversion, such as television or radio. *Diversion helps distract the focus from breathing.*
- Begin weaning procedures in the morning, when the client is well rested and alert; weaning may be discontinued overnight to provide rest. *The work of breathing increases during the weaning process; adequate rest is important.*
- When SIMV is used for weaning, decrease the SIMV rate by increments of two breaths per minute. *Slow reduction of ventilator support allows respiratory muscle reconditioning and gradual resumption of the work of breathing.*
- Avoid administering drugs that may depress respirations during the weaning process (except as ordered at night to facilitate rest when ventilator support is provided). *Sedatives or analgesics that depress respirations can impair the weaning process.*

**PRACTICE ALERT** *Frequently assess respiratory status following weaning and extubation. Keep an intubation kit readily available following extubation; be prepared for emergency reintubation. Laryngeal spasm or laryngeal edema may develop following extubation, necessitating reintubation to maintain respirations.* ■

- Keep oxygen at the bedside following weaning and extubation. *Supplemental oxygen may be necessary to maintain adequate blood and tissue oxygenation.*
- Provide pulmonary hygiene with percussion and postural drainage. *Maintaining patent airways and adequate alveolar ventilation is vital during the weaning process.*

### Home Care

When preparing the client who has recovered from ARDS and the family for home care, discuss the following topics.

- ARDS did not result from something they did or did not do, but developed as a consequence of serious illness. Provide factual information about ARDS.
- Maximal respiratory function following ARDS is usually achieved within 6 months; respiratory function may remain significantly impaired. This may necessitate changes in occupation, lifestyle, and family roles.

- Avoiding smoking and exposure to secondhand smoke and environmental pollutants is vital to prevent further lung damage.
- Obtain immunization for pneumococcal pneumonia and annual influenza immunizations to prevent further episodes of serious respiratory disease.

Provide referrals to home health and respiratory care services as indicated, as well as for occupational therapy and counseling as needed.

## Nursing Care Plan
## A Client with ARDS

Peggy Adamson is a 36-year-old single woman admitted to the hospital following a near-drowning in a local lake. On admission to the emergency department, Ms. Adamson is alert and oriented, having been rescued and resuscitated within 2 minutes of the accident. Rescuers report that she seemed to have aspirated "a lot" of water as she was water-skiing when the accident occurred. She is admitted to the intensive care unit for observation. Oxygen is started per nasal cannula at 6 L/min, intravenous fluids are administered to correct electrolyte imbalances, and 40 mg of furosemide (Lasix) is given intravenously for hypervolemia.

### ASSESSMENT

Nadia Mucha cares for Ms. Adamson the evening of the day after her admission. Throughout her stay, Ms. Adamson has remained alert and oriented with stable vital signs. Her respiratory rate has been 20 to 24 per minute, with scattered crackles, oxygen saturations of around 94%, and a $PO_2$ of 75 to 80 mmHg on 6 L/min of oxygen. Her pulse has been 96 to 100 and regular. On her initial assessment, Ms. Mucha notes that Ms. Adamson seems apprehensive and anxious. Although her blood pressure is 116/74, unchanged from previous levels, her heart rate is up to 106 and respiratory rate is 28 per minute. Her lungs have scattered crackles but good breath sounds throughout, unchanged from previous assessments. Ms. Adamson's oxygen saturation has dropped to 84%, so Ms. Mucha orders ABGs and increases the oxygen to 8 L/min. ABG results show $PO_2$ 65 mmHg and respiratory alkalosis pH 7.48, and $PCO_2$ 32 mmHg.

Ms. Mucha orders a portable chest X-ray and notifies the physician of the arterial blood gas results and the change in Ms. Adamson's status. The physician orders a nonrebreather mask at 8 L/min and repeat ABGs in 1 hour. The chest X-ray reveals scattered infiltrates and a normal heart size.

Ms. Adamson's oxygen saturation continues to fall, and subsequent blood gases show a $PO_2$ of 55 mmHg. The attending physician diagnoses probable ARDS and orders nasotracheal intubation and mechanical ventilation.

### DIAGNOSES

- *Ineffective breathing pattern* related to anxiety
- *Impaired gas exchange* related to effects of near-drowning
- *Anxiety* related to hypoxemia
- *Risk for decreased cardiac output* related to mechanical ventilation
- *Risk for injury* related to endotracheal intubation

### EXPECTED OUTCOMES

- Breathe effectively with the mechanical ventilator.

- Demonstrate improved oxygen saturation, $ETCO_2$, and ABG values.
- Express fears related to intubation and mechanical ventilation.
- Demonstrate reduced anxiety levels (relaxed facial expression, ability to rest).
- Maintain adequate cardiac output and tissue perfusion.
- Tolerate endotracheal intubation and mechanical ventilation without evidence of infection or barotrauma.

### PLANNING AND IMPLEMENTATION

- Obtain all necessary supplies and notify respiratory therapy and radiology in preparation for intubation and mechanical ventilation.
- Explain the purpose and procedure of intubation.
- Provide an opportunity to express fears related to intubation and mechanical ventilation; answer questions and provide reassurance.
- Discuss communication strategies while intubated; obtain a magic slate.
- Administer analgesics and/or sedatives as ordered.
- Monitor oxygen saturation and $ETCO_2$ levels every 30 to 60 minutes initially after instituting mechanical ventilation; report changes to the physician.
- Obtain ABGs as ordered or indicated; monitor and report results.
- Suction via endotracheal tube as needed to maintain clear airways.
- Allow periods of uninterrupted rest.
- Monitor vital signs every 1 to 2 hours.
- Assess skin color, capillary refill, and the presence of edema every 4 hours.
- Monitor urine output hourly; report output of less than 30 mL per hour.
- Assess lung sounds and chest excursion every 1 to 2 hours.

### EVALUATION

Ms. Adamson is intubated and placed on a volume-cycled ventilator at 50% $FIO_2$ and a tidal volume of 700 mL in the assist-control mode at 16 breaths per minute. She has difficulty working with the ventilator initially, so a fentanyl drip is ordered to reduce her anxiety. Ms. Adamson's oxygen saturation, $ETCO_2$, and ABG results do not begin to improve until 5 mmHg of PEEP is added to ventilator settings. After 3 days of mechanical ventilation with PEEP and aggressive fluid and diuretic therapy, Ms. Adamson begins to improve. She is placed on SIMV, and over the course of another 3 days she is gradually weaned off the ventilator to a face mask with CPAP. She eventually recovers fully, with minimal apparent long-term effects.

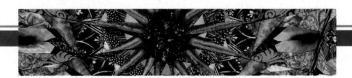

## Nursing Care Plan

## A Client with ARDS *(continued)*

### Critical Thinking in the Nursing Process

1. Endotracheal intubation and mechanical ventilation were effective in supporting Ms. Adamson's respiratory status as she recovered from ARDS. Discuss a possible sequence of events had it not been possible to wean her from the ventilator.
2. How might the presentation and management of an acute episode of respiratory failure due to ARDS differ from respiratory failure related to COPD?

3. What measures can nurses take to prevent the development of ARDS?
4. Develop a nursing care plan for Ms. Adamson for the nursing diagnosis, *Powerlessness* related to endotracheal intubation and mechanical ventilation.

See Evaluating Your Response in Appendix C.

## EXPLORE MediaLink

NCLEX review questions, case studies, care plan activities, MediaLink applications, and other interactive resources for this chapter can be found on the Companion Website at www.prenhall.com/lemone.

Click on Chapter 36 to select the activities for this chapter. For animations, video clips, more NCLEX review questions, and an audio glossary, access the Student CD-ROM accompanying this textbook.

## TEST YOURSELF

1. Admitting orders for a client with acute bacterial pneumonia include an intravenous antibiotic every 8 hours, oxygen per nasal cannula at 5 L/min, continuous pulse oximetry monitoring, bedrest with bathroom privileges and chair at bedside as desired, diet as tolerated, sputum specimen for C&S, CBC, urinalysis, and chemisty panel. Which order should the nurse carry out first?

    a. Start the oxygen per nasal cannula
    b. Insert an intravenous catheter and start the prescribed antibiotic
    c. Provide a dinner tray to the client
    d. Obtain the sputum specimen

2. All of the following nursing diagnoses are appropriate for a client with an acute asthma attack. Which is of highest priority?

    a. *Anxiety* related to difficulty breathing
    b. *Ineffective airway clearance* related to bronchoconstriction and increased mucous production
    c. *Ineffective breathing pattern* related to anxiety
    d. *Ineffective health maintenance* related of lack of knowledge about attack triggers and appropriate use of medications

3. Which of the following would be an expected assessment finding in a client admitted with chronic obstructive airway disease?

    a. AP chest diameter equal to or greater than lateral chest diameter
    b. Mental confusion and lethargy

    c. Three+ pitting edema of ankles and lower legs
    d. Oxygen saturation readings of 85% or less

4. Which of the following statements made by a client with a new diagnosis of lung cancer would indicate that the nurse's teaching has been effective?

    a. "Well, since I'm going to die anyway, I may as well go home, put my affairs in order, and spend the rest of my time in the easy chair."
    b. "I understand that because the cancer has already spread, I will be undergoing aggressive cancer treatment for the next several years to beat this thing."
    c. "Even though I can't undo the damage caused by cigarette smoking, I will try to quit to prevent further damage to my lungs."
    d. "Having the 'big C' is very scary; I'm just glad it is one of the more curable forms of cancer."

5. The nurse caring for a client undergoing mechanical ventilation for acute respiratory failure plans and implements which of the following measures to help maintain effective alveolar ventilation?

    a. Keeps the client in supine position
    b. Increases the tidal volume on the ventilator
    c. Maintains ordered oxygen concentration
    d. Performs endotracheal suctioning as indicated

See Test Yourself answers in Appendix C.

# BIBLIOGRAPHY

Ackley, B. J., & Ladwig, G. B. (2002). *Nursing diagnosis handbook: A guide to planning care* (5th ed.). St. Louis: Mosby.

Adatsi, G. (1999). Health going up in smoke: How can you prevent it? *American Journal of Nursing, 99*(3), 63–64, 66, 67–68.

Adiutori, D. M. (2000). Primary pulmonary hypertension: A review for advanced practice nurses. *MEDSURG Nursing, 9*(5), 255–264.

American Cancer Society. (2002). *Cancer facts and figures 2002.* Atlanta: Author.

Belza, B., Steele, B. G., Hunziker, J., Lakshminaryan, S., Holt, L., & Buchner, D. M. (2001). Correlates of physical activity in chronic obstructive pulmonary disease. *Nursing Research, 50*(4), 195–202.

Braunwald, E., Fauci, A. S., Kasper, D. L., Hauser, S. L., Longo, D. L., & Jameson, J. L. (2001). *Harrison's principles of internal medicine* (15th ed.). New York: McGraw-Hill.

Carroll, P. (2000). Exploring chest drain options. *RN, 63*(10), 50–54.

Centers for Disease Control and Prevention. (2003a). *Guidelines and recommendations. Interim domestic guidance for management of exposures to severe acute respiratory syndrome (SARS) for healthcare and other institutional settings.* Author: Department of Health and Human Services.

_____. (2003b). *Guidelines and recommendations. Interim guidance on infection control precautions for patients with suspected severe acute respiratory syndrome (SARS) and close contacts in households.* Author: Department of Health and Human Services.

_____. (2003c). *Fact sheet. Basic information about SARS.* Author: Department of Health and Human Services.

Chernecky, C. (2001). Pulmonary complications in patients with cancer. *American Journal of Nursing, 101*(5), 24A, 24E, 24G–24H.

Deglin, J. H., & Vallerand, A. H. (2003). *Davis's drug guide for nurses* (8th ed.). Philadelphia: F. A. Davis.

Dest, V. (2000). Ocology today: Lung cancer. *RN, 63*(5), 32–34, 36, 38.

Dunn, N. A. (2001). Keeping COPD patients out of the ED. *RN, 64*(2), 33–37.

Evans, T. (2000). Neuromuscular blockade: When and how. *RN, 63*(5), 56–60.

Fontaine, K. L. (2000). *Healing practices: Alternative therapies for nursing.* Upper Saddle River, NJ: Prentice Hall Health.

Goldsmith, C., & Haban, M. (2002). Lung cancer: A preventable tragedy. *NurseWeek, 3*(2), 17–18.

Goodfellow, L. T., & Jones, M. (2002). Bronchial hygiene therapy. *American Journal of Nursing, 102*(1), 37–43.

Hayes, D. D. (2001). Stemming the tide of pleural effusions. *Nursing2001, 31*(5), 49–52.

Higgins, P. A. (1998). Patient perception of fatigue while undergoing long-term mechanical ventilation: Incidence and associated factors. *Heart & Lung, 27*(3), 177–183.

Johnson, M., Bulechek, G., Dochterman, J. M., Maas, M., & Moorhead, S. (2001). *Nursing diagnoses, outcomes, & interventions.* St. Louis: Mosby.

Johnson, M., Maas, M., & Moorhead, S. (Eds.). (2000). *Nursing outcomes classification (NOC)* (2nd ed.). St. Louis: Mosby.

Kuhn, M. A. (1999). *Complementary therapies for health care providers.* Philadelphia: Lippincott.

LaDuke, S. (2001). Terminal dyspnea & palliative care. *American Journal of Nursing, 101*(11), 26–31.

Lehne, R. A. (2001). *Pharmacology for nursing care* (4th ed.). Philadelphia: Saunders.

Leifer, G. (2001). Hyperbaric oxygen therapy. *American Journal of Nursing, 101*(8), 26–34.

Lenaghan, N. A. (2000). The nurse's role in smoking cessation. *MEDSURG Nursing, 9*(6), 298–302.

Little, C. (2001). What you need to know about chronic bronchitis. *Nursing2001, 31*(9), 52–55.

Malarkey, L. M., & McMorrow, M. E. (2000). *Nurse's manual of laboratory tests and diagnostic procedures* (2nd ed.). Philadelphia: Saunders.

Marion, B. S. (2001). A turn for the better: 'Prone positioning' of patients with ARDS. *American Journal of Nursing, 101*(5), 26–34.

Martin, B., Llewellyn, J., Faut-Callahan, M., & Meyer, P. (2000). The use of telemetric oximetry in the clinical setting. *MEDSURG Nursing, 9*(2), 71–76.

McCance, K. L., & Huether, S. E. (2002). *Pathophysiology: The biologic basis for disease in adults and children* (4th ed.). St. Louis: Mosby.

McCloskey, J. C., & Bulechek, G. M. (Eds.) (2000). *Nursing interventions classification (NIC)* (3rd ed.). St. Louis: Mosby.

Miracle, V., & Winston, M. (2000). Take the wind out of asthma. *Nursing2000, 30*(8), 34–41.

Morrison, C., & Lew, E. (2001). Aspergillosis. *American Journal of Nursing, 101*(8), 40–48.

National Center for HIV, STD, and TB Prevention, Division of Tuberculosis Elimination. (2002). *Surveillance reports. Reported tuberculosis in the United States 2001.* Atlanta, GA: Centers for Disease Control and Prevention.

National Heart, Lung, and Blood Institute, National Institutes of Health. (2002). *Morbidity & mortality: 2002 chart book of cardiovascular, lung, and blood diseases.* Bethesda, MD: Author.

North American Nursing Diagnosis Association. (2001). *NANDA nursing diagnoses: Definitions & classification 2001–2002.* Philadelphia: NANDA.

Owen, C. L. (1999). New directions in asthma management. *American Journal of Nursing, 99*(3), 26–33.

Persell, D. J., Arangie, P., Young, C., Stokes, E. N., Payne, W. C., Skorga, P., & Gilbert-Palmer, D. (2002). Preparing for bioterrorism. *Nursing, 32*(2), 37–43.

Pope, B. B. (2002). Patient education series. Asthma. *Nursing2002, 32*(5), 44–45.

Porth, C. M. (2002). *Pathophysiology: Concepts of altered health states* (6th ed.). Philadelphia: Lippincott.

Ruppert, R. A. (1999). The last smoke. *American Journal of Nursing, 99*(11), 26–32.

Schultz, T. R. (2002). Straight talk about community-acquired pneumonia. *Nursing2002, 32*(1), 46–49.

Sellers, K. F., Hargrove, B., & Jenkins, P. (2000). Asthma disease management programs improve clinical and economic outcomes. *MEDSURG Nursing, 9*(4), 201–203, 207.

Tierney, L. M., McPhee, S. J., & Papadakis, M. A. (2001). *Current medical diagnosis & treatment* (40th ed.). New York: Lange Medical Books/McGraw-Hill.

Trogger, D. A., & Brenner, P. S. (2001). Metered dose inhalers. *American Journal of Nursing, 101*(10), 26–32.

Trudeau, M. E., & Solano-McGuire, S. M. (1999). Evaluating the quality of COPD care. *American Journal of Nursing, 99*(3), 47–50.

Truesdell, S. (2000). Helping patients with COPD manage episodes of acute shortness of breath. *MEDSURG Nursing, 9*(4), 178–182.

Urden, L. D., Stacy, K. M., & Lough, M. E. (2002). *Thelan's critical care nursing: Diagnosis and management* (4th ed.). St. Louis: Mosby.

Way, L. W., & Doherty, G. M. (2003). *Current surgical diagnosis & treatment* (11th ed.). New York: Lange Medical Books/McGraw-Hill.

Whitney, E. N., & Rolfes, S. R. (2002). *Understanding nutrition* (9th ed.). Belmont, CA: Wadsworth.

Wilkinson, J. M. (2000). *Nursing diagnosis handbook with NIC interventions and NOC outcomes* (7th ed.). Upper Saddle River, NJ: Prentice Hall Health.

Woods, S. L., Froelicher, E. S. S., & Motzer, S. U. (2000). *Cardiac nursing* (4th ed.). Philadelphia: Lippincott.

World Health Organization. (2003). Cumulative number of reported probable cases of severe acute respiratory syndrome (SARS). *Communicable disease surveillance & response (CSR).* Author.

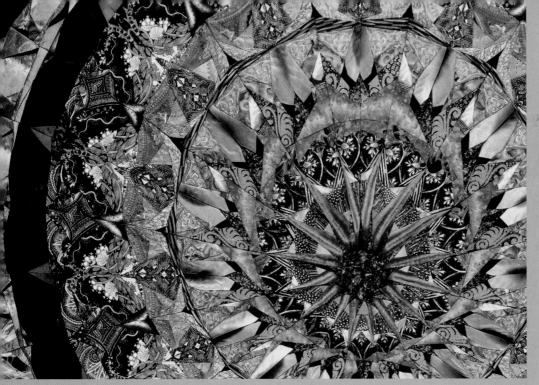

# RESPONSES TO ALTERED MUSCULOSKELETAL FUNCTION

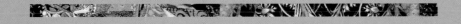

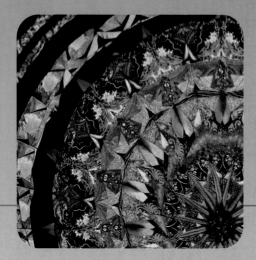

# Assessing Clients with Musculoskeletal Disorders

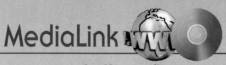

## MediaLink

**www.prenhall.com/lemone**

Additional resources for this chapter can be found on the Student CD-ROM accompanying this textbook, and on the Companion Website at www.prenhall.com/lemone. Click on Chapter 37 to select the activities for this chapter.

**CD-ROM**
• Audio Glossary
• NCLEX Review

*Animation*
• Musculoskeletal A&P

**Companion Website**
• More NCLEX Review
• Functional Health Pattern Assessment
• Case Study
   Knee Pain

## LEARNING OUTCOMES

After completing this chapter, you will be able to:

▪ Review the anatomy and physiology of the musculoskeletal system.

▪ Describe the normal movements allowed by synovial joints.

▪ Identify specific topics for consideration during a health history interview of the client with health problems involving the musculoskeletal system.

▪ Describe physical assessment techniques for musculoskeletal function.

▪ Identify abnormal findings that may indicate impairment of the musculoskeletal system.

The tissues and structures of the musculoskeletal system perform many functions, including support, protection, and movement. The musculoskeletal system has two subsystems: the bones and joints of the skeleton, and the skeletal muscles. These subsystems work together to allow the body to perform both gross, simple movements such as closing a door, and fine, complex movements such as repairing a watch.

## REVIEW OF ANATOMY AND PHYSIOLOGY

### The Skeleton

The human skeleton is made up of 206 bones (Figure 37–1 ■). The axial skeleton includes the bones of the skull, the ribs and sternum, and the vertebral column. The appendicular skeleton consists of all the bones of the limbs, the shoulder girdles, and the pelvic girdle.

Bones form the body's structure and provide support for soft tissues. They also protect vital organs from injury and serve to move body parts by providing points of attachment for muscles. Bones also store minerals and serve as a site for *hematopoiesis* (blood cell formation).

Bone cells include osteoblasts (cells that form bone), osteocytes (cells that maintain bone matrix), and osteoclasts (cells that resorb bone). Bone matrix is the extracellular element of bone tissue; it consists of collagen fibers, minerals (primarily calcium and phosphate), proteins, carbohydrates, and ground substance. Ground substance is a gelatinous material that facilitates diffusion of nutrients, wastes, and gases between the blood vessels and bone tissue. Bones are covered with **periosteum,** a double-layered connective tissue. The outer layer of the periosteum contains blood vessels and nerves; the inner layer is anchored to the bone.

Bones consist of a rigid connective tissue called osseous tissue, of which there are two types: Compact bone is smooth and dense; spongy bone contains spaces between meshworks of bone. Both types contain the same elements and are found in almost all bones of the body.

The basic structural unit of compact bone is the Haversian system (also called an osteon). The Haversian system consists of a central canal, called the Haversian canal; concentric layers of bone matrix, called lamellae; spaces between the lamellae, called lacunae; osteocytes within the lacunae; and small channels, called canaliculi (Figure 37–2 ■).

Spongy bone has no Haversian systems. Instead, the lamellae are arranged in concentric layers called trabeculae which branch and join to form meshworks. The spongy sections of long bones and flat bones contain tissue for hematopoiesis. In the adult, these sections, called red marrow cavities, are present in the spongy center of flat bones (especially the sternum) and in only two long bones: the humerus and the head of the femur. This red marrow is active in hematopoiesis in adults.

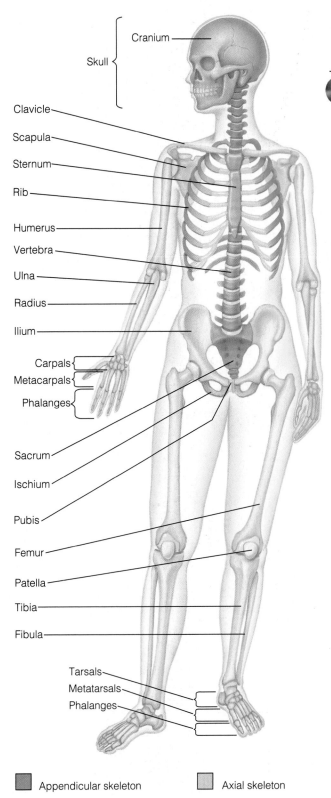

Appendicular skeleton    Axial skeleton

**Figure 37–1** ■ Bones of the human skeleton.

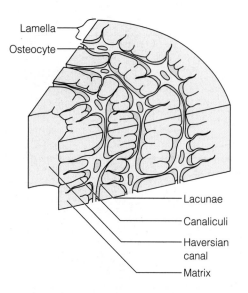

Lamella
Osteocyte
Lacunae
Canaliculi
Haversian canal
Matrix

**Figure 37–2** ■ The microscopic structure of compact bone.

Bones are classified by shape (Figure 37–3 ■):

- Long bones are longer than they are wide. They have a midportion, or shaft, called a **diaphysis** and two broad ends, called **epiphyses.** The diaphysis is compact bone and contains the marrow cavity, which is lined with endosteum. Each epiphysis is spongy bone covered by a thin layer of compact bone. Long bones include the bones of the arms and legs, fingers, and toes.
- Short bones, also called cuboid bones, are spongy bone covered by compact bone. They include the bones of the wrist and ankle.
- Flat bones are thin and flat, and most are curved. Their disclike structure consists of a layer of spongy bone between two thin layers of compact bone. Flat bones include most bones of the skull, the sternum, and the ribs.
- Irregular bones are of various shapes and sizes and, like flat bones, are plates of compact bone with spongy bone between. Irregular bones include the vertebrae, the scapulae, and the bones of the pelvic girdle.

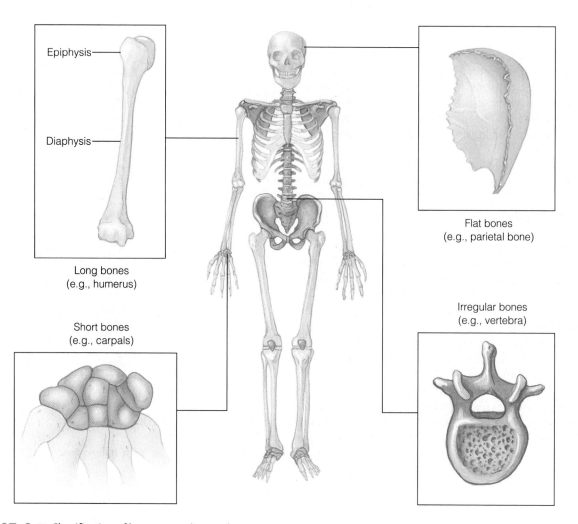

Epiphysis

Diaphysis

Long bones
(e.g., humerus)

Short bones
(e.g., carpals)

Flat bones
(e.g., parietal bone)

Irregular bones
(e.g., vertebra)

**Figure 37–3** ■ Classification of bones according to shape.

## Bone Remodeling in Adults

Although the bones of adults do not normally increase in length and size, constant remodeling of bones, as well as repair of damaged bone tissue, occurs throughout life. In the bone re-modeling process, bone resorption and bone deposit occur at all periosteal and endosteal surfaces. Hormones and forces that put stress on the bones regulate this process, which involves a combined action of the osteocytes, osteoclasts, and osteoblasts. Bones that are in use, and are therefore subjected to stress, in-crease their osteoblastic activity to increase ossification (the development of bone). Bones that are inactive undergo in-creased osteoclast activity and bone resorption.

The hormonal stimulus for bone remodeling is controlled by a negative feedback mechanism that regulates blood calcium levels. This stimulus involves the interaction of parathyroid hormone (PTH) from the parathyroid glands and calcitonin from the thyroid gland. When blood levels of calcium decrease, PTH is released; PTH then stimulates osteoclast activity and bone resorption so that calcium is released from the bone ma-trix. As a result, blood levels of calcium rise, and the stimulus for PTH release ends. Rising blood calcium levels stimulate the secretion of calcitonin, inhibit bone resorption, and cause the deposit of calcium salts in the bone matrix. Thus, bones regu-late blood calcium levels. Calcium ions are necessary for the transmission of nerve impulses, the release of neurotransmit-ters, muscle contraction, blood clotting, glandular secretion, and cell division. Of the body's 1200 to 1400 g of calcium, over 99% is present as bone minerals.

Bone remodeling is also regulated by the response of bones to gravitational pull and to mechanical stress from the pull of mus-cles. Although the exact mechanism is not fully understood, it is known that bones that undergo increased stress are heavier and larger. This finding supports Wolff's law, which states that bone develops and remodels itself to resist the stresses placed on it.

The process of bone repair following a fracture is discussed in Chapter 38.

## Joints, Ligaments, and Tendons

**Joints,** or **articulations,** are regions where two or more bones meet. Joints hold the bones of the skeleton together while al-lowing the body to move. Joints may be classified by function as synarthroses, amphiarthroses, or diarthroses. Table 37–1 de-scribes each of these types.

Joints are also classified by structure as fibrous, cartilagi-nous, or synovial. Fibrous joints permit little or no movement, because the articulating bones are joined either by short con-nective tissue fibers that bind the bones together, as with the sutures of the skull, or by short cords of fibrous tissue called ligaments (discussed on the next page), which permit slight give but no true movement.

Some cartilaginous joints, such as the sternocostal joints of the rib cage, are composed of hyaline cartilage growths that fuse together the articulating bone ends. These joints are im-mobile. In other cartilaginous joints, such as the intervertebral discs, the hyaline cartilage fuses to an intervening plate of flex-ible fibrocartilage. This structural feature accounts for the flex-ibility of the vertebral column.

Bones in synovial joints are enclosed by a cavity that is filled with synovial fluid, a filtrate of blood plasma. These joints are freely movable. Synovial joints are found at all artic-ulations of the limbs. They have several characteristics:

- The articular surfaces are covered with articular cartilage.
- The joint cavity is enclosed by a tough, fibrous, double-layered articular capsule; internally, the cavity is lined with a synovial membrane that covers all surfaces not covered by the articular cartilage.
- Synovial fluid fills the free spaces of the joint capsule, en-hancing the smooth movement of the articulating bones.

Synovial joints allow many kinds of movements, listed and described in Table 37–2.

### TABLE 37–1   Functional Classification of Joints

| Type | Description | Examples |
|------|-------------|----------|
| Synarthrosis | Immovable joint | Skull sutures Epiphyseal plates Joint between first rib and manubrium of sternum |
| Amphiarthrosis | Slightly movable joint | Vertebral joints Joint of the pubic symphysis |
| Diarthrosis | Freely movable joint | Joints of the limbs Shoulder joints Hip joints |

### TABLE 37–2   Movements Allowed by Synovial Joints

| Movement | Description |
|----------|-------------|
| Abduction | Move limb away from body midline |
| Adduction | Move limb toward body midline |
| Extension | Straighten limbs at joint |
| Flexion | Bend limbs at joint |
| Dorsiflexion | Bend ankle to bring top of foot toward shin |
| Plantar flexion | Straighten ankle to point toes down |
| Pronation | Turn forearm to place palm down |
| Supination | Turn forearm to place palm up |
| Eversion | Turn out |
| Inversion | Turn in |
| Circumduction | Move in circle |
| Internal rotation | Move inward on a central axis |
| External rotation | Move outward on a central axis |
| Protraction | Move forward and parallel to ground |
| Retraction | Move backward and parallel to ground |

The fibrous capsules that surround synovial joints are supported by ligaments, dense bands of connective tissue that connect bones to bones. Ligaments limit or enhance movement, provide joint stability, and enhance joint strength. Tendons are fibrous connective tissue bands that connect muscles to the periosteum of bones and enable the bones to move when skeletal muscles contract. When muscles contract, increased pressure causes the tendon to pull, push, or rotate the bone to which it is connected.

**Bursae** are small sacs of synovial fluid that cushion and protect bony areas that are at high risk for friction, such as the knee and the shoulder. Tendon sheaths are a form of bursae, but they are wrapped around tendons in high-friction areas.

## Muscles

The three types of muscle tissue in the body are skeletal muscle, smooth muscle, and cardiac muscle (Table 37–3). This discussion focuses on skeletal muscle, the only muscle that allows musculoskeletal function.

Skeletal muscle cells have typical functional properties:

- *Excitability:* the ability to receive and respond to a stimulus. The stimulus is usually a neurotransmitter released by a neuron, and the response is the generation and transmission of an action potential along the plasma membrane of the muscle cell. (Chapter 40 discusses action potentials.)
- *Contractibility:* the ability to respond to a stimulus by forcibly shortening.
- *Extensibility:* the ability to respond to a stimulus by extending and relaxing; muscle fibers shorten when they contract and extend when they relax.
- *Elasticity:* the ability to resume its resting length after it has shortened or lengthened.

Skeletal muscles are thick bundles of parallel multinucleated contractile cells called fibers. Each single muscle fiber is itself a bundle of smaller structures called myofibrils. The myofibrils have alternating light and dark bands that give skeletal muscle its striated (striped) appearance under an electron microscope. Myofibrils are strands of smaller repeating units called sarcomeres, which consist of thick filaments of myosin and thin filaments of actin, proteins that contribute to muscle contraction.

Skeletal muscle movement is triggered when motor neurons release acetylcholine, a neurotransmitter that alters the permeability of the muscle fiber. Sodium ions enter the fiber, producing an action potential that causes muscle contraction. The more fibers that contract, the stronger the contraction of the entire muscle.

Prolonged strenuous activity causes continuous nerve impulses and eventually results in a buildup of lactic acid and reduced energy in the muscle, or muscle fatigue. However, continuous nerve impulses are also responsible for maintaining muscle tone. Lack of use results in muscle atrophy, whereas regular exercise increases the size and strength of muscles.

Skeletal muscles attach to and cover the bones of the skeleton. Skeletal muscles promote body movement, help maintain posture, and produce body heat. They may be moved by conscious, voluntary control or by reflex activity. The body has approximately 600 skeletal muscles (Figure 37–4 ■).

## ASSESSING MUSCULOSKELETAL FUNCTION

The function of the musculoskeletal system is assessed by both a health assessment interview to collect subjective data and a physical assessment to collect objective data.

### Health Assessment Interview

This section provides guidelines for collecting subjective data through a health assessment interview specific to musculoskeletal function. An assessment interview to determine problems with musculoskeletal function may be conducted as part of a health screening or as part of a total health assessment, or it may focus on a chief complaint (such as pain, swelling, or limited mobility). Health problems affecting the neurologic system may manifest as musculoskeletal function problems; an assessment of both systems may be necessary. (See Chapter 40 for assessment of the neurologic system.) If the client has a health problem involving the bones or muscles, analyze its onset, characteristics and course, severity, precipitating and relieving factors, and any associated manifestations, noting the timing and circumstances. For example, ask the client:

- Describe the pain you have had in your elbow. Does the pain increase with movement? Have you noticed any redness or swelling?
- Did you injure your ankle before you began to experience difficulty walking?
- Is your pain worse in the morning, or does it get worse through the day?

The primary manifestations of altered function of the musculoskeletal system are pain and limited mobility. Specific descriptors of the pain, its location, and its nature are important. Other significant information includes associated manifestations, such as fever, fatigue, changes in weight, rash, and/or swelling. Also collect information about the client's lifestyle: type of employment, ability to carry out activities of daily living (ADLs) and provide self-care, exercise or participation in sports, use of alcohol or drugs, and nutrition. Explore past injuries and measures to self-treat pain (such as over-the-counter medications, prescribed medications, application of heat or cold, splinting, wrapping, or rest).

| TABLE 37–3 | Types of Body Muscle | |
|---|---|---|
| **Type** | **Description** | **Examples** |
| Skeletal | Striated, voluntary muscle (can consciously move) | Biceps, triceps, deltoid, gluteus maximus |
| Smooth | Nonstriated, involuntary muscle (cannot consciously move) | Muscles in the walls of the bladder, stomach, and bronchi |
| Cardiac | Striated, involuntary muscle | Heart muscle |

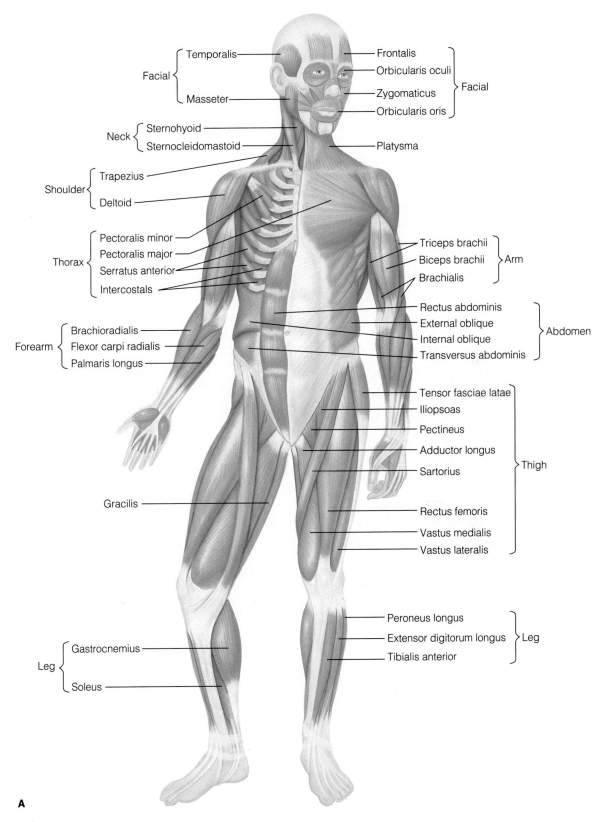

**Figure 37–4 ■** *A*, Muscles of the anterior body.

*(Figure continues on page 1184)*

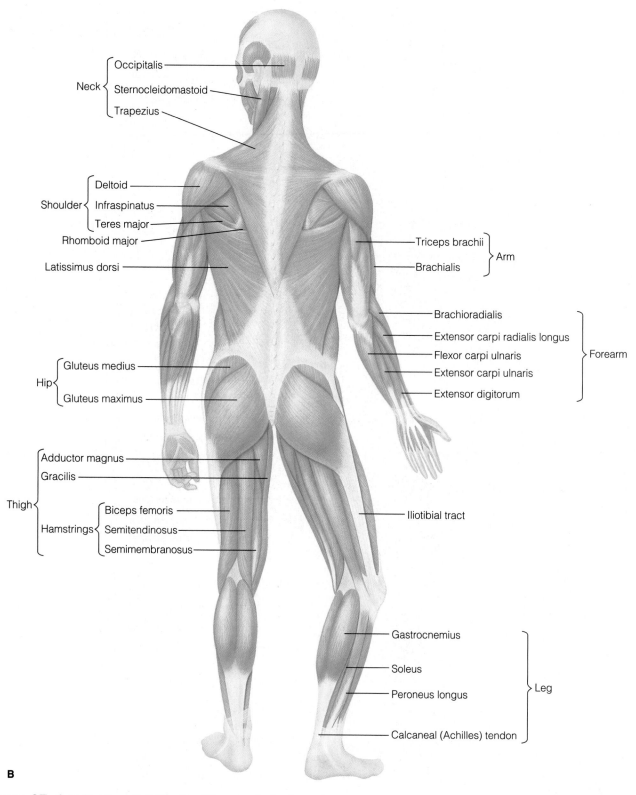

Neck
- Occipitalis
- Sternocleidomastoid
- Trapezius

Shoulder
- Deltoid
- Infraspinatus
- Teres major

Rhomboid major

Latissimus dorsi

Triceps brachii
Brachialis
} Arm

Brachioradialis
Extensor carpi radialis longus
Flexor carpi ulnaris
Extensor carpi ulnaris
Extensor digitorum
} Forearm

Hip
- Gluteus medius
- Gluteus maximus

Thigh
- Adductor magnus
- Gracilis
- Hamstrings
  - Biceps femoris
  - Semitendinosus
  - Semimembranosus

Iliotibial tract

Gastrocnemius
Soleus
Peroneus longus
Calcaneal (Achilles) tendon
} Leg

**B**

**Figure 37–4** ■ (Continued) *B,* Muscles of the posterior body.

Other questions and leading statements, categorized by functional health patterns, can be found on the Companion Website.

## Physical Assessment

Physical assessment of the musculoskeletal system is conducted through inspection, palpation, and measurement of muscle mass and range of motion. The client should be comfortably dressed in clothing that lets you see the movement of all joints clearly. The client may be standing, sitting, or lying down; the sequence of the examination should be such that the client does not have frequent position changes. An assessment of the older adult, the client in pain, or the client who is weak may take extra time.

The equipment necessary for assessing the musculoskeletal system is a tape measure to determine muscle size and a goniometer to measure joint range of motion (ROM). Prior to the examination, collect all equipment and explain the techniques to decrease the client's anxiety.

The general sequence for a musculoskeletal examination follows:

1. Begin the examination with an assessment of the client's gait and posture. Observe how the client walks, sits, and/or moves about in bed.
2. Inspect and palpate the client's bones for any obvious deformity or changes in size or shape. Palpation also will elicit tenderness or pain.
3. Measure the extremities for length and circumference. Before taking measurements, make sure the client is lying in a comfortable position. Remember to compare limbs bilaterally.
4. Assess muscle mass by first inspecting for obvious increase or decrease in size. Assess and document muscle strength on a scale of 0 to 5 (Table 37–4). Box 37–1 provides client instructions for testing the strength of various muscles.
5. Assess joints for swelling, pain, redness, warmth, crepitus, and ROM. Only assess the ROM of every joint if the client has a specific musculoskeletal problem; however, assessing one or more joints is a common part of nursing care. Use a goniometer for precise measurements of joint ROM (Figure 37–5 ■). This device has a pointer joined to a protractor at 0 degrees. These two arms are placed along articulating bones, and the angle of joint movement is recorded in degrees.

### BOX 37–1 ■ Guidelines for Determining Muscle Strength

In adults, muscles are usually strong and equally strong bilaterally. However, neuromuscular diseases, disuse, metabolic disorders, or infections can cause muscle weakness. Muscle strength is expected to be greater in the dominant arm and leg. In most instances (and especially when moving digits and extremities), the nurse provides resistance by pushing in the opposite direction.

The muscles listed below are routinely tested. Instructions for clients are also provided:

| Muscle | Client Instructions |
|---|---|
| Ocular muscles and lids | Close eyes tightly. |
| Finger muscles | Shake hands. |
| | Make a fist. |
| | Spread fingers. |
| Facial muscles | Blow out cheeks. |
| | Stick out tongue. |
| Hip muscles | Raise straight leg while supine. |
| Neck muscles | Bend head forward and backward. |
| Gluteal and leg muscles | Alternately cross legs while sitting. |
| Deltoid muscles | Hold arms up. |
| Biceps muscle | Bend the arm. |
| Quadriceps muscle | Straighten leg. |
| Triceps muscle | Straighten the arm. |
| Wrist muscles | Bend hand forward and backward. |
| Ankle and foot muscles | Bend foot up and down. |

### TABLE 37–4 Muscle Grading Scale

| Grading Scale | Assessment Description |
|---|---|
| 0 | (No visible) contraction; paralysis |
| 1 | Can feel contraction of muscle but there is no movement of limb |
| 2 | Passive ROM |
| 3 | Full ROM against gravity |
| 4 | Full ROM against some resistance |
| 5 | Full ROM against full resistance |

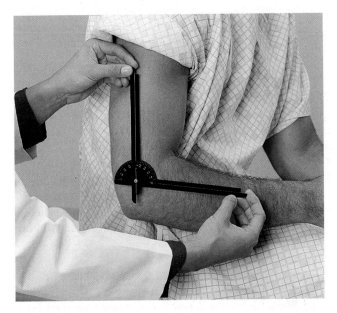

**Figure 37–5** ■ Using a goniometer to measure joint ROM.

## Gait and Body Posture Assessment with Abnormal Findings (✓)

- Inspect gait and body posture.
  - ✓ Joint stiffness, pain, deformities, and muscle weakness can cause changes in gait and posture.
- Inspect the spine for curvature. Ask the client to stand and bend back slowly as far as possible, bend slowly to the right and then to the left as far as possible, turn slowly to the right and left in a circular motion, and bend forward slowly and try to touch fingers to toes.
  - ✓ With herniated lumbar discs, the lumbar curve flattens and spinal mobility is decreased.
  - ✓ An increased lumbar curve, called **lordosis,** may be seen in obesity or pregnancy.
  - ✓ A lateral, S-shaped curvature of the spine is called **scoliosis.** Functional scoliosis usually is a compensatory response to painful paravertebral muscles, herniated discs, or discrepancy in leg length. It disappears with forward flexion. Structural scoliosis is often congenital and tends to appear during adolescence. It is accentuated with forward bending.
  - ✓ **Kyphosis** is an exaggerated thoracic curvature of the spine common in older adults.

## Joint Assessment with Abnormal Findings (✓)

- Inspect the joints for deformity, swelling, and redness.
  - ✓ Diseases of the joints may be manifested by such deformities as tissue loss, tissue overgrowth, or contractures, irreversible shortenings of muscles and tendons.
  - ✓ Edema in a joint may cause obvious bulging.
  - ✓ Redness, swelling, and pain are evidence of an inflammation or infection in the joint.
- Palpate the joints for tenderness, warmth, crepitation, consistency, and muscle mass.
  - ✓ Inflammation and injury cause joint pain.
  - ✓ Arthritis, bursitis, tendonitis, and osteomyelitis (infection of a bone) result in painful, hot joints.
  - ✓ **Crepitation** (a grating sound) is present in a joint when the articulating surfaces have lost their cartilage, such as in arthritis.

## Range-of-Motion Assessment with Abnormal Findings (✓)

Assess joint ROM by asking the client to perform activities specific to:

- *Temporomandibular joint:* "Open your mouth wide, and then close your mouth." (As the client opens and closes the mouth, palpate the temporomandibular joints with your index and middle fingers, as shown in Figure 37–6 ■.)
  - ✓ Clicking or popping noises, decreased ROM, pain, and swelling may indicate temporomandibular joint syndrome or, in rare cases, osteoarthritis.
- *Cervical spine:*
  45-degree flexion: "Touch your chin to your chest."
  55-degree extension: "Look at the ceiling."
  40-degree lateral bending: "Try to touch your right ear to your right shoulder." Repeat with the left side
  70-degree rotation: "Try to touch your chin to each shoulder."

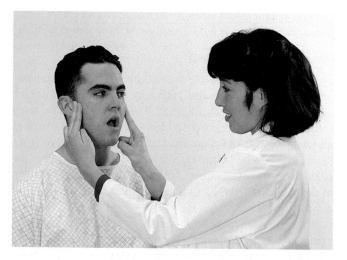

**Figure 37–6** ■ Palpating the temporomandibular joints.

  - ✓ Neck pain and limited extension with lateral bending are seen with herniated cervical discs and in cervical spondylosis.
  - ✓ An immobile neck with head and neck thrust forward is seen with ankylosing spondylitis.
- *Lumbar spine:*
  75- to 90-degree flexion: "Touch your toes with your fingers" (Figure 37–7A ■).
  30-degree extension: "Bend backward slowly."
  35-degree lateral bending: "Bend right and left" (Figure 37–7B).
  30-degree rotation: "Twist your shoulders right and left" (Figure 37–7C).
  - ✓ Decreased movement or pain with movement may indicate an abnormal spinal curvature, arthritis, herniated disc, or spasm of paravertebral muscles.
- *Fingers:*
  Flexion: "Make a fist."
  Extension: "Open your hand."
  Abduction: "Spread your fingers."
  Adduction: "Close your fingers."
  - ✓ Flexion and extension of fingers is decreased in arthritis.
  - ✓ Heberden's nodes and Bouchard's nodes are hard, nontender nodules on the dorsolateral parts of the distal and proximal interphalangeal joints, respectively. They are common in osteoarthritis.
  - ✓ Stiff, painful, swollen finger joints are seen in acute rheumatoid arthritis.
  - ✓ Boutonnière and swan-neck deformities are seen in chronic rheumatoid arthritis.
  - ✓ Swollen finger joints with a white chalky discharge may be seen in chronic gout.
- *Wrists:*
  90-degree flexion: "Bend wrist down."
  70-degree extension: "Bend wrist up."
  55-degree ulnar deviation: "Bend wrist toward little finger."
  20-degree radial deviation: "Bend wrist toward thumb."
  - ✓ Bilateral chronic swelling in the wrist is seen in arthritis.

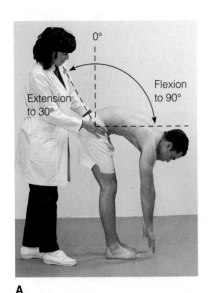
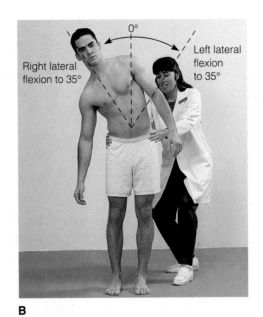
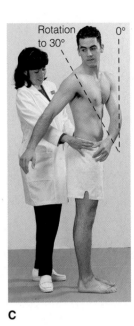

**A**  **B**  **C**

**Figure 37–7** ■ *A,* Forward flexion of spine. *B,* Lateral flexion of spine. *C,* Rotation of spine.

- *Elbows:*
  160-degree flexion: "Touch your hands to your shoulders."
  180-degree extension: "Straighten your elbows."
  90-degree supination: "Bend your elbows 90 degrees, and turn hands palm up."
  90-degree pronation: "Bend your elbows 90 degrees, and turn fists down."
  ✓ Swollen, tender, inflamed elbows are apparent in gouty arthritis and rheumatoid arthritis.
  ✓ Pain and tenderness at the lateral epicondyle occurs in tennis elbow.
- *Shoulders:*
  180-degree flexion: "Hold your arms straight up and out."
  50-degree hyperextension: "Put your straight arm behind your back."
  90-degree internal rotation: "Put your forearm behind your lower back."
  180-degree abduction: "Raise your straight arm up and out to your side."
  50-degree adduction: "Put your straight arm across your chest."
  ✓ Pain and tenderness over the biceps tendon occurs with tendinitis (inflammation of a tendon).
  ✓ The arm cannot be abducted fully when the supraspinatus tendon of the shoulder is ruptured.
  ✓ Pain and limited abduction is also seen with bursitis (inflammation of a bursa) and calcium deposits in this area.
- *Toes:*
  90-degree flexion: "Walk on your toes."
  ✓ The great toe is excessively abducted in hallux valgus.
  ✓ The joint above the great toe is swollen, inflamed, and painful in gouty arthritis.

✓ There is hyperextension of the metatarsophalangeal joint and flexion of the proximal interphalangeal joint with hammer toes.
- *Ankles:*
  20-degree dorsiflexion: "Point your foot to the ceiling."
  45-degree plantar flexion: "Point your foot to the floor."
  30-degree inversion: "Walk on the outside of your feet."
  20-degree eversion: "Walk on the inside of your feet."
  ✓ Contractures of the Achilles tendon may occur in clients with rheumatoid arthritis following prolonged bed rest.
- *Knees:*
  130-degree flexion: "Do a deep knee bend."
  180-degree extension: "Sit down and hold your legs straight out in front of you."
  ✓ Swelling over the suprapatellar pouch is seen with inflammation and fluid in the articular capsule of the knee. Synovitis is inflammation of the synovial membrane lining the articular capsule of a joint. It is common with knee trauma.
  ✓ Swelling over the patella is seen in bursitis.
- *Hips:* (The client is lying down.)
  120-degree flexion: "Bring bent knee up to your chest."
  30-degree hyperextension: "Lie on the abdomen, and lift up one leg at a time."
  45-degree abduction: "Hold your leg straight, and move it out to the side."
  40-degree internal rotation: "Bend your knee, and swing it toward your other leg."
  45-degree external rotation: "Bend your knee, and swing it out to the side."
  ✓ Movement of the hip is limited and/or painful in arthritis.

### Special Assessments with Abnormal Findings (✓)

- Perform *Phalen's test.* Ask the client to hold the wrist in acute flexion for 60 seconds (Figure 37–8 ■).

MediaLink | KNEE PAIN CASE STUDY

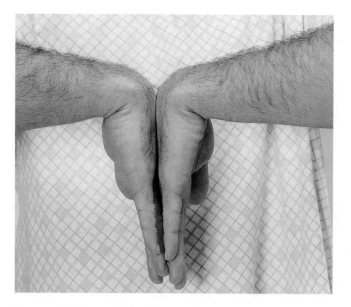

**Figure 37–8** ■ Phalen's test.

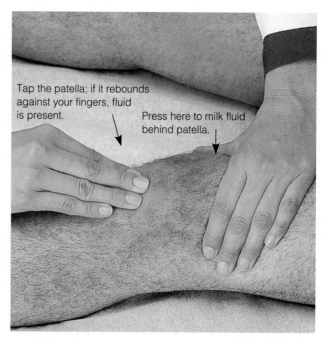

Tap the patella; if it rebounds against your fingers, fluid is present.

Press here to milk fluid behind patella.

**Figure 37–10** ■ Checking for ballottement.

✓ Numbness and burning in the fingers during Phalen's test may indicate carpal tunnel syndrome.

• Check for small amounts of fluid on the knee by assessing for a "bulge sign." Milk upward on the medial side of the knee, and then tap the lateral side of the patella (Figure 37–9 ■).

✓ A fluid bulge indicates increased fluid in the knee joint rather than soft tissue swelling.

• Check for larger amounts of fluid by assessing ballottement. Apply downward pressure on the knee with one hand while pushing the patella backward against the femur with the other hand (Figure 37–10 ■).

✓ Increased fluid will cause a tapping sound as the patella displaces the fluid and hits the femur.

• Perform *McMurray's test*. While reclining, ask the client to turn the flexed knee toward the center of the body. Stabilize the knee with one hand, and apply pressure on the lower leg with the other hand (Figure 37–11 ■).

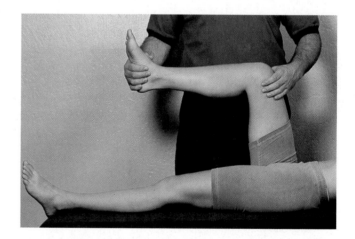

**Figure 37–11** ■ McMurray's test.

**Figure 37–9** ■ Checking for the bulge sign.

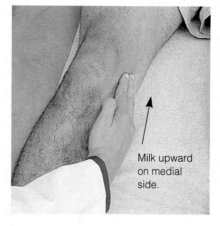

Milk upward on medial side.

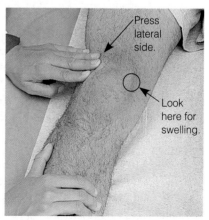

Press lateral side.

Look here for swelling.

✓ Pain, locking (inability to fully extend the knee), or a popping sound may indicate an injury to a meniscus, a disc of cartilaginous tissue in the knee.

• Perform the *Thomas test.* Ask the client to lie down and extend one leg while bringing the knee of the opposite leg to the chest (Figure 37–12 ■).

✓ A hip flexion contracture will cause the extended leg to rise off the table.

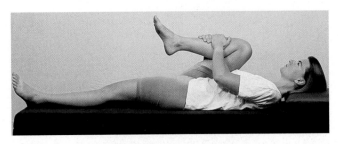

**Figure 37–12** ■ Thomas test for hip contracture.

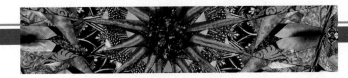

 **EXPLORE MediaLink**

NCLEX review questions, case studies, care plan activities, MediaLink applications, and other interactive resources for this chapter can be found on the Companion Website at www.prenhall.com/lemone.

Click on Chapter 37 to select the activities for this chapter. For animations, video clips, more NCLEX review questions, and an audio glossary, access the Student CD-ROM accompanying this textbook.

## TEST YOURSELF

1. What classification of bones has a diaphysis and epiphyses?
   a. Irregular bones
   b. Flat bones
   c. Long bones
   d. Short bones

2. The movement of a limb away from the body midline is:
   a. Abduction
   b. Adduction
   c. Extension
   d. Flexion

3. What would you ask the client to do in order to assess facial muscle strength?
   a. "Close your eyes tightly."
   b. "Stick out your tongue."
   c. "Bend your head forward."
   d. "Open your eyes widely."

4. What term is used to describe a grating sound when a joint is moved?
   a. Crackles
   b. Arthritis
   c. Synovitis
   d. Crepitation

5. What are the most common manifestations of musculoskeletal disorders?
   a. Pain and limited mobility
   b. Swelling and redness
   c. Cyanosis and decreased pulses
   d. Pallor and decreased ROM

See Test Yourself answers in Appendix C.

## BIBLIOGRAPHY

Andresen, G. (1998). Assessing the older patient. *RN, 61*(3), 46–56.

Bynum, D. (1997). Clinical snapshot: Gout. *American Journal of Nursing, 97*(7), 36–37.

Campbell-Giovaniello, K. (1997). Clinical snapshot: Plantar fasciitis. *American Journal of Nursing, 97*(9), 38–39.

Krug, B. (1997). Rheumatoid arthritis and osteoarthritis: A basic comparison. *Orthopedic Nursing, 16*(5), 73–75.

Ludwidk, R., Dieckman, B., & Snelson, C. (1999). Assessment of the geriatric orthopaedic trauma patient. *Orthopaedic Nursing, 18*(6), 11–20.

Mangini, M. (1998). Physical assessment of the musculoskeletal system. *Nursing Clinics of North America, 33*(4), 643–652.

McDougall, T. (1999). Orthopedic update: Assessment of limb injury. *Australian Emergency Nursing Journal, 2*(1), 26–28.

Neal, L. (1997). Basic musculoskeletal assessment: Tips for the home health nurse. *Home Healthcare Nurse, 15*(4), 227–235.

O'Hanlon-Nichols, T. (1998). A review of the adult musculoskeletal system: A guide to a key aspect of patient care. *American Journal of Nursing, 98*(6), 48–52.

Watson, R. (2001). Assessing the musculoskeletal system in older people. *Nursing Older People, 13*(5), 29–30.

Weber, J., & Kelley, J. (2002). *Health assessment in nursing* (2nd ed.) Philadelphia: Lippincott.

Wilson, S., & Giddens, J. (2001). *Health assessment for nursing practice.* St. Louis: Mosby.

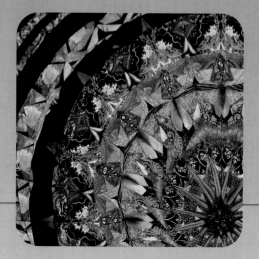

### CHAPTER 38

# Nursing Care of Clients with Musculoskeletal Trauma

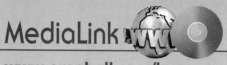

## www.prenhall.com/lemone

Additional resources for this chapter can be found on the Student CD-ROM accompanying this textbook, and on the Companion Website at www. prenhall.com/lemone. Click on Chapter 38 to select the activities for this chapter.

**CD-ROM**
• Audio Glossary
• NCLEX Review

*Animations*
• Bone Healing
• Fracture Repair

**Companion Website**
• More NCLEX Review
• Case Study
    A Client with Fractures
• Care Plan Activity
    Below-the-Knee Amputation
• MediaLink Application
    Preventing Musculoskeletal Injuries

## LEARNING OUTCOMES

After completing this chapter, you will be able to:

▪ Apply knowledge of normal anatomy, physiology, and assessments when providing care for clients with musculoskeletal trauma (see Chapter 37).

▪ Explain the factors that lead to musculoskeletal trauma and amputations.

▪ Describe the pathophysiology, manifestations, complications, and collaborative care for clients with contusions, strains, sprains, fractures, amputations, and repetitive use injury.

▪ Describe the stages of bone healing.

▪ Explain the purposes and related nursing interventions for casts, traction, and stump care.

▪ Use the nursing process as a framework for providing individualized care for clients who have experienced musculoskeletal trauma.

Musculoskeletal trauma is an injury to muscle, bone, or soft tissue that results from excessive external force. The external source transmits more kinetic energy than the tissue can absorb, and injury results. The severity of the trauma depends not only on the amount of force but also on the location of the impact, because different parts of the body can withstand different amounts of force. A wide variety of external sources can cause trauma, and the force involved can vary in severity (e.g., a step off the curb, a fall, being tackled in a football game, and a motor vehicle crash). See Chapter 6 ⊂⊃ for a detailed discussion of the results of different forces and types of injury from trauma.

Musculoskeletal injuries resulting from trauma include blunt tissue trauma, alterations in tendons and ligaments, and fractures of bones. Various forces that cause musculoskeletal trauma are typical for a specific environment, activity, or age group. For example, motorcycle crashes resulting in fractures of the distal tibia, midshaft femur, and radius are common in young men. Sports injuries, resulting from either overuse or acute trauma, are seen more often in adolescents and young adults. Falls are the most common cause of injury in people age 65 or older, with fractures of the vertebrae, proximal humerus, and hip seen most often (Porth, 2002).

Musculoskeletal trauma can result in mild or severe injuries. A client may experience a soft-tissue injury, a fracture, and/or a complete amputation. In addition, trauma to one part of the musculoskeletal system often produces dysfunction in adjacent structures. For example, a fracture of the femur prevents the adjacent muscles from abducting and adducting. Nursing care helps minimize the effects of trauma, prevents complications, and hastens restoration of function. The injury may require rehabilitation and temporary or permanent changes in lifestyle. This chapter discusses fractures, amputations, soft-tissue injuries, dislocations, and repetitive use injuries.

## TRAUMATIC INJURIES OF THE MUSCLES, LIGAMENTS, AND JOINTS

### THE CLIENT WITH A CONTUSION, STRAIN, OR SPRAIN

Contusion, strains, and sprains are among the most commonly reported injuries. They account for about 50% of work-related injuries, with lower back injuries the most commonly reported occupational injury. However, many sprains and strains are not work related, and often are not reported. The lower back and cervical region of the spine are the most common sites for muscle strains; the ankle is the most commonly sprained joint, usually caused by forced inversion of the foot.

## PATHOPHYSIOLOGY AND MANIFESTATIONS

A **contusion,** the least serious form of musculoskeletal injury, is bleeding into soft tissue that results from a blunt force, such as a kick or striking a body part against a hard object. The skin remains intact, but small blood vessels rupture and bleed into soft tissues. A contusion with a large amount of bleeding is referred to as a **hematoma.** The manifestations of a contusion include swelling and discoloration of the skin. The blood in the soft tissue initially results in a purple and blue color commonly referred to as a mark or bruise. As the blood begins to reabsorb, the mark becomes brown and then yellow, until it disappears.

A **strain** is a stretching injury to a muscle or a muscle-tendon unit caused by mechanical overloading. A muscle that is forced to extend past its elasticity will become strained. Lifting heavy objects without bending the knees, or a sudden acceleration-deceleration, as in a motor vehicle crash, can cause strains. The most common sites for a muscle strain are the lower back and cervical regions of the spine. The manifesta-

| BOX 38–1 | ■ Comparison of Sprains and Strains |

**Sprain**
- Defined as an injury to a ligament that results from a twisting motion.
- Can cause joint instability.
- Pain, edema, and swelling are present.
- Motion increases the joint pain.

**Strain**
- Defined as a microscopic tear in the muscle.
- Sharp or dull pain is present.
- Pain increases with isometric contraction of the muscle.
- Swelling and local tenderness are present.

tions of a strain include a sharp or dull pain that increases with isometric contraction of the muscle, swelling, and stiffness.

A **sprain** is an injury to a ligament surrounding a joint. Forces going in opposite directions cause the ligament to overstretch and/or tear. The ligaments may be incompletely or completely torn. Although any joint may be involved, sprains of the ankle and knee are most common. Manifestations include joint instability, discoloration, heat, pain, edema, and rapid swelling. Motion increases the joint pain. A comparison of sprains and strains is presented in Box 38–1.

## COLLABORATIVE CARE

Soft-tissue trauma is treated with measures that decrease swelling and alleviate pain. Severe sprains may require surgical repair. A splint may be applied to rest the injured area. Ice

is applied for the first 24 to 48 hours, after which heat can be applied. A compression dressing, such as an Ace bandage, may be applied. The injured extremity should be elevated to or above the level of the heart to increase venous return and decrease swelling. Ankle sprains may be immobilized with an air cast, with no limitations on weight bearing. A knee injury also requires a knee immobilizer. If the upper extremity is injured, a sling is provided. Physical therapy may be recommended during rehabilitation.

## Diagnostic Tests

The following diagnostic tests may be ordered when soft-tissue trauma is suspected:

- *X-rays* rule out a fracture before making a diagnosis of soft-tissue injury.
- *Magnetic resonance imaging (MRI)* is used if further assessment is necessary.

## Medications

Medications used to treat soft-tissue trauma include NSAIDs and analgesics.

## NURSING CARE

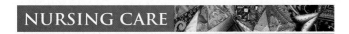

The nursing care of each client is individualized. A strain or sprain may not be as devastating to an attorney as it is to a professional athlete; therefore, the nurse should determine what the injury means to the particular client.

## Nursing Diagnoses and Interventions

Nursing diagnoses focus on providing information about self-care to decrease pain and return physical mobility to preinjury levels.

### Acute Pain

The pain that results from soft-tissue trauma is due primarily to the injury to the muscle or ligament and secondarily to bleeding and edema at the injury site.

- Teach the client the acronym RICE (rest, ice, compression, elevation) to care for the injury:
  - Rest the injured extremity. *Rest allows the injured muscle or ligament to heal.*
  - Apply ice to the injured area. *Cold causes vasoconstriction and decreases the pooling of blood in the injured area. Ice may also numb the tender area.*
  - Apply a compression dressing, such as an Ace bandage. *A compression dressing can decrease the formation of edema and thereby decrease pain.*
  - Elevate the extremity above the heart. *Elevating the extremity promotes venous return and decreases edema, which will decrease pain.*
- If pain is still present after 24 to 48 hours of applying ice, instruct the client to apply heat. *Heat increases blood flow and venous return and thereby decreases edema and pain.*

## Impaired Physical Mobility

Pain causes the client to avoid using or bearing weight with the injured extremity. Always observe the client's use of assistive devices; if the device is inappropriate, the client can face a greater risk of falling. The device may be appropriate, but the client may not be using it correctly or safely. As a person ages, muscle mass in the upper extremities declines. As a result, the older client with a sprained ankle may not be able to use crutches, because crutches require that the person distribute body weight along the upper extremities. Older clients may therefore find a walker more useful.

- Teach the correct use of crutches, walkers, canes, or slings if prescribed. *The correct technique increases safety and encourages use of these devices.*
- Encourage follow-up care. *Severe sprains may require further testing to determine if surgical intervention is indicated.*

## THE CLIENT WITH A JOINT DISLOCATION

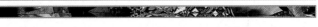

A **dislocation** of a joint is the loss of articulation of the bone ends in the joint capsule. Dislocations usually follow severe trauma, with the bone ends displaced or separated from their normal position in the joint capsule. They occur most frequently in the shoulder and acromioclavicular joints. A **subluxation** is a partial dislocation in which the bone ends are still partially in contact with each other.

## PATHOPHYSIOLOGY AND MANIFESTATIONS

Dislocations may be congenital, traumatic, or pathologic. Congenital dislocations are present at birth and are seen in the hip and knee. Traumatic dislocations result from falls, blows, or rotational injuries. Pathologic dislocations result from disease of the joint, including infection, rheumatoid arthritis, paralysis, and neuromuscular diseases. The manifestations of a dislocation include pain, deformity, and limited motion.

## COLLABORATIVE CARE

Care of the client with a dislocation focuses on relieving pain, correcting the dislocation, and preventing complications. The dislocation is diagnosed by physical examination and X-rays. The joint is reduced by means of manual traction.

Shoulder joint dislocations are reduced and immobilized in a sling for 3 weeks, after which time rehabilitation can begin. A dislocated hip requires immediate reduction in the emergency room to prevent necrosis of the femoral head and injury to the sciatic and femoral nerves. After reduction, the client is placed on bed rest. In some cases, traction is needed for several weeks. If a hip dislocation is accompanied by a fracture, the client will undergo surgery to increase mobility, decrease complications, and rapidly stabilize the joint.

## NURSING CARE

Nursing care of the client with a dislocation or subluxation is individualized to the cause of injury, the type of dislocation, and the age of the client.

### Nursing Diagnoses and Interventions

Nursing diagnoses focus on relieving pain (see previous section) and preventing complications.

#### Risk for Injury

The client with a dislocation requires frequent assessments to ensure that neurovascular compromise does not develop.

- Monitor neurovascular status by assessing pain, pulses, pallor, paralysis, and paresthesia. *Neurovascular compromise is indicated by increased pain, decreased or absent pulses, pale skin, inability to move a body part or extremity, and changes in sensation (such as "pins and needles" sensations, or loss of sense of sharp/dull touch).*
- Maintain immobilization after reduction. *Immobilization prevents the joint from dislocating again.*

### Home Care

Joint dislocations often tend to be recurring injuries for clients actively participating in contact sports and other vigorous physical activities. Younger adults have a 60% to 80% recurrence rate for anterior shoulder dislocations. Prolonged immobilization (for several weeks after the injury) and aggressive rehabilitation following the initial dislocation can reduce the risk of recurrent dislocation. The following topics should be addressed in preparing the client for home care.

- Importance of complying with the prescribed length of immobilization
- Skin care and ways to prevent skin-to-skin contact, particularly in the axillary area
- Prescribed rehabilitation exercises that will strengthen muscles and other supportive structures in the shoulder, decreasing the risk of future dislocations
- Alternatives to activities that precipitate recurrent dislocations
- Instructions or referrals to physical therapy if needed for further teaching about using assistive devices
- Referrals to physical and occupational therapy and home health services as needed

## TRAUMATIC INJURIES OF BONES

### THE CLIENT WITH A FRACTURE

A **fracture** is any break in the continuity of a bone. Fractures vary in severity according to the location and the type of fracture. Although fractures occur in all age groups, they are more common in people who have sustained trauma and in older clients.

### PATHOPHYSIOLOGY

Any of the 206 bones in the body can sustain a fracture. A fracture occurs when the bone is subjected to more kinetic energy than it can absorb. Fractures may result from a direct blow, a crushing force (compression), a sudden twisting motion (torsion), a severe muscle contraction, or disease that has weakened the bone (called a **pathologic fracture**). Two basic mechanisms produce fractures: direct force and indirect force. With direct force, the kinetic energy is applied at or near the site of the fracture. The bone cannot withstand the force. With indirect force, the kinetic energy is transmitted from the point of impact to a site where the bone is weaker. The fracture occurs at the weaker point.

Fractures are classified in the following ways:

- If the skin is intact, the fracture is considered a **closed** (or **simple) fracture.** If the skin integrity is interrupted, the fracture is considered an **open** (or **compound) fracture** (Figure 38–1 ■). An open fracture allows bacteria to enter the injured area and increases the risk of complications.

- The fracture line may be **oblique** (at a 45-degree angle to the bone) or **spiral** (curves around the bone). An **avulsed** fracture occurs when the fracture pulls bone and other tissues away from the point of attachment. It may also be described as **comminuted** (the bone breaks in many pieces), **compressed** (the bone is crushed), **impacted** (the broken bone

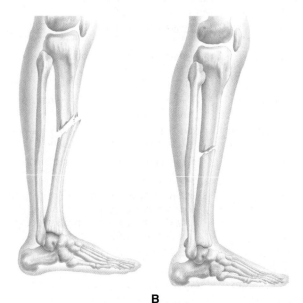

A                    B

**Figure 38–1** ■ *A*, An open fracture. *B*, A closed fracture.

MediaLink | FRACTURE CASE STUDY

ends are forced into each other), or **depressed** (the broken bone is forced inward).

- **Complete fractures** involve the entire width of the bone, whereas **incomplete fractures** do not involve the entire width of the bone.
- A **stable (nondisplaced) fracture** is one in which the bones maintain their anatomic alignment. An **unstable (displaced) fracture** occurs when the bones move out of correct anatomic alignment. If a fracture is displaced, immediate interventions are required to prevent further damage to soft tissue, muscle, and bone.
- Fractures may also be classified by point of reference on the bone, such as midshaft, middle third, and distal third. The point of reference may also be specific, such as intrarticular or diaphyseal.

## MANIFESTATIONS AND COMPLICATIONS

Fractures are often accompanied by soft tissue injuries that involve muscles, arteries, veins, nerves, or skin. The degree of soft-tissue involvement depends on the amount of energy or force transmitted to the area. Fracture manifestations and their causes are outlined in Table 38–1. The section following fracture healing describes manifestations and complications, with related collaborative and nursing care, for fractures of specific bones.

### Fracture Healing

Regardless of classification or type, fracture healing progresses over three phases: the inflammatory phase, the reparative phase, and the remodeling phase. See *Pathophysiology Illustrated* on the next page. The bleeding and inflammation that develop at the site of the fracture initiate the inflammatory phase. A hematoma forms between the fractured bone ends and around the bone surfaces. The osteocytes at the bone ends die as the hematoma clots, obstructing blood flow and depriving them of oxygen and nutrients. Necrosis of the cells heightens the inflammatory response, which in turn leads to vasodilation and edema. In addition, fibroblasts, lymphocytes, macrophages, and even osteoblasts from the bone migrate to the fracture site. Fibroblasts form a fibrin meshwork and promote the growth of granulation tissue and capillary buds. The lymphocytes and macrophages wall off the area, localizing and containing the inflammation. The capillary buds invade the fracture site and supply a source of nutrients to promote the formation of collagen. The collagen allows calcium to be deposited.

Once calcium is deposited, a callus begins to form. In this reparative phase, osteoblasts promote the formation of new bone, and osteoclasts destroy dead bone and assist in the synthesis of new bone. Collagen formation and calcium deposition continues. During the remodeling phase, excess callus is removed and new bone is laid down along the fracture line. Eventually, the fracture site is calcified, and the bone is reunited.

The age, physical condition of the client, and the type of fracture sustained influence the healing of fractures. Other factors influence bone healing either positively or negatively and may be grouped according to their local or systemic influence (Box 38–2). Healing time varies with the individual. An uncomplicated fracture of the arm or foot can heal in 6 to 8 weeks. A fractured vertebra will take at least 12 weeks to heal. A fractured hip may take from 12 to 16 weeks.

### TABLE 38–1   Manifestations of Fracture

| Manifestation | Cause |
| --- | --- |
| Deformity | Abnormal position of bones secondary to fracture and muscles pulling on fractured bone |
| Swelling | Edema from localization of serous fluid and bleeding |
| Pain/tenderness | Muscle spasm, direct tissue trauma, nerve pressure, movement of fractured bone |
| Numbness | Nerve damage or nerve entrapment |
| Guarding | Pain |
| Crepitus | Grating of bones or entrance of air in an open fracture. *Note:* Do not manipulate the extremity to elicit crepitus; doing so may cause additional damage. |
| Hypovolemic shock | Blood loss or associated injuries |
| Muscle spasms | Muscle contraction near the fracture |
| Ecchymosis | Extravasation of blood into the subcutaneous tissue |

### BOX 38–2 ■ Factors Influencing Bone Healing

**POSITIVE FACTORS**

**Local**
- Immobilization
- Timely correction of displacement
- Application of ice
- Electrical stimulation

**Systemic**
- Adequate amounts of growth hormone, vitamin D, and calcium
- Adequate blood supply
- Absence of infection or diseases
- Younger age
- Moderate activity level prior to injury

**NEGATIVE FACTORS**

**Local**
- Delay in correction of displacement
- Open fracture (increases risk of infection)
- Presence of foreign body at fracture site

**Systemic**
- Immunocompromised status
- Decreased circulation (as in diabetes or peripheral vascular disease)
- Malnutrition
- Osteoporosis
- Advanced age

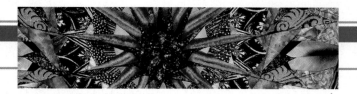

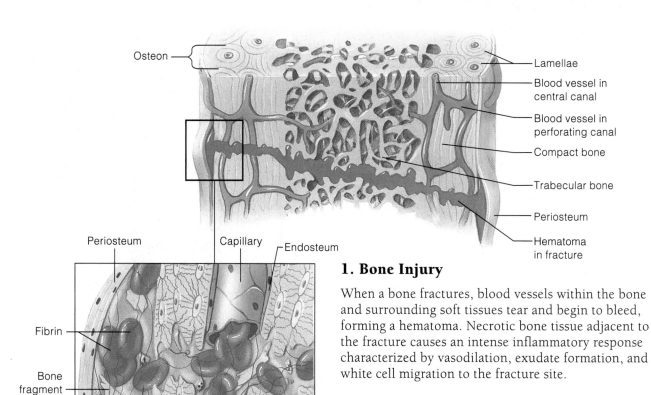

Osteon — Lamellae — Blood vessel in central canal — Blood vessel in perforating canal — Compact bone — Trabecular bone — Periosteum — Hematoma in fracture

Periosteum — Capillary — Endosteum

Fibrin

Bone fragment

Osteocyte

## 1. Bone Injury

When a bone fractures, blood vessels within the bone and surrounding soft tissues tear and begin to bleed, forming a hematoma. Necrotic bone tissue adjacent to the fracture causes an intense inflammatory response characterized by vasodilation, exudate formation, and white cell migration to the fracture site.

## 2. Fibrocartilaginous Callus Formation

Clotting factors within the hematoma form a fibrin meshwork. Within 48 hours, fibroblasts and new capillaries growing into the fracture form granulation tissue that gradually replaces the hematoma. Phagocytes begin to remove cell debris.

Osteoblasts, bone-forming cells, proliferate and migrate into the fracture site, forming a fibrocartilaginous callus. The osteoblasts build a web of collagen fibers from both sides of the fracture site that eventually unites to connect bone fragments, thus splinting the bone. Chondroblasts lay down patches of cartilage that provide a base for bone growth.

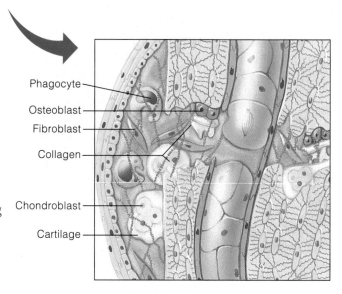

Phagocyte

Osteoblast

Fibroblast

Collagen

Chondroblast

Cartilage

*(continued on page 1196)*

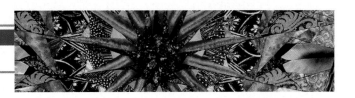

## 4. Bone Remodeling

Osteoblasts continue to form new woven bone, which is in turn organized into the lamellar structures of compact bone. Osteoclasts resorb excess callus as it is replaced by mature bone.

As the bone heals and is subjected to the mechanical stress of everyday use, osteoblasts and osteoclasts respond by remodeling the repair site along the lines of force. This ensures that the repaired section of bone eventually resembles the structure of the uninjured part.

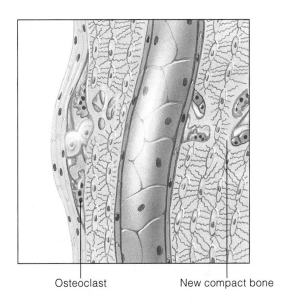

Osteoclast    New compact bone

## 3. Bony Callus Formation

Osteoblasts continue to proliferate and synthesize collagen fibers and bone matrix, which are gradually mineralized with calcium and mineral salts to form a spongey mass of woven bone. The trabeculae of woven bone bridge the fracture. Osteoclasts migrate to the repair site and begin removing excess bone in the callus. Bony callus formation usually continues for 2 to 3 months.

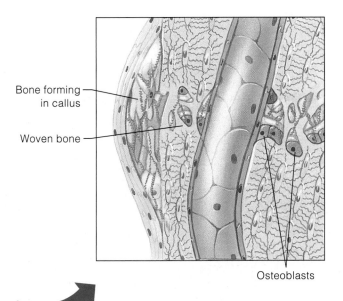

Bone forming in callus

Woven bone

Osteoblasts

## COLLABORATIVE CARE

A fracture requires treatment involving stabilizing the fractured bone(s), maintaining bone immobilization, preventing complications, and restoring function. The diagnosis of a fracture is primarily based on physical assessments and X-rays.

### Emergency Care

Emergency care of the client with a fracture includes immobilizing the fracture, maintaining tissue perfusion, and preventing infection. In the case of serious trauma, normal body alignment must be maintained and may involve cervical immobilization. Once the client is in a secure location, he or she is assessed for instability or deformity of the bone. If any deformity or instability is detected, the extremity is rapidly immobilized. Open wounds are covered with sterile dressings, and bleeding may be controlled with a pressure dressing. The extremities are assessed for the presence of pulses, movement, and sensation. The joint above and below the deformity is immobilized. Pulses, movement, and sensation are reevaluated after splinting.

The fracture is splinted to maintain normal anatomical alignment and prevent the fracture from dislocating. Splinting relieves pain and prevents further damage to the arteries, nerves, and bones. Splinting can be accomplished with air splints. If equipment is not available, the limb may be secured to the body. For example, an arm may be secured with a sling, or one leg may be strapped to the other leg.

### Diagnostic Tests

Diagnosis of a fracture begins with the history and initial assessment and usually is confirmed by radiographic tests. The following tests may be ordered:

- *X-rays* are commonly used to assess bones for fractures (Figure 38–2 ■).
- *Bone scan* may be necessary to determine if a fracture is present, indicated by an increased uptake, or a "hot spot."

- *Blood chemistry studies, complete blood count (CBC),* and *coagulation studies* may be used to assess blood loss, renal function, muscle breakdown, and the risk of excessive bleeding or clotting.

### Medications

Most clients with a fracture require pharmacologic interventions. The first and foremost intervention focuses on relieving pain. In the case of multiple fractures or fractures of large bones, narcotics are administered initially. As healing progresses, the client begins to take oral medication for pain. Pain management for the client with a fracture is described in Box 38–3.

Stool softeners may be administered to decrease the risk of constipation secondary to narcotics and immobility. Clients who have sustained trauma are often placed on antiulcer medications or antacids. NSAIDs may continue to be prescribed to decrease inflammation. Antibiotics may be administered prophylactically, particularly to clients with open or complex fractures. Anticoagulants may be prescribed to prevent deep vein thrombosis.

### Treatments

#### Surgery

Surgery is indicated in the client who has a fracture that requires direct visualization and repair, a fracture with common long-term complications, or a fracture that is severely comminuted and threatens vascular supply.

The simplest form of surgery is done by external fixation with an external fixator device. An external fixator consists of a frame connected to pins that are inserted perpendicular to the long axis of the bone (Figure 38–3 ■). The number of pins inserted varies with the type and site of the fracture, but in all cases the same number of pins is inserted above and below the fracture line. The pins require care similar to that of skeletal traction pins. The client is monitored for infection, and frequent neurovascular assessment is performed. The fixator increases independence while maintaining immobilization.

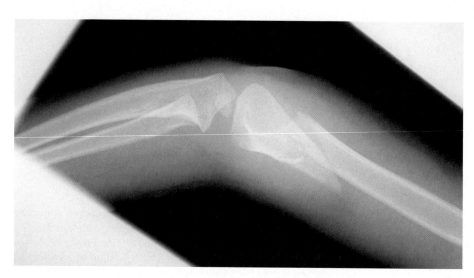

**Figure 38–2 ■** X-ray of an oblique fracture of the femur.

*Source: Charles Stewart and Associates.*

## BOX 38–3 ■ Pain Management in the Client with a Fracture

The client who has had musculoskeletal trauma from an accident or surgery experiences pain from many different causes:

- The interruption in the continuity of the bone itself
- Damage to ligaments and tendons
- Swelling of tissues around the trauma site
- Muscle spasms
- Tissue anoxia from swelling inside a cast, splint, or the muscle fascia sheath
- Hematoma formation
- Pressure over bony prominences from casts or splints

The pain is often severe and may be described as sharp, aching, or burning. Carefully assess any complaint of pain; pain may be an indication of a serious complication, such as compartment syndrome, decreased tissue perfusion and neurovascular impairment, or pressure ulcers. Do not administer analgesics until the location, character, and duration of pain has been carefully assessed. After the cause of the pain has been identified, the following nursing interventions may be implemented.

1. Administer prescribed analgesics, which may include NSAIDs and narcotic analgesics. For serious fractures or following orthopedic surgery, PCA or epidural methods of providing pain relief may be used. If medications are used on an as-needed basis, tell the client to request the medication before the pain is severe; alternatively, offer the medications at regular intervals for the first 24 to 48 hours. Reassure the client that addiction does not result from taking medications to relieve fracture or surgical pain. Most clients require only oral analgesics by the third or fourth day after orthopedic surgery. Refer to Chapter 4 ⊙⊙ for information about narcotic and nonnarcotic pain medications.

2. Elevate the involved extremity, and apply cold (if prescribed) to help decrease swelling.

3. Monitor and drain the accumulated fluids in any drainage devices to ensure patency and to decrease the possibility of hematoma formation.

4. Encourage the client to wiggle fingers and toes on an extremity in a cast or traction to improve venous return and decrease edema.

5. Assist the client to change positions to relieve pressure and use pillows to provide support.

6. Teach the client alternative methods of pain management, such as relaxation and guided imagery.

7. Notify the physician of unrelieved pain, which may indicate a serious complication such as compartment syndrome or neurovascular impairment.

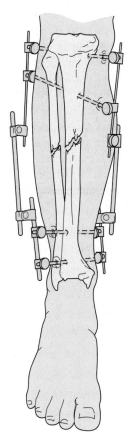

**Figure 38–3** ■ In external fixation, pins are placed through the bone above and below the fracture site to immobilize the bone. External fixation rods hold the pins in place.

Internal fixation can be accomplished through a surgical procedure called an *open reduction and internal fixation (ORIF)*. In this procedure, the fracture is reduced (placed in correct anatomic alignment) and nails, screws, plates, or pins are inserted to hold the bones in place (Figure 38–4 ■). Open fractures of the arms and legs are most commonly repaired in this way. Hip fractures in older clients are almost always repaired with ORIF to prevent complications and to allow early rehabilitation. Implications for postoperative nursing care are presented in Box 38–4.

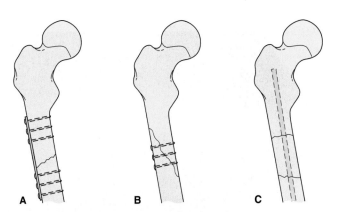

A   B   C

**Figure 38–4** ■ Internal fixation hardware is entirely within the body. *A,* Fixation of a short oblique fracture using a plate and screws above and below the fracture. *B,* Fixation of a long oblique fracture using screws through the fracture site. *C,* Fixation of a segmental fracture using a medullary nail.

**BOX 38–4**   ■ **Nursing Implications for Clients with Internal Fixation**

■ Expect the client to have sutures and at least one Hemovac drain.
■ Perform neurovascular assessments frequently.
■ Also assess the following:
  a. Wounds for drainage
  b. Hemovac for drainage of serosanguineous fluid
  c. Bowel sounds
  d. Lung sounds

■ Administer medications, such as analgesics and antibiotics, per physician's orders.
■ In hip fractures, place an abductor pillow between client's legs to prevent dislocation of the hip joint.
■ Arrange for physical and occupational therapy, as ordered.
■ Assist with weight-bearing program, if ordered.
■ Encourage early mobilization, coughing, and deep breathing, as appropriate, to help prevent complications.

## Traction

Muscle spasms usually accompany fractures and may pull bones out of alignment. **Traction** is the application of a straightening or pulling force to return or maintain the fractured bones in normal anatomic position. Weights are applied to maintain the necessary force. Types of traction are as follows:

• In **manual traction,** the hand directly applies the pulling force. Other common types of traction include straight traction, balanced suspension traction, skin traction, and skeletal traction (Figure 38–5 ■).
• **Straight traction** is a pulling force applied in a straight line to the injured body part resting on the bed. The most com-

mon type of straight traction is Buck's traction, in which the lower portion of the injured extremity is placed in a cradle-like sleeve. This sleeve is harnessed to itself, and a weight is hung from the bottom of a traction frame. The result is a force that pulls straight away from the body. This traction exerts its grabbing and pulling force through the client's skin. Therefore, this traction may be considered straight skin traction. The advantage of skin traction is the relative ease of use and ability to maintain comfort. The disadvantage is that the weight required to maintain normal body alignment or fracture alignment cannot exceed the tolerance of the skin, about 6 lb per extremity.

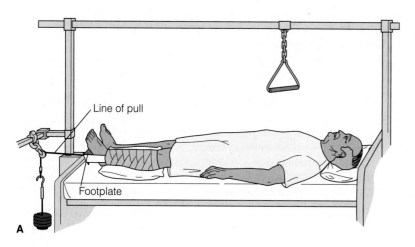

Line of pull

Footplate

**A**

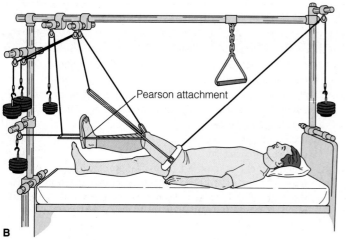

Pearson attachment

**B**

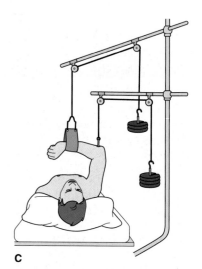

**C**

**Figure 38–5** ■ Traction is the application of a pulling force to maintain bone alignment during fracture healing. Different fractures require different types of traction. *A,* Skin traction (also called straight traction) such as Buck's traction shown here, is often used for hip fractures. *B,* Balanced suspension traction is commonly used for fractures of the femur. *C,* Skeletal traction, in which the pulling force is applied directly to the bone, may be used to treat fractures of the humerus.

- **Balanced suspension traction** involves more than one force of pull. Several forces work in unison to raise and support the client's injured extremity off the bed and pull it in a straight fashion away from the body. The advantage of this type of traction is that it increases mobility without threatening joint continuity. The disadvantage is that the increased use of multiple weights makes the client more likely to slide in the bed.
- **Skeletal traction** is the application of a pulling force through placement of pins into the bone. The client receives local anesthetic, and the pin is inserted in a twisting motion into the bone. This type of traction must be applied under sterile conditions because of the increased risk of infection. One or more pulling forces may be applied with skeletal traction. The advantage of this type of traction is that more weight can be used to maintain the proper anatomic alignment if necessary. The disadvantages include increased anxiety, increased risk of infection, and increased discomfort. Nursing implications for clients receiving traction are presented in Box 38–5.

## Casts

A **cast** is a rigid device applied to immobilize the injured bones and promote healing. The cast is applied to immobilize the joint above and the joint below the fractured bone so that the bone will not move during healing. A fracture is first reduced manually and a cast is then applied. Casts are applied on clients who have relatively stable fractures

The cast, which may be composed of plaster or fiberglass, is applied over a thin cushion of padding and molded to the normal contour of the body. The cast must be allowed to dry before any pressure is applied to it; simply palpating a wet cast with the fingertips will leave dents that may cause pressure sores. A plaster cast may require up to 48 hours to dry, whereas a fiberglass cast dries in less than 1 hour. The type of cast applied is determined by the location of the fracture (Figure 38–6 ■). Nursing implications for clients with casts are discussed in the box below. During follow-up appointments, the physician may X-ray the bone to assess alignment and healing, and possibly remove the cast for skin assessment.

---

### BOX 38–5 ■ Nursing Implications for Clients Receiving Traction

- In skeletal traction, never remove the weights.
- In skin traction, remove weights only when intermittent skin traction has been ordered to alleviate muscle spasm.
- For traction to be successful, a countertraction is necessary. In most instances, the countertraction is the client's weight. Therefore, do not wedge the client's foot or place it flush with the foot-board of the bed.
- Maintain the line of pull:
  a. Center the client on the bed.
  b. Ensure that weights hang freely and do not touch the floor.
- Ensure that nothing is lying on or obstructing the ropes. Do not allow the knots at the end of the rope to come into contact with the pulley.
- If a problem is detected, assist in repositioning. The area of the fracture must be stabilized when the client is repositioned.

- In skin traction:
  a. Frequently assess skin for evidence of pressure, shearing, or pending breakdown.
  b. Protect pressure sites with padding and protective dressings as indicated.
- In skeletal traction:
  a. Frequent skin assessments should include pin care per policy.
  b. Report signs of infection at the pin sites, such as redness, drainage, and increased tenderness.
  c. The client may require more frequent analgesic administration.
- Perform neurovascular assessments frequently.
- Assess for common complications of immobility, including formation of pressure ulcers, formation of renal calculi, deep vein thrombosis, pneumonia, paralytic ileus, and loss of appetite.
- Teach the client and family about the type and purpose of the traction.

---

# NURSING CARE OF THE CLIENT WITH A CAST

## NURSING RESPONSIBILITIES

- Perform frequent neurovascular assessments.
- Palpate the cast for "hot spots" that may indicate the presence of underlying infection.
- Report any drainage promptly.

## CLIENT AND FAMILY TEACHING

- Do not place any objects in the cast.
- If the cast is made of plaster, keep it dry.
- If the cast is made of fiberglass, dry it with a blow dryer on the cool setting if it becomes wet.
- Assess the injured extremity for coolness, changes in color, increased pain, increased swelling, and/or loss of sensation.

- Use a blow dryer on the cool setting to relieve itching by blowing cool air into the cast.
- If a sling is used, it should distribute the weight of the cast evenly around the neck. Do not roll the sling; this can impair circulation to the neck.
- If crutches are used, arrange for physical therapist to teach correct crutch walking.
- When the cast is removed, an oscillating cast remover will be used. A guard prevents the cast remover from penetrating past the depth of the cast, so it will not cut the client. It is noisy, and the client will feel vibration.

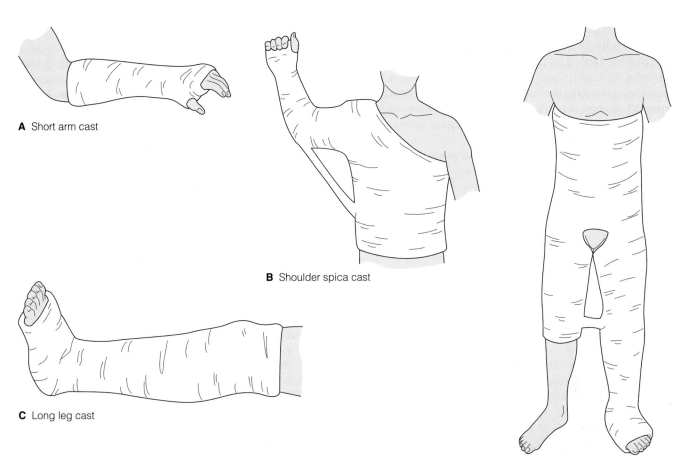

**A** Short arm cast

**B** Shoulder spica cast

**C** Long leg cast

**D** One-and-one half hip spica cast

**Figure 38–6** ■ Common types of casts used to immobilize fractures.

## Electrical Bone Stimulation

**Electrical bone stimulation** is the application of an electrical current at the fracture site. It is used to treat fractures that are not healing appropriately. The electrical stress increases the migration of osteoblasts and osteoclasts to the fracture site. Mineral deposition increases, promoting bone healing. Electrical bone stimulation can be accomplished invasively or noninvasively (Figure 38–7 ■). In invasive stimulation, the surgeon inserts a cathode and a lead wire at the fracture site. The lead wire is attached to an internal or external generator, which delivers electricity through the lead wire to the cathode 24 hours a day. In noninvasive inductive stimulation, a treatment coil encircles the cast or skin directly over the fracture site. The coil is attached to an external generator that runs on batteries. The electricity goes through the skin to the fracture site. The time period for external stimulation can vary from 3 to 10 hours per day. The client may be taught to self-administer the noninvasive electrical stimulation. Electrical bone stimulation is contraindicated in the presence of infection.

## Fracture Complications with Related Collaborative Care

Complications of musculoskeletal trauma are associated with pressure from edema and hemorrhage, development of fat emboli, deep vein thrombosis, infection, loss of skeletal integrity, or involvement of nerve fibers. Bone fragments may also result in further injury or complications.

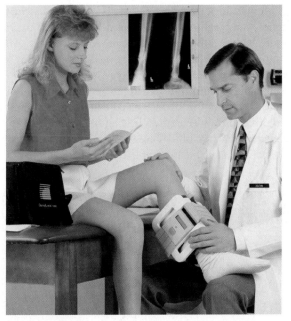

**Figure 38–7** ■ External electrical bone growth stimulator.

*Courtesy of Orthologic, Inc.*

## Compartment Syndrome

A compartment is a space enclosed by a fibrous membrane or fascia. The fascia lines the compartment within the limbs and is nonexpandable. Compartments within the limbs may enclose and support bones, nerves, and blood vessels. **Compartment syndrome** occurs when excess pressure in a limited space constricts the structures within a compartment, reducing circulation to muscles and nerves. Acute compartment syndrome may result from hemorrhage and edema within the compartment following a fracture or from a crush injury, or from external compression of the limb by a cast that is too tight. Increased pressure within the confined space of the compartment results in entrapment of nerves, blood vessels, and muscles.

Entrapment of the blood vessels limits tissue perfusion, beginning a cycle of events that may result in the loss of the limb. Inadequate oxygen supply causes cellular acidosis, which intensifies as cellular energy requirements are met through anaerobic metabolism. The capillaries inside the compartment dilate in an attempt to increase the supply of blood and oxygen. Additional blood and oxygen are not available, and plasma proteins leak out into the interstitial tissues. The interstitial tissue then pulls fluid in to balance the protein load. As a result, edema within the compartment increases. The edema causes further compression of the vascular network, and the cycle continues. Uninterrupted, this cycle threatens the client's limb and increases the risk of sepsis. Compartment syndrome usually develops within the first 48 hours of injury, when edema is at its peak. Manifestations of compartment syndrome are listed in the box below. It is important to note that arterial pulses may remain normal, even when pressure within the compartment is high enough to significantly impair tissue perfusion.

If compartment syndrome develops, interventions to alleviate pressure will be implemented; these may include removal of a tightly fitting cast. If the pressure is internal, a **fasciotomy,** a surgical intervention in which muscle fascia is cut to relieve pressure within the compartment, may be necessary. After a fasciotomy, the incision is left open, and passive ROM exercises are performed on the extremity.

Volkmann's contracture, a common complication of elbow fractures, can result from unresolved compartment syndrome. Arterial blood flow decreases, leading to ischemia, degeneration, and contracture of the muscle. Arm mobility is impaired, and the client is unable to completely extend the arm.

## Manifestations of Compartment Syndrome

### EARLY MANIFESTATIONS
- Pain
- Normal or decreased peripheral pulse

### LATER MANIFESTATIONS
- Cyanosis
- Tingling, loss of sensation (paresthesias)
- Weakness (paresis)
- Severe pain, especially when the extremity is passively flexed
- Eventual renal failure (due to release of myoglobin into the bloodstream; myoglobin molecule is too large for effective filtration and excretion by kidney and renal failure results)

## Fat Embolism Syndrome

Fat emboli occur when fat globules lodge in the pulmonary vascular bed or peripheral circulation. **Fat embolism syndrome (FES)** is characterized by neurologic dysfunction, pulmonary insufficiency, and a petechial rash on the chest, axilla, and upper arms. Long bone fractures and other major trauma are the principle risk factors for fat emboli; hip replacement surgery also poses a risk for FES.

When a bone is fractured, pressure within the bone marrow rises and exceeds capillary pressure; as a result, fat globules leave the bone marrow and enter the bloodstream. Another contributing factor may be the stress-induced release of catecholamine, which causes the rapid mobilization of fatty acids. Once the fat globules are released, they combine with platelets and travel to the brain, lungs, kidneys, and other organs, occluding small blood vessels and causing tissue ischemia.

Manifestations usually develop within a few hours to a week after injury. The manifestations result from the occlusion of the blood supply and the presence of fatty acids. Altered cerebral blood flow causes confusion and changes in level of consciousness. Pulmonary circulation may be disrupted, and free fatty acids damage the alveolar-capillary membrane. Pulmonary edema, impaired surfactant production, and atelectasis can result in significant respiratory insufficiency and manifestations of acute respiratory distress syndrome (ARDS) (see Chapter 36). Fat droplets activate the clotting cascade, causing thrombocytopenia. Petechiae (pin-sized purplish areas from bleeding under the skin) appearing on the skin, buccal membranes, and conjunctival sacs are thought to result from either microvascular clotting or the accompanying thrombocytopenia.

Early stabilization of long bone fractures is preventive for FES. Prompt identification and treatment of the syndrome are necessary to maintain adequate pulmonary function. In severe cases, the client may require intubation and mechanical ventilation to prevent hypoxemia. Fluid balance is closely monitored. Corticosteroids may be administered to decrease the inflammatory response of lung tissues, stabilize lipid membranes, and reduce bronchospasm (Porth, 2002).

## Deep Vein Thrombosis

A **deep vein thrombosis (DVT)** is a blood clot that forms along the intimal lining of a large vein. Three precursors linked to DVT formation are (1) venous stasis, or decreased blood flow, (2) injury to blood vessel walls, and (3) altered blood coagulation (Table 38–2). Any or all of these precursors can cause a DVT to form. Damage to the lining of the vein causes the platelets to aggregate or clump together, forming the thrombus. Fibrin, WBCs, and RBCs begin to cling to the thrombus, and a tail forms. This tail or the entire thrombus may dislodge and move to the brain, lungs, or heart. Five percent of DVTs dislodge and enter the pulmonary circulation to form a pulmonary embolus. If the thrombus remains in the vein, venous insufficiency may result from scarring and valve damage.

The best treatment for DVT is prevention. Early immobilization of the fracture and early ambulation of the client are imperative. The extremity should be elevated above the level of

| TABLE 38-2 | Precursors of Deep Vein Thrombosis |
|---|---|
| **Precursor** | **Implications for Fractures** |
| Decreased blood flow | Common in fracture clients, who are immobilized and less active. Bed rest alone can decrease venous flow by 50%. |
| Injury to blood vessel wall | May occur as a direct result of the force that caused the fracture or from surgical manipulation. |
| Altered blood coagulation | May result from active blood loss. The body's attempt to maintain homeostasis leads to increased production of platelets and clotting factor. |

the heart. Frequent assessments of the injured extremity may lead to early recognition of DVT and prevent the formation of pulmonary embolus. Prophylactic anticoagulant administration is also beneficial. Antiembolism stockings and compression boots also increase venous return and prevent stasis of blood. Constrictive clothing should be avoided.

If a DVT is present, there may be swelling, leg pain, tenderness, or cramping. Not all clients experience manifestations, however. For this reason, diagnostic tests, such as a venogram or Doppler ultrasound of lower extremities, may be required. A venogram requires intravenous administration of dye in the radiology department, whereas a Doppler ultrasound study is noninvasive and can be performed at the client's bedside. Doppler ultrasonography uses sound waves to form an image on a computer screen.

The diagnosis of DVT requires rapid intervention. The client is placed on bed rest for 5 to 7 days to prevent dislodgment of the clot. Thrombolytic agents, which dissolve the clot, may be administered. Heparin may be administered intravenously to prevent more clots from forming. A vena cava filter may be placed to prevent the existing clot from entering the pulmonary circulation and forming a pulmonary embolus. In extreme cases in which anticoagulation therapy is contraindicated, a thrombectomy (surgical removal of the clot) may be necessary. See Chapter 33 ⊙ for further discussion of DVT.

### Infection
Infection is more likely to occur in an open fracture than a closed fracture, but any complication that decreases blood supply increases the risk of infection. Infection may result from contamination at the time of injury or during surgery. *Pseudomonas, Staphylococcus,* or *Clostridium* organisms may invade the wound or bone. *Clostridium* infection is particularly serious because it may lead to severe gas gangrene and cellulitis, but any infection may delay healing and result in **osteomyelitis,** infection within the bone that can lead to tissue death and necrosis. (See Chapter 39 for a discussion of osteomyelitis.)

### Delayed Union and Nonunion
**Delayed union** is the prolonged healing of bones beyond the usual time period. Many factors may inhibit bone healing, including poor nutrition, inadequate immobilization, prolonged reduction time, infection, necrosis, age, immunosuppression,

and severe bone trauma resulting in multiple fragments. Delayed union is diagnosed by means of serial X-ray studies. It is important to note that X-ray findings may lag 1 to 2 weeks behind the healing process; for example, a client may be completely healed by week 13, but this fact may not be apparent on the X-ray until week 14.

Delayed union may lead to **nonunion,** which can cause persistent pain and movement at the fracture site. Nonunion may require surgical interventions, such as internal fixation and bone grafting. If infection is present, the bones are surgically debrided. Electrical stimulation of the fracture site may be as effective as bone grafting.

### Reflex Sympathetic Dystrophy
**Reflex sympathetic dystrophy** may occur after musculoskeletal or nerve trauma. This term refers to a group of poorly understood posttraumatic conditions involving persistent pain, hyperesthesias, swelling, changes in skin color and texture, changes in temperature, and decreased motion. Diagnosis is made by the client's history and physical examination. X-rays may demonstrate spotty osteoporosis, and bone scans may reveal increased uptake of radionucleide. Treatment with a sympathetic nervous system blocking agent often alleviates the symptoms.

## Fractures of Specific Bones or Bony Areas
### Fracture of the Skull
The skull may be fractured as a result of either a fall or a direct blow. The client must be assessed for neurologic damage and any loss of consciousness must be documented. A complete neurologic assessment is conducted: Pupillary reaction to light, movement and strength of all extremities, complaints of nausea and vomiting, level of consciousness and orientation to person, place, and time are noted. A displaced skull fracture, which is referred to as depressed, may press on the brain and cause neurologic damage. Brain injuries related to skull fractures are discussed in Chapter 42. ⊙

### Fracture of the Face
Fracture of the facial bones may result from a direct blow. The client presents with hematomas, pain, edema, and bony deformity. Nondisplaced fractures are monitored to ensure the airway is not compromised. The client is observed for any neurologic deficits. Severely displaced or multiple facial fractures are treated with open reduction and internal fixation with wires or plates.

Nursing care focuses on maintaining the airway by helping the client clear secretions from the oropharynx. The nurse monitors the client's breathing for increased effort or tachypnea and notifies the physician immediately if these findings are noted. Pain is treated with analgesics, and body image disturbances are addressed. If the client asks to see his or her face, the nurse should plan to stay with the client and answer questions while the client looks in a mirror.

### Fracture of the Spine
The spine can be injured in many ways, including sports injuries, falls, and motor vehicle crashes. The spine can be fractured in the cervical, thoracic, lumbar, or sacral area. The most

severe complication of spine fracture is injury to the spinal cord. A fracture to the vertebrae may cause the bones to become displaced and apply pressure on the spinal cord. This pressure on the spinal cord may result in permanent paralysis.

A nondisplaced cervical spinal fracture may be treated with a cervical collar or a halo immobilizing brace. The displaced cervical fracture is reduced by manual or skeletal traction and, eventually, application of a brace and/or surgical stabilization of the bones with plates and screws. Immobilization after a spinal fracture may last as long as 6 months. Chapter 41 ∞ discusses spinal fractures and spinal cord injury.

## Fracture of the Clavicle

A fracture of the clavicle commonly results from a direct blow or a fall. The most common location is midclavicular. A person with a midclavicular fracture typically assumes a protective slumping position to immobilize the arm and prevent shoulder movement. A less common fracture occurs along the distal third of the clavicle. This type of fracture may be associated with ligament damage. Injuries to the clavicle may be associated with skull or cervical fractures. The fractured bone, if displaced, may lacerate the subclavian vessels and result in hemorrhage. The fractured bone may also puncture the lung, resulting in a pneumothorax. Malunion may occur at the fracture site and result in asymmetry of the clavicles. Injury to the brachial plexus may result in numbness and decreased movement of the arm on the affected side.

A deformity may be observed or palpated along the clavicle. Treatment focuses on immobilizing the fractured bone in normal anatomic position by applying a clavicular strap (Figure 38–8 ■), or a surgical repair may be necessary.

## Fracture of the Humerus

The exact location of the fracture, the presence of displacement, and the results of the neurovascular examination determine the severity of a fracture of the humerus and the appropriate interventions. Treatment focuses on immobilizing the fractured bone in normal anatomic position. Common complications of humeral fracture include nerve and ligament damage, frozen or stiff joints, and malunion. Early interventions and follow-up may prevent permanent damage.

Fractures of the proximal humerus are common in older adults. A simple nondisplaced fracture of the proximal humerus (near the humeral head) with a normal neurovascular assessment can be safely treated with immobilization. A more com-

plicated displaced fracture of the proximal humerus with bone fragmentation requires surgical intervention. The more severe the fracture and damage to soft tissue, the more likely the range of motion of the shoulder will be impaired. Rehabilitative measures focus on increasing ROM.

The humerus may also fracture along the shaft, usually as a direct result of trauma. If the humeral shaft fracture is simple and nondisplaced, a hanging arm cast is applied. This cast maintains alignment of the fracture by using the pulling force of gravity; therefore, the client must be instructed not to rest the cast on anything to alleviate the weight. If the client is on bed rest, a hanging arm cast is not applied, because the arm would not be able to hang freely. Instead, the fracture is immobilized with external skeletal traction. This traction places the injured arm in an upright position over the face, and weights are hung off the distal portion of the humerus (see Figure 38–6C). Nursing implications for clients with fractures of the humerus are presented in Box 38–6.

## Fracture of the Elbow

The most common location of an elbow fracture is the distal humerus. Elbow fractures usually result from a fall or direct blow to the elbow. The client guards the injured extremity, holding the arm rigidly in a flexed position or an extended position. Because the radius, ulna, or humerus may be involved in the elbow fracture, all three bones must be visualized by X-ray.

Complications of an elbow fracture include nerve or artery damage and **hemarthrosis,** a collection of blood in the elbow joint. The most serious complication of an elbow fracture is **Volkmann's contracture,** which results from arterial occlusion and muscle ischemia. The client complains of forearm pain, impaired sensation, and loss of motor function. Rapid interventions are aimed at relieving pressure on the brachial artery and nerve and preventing muscle atrophy.

Nondisplaced elbow fractures are treated by immobilizing the fracture with a posterior splint or cast. The displaced fracture is first reduced and then immobilized. Nursing interventions focus on alleviating pain, maintaining immobilization, and educating clients in neurovascular assessments.

| BOX 38–6 | ■ Nursing Implications for Clients with Fractures of the Humerus |
| --- | --- |

- Perform neurovascular assessments frequently.
- Administer prescribed medications to alleviate pain.
- Encourage exercises for clients with a hanging cast.
  a. Finger exercises: Move each finger of the affected arm through complete range of motion.
  b. Pendulum shoulder exercises: Dangle the affected arm at the side, and move it forward and backward about 30 degrees in each direction.
- If client is discharged, instruct the client and family in cast care and sling application, neurovascular assessments, exercises, prescribed pain medications, and manifestations of complications.
- If client is admitted to the hospital, provide pre-operative teaching.

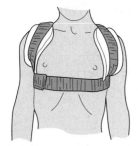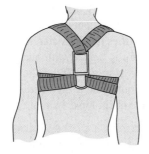

**Figure 38–8** ■ A clavicular strap is used to immobilize a clavicular fracture.

## Fracture of the Radius and/or Ulna

Fractures of the radius and ulna may occur as a result of either indirect injury, such as twisting or pulling on the arm, or direct injury, such as that resulting from a fall. The usual treatment of radius fractures depends on the location. The proximal radial head may be fractured from a fall on an outstretched hand. Blood commonly collects in the elbow joint and must be aspirated. If the fracture is nondisplaced, a sling is applied. If the fracture is displaced, surgical intervention is required. After surgical repair of a displaced fracture, the arm is splinted with a posterior plaster splint. The client avoids movement for the first week and then initiates movement gradually.

When both bones are broken, the fracture is usually displaced. The client complains of pain and inability to turn the palm of the hand up. A nondisplaced fracture is casted for about 6 weeks, and either a shorter cast or a brace is then applied for 6 more weeks. If the fracture is displaced, surgical intervention is performed. The physician reduces the fracture and may insert pins or screws to keep the bones in alignment. After the surgery, a cast is applied, and the client is encouraged to exercise the fingers.

Complications after a radius and/or ulnar fracture include compartment syndrome, delayed healing, and decreased wrist and finger movement. After surgery, the client also has an increased risk of infection. Nursing interventions focus on alleviating pain, maintaining immobilization, and educating clients in neurovascular assessments, the importance of elevation, and the need to inform the physician of changes in sensation or an increase in pain.

## Fractures in the Wrist and Hand

Wrist fractures often result from a fall onto an outstretched hand or onto the back of the hand. A common type of wrist fracture is **Colles's fracture,** in which the distal radius fractures after a fall onto an outstretched hand. The client with a wrist fracture presents with a bony deformity, pain, numbness, weakness, and decreased ROM of the fingers. The capillary refill and sensation of the hand must be assessed.

The hand is composed of many bones. Most commonly, the metacarpals and phalanges are involved in a hand fracture. The injuring mechanism in a hand fracture varies greatly from striking an object with a closed fist to closing a hand in a door. The client presents with complaints of pain, edema, and decreased ROM. The cause of the injury usually focuses the assessment on circulation, sensation, and ROM.

Comparative X-rays may be obtained to compare left and right wrists and hands. Complications of wrist and hand fractures are compartment syndrome, nerve damage, ligament damage, and delayed union. A wrist fracture is commonly treated with closed reduction, cast application, and elevation of the injured extremity. A hand fracture is splinted and elevated.

Nursing interventions focus on alleviating pain and educating the client in neurovascular assessments, the importance of elevation, and how to exercise the fingers to prevent stiffness. If the dominant hand is injured, the client will require assistance in performing ADLs.

## Fracture of the Ribs

Rib fractures commonly result from blunt chest trauma. The location of the fracture and involvement of underlying organs determine the severity of the injury. Fractures of the first through third ribs may result in injury to the subclavian artery or vein. Fractures of the lower ribs may result in spleen and liver injuries.

The client presents with a history of recent chest trauma. Typically, the client complains of pain along the lateral portion of the rib. Palpation of the rib reveals a bony deformity and increases pain. Deep inspiration also increases pain. The skin over the fracture site may be ecchymotic (bruised).

A complication of rib fractures is a **flail chest,** which results from the fracture of two or more adjacent ribs in two or more places and the formation of a free-floating segment that moves in the opposite direction of the rib cage. The bony instability impairs respirations (see Chapter 36). Treatment is aimed at stabilizing the flail segment and supporting respirations. Other complications of rib fractures include pneumothorax and/or hemothorax. The fractured rib may pierce the lung and injure it. The lower ribs may pierce the liver or spleen, resulting in intra-abdominal bleeding. Pneumonia may also develop from ineffective clearing of respiratory secretions.

A simple rib fracture is treated with pain medication and instructions for coughing, deep breathing, and splinting. The client is also instructed to return to the emergency room if shortness of breath develops. Nursing interventions focus on alleviating pain and teaching the client about splinting. Because deep inspiration increases pain, clients frequently avoid it. The client may be instructed to splint the injured rib with the hand or a pillow and take deep breaths and cough to decrease the chance of developing atelectasis. Incentive spirometry is encouraged.

## Fracture of the Pelvis

The client with a pelvic fracture presents with pain in the back or hip area. A single fracture in the pelvis is treated conservatively with bed rest on a firm mattress. Log rolling increases client comfort. A pelvic fracture with two fracture sites is considered unstable and treated with surgery. An external fixator may be applied to stabilize the pelvis. In the client who is not stable for surgery, a pelvic sling may be used. The pelvic sling stabilizes the pelvis and allows the client to move in bed with less pain. Common complications include hypovolemia, spinal injury, bladder injury, urethral injury, kidney damage, and gastrointestinal trauma.

Nursing care focuses on alleviating discomfort, maintaining immobilization, and preparing the client for surgery if necessary. The nurse monitors the client for increased heart rate, decreased blood pressure, and decreasing hemoglobin levels. These findings may indicate impending hypovolemia due to bleeding into the pelvis. Any blood in the urine should be reported to the physician; this may indicate kidney, bladder, or urethral damage.

## Fracture of the Shaft of the Femur

A large amount of force, such as from motor vehicle crashes, falls, or acts of violence, is required to fracture the shaft of the femur. Clients with femoral shaft fractures often have associated multiple trauma. A fracture of the femoral shaft is manifested by an edematous, deformed, painful thigh. The client is unable to move the hip or knee. Initial assessment focuses on the circulation and sensation present in the affected extremity. Pedal pulses and capillary refill in the affected extremity are compared to the unaffected extremity. Complications of a femoral shaft fracture include hypovolemia due to blood loss (which may be as great as 1.0 to 1.5 L), fat embolism, dislocation of the hip or knee, muscle atrophy, and ligament damage.

Treatment of fractures of the shaft of the femur initially includes skeletal traction to separate the bony fragments and reduce and immobilize the fracture. Depending on the location and severity of the fracture, traction may be followed by either external or internal fixation. Strength in the affected extremity is maintained through gluteal and quadricep exercises. ROM exercises for unaffected extremities are critical in preparation for ambulation. Although full weight bearing is usually restricted until X-rays demonstrate bone union, the client may be allowed to carry out non-weight-bearing activities with an assistive device.

The nurse assesses pulses in the extremity and compares them bilaterally. Sensation is evaluated by asking whether the client can feel touch and discriminate sharp from dull objects. Nursing interventions include providing pain medication, providing reassurance and decreasing anxiety, and assisting with exercises of the lower legs, feet, and toes.

### Fracture of the Hip

A hip fracture refers to a fracture of the femur at the head, neck, or trochanteric regions (Figure 38–9 ■). Hip fractures are classified as intracapsular or extracapsular. **Intracapsular fractures** involve the head or neck of the femur; **extracapsular fractures** involve the trochanteric region. The majority of hip fractures involve the neck or trochanteric regions. The femoral head and neck lie within the joint capsule and are not covered in periosteum; thus, they do not have a large blood supply. Fractures here usually fragment and may further decrease blood supply, increasing the risk of nonunion and avascular necrosis. The trochanteric region is covered in periosteum and therefore has more blood supply than the head or neck.

Hip fractures are a significant problem, causing the greatest number of deaths and most serious health problems of all fractures. Most are the result of falls, which account for 87% of all fractures for people 65 years or older (CDC, 2000). Statistics for hip fractures include the following:

- Approximately 75% to 80% of hip fractures are sustained by postmenopausal women, who have the highest incidence of osteoporosis.
- Most people with hip fractures are hospitalized for 2 weeks.
- Half of all older adults hospitalized for a hip fracture cannot return home or live independently after the fracture.
- By the year 2040, the number of hip fractures is expected to exceed 500,000, which reflects society's increasing older population. Factors contributing to falls include problems with gait and balance, neurological and musculoskeletal impairments, dementia, psychoactive medications, and visual impairments.

Hip fractures are common in older adults as a result of decreases in bone mass and the increased tendency to fall. Whether the femur breaks spontaneously and causes the fall or whether the fall causes the fracture is not always clear; regardless of the cause of the fracture, however, rapid interventions are required to prevent bone necrosis. Assessment findings commonly associated with a hip fracture are pain, shortening of the affected lower extremity, and external rotation. Rarely, the fracture dislocates posteriorly; if that occurs, the extremity may internally rotate.

A hip fracture may be treated with traction to decrease muscle spasms, followed by surgery; or surgery may be performed

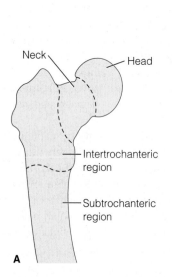
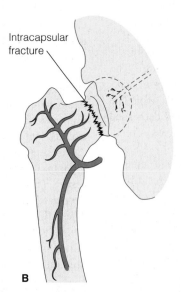
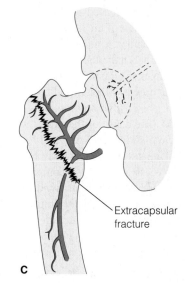

**Figure 38–9** ■ *A,* Regions where hip fractures may occur: the head of the femur, the neck of the femur, and the trochanteric regions of the femur. *B,* Intracapsular fractures occur across the head or neck of the femur. *C,* Extracapsular fractures occur across the trochanteric regions. Note how both intracapsular and extracapsular fractures disrupt the blood supply to the bone.

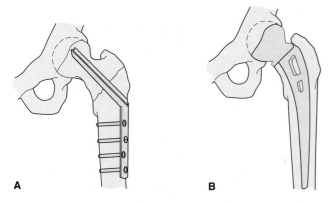

**Figure 38–10** ■ Surgical fixation of hip fractures. *A*, A surgical nail or screw used to stabilize an intertrochanteric fracture. *B*, Use of a hip prosthesis (artificial hip) to replace a damaged femoral head.

immediately or within the first 24 hours. The goal of surgery is to reduce and stabilize the fracture, thereby increasing mobility, decreasing pain, and preventing complications. Surgery usually consists of open reduction and internal fixation of the fracture. Fixation is accomplished by securing the femur in place with pins, screws, nails, or plates (Figure 38–10A ■). An open reduction and internal fixation works well for fractures in the trochanteric area. Fractures of the femoral neck frequently disrupt blood supply to the femoral head. If blood supply is disrupted, the surgeon will replace the femoral head with a prosthesis (Figure 38–10B). If the acetabulum has been damaged, the surgeon may insert a metal cup. Replacement of either the femoral head or the acetabulum with a prosthesis is called a hemiarthroplasty. Replacement of both the femoral head and the acetabulum is a total hip arthroplasty (THA), discussed in Chapter 39. Nursing care focuses on alleviating pain, maintaining circulation to the injured extremity, and increasing mobility.

### Fracture of the Tibia and/or Fibula

Fractures of the lower extremities often result from a fall on a flexed foot, a direct blow, or a twisting motion. The client presents with edema, pain, bony deformity, and a hematoma at the level of injury.

Circulation and sensation are assessed to rule out common complications of the fracture, including damage to the peroneal nerve or tibial artery, compartment syndrome, hemarthroses, and ligament damage. Peroneal nerve damage may be indicated by the client's inability to point the toe on the affected side upward. Tibial artery damage may be the cause of an absent dorsalis pedis pulse on the affected side. Compartment syndrome may be present if the client develops pain on passive movement and paresthesias. An edematous knee may indicate a collection of blood in the knee joint. Ligament damage may be present if the client cannot move the knee and/or ankle.

If the fracture is closed, a closed reduction and casting are frequently performed. A long leg cast that allows for partial weight bearing is used. Partial weight bearing usually is prescribed by the physician within 10 days of the fracture. A short leg cast will be applied in 3 to 4 weeks. If the fracture is open, either external fixation or open reduction and internal fixation

will be performed. After surgery, a cast may be applied, and weight bearing begins according to the physician's orders, usually in about 6 weeks.

Nursing care is designed to increase comfort, monitor neurovascular status, and prevent complications. The nurse instructs the client in cast care, the use of assistive devices, how to perform neurovascular assessment, and when to follow up with the physician.

### Fracture in the Ankle and Foot

The client with an ankle fracture presents with pain, limited ROM, hematoma, edema, and difficulty ambulating. Most ankle fractures are treated by closed reduction and casting. Open fractures are treated by surgical intervention and splinting.

The client with a foot fracture presents with similar symptoms; however, range of motion of the ankle is not usually affected. Most foot fractures are nondisplaced and treated with closed reduction and casting. More severe displaced foot fractures may require surgery and the placement of wires to maintain reduction of the fracture.

Nursing care focuses on increasing comfort, increasing mobility, and educating the client. Analgesia is given for pain. The extremity should be elevated, and ice can be applied. The client is taught cast care, neurovascular assessment, and crutch walking.

## NURSING CARE

In planning and implementing nursing care for the client with fractures, the nurse should consider the client's response to the traumatic experience. Although each client has individual needs, nursing care commonly focuses on client problems with pain, impaired physical mobility, impaired tissue perfusion, and neurovascular compromise.

### Health Promotion

Trauma prevention can save lives. Many communities are educating people of all ages, from grade-schoolers to older adults, in trauma prevention. Young adults face a high risk of sustaining trauma. They need to be taught the importance of safety equipment—such as automobile seat belts, bicycle helmets, football pads, proper footwear, protective eyewear, and hard hats—in preventing or decreasing the severity of injury from trauma. Older adults should have regular screenings for osteoporosis, activity levels, cognitive and affective disorders, sensory impairments, and risk for falls. Educational programs about workplace and farm safety, including information about ergonomic principles, can also help prevent musculoskeletal injuries.

Having a regular exercise program and avoiding obesity are important factors in maintaining good bone health in all adults. An adequate intake of calcium is essential to ensure proper growth, development, and maintenance of strong bones throughout life. It is important that women ensure good bone health prior to menopause, as the loss of estrogen during and after menopause decreases calcium use. Strong bones are formed by calcium intake and weight-bearing exercise, both of which are equally important in the postmenopausal woman.

## Meeting Individualized Needs

### TEACHING OLDER ADULTS TO PREVENT FALLS

- Begin a regular exercise program; lack of exercise leads to weakness and an increased chance of falling. Exercises that improve balance and coordination (such as tai chi) are the most helpful.
- Make your home safer:
  - Remove any items in your pathway, including from stairs, to avoid tripping.
  - Remove small throw rugs or use double-sided tape to keep rugs from slipping.
  - Place frequently used items within easy reach to avoid use of a step stool.
  - Install grab bars next to your toilet and in the tub or shower.
  - Use nonslip mats in the bathtub and on shower floors.
  - Improve lighting, using lamp shades or frosted bulbs to reduce glare.
  - Install handrails and lights in all staircases.
  - Wear shoes that give good support and have thin, nonslip soles. Avoid wearing slippers and athletic shoes with deep treads.
- Ask your health care provider to review your medications, including prescriptions and over-the-counter medications. Some medications or a combination of medications may cause dizziness or drowsiness, leading to falls.
- Have your vision checked by an eye doctor. Your glasses may no longer have the correct prescription, or you may have developed an eye condition such as cataracts or glaucoma that limits your vision.

Note. Adapted from *Preventing Falls Among Seniors* by Centers for Disease Control & Prevention, National Center for Injury Prevention & Control, 2002. Available www.cdc.gov/ncipc/duip/spotlite/falltips.htm

Older clients are at higher risk for musculoskeletal trauma due to falls. For these clients, home assessments must be performed and potential hazards removed. Specific teaching topics for preventing falls in older adults are outlined in the box above.

## Assessment

Collect the following data through the health history and physical examination (see Chapter 37).

- Health history: age, history of traumatic event, history of chronic illnesses, history of prior musculoskeletal injuries, medications (ask the older adult specifically about anticoagulants)
- Physical assessment: pain with movement, pulses, edema, skin color and temperature, deformity, range of motion, touch (These assessments include the five Ps of neurovascular assessment, as follows, included in both the initial assessment and ongoing focused assessments.)
  - *Pain.* Assess pain in the injured extremity by asking the client to grade it on a scale of 0 to 10, with 10 as the most severe pain.

- *Pulses.* Assess distal pulses beginning with the unaffected extremity. Compare the quality of pulses in the affected extremity to those of the unaffected extremity.
- *Pallor.* Observe for pallor and skin color in the injured extremity. Paleness and coolness may indicate arterial compromise, whereas warmth and a bluish tinge may indicate venous blood pooling.
- *Paralysis/Paresis.* Assess ability to move body parts distal to the fracture site. Inability to move indicates paralysis. Loss of muscle strength (weakness) when moving is paresis. A finding of limited range of motion may lead to early recognition of problems such as nerve damage and paralysis.
- *Paresthesia.* Ask the client if any change in sensation (paresthesia) has occurred.

## Nursing Diagnoses and Interventions

Nursing care for clients with fractures ranges from teaching for home care treatments provided in the emergency or urgent care department (such as manual reduction and cast application) to providing interventions to maintain health and decrease the risk of complications in clients with complex or multiple fractures. Teaching is also necessary for caregivers of the older adult who is discharged home or to a long-term care or rehabilitation facility following a fractured hip.

### Acute Pain

Pain is caused by soft tissue damage and is compounded by muscle spasms and swelling.

- Monitor vital signs. *Some analgesics decrease respiratory effort and blood pressure.*
- Ask the client to rate the pain on a scale of 0 to 10 (with 10 as the most severe pain) before and after any intervention. *This facilitates objective assessment of the effectiveness of the chosen pain relief strategy. Pain that increases in intensity or remains unrelieved with analgesics can indicate compartment syndrome.*
- For the client with a hip fracture, apply Buck's traction per physician's orders. *Buck's traction immobilizes the fracture and decreases pain and additional trauma.*
- Move the client gently and slowly. *Gentle moving helps to prevent the development of severe muscle spasms.*

**PRACTICE ALERT** *Supporting the extremity above and below the fracture (in the case of fracture in an extremity) can also decrease pain and muscle spasms.* ■

- Elevate the injured extremity above the level of the heart. *Elevating the extremity promotes venous return and decreases edema, which decreases pain.*
- Encourage distraction or other noninvasive methods of pain relief, such as deep breathing and relaxation. *Distraction, deep breathing, and relaxation help decrease the focus on the pain and may lessen the intensity of pain.*
- Administer pain medications as prescribed. For home care, explain the importance of taking pain medications before the pain is severe. *Analgesics alleviate pain by stimulating opiate receptor sites.*

## Risk for Peripheral Neurovascular Dysfunction

In the client with a fracture, compartment syndrome or deep vein thrombosis can impair circulation and, in turn, tissue perfusion.

- Assess the five Ps every 1 to 2 hours. Report abnormal findings immediately. *Unrelenting pain, pallor, diminished distal pulses, paresthesias, and paresis are strong indicators of compartment syndrome.*

> **PRACTICE ALERT**  *Pulses may remain strong, even in the presence of compartment syndrome.* ■

- Assess nailbeds for capillary refill. *Delayed capillary refill may indicate decreased tissue perfusion.*

> **PRACTICE ALERT**  *It may not be possible to accurately assess capillary refill in older adults who often have thickened, discolored nails. If so, test nearby skin.* ■

- Monitor the extremity for edema and swelling. *Excessive swelling and hematoma formation can compromise circulation.*
- Assess for deep, throbbing, unrelenting pain. *Pain that is not relieved by analgesics may indicate neurovascular compromise.*
- Assess the tightness of the cast. *Edema can cause the cast to become tight; a tight-fitting cast may lead to compartment syndrome or paralysis.*
- If cast is tight, be prepared to assist the physician with **bivalving** (Figure 38–11 ■). *Bivalving, the process of splitting the cast down both sides, alleviates pressure on the injured extremity.*

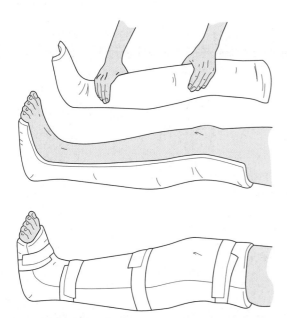

**Figure 38–11** ■ Bivalving is the process of splitting the cast down both sides to alleviate pressure on or allow visualization of the extremity.

- If compartment syndrome is suspected, assist the physician in measuring compartment pressure. Normal compartment pressure is 10 to 20 mmHg. *Compartment pressure greater than 30 mmHg indicates compartment syndrome.*
- Elevate the injured extremity above level of the heart. *Elevating the extremity increases venous return and decreases edema.*
- Administer anticoagulant per physician's order. *Prophylactic anticoagulation decreases the risk of clot formation.*

## Risk for Infection

The client who undergoes surgical repair will have a postoperative wound. Any break in skin integrity must be monitored for infection.

- Monitor vital signs and lab reports of WBCs. *Increases in pulse rate, respiratory rate, temperature, and WBCs may indicate infection.*
- Use sterile technique for dressing changes. *The initial postoperative dressing will be changed by the surgeon. The nurse must change all subsequent dressings without introducing organisms into the operative site.*
- Assess the wound for size, color, and the presence of any drainage. *Redness, swelling, and purulent drainage indicate infection.*
- Administer antibiotics per physician's orders. *Short-term prophylactic antibiotic administration inhibits bacterial reproduction and thereby helps prevent skin flora from entering the wound. Antibiotics are usually only administered for 24 hours.*

## Impaired Physical Mobility

The client who has experienced a fracture requires immobilization of the fractured bone(s). Immobilization alters normal gait and mobility. The client will need to use assistive devices such as crutches, canes, slings, or walkers.

- Teach or assist client with ROM exercises of the unaffected limbs. *ROM exercises help prevent muscle atrophy and maintain strength and joint function. Flexion and extension exercises prevent the development of foot drop, wrist drop, or frozen joints.*
- Teach isometric exercises, and encourage the client to perform them every 4 hours. *Isometric exercises help prevent muscle atrophy and force synovial fluid and nutrients into the cartilage.*
- Encourage ambulation when able; provide assistance as necessary. *Ambulation maintains and improves circulation, helps prevent muscle atrophy, and helps maintain bowel function*
- Teach and observe the client's use of assistive devices (such as canes, crutches, walkers, slings) in conjunction with the physical therapist. *Proper use of devices is necessary for safe ambulation and helps prevent the loss of joint function secondary to complications and falls.*
- Turn the client on bed rest every 2 hours. If the client is in traction, teach the client to shift his or her weight every hour. *Turning and shifting weight increase circulation and help prevent skin breakdown.*

## Risk for Disturbed Sensory Perception: Tactile

The client who has sustained a fracture is at risk for nerve injury from the initial trauma, as well as from complications such as compartment syndrome.

- Assess the ability to differentiate between sharp and dull touch and the presence of paresthesias and paralysis every 1 to 2 hours. *Paresthesias develop as a result of pressure on nerves and may indicate compartment syndrome.*

**PRACTICE ALERT**  *Paralysis is a late sign of nerve entrapment and requires that the physician be notified immediately.* ∎

- Elevate the injured extremity above the level of the heart. *Elevating the extremity decreases swelling and the risk of compartment syndrome and nerve entrapment.* Check the cast for fit. *A tightly fitting cast can decrease blood flow to distal tissues, compress nerves, and cause compartment syndrome.*
- Support the injured extremity above and below the fracture site when moving the client. *Supporting the injured extremity above and below the fracture site helps prevent displacement of bony fragments and decreases the risk of further nerve damage.*

## Using NANDA, NIC and NOC

Chart 38–1 shows links between NANDA nursing diagnosis, NIC, and NOC when caring for the client with a compound fracture.

## Home Care

Client and family teaching focuses on individualized needs. The type of fracture and its location determine how much teaching the client and family will require. For example, a client who has a simple nondisplaced tibial fracture may need to be taught only cast care and crutch walking. An older client who has sustained a hip fracture and requires surgical intervention, by contrast, has a wider array of teaching needs, including the use of an abduction pillow, proper bending, and proper sitting. Address the following topics for home care of the client who has fractured a hip.

- Encourage independence in ADLs (see the Nursing Research box on page 1211 for research in this area).
- Explain that the client should sit only on high chairs to prevent excess flexion of the hip; a high toilet seat can be added to a regular toilet seat.
- Encourage the client and family to equip the shower with a rail to aid stability and prevent falls.
- If a walker is needed, teach the client its proper use: Do not carry the walker, but lift it, advance it, and then take two steps, or use a rolling walker.
- If a cane is needed, instruct the client to use it on the affected side.
- Stress the importance of well-balanced meals, and explain all prescribed medications.

Clients who have experienced a fracture or who have had orthopedic surgery often require an extended period of immobilization or limited activities. Address the following topics for home care.

## CHART 38–1  NANDA, NIC, AND NOC LINKAGES

### The Client with a Compound Fracture

| NURSING DIAGNOSES | NURSING INTERVENTIONS | NURSING OUTCOMES |
|---|---|---|
| • Risk for Infection | • Infection Protection<br>• Wound Care | • Infection Status |
| • Acute Pain | • Analgesic Administration<br>• Heat/Cold Application<br>• Pain Management<br>• Simple Relaxation Therapy | • Comfort Level<br>• Symptom Severity |
| • Impaired Physical Mobility | • Exercise Promotion<br>• Self-Care Assistance<br>• Teaching: Prescribed Activity/Exercise<br>• Traction/Immobilization Care<br>• Cast Care: Wet<br>• Cast Care: Maintenance | • Mobility Level<br>• Self-Care: ADLs |
| • Risk for Peripheral Neurovascular Dysfunction | • Peripheral Sensation Management<br>• Circulatory Precautions<br>• Cast Care<br>• Embolus Precautions | • Circulation Status<br>• Neurologic Status<br>• Tissue Perfusion: Peripheral |

*Note.* Data from Nursing Outcomes Classification (NOC) *by M. Johnson & M. Maas (Eds.), 1997, St. Louis: Mosby;* Nursing Diagnoses: Definitions & Classification 2001–2002 *by North American Nursing Diagnosis Association, 2001, Philadelphia: NANDA;* Nursing Interventions Classification (NIC) *by J.C. McCloskey & G. M. Bulechek (Eds.), 2000, St. Louis: Mosby. Reprinted by permission.*

## Nursing Research

### Evidence-Based Practice for Care of the Older Adult with a Hip Fracture

Fracture of the hip often results in loss of independence and long-term disability. Postoperatively, helping the client regain independence in performing activities of daily living (ADLs) is a nursing care priority that often is inhibited by diminished cognitive status of the client. This study (Milisen, Abraham, & Broos, 1998) looked at the incidence of impaired cognition, its evolution, and its effects on functional status in 26 elderly clients with hip fracture. Nineteen of the 26 clients demonstrated some degree of cognitive impairment before and/or after surgery. The highest incidence of impaired cognition was seen during the postoperative period, with memory and psychomotor skills affected to the greatest degree. Additionally, clients with decreased cognition postoperatively remained more ADL-dependent than nonimpaired clients.

#### IMPLICATIONS FOR NURSING

Teaching and promoting independence in ADLs are important nursing care priorities for the client who experiences a fractured hip. However, the client who is cognitively impaired does not learn as effectively and is less able to regain the ability to independently perform ADLs following hip fracture. This study points out the importance of assessing the cognitive status of clients before and after surgery and using this information in planning nursing care activities. Nurses and other health care providers need to promote recovery in long-term care facilities as well as more effectively meet clients' needs in the home and community. In all settings, nurses must collaborate with other nurses and with other members of the health care team to facilitate continuity of care, teaching, and rehabilitation. Teaching for clients with memory impairment needs to be very focused, presented in brief sessions, and repeatedly reinforced. Despite all best efforts, it may be unrealistic to expect some clients to resume independent function in performing ADLs, at least during the initial postoperative period.

#### Critical Thinking in Client Care

1. Many people believe that a broken hip signals the onset of an older adult's decline until death. How can nurses change this perception?
2. If your client is an older adult who lives alone and has no available caregivers, what community resources can you recommend to provide care until independence is regained?
3. What factors do you think contribute to impaired cognition in the older adult who experiences a hip fracture and surgical stabilization or replacement?
4. You are caring for an 84-year-old woman with a fractured hip who is being discharged to a long-term care facility. She begins to cry and says, "I know I will die there; please don't let them send me there." What would you say to her?

---

- Do not try to scratch under a cast with a sharp object.
- Do not get a plaster cast wet.
- Follow the physician's order for weight bearing.
- Physical therapy departments or offices often can evaluate the home environment for safety and suggest modifications as needed. Physical therapists also teach crutch walking, limited weight bearing, transferring, and other activities.
- Home care agencies can teach wound care and provide ongoing monitoring of wound healing.
- Local medical equipment and supply sources rent or sell durable equipment such as crutches, walkers, wheelchairs, overhead trapeze units, shower chairs, elevated toilet seats, grab bars, and bedside commodes. Slings or braces may be purchased through medical equipment dealers.
- Local pharmacies are good resources for dressing supplies such as antiseptic solutions or ointments, dressings, and tape.
- Fitness equipment suppliers may be useful for rehabilitation needs such as hand or ankle weights for strengthening exercises.

## THE CLIENT WITH AN AMPUTATION

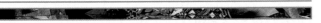

An **amputation** is the partial or total removal of a body part. Amputation may be the result of an acute process, such as a traumatic event, or a chronic condition, such as peripheral vascular disease or diabetes mellitus. Regardless of the cause, an amputation is devastating to the client. It is estimated that 350,000 people with amputations live in the United States, and that 135, 000 new amputations occur each year. In the United States, the most common causes of lower extremity amputations are disease (70%), trauma (22%), congenital or birth defects (4%), and tumors (4%). Upper extremity amputation is usually due to trauma or birth defect (Moss Rehab Resource Net, 2002).

The loss of all or part of an extremity has a significant physical and psychosocial effect on the client and family. Adaptation may take a long time and require much effort. A multidisciplinary health care team is necessary to meet the client's physical, spiritual, cultural, and emotional needs.

### CAUSES OF AMPUTATION

Peripheral vascular disease (PVD) is the major cause of amputation of the lower extremities (see Chapter 33). Common risk factors for the development of PVD include hypertension, diabetes, smoking, and hyperlipidemia. Peripheral neuropathy also places the person with diabetes at risk for amputation. In peripheral neuropathy, loss of sensation frequently leads to unrecognized injury and infection. Untreated infection may lead to gangrene and the need for amputation. These risks are fully discussed in Chapter 18.

Trauma is the major cause of amputation of the upper extremities. Upper extremity amputations represent a more

## Nursing Care Plan
## A Client with a Hip Fracture

Stella Carbolito is a 74-year-old Italian American with a history of osteoporosis. She is a widow and lives alone in a two-story row home. Mrs. Carbolito is retired and depends on a pension check and social security for her income. She takes pride in making all her own food from scratch.

While walking to the market one day, Mrs. Carbolito falls and fractures her left hip. She is transported by ambulance to the nearest hospital emergency department.

### ASSESSMENT

During the initial assessment at the ED, abnormal findings are that Mrs. Carbolito's left leg is shorter than her right leg and is externally rotated. Distal pulses are present and bilaterally strong; both legs are warm. Mrs. Carbolito complains of severe pain but states that no numbness or burning is present. She is able to wiggle the toes on her left leg and has full movement of her right leg. Initial vital signs are as follows: T 98.0°F (36.6°C), P 100, R 18, BP 120/58. Diagnostic tests include CBC, blood chemistry, and X-ray studies of the left hip and pelvis. The CBC reveals a hemoglobin of 11.0 g/dL and a normal WBC count. Blood chemistry findings are within normal limits. The X-ray reveals a fracture of the left femoral neck. Mrs. Carbolito is admitted to the hospital with an order for 10 lb of straight leg traction. An open reduction and internal fixation (ORIF) is planned for the following day.

### DIAGNOSIS

- *Acute pain* related to fractured left femoral neck and muscle spasms
- *Impaired physical mobility* related to bed rest and fractured left femoral neck
- *Risk for ineffective tissue perfusion* related to unstable bones and swelling
- *Risk for disturbed sensory perception: Tactile* related to the risk of nerve impairment

### EXPECTED OUTCOMES

- Verbalize a decrease in pain.
- Verbalize the purpose of traction and surgery
- Maintain normal neurovascular assessments.
- Demonstrate postoperative exercises.

### PLANNING AND IMPLEMENTATION

- Assess pain on a scale of 0 to 10 before and after implementing measures to reduce pain.
- Administer narcotics per the physician's order.
- Perform neurovascular assessment every 2 to 4 hours, and document findings.
- Apply straight leg traction per physician's order.
- Encourage deep breathing and relaxation techniques.
- Teach the purpose of traction and surgery.
- Teach the purpose of and the procedure for performing isometric and flexion/extension exercises.

### EVALUATION

Three days after surgery, Mrs. Carbolito is out of bed and in a chair. She verbalizes a decrease in pain. There have been no abnormal neurovascular assessments. She is able to independently perform isometric and flexion/extension exercises in both lower extremities. Discharge planning included referrals for home care. A home health nurse will visit, and the social worker at the hospital has ordered a trapeze for her bed, an elevated toilet seat, an elevated cushion for her chair, and a walker.

### Critical Thinking in the Nursing Process

1. What factors placed Mrs. Carbolito at risk for a hip fracture?
2. Mrs. Carbolito says, "I don't understand why they had to put that heavy thing on my leg before I went to surgery to get my hip fixed." What would you tell her? What preoperative factors might have decreased teaching effectiveness?
3. Describe how each of the following, if manifested by Mrs. Carbolito, would increase her risk for postoperative complications: urinary incontinence, weight more than 20% under normal for her height, chronic constipation. What nursing diagnoses and interventions would you include in her plan of care to decrease the risk?

See Evaluating Your Response in Appendix C.

---

serious threat to independence, because these limbs perform more specialized functions. The incidence of traumatic amputations is highest among young men. Most amputations in this group result from motor vehicle crashes or accidents involving machinery at work. The client may present to the trauma center with an injury that may be life threatening; significant loss of blood and tissue may have already occurred, and shock may develop. (See Chapter 6 ⊖⊃ for a discussion of shock and trauma.) Other traumatic events that may necessitate an amputation are frostbite, burns, or electrocution.

Amputations result from or are necessitated by interruption in blood flow, either acute or chronic. In acute trauma situations, the limb is partially or completely severed, and tissue death ensues. Replantation of fingers, small body parts, and entire limbs has been successful.

In the chronic disease processes, circulation is impaired, venous pooling begins, proteins leak into the interstitium, and edema develops. Edema increases the risk of injury and further decreases circulation. Stasis ulcers develop and readily become infected because impaired healing and altered immune processes allow bacteria to proliferate. The presence of progressive infection further compromises circulation and ultimately leads to gangrene (tissue death), which requires amputation.

## LEVELS OF AMPUTATION

The level of amputation is determined by local and systemic factors. Local factors include ischemia and gangrene; system factors include cardiovascular status, renal function, and sever-

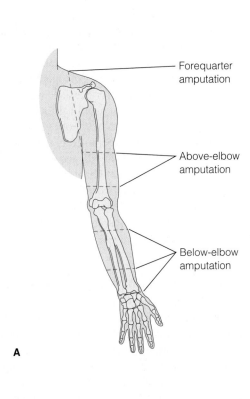

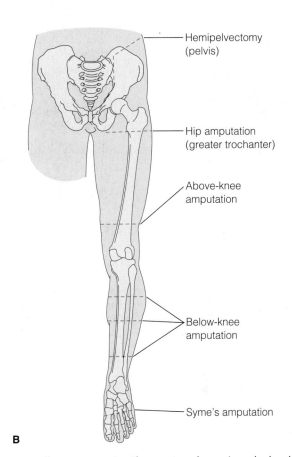

**Figure 38–12** ■ Common sites of amputation. *A,* The upper extremities. *B,* The lower extremities. The surgeon determines the level of amputation based on blood supply and tissue condition.

ity of diabetes mellitus. The goals are to alleviate symptoms, to maintain healthy tissue, and to increase functional outcome. When possible, the joints are preserved because they allow greater function of the extremity. Figure 38–12 ■ illustrates common sites of amputation.

## TYPES OF AMPUTATION

Amputations may be open (*guillotine*) or closed (*flap*). Open amputations are performed when infection is present. The wound is not closed but remains open to drain. When infection is no longer present, surgery is performed to close the wound. In closed amputations, the wound is closed with a flap of skin that is sutured in place over the stump. Terms used to refer to amputations are presented in Table 38–3.

## AMPUTATION SITE HEALING

For the prosthesis to fit well, the amputation site must heal properly. To promote healing, a rigid or compression dressing is applied to prevent infection and minimize edema. A rigid dressing is made by placing a cast on the stump and molding the stump to fit a prosthesis. A soft compression dressing is applied when frequent wound checks are necessary. When this type of dressing is used, a splint is sometimes applied to help mold the extremity to fit the prosthesis. After the wound is dressed, the client is encouraged to toughen the stump skin by

| TABLE 38–3 | Amputation Terms |
| --- | --- |
| **Term** | **Meaning** |
| Arm | Amputation of a portion of the arm, either above or below the elbow |
| Disarticulation | Amputation through a joint |
| Forequarter | Removal of the entire arm and disarticulation of the shoulder |
| Closed (flap) | Amputation in which a flap of skin is formed to cover the end of the wound |
| Open (guillotine) | Perpendicular cutting of the extremity in which the wound is left open; used when infection is present |
| Leg | Amputation below the knee (BK) |
| Thigh | Amputation above the knee (AK) |
| Finger or Toe | Amputation of one or all of the fingers or toes |
| Syme | Modified disarticulation of the ankle |
| Foot | Amputation of part of the foot and toes |

pushing it into first soft and then harder surfaces. The stump is wrapped in an Ace bandage to allow a conical shape to form and prevent edema. The bandage is applied from the distal to the proximal extremity (Figure 38–13 ■).

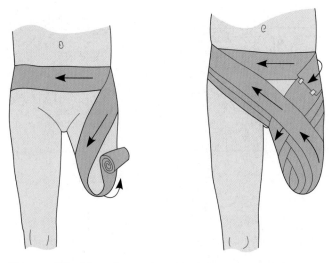

**Figure 38–13** ■ Stump dressings increase venous return, decrease edema, and help shape the stump for a prosthesis. With an above-knee amputation, a figure-eight bandage is started by bringing the bandage down over the stump and back up around the hips.

## COMPLICATIONS

Complications that may occur after an amputation include infection, delayed healing, chronic stump pain and phantom pain, and contracture.

### Infection

Generally, the client who suffers a traumatic amputation has a greater risk of infection than the person who has a planned amputation. However, even planned amputations carry a risk of infection. The client who is older, has diabetes mellitus, or suffers peripheral neurovascular compromise is at a particularly high risk for infection. Infection may present itself locally or systemically. Local manifestations of infection include drainage, odor, redness, positive wound cultures, and increased discomfort at the suture line. Systemic manifestations include fever, an increased heart rate, a decrease in blood pressure, chills, and positive wound or blood cultures.

### Delayed Healing

If infection is present or if the circulation remains compromised, delayed healing will result. Delayed healing occurs at a slower rate than expected. In older clients, other preexisting conditions can increase the risk of delayed healing. In clients of any age, electrolyte imbalances can contribute to delayed healing, as can a diet that lacks the proper nutrients to meet the body's increased metabolic demands. Smoking also compromises healing by causing vasoconstriction and decreasing blood flow to the stump. Deep vein thrombosis and compromised venous return, which may result from prolonged immobilization, are other potential factors. Decreased cardiac output decreases blood flow and thus also delays healing.

### Chronic Stump Pain and Phantom Pain

**Chronic stump pain** is the result of neuroma formation, causing severe burning pain. Interventions to relieve this pain include medications, nerve blocks, transcutaneous electrical nerve stimulation (TENS), and surgical stump reconstruction. **Phantom limb pain** is not the same as phantom limb sensation. A majority of amputees experience phantom limb sensation (sensations such as tingling, numbness, cramping or itching in the phantom foot or hand) early in the postoperative period. It is often self-limited, but may last for decades in some clients. When phantom limb sensation is painful, it is referred to as phantom limb pain. Although various theories have been proposed, the exact cause of this experience is unknown. Treatments include pain management, TENS, and a variety of surgical procedures. The management of phantom limb pain is often difficult for both clients and health care professionals. Clients with phantom limb pain often benefit from referral to a pain clinic for a comprehensive pain management program (Maher, Salmond, & Pellino, 2002).

### Contractures

A **contracture** is an abnormal flexion and fixation of a joint caused by muscle atrophy and shortening. Contracture of the joint above the amputation is a common complication. The client needs to be taught to extend the joint. The client with an above-the-knee amputation should lie prone for periods throughout the day. The client with a below-the-knee amputation should elevate the stump, keeping the knee extended. The same principles apply to the upper extremity. All joints should receive either active or passive ROM exercises every 2 to 4 hours. A trapeze frame should be added to the bed to encourage the client to change position every 2 hours. The client who has an upper extremity amputation should exercise both shoulders. Postural exercises can help prevent the client from hunching over secondary to the loss of weight on the affected side. The client with an above-the-knee amputation should not sit for prolonged periods of time; prolonged sitting can lead to hip contracture.

## COLLABORATIVE CARE

Multidisciplinary care is necessary for the client who has sustained an amputation. Physical therapy and occupational retraining are necessary, and the client may also benefit from the presence of clergy. The entire health care team must view both the positive and the negative effects of amputation; that is, they must see amputation as a means to increase the client's independence and to relieve symptoms. The client should be able to become familiar with the members of the health care team and their roles; this allows the client greater control over his or her care and rehabilitation and promotes independence.

### Diagnostic Tests

Preoperatively, the client has routine laboratory and diagnostic tests (see Chapter 7). Preoperative tests are performed to assess the circulation present in the limb at different levels and determine the level of viable tissue. Preoperative tests include:

- *Doppler flowmetry* to evaluate blood flow in the extremity.
- *Segmental blood pressure determinations* to evaluate the blood flow and vessel pressures in the extremity.

- *Transcutaneous partial pressure oxygen readings* to measure the oxygen delivery by blood vessels in the affected extremity.
- If revascularization with a bypass is planned in conjunction with the amputation, *angiography* is also performed.

Postoperative diagnostic tests include the following:

- *CBC* to determine hemoglobin and hematocrit levels. A sudden drop in these values may indicate hemorrhage. The WBC count is also monitored with a CBC; a sudden increase in the WBC may indicate the presence of infection.
- *Blood chemistries* measure electrolytes and reflect fluid balance.
- *Vascular Doppler ultrasonography* may be performed if a client is suspected of having a DVT.

## Medications

The client receives medications preoperatively, intraoperatively, and postoperatively. Preoperatively, the physician may prescribe intravenous antibiotics. Intraoperatively, anesthetic agents are administered. It also may be necessary to administer agents to control blood pressure during the surgery. Postoperatively, the client resumes any routinely prescribed medications and in addition may receive antibiotics and analgesics. Steroids may be administered to decrease swelling. A histamine $H_2$ antagonist may also be ordered to decrease the risk of peptic ulcer formation. Stool softeners may be administered to prevent constipation.

## Prosthesis

The type of prosthesis selected for the client with an amputation depends on the level of the amputation as well as the client's occupation and lifestyle. Each prosthesis is based on a detailed prosthetic prescription and is custom made for the client based on the specific characteristics of the stump. Most are made of plastic and foam materials. Many factors influence the client's use of the prosthesis, including the status of the remaining limb, cognitive status, cardiovascular status, preoperative activity level, and motivation to use the prosthesis (Maher, Salmond, & Pellino, 2002).

Clients with a lower extremity amputation are often fitted with early walking aids. These are pneumatic devices that fit over the stump and are used in the immediate postoperative period to allow early ambulation, decreased postoperative swelling, and improved morale. Clients may begin weight bearing as soon as 2 weeks after surgery. Clients with upper extremity amputations may be fitted for a prosthesis immediately after surgery. Rehabilitation of the client with an amputation is a team effort, involving the client, nurse, physician, physical therapist, occupational therapist, social worker, prosthetist, and vocational counselor.

## NURSING CARE

## Health Promotion

The goals of health promotion activities focus on preventing the progression of chronic diseases such as peripheral vascular disease and diabetes mellitus, and on safety. Clients with peripheral vascular disease from any cause need education about foot care and early recognition of decreased circulation. Education within both urban and rural populations should provide knowledge about working safely with farm and occupational machinery.

In addition, it is important that the public know what to do if a traumatic amputation occurs in the home, community, or workplace. The following guidelines may help preserve the amputated part until it can be surgically reattached:

- Keep the person in a prone position with the legs elevated.
- Apply firm pressure to the bleeding area, using a towel or article of clothing.
- Wrap the amputated part in a clean cloth. If possible, soak the cloth in saline (such as contact lens solution).
- Put the amputated part in a plastic bag and put the bag on ice. Do not let the amputated part come into direct contact with the ice or water.
- Send the amputated part to the emergency department with the injured person, and be sure the emergency personnel know what it is.

## Assessment

Collect the following data through the health history and physical examination. Further focused assessments are described in the nursing interventions below.

- Health history: mechanism of injury, current and past health problems, pain, occupation, activities of daily living, changes in sensation in the feet, cultural and/or religious guidelines for handling the amputated part
- Physical examination: bilateral neurovascular status of the extremities, bilateral capillary refill time, skin over the lower extremities (discoloration, edema, ulcerations, hair, gangrene)

## Nursing Diagnoses and Interventions

The goals of nursing care for a person with an amputation are to relieve pain, promote healing, prevent complications, support the client and family during the process of grieving and adaptation to alterations in body image, and restore mobility. Care is individualized, and the circumstances that led to the amputation (e.g., traumatic injury or disease) also must be addressed. Applying rehabilitation principles to nursing care is also important.

### Acute Pain

Pain from the surgical procedure can be compounded by muscle spasms, swelling, and phantom limb pain.

- Ask the client to rate the pain on a scale of 0 to 10 before and after any intervention. *This facilitates objective assessment of the effectiveness of the chosen pain relief strategy. Pain that increases in intensity or remains unrelieved with analgesics can indicate compartment syndrome.*
- Splint and support the injured area. *Splinting prevents additional injury by immobilizing the stump and decreasing edema while molding the stump for a good prosthetic fit.*
- Unless contraindicated, elevate the stump on a pillow for the first 24 hours after surgery. *Elevating the stump promotes venous return and decreases edema, which will decrease pain.*

MediaLink | AMPUTATION CARE PLAN

**PRACTICE ALERT** *Elevating the stump for long periods after the immediate postoperative period increases the risk for hip contractures.* ■

- Move and turn the client gently and slowly. *Gentle moving and turning prevents the development of severe muscle spasms.*
- Administer pain medications as prescribed. A PCA pump may be ordered by the physician. *Analgesics alleviate pain by stimulating opiate receptor sites. PCA pumps increase client control over and allow early relief of pain before it intensifies.*
- Encourage deep breathing and relaxation exercises. *These techniques increase the effectiveness of analgesics and modify the pain experience.*
- Reposition client every 2 hours; turning from side to side and onto abdomen. *Repositioning alleviates pressure from one area and distributes it throughout the body and helps prevent cramping of muscles.*

**PRACTICE ALERT** *Lying prone prevents hip contracture.* ■

## Risk for Infection
The client who has an amputation is at risk for wound infection. Early recognition of infection can lead to early treatment and prevent wound dehiscence.

- Assess the wound for redness, drainage, temperature, edema, and suture line approximation. *Redness is normal in the immediate postoperative period; if it persists, however, it can indicate infection. A hot area over the incision or increased drainage may also indicate infection.*
- Take the client's temperature at least once every 4 hours. *Increased body temperature may indicate infection.*
- Monitor white blood cell count. *The white blood cell count rises in the presence of infection.*
- Use aseptic technique to change the wound dressing. *Aseptic technique prevents the contamination of the wound with bacteria.*
- Administer antibiotics as ordered. *Antibiotics inhibit bacterial cell replication and help prevent or eradicate infection.*
- Teach the client stump-wrapping techniques. *Correctly wrapping the stump from the distal to proximal extremity increases venous return and prevents pooling of fluid, thereby reducing the chance of infection.*

## Risk for Impaired Skin Integrity
Stump care is essential, not only in the postoperative healing period, but also throughout life with a prosthesis. A variety of skin problems may be caused by a prosthesis, including epidermoid cysts, abrasions, blisters, and hair follicle infections. The client must be taught stump care prior to discharge.

- Each day, preferably at night, wash the stump with soap and warm water and dry thoroughly. Inspect the stump for redness, irritation, or abrasions. *It is essential to maintain intact skin to ensure successful use of the prosthesis.*

- Massage the end of the stump, beginning 3 weeks after surgery. *Massage helps desensitize the remaining part of the limb and prevents scar tissue formation. If the skin adheres to the underlying tissue, it will tear when stressed by wearing a prosthesis.*
- Expose any open areas of skin on the remaining part of the limb for 1 hour four times a day. *Air exposure promotes healing.*
- Change stump socks and elastic wraps each day. Wash these in mild soap and water, and allow to completely dry before using again. *Stump socks and elastic wraps must be kept clean and dry to prevent skin breakdown.*

## Risk for Dysfunctional Grieving
The client who has lost an extremity is at risk for dysfunctional grieving. Denial of the need for surgery and the inability to discuss feelings compound this risk.

- Encourage verbalization of feelings, using open-ended questions. *Asking open-ended questions allows the client to discuss feelings and communicates the listener's willingness to listen.*
- Actively listen and maintain eye contact. *Active listening and eye contact communicate respect for what the client is expressing.*
- Reflect on the client's feelings. *Reflection statements such as, "You seem angry," allow the client to recognize feelings and perhaps develop a plan for resolution.*
- Allow the client to have unlimited visiting hours, if possible. *Unlimited visiting hours allows increased social support.*
- If desired by the client, provide spiritual support by activities such as visits from a spiritual leader, prayer, and meditation. *These activities often provide support during the grieving process.*

## Disturbed Body Image
Although amputation is a reconstructive surgery, the client's body image will be disturbed. Risk for body image disturbance is higher in young trauma clients, in whom body image is a particularly important component of self-image.

- Encourage verbalization of feelings. *This allows the client to communicate concerns and fears and lets the client know the nurse is willing to listen.*
- Allow the client to wear clothing from home. *Familiar clothing provides emotional comfort and helps the client retain a sense of his or her own identity.*
- Encourage the client to look at the stump. *Looking at and touching the stump helps the client face his or her fear of the unknown and move from denial to acceptance.*
- Encourage the client to care for the stump. *Active participation in care increases self-esteem and independence.*
- Offer to have a fellow amputee visit the client. *A support person who has experienced the same change gives the client the hope that he or she can regain independence.*
- Encourage active participation in rehabilitation. *Active participation in rehabilitation increases independence and mobility.*

## Impaired Physical Mobility

If time allows, the client should begin strengthening muscles preoperatively. If the amputation is the result of an emergency, exercises begin within 24 to 48 hours of surgery. The return of independent mobility boosts self-esteem and promotes adaptation to amputation.

- Perform ROM exercises on all joints. *ROM exercises help prevent the development of joint contractures that limit mobility.*
- Maintain postoperative stump shrinkage devices. These may be elastic bandages, shrinker socks, elastic stockinette, or a rigid plaster cast. *Postoperative dressings decrease edema and shape the stump for prosthetic wear.*
- Turn and reposition the client every 2 hours. *The client with a lower extremity amputation should lie prone every 4 hours. Repositioning increases blood flow to muscles, forces synovial fluid into joints, and helps prevent contractures.*
- Reinforce teaching by the physical therapist in crutch walking or the use of assistive devices. *These devices increase mobility by balancing the client and facilitating ambulation.*
- Encourage active participation in physical therapy. *Physical therapy will fatigue the client in the early stage of healing. Encouragement may increase the client's participation in the physical therapy regimen and thereby increase activity tolerance.*

## Using NANDA, NIC and NOC

Chart 38–2 shows links between NANDA nursing diagnoses, NIC, and NOC when caring for the client with an amputation.

## Home Care

Client and family teaching focuses on stump care, prosthesis fitting and care, medications, assistive devices, exercises, rehabilitation, counseling, support services, and follow-up appointments. The depth of teaching depends on the cause and site of the amputation and the needs of the client. See the Meeting Individualized Needs box on page 1218.

Holistic nursing care is especially important for the older client with an amputation. The normal aging process decreases renal and liver function; hence, medications have longer half-lives. Altered circulation prolongs wound healing, and slowing of reflexes and alterations in gait may disrupt balance. A walker may be more appropriate than crutches, because older clients have less strength in the upper extremities. Safety issues, such as decreasing the risk for recurrent falls, must be addressed. The nurse should also assess the client's need for in-home assistance and make appropriate referrals to visiting nurses and home health aides.

In addition, suggest the following resources:

- The Amputee Coalition of America
- Amputee Resource Foundation of America

---

## CHART 38–2  NANDA, NIC, AND NOC LINKAGES

### The Client with an Amputation

| NURSING DIAGNOSES | NURSING INTERVENTIONS | NURSING OUTCOMES |
|---|---|---|
| • Risk for Infection | • Infection Protection<br>• Wound Care<br>• Vital Signs Monitoring | • Infection Status |
| • Impaired Skin Integrity | • Incision Site Care<br>• Amputation Care<br>• Exercise Promotion<br>• Prosthesis Care<br>• Skin Surveillance<br>• Wound Care | • Wound Healing: Primary Intention<br>• Wound Healing: Secondary Intention<br>• Tissue Integrity: Skin<br>• Immobility Consequences: Physiological |
| • Chronic Pain | • Pain Management<br>• Medication Management<br>• Progressive Muscle Relaxation<br>• Simple Relaxation Therapy | • Comfort Level<br>• Pain Control Behavior<br>• Symptom Severity<br>• Well-Being |
| • Disturbed Body Image | • Body Image Enhancement<br>• Amputation Care<br>• Wound Care<br>• Coping Enhancement<br>• Grief Work Facilitation | • Body Image<br>• Grief Resolution |

*Note. Data from Nursing Outcomes Classification (NOC) by M. Johnson & M. Maas (Eds.), 1997, St. Louis: Mosby; Nursing Diagnoses: Definitions & Classification 2001–2002 by North American Nursing Diagnosis Association, 2001, Philadelphia: NANDA; Nursing Interventions Classification (NIC) by J.C. McCloskey & G. M. Bulechek (Eds.), 2000, St. Louis: Mosby. Reprinted by permission.*

## Meeting Individualized Needs

### THE CLIENT WITH AN AMPUTATION

Amputation of a limb has significant long-term consequences for the client. The client will grieve the loss of a body part and must adjust to a new self-image. The client's ability to perform normal activities of daily living (ADLs) and to maintain his or her usual family and social roles may be significantly affected, at least initially. Depending on the client's occupation, job performance may be affected, necessitating a change of career.

The nurse may be responsible for involving multiple members of the health care team in the client's care and rehabilitation and coordinating their activities. Following an amputation, the client may need the services of any or all of the following:

- Social services to help with rehabilitative and financial arrangements
- Physical therapists to teach ambulation techniques, and to provide deep heat or massage
- Occupational therapists to assist the client in developing adaptive techniques to deal with the loss of a limb
- Prosthetists to develop a prosthesis for the missing limb that will meet the client's needs for ADLs and other activities
- Home health services for nursing care such as assessments and wound care
- Support group services to assist in adapting to the body image change and effects of amputation on ADLs

### Assessing for Home Care

Preparing the amputee for home care includes a careful assessment of the client, family and support services, and the home for possible barriers to the client's safety and independence.

Assess the client's acceptance of the amputation and knowledge base about care needs, any activity restrictions or special needs, and resources for home care. Discuss home management—who is responsible for household activities such as cleaning and cooking. Inquire about arrangements that have been made for home care activities and ADLs. Evaluate the client's use of prescription and nonprescription medications, paying particular attention to possible interactions and drugs that may affect the client's balance, mental alertness, or appetite. Ask about social habits, such as cigarette smoking, alcohol use, or other drug use, that may affect healing or the client's ability to provide self-care.

Assess the client's home environment for possible safety hazards or barriers to ambulation, such as:

- Scatter rugs
- Stairs between living areas of the house
- Presence of grab bars to facilitate toileting and bathing
- Access to clean water and other needs for wound care

### Teaching for Home Care

The new amputee needs a great deal of teaching to learn to adapt to loss of a limb, whether it is an upper or lower extremity that has been lost. Because the client must be ready to learn before teaching can be effective, use therapeutic communication techniques to encourage the client to verbalize feelings about the amputation and its effects. Use active listening and teach the client ways to reduce anxiety and deal with feelings of helplessness and loss. Encourage the client to participate in care of the stump to build self-esteem and reinforce teaching. Include the following in teaching for home care:

- Teach the client to wrap the stump appropriately in preparation for fitting the prosthesis.
- Discuss positioning of the stump. Contractures are a particular problem for clients with an above-knee amputation, and can interfere with ability to effectively use a prosthesis.
- Teach the client how to perform stump exercises to maintain joint mobility and muscle tone of the affected limb.
- Encourage the client to resume physical activities as soon as possible. This improves the client's health and well-being, as well as the client's self-esteem.
- Discuss household modifications to promote independence, such as grab bars in the bathroom, faucets with single-handle controls for water flow and temperature, and handheld shower heads and shower chairs for bathing.

---

## THE CLIENT WITH A REPETITIVE USE INJURY

Repeatedly twisting and turning the wrist, pronating and supinating the forearm, kneeling, or raising arms over the head can result in repetitive use injuries. Common repetitive use injuries include carpal tunnel syndrome, bursitis, and epicondylitis. Clients with repetitive use injuries pose a challenge to the health care team. Often these clients appear puzzled as they relate a history of manifestations that have worsened over time. They deny abrupt trauma and often worry about the ability to return to work. Repetitive use injuries are common. The number of worker's compensation claims for repetitive use injuries is steadily growing. The increase is believed to be a result of technology advances in the workplace.

## PATHOPHYSIOLOGY

### Carpal Tunnel Syndrome

The carpal tunnel is a canal through which flexor tendons and the median nerve pass from the wrist to the hand. The syndrome develops from narrowing of the tunnel and irritation of the median nerve. **Carpal tunnel syndrome** involves compression of the median nerve as a result of inflammation and swelling of the synovial lining of the tendon sheaths. The client complains of numbness and tingling of the thumb, index finger, and lateral ventral surface of the middle finger. The client may also complain of pain in this area that interferes with sleep and is alleviated by shaking or massaging the hand and fingers. The affected hand may become weak and the client may be unable to hold utensils or perform activities that require precision.

## Nursing Care Plan

## A Client with a Below-the-Knee Amputation

John Rocke is a 45-year-old divorcee with no children. He has a history of type one diabetes mellitus and poor control of blood glucose levels. Mr. Rocke is unemployed and currently receives unemployment compensation. He lives alone in a second-floor apartment. Mr. Rocke had developed gangrene in the toe and failed to seek prompt medical attention; as a result, a left below-the-knee amputation was necessary.

Mr. Rocke is in his second postoperative day and his vital signs are stable. The stump is splinted and has a soft dressing. The wound is approximating well without signs of infection. He has not performed ROM exercises or turning since his surgery, complaining of severe pain. When the nurse goes into the room, he yells, "Get out! I don't want anyone to see me like this." No one has visited him since his hospitalization. He is tolerating an 1800-kcal American Diabetes Association diet and is using a urinal independently. He has an order for meperidine (Demerol), 100 mg IM every 4 hours prn for pain, and cefazolin (Ancef), 1 g IV every 8 hours. He is on blood glucose coverage with regular insulin subcutaneously.

### ASSESSMENT

Jane Simmons, RN, has just come on duty. She notes that the client is upset and angry. Mr. Rocke will not let anyone enter the room to give him medication or assess his vital signs.

### DIAGNOSIS

- *Disturbed body image* related to amputation of a left lower leg
- *Dysfunctional grieving* related to anger and loss of left lower leg
- *Situational low self-esteem* related to appearance
- *Risk for injury from infection and contractures* related to refusal of care
- *Pain* related to surgery

### EXPECTED OUTCOMES

- Verbalize his feelings about the amputation.
- Allow the staff to monitor his vital signs and administer medications.

- Be allowed to control his pain with a PCA pump.
- Verbalize a decrease in pain.
- Verbalize the importance of turning.
- Turn every 2 hours.

### PLANNING AND IMPLEMENTATION

- Encourage verbalization of feelings.
- Actively listen to the client.
- Offer to arrange a visit with a fellow amputee.
- Ask the physician if the client can be placed on a PCA pump.
- Teach the client the importance of turning every 2 hours to prevent contractures.
- Encourage turning and lying prone.
- Teach the importance of antibiotics in preventing and treating infection.

### EVALUATION

One week after his surgery, Mr. Rocke is actively participating in his care. He has apologized for his behavior and has explained to Ms. Simmons that he was angry about the loss of his leg. He states, "I thought I knew what to expect, but I didn't."

### Critical Thinking in the Nursing Process

1. Once Mr. Rocke is ready to assist with his stump care, how would you proceed? Would you give him full responsibility for care and dressings, or would you gradually increase his participation? Why?
2. What factors in Mr. Rocke's home environment and medical history may make self-care more difficult? Do you expect Mr. Rocke to follow up on care after his discharge? Why or why not?
3. Mr. Rocke states, "Why should I exercise this leg—it was already cut off!" How would you respond? What is the purpose of exercising the stump?

See Evaluating Your Response in Appendix C.

---

Carpal tunnel syndrome is one of the three most common work-related injuries. The incidence is believed to be related directly to the number of people using computers. The incidence of carpal tunnel syndrome is higher in women, especially postmenopausal women.

## Bursitis

**Bursitis** is an inflammation of a bursa. A bursa is an enclosed sac found between muscles, tendons, and bony prominences. The bursae that commonly become inflamed are in the shoulder, hip, leg, and elbow. Constant friction between the bursa and the musculoskeletal tissue around it causes irritation, edema, and inflammation. Manifestations develop as the sac becomes engorged. The area around the sac is tender, and extension and flexion of the joint near the bursa produce pain. The inflamed bursa is hot, red, and edematous. The client guards the joint to decrease pain and may point to the area of the bursa when identifying joint tenderness.

## Epicondylitis

**Epicondylitis** is the inflammation of the tendon at its point of origin into the bone. Epicondylitis is also referred to as *tennis elbow* or *golfer's elbow*. The exact pathophysiology of epicondylitis is unknown. Current theories attribute inflammation of the tendon to microvascular trauma. Tears, bleeding, and edema are thought to cause avascularization and calcification of the tendon. Manifestations of epicondylitis include point tenderness, pain radiating down the dorsal surface of the forearm, and a history of repetitive use.

## COLLABORATIVE CARE

Medical management of repetitive use disorders focuses on relieving pain and increasing mobility. Once the diagnosis is made, treatment can range from conservative measures, such as rest and pharmacologic agents, to aggressive measures such as surgery.

## Diagnostic Tests

Carpal tunnel syndrome is diagnosed by the client's history and physical examination. History may reveal an occupation that involves areas such as computer work, jackhammer operation, mechanical work, or gymnastics. History of a radial bone fracture or rheumatoid arthritis also increases the risk of carpal tunnel syndrome. Tests specific for carpal tunnel include the Phalen test (see Chapter 37). ⊂⊃ Bursitis and epicondylitis are diagnosed by history and physical examination.

## Medications

The client with a repetitive use injury usually receives NSAIDs. Narcotics also may be administered for acute flare-ups and severe pain. For the client who has epicondylitis or carpal tunnel syndrome, corticosteroids may be injected into the joint.

## Treatments

### Conservative Management

The first steps in the care of all repetitive use injuries are to immobilize and rest the involved joint. The joint may be splinted, and ice may be applied in the first 24 to 48 hours to decrease pain and inflammation. Ice application may be followed by heat application every 4 hours.

### Surgery

Surgery is usually reserved for the client who does not obtain relief with conservative treatment. Surgery for carpal tunnel syndrome includes resection of the carpal ligament to enlarge the tunnel. In epicondylitis and bursitis, calcified deposits may be removed from the area surrounding the tendon or bursa.

## NURSING CARE

The nursing care of a client with a repetitive use injury focuses on relieving pain, teaching about the disease process and treatment, and improving physical mobility.

## Nursing Diagnoses and Interventions

### Acute Pain

Swelling and nerve inflammation lead to pain in the client with a repetitive use injury.

- Ask the client to rate the pain on a scale of 0 to 10 (with 10 being the most severe pain) before and after any intervention. *This facilitates objective assessment of the effectiveness of the chosen pain relief strategy.*
- Encourage the use of immobilizers. *Splinting maintains joint alignment and prevents pain due to movement of inflamed tissues.*
- Teach the client to apply ice and/or heat as prescribed. *Ice causes vasoconstriction and decreases the pooling of blood in the inflamed area. Ice may also numb the tender area. Heat decreases swelling by increasing venous return.*
- Encourage use of NSAIDs as prescribed. *NSAIDs decrease swelling by inhibiting prostaglandins.*
- Explain why treatment should not be abruptly discontinued. *Abrupt discontinuation of treatment may cause reinflammation of the injured area.*

### Impaired Physical Mobility

Joint pain and swelling can impair mobility.

- Suggest interventions to alleviate pain (such as using immobilizer and taking pain medications). *If the joint is pain free, the client will be more likely to take an active role in therapy.*
- Refer to a physical therapist for exercises. *The physical therapist can assist the client with exercise to prevent joint stiffness.*
- Suggest consultation with an occupational therapist. *Occupational therapy can help the client learn new ways to perform tasks to prevent recurring symptoms.*

## Home Care

Address the following topics for home care.

- Causes and treatments for repetitive use injury
- Rehabilitation to allow the client to return to a state of independence
- Ways to avoid unnecessary exposure to the activities that increase risk of redeveloping the injury. Suggest evaluation of the client's work environment by an environmental risk manager who can prescribe measures to reduce the risk of repetitive use injuries. Wrist supports or an ergonomic keyboard may be useful for the client who uses a computer extensively. Appropriate desk and chair height also are important in maintaining correct anatomical position while working.
- Information about sources for braces or other assistive devices.

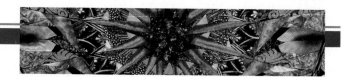

 EXPLORE MediaLink

## TEST YOURSELF

1. You are teaching a young adult how to provide self-care for a sprained ankle. You explain the reason for applying ice immediately after the injury is based on the principle that ice:

   a. Increases the diameter of blood vessels
   b. Decreases the diameter of blood vessels
   c. Is helpful in increasing white blood cells
   d. Lowers the blood pressure and pulse

2. A client with a compound, open fracture has been admitted to the emergency department and is scheduled for immediate surgery. Which of the following nursing diagnoses would be most appropriate in the immediate postoperative period?

   a. *Risk for posttrauma syndrome*
   b. *Impaired transfer ability*
   c. *Risk for infection*
   d. *Risk for falls*

3. While providing care to an older woman with a cast on her left lower arm (from below the elbow to above the fingers), you perform a neurovascular assessment. Which of the following assessments indicate a possible complication?

   a. Slightly edematous fingers

   b. Warm, pink skin above the cast
   c. Pale, cold fingers
   d. Pain rating of 2 on a 1 to 10 scale

4. At what position would you place the remaining extremity following a below-the-knee amputation during the first 24 hours after surgery?

   a. Elevated above the level of the heart
   b. Lower than the rest of the body
   c. Crossed over the intact extremity
   d. Level with the rest of the body

5. Your husband is cutting wood with a circular saw. He suddenly screams that he has cut off his finger. What would you do with the amputated finger?

   a. Don't worry about it; the important thing is to get him to the hospital
   b. Put it in a storage bag filled with warm water
   c. Tape it to his hand so the emergency personnel will know where it is
   d. Wrap it in a towel, put it in a plastic bag, and lay it on ice

See Test Yourself answers in Appendix C.

## BIBLIOGRAPHY

*Amputation.* (2001). Available www.hendrickhealth.org/healthy/0037150.html

*A parents guide to first aid. Amputation.* (2002). Available www.choa.org/first_aid/amputation.shtml.

Black, C. (1997). Wound management in patients with traumatic injuries. *Journal of Wound Care, 6*(5), 209–211.

Davis, P., & Barr, L. (1999). Principles of traction. *Journal of Orthopaedic Nursing, 3*(4), 222–227.

Electrical stimulation and bone healing. (2001). *Foot & Ankle Quarterly—The Seminar Journal, 14*(1), 1–37.

*Falls and hip fractures among older adults.* (2000). National Center for Injury Prevention & Control, CDC. Available www.cdc.gov/ncipc/factsheets/falls.htm

Hager, C. A., & Brncick, N. (1998). Fat embolism syndrome: A complication of orthopaedic trauma. *Orthopaedic Nursing, 17*(2), 41–43, 46, 58.

Hess, D. (1997). Employee perceived stress. Relationship to the development of repetitive strain injury symptoms. *AAOHN Journal, 45*(3), 115–123.

Johnson, M., & Maas, M. (Eds.). (1997). *Nursing outcomes classification (NOC).* St. Louis: Mosby.

Junge, T. (2000). Fat embolism: A complication of long bone fracture. *Surgical Technologist, 32*(11), 34–41.

Love, C. (2001). Using assisted walking devices. *Journal of Orthopaedic Nursing, 5*(1), 45–53.

Maher, A., Salmond, S., & Pellino, T. (2002). *Orthopedic nursing* (3rd ed.). Philadelphia: Saunders.

McCloskey, J. C., & Bulechek, G. M. (Eds.). (2000). *Nursing interventions classification (NIC)* (3rd ed.). St. Louis: Mosby.

Milisen, K., Abraham, I. L., & Broos, P. L. (1998). Postoperative variation in neurocognitive and functional status in elderly hip fracture patients. *Journal of Advanced Nursing, 27*(1), 59–67.

Mooney, N. (2001). Pain management in the orthopaedic patient. *Pain Management Nursing, 2*(1), 4–5.

Moss Rehab Resource Net. (2002). *Amputation fact sheet.* Available www.mossresourcenet.org/amputa.htm

North American Nursing Diagnosis Association. (2001). *NANDA nursing diagnoses: Definitions and classification, 2001–2002.* Philadelphia: Author.

National Center for Injury Prevention and Control. (2000). *Preventing falls among seniors.* Atlanta: Author.

O'Neill, M. (2001). Developing a clinically effective DVT prophylaxis protocol. *Journal of Orthopaedic Nursing, 5*(4), 186–191.

Pachucki-Hyde, L. (2001). Assessment of risk factors for osteoporosis and fracture. *Nursing Clinics of North America, 36*(3), 401–408.

Parsons, L., Krau, S., & Ward, K. (2001). Orthopedic trauma: Managing secondary medical problems. *Nursing Clinics of North America, 13*(3), 433–442.

Porth, C. M. (2002). *Pathophysiology: Concepts of altered health states* (6th ed.). Philadelphia: Lippincott.

Santy, J., & Mackintosh, C. (2001). A phenomenological study of pain following fractured shaft of femur. *Journal of Clinical Nursing, 10*(4), 521–527.

Scott, J. (1998). Mending broken bones. *Nursing Times, 94*(12), 28–30.

Shannon, M., Wilson, B., & Stang, C. (2002). *Health professionals drug guide 2002.* Upper Saddle River, NJ: Prentice Hall.

Sydell, W. (1999). Care of patients in casts. *Nursing Standard, 14*(8), 55.

Thompson, J., McFarland, G., Hirsch, J., & Tucker, S. (2002). *Mosby's clinical nursing* (5th ed.). St. Louis: Mosby.

Walls, M. (2002). Orthopedic trauma. *RN, 65*(7), 53–56.

Walsh, C. R., & McBryde, A. M., Jr. (1997). A joint protocol for home skeletal traction. *Orthopaedic Nursing, 16*(3), 28–33.

Weiss, S. A., & Lindell, B. (1996). Phantom limb pain and etiology of amputation in unilateral lower extremity amputees. *Journal of Pain and Symptom Management, 11*(1), 3–17.

Williams, M. A., Hughes, S. H., Bjorklund, B. C., & Oberst, M. T. (1996). Family caregiving in cases of hip fracture. *Rehabilitation Nursing, 21*(3), 124–131, 138.

Yarnold, B. (1999). Hip fracture: Caring for a fragile population. *American Journal of Nursing, 99*(2), 36–41.

Yetzer, E. A. (1996). Helping the patient through the experience of an amputation. *Orthopaedic Nursing, 15*(6), 45–49.

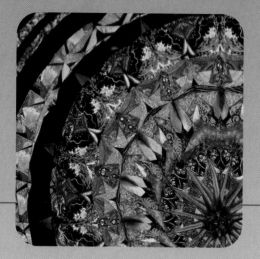

### CHAPTER 39

# Nursing Care of Clients with Musculoskeletal Disorders

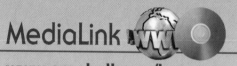

## MediaLink

### www.prenhall.com/lemone

Additional resources for this chapter can be found on the Student CD-ROM accompanying this textbook, and on the Companion Website at www.prenhall.com/lemone. Click on Chapter 39 to select the activities for this chapter.

**CD-ROM**
- Audio Glossary
- NCLEX Review

**Companion Website**
- More NCLEX Review
- Case Study
  Rheumatoid Arthritis
- Care Plan Activity
  Lower Back Pain
- MediaLink Application
  Osteoporosis Prevention

## LEARNING OUTCOMES

After completing this chapter, you will be able to:

- Apply knowledge of normal anatomy, physiology, and assessments when providing care for clients with musculoskeletal disorders (see Chapter 37).

- Explain the pathophysiology, manifestations, and complications of metabolic, degenerative, autoimmune, inflammatory, infectious, neoplastic, connective tissue, and structural musculoskeletal disorders.

- Describe the collaborative care, with related nursing care, of clients with musculoskeletal disorders.

- Provide appropriate nursing care for the client having musculoskeletal surgery.

- Use the nursing process as a framework for providing individualized care to clients with musculoskeletal disorders.

Various metabolic, autoimmune, inflammatory, degenerative, neoplastic, infectious, and structural disorders may affect the musculoskeletal system. Many of these diseases have significant physical, psychosocial, and financial consequences. When these problems occur, clients experience many different individualized responses to their altered health status. Nursing care is directed toward meeting physiologic needs, providing education, and ensuring psychologic support for the client and family.

**Arthritis,** meaning joint inflammation, and **arthralgia,** meaning joint pain, are terms used to describe many disease processes and manifestations involving the musculoskeletal system. These diseases affect not only the joints but also the connective tissues of the body. The various types of arthritis are discussed in this chapter in different sections, depending on the primary etiology of the disorder. Arthritis and other rheumatic disorders (various conditions that affect the musculoskeletal system) are widespread, affecting more than 33 million people in the United States. Arthritic disorders are a leading cause of disability; however, their very prevalence may lead the public and health care professionals to treat them as normal aging processes or discount the validity of the pain and disability experienced by the person with arthritis.

The etiology of most rheumatic disorders is not clear; in many cases, the pathophysiologic processes involved are often complex and poorly understood. Many are primary disorders; others occur as secondary processes associated with another disease. The wear and tear of aging, autoimmune processes, metabolic disorders, genetic factors, and infection are implicated as causative factors in some forms of rheumatic disease.

# METABOLIC DISORDERS

Metabolic bone disorders originate in the bone remodeling process, which normally involves a sequence of events of bone reabsorption and formation. In the adult, this process is primarily internal remodeling through replacement of trabecular bone. Adults replace about 25% of trabecular bone every 4 months through reabsorption of old bone by osteoclasts and formation of new bone by osetoblasts (Porth, 2002). Metabolic bone disorders may result from a variety of factors, including aging, calcium and phosphate imbalances, genetics, and changes in levels of hormones.

## THE CLIENT WITH OSTEOPOROSIS

**Osteoporosis,** literally defined as "porous bones," is a metabolic bone disorder characterized by loss of bone mass, increased bone fragility, and an increased risk of fractures. The reduced bone mass is caused by an imbalance of the processes that influence bone growth and maintenance. Although osteoporosis may result from an endocrine disorder or malignancy, it is most often associated with aging.

Osteoporosis is a health threat for an estimated 28 million Americans; 10 million people have osteoporosis and 18 million have low bone mass, increasing their risk for the disease (National Institute of Health [NIH], 2002). Although osteoporosis can occur at any age and in both men and women, it is most common in aging women. Approximately 50% of all women and 13% of men over the age of 50 will experience an osteoporosis-related fracture in their lifetime, most frequently in the hip, wrist, and vertebrae.

### RISK FACTORS

The risk of developing osteoporosis depends on how much bone mass is achieved between ages 25 and 35, and how much is lost later. Certain diseases, lifestyle habits, and ethnic backgrounds increase the risk of developing osteoporosis (see the Focus on Diversity box above). Many different variables affect one's risk of osteoporosis—some can be modified and others cannot. The risk factors are summarized in Box 39–1.

### Unmodifiable Risk Factors

Both men and women are susceptible to osteoporosis as they age, because the osteoblasts and osteoclasts undergo alterations

---

**Focus on Diversity**

**RISK AND INCIDENCE OF OSTEOPOROSIS IN PEOPLE AGE 50 OR OLDER**

- 20% of non-Hispanic white and Asian women are estimated to have osteoporosis; 52% have a low bone mass. In men, 7% have osteoporosis and 35% have low bone mass.
- 10% of Hispanic women are estimated to have osteoporosis, with another 49% having a low bone mass. In men, 3% have osteoporosis and 23% have low bone mass.
- 5% of African American women are estimated to have osteoporosis with an additional 35% having a lower bone mass. In men, 4% have osteoporosis; 19% have low bone mass.

---

**BOX 39–1 ■ Risk Factors for Osteoporosis**

***Unmodifiable Risk Factors***

- Age
- Female gender
- Race
- Genetic factors
- Endocrine disorders

***Modifiable Risk Factors***

- Calcium deficiency
- Estrogen deficiency
- Smoking
- High alcohol intake
- Sedentary lifestyle
- Medications

that diminish their activity. Women have a significantly higher risk for manifestations and complications of osteoporosis because their peak bone mass is 10% to 15% less than that of men. In addition, age-related bone loss begins earlier and proceeds more rapidly in women, beginning in the 30s and accelerating before menopause. Estrogen in women and testosterone in men appear to help prevent bone loss; decreasing levels of these hormones associated with aging contribute to bone loss. Age-related bone loss in men occurs 15 to 20 years later than in women and at a slower rate.

European Americans and Asians are at a higher risk for osteoporosis than African Americans, who have greater bone density (bone mass positively correlates with the amount of skin pigmentation). Premature osteoporosis is increasing in female athletes, who have a greater incidence of eating disorders and amenorrhea. Poor nutrition and intense physical training can result in a deficient production of estrogen. Decreased estrogen, combined with a lack of calcium and vitamin D, results in a loss of bone density (Porth, 2002).

Clients who have an endocrine disorder such as hyperthyroidism, hyperparathyroidism, Cushing's syndrome, or diabetes mellitus are at high risk for osteoporosis. These disorders affect the metabolism, in turn affecting nutritional status and bone mineralization.

## Modifiable Risk Factors

Modifiable risk factors include behaviors that place a person at risk for developing osteoporosis, as well as physical changes such as menopause whose contribution to osteoporosis can be modified by preventive strategies. Calcium deficiency is an important modifiable risk factor contributing to osteoporosis. Calcium is an essential mineral in the process of bone formation and other significant body functions. When there is an insufficient intake of calcium in the diet, the body compensates by removing calcium from the skeleton, weakening bone tissue. Acidosis, which may result from a high-protein diet, contributes to osteoporosis in two ways. Calcium is withdrawn from the bone as the kidneys attempt to buffer the excess acid. Acidosis also may directly stimulate osteoclast function. A high intake of diet soda with a high phosphate content also can deplete calcium stores (McCance & Huether, 2002).

With menopause and decreasing estrogen levels, bone loss accelerates in women. Estrogen promotes the activity of osteoblasts, increasing new bone formation. In addition, estrogen enhances calcium absorption and stimulates the thyroid gland to secrete calcitonin, a hormone that suppresses osteoclast activity and increases osteoblast activity. Estrogen replacement therapy (ERT) in postmenopausal women can reverse the bone changes that occur as estrogen levels decline in earlymenopause.

Cigarette smoking has long been identified as a risk factor for osteoporosis. Smoking decreases the blood supply to bones. Nicotine slows the production of osteoblasts and impairs the absorption of calcium, contributing to decreased bone density.

Excess alcohol intake is another risk factor for osteoporosis. Alcohol has a direct toxic effect on osteoblast activity, suppressing bone formation during periods of alcohol intoxication. In addition, heavy alcohol use may be associated with nutritional deficiencies that contribute to osteoporosis. Interestingly, moderate alcohol consumption in postmenopausal women actually may increase bone mineral content, possibly by increasing levels of estrogen and calcitonin.

Sedentary lifestyle is another modifiable risk factor that can cause osteoporosis. Weight-bearing exercise, such as walking, influences bone metabolism in several ways. The stress of this type of exercise causes an increase in blood flow to bones, which brings growth-producing nutrients to the cells. Walking causes an increase in osteoblast growth and activity.

Prolonged use of medications that increase calcium excretion, such as aluminum-containing antacids, corticosteroids, and anticonvulsants, increase the risk of developing osteoporosis. Heparin therapy increases bone resorption, and its prolonged use is associated with osteoporosis. Antiretroviral therapy for people with AIDS or HIV infection may cause decreased bone density and osteoporosis (Porth, 2002).

## PATHOPHYSIOLOGY

While the exact pathophysiology of osteoporosis is unclear, it is known to involve an imbalance of the activity of osteoblasts that form new bone and osteoclasts that resorb bone. Until age 35, when peak bone mass occurs, formation occurs more rapidly than does reabsorption. After peak bone mass is achieved, slightly more is lost than is gained (about 0.3% to 0.5% per year); this loss is accelerated if the diet is deficient in vitamin D and calcium. In women, bone loss increases after menopause (with loss of estrogen), then slows but does not stop at about age 60. Older women may have lost between 35% and 50% of their bone mass, older men may have lost between 20% and 35% (Mayo Clinic, 2002).

Osteoporosis affects the diaphysis (shaft of the bone) and the metaphysis (portion of the bone between the diaphysis and the epiphysis). The diameter of the bone increases, thinning the outer supporting cortex. As osteoporosis progresses, trabeculae are lost from cancellous bone (the spongy tissue of bone) and the outer cortex thins to the point that even minimal stress will fracture the bone (Porth, 2002).

## MANIFESTATIONS AND COMPLICATIONS

The most common manifestations of osteoporosis are loss of height, progressive curvature of the spine, low back pain, and fractures of the forearm, spine, or hip. Osteoporosis is often called the "silent disease," as bone loss occurs without symptoms.

The loss of height occurs as vertebral bodies collapse. Acute episodes generally are painful, with radiation of the pain around the flank into the abdomen. Vertebral collapse can occur with little or no stress; minimal movements such as bending, lifting, or jumping may precipitate the pain. In some clients, vertebral collapse may occur slowly, accompanied by little discomfort. Along with loss of height, characteristic dorsal kyphosis and cervical lordosis develop, accounting for the "dowager's hump" often associated with aging. The abdomen tends to protrude and knees and hips flex as the body attempts to maintain its center of gravity (Figure 39–1 ■).

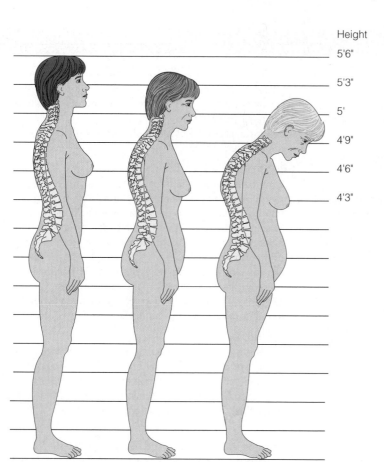

Height
5'6"
5'3"
5'
4'9"
4'6"
4'3"

Age    40    60    70

**Figure 39–1** ■ Spinal changes caused by osteoporosis. As the condition progresses, height can be reduced by as much as 7 inches.

Fractures are the most common complication of osteoporosis, with the disease being responsible for more than 1.5 million fractures each year. These include 700,000 vertebral compression fractures, 300,000 hip fractures, 250,000 wrist fractures, and 300,000 fractures at other sites (NIH, 2002). There may be no obvious manifestations of osteoporosis until fractures occur. Some fractures are spontaneous; others may result from everyday activities. While wrist and vertebral fractures have not been shown to increase disability or mortality, persistent pain and associated posture changes may restrict the client's activities or interfere with ADLs.

## COLLABORATIVE CARE

Care of the client with osteoporosis focuses on stopping or slowing the process, alleviating the symptoms, and preventing complications. Proper nutrition and exercise are important components of the treatment program.

### Diagnostic Tests

The manifestations of osteoporosis can mimic those of other bone disorders, so diagnostic tests are needed to differentiate osteoporosis from other problems

- *X-rays* provide a picture of skeletal structures; however, osteoporotic changes may not be seen until over 30% of the bone mass has been lost.

- *Quantitative computed tomography (QCT)* of the spine measures trabecular bone within vertebral bodies.
- *Dual-energy X-ray absorptiometry (DEXA)* measures bone density in the lumbar spine or hip and is considered to be highly accurate.
- *Ultrasound* transmits painless sound waves through the heel of the foot to measure bone density. This 1-minute test is not as sensitive as DEXA, but is accurate enough for screening purposes.
- *Alkaline phosphatase (AST)* may be elevated following a fracture.
- *Serum bone Gla-protein,* also called *osteocalcin,* can be used as a marker of osteoclastic activity and therefore is an indicator of the rate of bone turnover. This test is most useful to evaluate the effects of treatment, rather than as an indicator of the severity of the disease.

### Medications

Estrogen replacement therapy reduces bone loss, increases bone density in the spine and hip, and reduces the risk of fractures in postmenopausal women. It is particularly recommended for women who have undergone surgical menopause before age 50, and often is prescribed for women with other osteoporosis risk factors. Estrogen therapy alone is associated with an increased risk of endometrial cancer, so it usually is prescribed in combination with progestin (hormone replacement therapy or HRT). As discussed in Chapter 48, ☞ the

# Medication Administration

## The Client with Osteoporosis

### CALCIUM

Postmenopausal women, regardless if they take replacement estrogens, are encouraged to take calcium to prevent osteoporosis.

#### Nursing Responsibilities

- Help clients maintain an adequate dietary intake of calcium. The best dietary source is milk and other dairy products, including yogurt.
- Postmenopausal women who take estrogens need 1000 mg of calcium daily. Those who do not take estrogens need about 1500 mg daily to minimize osteoporosis.
- Identify alternate sources, such as skim milk and low-fat yogurt, oysters, canned sardines or salmon, beans, cauliflower, and dark-green leafy vegetables.

#### Client and Family Teaching

- Take calcium carbonate in divided doses 30 to 60 minutes before meals to allow for absorption.
- Take calcium citrate with meals to minimize gastrointestinal distress.

### CALCITONIN

    Calcitonin-salmon injection, synthetic
    Calcimar
    Miacalin (injection or nasal spray)

In postmenopausal osteoporosis, calcitonin prevents further bone loss and increases bone mass if the client consumes adequate amounts of calcium and vitamin D. Calcitonin may be used in postmenopausal women who cannot or will not take estrogen.

#### Nursing Responsibilities

- Calcitonin is protein in nature; both the parenteral and nasal spray forms may cause an anaphylactic-type allergic response. Observe the client for 20 minutes after administration; have appropriate emergency equipment and drugs available to treat anaphylaxis.
- Alternate nostrils daily when administering calcitonin nasal spray.
- Review medical history for conditions that contraindicate use of calcitonin products: hypersensitivity to salmon calcitonin and lactation (calcitonin is secreted in breast milk and may inhibit lactation).

- Observe for side effects: nausea and vomiting, anorexia, mild transient flushing of the palms of the hands and the soles of the feet, and urinary frequency.
- Teach the client the proper technique for handling and injecting the drug at home.

#### Client and Family Teaching

- Take the medication in the evening to minimize side effects.
- Warm nasal spray to room temperature before using.
- Rhinitis (runny nose) is the most common side effect with calcitonin nasal spray. Other possible side effects include sores, itching, or other nasal symptoms. Report nosebleeds to your primary care provider.
- Nausea and vomiting may occur during initial stages of therapy; they disappear as treatment continues.
- While taking the medication, be sure to consume adequate amounts of calcium and vitamin D.

### FLUORIDE

Fluoride is a mineral long recognized as essential for the normal formation of dentin and tooth enamel. Fluoride appears to decrease the solubility of bone mineral and therefore the rate of bone reabsorption. Its use in preventing and treating osteoporosis is relatively new but promising.

#### Nursing Responsibilities

- Monitor serum fluoride levels every 3 months.
- Have bone mineral density studies conducted at 6-month intervals to document progress of bone growth.

#### Client and Family Teaching

- Take sodium fluoride tablets after meals, and avoid milk or dairy products; these reduce gastrointestinal absorption of the medication.
- While taking fluoride, be sure to maintain an adequate calcium intake.
- Use fluoride mouth rinse immediately after brushing teeth and just before retiring at night. Do not swallow the rinse, and avoid eating or drinking for at least 30 minutes after use.
- Notify the physician if teeth become stained or mottled after repeated use of fluoride mouth rinse.

---

risks of HRT are believed to be too high for long-term therapy. The choice of using HRT to prevent osteoporosis is one that must be made between the woman and her health care provider.

Raloxifene (Evista) is a selective estrogen receptor modulator (SERM) that appears to prevent bone loss by mimicking estrogen's beneficial effects on bone density in postmenopausal women. It does not have the risks of estrogen. Hot flashes are a common side effect, and this drug should not be taken by a woman with a history of blood clots.

Alendronate (Fosamax), risedronate (Actonel), and etidronate (Didronel) are from the class of drugs known as biphosphonates. Biphosphonates are potent inhibitors of bone resorption that may be used to prevent and treat osteoporosis. They inhibit bone breakdown, preserve bone mass, and increase bone density in the

hip and vertebrae. These are especially useful for men, young adults, and to prevent or treat steroid-induced osteoporosis. The nursing implications of biphosphonates are found in the Medication Administration box on page 1232.

Calcitonin (Miacalcin) is a hormone that increases bone formation and decreases bone resorption. Calcitonin increases spinal bone density and reduces the risk of compression fractures; it may reduce the risk of hip fracture as well. Calcitonin usually is prescribed as a nasal spray, although it also is available in parenteral form. Because calcitonin is a protein, it can precipitate anaphylactic-type allergic responses. See the box above.

Sodium fluoride stimulates osteoblast activity, increasing bone formation. When used to treat osteoporosis, bone mass of

the spine increases and the risk of spinal fractures may be reduced. Fluoride therapy may, however, be associated with an increased risk of hip and other nonvertebral fractures. See the Medication Administration box on page 1226.

## NURSING CARE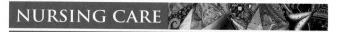

Osteoporosis is both preventable and treatable; therefore, nursing care focuses primarily on planning and implementing interventions to prevent the disease, its manifestations, and the resulting injuries. An important aspect of preventing osteoporosis is educating clients under age 35.

### Health Promotion

Health promotion activities to prevent or slow osteoporosis focus on calcium intake, exercise, and health-related behaviors.

#### Diet

For clients of all ages, stress the importance of maintaining a daily calcium intake that meets NIH recommendations (see Chapter 5). ⊂⊃ This is particularly important for adolescent girls and young adult women who may avoid eating many high-calcium foods such as dairy products because of concerns about weight. Optimal calcium intake before age 30 to 35 probably increases peak bone mass. Emphasize that lowfat (or nonfat) dairy products also contain calcium, although some fat in the product may enhance calcium absorption.

Milk and milk products are the best sources of calcium. The lactose in milk facilitates calcium absorption as well. Other food sources of calcium include sardines, clams, oysters, and salmon, as well as dark green, leafy vegetables such as broccoli, collard greens, bok choy, and spinach. For clients who avoid dairy products because of lactose intolerance or a vegetarian diet, suggest alternate sources.

Calcium supplements are available in many forms. Most supplements (including Tums) provide calcium carbonate in the range of 200 to 600 mg per tablet. Other forms of calcium, including citrate, gluconate, and lactate, generally provide a lower amount of elemental calcium per tablet. A combination of calcium with vitamin D is recommended, particularly for older adults who may have a vitamin D deficiency that impairs their ability to absorb and use calcium. (Calcium supplements are discussed in Chapter 5.) ⊂⊃

#### Exercise

Teach clients the importance of physical activity and weight-bearing exercises in preventing and slowing bone loss. Suggest that clients participate in regular exercise such as walking for at least 20 minutes four or more times a week. Inform clients that swimming and pool aerobic exercises are not as beneficial in maintaining bone density because of the lack of weight-bearing activity.

#### Healthy Behaviors

Behaviors that help prevent osteoporosis include not smoking, avoiding excessive alcohol intake, and limiting caffeine intake to two or three cups of coffee each day.

### Assessment

Collect the following data through the health history and physical examination (see Chapter 37).

- Health history: age, risk factors, history of fractures, smoking history, alcohol intake, medications, usual diet, menstrual history including menopause, usual exercise/activity level
- Physical examination: height, spinal curves, low back pain

### Nursing Diagnoses and Interventions

Nursing care of clients who have osteoporosis focuses on teaching about the disease process, helping maintain physical mobility and nutrition, and solving problems associated with pain and injury.

#### Health-Seeking Behaviors

At multiple points in the client's lifetime, nurses can provide vital information that will help clients use self-care strategies to reduce their risk of developing osteoporosis.

- Assess the client's health habits, including diet, exercise, smoking, and alcohol use. *The risk of developing osteoporosis in later life is affected by such things as diet, regular participation in weight-bearing exercise, and personal habits such as smoking and alcohol consumption.*
- Teach women and men of all ages about the importance of maintaining an adequate calcium intake. Provide a list of calcium-rich foods, and discuss the use of calcium supplements with clients who do not consume adequate dietary calcium. *Calcium needs vary during the course of a lifetime; however, many clients never consume adequate amounts of calcium. This affects their peak bone mass and the rate of bone loss with aging. Calcium in foods is more completely absorbed than that supplied by calcium supplements.*

> **PRACTICE ALERT** *Recommended calcium intake increases through the adult years as follows: age 19 to 50 = 1000 mg/day; age 51 to 64 = 12000 mg/day; age 65 and older = 1500 mg/day.* ■

- Discuss the importance of maintaining a regular schedule of weight-bearing exercise, either through an exercise program or regular physical activity. *Weight-bearing exercise promotes osteoblast activity, helping maintain bone strength and integrity.*
- Refer clients to smoking-cessation programs and alcohol treatment programs as appropriate. *Smoking interferes with estrogen's protective effects on bones, promoting bone loss. Excess alcohol intake affects the nutritional status of the client, increasing the risk of calcium and vitamin D deficiency.*
- Refer clients with significant risk factors for osteoporosis to primary care providers or clinics for bone-density evaluation as indicated. *Early identification and treatment of osteoporotic changes in bones can reduce the risk and possible long-term consequences of falls and fractures.*

#### Risk for Injury

Falls that would result in little or no injury in the healthy adult may cause fractures in the client with osteoporosis. Even

normal movements such as twisting, bending, lifting, or rising from bed can precipitate a vertebral fracture.

- Implement safety precautions as necessary for the client who is hospitalized or in a long-term care facility. Maintain the client's bed in low position; use side rails if indicated to prevent the client from getting up alone; provide nighttime lighting to toilet facilities. *Most falls are preventable, particularly in hospitals and long-term care facilities.*
- Avoid using restraints (if hospitalized or a resident in a long-term care facility) if at all possible. *Restraints may actually increase the client's risk of falling and increase the risk of injury associated with a fall.*

**PRACTICE ALERT** *Clients may fracture osteoporotic bones when pulling against restraints.* ■

- Teach clients who are able to participate in weight-bearing exercises to perform exercises at least three times a week for a sustained period of 30 to 40 minutes. The mechanical force of weight-bearing exercises promotes bone growth. *Bones weaken and demineralize without exercise. Walking is an easy, low-impact form of exercise. Swimming (including walking on the bottom of the pool) does not provide the needed weight-bearing activity.*
- Encourage older adults to use assistive devices to maintain independence in ADLs. *Walking sticks, canes, and other assistive devices encourage client independence and support activities that promote bone growth.*
- Teach older clients about safety and fall precautions. *A simple assessment of the client's home for safety and fall risks may reduce the risk of fractures and, in turn, the cost of hospitalization and potential disability and/or death.*
- Evaluate and closely monitor the client's medications. The reasons for, types of, and dosage of the client's medications should be evaluated, especially if the person has been falling frequently or has a change in mental status. *Falls may be related to the number of both prescribed and over-the-counter medications the client is taking.*

### Imbalanced Nutrition: Less Than Body Requirements

Most Americans do not maintain their recommended daily intake of calcium. Clients must therefore be made aware of the relationship between an adequate calcium intake and maintaining strong bones.

- Teach adolescents, pregnant or lactating women, and adults through age 35 to eat foods high in calcium and to maintain a daily calcium intake of 1200 to 1500 mg. *The National Institutes of Health recommend a daily calcium intake of 1200 to 1500 mg per day for adolescents and young adults, as well as for pregnant and lactating women.*
- Encourage postmenopausal women to maintain a calcium intake of 1000 to 1500 mg daily, either through diet or a calcium supplement. *Calcium needs for postmenopausal women vary, depending on age and estrogen therapy.*
- Teach clients taking calcium supplements the importance of taking the medication at the proper time and the side effects

that may occur. *Free hydrochloric acid is needed for calcium absorption. Calcium carbonate supplement (e.g., Tums) should be taken 30 to 60 minutes before meals to allow adequate absorption. Calcium citrate supplements should be taken with meals to prevent gastrointestinal distress.*

**PRACTICE ALERT** *Calcium supplements should be taken in divided doses (two to three times daily) for improved distribution.* ■

### Acute Pain

Advanced stages of osteoporosis can result in pain and immobilization. Acute pain usually results from a complicating fracture, especially a compression fracture of the vertebrae.

- Review activity tolerance and suggest modifications in exercise schedules as indicated. *Clients with osteoporosis should remain active and participate in weight-bearing exercises; however, the client's abilities and severity of the disease may warrant a modification in the exercise regimen.*
- Suggest anti-inflammatory pain medications for treatment of both acute and chronic phases of pain. Clients should be instructed in the amount and frequency as noted on the manufacturer's labels. *Continuous administration of ibuprofen or other NSAIDs can be useful to provide relief from pain.*

**PRACTICE ALERT** *Teach clients on long-term anti-inflammatory medications to watch for bright red bleeding from the stomach or dark black bowel movements.* ■

- Suggest the application of heat to relieve pain. *A heating pad may offer temporary pain relief. To avoid the "rebound effect," the heat should be removed every 20 to 30 minutes.*

### Using NANDA, NIC, and NOC

Chart 39–1 shows links between NANDA nursing diagnoses, NIC, and NOC when caring for the client with osteoporosis.

### Home Care

The client who has osteoporosis needs education on safety and preventing falls (see Chapter 38). In addition to home safety, outdoor safety is important too. Clients should be taught to use assistive devices for added stability, to wear rubber-soled shoes for traction, to walk on the grass when sidewalks are slippery, and to sprinkle salt or kitty litter on icy sidewalks in the winter.

Address the following topics when discussing home care.

- Resources for medical supplies and assistive devices
- Diet, exercise, and medications
- Pain management
- Maintaining good posture to help prevent stress on the spine
- Helpful resources:
  - National Osteoporosis Foundation
  - Osteoporosis and Related Bone Diseases National Resource Center (National Institutes of Health)
  - National Women's Health Resource Center
  - Older Women's League

## CHART 39–1  NANDA, NIC, AND NOC LINKAGES

### The Client with Osteoporosis

| NURSING DIAGNOSES | NURSING INTERVENTIONS | NURSING OUTCOMES |
|---|---|---|
| • Chronic Pain | • Medication Administration<br>• Pain Management | • Comfort Level<br>• Pain: Disruptive Effects |
| • Risk for Trauma | • Environmental Management: Safety<br>• Fall Prevention<br>• Health Education<br>• Teaching: Disease Process | • Risk Control<br>• Safety Behavior: Fall Prevention<br>• Self-Care: Activities of Daily Living |
| • Knowledge Deficit: Calcium Intake | • Teaching: Disease Process<br>• Teaching: Prescribed Diet<br>• Teaching: Prescribed Medications | • Knowledge: Disease Process<br>• Knowledge: Diet<br>• Knowledge: Prescribed Medications |

*Note: Data from Nursing Outcomes Classification (NOC) by M. Johnson & M. Maas (Eds.), 1997, St. Louis: Mosby; Nursing Diagnoses: Definitions & Classification 2001–2002 by North American Nursing Diagnosis Association, 2001, Philadelphia: NANDA; Nursing Interventions Classification (NIC) by J.C. McCloskey & G. M. Bulechek (Eds.), 2000, St. Louis: Mosby. Reprinted by permission.*

## Nursing Care Plan
## A Client with Osteoporosis

Nancy Bauer is a 53-year-old schoolteacher. She has been married for 36 years and has two children. Mrs. Bauer says she is 65 inches tall. She has smoked one pack of cigarettes a day for 30 years and drinks one to two glasses of wine with dinner each evening. She does not routinely exercise. Mrs. Bauer has had symptoms of menopause for 8 years, including hot flashes in the early years and mood swings of late. She has never been on hormone replacement therapy.

Mrs. Bauer is currently seeking medical advice for continuous low back pain. The pain is not relieved with an over-the-counter analgesic, and she frequently wakes up during the night because of the pain.

### ASSESSMENT

The nurse practitioner notes that Mrs. Bauer's vital signs are all within normal limits. She has full range of motion of all extremities and is able to stand and bend over, but she reports discomfort when returning to the upright position. Mrs. Bauer has a slightly pronounced "hump" on her upper back and is 1 inch shorter than her stated height on admission. Her muscle strength is symmetric and strong.

### DIAGNOSIS

- *Acute pain* of the lower spine related to vertebral compression
- *Deficient knowledge* related to osteoporosis and treatment to prevent further damage
- *Imbalanced nutrition: Less than body requirements* related to inadequate intake of calcium
- *Risk for injury* related to effects of change in bone structure secondary to osteoporosis

### EXPECTED OUTCOMES

- Verbalize a decrease in back pain.
- Be able to describe ways to treat her osteoporosis and prevent further complications.
- Verbalize an understanding of the current research and treatment regarding osteoporosis.

- Verbalize how stopping smoking can help prevent further progression of osteoporosis.
- Seek consultation for supplements and medications to prevent further bone loss.
- Design a program of physical activity to prevent complications of osteoporosis.
- Verbalize safety precautions to prevent fractures due to falls.

### PLANNING AND IMPLEMENTATION

- Teach back strengthening exercises.
- Refer to an osteoporosis support group, if available.
- Provide realistic, yet optimistic, feedback about loss of height and bone integrity and the potential outcomes of treatment.
- Assess current knowledge base, and correct misconceptions regarding treatment of osteoporosis.
- Provide current educational literature regarding treatment of osteoporosis.
- Instruct in dietary and calcium supplements that help prevent effects of osteoporosis.
- Discuss physical exercises that help prevent complications due to osteoporosis.
- Review safety and fall precautions, and provide literature regarding how to create a safe home environment.

### EVALUATION

On her return visit 6 months later, Mrs. Bauer reports that she feels much better. She is no longer irritable and does not experience mood swings, because she has been taking her prescribed hormone replacements for 6 months. She is eating products rich in calcium and taking a daily supplement of calcium with vitamin D. Mrs. Bauer has reduced her wine intake to one glass in the evening and now drinks decaffeinated coffee and tea. She also states that since she stopped smoking, she has been walking 30 to 45 minutes every day.

(continued on page 1230)

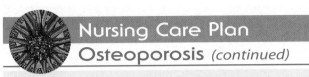

## Nursing Care Plan
### Osteoporosis (continued)

**Critical Thinking in the Nursing Process**

1. What is the rationale for stopping smoking and limiting caffeine and alcohol intake in the treatment of osteoporosis?
2. What foods would you encourage for clients at high risk for osteoporosis whose serum cholesterol and LDL/HDL ratios indicate a high risk for cardiovascular disease?
3. What physical activities would you consider beneficial in helping to prevent the effects of osteoporosis in the female client who is wheelchair bound or has limited mobility?
4. Develop a care plan for Mrs. Bauer for the nursing diagnosis, *Risk for trauma.*

See Evaluating Your Response in Appendix C.

## THE CLIENT WITH PAGET'S DISEASE

**Paget's disease,** also called **osteitis deformans,** is a progressive skeletal disorder that results from excessive metabolic activity in bone, with abnormal bone resorption and formation. This chronic remodeling results in the affected bones being larger and softer (McCance & Huether, 2002). This disorder affects the axial skeleton, especially the femur, pelvis, vertebrae, sacrum, sternum, and skull.

Paget's disease affects about 3% of the population over age 40, and the incidence doubles each 10 years after age 50. Paget's disease occurs more frequently in whites in continental Europe, England, Australia, New Zealand, and North America. It has a familial tendency and is slightly more common in men than in women (Porth, 2002).

## PATHOPHYSIOLOGY

The cause of Paget's disease is unknown; however, several theories have been proposed, including hormonal imbalance, vascular disorder, neoplasm, autoimmune disorder, and inborn error of connective tissue. Of people affected by Paget's disease, 20% to 30% have a family history of the disorder, suggesting a genetic linkage. A slow-activating viral infection also has been theorized as a cause of Paget's disease.

Paget's disease progresses slowly. It usually follows a two-stage process: an excessive amount of osteoclastic bone resorption, followed by excessive osteoblastic bone formation. The initial phase presents with an abnormal increase in osteoclasts. The bones increase in size and thickness because of the acceleration in bone resorption and regeneration, resulting in a thick layer of coarse bone with a rough and pitted outer surface (Porth, 2002). Resorption of cancellous bone occurs rapidly. As new bone tissue tries to replace the loss, fibrous tissue forms in the bone marrow. The bone is at first hyperemic and soft, and bowing occurs. When this excessive bone cell activity decreases, the result is a gain in bone mass, but the newly formed bone becomes hard and brittle. This brittleness may lead to fractures. Paget's disease varies in severity, and may involve one or many bones.

## MANIFESTATIONS AND COMPLICATIONS

Most clients with Paget's disease are asymptomatic, and the disease often is discovered when typical changes are seen on an incidental X-ray. Manifestations are often vague and depend on the specific area involved (see the box below). The most common complaint is localized pain of the long bones, spine, pelvis, and cranium. The pain is described as a mild to moderate deep ache that is aggravated by pressure and weight bearing. It is more noticeable at night or when the client is resting. The pain usually is due to metabolic bone activity, secondary degenerative osteoarthritis, fractures, or nerve impingement. Because of the increase in blood flow to pagetic bone, flushing and warmth of the overlying skin may be apparent.

Other complications of Paget's disease are as follows:

- Nerve palsy syndromes from involvement of the upper extremities
- Pathologic fractures from loss of bone structure
- Mental deterioration from compression of the brain when the skull is involved
- Compression of the spinal cord from affected cervical vertebra causing tetraplegia
- Cardiovascular disease, resulting from vasodilation of the vessels in the skin and subcutaneous tissues overlying the affected bones
- Osteogenic sarcoma (in about 1% of cases)

### Manifestations of Paget's Disease

**MUSCULOSKELETAL EFFECTS**
- Pain (in the long bones of lower extremities or joints)
- Deformity (enlargement of skull, bowing of lower extremities, and deformity of elbows and knees)
- Chalkstick-type fractures of lower extremities
- Pathologic fractures (especially of the tibia)
- Compression fractures
- Collapse of the vertebrae, resulting in kyphosis and loss of height
- Muscle weakness

**NEUROLOGIC EFFECTS**
- Hearing loss
- Spinal cord injuries
- Dementia
- Pain from spinal stenosis
- Bladder and/or bowel dysfunction

**CARDIOVASCULAR EFFECTS**
- High cardiac output
- Congestive heart failure
- Increased skin temperature over affected extremities

**METABOLIC EFFECTS**
- Symptoms of hypercalcemia in immobilized clients
- Hypercalciuria and renal calculi

TABLE 39–1  Differential Features of Osteoporosis, Osteomalacia, and Paget's Disease

| Differentiating Features | Osteoporosis | Osteomalacia | Paget's Disease |
|---|---|---|---|
| Pathophysiology | Resorption greater than bone formation | Inadequate mineralization of bone matrix | Excessive osteoclastic activity and formation of poor-quality bone |
| Calcium level (serum) | Normal | Low or normal | Normal or elevated (especially in immobilized clients) |
| Phosphate level (serum) | Normal | Low or normal | Normal |
| Parathyroid hormone level (serum) | Normal | High or normal | Normal |
| Alkaline phosphatase level (serum) | Normal | Elevated | Increased; not a reliable test for clients who have liver disease or are pregnant |
| Hydroxyproline (urine) | Not applicable | Not applicable | Increased |
| Radiographic findings | Osteopenia, fractures | Decreased bone density, radiolucent bands known as Looser's zones, or pseudofractures | "Punched-out" appearance of bone, increase in bone thickness, linear fractures, mosaic pattern of bone matrix |

## COLLABORATIVE CARE

Care of the client with Paget's disease focuses on relieving pain, suppressing bone cell activity if necessary, and preventing or minimizing the effects of complications. Many clients with Paget's disease are asymptomatic and do not require treatment. For more severely affected clients, pharmacologic agents are usually effective. Occasionally, surgery may be required.

### Diagnostic Tests

Many of the diagnostic tests that are useful for the diagnosis of osteoporosis are equally useful for clients with Paget's disease (Table 39–1). These include the following:

- *X-rays* illustrate localized areas of demineralization in the early stages, seen as "punched out" areas that lend a coarse, irregular appearance to the bone. In the later phase, X-rays show enlargement of the bones, tiny cracks in the long bones, and/or bowing of the weight-bearing bones.
- *Bone scan* will show areas of active Paget's disease.
- *CT scans* and *MRI* help identify possible causes of pain, including degenerative problems, spinal stenosis, or nerve root impingement.
- *Serum alkaline phosphatase* will show a steady rise as the disease progresses; the normal level (30 to 115 IU/L) may be elevated from high normal to over 3000 IU/L.
- *Urinary collagen pyridinoline testing* is a sensitive indicator of the rate of bone resorption.

### Medications

Clients who have mild symptoms often find relief using aspirin or NSAIDs, such as ibuprofen (Motrin) and indomethacin (Indocin). Clients who are experiencing manifestations and whose diagnostic test results are elevated are usually treated with an agent that retards bone resorption, such as calcitonin or a bisphosphonate.

Bisphosphonates such as alendronate (Fosamax), pamidronate (Aredia), and tiludronate (Skelid) are the primary treatments used for severe Paget's disease. These drugs inhibit bone resorption, possibly by attaching to the surface of the calcium/phosphate phase of bone and inhibiting osteoclast activity. They are safe, and usually are well tolerated by the client. In the United States, alendronate is available as an oral preparation, and pamidronate is available for intravenous administration. Oral preparations are poorly absorbed from the GI tract, and may cause gastric or esophageal irritation. Alendronate should be given with a full glass of water on an empty stomach, at least 30 minutes before other medications or food. Pamidronate is given as an intravenous infusion in D5W or normal saline. It is given for 3 successive days, generally promoting a rapid response with reduced urinary excretion of hydroxyproline and pyridinium and a fall in alkaline phosphatate. Intravenous pamidronate may cause flulike symptoms, but these generally are short-lived. Calcium supplements also are prescribed for clients receiving bisphosphonates. After bisphosphonate treatment, clients often experience remission of symptoms for a year or more. See the Medication Administration box on page 1232 for nursing implications.

Calcitonin inhibits osteoclastic resorption of bone. It also works as an analgesic for bone pain. The two derivatives of this medication are salmon (fish) and human. Salmon calcitonin (Calcimar) is generally preferred because it is inexpensive and widely available. Human calcitonin (Cibacalcin) is derived from human thyroid glands, which makes it more expensive and difficult to obtain. Both parenteral and nasal spray formulations of calcitonin are available (refer to the Medication Administration box on page 1226 for nursing implications).

### Surgery

Total hip or knee replacement is usually required when the client with Paget's disease develops degenerative arthritis of the hip or knee. These surgical procedures are usually performed

# Medication Administration

## The Client with Paget's Disease

### BISPHOSPHONATES

Alendronate (Fosamax)
Pamidronate (Aredia)
Tiludronate (Skelid)

The bisphosphonates inhibit bone resorption, increasing the mineral density of bones and reducing the incidence of fractures. They are also used both in the prevention and treatment of osteoporosis. When used for Paget's disease, bisphosphonates slow the accelerated bone turnover associated with this disease. Bone pain is relieved, and the incidence of pathologic fractures is reduced. Cardiac and vascular manifestations of the disease also improve.

### Nursing Responsibilities

- Administer alendronate with water when the client arises 30 minutes before food or other medications.
- Do not give foods high in calcium, vitamins with mineral supplements, or antacids within 2 hours of administering alendronate.
- Instruct the client to avoid lying down for 30 minutes after taking the drug.
- Assess renal function studies before initiating therapy; alendronate is not recommended for use in clients with renal insuffiency.
- Dilute the prescribed dose of pamidronate in 1000 mL of D5W or normal saline; infuse over at least 4 hours. Do not add to calcium-containing solutions such as Ringer's or lactated Ringer's solutions.
- Monitor the IV site for signs of thrombophlebitis.
- Assess the client for signs of electrolyte imbalance or other adverse responses such as a drug fever.

### Client and Family Teaching

- Take the medication as directed with clear water only. Consuming other beverages or food within 30 minutes of taking alendronate may interfere with its absorption and effectiveness.
- Do not lie down until after you have eaten breakfast. Alendronate can irritate the esophagus.
- Report symptoms such as new or worsening heart-burn, difficulty swallowing, or painful swallowing.
- Fever with or without chills may occur while receiving intravenous pamidronate; this will subside without treatment. Flu-like symptoms also may occur; these will subside within a week or so.
- Report any abnormal symptoms such as tingling around the mouth or numbness and tingling of the fingers or toes, which may indicate an imbalance of electrolytes in the blood.
- Take calcium and vitamin D supplements as instructed by your primary care provider.
- Response to these medications is gradual, and continues for months after the drug is stopped.

---

to address severe pain during weight bearing and impaired mobility. Neurologic manifestations related to spinal stenosis or nerve root compression may also require surgery.

## NURSING CARE

## Nursing Diagnoses and Interventions

The nursing interventions for the client with symptomatic Paget's disease focus on pain control, prevention of injury or fractures, and education regarding the disease process and prescribed therapies.

### Chronic Pain

The most common manifestation of Paget's disease is bone pain. This usually is the manifestation that prompts the client to seek health care.

- Assess the location and extent of the pain to determine the bone areas involved. *Bone pain in Paget's disease is poorly localized and is frequently described as "aching and deep."*
- Teach the client to take NSAIDs or aspirin on a regular basis as prescribed. *Pain is most noticeable at night or when the client is resting. The pain can become evident when it is aggravated by pressure and weight bearing.*
- Ensure correct placement of prescribed brace or corset. The client may be required to wear a light brace or corset to relieve back pain and provide support when assuming an upright position. *The client may need instruction in the correct application of the device and in the evaluation of pressure areas that may result from wearing the device.*
- Suggest referral for heat therapy and massage. *Heat therapy and massage can alleviate mild discomfort. Care should be taken when applying massage over areas prone to pathologic fractures.*

### Impaired Physical Mobility

Clients with Paget's disease need to maintain or improve mobility so that they can perform necessary self-care activities and prevent complications of immobility.

- Provide an assistive device for use when ambulating. *During the active phase of Paget's disease, the client is prone to fractures. Bone deformities, activity intolerance, fear of falling, and pain are all factors that may make the client more prone to falls. An assistive device can provide both physical and psychologic support during ambulation, permit the client to ambulate further, and provide a device for resting during the ambulation session.*
- Teach good body mechanics. *The client with bone deformities should avoid activities that require lifting and twisting.*

**PRACTICE ALERT** *Activities as seemingly simple as lifting a heavy box may result in a fracture in the client with Paget's disease.* ■

- Reinforce information about exercise protocols and activity regimens. *Exercise and activity protocols should be planned carefully to prevent injury and to minimize fatigue.*

## Home Care

Paget's disease, once diagnosed, can be frightening for the client and family. It is important that they understand that this is a treatable disease, and that many manifestations of the disease will be relieved with treatment. Inform the client that remissions of the disease often last for a year or more after effective treatment. The Paget Foundation should be suggested as a resource. Discuss the following topics.

- The importance of following the prescribed treatment regimen and keeping scheduled follow-up appointments
- Because it may take several weeks to notice a response to treatment, the importance of continuing therapy during this time and after a response is obtained
- If bisphosphonates such as alendronate or pamidronate are ordered, the importance of taking supplemental calcium to prevent low blood calcium levels
- The importance of remaining active
- Safety in the home and outdoor environment to prevent falls
- The need to report to the primary care provider any sudden pain or disability, even if no trauma has occurred, as pathologic fractures are possible

# THE CLIENT WITH GOUT

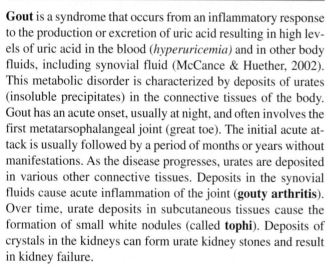

**Gout** is a syndrome that occurs from an inflammatory response to the production or excretion of uric acid resulting in high levels of uric acid in the blood (*hyperuricemia)* and in other body fluids, including synovial fluid (McCance & Huether, 2002). This metabolic disorder is characterized by deposits of urates (insoluble precipitates) in the connective tissues of the body. Gout has an acute onset, usually at night, and often involves the first metatarsophalangeal joint (great toe). The initial acute attack is usually followed by a period of months or years without manifestations. As the disease progresses, urates are deposited in various other connective tissues. Deposits in the synovial fluids cause acute inflammation of the joint (**gouty arthritis**). Over time, urate deposits in subcutaneous tissues cause the formation of small white nodules (called **tophi**). Deposits of crystals in the kidneys can form urate kidney stones and result in kidney failure.

Gout may occur as either a primary or secondary disorder. Primary gout is characterized by elevated serum uric acid levels resulting from either an inborn error of purine metabolism or a decrease in renal uric acid excretion due to an unknown cause. Purines are part of the structure of the nuclear compounds DNA and RNA; they also may be synthesized by the body. Impaired uric acid excretion leads to hyperuricemia in the majority of people with primary gout. In secondary gout, hyperuricemia occurs as a result of another disorder or treatment with certain medications. Disorders associated with rapid cell turnover, such as some malignancies (leukemia in particular), hemolytic anemia, and polycythemia, can increase purine metabolism. Chronic renal disease, hypertension, starvation, and diabetic ketoacidosis can interfere with

uric acid excretion, as can certain drugs, including some diuretics (such as furosemide, ethacrynic acid, and chlorothiazide), pyrazinamide, cyclosporin, ethambutol, and low-dose salicylates. Ethanol ingestion appears to interfere with uric acid excretion and to accelerate its synthesis. In addition, hospitalized clients with gout are at risk for an acute attack from changes in their diet, abdominal surgery, or medications (Tierney et al., 2001).

The peak age of onset of gout in men is between 40 and 50 years. It is rare in women before menopause. The disease is more common in Pacific Islanders.

## PATHOPHYSIOLOGY

Uric acid is the breakdown product of purine metabolism. Normally, a balance exists between its production and excretion, with approximately two-thirds of the amount produced each day excreted by the kidneys and the rest in the feces. The serum uric acid level is normally maintained between 3.4 and 7.0 mg/dL in men and 2.4 and 6.0 mg/dL in women. At levels greater than 7.0 mg/dL, the serum is saturated, and monosodium urate crystals may form. It is not known exactly how crystals of monosodium urate crystals are deposited in joints. Several mechanisms may be involved:

- Crystals tend to form in peripheral tissues of the body, where lower temperatures reduce the solubility of the uric acid.
- A decrease in extracellular fluid pH and reduced plasma protein binding of urate crystals are evident.
- Tissue trauma and a rapid change in uric acid levels may also lead to crystal deposition. A rapid increase in uric acid may occur with tissue trauma and release of cellular components.

The monosodium urate crystals may form in the synovial fluid or in the synovial membrane, cartilage, or other joint connective tissues. They may also form in the heart, earlobes, and kidneys. These crystals stimulate and continue the inflammatory process, during which neutrophils respond by ingesting the crystals. The neutrophils release their phagolysosomes, causing tissue damage, which perpetuates the inflammation.

## MANIFESTATIONS AND COMPLICATIONS

The manifestations of gout are hyperuricemia, recurrent attacks of inflammation of a single joint, tophi in and around the joint, renal disease, and renal stones. Unless treated, the manifestations of gout appear in three stages: asymptomatic hyperuricemia, acute gouty arthritis, and tophaceous gout.

### Asymptomatic Hyperuricemia

The first stage is asymptomatic hyperuricemia, with serum levels averaging 9 to 10 mg/dL. Most people with hyperuricemia do not progress to further stages of the disease.

### Acute Gouty Arthritis

The second state is acute gouty arthritis. The acute attack, usually affecting a single joint, occurs unexpectedly, often beginning at night. It may be triggered by trauma, alcohol ingestion, dietary excess, or a stressor such as surgery. It is often precipitated by an abrupt or sustained increase in uric acid levels. The

## Manifestations of Gout

### ACUTE GOUTY ARTHRITIS

- Usually monoarticular, affecting metatarsophalangeal joint of great toe, instep, ankle, knee, wrist, or elbow
- Acute pain
- Red, hot, swollen, and tender joint
- Fever, chills, malaise
- Elevated WBC and sedimentation rate

### CHRONIC TOPHACEOUS GOUT

- Tophi evident on joints, bursae, tendon sheaths, pressure points, helix of ear
- Joint stiffness, limited ROM, and deformity
- Ulceration of tophi with chalky discharge

affected joint becomes red, hot, swollen, and exquisitely painful and tender.

Approximately 50% of initial attacks of acute gouty arthritis occur in the metatarsophalangeal joint of the great toe. Other sites for acute attacks include the instep of the foot, ankles, heels, knees, wrists, fingers, and elbows. The pain, often intense, peaks within several hours and may be accompanied by fever and an elevated WBC and sedimentation rate. (See the box above.) The affected joints are swollen, the skin over the joint is warm and dusky red.

Acute attacks of gouty arthritis last from several hours up to several weeks and typically subside spontaneously. There are no long-lasting sequelae, and the client enters an asymptomatic period called the intercritical period. The intercritical period may last up to 10 years; however, approximately 60% of people experience a recurrent attack within 1 year. Successive attacks tend to last longer, occur with increasing frequency, and resolve less completely than the initial attack.

## Tophaceous (Chronic) Gout

Tophaceous or chronic gout occurs when hyperuricemia is not treated. The urate pool expands, and monosodium urate crystal deposits (tophi) develop in cartilage, synovial membranes, tendons, and soft tissues. They are seen most often in the helix of the ear; in tissues surrounding joints and bursae (especially around the elbows and knees); along tendons of the finger, toes, ankles, and wrists; on ulnar surfaces of the forearms; along the shins of the legs; and on other pressure points. The skin over tophi may ulcerate, exuding chalky material containing inflammatory cells and urate crystals. Tophi can also develop in the tissues of the heart and spinal epidura. Although tophi themselves are not painful, they may restrict joint movement and cause pain and deformities of the affected joints. Tophi may also compress nerves and erode and drain through the skin.

Kidney disease may occur in clients with untreated gout, particularly when hypertension is also present. Urate crystals are deposited in renal interstitial tissue. Uric acid crystals also form in the collecting tubules, renal pelvis, and ureter, forming stones. Renal stones are 1000 times more prevalent in people with primary gout (McCance & Huether, 2002).

The stones can range in size from a grain of sand to a massive structure filling the spaces of the kidney. Uric acid stones can potentially obstruct urine flow and lead to acute renal failure.

## COLLABORATIVE CARE

The classic presentation of acute gouty arthritis is so distinctive that the diagnosis can often be based on the client's history and physical examination. Treatment is directed toward terminating an acute attack, preventing recurrent attacks, and reversing or preventing complications resulting from crystal deposition in tissues and formation of uric acid kidney stones.

### Diagnostic Tests

Diagnostic testing is performed to establish an accurate diagnosis and direct long-term therapy.

- *Serum uric acid* is nearly always elevated (usually above 7.5 mg/dL) and is indicative of hyperuricemia.
- *WBC count* shows significant elevation, reaching levels as high as $20,000/mm^3$ during an acute attack.
- *Eosinophil sedimentation rate (ESR* or *sed rate)* is elevated during an acute attack from the acute inflammatory process that accompanies deposits of urate crystals in a joint.
- A *24-hour urine specimen* is analyzed to determine uric acid production and excretion.
- *Analysis of fluid* aspirated from the acutely inflamed joint or material aspirated from a tophus shows typical needle-shaped urate crystals, providing the definitive diagnosis of gout.

### Medications

Medications are used to terminate an acute attack, prevent further attacks, and reduce serum uric acid levels to prevent long-term sequelae of the disease. It is important to treat the acute attack of gouty arthritis before initiating treatment to reduce serum uric acid levels, because an abrupt decrease in serum uric acid may lead to further acute manifestations. Pharmacologic therapy is a mainstay of treatment in achieving these goals.

#### Acute Attack

NSAIDs are the treatment of choice for an acute attack of gout. Indomethacin (Indocin) is the most frequently used NSAID for gout, although others are equally effective. During an acute attack, indomethacin is usually prescribed at 50 mg every 8 hours until the client's manifestations have resolved. Other NSAIDs which may be prescribed include ibuprofen (Motrin), naproxen (Naprosyn, Anaprox), tolmetin sodium (Tolectin), piroxicam (Feldene), and sulindac (Clinoril). While extremely effective, NSAIDs are contraindicated for clients with active peptic ulcer disease, impaired renal function, or a history of hypersensitivity reactions to the drugs. (NSAIDS are fully described in Chapter 8.) 🔗

Colchicine can dramatically affect the course of an acute attack. Joint pain begins to diminish within 12 hours of the initiation of treatment and disappears within 2 days. Colchicine apparently acts by interrupting the cycle of urate crystal depo-

sition and inflammation in an acute attack of gout. It has no anti-inflammatory effect in other forms of arthritis, and its use is limited to gout. The use of colchicine is limited by significant side effects. When administered orally, the majority of clients develop significant abdominal cramping, diarrhea, nausea, or vomiting. Intravenous administration is limited by potential toxic effects including local pain, tissue damage if extravasation occurs during injection, bone marrow suppression, and disseminated intravascular coagulation (DIC). It is contraindicated for clients who have significant gastrointestinal, renal, hepatic, or cardiac disease.

Corticosteroids may also be prescribed for the client with acute gouty arthritis. If possible, the intra-articular route is preferred for monoarticular arthritis to avoid the multiple systemic effects of steroid therapy. When gout is polyarticular, corticosteroids may be administered either orally or intravenously.

Analgesics may also be prescribed during an acute episode of gouty arthritis. Either codeine or meperidine (Demerol) may be administered orally every 4 hours to manage the client's pain. Aspirin is avoided because it may interfere with uric acid excretion.

### Prophylactic Therapy

In clients at high risk for future attacks of acute gout, prophylactic therapy with daily colchicine may be initiated. Prophylaxis is particularly useful during the first 1 to 2 years of treatment with antihyperuricemic agents. Although colchicine does not affect the serum uric acid directly, it reduces the frequency of attacks by preventing crystal deposition within the joint. The doses required to achieve this effect are small, and few side effects are associated with therapy.

Treatment to reduce serum uric acid levels is typically initiated for clients with recurring gout, tophi, or renal damage. Asymptomatic hyperuricemic clients require no treatment. Uricosuric agents are used for clients who do not eliminate uric acid adequately; allopurinol is prescribed for clients who produce excessive amounts of uric acid. Uricosuric drugs block the tubular reabsorption of uric acid, promoting its excretion and reducing serum levels. These drugs reduce the frequency of acute attacks, particularly when administered with colchicine. Probenecid (Benemid) and sulfinpyrazone (Aprazone, Anturane, Zynol) are the primary uricosuric drugs employed.

Allopurinol (Zyloprim) is a xanthine oxidase inhibitor that lowers plasma uric acid levels and facilitates the mobilization of tophi. Because of its effectiveness in lowering serum uric acid levels, it may trigger an attack of acute gout. The nursing implications for medications used to treat gout are included on page 1236 in the Medication Administration box.

## Dietary Management

Dietary purines contribute only slightly to uric acid levels in the body, and no specific diet may be recommended. If a low-purine diet is recommended, the client should be taught that high purine foods include all meats and seafood, yeast, beans, peas, lentils, oatmeal, spinach, asparagus, cauliflower, and mushrooms. The obese client is advised to lose weight, but fasting is contraindicated for clients with gout. Alcohol intake and specific foods that tend to precipitate attacks are avoided.

## Other Treatments

During an acute attack of gouty arthritis, bed rest is prescribed. It is continued for approximately 24 hours after the attack has subsided, because early ambulation may bring about recurrence of acute manifestations (Tierney et al., 2001). The affected joint may be elevated, and hot or cold compresses may be applied for comfort.

A liberal fluid intake to maintain a daily urinary output of 2000 mL or more is recommended to increase urate excretion and reduce the risk of urinary stone formation. Urinary alkalinizing agents, such as sodium bicarbonate or potassium citrate, may be prescribed as well to minimize the risk of uric acid stones. It is important to monitor clients receiving these preparations carefully for signs of fluid and electrolyte or acid-base imbalances.

## NURSING CARE

Clients with gout provide self-care at home. Teaching focuses on self-management of pain and altered mobility.

## Nursing Diagnoses and Interventions

Pain is a primary focus for nursing interventions in the client experiencing an acute attack of gout. The client's mobility is also impaired during an acute attack, both because of discomfort and prescribed activity limitations.

### Acute Pain

The pain associated with an attack of acute gouty arthritis is intense and accompanied by exquisite tenderness of the affected joint. Measures to alleviate the pain are vital in the initial period until anti-inflammatory medications become effective and the acute inflammatory response is relieved. The following are important in teaching about pain relief.

- Position the affected joint for comfort. Elevate the joint or extremity (usually the foot) on a pillow, maintaining alignment. *Elevation and normal body alignment facilitate blood return from the affected joint, alleviating some of the edema.*
- Protect the affected joint from pressure, placing a foot cradle on the bed to keep bed covers off the foot. *A foot cradle keeps bed linens from applying pressure on the affected joint.*

**PRACTICE ALERT** *The affected joints are so painful that even the weight of a sheet can be unbearable.* ■

- Take anti-inflammatory and antigout medications as prescribed. In the initial period, colchicine may be given hourly. *These medications reduce the acute inflammatory response, gradually relieving discomfort.*

# Medication Administration

## The Client with Gout

### COLCHICINE

Colchicine is used to terminate an acute attack of gouty arthritis and to prevent recurrent episodes of the disease. Colchicine does not alter serum uric acid levels, but appears to interrupt the cycle of urate crystal deposition and inflammatory response. It may be administered either by mouth or intravenously. Colchicine is also available as a fixed-dose combination with a uricosuric agent, probenecid (Benemid). Only plain colchicine is used to treat an acute attack of gout; combination therapy is employed to prevent further attacks.

### Nursing Responsibilities

- Assess for possible contraindications to colchicine therapy, including serious gastrointestinal, renal, hepatic, or cardiac disease.
- Administer the following as ordered:
  - *Intravenous doses:* Give undiluted or diluted in up to 20 mL sterile normal saline for injection. Administer over a period of 2 to 5 minutes.
  - *Oral doses:* Give on an empty stomach to facilitate absorption.
- Evaluate for adverse effects, including abdominal cramping, nausea, vomiting, and diarrhea, and report promptly, because these side effects may necessitate discontinuation of the drug.

### Client and Family Teaching

- Drink 3 to 4 quarts of liquid per day.
- Report adverse responses, including gastrointestinal problems, fatigue, bleeding, easy bruising, or recurrent infections, to the physician.
- Do not drink alcohol.

### URICOSURIC DRUGS

  Probenecid (Benemid)
  Sulfinpyrazone (Anturane)

Probenecid is a uricosuric drug that inhibits the tubular reabsorption of urate, promoting the excretion of uric acid and decreasing serum uric acid levels. Sulfinpyrazone is a uricosuric drug that potentiates the renal excretion of uric acid, reducing serum uric acid levels. It is used to prevent recurrent attacks of acute gouty arthritis and treat chronic gout.

### Nursing Responsibilities

- Assess for prior hypersensitivity responses to this drug.
- Administer after meals or with milk to minimize gastric distress.
- Increase fluid intake to at least 3 L/day to prevent the formation of uric acid kidney calculi.
- Administer sodium bicarbonate or potassium citrate as ordered to maintain an alkaline urine.
- Do not administer aspirin to clients receiving probenecid because salicylates interfere with the action of the drug.
- Monitor clients receiving the following drugs concurrently with probenecid for increased or toxic effects: penicillin and related antibiotics, indomethacin, acetaminophen, naproxen, ketoprofen, meclofenamate, lorazepam, and rifampin.
- Monitor for possible adverse effects of probenecid, including headache, dizziness, hepatic necrosis, nausea and vomiting, renal colic, bone marrow depression, anaphylaxis, fever, hives, and pruritus.
- Administer sulfinpyrazone with meals or antacid to minimize gastric distress.

- Monitor clients taking sulfinpyrazone with other sulfa drugs for increased or toxic effects; monitor for hypoglycemia in clients receiving insulin or oral hypoglycemics concurrently, and monitor for bleeding or increased anticoagulant effect in clients receiving warfarin concurrently.
- Assess for contraindications to therapy with sulfinpyrazone, including active peptic ulcer disease, a history of hypersensitivity to phenylbutazone or other pyrazoles, or blood dyscrasias.

### Client and Family Teaching

- Do not take aspirin or products containing aspirin while taking probenecid. Use acetaminophen for relief of mild pain.
- Drink at least 3 quarts of fluids per day to minimize the risk of kidney stone formation.
- Take sulfinpyrazone with meals to minimize gastric distress, and report epigastric pain, nausea, or black stools to the physician promptly

### ALLOPURINOL (ZYLOPRIM)

Allopurinol acts on purine metabolism, reducing the production of uric acid and decreasing serum and urinary concentrations of uric acid. It is used for clients with manifestations of primary or secondary gout, including acute attacks, tophi, joint destruction, urinary stones, and nephropathy. It is not indicated for use in the treatment of asymptomatic hyperuricemia.

### Nursing Responsibilities

- Monitor intake and output and increase fluid intake to approximately 3 L/day.
- Monitor for desired effect of decreased serum uric acid levels, and for adverse effects such as nausea, diarrhea, and rash.
- Assess BUN and creatinine levels prior to the initiation of and during treatment with allopurinol. Report signs of impaired renal function such as an elevated BUN and creatinine, decreased urine output, and dilute or frothy urine to the physician.
- Administer with meals to minimize gastric distress.
- Monitor CBC periodically because allopurinol therapy may cause bone marrow depression.
- In clients receiving warfarin concurrently, monitor prothrombin times and be alert to evidence of bleeding, because allopurinol prolongs the half-life of warfarin.
- Monitor clients receiving chlorpropamide, cyclophosphamide, hydantoin, theophylline, vidarabine, or ACE inhibitors concurrently for increased drug effects.
- Discontinue the drug and notify the physician immediately if the client develops a rash. Rash and hypersensitivity responses occur more frequently in clients receiving ampicillin, amoxicillin, or thiazide diuretics.

### Client and Family Teaching

- Stop taking the drug and report any skin rash, painful urination, blood in the urine, eye irritation, or swelling of the lips or mouth to the physician immediately.
- Take the medication after meals to minimize gastric distress.
- Drink 3 to 4 quarts of fluid daily to maintain a urinary output greater than 2 L/day.
- Acute gouty attacks may occur during the initial stages of allopurinol therapy; continue therapy prescribed for attacks (such as colchicine) to minimize acute episodes.
- Do not take a double dose of medication if you miss a dose.

- Take analgesics as prescribed. *Supplemental analgesia may be necessary in the acute period until the inflammatory response is mediated.*
- Maintain bed rest. *It is important to immobilize the affected joint and promote rest to prevent exacerbation of joint inflammation.*

## Impaired Physical Mobility

Bed rest is prescribed to prevent further urate mobilization and joint inflammation as well as to protect the affected joint.

- Encourage active and passive ROM exercises of joints and muscle-tensing exercises on unaffected limbs. *These exercises help maintain joint mobility, muscle tone, and the client's sense of well-being.*
- When ambulation is allowed, suggest using a walker or cane as needed. *Weight bearing on the affected limb may be restricted until the inflammation is totally relieved.*
- Resume normal activities as allowed by the physician. *Initial acute attacks of gouty arthritis do not cause permanent damage to the affected joint, and the client can resume usual activities once the attack has subsided.*

## Home Care

Discuss the following topics with the client.

- *The disease and its manifestations.* Tell the client that initial attacks cause no permanent damage but that recurrent attacks can lead to permanent damage and joint destruction. Discuss other potential effects of continued hyperuricemia, including tophaceous deposits in subcutaneous and other connective tissues. Discuss the potential for kidney damage and kidney stones.
- *The rationale for and use of prescribed medication.* Stress the need to continue the medication until the physician discontinues it, even though the client is free of manifestations of gout.
- *The importance of a high intake of fluids each day and avoiding the use of alcohol.*

## THE CLIENT WITH OSTEOMALACIA

**Osteomalacia,** often referred to as *adult rickets,* is a metabolic bone disorder characterized by inadequate or delayed mineralization of bone matrix in mature compact and spongy bone. Bone mineralization requires adequate calcium and phosphate ions in extracellular fluid. When either of these ions is insufficient due to (1) inadequate calcium intake or decreased calcium absorption from the intestines because of insufficient vitamin D, and (2) increased renal losses or decreased intestinal absorption of phosphate, the bone matrix is not mineralized and cannot sustain weight bearing. Marked deformities of weight-bearing bone and pathologic fractures occur. The primary causes of osteomalacia are vitamin D deficiency and hypophosphatemia. Osteomalacia can be corrected with treatment.

Osteomalacia has been almost nonexistent in the United States because many foods are fortified with vitamin D, but its incidence is increasing among older adults, very-low-birth-weight infants, and people who adhere to strict vegetarian diets. It is a significant health problem in cultures whose diets tend to be deficient in calcium and vitamin D. Women in northern China, Japan, and northern India have a higher incidence of the disorder than men because of the combined effects of pregnancy, lactation, and more indoor confinement (Porth, 2002).

The major risk factors for vitamin D deficiency are a diet low in vitamin D, decreased endogenous production of vitamin D because of inadequate sun exposure, impaired intestinal absorption of fats (vitamin D is a fat-soluble vitamin), and disorders that interfere with the metabolism of vitamin D to its active forms. Gastrectomy and small bowel disorders may reduce the absorptive surface of the bowel to the extent that nutrients are not completely or adequately absorbed. Both vitamin D and calcium absorption may be affected. Hepatobiliary disorders that interfere with bile production and release, and chronic pancreatic insufficiency with inadequate pancreatic enzyme production, also can affect the absorption of fats and vitamin D from the bowel. Once absorbed, vitamin D is metabolized in the liver and the kidney to its active form; therefore, liver disorders such as cirrhosis and renal disorders can affect this activation. Certain drugs, such as isoniazid, rifampin, and anticonvulsants, accelerate vitamin D metabolism, resulting in less availability to the tissues. Renal excretion of vitamin D is increased in some kidney disorders such as nephrotic syndrome (Box 39–2).

---

### BOX 39–2  ■  Causes of Osteomalacia

**VITAMIN D DEFICIENCY**
- Inadequate dietary intake
- Lack of sun exposure
- Malabsorption from intestines: gastrectomy, small bowel disorders, gall bladder disease, chronic pancreatic insufficiency
- Renal or liver disorders
- Drug effects: isoniazid, rifampin, anticonvulsants

**PHOSPHATE DEPLETION**
- Inadequate intake
- Impaired absorption due to chronic antacid use
- Impaired renal tubular reabsorption due to either acquired or genetic disorders

**SYSTEMIC ACIDOSIS**
- Renal tubular acidosis
- Ureterosigmoidostomy
- Fanconi's syndrome

**BONE MINERALIZATION INHIBITORS**
- Hypophosphatasia
- Sodium fluoride or disodium etidronate (Didronel)
- Aluminum intoxication

**CHRONIC RENAL FAILURE**

**CALCIUM MALABSORPTION**

Hypophosphatemia can be the result of insufficient dietary intake, excessive losses through the urine or stool, or a shift into the cells. Alcohol abuse is the most common cause of hypophosphatemia, because of related dietary deficiencies, vomiting, antacid use, and increased renal excretion of phosphate. Ingesting large amounts of nonabsorbable antacids causes increased phosphate losses in the stool. Several acquired and genetic disorders cause increased losses of phosphate in the urine.

## PATHOPHYSIOLOGY AND MANIFESTATIONS

The two main causes of osteomalacia are (1) insufficient calcium absorption in the intestine due to a lack of calcium or resistance to the action of vitamin D and (2) increased losses of phosphorus through the urine (Porth, 2002). In its natural form, vitamin D is obtained from certain foods and ultraviolet radiation of the sun. Vitamin D maintains adequate serum levels of calcium and phosphate for normal mineralization of the bone. Vitamin D deficiency or resistance to its action disrupts the normal mineralization of the bone, causing softening of the bone.

Vitamin D is inactive when it is absorbed from the intestine or synthesized from exposure to ultraviolet light. For vitamin D to become active, a two-step process must occur. Vitamin D (and its metabolites) is transported in the blood to the liver, where it is converted to calcidiol. Calcidiol is then transported to the kidney and transformed to an active form, calcitriol.

The active form of vitamin D is needed for optimal absorption of calcium and phosphorus from the intestine. Calcium and phosphorus are transported in the blood to the bones for normal mineralization. If there is a lack of vitamin D, calcium and phosphorus are not absorbed from the intestine, and serum calcium and phosphorus levels therefore fall. A deficiency in these minerals in turn activates the parathyroid glands, with loss of calcium and phosphorus from bone. The continued loss of calcium and phosphate in the bone disrupts bone mineralization.

Impaired bone mineralization causes abnormalities in both spongy and compact bone. The osteoid (the soft, noncalcified part of the matrix) continues to be produced but is not mineralized. This abnormal buildup of demineralized bone leads to gross deformities of the long bones, spine, pelvis, and skull, because the bone is soft and unable to bear the weight and stress of body movement.

The manifestations of osteomalacia include bone pain and tenderness (see box in next column). As the disease progresses, fractures occur (Porth, 2002). In contrast to osteoporosis, osteomalacia is not associated with a significant occurrence of hip fractures. Instead, pathologic fractures occur in the commonly weakened areas (e.g., distal radius and proximal femur).

## COLLABORATIVE CARE

Once the specific cause is determined, appropriate therapy will correct the disorder. Osteomalacia may be difficult to differentiate from osteoporosis because the manifestations are very similar; however, certain diagnostic tests can help pinpoint its diagnosis.

### Manifestations of Osteomalacia

- Bone pain: May be vague and generalized at first, becoming more intense with activity as the disease progresses; occurs most frequently in the pelvis, long bones of the extremities, spine, and ribs.
- Difficulty changing from lying to sitting position, sitting to standing position, and so on.
- Muscle weakness: Frequently an early sign in severe cases.
- Waddling gait: May be due to pain and muscle weakness.
- Dorsal kyphosis: May occur in severe cases.
- Pathologic fractures

## Diagnostic Tests

A history of inadequate dietary intake, renal failure, or some malabsorption states may suggest osteomalacia. Table 39–1 compares the diagnostic findings of osteomalacia with those of osteoporosis and Paget's disease.

- *X-rays* demonstrate the effects of generalized bone demineralization: trabecular bone loss, cyst formation, compression fractures, bowing and bending deformities of the long bones, and osteoid deposits, particularly in the vertebral bodies and pelvis.
- *Serum calcium* level may be normal or low, depending on the cause of the disease. Calcium levels may be reduced when calcium absorption is impaired or in severe vitamin D deficiency. Secondary hypoparathyroidism may shift calcium from the bone into extracellular fluid, maintaining a normal serum calcium level.
- *Serum parathyroid hormone* is frequently elevated as a compensatory response to hypocalcemia in renal failure or vitamin D deficiency.
- *Serum alkaline phosphatase* level usually is elevated.

## Medications

Therapeutic management of osteomalacia depends on the cause of the disease. Because the causes are so diverse, it is difficult to generalize treatment. Most clients are placed on vitamin D therapy. Calcium and phosphate supplements also may be indicated. Radiologic evidence of healing often is apparent within weeks of initiating therapy.

## NURSING CARE

Managing the client with osteomalacia includes assessing the client's current dietary intake of vitamin D, calcium, and phosphorus and exposure to ultraviolet light. It also includes managing client responses to bone pain and tenderness, fractures, and muscle weakness.

Teaching is important not only for the client with osteomalacia, but also for people at risk for developing the disease. When milk and other dairy products began to be fortified with vitamin D, the incidence of childhood rickets decreased dramatically. Now many clients are unaware of the importance of vitamin D, calcium, and phosphorus to bone health.

Older adults as a group are at high risk for osteomalacia because of dietary deficiencies and possible physical mobility limitations that restrict their exposure to sunlight. Teach older adults about the importance of maintaining an adequate intake of milk and other dairy products that are not only rich in calcium and phosphorus, but also are fortified with vitamin D. Few other food sources provide enough vitamin D to meet recommended levels. Cod liver oil may be used as a supplement, as it contains significant amounts of vitamin D. Supplements are not recommended, however, for clients who get adequate vitamin D through dietary sources and sun exposure, because this fat-soluble vitamin may become toxic at high levels. Instruct clients who are taking supplements to report to their primary care provider symptoms such as anorexia, nausea and vomiting, frequent urination, muscle weakness, and constipation that may be indicative of hypervitaminosis D.

Instruct the client with osteomalacia about safety measures to prevent falls. Discuss the importance of eliminating scatter rugs and clutter from living areas to prevent tripping. Teach the client to place a night light in hallways and the bathroom to prevent falls associated with nighttime toileting. Suggest installing grab bars in the shower and tub and next to the toilet for safety.

Teach clients with bone pain and muscle weakness to use assistive devices such as walkers, canes, or crutches when ambulating. Provide referrals to physical therapy for teaching clients how to safely use these devices. Encourage clients to participate in a supervised exercise program such as water aerobics or tai chi to improve muscle strength and balance.

# DEGENERATIVE DISORDERS

Degenerative disorders, especially degenerative joint disease, are the most common form of arthritis in the older adult. Both primary and secondary forms are seen in adults of all ages. Primary or idiopathic osteoarthritis, the most common type, occurs without a clear precipitating factor. Secondary osteoarthritis is associated with an identifiable cause. For instance, it may be related to trauma to a joint, inflammation, skeletal disorders such as congenital hip dysplasia, or metabolic disorders. Regardless of cause, degenerative disorders of the joints and muscles can lead to impaired mobility and chronic pain. These problems may in turn cause disability, especially in the performance of ADLs by older adults.

## THE CLIENT WITH OSTEOARTHRITIS

**Osteoarthritis (OA)** (also labeled *degenerative joint disease*) is the most commonly occurring of all forms of arthritis. This disease is characterized by loss of articular cartilage in articulating joints and hypertrophy of the bones at the articular margins. OA may be idiopathic (without known cause) or secondary (associated with known risk factors). Idiopathic OA affects more than 60 million people in the United States, affecting adult men more than women until after age 55, when the incidence becomes twice as high in women (McCance & Huether, 2002) The joints most affected are in the hand, wrist, neck, lower back, hip, knee, ankles, and feet. Men are more likely than women to have hip OA, while postmenopausal women more often have hand OA.

Localized OA affects only one or two joints. Generalized OA affects three or more joints. Generalized OA may also be classified as nodal (involving the hand) or nonnodal (no hand involvement). Nodal OA may also affect the knees, hips, cer-

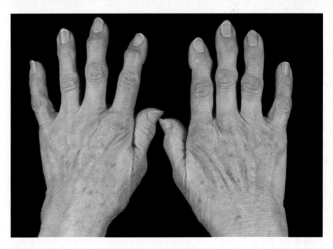

**Figure 39–2** ■ Typical interphalangeal joint changes associated with osteoarthritis.

*Source: L. Samsuri/Custom Medical Stock Photo.*

vical spine, and lumbar spine. Idiopathic OA most commonly affects the terminal interphalangeal joints (*Heberden's nodes*), and less often the proximal interphalangeal joints (*Bouchard's nodes*) (Figure 39–2 ■), the joints of the thumb, the hip, the knee, the metatarsophalangeal joint of the big toe, and the cervical and lumbar spine. Secondary OA may occur in any joint from an articular injury.

### RISK FACTORS

Idiopathic OA is associated with increasing age, with more than 90% of individuals affected by age 40 but few experiencing manifestations until after 50 or 60 (Maher, Salmond, & Pellino, 2002). It has been suggested that OA may be inherited as an autosomal recessive trait, with genetic defects that cause premature destruction of the joint cartilage. The causes of secondary OA include trauma, mechanical stress, inflammation of joint structures, joint instability, neurologic disorders, endocrine disorders, and selected medications.

Excessive weight contributes to the development of OA, especially in the hip and knee. Inactivity is another risk factor. Moderate recreational exercise has been shown to both decrease the chance of developing OA and the progression of manifestations when OA is present. People involved in strenuous, repetitive exercise (such as participating in sports) have an increased risk of developing secondary OA.

Other risk factors that are linked to OA are hormonal factors such as decreased estrogen in menopausal women, excessive growth hormone, and increased parathyroid hormone.

## PATHOPHYSIOLOGY

The cartilage that lines joints provides a smooth surface, so that the bones of the joint glide over one another without friction, and it distributes the load from one bone to the next, dissipating the mechanical stress that occurs with joint loading. This cartilage normally contains more than 70% water. More than 90% of its dry weight is collagen, which provides strength, and proteoglycans, which provide elasticity and stiffness to compression. Cartilage cells, the chondrocytes, nest in this meshwork of collagen and proteoglycans. Normal articular cartilage exudes some of its water with compression, providing lubrication for joint surfaces. This water is reabsorbed during relaxation of the joint.

In OA, proteoglycans and collagen are lost from the cartilage as a result of enzymatic degradation. The water content of the cartilage increases as the collagen matrix is destroyed. With the loss of proteoglycans and collagen fibers, the cartilage becomes yellow or brownish gray and loses its tensile strength. Surface ulcerations occur, and fissures develop in deeper layers of the cartilage. Eventually, large areas of articular cartilage are lost, and underlying bone is exposed. The bone thickens in exposed areas, reducing its ability to absorb energy in joint loading. Cysts can also develop in the bone. Cartilage-coated **osteophytes** (bony outgrowths often called "joint mice") change the anatomy of the joint. As these spurs or projections enlarge, small pieces may break off, leading to mild synovitis (inflammation of the synovial membrane).

## MANIFESTATIONS AND COMPLICATIONS

The onset of OA is usually gradual and insidious, and the course slowly progressive. Pain and stiffness in one or more joints (usually weight bearing) are the first manifestations of OA. The pain is localized to the affected joints and may be described as a deep ache. It typically is aggravated by use or motion of the joint and relieved by rest, although it may become persistent as the disease progresses. Pain at night may be accompanied by paresthesias (numbness, tingling). Pain may also be referred to other parts of the body; for example, OA of the lumbosacral spine may cause severe pain along the path of the sciatic nerve. Following periods of immobility, such as sleeping all night or after a long automobile ride, involved joints may stiffen. Usually only a few minutes of activity are neces-

| TABLE 39–2 | Manifestations of Osteoarthritis |
|---|---|
| **Affected Site** | **Manifestations** |
| Interphalangeal joints | • *Heberden's nodes*—bony enlargements of distal joints; may cause pain, redness, swelling<br>• *Bouchard's nodes*—bony enlargement of proximal joints |
| First carpometacarpal | • Swelling, tenderness at base of thumb<br>• Crepitus with movement<br>• "Squared" appearance of joint |
| Spine | • Localized pain and stiffness<br>• Muscle spasm<br>• Limited range of motion<br>• Nerve root compression with radicular pain and motor weakness |
| Hips | • Pain referred to inguinal area, buttock, thigh, or knee<br>• Loss of internal rotation<br>• Limited extension, adduction, and flexion |
| Knees | • Pain and bony enlargement<br>• Effusions<br>• Crepitus<br>• Instability and deformity with advanced disease |

sary to relieve the stiffness. Range of motion of the joint decreases as the disease progresses, and grating or crepitus may be noted during movement. Bony overgrowth may cause joint enlargement, and flexion contractures may occur because of joint instability. In OA, enlarged joints are characteristically bony-hard and cool on palpation. Manifestations specific to affected joints are outlined in Table 39–2.

OA of the spine may involve the vertebral bodies and intervertebral disks, the diarthrodial joints, or both. Spondylosis is degenerative disk disease. As the intervertebral disks degenerate, disk space between the vertebrae is lost. Degenerative disk disease may be complicated by herniated disk, the protrusion of the nucleus pulposus of the disk. Herniation usually occurs in a lateral direction, potentially compressing nerve roots and causing radicular (distributed along the nerve) pain and muscle weakness. See Chapter 41 for further discussion of disk disorders.

Disk degeneration and joint space narrowing alter the mechanics of the spinal column, promoting osteoarthritic changes in the articular processes (the facet joints) of the vertebrae. The cartilage covering the inferior and superior articular processes degenerates, causing localized pain, stiffness, muscle spasm, and limited range of motion. Osteophytes may form on articular processes, further contributing to pain and muscle spasm.

The presentation of OA in older clients is similar to that in younger adults. However, in this population, the risk of debilitation because of OA is greater, and the disease may progress faster. In addition, pain, stiffness, and limited range of motion increase the risk of falls and fractures in the older adult.

# COLLABORATIVE CARE

At this time, no treatment is available to arrest the process of joint degeneration. Appropriate management, however, is important to relieve pain and maintain the client's function and mobility.

## Diagnostic Tests

The diagnosis of OA is generally based on the client's history and physical examination and X-rays of affected joints. Characteristic changes of OA are visible in X-ray studies of affected joints. Initially, irregular joint space narrowing is seen. Progressive changes include increased density of subchondral (under cartilage) bone, osteophyte formation at the joint periphery, and the formation of cysts in the bone.

## Medications

The pain of OA often can be managed through the use of analgesics such as aspirin or acetaminophen. Acetaminophen is generally preferred for use in older clients because it has fewer toxic side effects. NSAIDs may also be prescribed. These medications are discussed in more detail in Chapter 8. ⊂⊃ Capsaicin cream can reduce joint pain and tenderness when applied topically to affected joints.

Medications that have proven effective in decreasing the pain and stiffness of OA are the NSAID COX-2 inhibitors meloxicam (Mobic), celecoxib (Celebrex), and rofecoxib (Vioxx). These medications provide analgesic/anti-inflammatory effects comparable to conventional NSAIDS, but have fewer adverse effects on the gastrointestinal and renal systems. Clients should be taught to report any signs of gastrointestinal bleeding to their health care providers. If meloxicam is prescribed, teach the client that it may decrease the effectiveness of ACE inhibitors and diuretics, may increase lithium levels and toxicity, and there is a risk of increased bleeding if taken at the same time as aspirin, warfarin, and the herbs feverfew, garlic, ginger, and ginko.

Potent anti-inflammatory medications, such as systemic corticosteroids, are seldom prescribed for clients with OA, although intra-articular corticosteroid injections may be used. With intra-articular injections, a long-acting corticosteroid medication, often mixed with a local anesthetic such as lidocaine, is injected directly into the joint space of the affected joints. Although this procedure may provide marked pain relief, it can hasten the rate of cartilage breakdown if performed more frequently than every 4 to 6 months.

## Conservative Treatment

Conservative treatment may include any or all of the following:

- Physical therapy for ROM exercises
- Resting the involved joint
- Using a cane, crutches, or a walker
- Weight loss, if indicated
- Analgesic and anti-inflammatory medications

## Surgery

Surgical procedures can provide dramatic results for clients with significant chronic pain and loss of joint function. Although elective surgical procedures are frequently avoided in the older adult, even aged clients can benefit significantly if they do not have a chronic medical condition that contraindicates surgery.

### Arthroscopy

Although arthroscopic debridement and lavage of involved joints has been used, certain questions exist about its effectiveness and thus research is ongoing (Reuters Health, 2002).

### Osteotomy

An **osteotomy,** an incision into or transection of the bone, may be performed to realign an affected joint, particularly when significant bony overgrowth or osteophyte formation has occurred. This procedure may also be used to shift the joint load toward areas of less severely damaged cartilage. Although osteotomy does not halt the process of OA, it may have a beneficial effect on joint function and pain, delaying the need for a joint replacement by several years.

### Joint Arthroplasty

A **joint arthroplasty** is the reconstruction or replacement of a joint. Arthroplasty is usually indicated when the client has severely restricted joint mobility and pain at rest. Pain is virtually eliminated, and the function of the joint is generally improved. Arthroplasty may involve partial joint replacement or reshaping of the bones of a joint. For most clients with OA, both surfaces of the affected joint are replaced with prosthetic parts in a procedure known as a **total joint replacement.** Joints that may be replaced include the hip, knee, shoulder, elbow, ankle, wrist, and joints of the fingers and toes.

In a total joint replacement, some or all of the synovium, cartilage, and bone on both sides of the joint are removed. A metallic prosthesis is inserted to replace one joint surface (generally the load-end or distal portion of a weight-bearing joint). The other joint surface is replaced by a silicone-lined ceramic or plastic prosthesis.

Most prosthetic joints are uncemented, that is, made of porous ceramic and metal components inserted so that they fit tightly into existing bone. The implant is secured by new bone growth into the prosthesis, a process that requires approximately 6 weeks. Although a longer non-weight-bearing period is necessary initially until the prosthesis is fixed in place by the bony growth, the implant appears to have a longer useful life span than cemented prostheses. In a cemented joint replacement, methyl methacrylate (a pliable polymer that hardens to hold the prosthesis in place) is used to secure the prosthesis to existing bone. Although the client is able to resume normal activities more rapidly following a cemented joint replacement, methyl methacrylate initiates an inflammatory response, and the joint eventually loosens.

- In a *total hip replacement,* the articular surfaces of the acetabulum and femoral head are replaced. The entire head of the femur and part of the femoral neck are removed and replaced with a prosthesis (Figure 39–3 ■). The acetabulum is remodeled, and a prosthesis of high-molecular-weight polyethylene is inserted. The success rate for total hip replacement is reported to be greater than 90%. Approximately 250,000 total hip replacements are done each year in the United States; most are for treatment of OA (McCance & Huether, 2002). Potential problems associated with a total hip replacement include dislocation within the prosthesis, loosening of joint components from surrounding bone, and infection. If recurrent or ineffectively treated, these complications may necessitate removal of the prosthesis, resulting in severe shortening of the extremity and an unstable hip joint.

- *Total knee replacement* is performed if the client has intractable pain and X-ray films show evidence of arthritis of the knee. Several prosthetic devices involving removal of varying amounts of bone are available for knee joint replacement (Figure 39–4 ■). The femoral side of the joint is replaced with a metallic surface, and the tibial side with polyethylene. More than 80% of clients obtain significant or total relief of pain with a total knee replacement. They must, however, engage in a vigorous program of rehabilitation to achieve the best results. Joint failure is more common with knee replacement than with a total hip replacement. Loosened joint components, often on the tibial side, are the most common cause of failure.
- *Total shoulder replacement* is indicated for unremitting pain and marked limitation of range of motion because of arthritic involvement of both the humeral and glenoid joint surfaces of the shoulder. The joint is immobilized in a sling or abduction splint for 2 to 3 weeks following arthroplasty. Dislocation, loosening of the prosthesis, and infection are potential problems associated with total shoulder replacement.
- *Total elbow replacement* involves replacement of the humeral and ulnar surfaces of the elbow joint with a metal and polyethylene prosthesis. Pain and disabling stiffness of

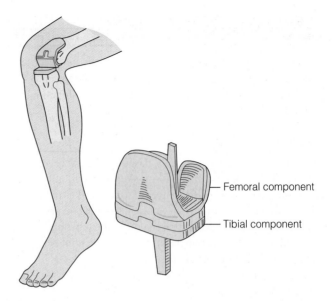

**Figure 39–4** ■ Total knee replacement.

the joint are indications for an elbow arthroplasty. Complications, including dislocation, fracture, tricep weakness, loosening, and infection, occur frequently.

Infection is the major complication associated with total joint replacement. Not only does infection interfere with healing and prolong recovery, but also it may necessitate removal of the prosthesis and may lead to loss of joint function. Other potential complications include circulatory impairment to the affected limb, thromboembolism, nerve damage, and dislocation of the joint.

Nursing care for the client undergoing total joint replacement is outlined on pages 1243–1244. Refer to Chapter 7 <a> for further discussion of care for the client undergoing surgery.

## Complementary Therapies

The following complementary therapies are examples of those that may be used by people with OA to relieve pain and stiffness (Springhouse, 1998).

- Bioelectromagnetic therapy
- Eliminating nightshade foods such as potatoes, tomatoes, peppers, eggplant, tobacco
- Taking nutritional supplements, such as boron, zinc, copper, selenium, manganese, flavonoids, evening primrose oil
- Herbal therapy
- Osteopathic manipulation
- Vitamin therapy
- Yoga

## NURSING CARE

OA is a chronic process for which there is no cure. The focus of nursing care for the client with OA is providing comfort, helping maintain mobility and ADLs, and assisting with adaptations to maintain life roles.

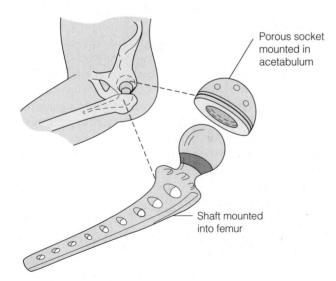

Porous socket mounted in acetabulum

Shaft mounted into femur

**Figure 39–3** ■ Total hip prosthesis.

# NURSING CARE OF THE CLIENT HAVING TOTAL JOINT REPLACEMENT

## PREOPERATIVE CARE

- Assess the client's knowledge and understanding of the planned operative procedure. Provide further explanations and clarification as needed. *It is important that the client have a clear and realistic understanding of the surgical procedure and expected results. Knowledge decreases anxiety and increases the client's ability to assist with postoperative care procedures.*

- Obtain a nursing history and physical assessment, including range of motion of the affected joints. *This information not only allows nurses to tailor care to the needs of the individual but also serves as a baseline for comparison of postoperative assessment data.*

- Explain necessary postoperative activity restrictions. Teach how to use the overhead trapeze for changing positions. *The client who learns and practices moving techniques before surgery can use them more effectively in the postoperative period.*

- Provide or reinforce teaching of postoperative exercises specific to the joint on which surgery is to be performed. *Exercises are prescribed postoperatively to (a) strengthen muscles providing joint stability and support, (b) prevent muscle atrophy and joint contractures; and (c) prevent venous stasis and possible thromboembolism.*

- Teach respiratory hygiene procedures such as the use of incentive spirometry, coughing, and deep breathing. *Adequate respiratory hygiene is imperative for all clients undergoing joint replacement to prevent respiratory complications associated with immobility and the effects of anesthesia. In addition, many clients undergoing total joint replacement are elderly and may have reduced mucociliary clearance.*

- Discuss postoperative pain control measures, including use of patient-controlled analgesia (PCA) or epidural infusion as appropriate. *It is important for the client to understand the purpose and use of postoperative pain control measures to allow early mobility and reduce complications associated with immobility.*

- Teach or provide prescribed preoperative skin preparation such as shower, shampoo, and skin scrub with antibacterial solution. *These measures help reduce transient bacteria that may be introduced into the surgical site.*

- Administer intravenous antibiotic as ordered. *Antibiotic therapy is initiated before or during surgery and continued postoperatively to further reduce the risk of infection.*

## POSTOPERATIVE CARE

- Check vital signs, including temperature and level of consciousness, every 4 hours or more frequently as indicated. Report significant changes to the physician. *These routine assessments provide information about the client's cardiovascular status and can give early indications of complications such as excessive bleeding, fluid volume deficit, and infection.*

- Perform neurovascular checks (color, temperature, pulses and capillary refill, movement, and sensation) on the affected limb hourly for the first 12 to 24 hours, then every 2 to 4 hours. Report abnormal findings to the physician immediately. *Surgery can disrupt the blood supply to or innervation of the af-*

*fected extremity. If so, rapid intervention is important to preserve the function of the extremity.*

- Monitor incisional bleeding by emptying and recording suction drainage every 4 hours and assessing the dressing frequently. *Significant blood loss can occur with a total joint replacement, particularly a total hip replacement.*

- Reinforce the dressing as needed. *The dressing is usually changed 24 to 48 hours after surgery but may need reinforcement if excess bleeding occurs.*

- Maintain intravenous infusion and accurate intake and output records during the initial postoperative period. *The client is at risk for fluid volume deficit in the initial postoperative period because of blood and fluid loss during surgery, as well as the effects of the anesthetic.*

- Maintain bed rest and prescribed position of the affected extremity using a sling, abduction splint, brace, immobilizer, or other prescribed device. *Proper positioning of the affected extremity is vital in the initial postoperative period so that the joint prosthesis does not become dislocated or displaced.*

- Help the client shift position at least every 2 hours while on bed rest. *Shifting of position helps prevent pressure sores and other complications of immobility.*

- Remind the client to use the incentive spirometer, to cough, and to breathe deeply at least every 2 hours. *These measures are important to prevent respiratory complications such as pneumonia.*

- Assess the client's level of comfort frequently. Maintain PCA, epidural infusion, or other prescribed analgesia to promote comfort. *Adequate pain management promotes healing and mobility.*

- Help the client get out of bed as soon as allowed. Teach and reinforce the use of techniques to prevent weight bearing on the affected extremity, such as the over-head trapeze, pivot turning, and toe-touch. *Early mobility prevents complications such as pneumonia and thromboembolism, but appropriate techniques must be used to prevent injury to the operative site.*

- Initiate physical therapy and exercises as prescribed for the specific joint replaced, such as quadriceps setting, leg raising, and passive and active range-of-motion exercises. *These exercises help prevent muscle atrophy and thromboembolism and strengthen the muscles of the affected extremity so that it can support the prosthetic joint.*

- Use sequential compression devices or antiembolism stockings as prescribed. *These help prevent thromboembolism and pulmonary embolus for the client who must remain immobile following surgery.*

- For the client with a total hip replacement, prevent hip flexion of greater than 90 degrees or adduction of the affected leg. Provide a seat riser for the toilet or commode. *These measures prevent dislocation of the joint.*

- Assess the client with a total hip replacement for signs of prosthesis dislocation, including pain in the affected hip or shortening and internal rotation of the affected leg.

*(continued on page 1244)*

## NURSING CARE OF THE CLIENT HAVING TOTAL JOINT REPLACEMENT (continued)

- For the client with a total knee replacement, use a continuous passive range-of-motion (CPM) device or range-of-motion exercises as prescribed. *Dislocation is not a problem with a knee replacement, and more emphasis is placed on range-of-motion exercises in the early postoperative period.*
- Maintain fluid intake and encourage a high-fiber diet. Administer stool softeners or rectal suppositories as needed. *Immobility contributes to the potential problem of constipation; these measures help maintain regular fecal elimination.*
- Encourage consumption of a well-balanced diet with adequate protein. *Adequate nutrition promotes tissue healing.*
- Teach or reinforce postdischarge exercises and activity restrictions. Emphasize the importance of scheduled follow-up physi-

cian visits. *Clients are discharged from the acute care facility before healing is complete. Exercises are prescribed and activities are resumed gradually to protect the integrity of the joint replacement and prevent contractures.*
- For those clients needing additional direct care after discharge, arrange placement in a long-term care or rehabilitation facility. *Activity restrictions may preclude discharge to home for some clients.*
- Make referrals as needed to home health agencies and physical therapy. *Clients often require home health care for both nursing care needs and continued physical therapy following discharge from acute or long-term care.*

## Health Promotion

Although OA cannot be prevented, maintaining a normal weight and having a program of regular, moderate exercise will reduce risk factors. Glucosamine and chrondroitin are popular nutritional supplements for OA that are increasingly popular and have been found to be of benefit in reducing manifestations. Clients should discuss these supplements with their health care provider before using them.

## Assessment

Collect the following data through the health history and physical examination (see Chapter 37).

- Health history: family history of OA, occupation, recreational activities, joint pain and stiffness, ability to carry out ADLs and self-care activities
- Physical assessment: height/weight; gait, joints: symmetry, size, shape, color, appearance, temperature, pain, crepitus, range of motion, Heberden's nodes, Bouchard's nodes

## Nursing Diagnoses and Interventions

### Chronic Pain

Pain is a primary manifestation of OA. As joint tissues degenerate and changes in joint structure occur, the amount of discomfort generally increases. The pain associated with OA increases with activity and tends to be relieved with rest. Nonpharmacologic comfort measures are appropriate, with mild analgesics used to supplement these as needed.

- Monitor the client's level of pain, including intensity, location, quality, and aggravating and relieving factors. *Accurate assessment of pain provides a basis for evaluation of the effect of interventions.*
- Teach clients to take prescribed analgesic or anti-inflammatory medication as needed. *Analgesics reduce the perception of pain and may decrease muscle spasm as well. Anti-inflammatory medication may be ordered to decrease local inflammatory response in affected joints.*
- Encourage rest of painful joints. *The pain of OA is often relieved by joint rest.*

- Suggest applying heat to painful joints using the shower, a tub or sitz bath, warm packs, hot wax baths, heated gloves, or diathermy, which uses high-frequency electrical currents to generate heat. *Heat application reduces accompanying muscle spasm, relieving pain. Moist heat penetrates deeper than dry heat; diathermy delivers heat directly to lesions in deeper body tissues.*
- Emphasize the importance of proper posture and good body mechanics for walking, sitting, lifting, and moving. *Good body mechanics and posture reduce stress on affected joints.*
- Encourage the overweight client to reduce. *Excess weight places abnormal stress on joints, particularly the knees.*
- Teach the client to use splints or other devices on affected joints as needed. *These assistive devices help maintain the correct anatomic position of the joint and relieve stress.*
- Encourage the client to use nonpharmacologic pain relief measures such as progressive relaxation, meditation, visualization, and distraction. *These adjunctive pain relief measures can reduce the client's reliance on analgesics and increase comfort.*

### Impaired Physical Mobility

As intra-articular cartilage degenerates and joint structures are altered, the client with OA experiences pain, stiffness, and decreased range of motion in affected joints. When the spine, large weight-bearing joints of the hips and knees, or the ankles and feet are affected, physical mobility can be significantly reduced.

- Assess the range of motion of affected joints. *Assessing joint mobility is important as a basis for planning appropriate interventions.*
- Perform a functional mobility assessment, evaluating the client's gait, ability to sit and rise from sitting, ability to step into and out of the tub or shower, and negotiation of stairs. *The functional assessment provides vital data about the client's ability to maintain ADLs.*
- Teach the client active and passive ROM exercises as well as isometric, progressive resistance, and low-impact aerobic exercises. *Active ROM exercises help maintain muscle tone and mobility of affected joints and prevent contractures.*

*Isometric and progressive resistance exercises improve muscle tone and strength; aerobic exercise improves endurance and cardiovascular fitness.*

**PRACTICE ALERT** *The older woman with OA may be more willing to take part in weight-bearing exercises if she does so as part of a group or organized activity.* ■

- Suggest the client take analgesics or other pain relief measures prior to exercise or ambulation. *With decreased pain, the client is able to perform exercises better and ambulate greater distances.*
- Encourage the client to plan periods of rest during the day. *Rest helps reduce fatigue, pain, and joint stress.*
- Teach the client how to use ambulatory aids such as a cane or walker as prescribed. *These devices help relieve some weight bearing and stress on affected joints.*

### Self-Care Deficit

Just as OA of the lower extremities can reduce the client's mobility, OA of the upper extremities (the wrist, hand, and finger joints in particular) can significantly interfere with performance of ADLs such as cooking and brushing the hair. When the lower extremities are affected, bathing and toileting can be difficult.

- Perform a functional assessment of the upper and lower extremities. For upper extremities, assess the ability to touch the back of the head, and to hold and use small items such as eating utensils. *The functional assessment provides important data about the client's ability to provide self-care.*
- Assess the client's home setting to determine the need for assistive devices such as handrails, grab bars, walk-in shower stall, or shower chair and handheld showerhead. *Many assistive devices are relatively easy and inexpensive to obtain and can significantly improve the client's independence in performing ADLs.*

- Assist the client in obtaining other assistive devices such as long-handled shoehorns, zipper grabbers, long-handled tongs or grippers for retrieving items from the floor, jar openers, and special eating utensils. *These devices can prolong independence in performing ADLs.*

## Using NANDA, NIC, and NOC

Chart 39–2 shows links between NANDA nursing diagnoses, NIC, and NOC when caring for the client with OA.

## Home Care

Because of the chronicity of OA, clients and their families need appropriate teaching to manage the disease and its consequences effectively. Much of the teaching focus is on preservation of joint function and mobility. Discuss the following topics.

- Safeguard against hazards to safe mobility, such as scatter rugs. Encourage installation of safety devices such as hand rails and grab bars.
- Understand the disease process and its chronic degenerative nature.
- Learn exercise techniques, including range of motion, isometric, postural, stretching, and strengthening, to maintain healthy cartilage, preserve range of motion, and develop supportive muscles and tendons. A walking program is beneficial for clients with OA of the knee.
- Do not overuse or stress affected joints with heavy lifting, excessive stair climbing or bending, or other repetitive actions.
- Balance exercise with rest of affected joints through the use of whole body rest, splints, or assistive devices. In addition, sit in a straight chair without slumping; avoid soft chairs or recliners and sleep on a firm mattress or use a bed board.
- Use pain relief measures including prescribed or over-the-counter analgesic medications, and nonpharmacologic pain relief measures such as heat, rest, massage, relaxation, and meditation.

---

### CHART 39–2 NANDA, NIC, AND NOC LINKAGES

#### The Client with Osteoarthritis

| NURSING DIAGNOSES | NURSING INTERVENTIONS | NURSING OUTCOMES |
|---|---|---|
| • Chronic Pain | • Medication Administration<br>• Pain Management<br>• Heat/Cold Application | • Comfort Level<br>• Pain: Disruptive Effects |
| • Impaired Physical Mobility | • Mobility Level<br>• Exercise Therapy: Joint Mobility<br>• Exercise Therapy: Ambulation | • Ambulation: Walking<br>• Joint Movement: Active |
| • Knowledge Deficit: Weight Loss | • Teaching: Prescribed Diet<br>• Nutrition Management<br>• Weight Management | • Knowledge: Diet |

*Note: Data from Nursing Outcomes Classification (NOC) by M. Johnson & M. Maas (Eds.), 1997, St. Louis: Mosby; Nursing Diagnoses: Definitions & Classification 2001–2002 by North American Nursing Diagnosis Association, 2001, Philadelphia: NANDA; Nursing Interventions Classification (NIC) by J.C. McCloskey & G. M. Bulechek (Eds.), 2000, St. Louis: Mosby. Reprinted by permission.*

## Nursing Care Plan
## A Client with Osteoarthritis

Robert Cerulli is a 72-year-old retired commercial fisherman who has experienced arthritic pain in his hips for the past 10 to 15 years. Over the past year, the pain in his right hip has become severe, prompting him to seek medical attention. Significant degenerative changes in both hip joints are noted on X-ray films. The physician recommends a total replacement of the right hip, and total replacement of the left hip to follow in 6 to 12 months. Mr. Cerulli has preoperative teaching and tests the afternoon prior to his surgery, scheduled for 0800 the following morning.

### ASSESSMENT

Christie Phlaugh, RN, completes a nursing history and examination of Mr. Cerulli on admission. Reviewing his medical record, she notes that Mr. Cerulli has mild Parkinson's disease and is taking carbidopa/levodopa (Sinemet 25-100) four times a day to control his symptoms. No other chronic medical conditions have been reported. Mr. Cerulli says he has been essentially healthy his entire life. He has no known allergies to medications, has never smoked, and consumes only small amounts of alcohol.

On examination of Mr. Cerulli, Ms. Phlaugh notes that he is alert and oriented. His vital signs are BP 116/64, P 68 regular, R 18, T 97.4°F (36.3°C) PO. Peripheral pulses are strong and equal in the upper extremities, and slightly weaker but equal in the lower extremities. His feet are cool to touch but have immediate capillary refill. He has full ROM of his shoulders, elbows, and wrists. The ROM of both hips is significantly restricted. Hip flexion beyond 90 degrees prompts pain on both sides. Both flexion and extension of the knees are limited slightly. Mr. Cerulli walks with a limp, favoring his right hip, and has a shuffling gait.

Preoperative laboratory studies including CBC, coagulation studies, chemistry panel, and urinalysis show a serum creatinine of 1.7 mg/dL and BUN of 30 mg/dL, with no other abnormal values noted. His ECG and chest X-ray show no apparent pathologies. Cefazolin (Ancef) 500 mg is to be administered intravenously at 0600 prior to surgery, and Mr. Cerulli is to shower and shampoo with antibacterial soap at bedtime. The physical therapist meets with Mr. Cerulli to evaluate his mobility and begin teaching him about postoperative weight-bearing restrictions.

### DIAGNOSIS (Postoperative)

- *Acute pain* related to surgical incision
- *Impaired physical mobility* related to activity and weight-bearing restrictions
- *Risk for infection* related to disruption in skin integrity
- *Risk for ineffective tissue perfusion, right leg* related to vascular disruption and edema

### EXPECTED OUTCOMES

- Maintain an adequate level of comfort postoperatively as demonstrated by:
  - The ability to move easily within restrictions.
  - Compliance with instructions to cough and breathe deeply.
  - Verbal expressions of comfort.
- Remain free of adverse consequences of immobility such as pneumonia, pressure areas, thromboembolism, or contracture.
- Remain free of infection.

- Maintain adequate perfusion of affected leg.
- Remain free of injury postoperatively.

### PLANNING AND IMPLEMENTATION

- Assess pain at least hourly during first 24 to 48 hours postoperatively, and as needed thereafter.
- Instruct in the use of patient-controlled analgesia (PCA) and monitor its effectiveness.
- Help change position at least every 2 hours; encourage the use of the overhead trapeze to shift positions frequently.
- Maintain sequential compression device and antiembolic stocking as ordered; remove for 1 hour daily.
- Encourage the use of the incentive spirometer hourly for first 24 hours, then at least every 2 hours while awake.
- Assist out of bed three times a day after the first 24 hours.
- Maintain abduction of the right hip with pillows.
- Perform passive ROM exercises of unaffected extremities every shift.
- Encourage frequent quadriceps-setting exercises and plantar and dorsiflexion of feet.
- Assess the surgical site frequently; report signs of excess bleeding or inflammation.
- Monitor temperature every 4 hours.
- Assess pulses, color, movement, and sensation of right foot hourly for the first 24 hours, then every 2 hours for 24 hours, then every 4 hours.

### EVALUATION

Mr. Cerulli returns to the orthopedic unit from the postanesthesia care unit. He becomes confused and disoriented during the first 36 hours after surgery, but his orientation and thought processes gradually clear. His family has stayed with him, and he has not experienced injury or other adverse consequences from his confusion. Otherwise, Mr. Cerulli has had an uneventful postoperative recovery. Six days after surgery, he is transferred to an extended care rehabilitation facility for further therapy until he is able to ambulate with partial weight bearing on his affected leg. He returns home 5 weeks after surgery, able to use a walker for ambulation. Arrangements are made for an overbed trapeze, elevated toilet seat, and shower chair in his home. A home health nurse and physical therapist visit Mr. and Mrs. Cerulli weekly for a month following his discharge. During this time he gradually resumes full weight bearing. Mr. Cerulli expresses pleasure with the relief of his hip pain and says he has no fear of having his left hip replaced in the future.

### Critical Thinking in the Nursing Process

1. Mr. Cerulli's preoperative laboratory work showed a modest elevation in his serum creatinine and BUN. What do these studies indicate? How might these changes affect nursing responsibilities related to medication administration for Mr. Cerulli?
2. Mr. Cerulli became confused postoperatively. What factors in his history might have alerted the nurses to this possibility? How might anesthesia and postoperative analgesics have contributed to his confusion?
3. Develop a care plan for Mr. Cerulli using the nursing diagnosis, *Acute confusion*.

See Evaluating Your Response in Appendix C.

- For the client who has had a total joint replacement, discuss the following:
  - Use and weight bearing of the affected limb
  - Proper use of splints, braces, slings, or other devices to maintain the desired limb position during healing
  - Appropriate environmental modifications, such as an overhead trapeze for getting out of bed, elevated toilet seats, and types of chairs to use and avoid when sitting
  - Prescribed exercises
  - Use of assistive devices for ambulation, such as crutches or a walker
  - Possible complications, including signs of infection or dislocation, and the need to notify the physician promptly if these occur.
- Make referrals to home care, physical or occupational therapy, or other community agencies as indicated.

## THE CLIENT WITH MUSCULAR DYSTROPHY

**Muscular dystrophy (MD)** is a group of inherited muscle diseases that cause progressive muscle degeneration and wasting. The differences in the types of MD relate to the age at onset, the gender affected by the disorder, the muscles involved, and the rate at which the disease progresses. These factors are summarized in Table 39–3. In the majority of cases of MD, there is a positive family history.

The most common form of MD, Duchenne's muscular dystrophy, is inherited as a recessive single gene defect on the X chromosome (a sex-linked recessive disorder), and is transmitted from the mother to male children (Porth, 2002). This disorder affects males exclusively and occurs in 1 of 3500 live male births. It can be recognized early in pregnancy in about 95% of cases by genetic studies; or in late pregnancy through amniocentesis. Genetic counseling cannot be reliably used to prevent this disease because there is no way to determine if the woman carries the defective gene. The manifestations appear in early childhood, with the average lifespan being about 15 years after onset.

Other types of MD have an onset at any age, and a slow progression with a normal lifespan.

## PATHOPHYSIOLOGY AND MANIFESTATIONS

The basic defect in MD is unknown; however, three theories have been proposed. The *vascular* and *neurogenic theories* suggest that the cause is a lack of blood supply to the muscle or a disturbance in the interaction between the nerve and muscle. The *membrane theory* suggests that an alteration in the cell membranes of the muscle causes them to degenerate. Recent genetic studies have shown a deficiency in the amount of dystrophin, a muscle membrane protein, in clients with Duchenne's MD. Dystrophin plays an important role in protecting the muscle against mechanical stresses.

All forms of MD exhibit manifestations of muscle weakness. The specific muscles involved depend on the type of MD. As the disease progresses, the person develops difficulty with ambulation and eventually becomes wheelchair-bound and finally bed-bound. Cardiac abnormalities, endocrine abnormalities, and mental retardation may also be involved.

## COLLABORATIVE CARE

Because there is no cure or specific treatment for MD, care focuses on preserving and promoting mobility. A multidisciplinary approach, involving many members of the health care team, is necessary to meet the physical and psychologic needs of these clients and their families.

TABLE 39–3  Types of Muscular Dystrophy

| Type | Sex and Age at Onset | Clinical Manifestations | Progression |
|------|----------------------|-------------------------|-------------|
| Duchenne | Males Age 3 to 5 | Weakness of pelvic and shoulder girdles Waddling gait Toe walking Lordosis Cardiac abnormalities Low IQ in 50% of cases | Rapid; client usually confined to wheelchair by age 15; death occurs by age 20 |
| Myotonic | Males and females Any age | Myotonia of hand muscles Muscular weakness of arms and legs Cardiac abnormalities Endocrine abnormalities Mental retardation (common) | Slow; death usually occurs in early 50s |
| Becker's | Males Age 5 to 20 | Weakness of pelvic and shoulder girdles | Slow; client usually confined to wheelchair at 25 years after onset; normal life span |
| Facioscapulohumeral | Males and females Age 10 to 20 | Weakness of face and shoulder girdles | Slow; normal life span |
| Limb-girdle | Males and females Age 20 to 40 | Weakness of shoulder and pelvic girdles | Extremely variable; usually slow |

Diagnosis and classification of the muscular dystrophies are most often based on the manifestations and the pattern of muscle involvement. Biochemical examination, muscle biopsy, and electromyography confirm the diagnosis. Tests include the following:

- *Creatine kinase* (CK-MM, the isoenzyme found in skeletal muscle) is elevated in the client with suspected MD.
- *Muscle biopsy* will show fibrous connective tissue and fatty deposits that displace functional muscle fibers.
- *Electromyogram* (EMG) readings show a decrease in amplitude.

## NURSING CARE

Nursing care for a client with MD focuses on promoting independence and mobility and providing psychologic support for both the client and family. A holistic approach is essential in planning and implementing care.

### Nursing Diagnoses and Interventions

#### Self-Care Deficit

The progressive muscle weakness that is associated with MD impairs the client's ability to perform self-care. Nursing interventions with rationales follow:

- Provide clients and family with supportive care during the progress of the disease. *The goal of treatment is to prolong each functional stage and delay or prevent deformity. When transition from ambulation to a wheelchair occurs, depression and grief may occur.*
- Promote independence. Encourage tasks the client can accomplish rather than letting the client struggle with tasks that may prove frustrating. *All forms of MD result in progressive muscle weakness. Management of the disease is directed toward keeping the client as functional as possible while preventing any deformities.*

### Home Care

Teaching of the client with MD focuses on maintaining function and independence and preventing deformities. Teach prescribed exercises such as stretching and counterposturing exercises. For the client with braces, discuss skin care and ways to prevent irritation under the brace. Because the client may have weakness involving muscles of respiration, instruct the client on ways to prevent respiratory infections, such as avoiding crowds during flu season and being immunized against pneumococcal pneumonia and influenza. Provide information about support services and organizations such as the Muscular Dystrophy Association.

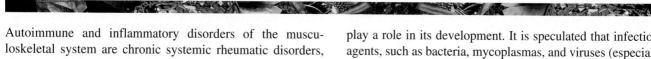

# AUTOIMMUNE AND INFLAMMATORY DISORDERS

Autoimmune and inflammatory disorders of the musculoskeletal system are chronic systemic rheumatic disorders, characterized by diffuse inflammatory lesions and degenerative changes in connective tissues. The disorders have similar clinical features and may affect many of the same structures and organs.

## THE CLIENT WITH RHEUMATOID ARTHRITIS

**Rheumatoid arthritis (RA)** is a chronic systemic autoimmune disease that causes inflammation of connective tissue, primarily in the joints. It is found worldwide, affecting 1% to 2% of the total population and all races. It affects 3 times as many women as men. The onset of RA occurs most frequently between the ages of 20 and 40 years. Its course and severity are variable, and the range of manifestations is broad. Manifestations of RA may be minimal, with mild inflammation of only a few joints and little structural damage, or relentlessly progressive, with multiple inflamed joints and marked deformity. Most clients exhibit a pattern of symmetric involvement of multiple peripheral joints and periods of remission and exacerbation.

The cause of RA is unknown. A combination of genetic, environmental, hormonal, and reproductive factors are thought to play a role in its development. It is speculated that infectious agents, such as bacteria, mycoplasmas, and viruses (especially Epstein-Barr virus) may play a role in initiating the autoimmune processes present in RA.

The course of RA is variable and fluctuating. Remissions are most likely to occur in the first year of the disease. The rate at which joint deformities develop is not constant. Disease progression is fastest during the first 6 years, slowing thereafter. RA contributes to disability and a tendency to shorten life expectancy.

The incidence of RA increases with age up to about 70 years. Although the onset and manifestations of RA are much the same in older and younger clients, differentiating between RA and OA in the older adult may be difficult at times. It is important to establish an accurate diagnosis, however, because the management of these disorders differs significantly. Clinical features distinguishing RA from OA are listed in Table 39–4.

For older clients, RA is managed much as it is for younger people. However, prolonged bed rest or inactivity is not prescribed for acute episodes, because it may result in irreversible immobility in the older adult. Also, pharmacologic therapy is used with greater caution because of the increased risk of toxicity. In many cases, less emphasis is placed on preventing joint deformity and more emphasis on maintaining function for the older client with RA.

TABLE 39-4    A Comparison of the Manifestations of Rheumatoid Arthritis and Osteoarthritis

| Feature | Rheumatoid Arthritis | Osteoarthritis |
|---|---|---|
| Onset | Usually insidious, may be abrupt | Insidious |
| Course | Generally progressive, characterized by remissions and exacerbations | Slowly progressive |
| Pain and stiffness | Predominant on arising, lasting >1 hour; also occurs after prolonged inactivity | Pain with activity; stiffness following periods of immobility generally relieved within minutes |
| Affected joints | • Appear red, hot, swollen; "boggy" and tender to palpation; decreased ROM, weakness<br>• Multiple joints affected in symmetric pattern; PIP, MCP, wrists, knees, ankles, and toes often involved | • Affected joints may appear swollen; cool and bony hard on palpation; decreased ROM<br>• One or several joints affected including hips, knees, lumbar and cervical spine, PIP and DIP, wrist, and 1st MTP joint |
| Systemic manifestations | Fatigue, weakness, anorexia, weight loss, fever; rheumatoid nodules; anemia | Fatigue |

## PATHOPHYSIOLOGY

It is believed that long-term exposure to an unidentified antigen causes an aberrant immune response in a genetically susceptible host. As a result, normal antibodies (immunoglobulins) become autoantibodies and attack host tissues. These transformed antibodies, usually present in people with RA, are called **rheumatoid factors (RFs).** The self-produced antibodies bind with their target antigens in blood and synovial membranes, forming immune complexes (see Chapter 9 ⊂⊃ for further information about autoimmune processes).

The damage to cartilage that occurs in RA is the result of at least three processes (McCance & Huether, 2002):

- Neutrophils, T cells, and other synovial fluid cells are activated and degrade the surface layer of the articular cartilage.
- Cytokines (especially interleukin-1 and tumor necrosis factor alpha) cause the chondrocytes to attack the cartilage.
- The synovium digests nearby cartilage, releasing inflammatory molecules containing interleukin-1 and tumor necrosis factor alpha.

Leukocytes are attracted to the synovial membrane from the circulation, where neutrophils and macrophages ingest the immune complexes and release enzymes that degrade synovial tissue and articular cartilage. Activation of B and T lymphocytes results in increased production of rheumatoid factors and enzymes that increase and continue the inflammatory process.

The synovial membrane is damaged by the inflammatory and immune processes. It swells from infiltration of the leukocytes and thickens as cells proliferate and abnormally enlarge. The inflammation spreads and involves synovial blood vessels. Small venules are occluded and vascular flow to the synovial tissue decreases. As blood flow decreases and metabolic needs increase (from the increased number and size of cells), hypoxia and metabolic acidosis occur. Acidosis stimulates synovial cells to release hydrolytic enzymes into surrounding tissues, starting erosion of the articular cartilage and inflammation of the supporting ligaments and tendons.

The inflammation also causes hemorrhage, coagulation, and deposits of fibrin on the synovial membrane, in the intracellu-

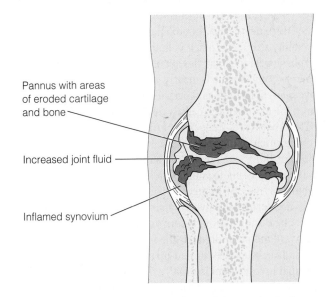

Pannus with areas of eroded cartilage and bone

Increased joint fluid

Inflamed synovium

**Figure 39–5 ■** Joint inflammation and destruction in rheumatoid arthritis. Note synovial inflammation with pannus formation and the erosion of cartilage and underlying bone.

lar matrix, and in the synovial fluid. Fibrin develops into granulation tissue (**pannus**) over denuded areas of the synovial membrane. The formation of pannus leads to scar tissue formation that immobilizes the joint (Figure 39–5 ■).

### Joint Manifestations

The onset of RA is typically insidious, although it may be acute (precipitated by a stressor such as infection, surgery, or trauma). Joint manifestations are often preceded by systemic manifestations of inflammation, including fatigue, anorexia, weight loss, and nonspecific aching and stiffness. Clients report joint swelling with associated stiffness, warmth, tenderness, and pain. The pattern of joint involvement is typically polyarticular (involving multiple joints) and symmetric. The proximal interphalangeal (PIP) and metacarpophalangeal (MCP) joints of the fingers, the wrists, the knees, the ankles, and the toes are most frequently involved, although RA can

MediaLink | RHEUMATOID ARTHRITIS CASE STUDY

affect any joint. Stiffness is most pronounced in the morning, lasting more than 1 hour. It may also occur with prolonged rest during the day and may be more severe following strenuous activity. Swollen, inflamed joints feel "boggy" or spongelike on palpation because of synovial edema. Range of motion is limited in affected joints, and weakness may be evident.

The persistent inflammation of RA causes deformities of the joint itself and supporting structures such as ligaments, tendons, and muscles. As the joint is destroyed, ligaments, tendons, and the joint capsule are weakened or destroyed. Joint cartilage and bone are also destroyed. Weakening or destruction of these supporting structures results in lack of opposition to muscle pull, causing deformity.

Characteristic changes in the hands and fingers include ulnar deviation of the fingers and subluxation at the MCP joints. Swan-neck deformity is characterized by hyperextension of the PIP joint with compensatory flexion of the distal interphalangeal (DIP) joints. A flexion deformity of the PIP joints with extension of the DIP joint is called a boutonnière deformity (Figure 39–6 ■). The ability to effect a pinch is limited by hyperextension of the interphalangeal joint and flexion of the MCP joint of the thumb.

Wrist involvement is nearly universal, leading to limited movement, deformity, and carpal tunnel syndrome. Inflammation of the elbows often causes flexion contracture.

The knees are frequently affected in RA, with visible swelling often obliterating normal contours. Instability of the knee joint along with quadriceps atrophy, contractures, and valgus (knock-knee) deformities can lead to significant disability. Ambulation may be limited by pain and deformities when the ankles and feet are involved. Typical deformities of the feet and toes include subluxation, hallux valgus (deviation of the great toe toward the other digits of the foot), lateral deviation of the toes, and cock-up toes (turned-up toes).

Spinal involvement is usually limited to the cervical vertebrae. Neck pain is common, and neurologic complications can occur.

## Extra-Articular Manifestations

RA is a systemic disease with a variety of extra-articular manifestations. These are seen particularly in clients with high levels of circulating rheumatoid factor. Fatigue, weakness, anorexia, weight loss, and low-grade fever are common when the disease is active. Anemia resistant to iron therapy frequently affects clients with RA. Skeletal muscle atrophy is common, usually most apparent in the musculature around affected joints.

Rheumatoid nodules may develop, usually in subcutaneous tissue in areas subject to pressure: on the forearm, olecranon bursa, over the MCP joints, and on the toes. Rheumatoid nodules are granulomatous lesions that are firm and either movable or fixed. They may also be found in viscera, including the heart, lungs, intestinal tract, and dura.

Other possible extra-articular manifestations of RA include subcutaneous nodules, pleural effusion, vasculitis, pericarditis, and splenomegly (enlargement of the spleen). The *Multisystem Effects of RA* are illustrated on page 1251.

## COLLABORATIVE CARE

The diagnosis of RA is based on the client's history, physical assessment, and diagnostic tests. Diagnostic criteria developed by the American Rheumatism Association are used as well (Box 39–3). At least four of seven criteria must be present to establish the diagnosis.

Once the diagnosis of RA has been established, the goals of therapy are to:

- Relieve pain.
- Reduce inflammation.
- Slow or stop joint damage.
- Improve well-being and ability to function.

No cure currently exists for RA; the goal of treatment is to relieve its manifestations. A multidisciplinary approach is used, with a balance of rest, exercise, physical therapy, and suppression of the inflammatory processes.

Because a cure is not available and traditional therapies are not always fully effective, the client with RA is vulnerable to quackery. Many nontraditional treatments, including diets, topical preparations, vaccines, hormones, plant extracts, and copper bracelets, have been put forth. These treatments are often costly, and none has been shown to be effective.

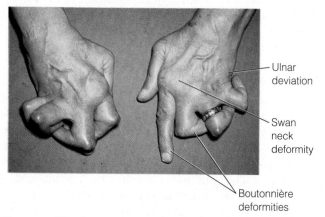

**Figure 39–6** ■ Typical hand deformities associated with rheumatoid arthritis.

Ulnar deviation

Swan neck deformity

Boutonnière deformities

*Source: Biophoto Associates/Photo Researchers, Inc.*

| BOX 39–3 ■ Diagnostic Criteria for Rheumatoid Arthritis |
|---|

■ Morning stiffness lasting for at least 1 hour and persisting over at least 6 weeks
■ Arthritis with swelling or effusion of three or more joints persisting for at least 6 weeks
■ Arthritis of wrist, MCP, or PIP joints persisting for at least 6 weeks
■ Symmetric arthritis with simultaneous involvement of corresponding joints on both sides of the body
■ Rheumatoid nodules
■ Positive serum rheumatoid factor
■ Characteristic radiologic changes of rheumatoid arthritis noted in hands and wrists

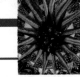

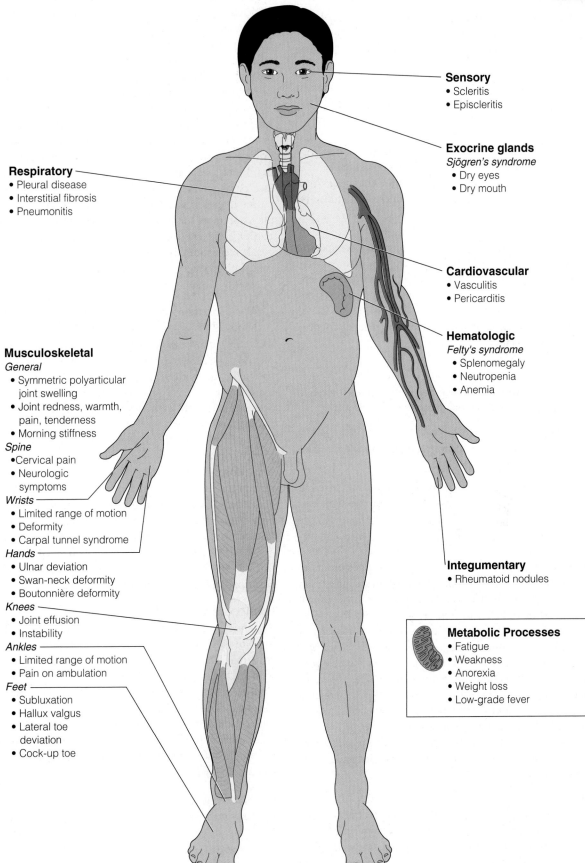

**Sensory**
- Scleritis
- Episcleritis

**Exocrine glands**
*Sjögren's syndrome*
- Dry eyes
- Dry mouth

**Respiratory**
- Pleural disease
- Interstitial fibrosis
- Pneumonitis

**Cardiovascular**
- Vasculitis
- Pericarditis

**Hematologic**
*Felty's syndrome*
- Splenomegaly
- Neutropenia
- Anemia

**Musculoskeletal**
*General*
- Symmetric polyarticular joint swelling
- Joint redness, warmth, pain, tenderness
- Morning stiffness

*Spine*
- Cervical pain
- Neurologic symptoms

*Wrists*
- Limited range of motion
- Deformity
- Carpal tunnel syndrome

*Hands*
- Ulnar deviation
- Swan-neck deformity
- Boutonnière deformity

*Knees*
- Joint effusion
- Instability

*Ankles*
- Limited range of motion
- Pain on ambulation

*Feet*
- Subluxation
- Hallux valgus
- Lateral toe deviation
- Cock-up toe

**Integumentary**
- Rheumatoid nodules

**Metabolic Processes**
- Fatigue
- Weakness
- Anorexia
- Weight loss
- Low-grade fever

## Diagnostic Tests

Diagnostic tests are used to help establish the diagnosis of RA, although no test specific to the disease is available. Testing is also used to rule out other forms of arthritis and connective tissue disorders.

- *Rheumatoid factors* (RFs), autoantibodies to IgG, are present in approximately 75% of people with RA. High levels of RF are often associated with severe RA.
- *Erythrocyte sedimentation rate (ESR)* is typically elevated and is often used as an indicator of disease and inflammatory activity when evaluating the effectiveness of treatment.
- *Synovial fluid examination* will demonstrate changes associated with inflammation, including increased turbidity (cloudiness), decreased viscosity, increased protein levels, and 3000 to 50,000 WBCs.
- *X-rays* of affected joints are taken, and are the most specific for diagnosis of RA. Early in the disease, few changes may be evident other than soft-tissue swelling and joint effusions. As the disease progresses, joint space narrowing and erosions are seen.
- *CBC* usually shows moderate anemia. The platelet count is often elevated.

## Treatments

The primary objectives in treating RA are to reduce pain and inflammation, preserve function, and prevent deformity.

### Medications

Four general approaches are used in the pharmacologic management of clients with RA.

- Aspirin and other NSAIDs and mild analgesics are used to reduce the inflammatory process and manage the signs and symptoms of the disease. Although these drugs may relieve manifestations of RA, they appear to have little effect on disease progression.
- The second approach uses low-dose oral corticosteroids to reduce pain and inflammation. Recent studies suggest that low-dose oral corticosteroids also may slow the development and progression of bone erosions associated with RA.
- A diverse group of drugs classified as disease-modifying or slow-acting antirheumatic drugs are employed in the third approach to treating RA. These drugs, which include gold compounds, D-penicillamine, antimalarial agents, and sulfasalazine, appear to alter the course of the disease, reducing its destruction of joints. Immunosuppressive and cytotoxic drugs are included in this category as well.
- Intra-articular corticosteroids may be used to provide temporary relief in clients for whom other therapies have failed to control inflammation.

### Aspirin

Aspirin is often the first drug prescribed in the treatment of RA unless its use is contraindicated for the client. Aspirin is an inexpensive and effective anti-inflammatory and analgesic agent. The dose of aspirin required to achieve a therapeutic blood level of 15 to 30 mg/dL and its full anti-inflammatory effect is approximately 4 g per day in divided doses (three or four 5 g [325 mg] tablets qid). This effective dose is just under the toxic dose, which produces tinnitus and hearing loss. The client may be instructed to increase the dose of aspirin gradually until either maximal improvement or toxicity occurs. If tinnitus develops, the client reduces the dose by two to three tablets per day until the tinnitus stops.

Gastrointestinal side effects and interference with platelet function are the greatest hazards of aspirin therapy. Clients are instructed to take aspirin with meals, milk, or antacids to minimize gastrointestinal distress and reduce the risk of GI bleeding. Enteric-coated forms of aspirin and nonacetylated salicylate compounds produce less gastric distress than plain or buffered aspirin and reduce the risk of gastric ulceration, but they are more expensive. Salsalate (Disalcid, Mono-Gesic, Salflex) and choline magnesium trisalicylate (Trilisate, Tricosal) are examples of nonacetylated salicylate products. All salicylate products are contraindicated for clients with a history of aspirin allergy.

### Other Nonsteroidal Anti-Inflammatory Drugs

A number of other nonsteroidal anti-inflammatory drugs (NSAIDs) are available for use in the management of RA if aspirin is not tolerated or effective. All NSAIDs act by inhibiting prostaglandin synthesis. Although the efficacy of all NSAIDs, including aspirin, is equivalent, client responses are individual. Several trials of different NSAIDs may be necessary to find the most effective drug.

Some NSAIDs are considerably more expensive than aspirin but may cause less gastrointestinal distress and require fewer doses per day. Gastric irritation, ulceration, and bleeding remain the most common toxic effects of NSAIDs. They can also affect the lower intestinal tract, leading to perforation or aggravation of inflammatory bowel disorders. All NSAIDs can also be toxic to the kidneys.

NSAIDs commonly prescribed for clients with RA are listed in Table 39–5. Nursing implications of their administration are described in Chapter 8. ⊘⊘

### Corticosteroids

Systemic corticosteroids can dramatically relieve the symptoms of RA and appear to slow the progression of joint destruction. The long-term use of corticosteroids is associated with multiple side effects, such as poor wound healing, increased risk of infection, osteoporosis, and gastrointestinal bleeding. Severe rebound manifestations can occur when these medications are discontinued. For these reasons, the use of systemic corticosteroids is limited to low dosages daily. The nursing implications for corticosteroid therapy are discussed in Chapter 9. ⊘⊘

### Disease-Modifying Drugs

Disease-modifying drugs are a diverse group of medications including drugs that modify immune and inflammatory responses, gold salts, antimalarial agents, sulfasalazine, and D-penicillamine (Table 39–6). They share characteristics that make them useful in the treatment of RA. Although beneficial

**TABLE 39-5** Examples of Nonsteroidal Anti-Inflammatory Drugs Used to Treat Rheumatoid Arthritis

| Drug | Average Dose | Comments and Precautions |
|---|---|---|
| Aspirin | 600–900 mg 4 to 6 times daily | Least expensive NSAID; associated with risk of GI ulceration, bleeding, and possible hemorrhage; may cause hepatotoxicity |
| Diclofenac (Voltaren) | 50 mg tid or qid; or 75 mg bid | Expensive; risk of hepatotoxicity |
| Etodolac (Lodine) | 200–400 mg q6h | Expensive; may have less gastrointestinal toxicity |
| Fenoprofen (Nalfon) | 300–600 mg tid or qid | Should not be administered to clients with impaired renal function; risk of GU effects such as dysuria, cystitis, hematuria, acute interstitial nephritis, and nephrotic syndrome |
| Flurbiprofen (Ansaid) | 50–100 mg tid or qid, not to exceed 300 mg/day | Expensive |
| Ibuprofen (Motrin, Advil, others) | 300 mg qid; 400–800 mg tid or qid | Available in prescription and over-the-counter forms; less gastric distress reported than with aspirin or indomethacin; discontinue if visual disturbances develop |
| Indomethacin (Indocin) | 25–50 mg bid or tid | A potent NSAID used for moderate to severe RA and acute episodes of chronic disease; higher incidence of adverse GI effects and CNS effects such as headache, dizziness, and depression |
| Ketoprofen (Orudis) | 50–75 mg tid or qid | Expensive; older adults and clients with renal insufficiency require lower doses |
| Meclofenamate sodium (Meclomen) | 100 mg bid to qid | Increased risk of adverse effects in older adults; GI effects include diarrhea and abdominal pain; anemia may develop during therapy |
| Nabumetone (Relafen) | 1000–2000 mg per day | Most common adverse effects include diarrhea, dyspepsia, and abdominal pain |
| Naproxen (Aleve, Anaprox, Naprosyn) | 250–500 mg bid | Available in prescription and over-the-counter preparations |
| Oxaprozin (Daypro) | 1200 mg daily | Expensive; risk of severe hepatotoxicity; rash may occur |
| Piroxicam (Feldene) | 20 mg daily in a single or divided dose | Expensive; GI side effects including stomatitis, anorexia, and gastric distress may occur more frequently than with other NSAIDs |
| Sulindac (Clinoril) | 150–200 mg bid | May be safer for use than other NSAIDs in clients with chronic renal disease; rare fatal hypersensitivity reaction with fever, liver function abnormalities, and severe skin reaction |
| Tolmetin (Tolectin) | 200–600 mg tid | Expensive; may have higher rate of side effects including GI distress, headache, dizziness, elevated blood pressure, edema, and weight gain |

effects are not apparent for several weeks or months following the initiation of therapy, they can produce not only clinical improvement but also evidence of decreased disease activity. Because their anti-inflammatory effect is minimal, NSAIDs are continued during therapy. As many as two-thirds of clients taking disease-modifying drugs show improvement, although these drugs have not been shown to slow bone erosion or facilitate healing. All of these drugs are fairly toxic, and close monitoring is necessary during the course of therapy.

Drugs that modify the autoimmune and inflammatory responses in clients with RA include leflunomide (Arava) and etanercept (Enbrel). Leflunomide reversibly inhibits an enzyme involved in the autoimmune process and etanercept inhibits the binding of tumor necrosis factor to receptor sites.

Gold salts may be administered by mouth, but the intramuscular route is preferred because it is more effective. The mode of action of gold is unknown, but it may produce clinical remission in some clients and decrease new bony erosions. Weekly therapy is continued until significant improvement is noted unless toxic reactions occur. Clients experiencing benefit from gold therapy may be continued on monthly injections

for several years. About 30% of clients on gold therapy experience toxic reactions, including dermatitis, stomatitis, bone marrow depression, and proteinuria. Mild skin reactions do not always necessitate discontinuation of therapy. CBC and urinalysis are monitored throughout treatment with gold to assess for more severe toxic responses.

Hydroxychloroquine (Plaquenil) is an antimalarial agent sometimes employed in the treatment of RA. Three to 6 months of therapy is required to achieve the desired response, and many clients do not experience significant benefit. Although hydroxychloroquine has a relatively low toxicity, it can cause pigmentary retinitis and vision loss. Clients receiving this drug require a thorough vision examination every 6 months.

Sulfasalazine, a drug regularly prescribed for chronic inflammatory bowel disease, may also be prescribed for RA. See Chapter 23 ⊙ for further discussion of this drug and its nursing implications. For clients not responding to the above preparations, penicillamine may be prescribed. Although this agent may be effective in the management of RA, toxic reactions are common and can be severe, including bone marrow suppression, proteinuria, and nephrosis.

**TABLE 39–6   Disease-Modifying Drugs Used to Treat Rheumatoid Arthritis**

| Class/Medications | Usual Dose | Adverse Effects | Comments/Nursing Responsibilities |
|---|---|---|---|
| Gold salts: Gold sodium thiomalate (Myochrysine) Aurothioglucose (Solganal) Auranofin (Ridaura Capsules) | Parenteral: 1st dose 10 mg; 2nd dose 25 mg, then 50 mg weekly IM Oral: 6 mg daily | • Pruritus, dermatitis • Stomatitis, metallic taste • Renal toxicity • Blood dyscrasias • Gastrointestinal distress | • Frequent UA and CBC • Monitor client after injection for flushing, fainting, dizziness, sweating, possible anaphylactic reaction |
| Antimalarial: Hydroxychloroquine (Plaquenil) | 200–600 mg daily with meals | • CNS reactions including irritability, nightmares, psychoses • Retinopathy • Alopecia, pruritus • Blood dyscrasias • GI disturbances | • Should not be used during pregnancy • Regular ophthalmologic examination required |
| Sulfasalazine (Azulfidine) | 2 g/day in divided doses with meals | • Anorexia, nausea, vomiting, gastric distress • Decreased sperm count • Headache • Rash • Blood dyscrasias • Hypersensitivity responses including Stevens-Johnson syndrome • CNS, liver, and renal toxicity | • Administer in evenly divided doses • Maintain high fluid intake • May cause yellow-orange skin or urine discoloration • Regular CBCs necessary |
| Penicillamine (Cuprimine, Depen Titratable) | 125–250 mg/day initially, slowly increased to a total of 1000–1500 mg/day | • Skin rashes • Fever • Gastrointestinal distress • Oral ulcers, loss of taste • Fever • Bone marrow depression with thrombocytopenia, leukopenia, anemia • Renal toxicity • May induce immune complex disorders such as Goodpasture's syndrome and myasthenia gravis | • Regular CBC and UA necessary • Administer on an empty stomach • Discontinue during pregnancy • May require 2 to 3 months of therapy before benefit is seen |

## Immunosuppressive Therapy

Immunosuppressive or cytotoxic drugs are increasingly employed in the management of RA. Indeed, many now consider methotrexate the treatment of choice for clients with aggressive RA. Methotrexate may be used along with NSAIDs in the initial treatment plan. A weekly dose can produce a beneficial effect in as few as 2 to 4 weeks. Gastric irritation and stomatitis are the most frequent side effects associated with methotrexate. Alcoholism, diabetes, obesity, advanced age, and renal disease increase the risk of toxic effects (hepatotoxicity, bone marrow suppression, interstitial pneumonitis).

Other immunosuppressive agents such as cyclosporine, azathioprine, and monoclonal antibodies have also been employed in the treatment of clients with severe, progressive, crippling disease who have failed to respond to other measures.

## Rest and Exercise

A balanced program of rest and exercise is an important component in the management of clients with RA. During an acute exacerbation of the disease, the client may be hospitalized, or a short period of complete bed rest may be prescribed. For most clients, regular rest periods during the day are beneficial to reduce manifestations of the disease. Additionally, splinting of inflamed joints reduces unwanted motion and provides local joint rest. A variety of orthotic devices are available to reduce joint strain and help maintain function.

Rest must be balanced with a program of physical therapy and exercise to maintain muscle strength and joint mobility. Range-of-motion exercises are prescribed to maintain joint function and prevent contractures. Isometric exercises are used to improve muscle strength without increasing joint stress. Isotonic exercises also help improve muscle strength and preserve function. Low-impact aerobic exercises, such as swimming and walking, have been shown to benefit clients with RA without adversely affecting joint inflammation or prompting acute episodes.

## Physical and Occupational Therapy

Physical and occupational therapists can design and monitor individualized activity and rest programs.

## Heat and Cold

Heat and cold are used for their analgesic and muscle-relaxing effects. Moist heat is generally the most effective, and can be provided by a tub bath. Joint pain is relieved in some clients through the application of cold.

## Assistive Devices and Splints

Assistive devices, such as a cane, walker, or raised toilet seat, are most useful for clients with significant hip or knee arthritis. Splints provide joint rest and prevent contractures. Night splints for the hands and/or wrists should maintain the extremity in a position of maximum function. The best "splint" for the hip is lying prone for several hours a day on a firm bed. In general, splints should be applied for the shortest period needed, should be made of lightweight materials, and should be easily removed to perform ROM exercises once or twice a day.

## Diet

For most clients with RA, an ordinary, well-balanced diet is recommended. Some clients may benefit from substitution of usual dietary fat with omega-3 fatty acids found in certain fish oils.

## Surgery

Surgical intervention may be employed for the client with RA at a variety of disease stages. Early in the course of the disease, synovectomy, excision of synovial membrane, can provide temporary relief of inflammation, relieve pain, and slow the destructive process, helping to preserve joint function. Arthrodesis, joint fusion, may be used to stabilize joints such as cervical vertebrae, wrists, and ankles. Arthroplasty, or total joint replacement, may be necessary in cases of gross deformity and joint destruction. Total joint replacement and nursing care needs of clients undergoing this surgery are discussed in the preceding section on OA.

## Other Therapies

Several newer treatments that are not yet in widespread use may be employed in clients with progressive RA. These experimental therapies are directed toward ameliorating the underlying immunologic process. Plasmapheresis has been used to remove circulating antibodies, moderating the autoimmune response. Total lymphoid irradiation decreases total lymphocyte levels, although serious adverse effects are associated with this treatment, and its continued efficacy has not been established.

## NURSING CARE

Clients with chronic, progressive, systemic disorders such as RA have multiple nursing care needs involving all functional health patterns. Physical manifestations of the disease often result in acute and chronic pain, fatigue, impaired mobility, and difficulty performing routine tasks. The disease also has many psychosocial effects. The client has an incurable chronic disease that may lead to severe crippling. Pain and fatigue can interfere with the client's ability to perform expected roles, such as home maintenance or job responsibilities. Even though the

client's hands may appear swollen, other people may not understand the systemic nature of the disease or realize the difference between RA and OA.

## Health Promotion

People with RA have control of their lives by becoming arthritis self-managers. They can help prevent deformities and the effects of arthritis by following prescriptions for exercise, rest, weight management, posture, and positioning. The following suggestions are outlined by the Moss Rehab Resource Net (2002).

- Never attempt an activity that cannot be stopped immediately if it proves to be beyond your power to complete it.
- Respect pain as a warning signal. When you experience pain, change your method of doing things, use equipment or tools if necessary, and take intermittent rest periods.
- Use the strongest joints available for an activity. For example, use the palm of your hand or the crook of your elbow instead of fingers for grasping while carrying.
- Avoid stress toward a position of deformity, such as when the fingers drift toward the little finger. For example, open a jar with your right hand and close a jar with your left hand.
- Avoid activities that need a tight grip, such as writing, wringing, and unscrewing.

## Assessment

Collect the following data through the health history and physical examination (see Chapter 37).

- Health history: pain, stiffness, fatigue, joint problems: location, duration, onset, effect on function, fever, sleep patterns, past illnesses or surgery, ability to carry out ADLs and self-care activities
- Physical assessment: height/weight; gait, joints: symmetry, size, shape, color, appearance, temperature, range of motion, pain; skin: nodules, purpura; respiratory: cough, crackles; cardiovascular: pericardial friction rub, apical bradycardia, $S_3$.

## Nursing Diagnoses and Interventions

Many nursing diagnoses may be appropriate for the client with RA. This section focuses on those related to its predominant manifestations and their effect on the client's life.

### Chronic Pain

Pain is a constant feature of RA when the disease is active. Pain accompanies both acute inflammation and lower levels of chronic inflammation. Some clients say the pain in joints and surrounding tissue is like a deep, constant toothache. Pain can significantly affect the client's ability to provide self-care and maintain daily activities. It also contributes to the client's fatigue.

- Monitor the level of pain and duration of morning stiffness. *Pain and morning stiffness are indicators of disease activity. Increased pain may necessitate changes in the therapeutic treatment plan.*
- Encourage the client to relate pain to activity level and adjust activities accordingly. Teach the importance of joint and whole-body rest in relieving pain. *Pain is an indicator of*

*excess stress on inflamed joints. Increasing pain indicates a need to decrease activity levels.*

- Teach the use of heat and cold applications to provide pain relief. The client may apply heat by showering or taking tub baths, or using warm compresses or other local applications such as paraffin dips. For clients who find that heat increases pain and swelling during periods of acute inflammation, cold packs may be more effective. *Both heat and cold have analgesic effects and can help relieve associated muscle spasms.*
- Teach about the use of prescribed anti-inflammatory medications and the relationship of pain and inflammation. *Anti-inflammatory agents reduce chemical mediators of inflammation and swelling, relieving pain.*
- Encourage using other nonpharmacologic pain relief measures such as visualization, distraction, meditation, and progressive relaxation techniques. *These techniques can reduce muscle tension and help the client focus away from the pain, decreasing the intensity of the pain experience.*

## Fatigue

The pain and chronic inflammatory processes associated with RA lead to fatigue. Other factors contribute as well. Discomfort often disrupts the client's sleep patterns. Anemia, muscle atrophy, and poor nutrition also play a role in the development of fatigue. The client with RA may experience depression or hopelessness, with associated manifestations of fatigue. (See the box in next column for related nursing research).

- Encourage a balance of periods of activity with periods of rest. *Both joint and whole-body rest are important to reduce the inflammatory response.*
- Stress the importance of planned rest periods during the day. *Rest is vital during acute exacerbations of the disease but also important to maintain the client in remission.*
- Help in prioritizing activities, performing the most important ones early in the day. *Assigning priorities helps the client avoid performing relatively unimportant activities at the expense of more meaningful and important ones.*
- Encourage regular physical activity in addition to prescribed ROM exercises. *Aerobic exercise promotes a sense of well-being and restful sleep patterns.*
- Refer to counseling or support groups. *Counseling and support groups can help the client develop effective coping strategies and deal with depression and hopelessness.*

## Ineffective Role Performance

Fatigue, pain, and the crippling effects of RA can interfere with the client's ability to pursue a career and fill other life roles, such as parent, spouse, or homemaker. As the client's role changes, so must the roles of other family members. This can contribute to changes in family processes, increased stress in the family, and further difficulty coping with the effects of the disease.

- Discuss the effects of the disease on the client's career and other life roles. Encourage the client to identify changes brought on by the disease. *Discussion helps the client to accept the changes and begin to identify strategies for coping with them.*
- Encourage the client and family to discuss their feelings about role changes and grieve lost roles or abilities. *Verbal-*

## Nursing Research

### Evidence-Based Practice for Fatigue in Clients with Rheumatoid Arthritis

Fatigue is a common systemic manifestation of rheumatoid arthritis (RA) that can interfere with clients' ability to maintain independence, their family roles, sense of well-being, and self esteem. In this study, researchers evaluated the effects of 12 weeks of low-impact aerobic exercise on fatigue, aerobic fitness, and disease activity in a group of 25 adults with rheumatoid arthritis (Neuberger et al., 1997). Study results showed that subjects who participated in aerobic exercise more frequently reported decreased fatigue, while those who participated less frequently reported increased fatigue. All subjects benefited from increased aerobic fitness, increased grip strength and decreased pain. Interestingly, measures of increased disease activity, including number of involved joints and sedimentation rate (erythrocyte sedimentation rate or ESR), remained stable or improved during the course of the study.

#### IMPLICATIONS FOR NURSING
Nurses and other health care providers should encourage clients with rheumatoid arthritis to maintain a regular schedule of activities such as walking, swimming, and other activities that place relatively little stress on joints. Regular activity improves the client's overall health and general fitness. It may help reduce disease activity, and promotes comfort and restful sleep. These can reduce fatigue and improve the client's functional capacity.

#### Critical Thinking in Client Care
1. How do you think regular low-impact aerobic exercise works to reduce disease activity in the client with rheumatoid arthritis?
2. Develop an exercise/activity plan for a client with RA that takes the disease manifestations into consideration and minimizes stress on affected joints.
3. What measures can the nurse recommend to promote comfort and uninterrupted, restful sleep for the client with RA?

*ization allows family members to validate and accept feelings about losses and changes, thus helping them to move into new roles.*

- Listen actively to concerns expressed by the client and family members; acknowledge the validity of concerns about the disease, prescribed treatment, and the prognosis. *Demonstrating acceptance of these feelings and concerns promotes trust and validates their reality.*

**PRACTICE ALERT** *Remember that grief resolution takes time and that clients may respond to loss with anger.* ■

- Help the client and family identify strengths they can use to cope with role changes. *Identifying strengths helps the client and family to consider role changes that maintain self-esteem and dignity.*
- Encourage the client to make decisions and assume personal responsibility for disease management. *Clients who assume*

*a personal and active role in managing their disease maintain a greater sense of self-control and self-esteem.*
- Encourage the client to maintain life roles as far as the disease allows. *Maintaining roles helps the client continue to feel useful and stay in contact with other people.*

### Disturbed Body Image

The acute and long-term effects of RA can affect the client's body image, leading to feelings of hopelessness and powerlessness, social withdrawal, and difficulty adapting to changes. When inflammation and joint deformity occur despite compliance, the client may have difficulty accepting the need to continue therapeutic measures, particularly those that have side effects or are costly or time consuming. In addition, unproven alternative treatment strategies and quackery may become increasingly attractive to the client.

- Demonstrate a caring, accepting attitude toward the client. *This attitude helps the client accept the physical changes brought on by the disease.*
- Encourage the client to talk about the effects of the disease, both physical effects and effects on life roles. *Verbalization helps the client identify feelings and gives the nurse opportunity to validate these feelings.*
- Encourage the client to maintain self-care and usual roles to the extent possible. Discuss the use of clothing and adaptive devices that promote independence. *Independence enhances the client's self-esteem.*
- Provide positive feedback for self-care activities and adaptive strategies. *Positive reinforcement encourages the client to continue adaptive measures and maintain independence.*

- Refer to self-help groups, support groups, and other agencies that provide assistive devices and literature. *These groups and agencies can help the client develop adaptive strategies to cope with the effects of RA, enhancing the client's self-concept, body image, and independence.*

### Using NANDA, NIC, and NOC

Chart 39–3 shows links between NANDA nursing diagnoses, NIC, and NOC when caring for the client with RA.

### Home Care

RA is typically a chronic, progressive disease. As with most diseases of this nature, involvement of the client and family in its management is vital. Education is an important nursing role in caring for clients with RA and their families. Address the following topics for home care of the client and for family members.

- Disease process and treatments, including rest and exercise
- Medications
- Management of stiffness and pain
- Energy conservation
- Use of assistive devices to maintain independence, including self-care aids such as handheld showers, long-handled brushes and shoe horns, and eating utensils with oversized or special handles
- Clothing options such as elastic waist pants without zippers, Velcro closures, zippers with large pull-tabs, and slip-on shoes
- How to apply splints and take care of skin
- Home and equipment modifications, such as a raised toilet seat, grab bars in the bathroom, a bath chair, or adapted counter heights for clients in a wheelchair

## CHART 39–3 NANDA, NIC, AND NOC LINKAGES

### The Client with Rheumatoid Arthritis

| NURSING DIAGNOSES | NURSING INTERVENTIONS | NURSING OUTCOMES |
|---|---|---|
| • Chronic Pain | • Medication Administration<br>• Pain Management<br>• Heat/Cold Application | • Comfort Level<br>• Pain: Disruptive Effects |
| • Fatigue | • Energy Management<br>• Sleep Enhancement | • Energy Conservation<br>• Rest |
| • Self-Care Deficit: Bathing/Hygiene; Dressing/Grooming; Feeding; Toileting | • Self-Care Assistance<br>• Teaching: Individual | • Self-Care: Activities of Daily Living<br>• Self-Care: Bathing/Hygiene; Dressing; Grooming; Eating; Toileting |
| • Powerlessness | • Emotional Support<br>• Self-Esteem Enhancement<br>• Environmental Management<br>• Self-Care Assistance<br>• Support Group | • Health Beliefs: Perceived Control<br>• Health Beliefs: Perceived Resources<br>• Social Support |
| • Ineffective Sexuality Patterns | • Teaching: Sexuality<br>• Sexual Counseling | • Body Image<br>• Self-Esteem |

*Note. Data from Nursing Outcomes Classification (NOC) by M. Johnson & M. Maas (Eds.), 1997, St. Louis: Mosby; Nursing Diagnoses: Definitions & Classification 2001–2002 by North American Nursing Diagnosis Association, 2001, Philadelphia: NANDA; Nursing Interventions Classification (NIC) by J.C. McCloskey & G. M. Bulechek (Eds.), 2000, St. Louis: Mosby. Reprinted by permission.*

- Physical therapy, occupational therapy, home health and homemaker services
- Helpful resources:
  - National Institute of Arthritis and Musculoskeletal and Skin Diseases

- American College of Rheumatology
- Arthritis Foundation
- American Physical Therapy Foundation
- American Chronic Pain Association

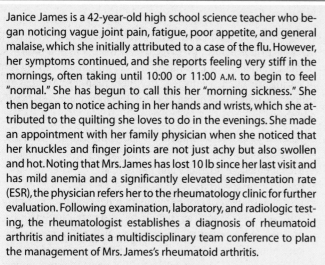

## Nursing Care Plan
## A Client with Rheumatoid Arthritis

Janice James is a 42-year-old high school science teacher who began noticing vague joint pain, fatigue, poor appetite, and general malaise, which she initially attributed to a case of the flu. However, her symptoms continued, and she reports feeling very stiff in the mornings, often taking until 10:00 or 11:00 A.M. to begin to feel "normal." She has begun to call this her "morning sickness." She then began to notice aching in her hands and wrists, which she attributed to the quilting she loves to do in the evenings. She made an appointment with her family physician when she noticed that her knuckles and finger joints are not just achy but also swollen and hot. Noting that Mrs. James has lost 10 lb since her last visit and has mild anemia and a significantly elevated sedimentation rate (ESR), the physician refers her to the rheumatology clinic for further evaluation. Following examination, laboratory, and radiologic testing, the rheumatologist establishes a diagnosis of rheumatoid arthritis and initiates a multidisciplinary team conference to plan the management of Mrs. James's rheumatoid arthritis.

### ASSESSMENT

Cathy Greenstein, RN, completes a nursing assessment of Mrs. James. She notes that Mrs. James is well groomed and answers questions readily but appears fatigued and ill. Mrs. James relates that her job has been extremely stressful because teacher layoffs have resulted in larger class sizes and fewer teaching assistants. Despite symptoms, she continues to teach full time, but says she feels unable to keep up with all her responsibilities due to her fatigue.

Mrs. James states that she is allergic to penicillin. Her past medical history reveals only the usual childhood diseases and three uncomplicated pregnancies, resulting in the births of her children, ages 14, 11, and 9. Physical assessment findings include. BP 124/78, P 82 regular, R 18, T 100.2°F (37.8°C) PO. Hands: swelling of the proximal interphalangeal (PIP) and metacarpophalangeal (MCP) joints of both hands; second and third PIP and second MCP joints on right hand are red, shiny, hot, spongy, and tender to palpation; able to extend fingers to 180 degrees but cannot make a complete fist with either hand, with flexion limited to less than 90 degrees; grip strength is weak bilaterally; wrist ROM is limited in all directions. Knees are swollen, and flexion is slightly limited; positive bulge sign in the right knee. Diagnostic findings are an ESR of 52 mm/hr, a hematocrit of 30%, and positive for rheumatoid factor. Few changes other than soft-tissue swelling are evident on hand and wrist X-rays.

### DIAGNOSIS

- *Chronic pain* related to joint inflammation
- *Impaired home maintenance* related to fatigue
- *Activity intolerance* related to the effects of inflammation
- *Deficient knowledge: Therapeutic regimen*

### EXPECTED OUTCOMES

- Verbalize effective pain management strategies.

- Use assistive devices to minimize joint stress with ADLs.
- Verbalize a plan to reduce responsibilities for home maintenance.
- Express a willingness to plan rest breaks during the day.
- Demonstrate understanding of the prescribed therapeutic regimen and its importance for both short- and long-term benefit.

### PLANNING AND IMPLEMENTATION

- Teach techniques for relieving pain and morning stiffness, including:
  - Scheduling NSAIDs at equal intervals throughout the day
  - Taking morning NSAID dose with milk and crackers approximately 30 minutes before rising
  - Performing ROM exercises in shower or bathtub
  - Applying local heat with paraffin dip or compress; using cold packs as needed
- Teach techniques to minimize joint stress while performing ADLs.
- Provide Arthritis Foundation literature and information.
- Discuss ways to delegate household tasks to other family members.
- Explore ways to incorporate 30-minute rest breaks into Mrs. James's work schedule.
- Provide information about the disease process and its manifestations, prescribed medications with desired and adverse effects, and the importance of balancing rest and activity.

### EVALUATION

The initial treatment regimen of aspirin, rest, exercise, and physical therapy succeeded in partially relieving the acute manifestations of rheumatoid arthritis in Mrs. James. Her "morning sickness" now lasts only about 45 minutes. However, complete remission has not been achieved. She has had difficulty scheduling rest periods at work and has had to struggle to delegate household tasks. "I don't look sick to the kids, and they seem to think housecleaning is a terrible imposition on their time. It's often easier to just do it myself than to fight about it. Besides, that way it gets done right." Mrs. James has faithfully followed the prescribed medication regimen and exercise routines, and she has kept her scheduled appointments and maintained contact with the treatment team.

### Critical Thinking in the Nursing Process

1. Mrs. James is 42 years old. Would your nursing interventions differ if she were 72 years old? If so, how.
2. Rheumatoid arthritis is a chronic illness. What are the physical, emotional, and economic implications of a chronic illness that results in chronic pain and deformity?
3. Develop a nursing care plan for Mrs. James using the nursing diagnosis, *Ineffective role performance*.

See Evaluating Your Response in Appendix C.

## THE CLIENT WITH ANKYLOSING SPONDYLITIS

**Ankylosing spondylitis** is a chronic inflammatory arthritis that primarily affects the axial skeleton, leading to pain and progressive stiffening and fusion of the spine. The incidence is greater in men than women and men have more severe disease. It is common in people of European ancestry and certain Native American tribes; it is rare in African Americans and people of Japanese descent. The onset of the disease is usually in the late teens and early 20s.

The cause of ankylosing spondylitis is unknown. As with the other spondylarthropathies, there is a strong genetic component. Approximately 90% of people with ankylosing spondylitis have the HLA-B27 antigen; about 8% of the general population have this antigen (Porth, 2002).

## PATHOPHYSIOLOGY AND MANIFESTATIONS

Early inflammatory changes often are first noted in the sacroiliac joints. As the cartilage erodes, joint margins ossify and are replaced by scar tissue. The joints of the spine are also affected, with inflammation of the cartilaginous joints, and gradual calcification and ossification that leads to ankylosis, or joint consolidation and immobility. Other organ systems may be affected as well, including the eyes, lungs, heart, and kidneys.

The onset of ankylosing spondylitis is usually gradual and insidious. Clients may have persistent or intermittent bouts of low back pain. The pain is worse at night, followed by morning stiffness that is relieved by activity. Pain may radiate to the buttocks, hips, or down the legs. As the disease progresses, back motion becomes limited, the lumbar curve is lost, and the thoracic curvature is accentuated (Figure 39–7 ■). In severe cases, the entire spine becomes fused, preventing any motion. Clients with ankylosing spondylitis may also experience some peripheral arthritis, primarily affecting the hip, shoulders, and knee joints. Systemic manifestations include anorexia, weight loss, fever, and fatigue. Many clients develop uveitis, inflammation of the iris and the middle, vascular layer of the eye.

For most clients with ankylosing spondylitis, the disease is intermittent with mild to moderate acute episodes. These clients have a good prognosis with little risk of severe disability.

## COLLABORATIVE CARE

Diagnostic testing shows an elevated ESR during periods of active disease and typically a positive HLA-B27 antigen. The diagnosis of ankylosing spondylitis is usually confirmed with X-ray examination of the sacroiliac joints and spine. The sacroiliac joint becomes blurred and gradually obliterated. As the disease progresses, vertebrae become squared, and disc spaces narrow.

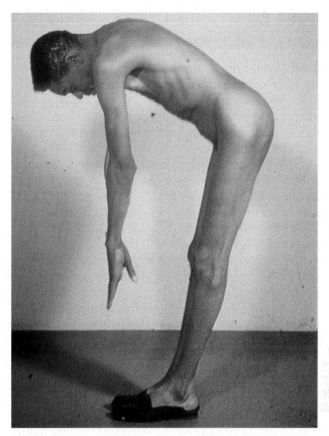

**Figure 39–7 ■** A client with ankylosing spondylitis. Note the flattened lumbar curve, exaggerated thoracic curvature, and flexion deformity of the neck.

*Source: American College of Rheumatology.*

As with other forms of arthritis, the management of ankylosing spondylitis is multidimensional. Physical therapy and daily exercises are important to maintain posture and joint range of motion. NSAIDs relieve pain and stiffness and allow the client to perform necessary exercises. Indomethacin (Indocin) is the NSAID most commonly used to treat ankylosing spondylitis. It may, however, have many adverse effects, including headache, nausea and vomiting, depression, and psychosis. Other drugs that may be prescribed include sulfasalazine (Azulfidine) and topical or intra-articular corticosteroids. Severe hip joint arthritis may necessitate total hip arthroplasty.

## NURSING CARE

The primary nursing role in ankylosing spondylitis is one of providing supportive care and education. To promote mobility, teach the client to take NSAIDs at regular intervals throughout the day with food, milk, or antacid. Encourage the client to maintain a fluid intake of 2500 mL or more per day. Suggest that the client perform exercises in the shower because warm, moist heat prompts mobility. Stress the importance of following the prescribed physical therapy and exercise program to maintain mobility.

## THE CLIENT WITH REACTIVE ARTHRITIS

**Reactive arthritis (Reiter's syndrome)** is an acute, nonpurulent inflammatory arthritis that complicates a bacterial infection of the genitourinary or gastrointestinal tracts. This type of arthritis most often affects young men who have an inherited HLA-B27 antigen. Reactive arthritis is often found in clients with HIV infection, although the reason for the association is not clear. The defining characteristics are arthropathy (usually of the lower extremity) and one of more of urethritis/cervicitis, dysentery, inflammatory eye disease, and disorders of the skin and mucous membranes (Maher, et al., 2002). Reactive arthritis is typically self-limited, although it can be recurrent or progressive.

Nonbacterial urethritis is often the initial manifestation of Reiter's syndrome. In women, urethritis and cervicitis may be asymptomatic. Conjunctivitis and inflammatory arthritis follow. The arthritis is usually asymmetric, affecting large weight-bearing joints such as the knees and ankles, the sacroiliac joints, or the spine. Mouth ulcers, inflammation of the glans penis, and skin lesions may occur. The heart and aorta may also be affected.

The diagnosis of reactive arthritis is generally based on the client's history and presenting symptoms. No test is specific for the disorder. Urethral or cervical cultures are obtained to rule out gonococcal infection. When Chlamydia is suspected, the client and sexual partner are treated with tetracycline or erythromycin. Reactive arthritis is treated symptomatically, usually with NSAIDs.

## NURSING CARE

Clients with reactive arthritis usually are seen in primary care settings such as a clinic or physician's office, making the nursing role primarily one of education. Teach the client about the association of the arthritis with the precipitating infection (if identified). Stress the importance of treating the infection effectively if it is still present. Use this opportunity to provide information about sexually transmitted diseases and protective measures to prevent their transmission. Discuss the usual self-limited nature of reactive arthritis, the appropriate use of prescribed NSAID preparations, and symptomatic relief measures such as application of heat and rest.

## THE CLIENT WITH SYSTEMIC LUPUS ERYTHEMATOSUS

**Systemic lupus erythematosus (SLE)** is a chronic inflammatory immune complex connective-tissue disease. It affects almost all body systems, including the musculoskeletal system. The manifestations of SLE are widely variable, thought to result from cell and tissue damage caused by deposition of antigen-antibody complexes in connective tissues. SLE affects multiple body systems, and it can range from a mild, episodic disorder to a rapidly fatal disease process.

Approximately 1 person in 2000 is affected by SLE, with women predominating by a ratio of 9:1 over men. The disease usually affects women of childbearing age (when the incidence is 30 times greater than in men) but it can occur at any age. It is more common in African Americans, Hispanics, and Asians than it is in Caucasians (Porth, 2002). The incidence is higher in some families.

Although the exact etiology of SLE is unknown, genetic, environmental, and hormonal factors play a role in its development. Twin studies and a familial pattern of the disease point to a genetic component, as does an increased incidence of other connective-tissue diseases in relatives of people with SLE. Certain human leukocyte antigen (HLA) genes are seen more frequently in people with SLE. Environmental factors such as viruses, bacterial antigens, chemicals, drugs, or ultraviolet light may play a role in activation of the pathologic mechanisms of the disease. In addition, it is felt that sex hormones may influence the development of SLE. Women with SLE have reduced levels of several active androgens that are known to inhibit antibody responses. Estrogens have been shown to enhance antibody responses and have an adverse effect in clients with SLE.

The course of SLE is mild and chronic in most clients, with periods of remission and exacerbation. The number and severity of exacerbations tend to decrease with time. In some clients, however, SLE is a virulent disease with significant organ system involvement.

Clients with active disease have an increased risk for infections, which are often opportunistic and severe. Infections such as pneumonia and septicemia are the leading cause of death in clients with SLE, followed by the effects of renal or central nervous system involvement.

## PATHOPHYSIOLOGY

The pathophysiology of SLE involves the production of a large variety of autoantibodies against normal body components such as nucleic acids, erythrocytes, coagulation proteins, lymphocytes, and platelets. Autoantibody production results from hyperreactivity of B cells (humoral response) because of disordered T-cell function (cellular immune response). The most characteristic autoantibodies in SLE are produced in response to nucleic acids, including DNA, histones, ribonucleoproteins, and other components of the cell nucleus.

SLE autoantibodies react with their corresponding antigen to form immune complexes, which are then deposited in the connective tissue of blood vessels, lymphatic vessels, and other tissues. The deposits trigger an inflammatory response leading to local tissue damage. The kidneys are a frequent site of complex deposition and damage; other tissues affected include the musculoskeletal system, brain, heart, spleen, lung, GI tract, skin, and peritoneum. The autoantibodies produced and their target tissue determine the manifestations of SLE.

A number of drugs can cause a syndrome that mimics lupus in clients with no other risk factors for the disease. Procainamide (Procan-SR, Pronestyl, others) and hydralazine (Apresoline, Hydralyn) are the most common drugs implicated, along with isoniazid (INH).

Renal and CNS manifestations of SLE rarely occur with drug-induced lupus, but arthritic and other systemic symptoms are common. Manifestations of drug-induced lupus usually resolve when the medication is discontinued.

## MANIFESTATIONS AND COMPLICATIONS

Typical early manifestations of SLE mimic those of rheumatoid arthritis, including systemic manifestations of fever, anorexia, malaise, and weight loss, and musculoskeletal manifestations of multiple arthralgias and symmetric polyarthritis. Joint symptoms affect more than 90% of clients with SLE. Although synovitis may be present, the arthritis associated with SLE is rarely deforming.

Most people affected by SLE have skin manifestations at some point during their disease. In fact, SLE was originally described as a skin disorder and named for the characteristic red butterfly rash across the cheeks and bridge of the nose (Figure 39–8 ■). Many clients with SLE are photosensitive; a diffuse maculopapular rash on skin exposed to the sun is also common. Other cutaneous manifestations include discoid lesions (raised, scaly, circular lesions with an erythematous rim), hives, erythematous fingertip lesions, and splinter hemorrhages. Alopecia is common in clients with SLE, although the hair usually grows back. Painless mucous membrane ulcerations may occur on the lips or in the mouth or nose.

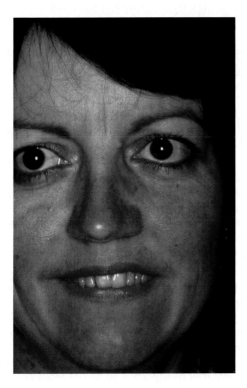

**Figure 39–8** ■ The butterfly rash of systemic lupus erythematosus.

*Source: Wellcome Trust/Custom Medical Stock Photo.*

Approximately 50% of people with SLE experience renal manifestations of the disease, including proteinuria, cellular casts, and nephrotic syndrome. Up to 10% develop renal failure as a result of the disease.

Hematologic abnormalities such as anemia, leukopenia, and thrombocytopenia are common with SLE. Cardiovascular disorders such as pericarditis, vasculitis, and Raynaud's phenomenon often occur. Less frequently, myocarditis, endocarditis, and venous or arterial thrombosis may develop. Pleurisy, pleural effusions, and lupus pneumonitis are common pulmonary manifestations of SLE.

Many clients with SLE develop transient nervous system involvement, often within the first year of the disease. Organic brain syndrome manifestations include decline in intellect, memory loss, and disorientation. Other possible neurologic manifestations include psychosis, seizures, depression, and stroke. Ocular manifestations of SLE include conjunctivitis, photophobia, and transient blindness due to retinal vasculitis.

Gastrointestinal symptoms of SLE, such as anorexia, nausea, abdominal pain, and diarrhea, may affect up to 45% of clients with the disease. The liver may be enlarged, and liver function tests may yield abnormal results.

Clients with SLE who become pregnant may experience abrupt onset of hypertension, edema, and proteinuria (a syndrome similar to pregnancy-induced hypertension). Midtrimester fetal death may result.

The *Multisystem Effects of SLE* are illustrated on page 1262.

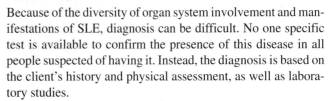

## COLLABORATIVE CARE

Because of the diversity of organ system involvement and manifestations of SLE, diagnosis can be difficult. No one specific test is available to confirm the presence of this disease in all people suspected of having it. Instead, the diagnosis is based on the client's history and physical assessment, as well as laboratory studies.

As with rheumatoid arthritis, effective management of SLE requires teamwork, with active participation by both the client and the physician. Communication, trust, and emotional support are especially important. Although there is no cure for SLE, the 10-year survival rate is greater than 70% among clients with this disease, which was once considered fatal in most cases.

### Diagnostic Tests

The multiple autoantibodies produced in SLE cause a number of abnormalities in laboratory studies.

- *Anti-DNA antibody testing* is a more specific indicator of SLE, because these antibodies are rarely found in any other disorder.
- *Eosinophil sedimentation rate (ESR)* is typically elevated, occasionally to >100 mm/hr.
- *Serum complement levels* are usually decreased as complement is consumed or "used up" by the development of antigen-antibody complexes.

## COLLABORATIVE CARE

There is no specific test to diagnose polymyositis. Autoantibodies may be identified in blood serum. Serum levels of muscle enzymes are elevated, particularly creatine kinase (CK) and aldolase levels. Biopsy of involved muscle shows patchy muscle fiber necrosis and the presence of inflammatory cells.

A combination of rest and corticosteroid therapy is prescribed for the client with polymyositis. Long-term corticosteroid therapy may be necessary to manage the disease. Immunosuppressive agents such as methotrexate, cyclophosphamide, and azathioprine may be used for clients who do not respond well to treatment with corticosteroids.

## NURSING CARE

The nursing role in caring for the client with polymyositis is supportive. Measures to promote comfort are important. Muscle weakness may interfere with the client's ability to provide self-care and manage health and home. The client may have difficulty with speech because of pharyngeal muscle weakness. Provide alternate means of communication as needed, and use patience in listening. Observe closely while the client eats, because aspiration is a potential problem. Modify the client's diet as needed to maintain nutrition and safety.

Education of the client and family is an important component of care. Emphasize the need to balance periods of rest and activity. Discuss skin care to prevent dryness and infection. Teach the client about prescribed medications and their short- and long-term side effects. Provide information about safety measures while eating. Encourage family members to become trained in performance of the Heimlich maneuver and CPR. Discuss signs of respiratory infection and other possible complications of polymyositis, including renal failure and malignancy.

## THE CLIENT WITH LYME DISEASE

**Lyme disease** is an inflammatory disorder caused by the spirochete *Borrelia burgdorferi,* which is transmitted primarily by ticks. It is the most commonly reported tick-borne illness in the United States. Geographically, Lyme disease is more prevalent in the mid-Atlantic, northeastern, and North Central regions of the United States (Tierney et al., 2001). It has also been reported throughout Europe, Asia, and Australia. Ticks that act as vectors for Lyme disease, primarily *Ixodes dammini, Ixodes pacificus,* and *Ixodes scapularis* in the United States, are usually carried by mice or deer, although other animals may be infected. The most frequent time of onset is the summer months.

## PATHOPHYSIOLOGY AND MANIFESTATIONS

Manifestations often are seen in the skin, musculoskeletal system, and central nervous system. The typical progression of Lyme disease is initially flulike manifestations and a skin rash; followed weeks or months later by Bell's palsy or meningitis, and months to years later, arthritis. This progression is highly individualized.

*Borrelia burgdorferi* enters the skin at the site of the tick bite. After an incubation period of up to 30 days, it migrates outward in the skin, forming a characteristic lesion called erythema migrans. It may also spread via lymph or blood to other skin sites, nodes, or organs. The inflammatory joint changes associated with Lyme disease closely resemble those of rheumatoid arthritis (vascular congestion, tissue infiltration by inflammatory cells, possible pannus formation, and erosion of cartilage and bone).

Erythema migrans is the initial manifestation of Lyme disease. This flat or slightly raised red lesion at the site of the tick bite expands over several days (up to a diameter of 50 cm), with the central area clearing as it expands. Systemic symptoms such as fatigue, malaise, fever, chills, and myalgias often accompany the initial lesion. As the disease spreads, secondary skin lesions develop, as do migratory musculoskeletal symptoms, including arthralgias, myalgias, and tendinitis. Persistent fatigue is common during this stage of the disease. Headache and stiff neck are characteristic neurologic manifestations.

With untreated infection, late manifestations can develop months to years after the initial infection. Chronic recurrent arthritis, primarily affecting large joints (especially the knee), is common. Permanent disability may result. Other effects that may be seen weeks to months after the initial infection include meningitis, encephalitis, and neuropathies, as well as cardiac manifestations including myocarditis and heart block.

## COLLABORATIVE CARE

Both manifestations and laboratory studies are used to establish the diagnosis of Lyme disease. Culture of the organism from tissues and body fluids is difficult and slow. Antibodies to *B. burgdorferi* can be detected by either ELISA (enzyme-linked immunosorbent assay) or Western blot methods within 2 to 4 weeks of the initial skin lesion.

The early diagnosis and proper antibiotic treatment of Lyme disease are important to preventing the complications of infection. A number of antibiotics may be used to treat Lyme disease, including doxycycline (Doxy-Caps, Vibramycin), tetracycline, amoxicillin (Amoxil), cefuroxime axetil (Ceftin), or erythromycin. Therapy may be continued for up to 1 month to ensure eradication of the organism from affected tissues. The nursing implications for various classes of antibiotics are summarized in Chapter 8. 

In addition to antibiotic treatment, aspirin or another NSAID may be prescribed for relief of arthritic symptoms. The affected joint may be splinted to rest the joint. When the knee is involved, weight bearing may be restricted and the use of crutches indicated.

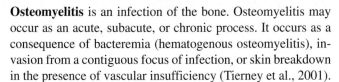

## NURSING CARE

Nursing care focuses on prevention of the disease. Many people do not protect themselves from tick bites. This protection is becoming increasingly important with a higher incidence of Lyme disease, due in part to an overpopulation of deer and the encroachment of the suburbs on once rural areas. Simple measures that can help prevent tick bites are as follows:

- Avoid tick-infested areas, especially in spring and summer, such as woods and rural areas with brush and tall weeds.

- Cover exposed skin with long-sleeved shirts and tuck pants into socks. Wearing high rubber boots may provide additional protection.
- Use insect repellents that contain DEET on clothing and exposed skin and apply permethrin to clothing prior to exposure.
- Inspect skin, especially in areas of tight-fitting clothing, after exposure. Transmission of the bacteria from the tick is unlikely to occur until 36 hours of tick attachment.
- Remove attached ticks with fine-tipped tweezers. Grasp the tick firmly as close to the skin as possible and pull the tick's body away from the skin. If the tick's head remains in the skin, it will not cause Lyme disease (the bacteria are in the tick's midgut). Clean the area with an antiseptic.

# INFECTIOUS DISORDERS

Infectious disorders are caused by a pathogen. These infections of bone and joints are often difficult to treat. Chronic infections may result in pain, deformity, and disability.

## THE CLIENT WITH OSTEOMYELITIS

**Osteomyelitis** is an infection of the bone. Osteomyelitis may occur as an acute, subacute, or chronic process. It occurs as a consequence of bacteremia (hematogenous osteomyelitis), invasion from a contiguous focus of infection, or skin breakdown in the presence of vascular insufficiency (Tierney et al., 2001).

Osteomyelitis can occur at any age, but adults over age 50 are more commonly affected. The older adult is at risk for osteomyelitis for several reasons. Immune function tends to decline with aging; the older adult also is more likely to have a chronic disease process that affects immune function. Circulatory status in the elderly often is compromised by atherosclerotic processes, impairing blood flow to the bone. Older adults have a higher risk of pressure ulcers because of circulatory, skin, sensation, and mobility changes associated with aging. Pressure ulcers that cannot be staged and treated because of eschar formation pose a particular risk. In addition, the older adult may not demonstrate typical signs of infection and inflammation, thus allowing an infectious process to become well established before it is detected.

## PATHOPHYSIOLOGY AND MANIFESTATIONS

The cause of osteomyelitis is usually bacterial; however, fungi, parasites, and viruses can also cause bone infection. *Staphylococcus aureus* is the most common infecting organism. Other organisms include *Escherichia coli, Pseudomonas, Klebsiella, Salmonella,* and *Proteus.*

Direct contamination of bone from an open wound, such as an open fracture or a gunshot or puncture wound, is the most common cause of osteomyelitis; osteomyelitis also may occur

as a complication of surgery. The third mode of entry for microorganisms that invade bone tissue is the extension from adjacent soft-tissue infection. Clients with venous stasis or arterial ulcers of the lower extremities or long-term complications of diabetes mellitus are good candidates for this type of bacterial invasion.

After entry, bacteria lodge and multiply in the bone, resulting in the inflammatory and immune system response. Phagocytes attempt to contain the infection, releasing enzymes in the process that destroy bone tissue. Pus forms, followed by edema and vascular congestion. The Haversian canals in the medullary (marrow) cavity of the bone allow the infection to travel to other segments of the bone. If the infection reaches the outer margin of the bone (Figure 39–9 ■), it raises the periosteum of the bone, spreading along the surface. Lifting of the periosteum from the cortex disrupts the blood vessels that enter the bone. Pressure increases, further compromising the vascular supply and leading to ischemia and eventual necrosis of the bone. Blood and antibiotics cannot reach the bone tissue once the pressure compromises the vascular and arteriolar systems. In addition, bacteria adhere to damaged bone, coating the underlying bone with a protective film that further impedes host defenses.

### Hematogenous Osteomyelitis

Hematogenous infections are caused by pathogens that are carried in the blood from sites of infection elsewhere in the body. Hematogenous osteomyelitis primarily affects older adults, people with sickle cell anemia, and intravenous drug users. The spine is the usual site of infection in adults. Pathogens enter the well-perfused vertebral bodies of adults via the spinal arteries. From there, the infection spreads into the disk space. The lumbar spine is involved more frequently than the thoracic or cervical spine. Urinary tract infections, soft-tissue infection, endocarditis, and infected intravenous sites are sources of pathogens.

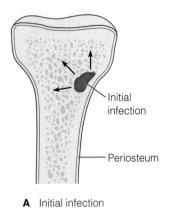

**A** Initial infection

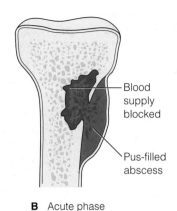

**B** Acute phase

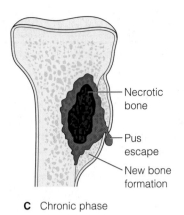

**C** Chronic phase

**Figure 39–9** ■ Osteomyelitis. *A,* Site of initial infection. Bacteria enter and multiply in the bone, and the inflammatory response is initiated. *B,* Acute phase, in which infection spreads to other parts of the bone. Pus forms, edema occurs, and the vascular supply is compromised. If the infection reaches the outer margin of the bone, the periosteum is lifted, and ischemia and necrosis eventually occur. *C,* Chronic phase. Necrotic bone separates, a new layer of bone forms around the necrotic bone, and a sinus develops to allow the wound to drain.

Clients with acute hematogenous osteomyelitis experience an acute onset of pain, tenderness, and fever. Soft-tissue swelling over the affected bone may be noted. The course of vertebral osteomyelitis in intravenous drug users often is subacute, with vague, dull pain in the affected region and a normal or low-grade fever. The pain intensifies over 2 to 3 months, and is accompanied by tenderness, muscle spasm, and limited range of motion.

## Osteomyelitis from a Contiguous Infection

Infections caused by an extension of infection from adjacent soft tissues fall into this category of osteomyelitis. The infection is a result of or complication of direct penetrating wounds, joint replacements, decubitus ulcers, and neurosurgery. This is the most common cause of osteomyelitis in adults.

## Manifestations of Osteomyelitis

### CARDIOVASCULAR EFFECTS
- Tachycardia

### GASTROINTESTINAL EFFECTS
- Nausea and vomiting
- Anorexia

### MUSCULOSKELETAL EFFECTS
- Limp in involved extremity
- Localized tenderness, especially in epiphyseal area

### INTEGUMENTARY EFFECTS
- Drainage and ulceration at involved site
- Swelling, erythema, and warmth at involved site
- Lymph node involvement, especially in the involved extremity

### OTHER EFFECTS
- High temperature with chills
- Abrupt onset of pain
- Malaise

The diagnosis of osteomyelitis often is not made until the infection has become chronic because the signs of acute infection may be masked by local tissue inflammation. Failure to heal a surgical wound or fracture or a developing sinus tract may be initial indicators of infection.

## Osteomyelitis Associated with Vascular Insufficiency

People with diabetes and peripheral vascular disease are at risk for developing osteomyelitis involving the feet. Diabetic neuropathy exposes the foot to trauma and pressure sores; the client may be unaware of the infection as it spreads into the bone. When tissue perfusion is poor, normal inflammatory responses and wound healing are impaired. The infection often is diagnosed when the client seeks treatment for a nonhealing sore, swollen toe, or acute cellulitis.

Manifestations of osteomyelitis vary according to the age of the client, the cause and site of involvement, and whether the infection is acute, subacute, or chronic (see box in left column).

## COLLABORATIVE CARE

The care of the client with osteomyelitis focuses on relieving pain, eliminating the infection, and preventing or minimizing complications. Early diagnosis is important to prevent bone necrosis by early antibiotic therapy. Most clients require both debridement of bone and a long period of antibiotic administration.

## Diagnostic Tests

The diagnosis of osteomyelitis is based on bone scans, magnetic resonance imaging, blood tests, and biopsy.

- *Magnetic resonance imaging (MRI)* can show epidural abscesses and other soft-tissue processes accompanying osteomyelitis.
- *Computed tomography (CT) scan* is used to detect sequestra, sinus tracts, and soft-tissue abscesses.

## Nursing Implications for Diagnostic Tests

### Bone Scan and Gallium Scan

#### BONE SCAN

##### Client Preparation

- Assess the client's understanding of the procedure, providing explanation, clarification, and emotional support as needed.
- Radioactive material (technetium-99m phosphate) is injected intravenously for 2 to 3 hours so that it concentrates in the bone.
- Observe the injection site for redness or swelling. If a hematoma forms, apply warm soaks to the area.
- Have the client drink four to six glasses of water in the 2- to 3-hour waiting period before the procedure to facilitate renal clearance of any circulating radioactive material.
- The client is not restricted to foods or fluids prior to the exam.
- Have the client empty the bladder prior to testing; a full bladder will mask the pelvic bones and make the client uncomfortable.
- The scan takes about 30 to 60 minutes to complete. The client must remain still during the scanning.
- The client may be active during the waiting period.
- A sedative should be ordered and administered to any client who may have difficulty lying quietly.

##### Postprocedure Care

- No specific care is needed after the procedure.

##### Client and Family Teaching

- Remove jewelry or any metal objects that may hide X-ray visualization of the bones.

- The scanner machine moves over the body and detects radiation emitted by the skeleton. X-ray films are prepared, showing a two-dimensional view of the skeleton. You may have to be repositioned several times.
- The scanning machine makes a clicking sound.
- Drinking liquids and frequent activity in the first 6 hours after the procedure help reduce excess radiation to the bladder and gonads.
- Family members will not be affected by the radionuclide, nor will urine or feces need special handling before, during, or after the procedure.

#### GALLIUM SCAN

##### Client Preparation

- Prepare as for a bone scan.
- Radioactive material, gallium-67, is injected intravenously 24 to 72 hours prior to the examination.
- Gallium is used because of its high affinity for soft-tissue abscesses.

##### Postprocedure Care

- Additional imaging may be performed at 24-hour intervals to differentiate normal activity from pathologic concentrations.
- No specific care is needed after the procedure.

##### Client and Family Teaching

- Refer to bone scan discussion.
- After a gallium scan, X-ray films may be obtained in 24-hour intervals for comparative results.

---

- *Radionucleotide bone scans* help determine if infection is active and differentiate between infectious and noninflammatory bone changes. Nursing care for clients having these procedures is described in the box above.
- *Ultrasound* can detect subperiosteal fluid collections, abscesses, and periosteal thickening and elevation associated with osteomyelitis.
- *Erythrocyte sedimentation rate (ESR)* and *WBC* are elevated in an acute infection.
- *Blood and tissue cultures* (from affected bone or soft tissue) are obtained to identify the infecting organism and direct antibiotic therapy.

### Medications

Antibiotic therapy is mandatory to prevent acute osteomyelitis from progressing to the chronic phase. Parenteral antibiotic therapy begins as soon as cultures (blood and/or wound) are obtained. A penicillinase-resistant semisynthetic penicillin (e.g, methacillin, oxacillin) may be given until the culture and sensitivity results are known. These antibiotics are used initially because many cases of osteomyelitis are caused by *Staphylococcus aureus.* When the detailed sensitivity report is obtained from the cultures, more definitive antibiotics are prescribed.

For the client with acute or chronic osteomyelitis, antibiotics are continued for 4 to 6 weeks. Intravenous antibiotic adminis-

tration or oral therapy is common. Oral therapy with twice-daily ciprofloxacin has been shown to be as effective as parenteral therapy for treating adult clients with chronic osteomyelitis caused by susceptible organisms (Tierney et al., 2001).

### Surgery

Needle aspiration or percutaneous needle biopsy may be performed to obtain a specimen in acute osteomyelitis. Surgery may be performed to obtain a specimen of the infectious agent, to debride the area, or both.

Surgical debridement is the primary treatment for the client with chronic osteomyelitis. The periosteum is excised and the cortex is drilled to release the pressure from accumulated pus. During this procedure, cultures may be obtained and sent to the laboratory for analysis. The wound holes are irrigated, and the wound is then closed. The cavity may be kept clean by inserting drainage tubes that are connected to an irrigation and suction system.

Postoperatively, the nurse is responsible for instilling and removing dilute antibiotic solutions through the drainage tubes. See the Nursing Care box on page 1270 for related nursing care.

A musculocutaneous (myocutaneous) flap is another approach used for the treatment of the dead space caused by extensive debridement of the infected site. The procedure involves moving or rotating a muscle and the section of skin fed

## NURSING CARE OF THE CLIENT UNDERGOING SURGICAL DEBRIDEMENT FOR OSTEOMYELITIS

### PREOPERATIVE CARE

- Discuss the impending surgery, the client's concerns regarding surgery and its risks, and what steps will be taken if surgery is ineffective. *Open discussion and active listening are important means of gaining the client's trust and encouraging the client to express concerns about the outcome of the surgery. Surgery is frequently performed when 36 to 48 hours of antimicrobial therapy yields no improvement and when prolonged bacteremia and evidence of an abscess formation are present. The periosteum is excised, allowing access to the purulent material in the infected area. If pus is not apparent, several holes may be drilled into the bone. In some cases, irrigation tubes are inserted and connected to an elaborate system for postoperative antimicrobial therapy.*
- Clients may need extensive antimicrobial treatment postoperatively if an irrigation system is surgically implanted. Before the procedure, explain to the client that bed rest and an extended period of treatment in the hospital are imperative. *Clients who understand the events that may occur postoperatively may be more accepting of the required restrictions.*

### POSTOPERATIVE CARE

- Provide meticulous care of the dressing and/or irrigation setup. *Frequently, the irrigation tubes are connected to a 3-way stopcock, which allows irrigation and drainage of the debrided area without separating the tube from the collection device. Nurses need to be extremely cautious and adhere to strict sterile technique.*
- Assess the client for manifestations of further infection. *Although the client will receive antimicrobial agents, it is important to assess the client continually for sudden spikes in temperature, pain at the involved site, and other indications of superinfection.*

### CLIENT AND FAMILY TEACHING

- While receiving antimicrobial agents, be sure to drink adequate amounts of fluid and eat a high-calorie diet to minimize the risks for damage to the kidneys, yeast infection, and adverse gastrointestinal effects.

---

by the arteries from that muscle into the cavity created by the surgery. A skin graft is performed later.

## NURSING CARE

The client with chronic osteomyelitis faces frequent and lengthy hospitalizations and/or treatment modalities. The prognosis is uncertain, and functional deficits and amputation are a constant concern. The ongoing expenses, loss of financial support, and role changes within the family are also nursing concerns.

### Nursing Diagnoses and Interventions

Nursing diagnoses associated with acute osteomyelitis focus on preventing the transmission of infection and problems due to immobility. Providing comfort and client teaching are also very important.

### Risk for Infection

Compromised immune status places the client with osteomyelitis at risk for superinfection. An inadequate kcal intake is an additional factor that contributes to the risk.

- Maintain strict handwashing practices. *Meticulous handwashing helps prevent the spread of infection by minimizing the entry of organisms into susceptible clients.*

**PRACTICE ALERT** *Careful handwashing before and after direct care is essential even if gloves are worn.* ■

- Administer antimicrobial therapy at specified time intervals. *Optimal blood levels of antibiotic therapy are mandatory in clients with infectious processes.*

- Maintain the client's optimal dietary kcal and protein intake. *High kcal and protein intake provide the client with sufficient nutritional support for the body's needs during the stressful event of the inflammatory process.*

### Hyperthermia

The infection and associated inflammatory process can cause fever in the client with osteomyelitis.

- Monitor temperature every 4 hours and when client reports chills and/or fever. Blood cultures are frequently ordered when an acute elevation of temperature occurs. *A sudden rise in temperature in clients with either acute or chronic osteomyelitis may indicate inadequate antimicrobial management.*
- Maintain a cool environment and provide light clothing and bedding during temperature elevation. *Proper environmental conditions and clothing enhance the evaporative process during acute temperature elevation and promote comfort.*
- Ensure a daily fluid intake of 2000 to 3000 mL. Dehydration may result from evaporative fluid losses during acute temperature elevations. Furthermore, clients taking large doses of antibiotic therapy may experience fluid loss through excessive diarrhea, as a side effect of the therapy. *Fluid replacement is necessary during this time to prevent further dehydration.*

### Impaired Physical Mobility

Pain, infection, inflammation, and the use of immobilizers can all impair the mobility of the client with osteomyelitis.

- Maintain the affected limb in functional position when immobilized. *The client may hesitate to move the involved extremity because of continuous pain; therefore, the extremity must be maintained in functional position to avoid flexion contracture.*

- Maintain rest, and avoid subjecting the affected extremity to weight-bearing activities. *The involved extremity must be immobilized to avoid pathologic fractures caused by stress on the weakened bone.*
- Ensure active or passive ROM exercises every 4 hours. *Flexion contracture occurs when the client remains immobile or when there is only minimal joint movement. Consult a physical therapist for plan of exercises to avoid contracture.*

### Acute Pain

The client with osteomyelitis experience pain due to swelling.

- Use a splint or immobilizer when the client experiences acute pain from swelling. *Splinting or immobilizing the involved extremity provides support and reduces pain caused by movement.*
- Ask the physician to order scheduled administration of narcotic and nonnarcotic analgesics on a 24-hour basis rather than as needed. *The use of 24-hour administration allows blood levels of pain-relieving medications to remain constant.*

**PRACTICE ALERT** *Clients are often reluctant to ask for a prn pain medication, allowing the pain to reach a level that is difficult to manage.* ■

- Use nonpharmacologic strategies (e.g., distraction, relaxation techniques) for pain management. *Pain of the muscles and joints may be controlled through nonpharmacologic interventions. Warm moist packs, warm baths, or heating pads to the involved extremity provide comfort due to vasodilation.*
- Avoid excessive manipulation of the involved area; handle the area gently. Carefully assess the client for guarding, limping, or unwillingness to move the affected part. Communicate to other health care professionals the client's preferences for assistive devices and means of manipulating the involved area. *Gentle handling and minimal manipulation help reduce pain.*

### Anxiety

The long-term nature of the disease can cause feelings of anxiety in the client with osteomyelitis.

- While the client is in the hospital, provide information regarding the disease process and diagnostic tests. *An understanding of the disease process and the diagnostic and treatment modalities minimizes anxiety.*
- Inform the client about ways to maximize the treatment phases for the disease process. *The nurse should enable the client to participate fully in the treatment plan so that maximum results can be obtained. Clients need to understand that their adherence to the prescribed antibiotic therapy is essential.*

### Home Care

Although clients may be hospitalized for acute treatment and surgery, most care is provided at home. Home health services can provide intravenous medications, if prescribed. Discuss the following topics for home care.

- The importance of careful handwashing, especially after toileting and dressing changes
- The importance of taking all antibiotics as prescribed. Include information about helping prevent the yeast infections (of the mouth or vagina) often associated with prolonged antibiotic therapy by eating 8 oz of live-culture yogurt each day.
- The need to take pain medications on a regular basis to prevent pain from becoming severe. Provide information about how to deal with side effects, such as constipation, by increasing fluid and fiber intake.
- How to perform wound care and sources for needed equipment and supplies
- Rest or limited weight bearing for the affected extremity or body part. Teach how to avoid complications associated with prolonged immobilization, such as frequently shifting position, keeping skin and linens clean and dry, and doing active ROM exercises for unaffected joints.
- The importance of maintaining good nutrition. An adequate supply of kilocalories, protein, and other nutrients is necessary for immune function and healing. Suggest frequent small meals and using nutritional supplements such as Ensure to help maintain nutritional intake.

## THE CLIENT WITH SEPTIC ARTHRITIS

**Septic arthritis** can develop if a joint space is invaded by a pathogen. The primary risk factors for septic arthritis are persistent bacteremia (bacteria in the blood) (e.g., due to use of injectable drugs, endocarditis) and previous joint damage (e.g., due to trauma or rheumatoid arthritis). Arthroscopic surgery and total joint replacements which allow potential direct contamination of the joint are additional risk factors (Tierney et al., 2001).

## PATHOPHYSIOLOGY AND MANIFESTATIONS

The most common bacteria implicated in septic arthritis include *gonococci, Staphylococcus aureus,* and *streptococci.* Infections by gram-negative bacteria such as *E. coli* and *Pseudomonas* are seen with increasing frequency, particularly in people who inject recreational drugs or are immunocompromised (Tierney et al., 2001).

Infection of the joint leads to inflammation with resulting synovitis and joint effusion. Abscesses may form in synovial tissues or bone underlying joint cartilage. If not treated promptly and effectively, septic arthritis can lead to destruction of the affected joint. A single joint, often the knee, is usually affected. Septic arthritis may also affect other joints such as the shoulder, wrist, hip, fingers, or elbow.

The onset of septic arthritis is typically abrupt, marked by pain and stiffness of the infected joint. The joint appears red and swollen, and is hot and tender to the touch. Effusion (increased fluid within the joint space) is usually present. Systemic manifestations of infection, such as chills and fever, often accompany local manifestations, although these may be muted if the client is taking anti-inflammatory medications.

## COLLABORATIVE CARE

Septic arthritis is a medical emergency requiring prompt treatment to preserve joint function. When it is suspected, the affected joint is aspirated and fluid sent for Gram stain and culture. Cultures also are obtained from all likely sources of the infection, including blood, sputum, or wounds. The synovial fluid culture is always positive in nongonococcal septic arthritis but often is negative for bacteria in early gonococcal arthritis. Infected synovial fluid usually is cloudy, with a high WBC count and a low glucose level. Joint X-ray films are often normal in the initial stages, but soon show demineralization, bony erosions, and joint space narrowing.

The infected joint is treated with rest, immobilization, and elevation along with systemic antibiotic therapy. Therapy with a broad-spectrum parenteral antibiotic is initiated before the results of culture are obtained. The medication may be changed or adjusted once the organism has been identified. Antibiotic therapy is continued for at least 2 weeks after inflammatory signs and symptoms have abated. Frequent joint aspirations may be performed to remove excess fluid and pus, and to evaluate for the continued presence of bacteria. Surgical drainage may be performed if the hip joint is involved (because of the difficulty of aspirating this joint) or when medical therapy does not rapidly eliminate bacteria from the synovial fluid. Physical therapy is implemented during the recovery period to ensure maintenance of optimal joint function.

## NURSING CARE

Septic arthritis can be frightening to the client who experiences a sudden onset of joint pain and swelling and is faced with the possibility of rapid functional loss of movement. Nursing care is both supportive and educative. Clients may be hospitalized for initial treatment with intravenous antibiotics. It is important to monitor the client's response to therapy, including systemic manifestations such as fever. Position the affected joint appropriately, using pillows to elevate it as needed. Splints or traction may be used to immobilize the joint. Warm compresses may be ordered for comfort. Active ROM exercises preserve joint mobility and should be initiated as soon as the physician allows.

The client with septic arthritis needs information about the disorder, its etiology, and its treatment. Teach the client how organisms may gain entry into the joint space. Discuss the role that the use of injected drugs and sexually transmitted diseases play in septic arthritis, and means to prevent infection as appropriate (e.g., using clean "works," practicing safer sex). Refer the client to a drug treatment program if necessary. Emphasize the importance of complying with all aspects of the treatment plan to prevent joint destruction and disability.

# NEOPLASTIC DISORDERS

Bone tumors, or neoplasms of skeletal tissue, may be either primary (arising in the bone itself) or metastatic (seeded from a tumor elsewhere in the body). Like other tumors, bone tumors can be either benign or malignant.

## THE CLIENT WITH BONE TUMORS

Benign bone tumors tend to grow slowly and do not often destroy surrounding tissues. Malignant tumors grow rapidly and metastasize. Primary malignant tumors of the bone are rare, accounting for only about 1% of all adult cancers (Porth, 2002). Virtually every malignant tumor can metastasize to bone. However, the most common metastatic bone tumors originate from primary tumors of the prostate, breast, kidney, thyroid, and lung.

Primary bone tumors arise from bone tissue itself, that is, cartilage (chondogenic), bone (osteogenic), collagen (collagenic), and bone marrow cells (myelogenic). The tissue type, neoplasm classification, sites, and incidence of the most common primary bone tumors are summarized in Table 39–7. The focus for discussion in this section is care of the client with a primary bone tumor.

## PATHOPHYSIOLOGY AND MANIFESTATIONS

The etiology of bone tumors is unknown, but there is a connection between increased bone activity and the development of primary bone tumors. Bone tumors frequently occur when primary bone growth is at its peak in adolescence or is overstimulated during disease, such as Paget's disease.

Primary tumors cause bone breakdown, called *osteolysis,* which weakens the bone, resulting in bone fractures. Normal bone adjacent to the tumor responds to tumor pressure by altering its normal pattern of remodeling. The bone's surface becomes altered, and the contours enlarge in the area of the tumor growth.

Malignant bone tumors invade and destroy adjacent bone tissue by producing substances that promote bone resorption or by interfering with a bone's blood supply. Benign bone tumors, unlike malignant ones, have a symmetric, controlled growth pattern. As they grow, they push against neighboring bone tissue. This weakens the bone's structure until it becomes unable to withstand the stress of ordinary use and frequently causes pathologic fracture.

The three main manifestations of bone tumors are pain, a mass, and impaired function. The manifestations of bone tu-

TABLE 39–7 Description of Common Primary Bone Tumors

| Tissue Type | Benign | Malignant | Site | Incidence |
|---|---|---|---|---|
| Chondrogenic (cartilage-forming tumors) | Osteochondroma— most common benign tumor | | Pelvis, scapula, ribs | Higher in males |
| | Chondroma | | Hands, feet, ribs, spine, sternum, or long bones | Age 30 to 50<br>Higher in males |
| | | Chondrosarcoma | Femur, pelvis, ribs, head (epiphysis) of long bones | 13% of malignant bone tumors<br>Middle age and older<br>Higher in males |
| Osteogenic (bone-forming tumors) | Osteoid Osteoma | | Shaft (diaphysis) of long bones, i.e., femur, tibia | Age 20 to 30<br>Higher in males |
| | | Osteosarcoma— most common malignant tumor | Long bones, knee | 38% of malignant bone tumors<br>Predominant in adolescents and people 50 to 60 |
| Collagenic (collagen-forming tumors) | | Fibrosarcoma | Femur, tibia | 4% of malignant bone tumors<br>Wide age distribution, but usually occurs in people 40 to 50<br>Higher in females |
| Myelogenic (tumors of bone marrow cells) | Giant cell tumor | | Shaft (diaphysis) of long bones, i.e., femur, tibia, radius, humerus | 4% to 5% of bone tumors<br>Wide age distribution<br>Higher in females |

mors are usually associated with a history of a fall or blow to the extremity that brings the mass to the client's attention. The injury, rather than the growth itself, usually causes the client to seek medical attention. Manifestations of bone tumors are listed in the box below.

## COLLABORATIVE CARE

Care of the client with bone tumors focuses on prompt diagnosis, removal of the tumor, prevention of complications, and client education.

## Manifestations of Neoplasms of the Musculoskeletal System

### BONY SARCOMAS

**Site**
Upper or lower extremity or pelvis

**Manifestations**
- Worsening deep bony pain due to inflammation or weakness of bone
- Pain at night or during rest that may radiate and become severe
- Muscular weakness or atrophy due to pain

Metaphysis of distal femur, proximal tibia, proximal humerus, and pelvis
- Soft-tissue mass extending from bone with erythematous or warm skin over tissue mass
- Alternation in ability to perform activities of daily living
- Fever

### SOFT TISSUE SARCOMAS

**Site**
Upper or lower extremity and pelvis

**Manifestations**
- Enlarging firm mass with irregular borders, which causes pain in surrounding soft-tissue structures

Thigh, shoulder, and pelvis
- Erythema or warmth and venous dilation over skin
- Muscular weakness and atrophy with limited range of motion, alteration in ability to perform activities of daily living, and alteration in gait
- Paresthesia with neurologic involvement and distal swelling
- Palpable local lymph nodes resulting from inflammation of tumor

Pelvis
- Above manifestations, plus altered bowel and bladder habits or pain with intercourse
- Weakening of muscles due to lumbosacral nerve involvement

## Diagnostic Tests

The diagnosis of bone tumors is critical to the survival of the client and possible preservation of the affected limb. The following tests may be performed.

- *X-rays* show the location of the tumors and the extent of bone involvement. Benign tumors are characterized by sharp margins that are clearly separate from the surrounding normal bone. Metastatic bone destruction has a characteristic "moth-eaten" pattern in which the growth has a less-defined margin that cannot be separated from the normal bone.
- *CT scan* is useful in evaluating the extent of tumor invasion into bone, soft tissues, and neurovascular structures.
- *MRI* is used to determine the extent of tumor invasion of surrounding tissue, to determine the response of bone tumors to radiation or chemotherapy, and to detect recurrent disease.
- *Percutaneous needle biopsy* or *needle biopsy* at the time of surgery is used to determine the exact type of bone tumor.
- *Serum alkaline phosphatase* is elevated in the client with a malignant bone tumor.
- *RBC count* is elevated.
- *Serum calcium* is elevated when there is massive bone destruction.

## Chemotherapy

Chemotherapeutic agents are administered to shrink the tumor before surgery, to control recurrence of tumor growth after surgery, or to treat metastasis of the tumor. Chemotherapeutic agents used to treat bone tumors are listed in Box 39–4. See Chapter 10 ⊂⊃ for further discussion of chemotherapy and its nursing implications.

## Radiation Therapy

Radiation therapy may be used in combination with chemotherapy. Radiation therapy is frequently applied to metastatic bone carcinomas as a method of pain control. It is also used to eliminate bony tumors or to eliminate any remaining tumor after a surgical procedure. Radiation therapy is discussed in Chapter 10.

## Surgery

The goal of surgery for the treatment of primary bone tumors is to eliminate the tumor completely. Tumors are removed either by excising the tumor itself or by amputating the affected limb. The type of procedure varies from removing the tumor only, to removing the tumor along with a small margin of normal tissue surrounding the tumor, to removing the tumor and a wide zone of normal tissue, to removing the tumor and part or all of the bone in which it lies. Cadaver allografts or metal prostheses often are used to replace missing bone, avoiding amputation. Care of the client undergoing amputation is discussed in Chapter 38.

## NURSING CARE

Nursing care for the client with bone tumors requires innovative actions from the time of diagnosis through the rehabilitation phase. In the acute phase, problems associated with pain, lack of knowledge, immobility, coping, and anxiety are foremost. If the client develops complications from treatment or if a malignancy metastasizes, problems related to home health maintenance management, self-concept, and prevention of further complications become more prominent.

### Nursing Diagnoses and Interventions

#### Risk for Injury

In the client with a bone tumor, changes in bone tissue can cause pathologic fractures.

- Instruct clients in ways to avoid falls or injury to the tumor site. *Pathologic fractures may occur at the tumor site because bone destruction can weaken the area.*
- Provide referral to physical or occupational therapy for fitting of and teaching about assistive devices for ambulating, such as a cane, crutches, or a walker. *Assistive devices can reduce the risk of falling when the client has significant weakness of an extremity or when balance has been affected by treatment of the disease.*

#### Acute and Chronic Pain

In the client with a bone tumor, pain may be related to direct invasion of the tumor or to pathologic fractures.

- Develop strategies for controlling both acute pain (from surgery, fracture, or inflammation) and chronic pain (from progression of the disease). *Analgesics combined with nonpharmacologic methods of pain control provide optimum relief of pain. Chronic pain, when mild in nature, is best managed with NSAIDs or aspirin. Moderate pain is best managed with a combination of codeine and NSAIDs. Severe pain is best relieved with long-acting or sustained relief narcotic analgesics.*
- Provide assistive devices (e.g., canes, walkers, crutches) when the client ambulates. *Assistive devices lessen the pain by supporting weight bearing during ambulation.*
- Provide regular rest periods between therapeutic activities. *Therapy should be performed at a time of maximum comfort for the client to increase mobility.*

#### Impaired Physical Mobility

Pain, muscle wasting, or surgical procedures can impair the physical mobility of the client with a bone tumor.

- Begin muscle strengthening and active and passive ROM exercises immediately after surgery. A continuous passive motion (CPM) machine may be used after surgical proce-

---

| BOX 39–4 | ■ Chemotherapeutic Agents Used for Musculoskeletal Neoplasms |
|---|---|

| **Alkylating Agents** | **Antimetabolites** |
|---|---|
| Ifosfamide | Methotrexate |
| Cyclophosphamide | |
| | **Plant Alkaloids** |
| **Antibiotics** | Vincristine |
| Doxorubicin | |
| Bleomycin | **Synthetic Agents** |
| | Cisplatin |

dures to either upper or lower extremities. *Muscle strengthening exercises must be encouraged as soon as possible to prevent muscle wasting and shorten the rehabilitation period.*

- Encourage exercises that help strengthen the triceps muscles. *The triceps are the major muscles in the arms and must be strengthened to assist in use of crutches or other assistive devices.*
- For the client who has undergone an amputation of a lower extremity, encourage quadriceps and gluteal setting exercises and leg raises. *These exercises will benefit the client when the rehabilitation period begins.*
- Teach clients how to use the trapeze correctly. Clients can use the trapeze to reposition themselves while supine, get out of bed, and assist the nurse's efforts to reposition them in bed and perform other activities. *Use of the trapeze helps strengthen the biceps of the arm.*

### Decisional Conflict

Knowledge deficit about diagnosis and treatment regimen can impair the client's ability to make informed decisions about the treatment plan.

- Explain issues related to diagnosis, radiologic evaluation, biopsy, surgery, chemotherapy, radiation therapy, potential complications, alternative therapies, risks, benefits, nursing management, discharge plans, home care, and long-term treatment and follow-up. *The client requires this information in order to make informed decisions about treatment.*

### Home Care

The client with a primary bone tumor needs information about the disease, its potential consequences, and treatment options. Present information in a matter-of-fact manner, taking time to listen to and address the client's and family's concerns. Discuss expected effects and potential side effects of surgery, chemotherapy, and radiation therapy. Provide information about how to minimize side effects. Teach the postsurgical client about wound care, demonstrating dressing changes and stump care (if amputation has occurred). Provide the client with a list of local resources for obtaining supplies. Discuss activity and weight-bearing restrictions. Refer the client to physical therapy for teaching about ambulation and appropriate muscle-group strengthening exercises. Ensure that the client who has experienced an amputation is working with or has a referral to a prosthetic specialist. For the client with metastatic disease, discuss hospice services and support groups for clients with cancer.

## CONNECTIVE TISSUE DISORDERS

Connective tissue is the most abundant and widely distributed body tissue. It not only connects body parts but also provides support; forms bones, cartilage, and the walls of blood vessels; and attaches muscles to bones. Connective tissue consists of three elements: (1) long fibers embedded in a (2) noncellular ground substance, and (3) cells specific to the class of connective tissue. Fibers made up primarily of collagen, a protein, are the most abundant in connective tissue.

Connective-tissue disorders, also known as collagen diseases, are a group of immune-mediated disorders. Although they appear to have a genetic component, their cause is unknown. Because connective tissue and collagen are widely distributed in many varied tissues, these are systemic diseases with diverse manifestations.

### THE CLIENT WITH SYSTEMIC SCLEROSIS (SCLERODERMA)

**Systemic sclerosis,** also known as **scleroderma** ("hardening of the skin"), is a chronic disease characterized by the formation of excess fibrous connective tissue and diffuse fibrosis of the skin and internal organs. The cause of scleroderma is unknown, although genetic, immune, and environmental factors are thought to play a role. Although this uncommon disease is distributed worldwide, a higher incidence is noted in coal and gold miners and in people exposed to certain chemicals such as polyvinyl chloride, epoxy resins, and aromatic hydrocarbons. It affects women more often than men by a ratio of approximately 3:1. The onset of scleroderma typically occurs between the ages of 30 and 50 years (Tierney et al., 2001).

### PATHOPHYSIOLOGY

Abnormalities in cellular immune function are believed to contribute to the development of scleroderma. Abnormal proliferation of fibrous connective tissue occurs in affected tissues, including the skin, blood vessels, lungs, kidneys, and other organs.

Scleroderma may be either localized, affecting the skin only, or generalized (systemic sclerosis), with both skin and visceral organ involvement. Eighty percent of people with generalized disease have limited involvement, frequently manifested by CREST syndrome, a combination of calcinosis (abnormal calcium salt deposition in the tissues), Raynaud's phenomenon, esophageal dysfunction, sclerodactyly (localized scleroderma of the fingers), and telangiectasia (dilated, superficial blood vessels). The remainder of clients with generalized systemic sclerosis have a diffuse form of the disease and a higher risk of visceral organ involvement.

### MANIFESTATIONS AND COMPLICATIONS

The initial manifestations of systemic sclerosis are usually noted in the skin, which thickens markedly. Diffuse, nonpitting swelling also is noted. As the disease progresses, the skin begins to atrophy, becoming taut, shiny, and hyperpigmented

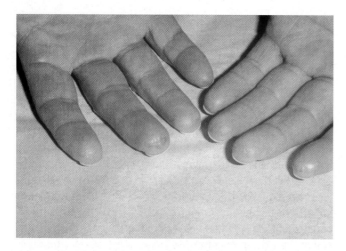

**Figure 39–10** ■ Characteristic skin changes of scleroderma.

*Source: Logical Images/Custom Medical Stock Photo.*

(Figure 39–10 ■). Facial skin tightening leads to loss of skin lines and a pursed-lip appearance. Skin tightness may limit mobility, particularly of the face and hands. Other skin manifestations include telangiectasias (flat, red areas caused by dilation of small blood vessels, usually noted on the face, hands, and in the mouth) and calcium deposits, usually noted around joints.

Arthralgias and Raynaud's phenomenon also are common early manifestations of systemic sclerosis. Raynaud's phenomenon (intermittent attacks of small artery vasospasm) is characterized by pallor of the fingers followed by cyanosis, and then reactive hyperemia with redness. Attacks are usually triggered by cold temperatures.

The client with visceral organ involvement may have varied symptoms. Dysphagia is common, because the motility of the esophagus is affected. Pulmonary involvement can lead to exertional dyspnea due to impaired gas exchange and right-sided heart failure due to pulmonary hypertension. Involvement of the heart may cause manifestations of pericarditis and dysrhythmias. Diarrhea or constipation, abdominal cramping, and malabsorption can occur when the GI tract is affected. Renal effects can lead to proteinuria, hematuria, hypertension, and renal failure.

The prognosis for localized and limited scleroderma is good; many clients have a normal life span. The course of diffuse systemic sclerosis is highly variable. This disease is usually progressive; complete remission is rare.

## COLLABORATIVE CARE

The manifestations of systemic sclerosis often allow diagnosis with little or no testing. No cure is currently available; treatment is symptomatic and supportive.

### Diagnostic Tests

No single test is specific for systemic sclerosis. The following tests may be ordered.

- *ESR* is typically elevated because of the chronic inflammatory process.

- *CBC* will typically find anemia because of the chronic disease process and its effects on various organs.
- *Gammaglobulin levels* are often high, and *antinuclear antibodies* and *rheumatoid factor* may be present in low levels.
- *Skin biopsy* may be performed to confirm the diagnosis.

### Medications

Medications to treat systemic sclerosis are chosen based on the client's symptoms. Immunosuppressive agents and corticosteroids are of limited benefit, but may be used to slow or prevent pulmonary fibrosis and in life-threatening disease. Penicillamine may be used to treat scleroderma and pulmonary fibrosis. Calcium channel blockers such as nifedipine (Procardia) or alpha-adrenergic blockers such as prazosin (Minipress) may be prescribed for clients with Raynaud's phenomenon. When manifestations of esophagitis accompany systemic sclerosis, $H_2$-receptor blockers such as cimetidine (Tagamet) or ranitidine (Zantac), antacids, or omeprazole (Prilosec), which blocks all gastric secretion, may be ordered. Tetracycline or another broad-spectrum antibiotic may be prescribed to suppress intestinal flora and relieve symptoms of malabsorption. Clients with kidney disease are usually treated with angiotensin-converting enzyme (ACE) inhibitors such as captopril (Capoten) to control hypertension and preserve renal function. End-stage kidney disease is managed with dialysis and transplantation.

### Physical Therapy

Physical therapy is an important part of the management of systemic sclerosis to maintain mobility of affected tissues, the hands and face in particular. Because the mouth opening becomes increasingly smaller as the disease progresses, stretching and strengthening of facial muscles can be vital to maintaining oral food intake.

## NURSING CARE

Nursing care needs of clients with systemic sclerosis are individualized to the effects and manifestations of the disease, with interventions summarized in the following discussion.

### Nursing Interventions

Skin manifestations are present to some degree in nearly all clients with scleroderma. Nursing care related to the skin focuses on maintaining skin integrity and flexibility. Measures to maintain supple skin are important, because elasticity cannot be regained once it is lost. Apply moisturizers to prevent dryness and cracking. Protect the skin where it is stretched taut over joints or bony prominences. Perform ROM exercises to help prevent joint contractures due to increasingly tight skin.

Difficulty swallowing and recurrent esophagitis may interfere with the client's nutritional status. Provide small, frequent meals. Consult with the dietitian and the client to determine which foods are easy to swallow. Keep the client in a sitting or Fowler's position after meals to minimize esophageal reflux. Elevate the head of the bed at night as well.

The dermatologic and systemic effects of the disease may have significant psychologic effects on the client, leading to feelings of helplessness and hopelessness, and self-esteem disturbance. Establish an atmosphere of trust with the client. Listen actively and acknowledge concerns about the disease and its effects on the client's life and appearance. Encourage the client to share these concerns with family members and significant others. Provide referral to social services or counseling as appropriate.

The client with predominant pulmonary disease has nursing care needs similar to those of other clients with restrictive respiratory disorders (see Chapter 36). If the client with systemic sclerosis has impaired renal function, nursing care is similar to that for clients with chronic renal failure (see Chapter 27).

## Home Care

Teach the client with systemic sclerosis about the disease and introduce measures to help manage its effects. Stress the importance of good skin care and physical therapy exercises to maintain mobility, particularly of the hands and face. Discuss the need to avoid chilling (local and whole body) to prevent episodes of Raynaud's phenomenon. Teach the role of proper dress: loose, warm clothing, gloves, and warm stockings in the winter. Stress the need to stop smoking because of the vasoconstrictive effect of nicotine and the respiratory effects of the disease. Provide the client with information about manifestations of disease progression and organ involvement. Teach the client to report new or worsening symptoms to the physician. In addition, suggest the following resources.

- National Arthritis and Musculoskeletal and Skin Diseases, National Institutes of Health
- Scleroderma Foundation, Inc.
- Scleroderma Research Foundation

## THE CLIENT WITH SJÖGREN'S SYNDROME

**Sjögren's syndrome** is an autoimmune disorder that causes inflammation and dysfunction of exocrine glands throughout the body. Sjögren's syndrome primarily affects women, with a ratio of women to men at 9:1 The highest incidence is between the ages of 40 and 60 years. Although it can occur as a primary disorder, Sjogren's syndrome is often associated with other rheumatic disease, including rheumatoid arthritis, systemic lupus erythematosus, primary biliary cirrhosis, scleroderma, Hashimoto's thyroiditis, and interstitial pulmonary fibrosis (Tierney et al., 2001).

## PATHOPHYSIOLOGY

In this disease, exocrine glands in many areas of the body are destroyed by the infiltration of lymphocytes and deposition of immune complexes. The salivary and lacrimal glands are particularly affected, leading to the characteristic manifestations of *xerophthalmia* (dry eyes) and *xerostomia* (dry mouth). Clients often experience dry, gritty-feeling eyes and may de-

velop corneal ulcerations. Mucosal dryness affects taste, smell, chewing, and swallowing and leads to increased dental caries. Parotid gland enlargement is common. Excess dryness can also affect the nose, throat, larynx, bronchi, vagina, and skin. Systemic effects of Sjögren's syndrome include arthritis, dysphagia, pancreatitis, pleuritis, neurologic manifestations including migraine, and vasculitis. Nephritis may occur, but renal failure rarely results. Clients with Sjögren's syndrome have a greatly increased risk of developing malignant lymphoma.

## COLLABORATIVE CARE

The diagnosis of Sjögren's syndrome is often based on the client's history and clinical presentation. Schirmer's test, which measures the quantity of tears secreted in a 5-minute period in response to irritation, ocular staining, and slit-lamp examination of the eye, may be performed. A definitive diagnosis can be made by biopsy of either the lacrimal or salivary gland.

Treatment is supportive. Artificial tears are used to decrease eye irritation and dryness. The client can keep the mouth moist by drinking fluids, using a saliva substitute, and chewing sugarless gum. Medications that increase mouth dryness, such as atropine and decongestants, should be avoided.

## NURSING CARE

Nurses caring for clients with Sjögren's syndrome need to promote and teach measures to protect the client's eyes and oral mucosa. Instill artificial tears as needed. Encourage the client to sip fluids throughout the day. Provide frequent oral hygiene, particularly before and after meals. Ensure that the client has sufficient fluids to drink during meals, because fluids help with chewing and swallowing.

## THE CLIENT WITH FIBROMYALGIA

**Fibromyalgia** is a common rheumatic syndrome characterized by musculoskeletal pain, stiffness, and tenderness. Fibromyalgia affects from 3% to 10% of the general population, and is found most commonly in women between 20 years and 50 years (Tierney et al., 2002). The cause is unknown, but possible etiologies include sleep disorders, depression, infections, and an altered perception of normal stimuli. Fibromyalgia can be a complication of hypothyroidism, rheumatoid arthritis, or (in men) sleep apnea. It closely resembles chronic fatigue syndrome, except that musculoskeletal pain is predominant in fibromyalgia, whereas fatigue is a more significant feature of chronic fatigue syndrome.

## PATHOPHYSIOLOGY AND MANIFESTATIONS

No inflammatory, structural, or physiologic muscle changes have been demonstrated in fibromyalgia. A gradual onset of chronic, achy muscle pain is typical, although the onset may be sudden, occasionally following a viral illness. The pain may be localized or involve the entire body. The neck, spine, shoulders, and hips are often affected. Pain is produced by palpating localized "tender points" (for example, on the trapezius, medial fat pad of the knee, and the lateral epicondyle of the elbow). Local tightness or muscle spasm may also occur. Systemic manifestations of fibromyalgia include fatigue, sleep disruptions, headaches, and an irritable bowel. Pain and fatigue are aggravated by exertion.

## COLLABORATIVE CARE

The diagnosis of fibromyalgia is based on the history and physical assessment. There are no laboratory or diagnostic tests for the disorder, although tests may be performed to rule out other rheumatic disorders, such as rheumatoid arthritis or systemic lupus erythematosus. Fibromyalgia also may occur as a complication of hypothyroidism, so thyroid function studies are performed. Criteria for diagnosis of fibromyalgia, developed by The American College of Rheumatology, are that the person must have widespread pain in combination with tenderness in at least 11 of the 18 specific tender point sites.

This disorder may resolve spontaneously or become chronic and recurrent. The client with fibromyalgia needs reassurance of the benign nature of the disorder along with validation of its reality. Other therapeutic measures include local heat applications, massage, stretching exercises, and sleep improvement. Amitriptyline, a tricyclic antidepressant, has been shown to promote better sleep and relieve manifestations of fibromyalgia. NSAIDs have not been effective in its treatment.

## NURSING CARE

Nursing care for clients with fibromyalgia is supportive and educational, provided in community settings such as clinics and other primary care settings. It is important to validate clients' concerns and reassure them that their symptoms are not "all in the head." This syndrome is recognizable and manageable; its course is not progressive. Teach clients about the disorder, and reassure them that it resolves uneventfully in most instances. Provide verbal and written instructions about the use of heat, exercise, stress-reduction techniques, and prescribed medications to relieve its manifestations. In addition, suggest the following resources:

- Fibromyalgia Network
- National Fibromyalgia Awareness Campaign

# STRUCTURAL DISORDERS

Structural disorders of the musculoskeletal system most commonly affect the spine. The disorders discussed in this section are spinal deformities and low back pain.

## THE CLIENT WITH SPINAL DEFORMITIES

Scoliosis and kyphosis are the two most common deformities of the spinal column. **Scoliosis** is a lateral curvature of the spine. **Kyphosis** is excessive angulation of the normal posterior curve of the thoracic spine (Figure 39–11 ■).

An estimated 500,000 adults in the United States are affected by scoliosis. It usually is diagnosed in adolescence, with girls affected more than boys by an 8:1 margin. Idiopathic scoliosis is the most common form of the disorder, accounting for approximately 75% of cases. Congenital and neuromuscular disorders such as cerebral palsy, poliomyelitis, and MD account for the rest (Porth, 2002).

Kyphosis can be caused by a variety of congenital conditions or childhood disorders. Detailed discussions of the causes and treatment of scoliosis and kyphosis in younger clients can be found in pediatric nursing textbooks. This discussion focuses on the nursing care of adults with these disorders.

The manifestations of scoliosis and kyphosis are listed in the box on page 1279.

## PATHOPHYSIOLOGY AND MANIFESTATIONS
### Scoliosis

Scoliosis is classified as *postural* when the small curve corrects with bending, and *structural* when the curve does not correct with bending (Porth, 2002). Most clients requiring treatment have structural scoliosis, a curve caused by a fixed deformity.

The lateral curve that occurs in scoliosis is usually evident in the thoracic, lumbar, or thoracolumbar regions of the spine. The vertebral bodies in these spinal regions can be rotated as well as curved to one side or the other.

As scoliosis emerges, the soft tissues (muscles and ligaments) shorten on the concave side of the curvature. Over time, progressive deformities of the vertebral column and ribs develop, causing one-sided compression of the vertebral bodies. The degree of compression and twisting varies according to the location of each vertebra within the curved portion of the spine.

If the lateral curvature is less than 40 degrees when the client's spine reaches maturity, the risk of further progression during adult life is small. However, the spine becomes unstable if the lateral curvature is greater than 50 degrees, and curvature likely will worsen throughout the client's lifetime.

Scoliosis is usually first noted by the deformity it causes, such as one shoulder that is higher than the other, a prominent hip, or a projecting scapula. Pain is present in severe cases, usually in the lumbar region. Pain also may be caused by pressure on the ribs or the crest of the ilium. Shortness of breath may re-

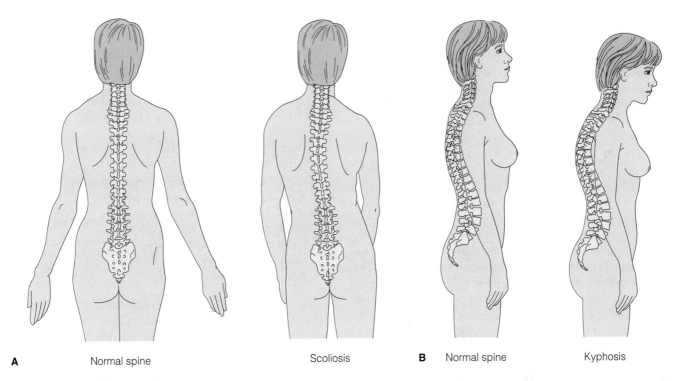

A   Normal spine                      Scoliosis          B   Normal spine          Kyphosis

**Figure 39–11** ■ Common deformities of the spinal column: *A,* Scoliosis is a lateral curvature of the spine. *B,* Kyphosis is an exaggerated posterior curvature of the thoracic spine.

## Manifestations of Scoliosis and Kyphosis

### SCOLIOSIS

- Asymmetry of shoulders, scapulae, waist creases
- Prominence of the thoracic ribs or paravertebral muscles on forward bend
- Lateral curvature and vertebral rotation on posteroanterior X-ray film

### SEVERE SCOLIOSIS

- Back pain
- Shortness of breath
- Anorexia, nausea

### KYPHOSIS

- Posterior rounding at the thoracic level
- Kyphotic curve of over 45 degrees on X-ray film

sult from diminished chest expansion, and gastrointestinal disturbances because of crowding of the abdominal organs.

## Kyphosis

Like scoliosis, kyphosis is classified as postural or structural. Postural kyphosis is caused by a slumping posture. Structural kyphosis may result from congenital malformations or pediatric disorders such as rickets or poliomyelitis. However, kyphosis also may occur during adulthood from vertebral tuberculosis and Paget's disease or from metabolic disorders such as osteoporosis and osteomalacia. The condition can also

result from the surgical removal or radiation of intervertebral discs for the treatment of spinal cord tumors or cysts.

The manifestations of kyphosis include moderate back pain and increased curvature of the thoracic spine as viewed from the side ("hunchback"). Impaired mobility and respiratory problems may occur in cases of severe curvature.

## COLLABORATIVE CARE

Diagnosis of scoliosis and kyphosis is important to prevent severe spinal deformity in the adult. The client stands with the arms relaxed and hanging freely at the sides while the examiner evaluates the client from both the back and the front for symmetry of the shoulders, scapulae, waist creases, and the length of the arms. The client then bends forward, and the examiner observes for prominence of the thoracic ribs or vertebral muscles. The client is then viewed from the side while the screener looks for increased thoracic rounding or lumbar swayback.

A scoliometer is used to quantify the prominence of any curvatures noted during the examination. The scoliometer is placed at the apex of the curvature. A reading of greater than 10 degrees requires referral to a physician (Porth, 2002).

### Diagnostic Tests

Upright posteroanterior and lateral radiographs are used to confirm the diagnosis of curvature of the spine. For the client with scoliosis, the degree of curve is measured by determining the amount of lateral deviation to the left or right. For the client with kyphosis, anteroposterior and lateral views typically reveal wedging of the vertebrae.

## Conservative Treatment

Braces, electrical stimulation, and traction may be used to prevent progression of scoliosis and kyphosis in younger clients whose skeletons have not yet matured. Unfortunately, these approaches are ineffective in the adult client. Conservative treatment for adults with scoliosis and kyphosis may include weight reduction, active and passive exercises, and the use of braces for support.

## Surgery

For adolescents and adults, the use of surgery to correct spinal deformities depends on factors such as the degree of curvature and the client's overall physical, emotional, and neurologic status. Even with surgery, it is not possible to correct the abnormal curvature completely. The surgical procedure involves attaching metal reinforcing rods to the vertebrae, and is usually performed using an anterior approach, although more severe curvature may require both an anterior and a posterior approach. The types of straightening devices used most frequently use bilateral rods with wire hooks or screws that stabilize the spine and correct the deformity.

## NURSING CARE

Nursing interventions focus on minimizing the risk for injury and neurologic impairment.

## Nursing Diagnoses and Interventions

### Risk for Injury

Clients with spinal deformities are at risk for injury from several sources, including structural aspects of bracing both prior to and after surgical intervention, dislocation of hooks and rods resulting from improper alignment or movement of the back, and changes in body position after prolonged immobilization.

- Assess the environment for safety hazards. *The client needs to learn to use the handrail on stairways and take precautions when walking on slippery surfaces or areas with throw rugs.*

**PRACTICE ALERT** *Some braces do not allow the client to flex or hyperextend the spinal column.* ■

- Teach the clients ways to reduce irritation of skin surfaces beneath the brace: wearing a smooth cotton T-shirt or cotton tube under the brace at all times, changing undergarments at least once daily, and washing them with a mild soap. Undergarments should be changed more frequently in warmer weather. *The client wearing a brace is especially prone to skin breakdown and must take precautions to prevent it.*

**PRACTICE ALERT** *Teach the client to avoid lotion and body powders; they may irritate the skin.* ■

- Teach the client to loosen the brace during meals and for the first 30 minutes after each meal. *Clients have difficulty eating if the brace is tight. Loosening the brace after each meal will allow adequate nutritional intake and promote comfort.*
- Teach clients how to apply the brace, and explain ambulatory restrictions. *Clients requiring a brace need to learn how to apply the brace prior to ambulating. Ambulation is frequently restricted to walking rather than sitting for long periods.*
- Turn clients who have undergone spinal surgery by using the log-rolling technique. Clients require a position change at least every 2 hours. *The use of a turnsheet and sufficient assistance allow the nurse to maintain the client's proper body alignment during the turning procedure.*
- Use a fracture bedpan following surgery. *The fracture bedpan provides minimal misalignment of spine and thus ensures comfort.*

### Risk for Peripheral Neurovascular Dysfunction

Surgical procedures can lead to neurologic impairment in the client with a spinal deformity.

- Assess the movement and sensation of lower extremities every 2 hours for the first 8 hours then every shift and as needed. *Neurologic assessment related to sensation and movement of the lower extremities is necessary because the surgical procedure is in close proximity to spinal nerves. Swelling of the surgical site can impinge on the spinal nerves and cause a loss of sensation.*

## Home Care

Clients with structural scoliosis or kyphosis need reassurance that the condition was not caused by poor posture. If a brace is prescribed to relieve pain and other symptoms associated with the disorder, provide verbal and written instructions for wearing the brace, such as the number of hours per day it is to be worn and activity restrictions to follow when wearing or not wearing the brace. Teach the client how to protect and care for skin under the brace.

Surgical clients need postoperative teaching regarding site care and activities. Clients who have spinal surgery often are allowed to ambulate fairly rapidly after surgery, but sitting may be restricted because of the stresses it places on the spine. Instruct the client to notify the physician if numbness, tingling, pain, or weakness of an extremity develop after surgery.

Discuss the importance of not smoking and of avoiding respiratory infections for clients with scoliosis or kyphosis that restrict respiratory excursion. Encourage these clients to obtain pneumococcal pneumonia and influenza immunizations.

## THE CLIENT WITH LOW BACK PAIN

Acute or chronic low back pain involves the lumbar, lumbosacral, or sacroiliac areas of the back. In most cases, low back pain is due to strains in the muscles and tendons of the back caused by abnormal stress or overuse. Low back pain

| BOX 39–5 ■ Factors Associated with Back Pain |
| --- |

**MECHANICAL INJURY OR TRAUMA**
- Muscle strain or spasm
- Compression fracture
- Lumbar disc disease

**DEGENERATIVE DISORDERS**
- Spondylosis
- Spinal stenosis
- Osteoarthritis

**SYSTEMIC DISORDERS**
- Osteomyelitis
- Osteoporosis or osteomalacia
- Neoplasms, primary or metastatic

**REFERRED PAIN**
- Gastrointestinal disorders
- Genitourinary disorders
- Gynecologic disorders
- Abdominal aortic aneurysm
- Hip pathology

**OTHER**
- Fibromyalgia
- Psychiatric syndromes
- Chronic anxiety
- Depression

caused by degenerative disc disease and herniated vertebral discs is covered in Chapter 41. ∞

## PATHOPHYSIOLOGY AND MANIFESTATIONS

The pathophysiology of back pain varies with its many causes (Box 39–5). In general, the five types of back pain are as follows:

- Local pain is caused by compression or irritation of sensory nerves. Fractures, strains, and sprains are common causes of local pain; tumors also may press on pain-sensitive structures.
- Referred pain may originate from abdominal or pelvic viscera.
- Pain of spinal origin, that is, pain associated with pathology of the spine such as disk disease or arthritis, may be referred to other structures such as the buttocks, groin, or legs.
- Radicular back pain is sharp, radiating from the back to the leg along a nerve root. This pain may be aggravated by movements such as coughing, sneezing, or sitting.
- Muscle spasm pain is associated with many spine disorders, although its origin may be unclear. This type of back pain is dull and may be accompanied by abnormal posture and taut spinal muscles.

Clients with low back pain report pain ranging from mild discomfort lasting a few hours to chronic debilitating pain. Acute pain is usually caused when the client participates in an activity that is not usually pursued, such as unusual lifting or bending, playing an active sport, or shoveling snow. Manifestations are presented in the box in the next column.

## Manifestations of Low Back Pain

**ALTERATIONS IN GAIT AND FLEXION**
- Walking in a stiff, flexed state
- Inability to bend at waist
- Limp, which may indicate impairment of the sciatic nerve

**NEUROLOGIC INVOLVEMENT**
- When tested for light and deep touch with a pin and cotton ball, may feel sensations in both limbs but experience a stronger sensation in the unaffected side
- Loss of both bowel and bladder control due to involvement of the sacral nerve

**PAIN**
- Pain in the affected leg when walking on heel or toes
- Continuous, knifelike localized pain in muscles close to the affected disk
- Pain that radiates down posterior of leg
- Sharp, burning pain in the posterior thigh or calf
- Pain in middle of buttock
- Tenderness when muscle close to the affected disc is palpated
- Severe pain with straight leg-raising maneuver

## COLLABORATIVE CARE

Care of the client with low back pain focuses on relieving pain, correcting the condition if possible, preventing complications, and educating the client.

### Diagnostic Tests

The choice of diagnostic tests for the client with low back pain depends on the suspected diagnoses, clinical findings, and history. Current guidelines for care recommend that radiography, CT scans, and MRI be used only with clinical signs of a potentially serious underlying condition. They also state that diagnostic testing may be considered if pain and other manifestations continue to limit the client after 4 weeks of conservative treatment.

### Medications

The medications of choice for low back pain include NSAIDs and analgesics. NSAIDs block prostaglandin production and reduce inflammation, thus relieving the pain. Muscle relaxants, such as cyclobenzaprine (Flexeril), methocarbamol (Robaxin), or carisoprodol (Soma) may be used, but little evidence supports their efficacy.

Epidural steroid injections may be used to help reduce intense, intractable pain. A steroid solution is injected into the epidural space, which helps decrease the swelling and inflammation of the spinal nerves.

### Conservative Treatment

The majority of clients with acute low back pain need only a short-term treatment regimen. Limited rest, combined with appropriate exercise and education, is often the primary method of treatment. There is no evidence that activity is harmful or aggravating to the source of pain. In fact, increased activity promotes bone and muscle strength and may increase endorphin levels. Therefore, active rehabilitation helps to restore function and reduce pain.

Pain may be relieved by an ice bag or hot water bottle (or heating pad) applied to the back. Exercise programs are helpful provided that the client begins gradually and increases activity gradually as the recovery process continues. Physical therapy procedures include diathermy (deep heat therapy), ultrasonography, hydrotherapy, and transcutaneous electrical nerve stimluation (TENS) units. These therapies reduce the muscle spasms and pain temporarily. They are frequently used in combination with exercise to provide early mobilization for the client.

# NURSING CARE

Nursing care of the client with low back pain focuses on relieving the pain. In addition, most clients have very little understanding of the anatomy of the spine, the reasons for the pain, the choices for treatment, and the importance of self-management. Therefore, education is another essential aspect of treating low back pain.

## Health Promotion

Recommendations for preventing back pain from the National Institute of Neurological Disorders and Stroke (2001) include:

- Have a regular exercise program.
- Stretch before working in the yard, jogging, and playing sport.
- Quit smoking.
- Lose weight.
- Maintain a correct posture.
- Use supportive seats when driving.
- Lift by bending at the knees rather than at the waist.
- Reduce emotional stress that causes muscle tension.

In industrial and work settings, nurses should be alert for situations that increase the risk of back pain and injury. Office workers should have chairs with appropriate seat height and length and back support. Modifications of work space or machinery may be necessary for industrial workers to avoid excess stresses on back muscles. Finally, it is important to remember that back pain is a leading cause of lost work time for nurses themselves. Remind coworkers to use good body mechanics and to seek help when lifting or moving clients.

## Nursing Diagnoses and Interventions

### Acute Pain

Muscle spasms and inflammation are among the contributing factors of low back pain.

- Teach the client appropriate comfort measures. *Every client with low back pain has discomfort due to muscle spasms and/or inflammation due to nerve compression, surgery, or irritation from a brace.*
- Instruct the client to take NSAIDs or analgesics on a routine schedule rather than as needed. *Maintaining a constant blood level of the NSAIDs or analgesics reduces inflammation and provides continuous pain relief.*

### Deficient Knowledge

The client with low back pain requires information regarding treatment modalities.

- Encourage clients to remain on bed rest for a limited period. *There is little scientific evidence to show that bed rest is beneficial, but there is ample evidence about the adverse effects of bed rest. Prolonged rest can lead to depression, loss of work, and difficulty in initiating rehabilitation.*
- Teach the client about the "rebound phenomenon" of prolonged heat or ice therapy. *Ice remaining on the skin longer than 15 minutes or heat longer than 30 minutes causes a reverse effect known as the rebound phenomenon. For example, heat produces maximum vasodilation in 20 to 30 minutes. Continuation of the application beyond 30 to 45 minutes causes tissue congestion, and the blood vessels constrict. Likewise, with cold application, maximum vasoconstriction occurs when the skin reaches a temperature of $60°F (15°C)$. Prolonged cold can create a drop in temperature, at which time vasodilation occurs.*
- Provide instructions about appropriate back exercises such as partial sit-ups with the knees bent and knee-chest exercises to stretch hamstrings and spinal muscles. Each exercise should be done 5 times and gradually increased to 10 times. Advise the client to discontinue any exercise that is painful and to seek professional advice before continuing the exercise. *Repetition of prescribed back exercises, such as the pelvic tilt, partial sit-ups, and back rolls, will strengthen the muscles that protect the spine and thus prevent back strain.*

### Risk for Impaired Adjustment

In the client with low back pain, the need for lifestyle changes may lead to impaired adjustment.

- Teach the client to use appropriate body mechanics in lifting and reaching. The client should be instructed to plan the lift, keep the object being lifted close to the body, and avoid twisting when lifting. Encourage the client to obtain help when lifting. *An item is considered excessively heavy if it equals 35% of the lifter's body weight.*
- Instruct the client to modify the workplace or environment to minimize stress to the lower back. *Lumbar supports in chairs, adjustment of chair or table height, and rubber floor mats help prevent back strain or injury.*
- Encourage obese clients to lose weight. *The trunk of the body must carry excess weight when the client is obese. Obese people are farther away from the objects they lift because of their greater abdominal girth. They may also have more difficulty squatting to lift. The greater the distance between an object and the client's center of gravity, the higher the risk for straining the lower back.*
- Encourage the client to stop smoking. *Research indicates that smoking decreases blood oxygenation to the disc and thereby interferes with repair of the disc and causes premature aging and degeneration. Smokers also cough frequently,*

*which increases the number of pounds of pressure on the disc, increasing disc stress.*

- Instruct client to refrain from prolonged standing or sitting, lying prone, and wearing high heels. *These activities exacerbate back pain.*

## Home Care

Back pain is a common problem in the United States and other industrialized countries. Nurses can have an effect on this significant problem by teaching health practices to prevent back injury to clients of all ages. Teach clients how to safely lift, bend, and turn when engaging in physical activity. Stress the importance of using large muscle groups of the legs to lift rather than bending and lifting with the smaller muscles of the back. Teach other aspects of good body mechanics, including posture, sleeping on a firm mattress, and sitting in chairs that provide good support. Discuss the positive effect of maintaining optimal body weight and good physical fitness.

# THE CLIENT WITH COMMON FOOT DISORDERS

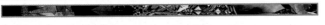

Hallux valgus, hammertoe, and Morton's neuroma are common foot disorders that cause pain or difficulty in walking. All three disorders may be caused by wearing poorly fitting or confining shoes. For this reason, these disorders are more prevalent among women.

## PATHOPHYSIOLOGY

### Hallux Valgus

**Hallux valgus,** commonly called a **bunion,** is the enlargement and lateral displacement of the first metatarsal (the great toe) (Figure 39–12 ■). Hallux valgus develops when chronic pressure against the great toe causes the connective tissue in the sole of the foot to lengthen so that the stabilizing action of the great toe is gradually lost. The toe bends laterally away from the midline of the body, and the metatarsophalangeal joint (MTP) is exposed to friction during walking and becomes en-

larged. As the deformity progresses, calluses form over the metatarsal head, and bursitis develops in the MTP. In severe cases, the lateral displacement of the great toe may approach 70 to 90 degrees, and the second toe may be forced upward, causing hammertoe. Although bunions may be a congenital disorder, most are caused by wearing pointed, narrow-toed shoes or high heels.

Hallux valgus is obvious on physical examination of the foot. The client may report an inability to fit into shoes. Often, the client may report joint pain or pain around calluses. In advanced or severe cases, the first metatarsal joint may have limited range of motion, particularly in dorsiflexion, and crepitus (crackling or popping) may occur during joint movement.

### Hammertoe

**Hammertoe** (claw toe) is the dorsiflexion of the first phalanx with accompanying plantar flexion of the second and third phalanges (Figure 39–13 ■). The condition may affect any toe, but the second toe is most commonly affected. As the deformity begins, clients experience mild inflammation of the synovial membranes of the involved joints. As the deformity progresses, the dorsiflexed joint rubs against the overlying shoe, causing painful corns to develop.

### Morton's Neuroma

**Morton's neuroma** is a tumorlike mass formed within the neurovascular bundle of the intermetatarsal spaces (Figure 39–14 ■). The neuromas usually occur in only one foot, most frequently in the third web space. Like other common foot disorders, Morton's neuroma usually is caused by wearing tight, confining shoes. The condition develops when repeated compression of the toes causes irritation and scarring of tissues surrounding the plantar digital nerve. The affected nerve becomes inflamed and swells. After repeated episodes of inflammation, the nerve fibers become fibrotic, and a neuroma forms.

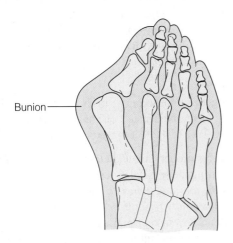

Bunion

**Figure 39–12** ■ Hallux valgus (bunion).

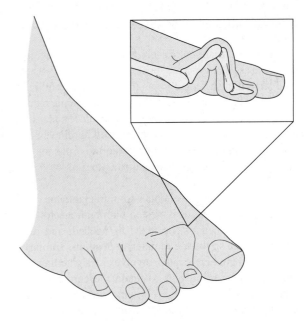

**Figure 39–13** ■ Hammertoe.

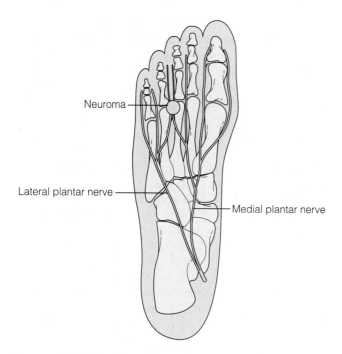

**Figure 39–14** ■ Morton's neuroma.

Manifestations include a burning pain at the web space of the affected foot that radiates into the tips of the involved toes. Weight bearing usually worsens any symptoms; removing the shoe and massaging the foot often relieves the pain. The neuroma may present as a palpable mass between the affected toes. The area over the neuroma usually is tender.

## COLLABORATIVE CARE

Care of the client with common foot disorders such as hallux valgus, hammertoe, and Morton's neuroma focuses on relieving pain, correcting the structural deformity, and preventing reoccurrence. In most cases, all three conditions are diagnosed by inspection; X-ray films of the affected foot are taken if the need for surgery arises.

Conservative treatment for common foot disorders usually involves the use of corrective shoes. Orthotic devices that cushion and stretch the affected joints may be placed within shoes or between the client's toes. For Morton's neuroma, metatarsal pads are used to spread the client's toes and decompress the affected nerve. Analgesics may be prescribed to relieve pain and inflammation. In severe cases, corticosteroid drugs may be injected into the affected joints or surrounding tissue to relieve acute inflammation.

Surgery is reserved for clients with intractable toe deformities or pain. Hallux valgus is treated with bunionectomy; ligaments are lengthened or shortened as needed, and pins are drilled into place so the toe remains in position. Similarly, the correction of hammertoe also involves straightening the affected toe and inserting pins to retain the correction. A cast may be applied over the foot following surgery to correct toe deformities. Surgery for Morton's neuroma causes loss of sen-

sation to a portion of the foot because removing the neuroma involves cutting out a portion of the plantar nerve.

## NURSING CARE

Nursing care for clients with these foot deformities focuses on the same areas because the conservative treatment and preoperative and postoperative interventions are similar.

### Nursing Diagnoses and Interventions

Pain relief, prevention of infection, and client education are important components of the nursing care of these clients.

#### Chronic Pain

In the client with a foot deformity, constant pressure of footwear over the involved joint can cause pain.

- Instruct clients to wear corrective footwear to assist in the conservative treatment of foot problems. *Pain related to foot problems can result from improper footwear that does not provide proper toe room; in addition, heels higher than 1 inch can cause constant flexion and hyperextension problems. In some instances, the client must purchase special shoes or orthotics to ensure correct fit and relief of symptoms. Shoes that fit well and provide enough foot space laterally and dorsally, such as running shoes, are recommended.*

- Provide clients with information about available resources that can help them obtain a proper shoe fit. *Shoe stores have devices for stretching the shoe at the pressure area, but the customer must purchase the shoe before the stretching is done. Shoe repair shops charge a reasonable fee for stretching a shoe. Fabric shoes are the most comfortable shoes for the aged client with bunions because fabric stretches more readily than leather or other synthetic materials.*

- Suggest purchasing appropriate pads to wear over painful bunions, calluses/corns, and the ball of the foot. *Protective pads are manufactured for specific foot problems; these include bunion pads, corn pads, and metatarsal pads.*

- Instruct clients to remove pads and inspect the skin every other day. Clients who have difficulty reaching or observing the involved foot should ask another person to do the inspection for them. *It is very important to emphasize the need for inspection to clients who have experienced loss of sensation of the feet due to such disorders as diabetes and chronic peripheral vascular disease.*

#### Risk for Infection

Like all surgeries, foot surgery carries a risk of infection. This risk may be increased because of impaired peripheral circulation and exposure of the feet to the environment.

- Teach clients proper care and cleaning of exposed pins implanted during the surgical procedure. *Pins inserted into soft tissue of the toes and bones are prone to becoming infected and can potentially result in osteomyelitis.*

- Teach clients how to keep pins and casts dry while bathing or ambulating in inclement weather. Clients must wear a plastic bag over the cast or pins when bathing or walking in rain or snow. *When casts or pins are exposed in water, infection may result.*

## Home Care

For clients in all age groups, teach the importance of well-fitting footwear. Discuss the long-term effects of wearing high-heeled shoes with constricting toes with women in particular. Suggest alternatives for stylish footwear, and encourage clients to wear supportive and nonrestrictive footwear at all times. Discuss the possible effects of bunions on balance, and talk about safety measures to prevent falls and injury. Teach clients techniques to relieve pressure on affected joints.

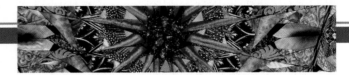

 **EXPLORE MediaLink**

NCLEX review questions, case studies, care plan activities, MediaLink applications, and other interactive resources for this chapter can be found on the Companion Website at www.prenhall.com/lemone.

Click on Chapter 39 to select the activities for this chapter. For animations, video clips, more NCLEX review questions, and an audio glossary, access the Student CD-ROM accompanying this textbook.

## TEST YOURSELF

1. Although all of the following nursing diagnoses are important when planning care for the client with osteoporosis, which is most significant in terms of long-term disability?

    a. *Chronic pain*
    b. *Risk for falls*
    c. *Activity intolerance*
    d. *Acute pain*

2. You are preparing a teaching plan for a woman with osteoarthritis. Which group of medications should you be prepared to discuss?

    a. Opioids
    b. Antibiotics
    c. Hormones
    d. NSAIDs

3. A postoperative nursing care plan for a client who has had a total knee replacement includes monitoring vital signs and laboratory results. The rationale for these interventions is to:

    a. Reassure the client that blood pressure and pulse are fine
    b. Promote rapport between the client and the health care providers

    c. Ensure adequate circulation to the involved extremity
    d. Prevent the progression of infection (the most common complication)

4. When comparing osteoarthritis and rheumatoid arthritis, what assessment finding would be different in the client with rheumatoid arthritis?

    a. Health history includes general feeling of sickness
    b. Abnormal joint findings are limited to the hands
    c. Stiffness is relieved by activity
    d. Herberden nodes are located on the finger joints

5. *Ineffective protection* is an appropriate nursing diagnosis for the client with SLE. What would be your most important intervention for the hospitalized client?

    a. Monitor laboratory findings
    b. Provide appropriate skin care
    c. Practice careful handwashing
    d. Administer prescribed medications

See Test Yourself answers in Appendix C.

## BIBLIOGRAPHY

Adler, P., Good, M., Roberts, B., & Snyder, S. (2000). Abstract: The effects of Tai Chi on older adults with chronic arthritis pain. *Journal of Nursing Scholarship, 32*(4), 377.

American Cancer Society. (2001). *What is bone cancer?* Available www.cancer.org

Barbieri, R. L. (1998). A step-by-step approach to osteoporosis treatment. *Patient Care, 32*(8), 138–147.

Curry, L., & Hogstel, M. (2002). Osteoporosis. *American Journal of Nursing, 102*(1), 26–33.

Delmas, P. D., & Meunier, P. J. (1997). The management of Paget's disease of bone. *The New England Journal of Medicine, 336*(8), 558–567.

Drugay, M. (1997). Breaking the silence: A health promotion approach to osteoporosis. *Journal of Gerontological Nursing, 23*(6), 36–43.

Garfin, J., & Garfin, S. (2002). Low back pain: Exercises to prevent recurrence. *Consultant, 42*(3), 357–358.

Hill, N., & Davis, P. (2000). Nursing care of total joint replacement. *Journal of Orthopaedic Nursing, 4*(1), 41–45.

Holmes, S. (1998). Osteoporosis: The hidden illness. *Nursing Times, 94*(1), 20–23.

Johnson, M., & Maas, M. (Eds.). (1997). *Nursing outcomes classification (NOC).* St. Louis: Mosby.

Katz, W. A., & Sherman, C. (1998). Osteoporosis: The role of exercise in optimal management. *The Physician and Sportsmedicine, 26*(2), 33–41.

Kee, C. C., McCoy, S., Rouser, G., Booth, L. A., & Harris, S. (1998). Perspectives on the nursing management of osteoarthritis. *Geriatric Nursing, 19*(1), 19–26.

Kee, J. (2001). *Handbook of laboratory and diagnostic tests with nursing implications* (4th ed.). Upper Saddle River, NJ: Prentice Hall.

Krug, B. (1997). Rheumatoid arthritis and osteoarthritis: A basic comparison. *Orthopaedic Nursing, 16*(5), 73–75.

Mahat, G. (1997). Perceived stressors and coping strategies among individuals with rheumatoid arthritis. *Journal of Advanced Nursing, 25*(6), 1144–1150.

Maher, A., Salmond, S., & Pellino, T. (2002). *Orthopaedic nursing* (3rd ed.). Philadelphia: Saunders.

Mayo Clinic. (2002). *Osteoporosis.* Available www.mayoclinic.com/invoke.cfm?id=DS00128

Matula, P., & Shollenberger, D. (1999). Total joint project: Acute care to home care. *MEDSURG Nursing, 8*(2), 92–98.

McCance, K., & Huether, S. (2002). *Pathophysiology: The biologic basis for disease in adults & children* (4th ed.). St. Louis: Mosby.

McCloskey, J., & Bulechek, G. (Eds.). (2000). *Nursing interventions classification (NIC)* (3rd ed.). St. Louis: Mosby.

Mooney, N. (2001). Pain management in the orthopaedic patient. *Pain Management Nursing, 2*(1), 4–5.

Moss Rehab Resource Net. (2002). *Arthritis fact sheet.* Available www.mossresourcenet.org/arthritis.htm

National Center for Chronic Disease Prevention and Health Promotion. (2002). *Arthritis.* Available www.cdc.gov/ncedphp/arthritis/index.htm

National Center for Chronic Disease Prevention and Health Promotion. (2002). *Chronic diseases and conditions: Arthritis.* Available www.cdc.gov/needphp/major.htm

National Center for Chronic Disease Prevention and Health Promotion. (2002). *Healthy aging: Preventing disease and improving quality of life among older Americans.* Available www.cdc.gov/nccdphp/aag-aging.htm

National Institute of Arthritis and Musculoskeletal and Skin Diseases. (2002). *Questions and answers about fibromyalgia.* Available www.niams.nih.gov/i/topics/fibromyalgia/fibrofs.htm

National Institute of Neurological Disorders and Stroke. (2001). *NINDS back pain information page.* Available www.ninds.nih.gov/health_and_medical disorders/back pain_doc.htm

National Institutes of Health. (2002). *Osteoporosis overview.* Available www.osteo.org/osteo.html

Neuberger, G. B., Press, A. N., Lindsley, H. B., Hinton, R., Cagle, P. E., Carlson, K., Scott, S., Dahl, J., & Kramer, B. (1997). Effects of exercise on fatigue, aerobic fitness, and disease activity measures in persons with rheumatoid arthritis. *Research in Nursing and Health, 20*(3), 195–204.

North American Nursing Diagnosis Association. (2001). *Nursing diagnoses: Definitions and classification, 2001–2002.* Philadelphia: Author.

Overdorf, J., Pachuki-Hyde, L., Kressenich, C., McClung, B., & Lucasey, C. (2001). Osteoporosis: There's so much we can do. *RN, 64*(12), 30–35,

Pachucki-Hyde, L. (2001). Assessment of risk factors for osteoporosis and fracture. *Nursing Clinics of North America, 36*(3), 401–408.

Porth, C. M. (2002). *Pathophysiology: Concepts of altered health states* (6th ed.). Philadelphia: Lippincott.

Raak, R., & Wahren L. (2002). Background pain in fribromyalgia patients affecting clinical examination of the skin. *Journal of Clinical Nursing, 11*(1), 58–64.

Ramsburg, K. (2000). Rheumatoid arthritis. *American Journal of Nursing, 100*(11), 40–43.

Reuters Health. (2002). *Arthroscopic surgery for knee arthritis doubted.* Available www.reutershealth.com

Rizzoli, R., Schaad, M., & Uebelhart, B. (2001). Osteoporosis in men. *Nursing Clinics of North America, 36*(3), 467–479.

Rossiter, R. (2000). Understanding the special needs of the patient with scleroderma. *Australian Nursing Journal, 8*(3), Insert 1–4 (27–30).

Ryan, S. (1996). The role of the nurse in the management of scleroderma. *Nursing Standard, 10*(48), 39–42.

Sedlak, C., & Dohehy, M. (2000). Fashion tips for women with osteoporosis. *Orthopedic Nursing, 19*(5), 31–35.

Shannon, M., Wilson, B., & Stang, C. (2002). *Health professional's drug guide 2002.* Upper Saddle River, NJ: Prentice Hall.

Solomon, J. (1998). Osteoporosis. When supports weaken. *RN, 61*(5), 37–40.

Springhouse. (1998). *Nurse's handbook of alternative & complementary therapies.* Springhouse, PA: Springhouse Corp.

Tierney, L. M., McPhee, S. J., & Papadakis, M. A. (Eds.). (2001). *Current medical diagnosis & treatment (40th ed.).* Stamford, CT: Appleton & Lange.

Weinstein, R. S. (1997). Advances in the treatment of Paget's bone disease. *Hospital Practice, 32*(3), 63–76.

Wright, A. (1998). Nursing interventions with advanced osteoporosis. *Home Healthcare Nurse, 16*(3), 144–151.

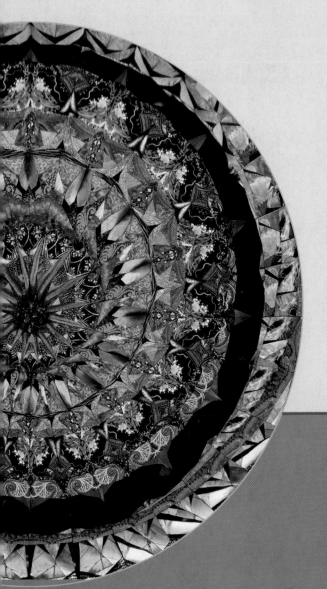

# COGNITIVE AND PERCEPTUAL PATTERNS

Unit 12
Responses to Altered Neurologic Function
Unit 13
Responses to Altered Visual and Auditory
Function

# Functional Health Patterns with Related Nursing Diagnoses

## HEALTH PERCEPTION HEALTH MANAGEMENT
- Perceived health status
- Perceived health management
- Health care behaviors: health promotion and illness prevention activities, medical treatments, follow-up care

## VALUE-BELIEF
- Values, goals, or beliefs (including spirituality) that guide choices or decisions
- Perceived conflicts in values, beliefs, or expectations that are health related

## COPING-STRESS-TOLERANCE
- Capacity to resist challenges to self-integrity
- Methods of handling stress
- Support systems
- Perceived ability to control and manage situations

## NUTRITIONAL-METABOLIC
- Daily consumption of food and fluids
- Favorite foods
- Use of dietary supplements
- Skin lesions and ability to heal
- Condition of the integument
- Weight, height, temperature

## Part 5
### Cognitive-Perceptual Patterns
### NANDA Nursing Diagnoses

- Acute Confusion
- Decreased Intracranial Adaptive Capacity
- Autonomic Dysreflexia
- Risk for Autonomic Dysreflexia
- Chronic Confusion
- Impaired Verbal Communication
- Acute Pain
- Chronic Pain
- Impaired Memory
- Unilateral Neglect
- Risk for Peripheral Neurovascular Dysfunction
- Risk for Post-Trauma Syndrome
- Ineffective Protection
- Disturbed Sensory Perception
- Disturbed Thought Processes
- Decisional Conflict
- Risk for Trauma
- Wandering
- Unilateral Neglect
- Impaired Environmental Interpretation Syndrome

## SEXUALITY-REPRODUCTIVE
- Satisfaction with sexuality or sexual relationships
- Reproductive pattern
- Female menstrual and perimeno-pausal history

## ELIMINATION
- Patterns of bowel and urinary excretion
- Perceived regularity or irregularity of elimination
- Use of laxatives or routines
- Changes in time, modes, quality or quantity of excretions
- Use of devices for control

## ROLE-RELATIONSHIP
- Perception of major roles, relationships, and responsibilities in current life situation
- Satisfaction with or disturbances in roles and relationships

## ACTIVITY-EXERCISE
- Patterns of personally relevant exercise, activity, leisure, and recreation
- ADLs which require energy expenditure
- Factors that interfere with the desired pattern (e.g., illness or injury)

## SELF-PERCEPTION–SELF-CONCEPT
- Attitudes about self
- Perceived abilities, worth, self-image, emotions
- Body posture and movement, eye contact, voice and speech patterns

## SLEEP-REST
- Patterns of sleep and rest-/relaxation in a 24-hr period
- Perceptions of quality and quantity of sleep and rest
- Use of sleep aids and routines

## COGNITIVE-PERCEPTUAL
- Adequacy of vision, hearing, taste, touch, smell
- Pain perception and management
- Language, judgment, memory, decisions

*Reprinted from Nursing Diagnosis: Process and Application, 3rd ed., by M. Gordon, pp. 80–96, Copyright © 1994, with permission from Elsevier Science.*

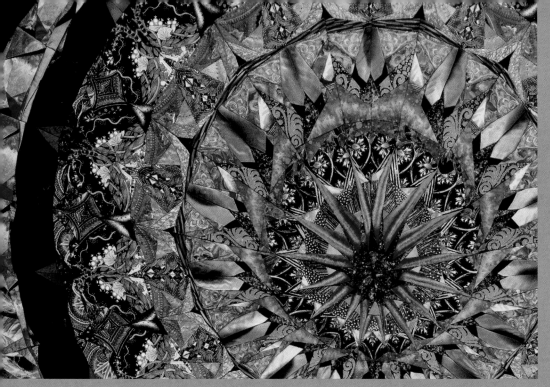

# RESPONSES TO ALTERED NEUROLOGIC FUNCTION

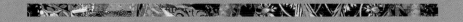

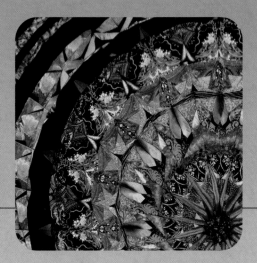

# Assessing Clients with Neurologic Disorders

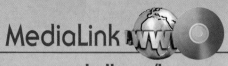

## MediaLink

**www.prenhall.com/lemone**

Additional resources for this chapter can be found on the Student CD-ROM accompanying this textbook, and on the Companion Website at www. prenhall.com/lemone. Click on Chapter 40 to select the activities for this chapter.

**CD-ROM**
- Audio Glossary
- NCLEX Review

*Animation*
- Nervous System A&P

*Video*
- Extrapyramidal Signs

**Companion Website**
- More NCLEX Review
- Functional Health Pattern Assessment
- Case Study
    Assessing an Unconscious Client

## LEARNING OUTCOMES

After completing this chapter, you will be able to:

- Review the anatomy and physiology of the nervous system.

- Identify specific topics for consideration during a health history assessment interview of the client with neurologic disorders.

- Describe assessment of neurologic function, including examinations of mental status, cranial nerves, sensory nerves, motor nerves, cerebellar function, and reflexes.

- Describe special neurologic examinations for clients with suspected meningeal irritation and for comatose clients.

- Identify abnormal findings that may indicate impairment of neurologic function.

The nervous system regulates and integrates all body functions, mental abilities, and emotions. It collects information from the internal and external environments as sensory input, processes and interprets the input, and causes responses that are manifested as motor or sensory output.

## REVIEW OF ANATOMY AND PHYSIOLOGY

The nervous system is divided into two regions: the central nervous system (CNS), which consists of the brain and spinal cord, and the peripheral nervous system (PNS), which consists of the cranial nerves, the spinal nerves, and the autonomic nervous system. These two highly integrated regions consist of just two types of cells: neurons, which receive impulses and send them on to other cells, and neuroglia, which protect and nourish the neurons.

### Neurons

Each neuron consists of a dendrite, a cell body, and an axon. The dendrite is a short process (projection) from the cell body that conducts impulses toward (afferent) the cell body. Cell bodies, most of which are located within the CNS, are clustered in ganglia or nuclei. The cell bodies and dendrites comprise what is often called the gray matter of the CNS. The axon, a long process, conducts impulses away (efferent) from the cell body. Many axons are covered with a myelin sheath, a white lipid substance. It is interrupted at intervals in unmyelinated areas called nodes of Ranvier, which allow movement of ions between the axon and the extracellular fluid. The myelin sheath serves to increase the speed of nerve impulse conduction in axons and is essential for the survival of larger nerve processes. Myelinated nerve fibers comprise the white matter of the brain and spinal cord.

### Action Potentials

Action potentials are impulses (movements of electrical charge along an axon membrane) that allow neurons to communicate with other neurons and body cells. They are initiated by stimuli and propagated by the rapid movement of charged ions through the cell membrane. When a neuron reaches a certain level of stimulation, an electrical impulse is generated and conducted along the length of its axon. The movement of impulses to and from the CNS is made possible by afferent and efferent neurons. Afferent, or sensory, neurons have receptors in skin, muscles, and other organs and relay impulses to the CNS. Efferent, or motor, neurons transmit impulses from the CNS to cause some type of action.

Nerve impulses occur when a stimulus reaches a point great enough to generate a change in electrical charge across the cell membrane of a neuron. A neuron that is not involved in impulse conduction is in a resting, or polarized, state, in which the number of positive ions in the fluid outside of the cell membrane is greater than in the fluid within the cell. The chief regulators of membrane potential are sodium and potassium: Sodium is the major positive ion in the extracellular fluid, and potassium is the major positive ion in the intracellular fluid. In response to an electrical stimulus, the cell membrane becomes permeable to sodium, which moves into the cell. This changes the polar-

ity of the cell membrane, and the neuron is said to depolarize. This event stimulates an action potential, or a nerve impulse, to travel down the axon. When the charges and ions return to their original resting state, the neuron is repolarized. The events in an action potential are as follows:

- Initially, sodium permeability increases. As the membrane is depolarized, sodium channels open and sodium rushes into the cell to a point of depolarization (the inside of the cell becomes less negative in comparison to the outside of the cell).
- This is followed by a decrease in sodium permeability, lasting only about 1 millisecond. The sodium gates close and the sodium influx stops.
- The final event is an increase in potassium permeability. The potassium gates open, potassium rushes out of the cell, and the cell interior becomes progressively less positive. The membrane potential moves back to its resting state and is repolarized.

The action potential is generated only at the point of the stimulus; but once generated, it is propagated along the entire length of the axon regardless if the stimulus continues. Conduction of the impulse is rapid in myelinated fibers, with the action potential "jumping" from one node of Ranvier to the next. The conduction of the impulse is slower in unmyelinated fibers.

### Neurotransmitters

Neurotransmitters are the chemical messengers of the nervous system. When the action potential reaches the end of the axon at the presynaptic terminal, a neurotransmitter is released and travels across the synaptic cleft to bind with receptors in the postsynaptic neuron dendrite or cell body. The neurotransmitter may either be inhibitory or excitatory. The excitatory neurotransmitter is almost always acetylcholine (ACh), which is rapidly degraded by the enzyme acetylcholinesterase. Norepinephrine (NE) is another major neurotransmitter. It may be either excitatory or inhibitory.

Nerves that transmit impulses through the release of ACh are called cholinergic. Receptors that bind ACh are found in the viscera, skeletal muscle cells, and the adrenal medulla (where they stimulate the release of epinephrine). The effect of ACh binding may be either to stimulate or to inhibit a response.

Nerves that transmit impulses through the release of NE are called adrenergic. Receptors that bind NE are found in the heart, lungs, kidneys, blood vessels, and all target organs stimulated by the sympathetic division except the heart. Adrenergic receptors are further divided into alpha and beta types. Alpha-adrenergic receptors help control such varied functions as arterial vasoconstriction and pupil dilation. Beta-adrenergic fibers may be either beta$_1$ or beta$_2$ receptors. Beta$_1$ receptors are found in the heart, where they regulate the rate and force of contraction. Beta$_2$ receptors are found in receptor cells of the lungs, arteries, liver, and uterus; they help regulate bronchial diameter, arterial diameter, and glycogenesis. Generally, binding of NE to alpha receptors stimulates a response, whereas binding to beta receptors inhibits a response.

Other neurotransmitters include gamma aminobutyric acid (GABA), which inhibits CNS function; dopamine, which may be inhibitory or excitatory and helps control fine movement and emotions; and serotonin, which is usually inhibitory and controls sleep, hunger, and behavior and also affects consciousness.

## The Central Nervous System

The central nervous system (CNS) consists of the brain and spinal cord, highly evolved clusters of neurons which act to accept, interconnect, interpret, and generate a response to nerve impulses originating throughout the body.

### The Brain

The brain is the control center of the nervous system and also generates thoughts, emotions, and speech. Averaging 3 to 4 lb in weight, the brain is surrounded by the skull, a bony structure that provides support and protection. The brain has four major regions: the cerebrum, the diencephalon, the brainstem, and the cerebellum (Figure 40–1 ■). The general functions of these regions are summarized in Table 40–1.

The two hemispheres of the cerebrum account for almost 60% of brain weight. The surface of the cerebrum is folded into elevated ridges of tissue called gyri, which are separated by shallow grooves called sulci. Deep grooves called fissures further divide the surface of the cerebrum. The longitudinal fissure separates the hemispheres, and the transverse fissure separates the cerebrum from the cerebellum. In addition, each cerebral hemisphere is divided into frontal, parietal, temporal, and occipital lobes (Figure 40–2 ■).

The cerebral hemispheres are connected by a thick band of nerve fibers called the corpus callosum, which allows communication between the two hemispheres. Each hemisphere receives sensory and motor impulses from the opposite side of the body. One of the cerebral hemispheres tends to develop

| TABLE 40–1 | General Functions of the Four Regions of the Brain |
|---|---|
| **Region** | **Functions** |
| Cerebrum | Interprets sensory input. Controls skeletal muscle activity. Processes intellect and emotions. Contains skills memory. |
| Diencephalon | Conducts sensory and motor impulses. Regulates autonomic nervous system. Regulates and produces hormones. Mediates emotional responses. |
| Brainstem | Serves as conduction pathway. Serves as site of decussation of tracts. Contains respiratory nuclei. Helps regulate skeletal muscles. |
| Cerebellum | Processes information. Provides information necessary for balance, posture, and coordinated muscle movement. |

more than the other. Most people have a more highly developed left hemisphere, which is responsible for the control of language. The right hemisphere has greater control over nonverbal perceptual functions.

The cerebral cortex is the outer surface of the cerebrum. It consists of neuron cell bodies, unmyelinated fibers, neuroglia, and blood vessels. The functions of the different lobes of the cerebrum and the specific areas of the cerebral cortex are shown in Figure 40–2 and listed in Table 40–2.

The diencephalon is embedded in the cerebrum superior to the brainstem. It consists of the thalamus, hypothalamus, and epithalamus (see Figure 40–1). The thalamus begins to process sensory impulses before they ascend to the cerebral cortex. It

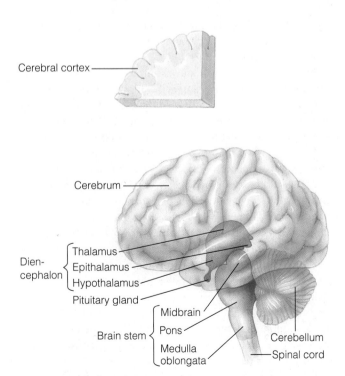

**Figure 40–1** ■ The four major regions of the brain.

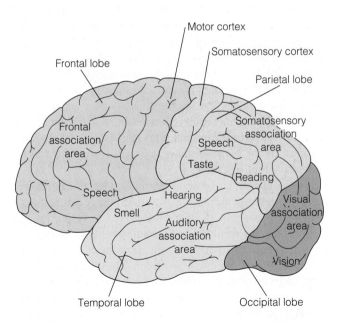

**Figure 40–2** ■ Lobes of the cerebrum and functional areas of the cerebral cortex.

**TABLE 40–2**  Functions of Lobes of the Cerebrum and Areas of the Cerebral Cortex

| Area | Functions |
|---|---|
| Parietal lobe (somatic sensory area of cerebral cortex) | Promotes recognition of pain, coldness, and light touch. The left side receives input from the right side of the body, and vice versa. |
| Occipital lobe | Receives and interprets visual stimuli. |
| Temporal lobe | Receives and interprets olfactory and auditory stimuli. |
| Frontal lobe | Controls movements of voluntary muscles. |
| Primary motor area | Facilitates voluntary movement of skeletal muscles. |
| Speech area | Promotes understanding of spoken and written words. |
| Motor speech area (Broca's area) | Promotes vocalization of words. |

serves as a sorting, processing, and relay station for input into the cortical region. The hypothalamus, located inferior to the thalamus, regulates temperature, water metabolism, appetite, emotional expressions, part of the sleep-wake cycle, and thirst. The epithalamus forms the dorsal part of the diencephalon and includes the pineal body, which is part of the endocrine system that affects growth and development.

**BRAINSTEM.**  The brainstem consists of the midbrain, pons, and medulla oblongata (see Figure 40–1). The midbrain is a center for auditory and visual reflexes. In addition, it functions as a nerve pathway between the cerebral hemispheres and lower brain. The pons is located just below the midbrain. It consists mostly of fiber tracts, but it also contains nuclei that control respiration. The medulla oblongata, located at the base of the brainstem, is continuous with the superior portion of the spinal cord. Nuclei of the medulla oblongata play an important role in controlling cardiac rate, blood pressure, respiration, and swallowing.

The cerebellum is connected to the midbrain, pons, and medulla. Its functions include coordination of skeletal muscle activity, maintenance of balance, and control of fine movements.

**VENTRICLES.**  The brain contains four ventricles, which are chambers filled with cerebrospinal fluid (CSF). They are linked by ducts that allow the CSF to circulate. One lateral ventricle is located within each hemisphere. These communicate with the third ventricle through the foramen of Monro. The third ventricle communicates with the fourth ventricle through the cerebral aqueduct that runs through the midbrain. The cerebral aqueduct is continuous with the central canal of the spinal cord.

**CEREBROSPINAL FLUID.**  A clear and colorless liquid, cerebrospinal fluid (CSF) is formed by the choroid plexus, which are groups of capillaries located in the brain ventricles. It consists of 99% water and contains protein, sodium, chloride, potassium, bicarbonate, and glucose. The usual amount of CSF

ranges from 80 to 200 mL, averaging about 150 mL, and is replaced several times each day. It is absorbed by arachnoid villi. CSF is normally produced and absorbed in equal amounts. CSF circulates from the lateral ventricles of the cerebral hemispheres into the third ventricle, through the midbrain, and into the fourth ventricle. Some CSF flows down the center of the spinal cord as the rest of it circulates into the subarachnoid space and returns to the blood through the arachnoid villi. CSF forms a cushion for the brain tissue, protects the brain and spinal cord from trauma, helps provide nourishment for the brain, and removes waste products of cerebrospinal cellular metabolism.

**MENINGES.**  The CNS is covered and protected by three connective tissue membranes called meninges. The meninges form divisions within the skull, enclose venous sinuses, and contain CSF. The meninges have three layers (Figure 40–3 ■). The outermost layer is attached to the inner surface of the skull, and the innermost layer is the most external brain covering. The outermost, double layer is the dura mater. The middle layer is the arachnoid mater. It forms a space that contains CSF and is the site of all major cerebral blood vessels. The innermost layer, the pia mater, clings to the brain itself and is filled with small blood vessels.

### Cerebral Circulation and the Blood-Brain Barrier
The cerebral hemispheres receive their blood supply from the anterior and middle internal cerebral arteries. These two arteries are branches of the common carotid arteries. The brainstem and cerebellum receive their blood supply from the basilar

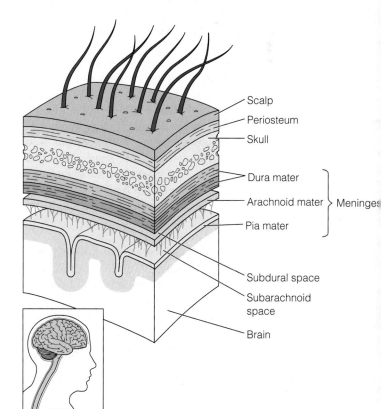

**Figure 40–3** ■ Anatomy of the meninges.

**Figure 40–4** ■ Major arteries serving the brain and the circle of Willis.

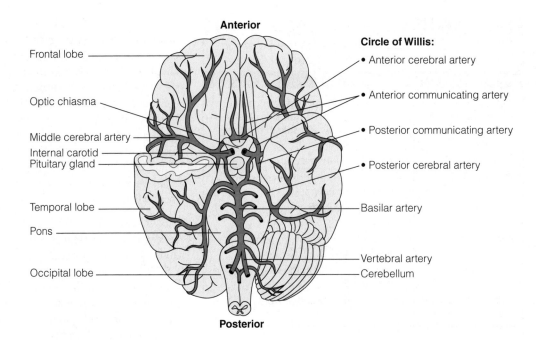

**Anterior**

Frontal lobe

Optic chiasma

Middle cerebral artery

Internal carotid

Pituitary gland

Temporal lobe

Pons

Occipital lobe

**Posterior**

**Circle of Willis:**

• Anterior cerebral artery

• Anterior communicating artery

• Posterior communicating artery

• Posterior cerebral artery

Basilar artery

Vertebral artery

Cerebellum

artery. The posterior cerebrum receives blood from the posterior cerebral arteries. These major arteries are connected by small anterior and posterior communicating arteries, which form a circle of connected blood vessels called the circle of Willis (Figure 40–4 ■). This circle serves as a protective device, providing alternative routes for brain tissues to receive their blood supply. The brain receives about 750 mL of blood each minute and uses 20% of the body's total oxygen uptake. The large amount of oxygen is necessary for metabolism of glucose, which is the brain's sole source of energy.

The capillaries in the brain have low permeability because the cells that compose their walls join at very tight junctions and are surrounded by a basement membrane and by the processes of supporting cells in the brain (called astrocytes). As a result, the brain is protected from many harmful substances in the blood. This blood-brain barrier allows lipids, glucose, some amino acids, water, carbon dioxide, and oxygen to pass through it, thus maintaining a controlled environment. Substances such as urea, creatinine, proteins, some toxins, and most antibiotics cannot pass this barrier and enter brain tissue. However, injury to or infection of the brain may cause increased permeability of the blood-brain barrier, altering concentrations of proteins, water, and electrolytes.

### The Limbic System and the Reticular Formation

The limbic system and the reticular formation are functional brain systems. These systems, made of networks of neurons, communicate across areas of the brain.

The limbic system consists of structures that form a ring of tissue in the medial side of each hemisphere, surrounding the upper portion of the brainstem and corpus callosum. The limbic system integrates and modulates input to make up the affective part of the brain, providing emotional and behavioral responses to environmental stimuli.

The reticular formation is located through the central core of the medulla oblongata, pons, and midbrain. This system has

widespread connections throughout the brain and relays sensory input from all body systems to all levels of the brain. The reticular formation includes the reticular activating system (RAS). The RAS is a stimulating system for the cerebral cortex, keeping it alert and responsive to incoming sensory stimuli while filtering out repetitive or unwanted stimuli. The sleep center inhibits activity of the RAS and drugs and alcohol may depress it. Other parts of the reticular formation include motor nuclei that help maintain muscle tone and coordinated movements through interconnections with spinal nerves, and the vasomotor and cardiovascular regulatory centers, which are part of autonomic regulation of the cardiovascular system.

### The Spinal Cord

The spinal cord is surrounded and protected by 33 vertebrae, including 7 cervical, 12 thoracic, 5 lumbar, 5 sacral, and 4 fused vertebrae, which form the coccyx. Each vertebra consists of a body and a vertebral arch formed by projections from the body. This arch encloses a space called the vertebral foramen. The vertebral foramina of all the vertebrae form the vertebral canal through which the spinal cord passes. Intervertebral foramina are spaces between the vertebrae through which spinal nerve roots pass as they exit the vertebral column.

Intervertebral discs are located between each of the movable vertebrae. Each disc is made of a thick capsule surrounding a gelatinous core called the nucleus pulposus. Ligaments that provide mobility and protection surround the vertebral column, which is discussed in greater detail in Chapter 42. ⊂⊃

The spinal cord extends from the medulla to the level of the first lumbar vertebra (Figure 40–5 ■). It serves as a center for conducting messages to and from the brain and as a reflex center. The spinal cord is about 17 inches (42 cm) long and 0.75 inch (1.8 cm) thick. The cord is protected by the vertebrae, the meninges, and cerebrospinal fluid. The gray matter of the cord is on the inside, and the white matter is on the outside (the reverse of the arrangement in the brain).

The roots of 31 pairs of spinal nerves, divided into the cervical, thoracic, and lumbar nerves, arise from the cord (see Figure 40–5). Each separates into posterior (sensory) and anterior (motor) roots. Damage to the posterior roots results in loss of sensation, whereas damage to the anterior root results in flaccid paralysis.

## Functions of the Spinal Cord and Spinal Roots

Messages to and from the brain are conducted via ascending (sensory) pathways and descending (motor) pathways (Figure 40–6 ■). The major ascending tracts are the lateral and anterior spinothalamic tracts, which carry sensations for pain, temperature, and crude touch; and the posterior tracts, called the fasciculus gracilis and fasciculus cuneatus, which carry sensations for fine touch, position, and vibration. The lateral and anterior corticospinal (pyramidal) tracts are descending tracts consisting of fibers that originate in the motor cortex of the brain and travel to the brainstem and then down the spinal cord. They mediate voluntary purposeful movements and stimulate certain muscular actions while inhibiting others. They also carry fibers that inhibit muscle tone. The rubrospinal, anterior and lateral reticulospinal, and tectospinal (extrapyramidal) tracts include the pathways between the cerebral cortex, basal ganglia, brainstem, and spinal cord outside the pyramidal tract. They maintain muscle tone and gross body movements.

## Upper and Lower Motor Neurons

Upper motor neurons, such as those of the corticospinal and extrapyramidal tract, carry impulses from the cerebral cortex to the anterior gray column of the spinal cord. Damage to upper motor neurons results in increased muscle tone, decreased muscle strength, decreased coordination, and hyperactive reflexes. Lower motor neurons, such as the peripheral and cranial nerves, begin in the anterior gray column of the spinal cord and end in the muscle. These are the "final common pathways." Damage to lower motor neurons results in decreased muscle tone and loss of reflexes.

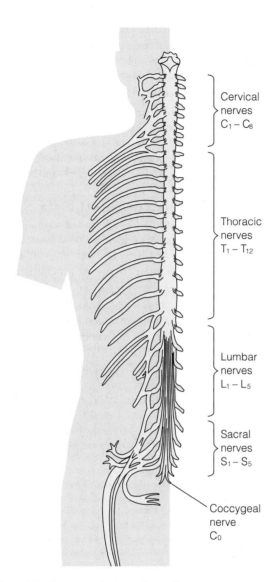

**Figure 40–5** ■ Distribution of spinal nerves.

Cervical nerves $C_1 - C_8$

Thoracic nerves $T_1 - T_{12}$

Lumbar nerves $L_1 - L_5$

Sacral nerves $S_1 - S_5$

Coccygeal nerve $C_0$

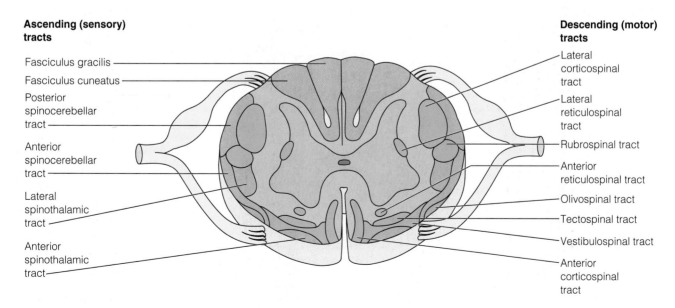

**Ascending (sensory) tracts**

Fasciculus gracilis
Fasciculus cuneatus
Posterior spinocerebellar tract
Anterior spinocerebellar tract
Lateral spinothalamic tract
Anterior spinothalamic tract

**Descending (motor) tracts**

Lateral corticospinal tract
Lateral reticulospinal tract
Rubrospinal tract
Anterior reticulospinal tract
Olivospinal tract
Tectospinal tract
Vestibulospinal tract
Anterior corticospinal tract

**Figure 40–6** ■ Ascending and descending tracts of the spinal cord.

## The Peripheral Nervous System

The peripheral nervous system (PNS) links the CNS with the rest of the body. It is responsible for receiving and transmitting information from and about the external environment. The PNS consists of nerves, ganglia (groups of nerve cells), and sensory receptors located outside—or peripheral to—the brain and spinal cord. The PNS is divided into a sensory (afferent) division and a motor (efferent) division. Most nerves of the PNS contain fibers for both divisions and all are classified regionally as either spinal nerves or cranial nerves.

### Spinal Nerves

The 31 pairs of spinal nerves (see Figure 40–5) are named by their location:

- Cervical nerves: 8 pairs
- Thoracic nerves: 12 pairs
- Lumbar nerves: 5 pairs
- Sacral nerves: 5 pairs
- Coccygeal nerves: 1 pair

Spinal nerves exit the vertebral column through intervertebral foramina to travel to the body regions they serve. The spinal cord does not reach the end of the vertebral column; as a result, the lumbar and sacral nerve roots travel inferiorly through the vertebral canal for some distance before exiting the vertebral column through their associated intervertebral foramina. This collection of descending nerve roots is called the cauda equina.

Each spinal nerve contains both sensory and motor fibers. The sensory fibers are located in the dorsal root, and their cell bodies are located within the dorsal root ganglion. The motor fibers are located in the ventral root, and their cell bodies are located within the spinal cord. The dorsal and ventral roots merge outside the vertebral canal just past the dorsal root ganglion, forming a spinal nerve. Each spinal nerve further divides into branches called rami.

The ventral rami of the cervical, brachial, lumbar, and sacral regions form complex clusters of nerves called plexuses. The main spinal nerve plexuses innervate the skin and the underlying muscles of the arms and legs. For example, the cervical plexus innervates the diaphragm through the phrenic nerve; the brachial plexus innervates the upper extremities through the median, ulnar, and radial nerves; and the lumbar plexus innervates the anterior thigh through the femoral nerve.

An area of skin innervated by cutaneous branches of a single spinal nerve is called a dermatome. The dorsal roots of the spinal nerves carry sensations from these specific dermatomes. Dermatomes provide anatomical landmarks that are useful for locating neurologic lesions (Figure 40–7 ■).

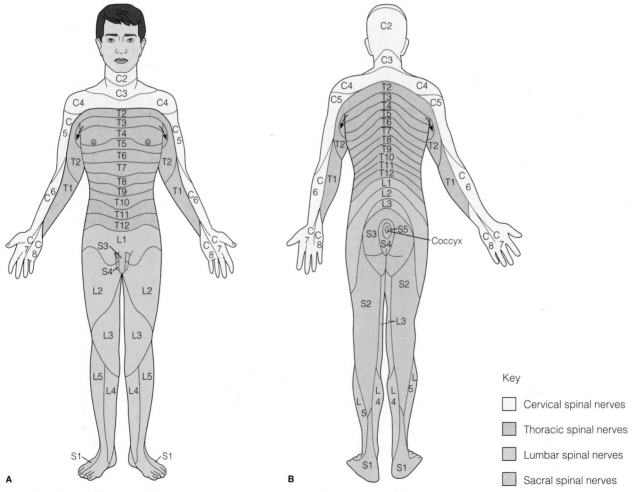

**Figure 40–7** ■ *A,* Anterior, and *B,* posterior dermatomes of the body.

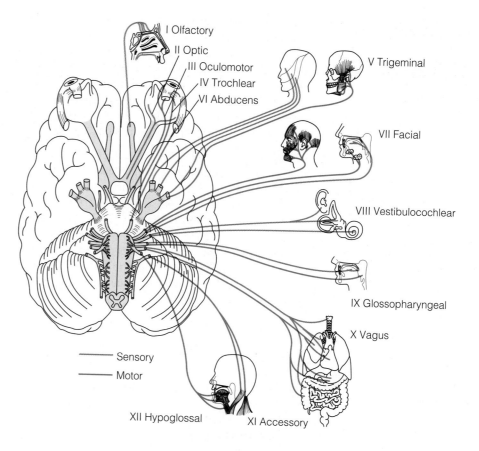

**Figure 40-8** ■ Cranial nerves.

## Cranial Nerves

Twelve pairs of cranial nerves originate in the forebrain and brainstem (Figure 40–8 ■). The vagus nerve extends into the ventral body cavity, but the 11 other pairs innervate only head and neck regions. Although most are mixed nerves, three pairs (olfactory, optic, and vestibulocochlear) are solely sensory. The cranial nerves and their related functions are listed in Table 40–3.

## Reflexes

A reflex is a rapid, involuntary, predictable motor response to a stimulus. Reflexes are categorized as either somatic or autonomic. *Somatic reflexes* result in skeletal muscle contraction. *Autonomic reflexes* activate cardiac muscle, smooth muscle, and glands. A reflex occurs over a pathway called a reflex arc.

The essential components of a *reflex arc* are a receptor, a sensory neuron to carry afferent impulses to the CNS, an integration center in the spinal cord or brain, a motor neuron to carry efferent impulses, and an effector (the tissue that responds by contracting or secreting) (Figure 40–9 ■).

Somatic reflexes mediated by the spinal cord are called *spinal reflexes.* Many spinal reflexes occur without impulses traveling to and from the brain, with the cord serving as the integration center, while others require brain activity and modulation. *Deep-tendon reflexes (DTRs)* occur in response to muscle contraction and cause muscle relaxation and lengthening. DTRs depend on intact sensory and motor nerve roots, functional synapses in the spinal cord, a functional neuromuscular

junction, and a competent muscle. Thus, an abnormal deep-tendon reflex could indicate a variety of health problems, including a lesion of a spinal nerve. Flexor, or withdrawal, reflexes are caused by actual or perceived painful stimuli and result in withdrawal of the part of the body that is threatened. Superficial responses result from gentle cutaneous stimulation. These responses depend on functional upper motor pathways and on an intact reflex arc.

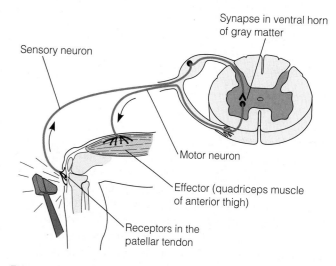

**Figure 40-9** ■ A typical reflex arc of a spinal nerve. In the two-neuron reflex arc, the stimulus is transferred from the sensory neuron directly to the motor neuron at the point of synapse in the spinal cord.

| TABLE 40-3 | Cranial Nerves |
|------------|----------------|
| **Name** | **Function** |
| I Olfactory | Sense of smell |
| II Optic | Vision |
| III Oculomotor | Eyeball movement<br>Raising of upper eyelid<br>Constriction of pupil<br>Proprioception |
| IV Trochlear | Eyeball movement |
| V Trigeminal | Sensation of the upper scalp, upper eyelid, nose, nasal cavity, cornea, and lacrimal gland<br>Sensation of the palate, upper teeth, cheek, top lip, lower eyelid, and scalp<br>Sensation of the tongue, lower teeth, chin, and temporal scalp<br>Chewing |
| VI Abducens | Lateral movement of the eyeball |
| VII Facial | Movement of facial muscles<br>Secretions of lacrimal, nasal, submandibular, and sublingual glands<br>Sensation of taste |
| VIII Vestibulocochlear | Sense of equilibrium<br>Sense of hearing |
| IX Glossopharyngeal | Swallowing<br>Gag reflex<br>Secretions of parotid salivary gland<br>Sense of taste<br>Touch, pressure, and pain from pharynx and posterior tongue<br>Pressure from carotid arteries<br>Receptors to regulate blood pressure |
| X Vagus | Swallowing<br>Regulation of cardiac rate<br>Regulation of respirations<br>Digestion<br>Sensation from thoracic and abdominal organs<br>Proprioception<br>Sense of taste |
| XI Accessory | Movement of head and neck<br>Proprioception |
| XII Hypoglossal | Movement of tongue for speech and swallowing |

## The Autonomic Nervous System

The autonomic nervous system (ANS) is a division of the PNS that regulates the internal environment of the body. It is also called the general visceral motor system, because it consists of motor neurons that innervate the body's viscera. Whereas skeletal muscle activity is regulated by a division of the PNS called the somatic nervous system, the ANS regulates the activity of cardiac muscle, smooth muscle, and glands.

The reticular formation in the brainstem is the primary controller of the ANS. Stimulation of centers in the medulla initiates reflexes that regulate cardiac rate, blood vessel diameter, and gastrointestinal function.

The ANS has sympathetic and parasympathetic divisions. Although fibers from both divisions affect the same structures, the actions of the two divisions are opposite in effect, and they serve to counterbalance each other. The major neurotransmitters for impulse transmission in the ANS are acetylcholine and norepinephrine. Acetylcholine is the primary neurotransmitter of the parasympathetic division. Norepinephrine is the primary neurotransmitter of the sympathetic division.

**SYMPATHETIC DIVISION.** The sympathetic division of the ANS prepares the body to handle situations that are perceived as harmful or stressful and to participate in strenuous activity. Cell bodies for this division arise in the lateral horns of the spinal cord in the area from $T_1$ through $L_2$. The fibers separate after leaving the cord, and form a chain of ganglia that extends from the neck to the pelvis. Long fibers then extend to the organs that are supplied by the sympathetic division. Stimulation of the sympathetic division can exert the following effects on target organs or tissues.

- Dilated pupils
- Inhibited secretions
- Copious production of sweat (**diaphoresis**)
- Increased rate and force of heartbeat
- Vasodilation of the coronary arteries
- Dilation of the bronchioles
- Decreased digestion
- Increased release of glucose by the liver
- Decreased urine output
- Vasoconstriction of arteries
- Vasoconstriction of abdominal and skin blood vessels
- Increased blood clotting
- Increased metabolic rate
- Increased mental alertness

**PARASYMPATHETIC DIVISION.** The parasympathetic division of the ANS operates during nonstressful situations. Cell bodies for this division are located in the brainstem (for the cranial nerves) and in the lateral gray matter of $S_2$ through $S_4$. Other than the fibers supplying the cranial nerves III, VII, IX, and X, the fibers are carried by the vagus nerve to body tissues, thoracic organs, and visceral organs. Stimulation of the parasympathetic division of the ANS produces the following effects.

- Constriction of pupils
- Stimulation of glandular secretions
- Decreased heart rate
- Vasoconstriction of coronary arteries
- Constriction of the bronchioles
- Increased peristalsis and secretion of gastrointestinal fluid

## ASSESSING NEUROLOGIC FUNCTION

The client's neurologic system is assessed by both a health assessment interview to collect subjective data and a physical assessment to collect objective data.

### Health Assessment Interview

This section provides guidelines for collecting subjective data through a health assessment interview specific to the functions

## TABLE 40-4  Glasgow Coma Scale

| Assessment | Response | Score* |
|---|---|---|
| **Eyes open** (Record C if eyes are closed by swelling.) | Spontaneously | 4 |
| | To speech | 3 |
| | To pain | 2 |
| | No response | 1 |
| **Best motor response** (Record best upper arm response.) | Obeys commands | 6 |
| | Localizes pain | 5 |
| | Flexion-withdrawal | 4 |
| | Abnormal flexion | 3 |
| | Abnormal extension | 2 |
| | No response | 1 |
| **Best verbal response** (Record T if an endotracheal or tracheostomy tube is in place.) | Oriented | 5 |
| | Confused | 4 |
| | Inappropriate words | 3 |
| | Incomprehensible sounds | 2 |
| | No response | 1 |
| **Total Score:** | | — |

*A higher score indicates a higher level of functioning.

of the neurologic system. If the client's level of consciousness is altered, the nurse may need to rely on family members for information. The client's level of consciousness may be assessed by using the Glasgow Coma Scale, found in Table 40–4.

An interview to assess neurologic function may focus on a chief complaint or may be done as part of a total health assessment. If the client has a health problem involving any component of neurologic function, analyze its onset, characteristics and course, severity, precipitating and relieving factors, and any associated symptoms, noting the timing and circumstances. For example, ask the client the following:

- Describe the location and intensity of the pain you have experienced in your left leg. Is it made worse by coughing, sneezing, or walking?
- When did you first notice that you were having numbness in your fingers?
- Describe the difficulty you have when you try to walk.

Questions about present health status include information about numbness, tingling sensations, tremors, problems with coordination or balance, or loss of movement in any part of the body. Ask the client about difficulty with speaking, seeing, hearing, tasting, or detecting odors. In addition, elicit information about memory, feeling state (such as anxiety or depression), recent changes in sleep patterns, ability to perform self-care and activities of daily living, sexual activity, and weight. If the client is taking prescribed or over-the-counter medications, ask about the type and purpose, as well as the frequency and duration of use.

Ask about any past history of seizures, fainting, dizziness, headaches, and any trauma, tumors, or surgery of the brain, spinal cord, or nerves. Discuss illnesses that may cause neurologic manifestations, including cardiac disease, strokes, pernicious anemia, sinus infections, liver disease, and/or renal failure. Also ask the client about family history of neurologic health

problems, diabetes mellitus, hypertension, seizures, or mental health problems.

Question the client about occupational hazards, such as exposure to toxic chemicals or materials, use of protective headgear, and the amount of time spent performing repetitive motions (e.g., data entry and assembly). Ask questions about self-care to assess the client's diet and use of tobacco, drugs, or alcohol, and ask whether the client wears a helmet when riding a bike or motorcycle or participating in contact sports.

Interview questions categorized by functional health patterns can be found on the Companion Website.

## Physical Assessment

Physical assessment of the client begins when the nurse first meets the client and makes an overall evaluation of the client's mental and physical status. The mental status examination is conducted with both the nurse and the client seated. The rest of the neurologic examination may be performed with the client either sitting or standing.

The neurologic system is assessed through inspection, palpation, and percussion (with a reflex hammer). When conducting the mental status and cognitive portions of the examination, be aware that fatigue or illness may alter findings. Provide rest periods for the client as needed. When interpreting findings, consider the client's age, educational background, and cultural orientation.

Collect the equipment necessary for this assessment: a cotton ball and safety pin, tongue blade, tuning fork, ophthalmoscope, reflex hammer, pencil and paper, printed materials, and substances to test the senses of smell and taste. The assessment should take place in a private, comfortable setting. Ask the client to remove outer clothing, shoes, and stockings. Provide a gown for the client to wear. It is important to explain to the client that the neurologic examination is lengthy and may consist of questions and requests that seem strange to the client. Explain the rationale for each part of the examination.

A brief version of this physical assessment, often referred to as a *neuro check,* may be performed in a shorter time period when a client requires frequent ongoing assessments of neurologic status (Box 40–1).

### Mental Status Assessment with Abnormal Findings (✓)

- Assess appearance.
- Observe dress, hygiene, and grooming.

### BOX 40–1  ■ Abbreviated Neurologic Assessment (Neuro Check)

1. Assess level of consciousness (response to auditory and/or tactile stimulus).
2. Obtain vital signs (BP, P, R).
3. Check pupillary response to light.
4. Assess strength of hand grip and movement of extremities bilaterally.
5. Determine ability to sense touch/pain in extremities.

MediaLink | FUNCTIONAL HEALTH PATTERN ASSESSMENT

- Observe gait and posture.
  - ✓ Unilateral neglect (inattention to one side of body) may occur with some strokes of the middle cerebral artery. Poor hygiene and grooming may be seen in clients with dementing disorders.
  - ✓ Abnormal gait and posture may be seen in transient ischemic attacks (TIAs), strokes, and Parkinson's disease.
- Assess behavior.
  - Observe client's actions and affect.
  - Note the content and quality of speech.
  - Note level of consciousness. Use the Glasgow Coma Scale (see Table 40–4) to document findings. Scores may range from 3 (deeply comatose) to 15 (alert and oriented).
  - ✓ Emotional swings or changes in personality may be observed with strokes of the anterior cerebral artery.
  - ✓ The face appears masklike (very little expressive movement of facial muscles) in clients with Parkinson's disease.
  - ✓ Apathy is seen in dementing disorders.
  - ✓ Aphasia (defective or absent language function) may occur in TIAs. Receptive aphasia (inability to understand verbal or written language) is often noted in strokes of the posterior or anterior cerebral artery. Aphasias are seen with damage to the left cerebral cortex. Aphasias are more often seen with strokes of the right hemisphere than the left hemisphere.
  - ✓ Dysphonia (change in the tone of the voice) is common in strokes of the posterior inferior cerebral artery. Dysphonia is seen with paralysis of the vocal cords (cranial nerve X).
  - ✓ Dysarthria (difficulty speaking) is seen with lesions of upper and lower motor neurons, the cerebellum, and the extrapyramidal tract. It is also seen in strokes of the anterior inferior and superior cerebral arteries.
  - ✓ Damage to the brainstem and/or cerebral cortex may alter level of consciousness.
  - ✓ Drowsiness and decreased level of consciousness may be associated with brain trauma, infections, TIAs, stroke, and brain tumors.
  - ✓ Level of consciousness is usually altered and may progress to coma with stroke of the middle cerebral artery.
  - ✓ Confusion and coma may be seen in clients with strokes affecting the vertebralbasilar arteries.
- Assess cognitive function.
  - Note orientation to time, place, and person.
  - Note attention span and recent and remote memory. Ask the client to:
    1. Repeat five to seven numbers.
    2. Recall three items after 5 minutes.
    3. Recall his or her address, breakfast, or birthday.
  - Assess thought processes (both content and perceptions) by noting responses to questions.
  - Note ability to understand what is said and to express thoughts.
  - Note ability to make logical and safe judgments.
  - ✓ Disorientation to time and place may occur in clients with stroke of the right cerebral hemisphere.
  - ✓ Memory deficits are often seen with strokes of the anterior cerebral artery and vertebralbasilar artery.

- ✓ Perceptual deficits may be seen in strokes of the middle cerebral artery. These same deficits may occur following brain trauma and in dementing disorders.
- ✓ Impaired cognition is often noted with strokes of the middle cerebral artery, cerebral trauma, and brain tumors.

## Cranial Nerve Assessments with Possible Abnormal Findings (✓)

- Test CN I (olfactory).
- Note client's ability to smell scents (e.g., soap, coffee) with each nostril. This test is usually done only if a problem with the ability to smell is reported.
  - ✓ Anosmia (an inability to smell) may be seen with lesions of the frontal lobe and may also occur with impaired blood flow to the middle cerebral artery.
- Test CN II (optic).
  - Assess vision with Snellen chart (see Chapter 44 ∞ for guidelines).
  - ✓ Blindness in one eye may be seen with strokes of the internal carotid artery or with TIAs. Impaired vision or blindness in one side of both eyes (homonymous hemianopia) is associated with blockage of the posterior cerebral artery.
  - ✓ Impaired vision may also be seen with strokes of the anterior cerebral artery and brain tumors.
  - ✓ Blindness or double vision may be noted with involvement of the vertebralbasilar arteries. Double or blurred vision may also occur with TIAs.
  - ✓ Papilledema (swelling of the optic nerve) occurs with increased intracranial pressure.
- Test CN III, IV, and VI (oculomotor, trochlear, and abducens).
  - Assess extraocular movements by asking the client to follow your finger as you write an *H* in the air (see Chapter 44).
  - Assess PERRL ("pupils equally round and reactive to light") by covering one eye at a time and shining a bright light directly into the uncovered eye (use a penlight or the ophthalmoscope). See Chapter 44 for more detailed assessment guidelines.
  - Assess for ptosis (drooping eyelids).
  - ✓ Nystagmus (involuntary eye movement) may be seen with strokes of the anterior, inferior, and superior cerebellar arteries. Constricted pupils are associated with impaired blood flow to the vertebralbasilar arteries. Ptosis (also called Horner's syndrome) occurs with strokes of the posterior inferior cerebellar artery, myasthenia gravis, and palsy of CN III.
- Test CN V (trigeminal).
  - Assess ability to feel light, dull, and sharp sensations on the face. With the client's eyes closed, check whether sensation is the same on both sides of the face. Stroke the cheek with a wisp of cotton for light touch, with a closed safety pin for dull touch, and with a tongue blade for sharp touch. If the sharp point of a safety pin is used to assess sharp touch, be sure to avoid scratching the surface of the skin, and discard the pin after it is used.
  - Assess the corneal reflex by touching the corneal surface with a wisp of cotton. This reflex is tested on unconscious clients. Normally the client blinks.

✓ Changes in facial sensations are noted with impaired blood flow to the carotid artery.

✓ Decreased sensations to the face and cornea on the same side of the body occur with strokes of the posterior inferior cerebral artery.

✓ Lip and mouth numbness occur with strokes of the vertebralbasilar artery.

✓ Loss of facial sensation or contraction of the masseter and temporal muscles is seen with lesions of CN V.

✓ Severe facial pain is seen with trigeminal neuralgia (tic douloureux).

✓ The corneal reflex may be impaired with lesions of CN V or VII.

- Test CN VII (facial).
  - Assess ability to taste sweet, sour, and salt on the anterior two-thirds of the tongue by asking the client to stick out the tongue and applying a salty, sweet, or sour substance.
  - Assess ability to frown, show teeth, blow out cheeks, raise eyebrows, smile, and close eyes tightly.
  - ✓ Loss of ability to taste may occur with brain tumors or with nerve impairment.
  - ✓ Asymmetry or decreased movement of facial muscles is noted with lesions of the upper and lower motor neurons.
  - ✓ Paralysis of the lower motor neurons results in the inability to close eyes, a flat nasolabial fold, paralysis of lower face, and inability to wrinkle forehead.
  - ✓ Paralysis of the upper motor neurons results in weakness of eyelids and paralysis of lower face.
  - ✓ Pain, paralysis, and sagging of facial muscles is seen on the affected side in Bell's palsy.
- Test CN VIII (acoustic).
  - Assess ability to hear the ticking of a watch and whispered and spoken words (see Chapter 44).
  - ✓ Decreased hearing or deafness may occur with strokes of the vertebralbasilar arteries and/or tumors of CN VIII.
- Test CN IX and X (glossopharyngeal and vagus).
  - Observe client swallowing a small drink of water.
  - Observe for a symmetrical rise of the soft palate and uvula as the client says "ah."
  - Assess gag reflex by touching back of client's throat with tongue blade.
  - Assess ability to taste salty, sweet, and sour substances on the posterior third of the tongue (see previous description).
  - ✓ **Dysphagia** (difficulty swallowing) is common with impaired blood flow to the vertebralbasilar arteries and to the posterior inferior, anterior inferior, or superior cerebellar arteries.
  - ✓ Unilateral loss of the gag reflex occurs with lesions of CN IX and X.
- Test CN XI (spinal accessory).
  - Assess the client's ability to shrug the shoulders and turn head against resistance: Ask the client to turn the head to one side against the resistance of your hand; ask the client to shrug the shoulders while you exert downward pressure. Observe symmetry, strength, and size of muscles.
  - ✓ Muscle weakness is noted with lower motor neuron disease. Contralateral hemiparesis is seen with strokes affecting the middle or internal carotid artery.

- Test CN XII (hypoglossal).
  - Assess the client's ability to stick out the tongue and move the tongue from side to side against resistance of a tongue blade.
  - ✓ Atrophy and **fasciculations** (twitches) of the tongue are seen in lower motor neuron disease. The tongue may deviate toward involved side of the body.

### Sensory Function Assessments with Abnormal Findings (✓)

- Assess ability to perceive various sensations.
  - Touch both sides of various parts of the body (the chest, abdomen, arms, and legs) with one or more of the following:
    1. Cotton wisp
    2. Sharp object
    3. Dull object
    4. Vibrating tuning fork placed on bony prominences
  - ✓ Decreased sensation of pain occurs with injury to the spinothalamic tract.
  - ✓ Decreased vibratory sensations are seen with injuries to the posterior column tract.
  - ✓ Transient numbness of face, arm, or hand is seen with TIAs.
  - ✓ Sensory loss on one side of the body is seen with lesions of higher pathways to the spinal cord.
  - ✓ Bilateral sensory loss is seen in polyneuropathy. Sensations are impaired with strokes, brain tumors, and spinal cord trauma or compression.
- Assess sense of position (**kinesthesia**).
  - Move the client's finger or big toe up or down. Ask the client to describe the movement.
  - ✓ Lesions of the posterior column of the spinal cord may affect sense of position.
- Assess ability to discriminate fine touch.
  - Ask the client to identify:
    1. Object in hand, such as a coin or key (tests stereognosis).
    2. Number written on hand (tests graphesthesia) (Figure 40–10 ■).

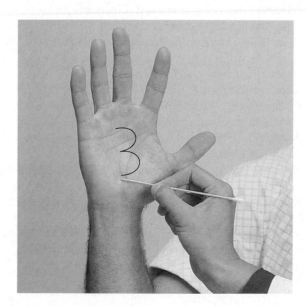

**Figure 40–10** ■ Testing graphesthesia.

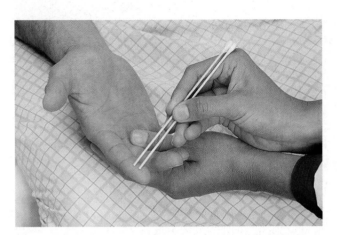

**Figure 40–11** ■ Testing two-point discrimination.

3. Two points of simultaneous pinpricks on the hand (tests two-point discrimination) (Figure 40–11 ■).
4. Where he/she is being touched (tests localization).
5. How many sensations are felt when touched simultaneously on both sides of the body (tests extinction).
✓ Inability to discriminate fine touch (stereognosis, graphesthesia, two points, point localization and extinction) may occur with injury to the posterior columns or sensory cortex.

## Motor Function Assessments with Abnormal Findings (✓)

• Assess bilateral symmetry and size of muscles.
✓ Atrophy of muscles is seen with disease of the lower motor neurons.
• Assess for **tremors** (rhythmic movements) and fasciculations. Observe movements as client is at rest (not making a purposeful movement) and with activity (making a purposeful movement, such as reaching for a glass of water).
✓ Tremors that occur with activity are seen in multiple sclerosis and disease of the cerebellar system.
✓ Tremors that occur at rest and disappear with movement are common in Parkinson's disease.
✓ Fasciculations occur in disease or trauma to the lower motor neurons, as a side effect of medications, in fever, in sodium deficiency, and in uremia.
• Assess muscle tone.
✓ Muscle tone is decreased (**flaccidity**) in disease or trauma of the lower motor neurons and early stroke.
✓ Muscle tone is increased (**spasticity**) in disease of the corticospinal motor tract.
✓ Muscles are rigid in disease of the extrapyramidal motor tract.
✓ Muscles move in small, regular jerky movements (cogwheel rigidity) in Parkinson's disease.
• Assess bilateral muscle strength and movement. The following criteria for recording the grading of muscle strength are often used.
0 = no contraction
1 = trace of contraction
2 = active movement with gravity

3 = active movement against gravity
4 = active movement against gravity and resistance
5 = normal power

Ask the client to:

1. Squeeze your hands.
2. Push feet against the resistance of your hands.
3. Raise both legs off the bed.
✓ Weakness of the arms, legs, or hands is often seen with TIAs. **Hemiplegia** (paralysis of one-half of the body vertically) is noted with strokes of the internal carotid artery and posterior cerebral artery.
✓ Weakness of extremities is often noted with strokes of the vertebralbasilar arteries.
✓ Flaccid paralysis is noted with strokes of the anterior spinal artery.
✓ Paralysis or decreased movement is seen in multiple sclerosis and myasthenia gravis.
✓ There is total loss of motor function below the level of injury in complete spinal cord transection and in injuries to the anterior portion of the spinal cord.
✓ Spasticity of muscles may occur as a result of incomplete spinal cord injuries.

## Cerebellar Function Assessments with Abnormal Findings (✓)

• Assess the gait. Ask the client to walk normally, then in a heel-to-toe fashion, then on toes, and finally on heels.
• Perform Romberg's test: Ask the client to stand with the feet together and eyes closed. (Stand close to client to prevent falling). There should be minimal swaying for up to 20 seconds.
✓ **Ataxia** is a lack of coordination and a clumsiness of movements, with staggering, wide-based, and unbalanced gait. Ataxia is often seen with anterior strokes and cerebellar tumors. Swaying and falling is seen in cerebellar ataxia. Inability to walk on toes, then heels may indicate disease of the upper motor neurons.
✓ Spastic hemiparesis is often associated with strokes or upper motor neuron disease. The client walks with one leg stiffly dragging while the other leg circles out and forward. One arm is held flexed and close to the side.
✓ Steppage gait is noted with disease of the lower motor neurons. The client drags or lifts the foot high, then slaps the foot onto the floor. The client cannot walk on the heels.
✓ Sensory ataxia may be associated with polyneuropathy or damage to the posterior columns. The client walks on the heels before bringing down the toes and the feet are held wide apart. Gait worsens with the eyes closed.
✓ Parkinsonian gait is often seen in Parkinson's disease. The client stoops over while walking and shuffles the feet. The arms are held close to the side.
✓ A positive Romberg's test may be seen in cerebellar ataxia.
• Assess coordination.
• Observe ability to pat knees, alternating front and back of hands and increasing speed.
• Observe ability to touch each finger of one hand to the thumb.

MediaLink | EXTRAPYRAMIDAL SIGNS VIDEO

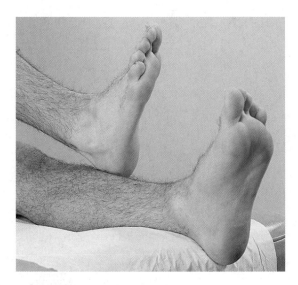

**Figure 40–12** ■ Heel-to-shin test.

- Observe ability to touch the nose, then one of your fingers, then the nose again.
- Observe ability to run each heel down each shin, while in a supine position (Figure 40–12 ■).
  ✓ Ataxic movements are apparent in cerebellar disease.

## Reflex Assessments with Abnormal Findings (✓)

A reflex hammer is used to strike the tendon of various reflex sites. To test deep-tendon reflexes, ask the client to lock the fingers of both hands together and then pull; this encourages relaxation and promotes reflexes of lower extremities. Superficial reflexes are assessed by lightly stroking the area with the end of a tongue blade. The following criteria for recording reflexes are often used. A score of 2 is considered normal.

0 = absent or no response
1 = hypoactive; weaker than normal (+)
2 = normal (++)
3 = stronger than normal (+++)
4 = hyperactive (++++)

- Assess the patellar, biceps, brachioradialis, triceps, and achilles deep-tendon reflexes (Figure 40–13 ■).
  ✓ Hyperactive reflexes are present with lesions of upper motor neurons.
  ✓ Decreased reflexes are present with lower motor neuron involvement.
- Assess for clonus by dorsiflexing the client's foot.
  ✓ **Clonus,** a hyperactive, rhythmic dorsiflexion and plantar flexion of the foot, is noted with upper motor neuron disease.

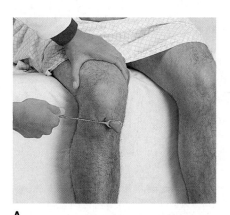

**A**

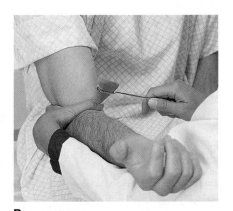

**B**

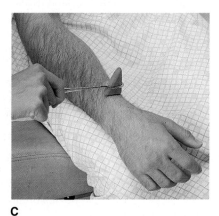

**C**

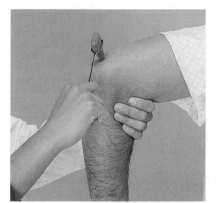

**D**

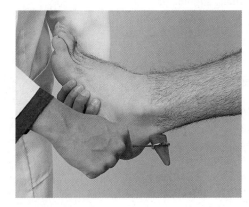

**E**

**Figure 40–13** ■ Deep-tendon reflexes. *A,* Using reinforcement technique to test the patellar reflex. *B,* Biceps reflex. *C,* Brachioradialis reflex. *D,* Triceps reflex. *E,* Achilles reflex.

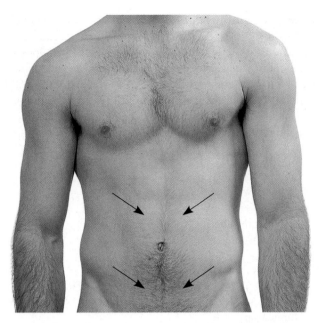

**Figure 40–14** ■ Location of superficial abdominal reflexes.

- Assess the superficial abdominal and cremasteric reflexes.
  - Abdominal reflex: Lightly stroke the abdomen with a tongue blade from the side to the midline. Normally the side of the abdomen being stroked will contract (Figure 40–14 ■).
  - Cremasteric reflex: Lightly stroke the inner thigh of the male client with a tongue blade. Normally, the testicle on the side being stroked will rise.
  - ✓ Superficial reflexes may be absent with disease of the lower and upper motor neurons.
- Assess the Babinski reflex (Figure 40–15 ■).
  - ✓ Dorsiflexion of the big toe and fanning of the other toes is seen with upper motor neuron disease of the pyramidal tract.

## Special Neurologic Assessments with Abnormal Findings (✓)

- Assess for Brudzinski's sign. With the client supine, flex the head to the chest (Figure 40–16 ■).
  - ✓ Pain, resistance, and flexion of hips and knees occur with meningeal irritation.
- Assess for Kernig's sign. With the client supine, flex the knees and hips, then straighten the knee (Figure 40–17 ■).
  - ✓ Excessive pain and/or resistance occurs with meningeal irritation.
- Assess for abnormal postures.
  - Observe for **decorticate posturing,** in which the upper arms are close to the sides; the elbows, wrists, and fingers are flexed; the legs are extended with internal rotation; and the feet are plantar flexed (Figure 40–18 ■).
  - Observe for **decerebrate posturing,** in which the neck is extended, with the jaw clenched; the arms are pronated, extended, and close to the sides; the legs are extended straight out; and the feet are plantar flexed (Figure 40–19 ■).
  - ✓ Decorticate posturing occurs with lesions of the corticospinal tracts.
  - ✓ Decerebrate posturing occurs with lesions of the midbrain, pons, or diencephalon.

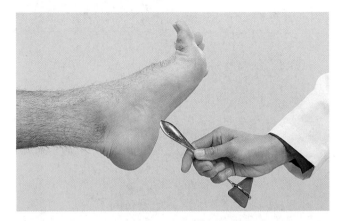

**Figure 40–15** ■ Testing for the Babinski reflex.

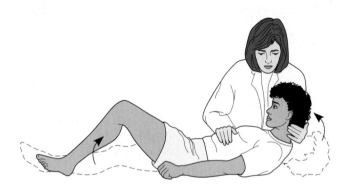

**Figure 40–16** ■ Testing for Brudzinski's sign.

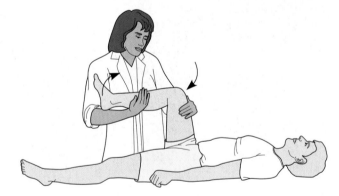

**Figure 40–17** ■ Testing for Kernig's sign.

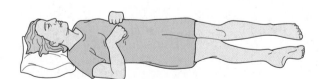

**Figure 40–18** ■ Decorticate posturing.

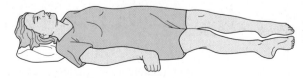

**Figure 40–19** ■ Decerebrate posturing.

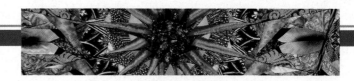

 EXPLORE MediaLink

NCLEX review questions, case studies, care plan activities, MediaLink applications, and other interactive resources for this chapter can be found on the Companion Website at www.prenhall.com/lemone.

Click on Chapter 40 to select the activities for this chapter. For animations, video clips, more NCLEX review questions, and an audio glossary, access the Student CD-ROM accompanying this textbook.

## TEST YOURSELF

1. What component of the brain protects it from harmful substances?

   a. The circulation of cerebrospinal fluid
   b. The large oxygen demand
   c. The structure of neurons
   d. The blood-brain barrier

2. What pathophysiology results from damage to the lower motor neurons?

   a. Loss of cognitive ability
   b. Inability to communicate verbally
   c. Loss of reflexes
   d. Decreasing levels of consciousness

3. Which of the physical assessment techniques is **not** used in the neurologic examination?

   a. Inspection
   b. Auscultation
   c. Percussion
   d. Palpation

4. What would you need to assess function of cranial nerve V (trigeminal)?

   a. Cotton ball and safety pin
   b. Stethoscope with bell and diaphragm
   c. Measuring tape and pencil
   d. Various scents, such as coffee and vanilla

5. Which position best describes decorticate posturing?

   a. Neck extended, arms extended and pronated, feet plantar flexed
   b. Arms close to sides, elbows and wrists flexed, legs extended
   c. In prone position with arms and knees sharply flexed
   d. In supine position, spine extended, legs extended

See Test Yourself answers in Appendix C.

## BIBLIOGRAPHY

Jagoda, A., & Riggio, S. (1999). The rapid neurologic examination, part 1. History, mental status, cranial nerves. An orderly search identifies problems requiring immediate care. *Journal of Critical Illness, 14*(6), 325–331.

Maher, L. (2000). A quick neurologic examination. *Patient Care, 34*(3), 161–162, 165–168, 171–172.

O'Hanlon-Nichols, T. (1999). Neurologic assessment. *American Journal of Nursing, 99*(6), 44–50.

Riggio, S., & Jagoda A. (1999). The rapid neurologic examination, part 2: Movement, reflexes, sensation, balance. Know the signs that lead to the site of the pathologic process. *Journal of Critical Illness, 14*(7), 368–372.

Weber, J., & Kelley, J. (2002). *Health assessment in nursing* (2nd ed.). Philadelphia: Lippincott.

### CHAPTER 41

# Nursing Care of Clients with Cerebrovascular and Spinal Cord Disorders

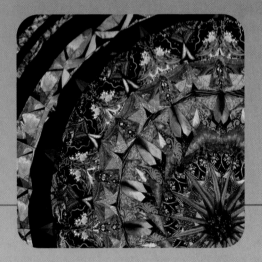

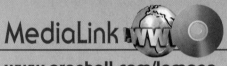

## MediaLink

## www.prenhall.com/lemone

Additional resources for this chapter can be found on the Student CD-ROM accompanying this textbook, and on the Companion Website at www. prenhall.com/lemone. Click on Chapter 41 to select the activities for this chapter.

**CD-ROM**
- Audio Glossary
- NCLEX Review

**Companion Website**
- More NCLEX Review
- Case Study
  Spinal Cord Injury
- Care Plan Activity
  Hemorrhagic Stroke

## LEARNING OUTCOMES

After completing this chapter, you will be able to:

- Apply knowledge of normal neurologic anatomy and physiology and assessments when providing nursing care for clients with cerebrovascular and spinal cord disorders (see Chapter 40).

- Identify factors responsible for disorders in cerebral blood flow.

- Explain the pathophysiologic effects, manifestations, and complications of alterations in cerebral blood flow due to thrombi, emboli, hemorrhage, aneurysm, and arteriovenous malformation.

- Identify factors responsible for spinal cord injuries.

- Discuss the pathophysiologic effects of injuries of the spinal cord by level of injury.

- Describe the causes and manifestations of cervical and lumbar herniated intervertebral disks.

- Discuss the types and manifestations of spinal cord tumors.

- Explain the collaborative care of clients with cerebrovascular and spinal cord disorders.

- Use the nursing process as a framework for providing individualized care to clients with cerebrovascular and spinal cord disorders.

The health problems discussed in this chapter result from alterations in cerebral blood flow and from disorders of the spinal cord. Disorders of the spinal cord and brain affect an estimated 50 million Americans, costing the American public more than $400 billion a year in direct health care costs and indirect lifetime costs. Clients with disorders of cerebral blood flow and the spinal cord experience a wide variety of neurologic deficits that affect cognitive and perceptual health patterns.

Nursing care for clients with these disorders is tailored to meet the needs of the client and is individualized according to the client's responses to alterations in intracranial and spinal cord structure and function. This chapter's discussion of nursing care includes consideration of acute and long-term health care needs.

# CEREBROVASCULAR DISORDERS

## THE CLIENT WITH A STROKE

A **stroke (cerebral vascular accident, CVA),** also referred to as a *brain attack,* is a condition in which neurologic deficits result from decreased blood flow to a localized area of the brain. Strokes may be *ischemic* (when blood supply to a part of the brain is suddenly interrupted by a thrombus or embolus) or *hemorrhagic* (when a blood vessel breaks open, spilling blood into spaces surrounding neurons). The neurologic deficits caused by ischemia and the resultant necrosis of cells in the brain vary according to the area of the brain involved, the size of the affected area, and the length of time blood flow is decreased or stopped. A major loss of blood supply to the brain can cause severe disability or death. When the duration of decreased blood flow is short and the anatomical area involved is small, the person may not be aware that damage has been done.

### INCIDENCE AND PREVALENCE

Strokes are the third leading cause of death in North America, where approximately 600,000 people suffer a stroke each year. Of those, 160,000 die, and many clients who survive are left with some type of functional impairment (Porth, 2002). The highest incidence occurs in people over 65 years of age. However, 28% of cerebral vascular accidents occur in people under the age of 65, and strokes occur in every age group. They occur more frequently in men than women.

### Risk Factors

Certain diseases, lifestyle habits, and ethnic backgrounds increase the risk of a stroke (see the box below), including:

### Focus on Diversity

#### RISK AND INCIDENCE OF CVA

- CVAs are more common in the African American population, probably because of an increased incidence of hypertension in individuals of African descent. An additional factor is sickle cell anemia, specific to this race.
- The incidence of hemorrhagic CVAs is highest in Asians (especially the Japanese).

- *Hypertension.* Increased systolic and diastolic blood pressure is associated with damage to all blood vessels, including the cerebral vessels.
- *Diabetes mellitus.* Diabetes leads to vascular changes in both the systemic and cerebral circulation and increases the risk of hypertension.
- *Sickle cell disease.* Changes in the shape of the red blood cells increase blood viscosity and produce erythrocyte clumps that may occlude small cerebral vessels.
- *Substance abuse.* The injection of unpurified substances increases the risk for a stroke, and abuse of certain drugs can decrease cerebral blood flow and increase the risk for intracranial hemorrhage. Substances associated with strokes include alcohol, nicotine, heroin, amphetamines, and cocaine.
- *Atherosclerosis.* Occlusion of cerebral vessels by atherosclerotic plaque impairs or obstructs blood flow to specific areas of the brain.

Other risk factors include a family history of obesity, a sedentary lifestyle, hyperlipidemia, atrial fibrillation, cardiac disease, cigarette smoking, and previous transient ischemic attacks. Risk factors specific to women are oral contraceptive use, pregnancy, and menopause.

### Overview of Normal Cerebral Blood Flow

The brain, which makes up only 2% of total body weight, receives approximately 20% of the cardiac output each minute (about 750 mL) and accounts for 20% of the body's oxygen consumption. Brain function depends on a consistent blood and oxygen supply. When cerebral blood flow is decreased or interrupted, the resulting ischemia may lead to death of brain cells and pathophysiologic alterations (Porth, 2002).

The brain is supplied with blood from the internal carotid arteries (anteriorly) and the vertebral arteries (posteriorly) (see Figure 40–4 on page 1294). Two sets of veins drain cerebral blood into venous plexuses and dural sinuses and then into the internal jugular veins at the base of the skull. The veins in the cerebral system do not have valves; therefore, the direction of flow depends on gravity or pressure differences between the venous sinuses and the extracranial veins.

Activities that increase intrathoracic pressure (such as sneezing, coughing, straining to have a bowel movement, or vomiting) also briefly increase intracranial pressure. This increased intracranial pressure occurs because the increased intrathoracic pressure is transmitted through the internal jugular veins and the dural sinuses.

Cerebral blood flow, especially in the deep cerebral vessels, is largely self-regulated by the brain to meet metabolic needs. This self-regulation (also called *autoregulation*) allows the brain to maintain a constant blood flow despite changes in systemic blood pressure. However, autoregulation is not effective when systemic blood pressure falls below 50 mmHg or rises above 160 mmHg. In the latter case, the increased systemic pressure (as in hypertension) causes an increase in cerebral blood flow with resultant overdistention of cerebral vessels. Cerebral blood flow is affected by concentrations of carbon dioxide, oxygen, and hydrogen ions. Cerebral blood flow increases in response to increased carbon dioxide concentrations, increased hydrogen ion concentrations, and decreased oxygen concentrations.

## PATHOPHYSIOLOGY

A stroke is characterized by a gradual or rapid onset of neurologic deficits due to compromised cerebral blood flow. Strokes may result from a variety of problems, including transient ischemic attack (TIA), cerebral thrombosis, cerebral embolism, and cerebral hemorrhage.

When blood flow to and oxygenation of cerebral neurons are decreased or interrupted, pathophysiologic changes at the cellular level take place in 4 to 5 minutes. Cellular metabolism ceases as glucose, glycogen, and adenosine triphosphate (ATP) are depleted and the sodium-potassium pump fails. Cells swell as sodium draws water into the cell. Cerebral blood vessel walls also swell, further decreasing blood flow. Even if circulation is restored, vasospasm and increased blood viscosity can continue to impede blood flow. Severe or prolonged ischemia leads to cellular death. A central core of dead or dying cells is surrounded by a band of minimally perfused cells, called the *penumbra*. Although cells in the penumbra have impaired metabolic activities, their structural integrity is maintained. The survival of these cells depends on a timely return of adequate circulation, the volume of toxic products released by adjacent dying cells, the degree of cerebral edema, and alterations in local blood flow. The potential survival of cells in the penumbra has led to the use of thrombolytic agents in the early treatment of ischemic stroke (Porth, 2002).

The neurologic deficits that occur as a result of a stroke can often be used to identify its location. Because the sensory-motor pathways cross at the junction of the medulla and spinal cord (decussation), strokes lead to loss or impairment of sensory-motor functions on the side of the body opposite the side of the brain that is damaged. This effect, known as a **contralateral deficit,** causes a stroke in the right hemisphere of the brain to be manifested by deficits in the left side of the body (and vice versa).

### Ischemic Stroke

Ischemic strokes result from cerebrovascular obstruction by thrombosis or emboli. They include TIAs, thrombotic stroke, and embolic stroke.

### Transient Ischemic Attack

A **transient ischemic attack (TIA)** is a brief period of localized cerebral ischemia that causes neurologic deficits lasting for less than 24 hours (usually less than 1 to 2 hours) (Porth, 2002). The deficits may be present for only minutes or may last for hours. TIAs are often warning signals of an ischemic thrombotic stroke. One or many TIAs may precede a stroke, with the time between the TIA and a stroke ranging from hours to months.

The etiology of TIA includes inflammatory artery disorders, sickle cell anemia, atherosclerotic changes in cerebral vessels, thrombosis, and emboli. Transient cerebral ischemia may also occur as a result of subclavian steal syndrome, a relatively rare pathophysiologic process in which blood that normally flows from the vertebral arteries into the circulation of the brain changes direction and flows from the vertebral arteries into the arteries of the arm. This reverse flow occurs when the arm is exercised and the subclavian artery is occluded.

Neurologic manifestations of a TIA vary according to the location and size of the cerebral vessel involved. Manifestations have a sudden onset and often disappear within minutes or hours. Commonly occurring deficits include contralateral numbness or weakness of the hand, forearm, and corner of the mouth (due to middle cerebral artery involvement); aphasia (due to ischemia of the left hemisphere); and visual disturbances such as blurring (due to involvement of the posterior cerebral artery) (Porth, 2002).

### Thrombotic Stroke

A **thrombotic stroke** is caused by occlusion of a large cerebral vessel by a thrombus (a blood clot). Thrombotic CVAs most often occur in older people who are resting or sleeping. The blood pressure is lower during sleep, so there is less pressure to push the blood through an already narrowed arterial lumen, and ischemia may result.

Thrombi tend to form in large arteries that bifurcate and have narrowed lumens as a result of deposits of atherosclerotic plaque. The plaque involves the intima of the arteries, causing the internal elastic lamina to become thin and frayed with exposure of underlying connective tissue. This structural change causes platelets to adhere to the rough surface and release the enzyme adenosine diphosphate. This enzyme initiates the clotting sequence, and the thrombus forms. A thrombus may remain in place and continue to enlarge, completely occluding the lumen of the vessel, or a part of it may break off and become an embolus.

The most common locations of thrombi are the internal carotid artery, the vertebral arteries, and the junction of the vertebral and basilar arteries. Thrombotic strokes affecting the smaller cerebral vessels are called **lacunar strokes,** because the infarcted areas slough off, leaving a small cavity or "lake" in the brain tissue. A thrombotic stroke usually affects only one region of the brain that is supplied by a single cerebral artery.

A thrombotic stroke occurs rapidly but progresses slowly. It often begins with a TIA, and continues to worsen over 1 to 2 days; the condition is called a stroke-in-evolution. When maximum neurologic deficit has been reached, usually in 3 days, the condition is called a completed stroke. At that time, the damaged area is edematous and necrotic.

## Embolic Stroke

An **embolic stroke** occurs when a blood clot or clump of matter traveling through the cerebral blood vessels becomes lodged in a vessel too narrow to permit further movement. The area of the brain supplied by the blocked vessel becomes ischemic. The most frequent sites of cerebral emboli are at bifurcations of vessels, particularly those of the carotid and middle cerebral arteries. This type of stroke is typically seen in clients who are younger than those experiencing thrombotic strokes and occurs when the client is awake and active.

Many embolic strokes originate from a thrombus in the left chambers of the heart, formed during atrial fibrillation. These are referred to as *cardiogenic embolic strokes.* Emboli result when parts of the thrombus break off and are carried through the arterial system to the brain. Cerebral emboli may also be due to carotid artery atherosclerotic plaque, bacterial endocarditis, recent myocardial infarction, rheumatic heart disease, and ventricular aneurysm.

An embolic stroke has a sudden onset and causes immediate deficits. If the embolus breaks up into smaller fragments and is absorbed by the body, symptoms will disappear in a few hours to a few days. If the embolus is not absorbed, symptoms will persist. Even if the embolus is absorbed, the vessel wall where the embolus lodges may be weakened, increasing the potential for cerebral hemorrhage.

## Hemorrhagic Stroke

A **hemorrhagic stroke,** or **intracranial hemorrhage,** occurs when a cerebral blood vessel ruptures. It occurs most often in people with sustained increase in systolic-diastolic pressure. Intracranial hemorrhage usually occurs suddenly, often when the affected person is engaged in some activity. Although hypertension is the most common cause, a variety of factors may contribute to a hemorrhagic stroke, including ruptured intracranial aneurysms, trauma, erosion of blood vessels by tumors, arteriovenous malformations, anticoagulant therapy, and blood disorders. Of all forms of stroke, this form is most often fatal.

As a result of the blood vessel rupture, blood enters the brain tissue, the cerebral ventricles, or the subarachnoid space, compressing adjacent tissues and causing blood vessel spasm and cerebral edema. Blood in the ventricles or subarachnoid space irritates the meninges and brain tissue, causing an inflammatory reaction and impairing absorption and circulation of cerebral spinal fluid.

The onset of manifestations from a hemorrhagic stroke is rapid. Manifestations depend on the location of the hemorrhage, but may include vomiting, headache, seizures, hemiplegia, and loss of consciousness. Pressure on the brain tissue from increased intracranial pressure (discussed in Chapter 42) may cause coma and death.

## MANIFESTATIONS AND COMPLICATIONS

Manifestations and complications of a stroke vary according to the cerebral artery involved and the area of the brain affected.

---

### Manifestations of a Stroke by Involved Cerebral Vessel

**INTERNAL CAROTID ARTERY**

- Contralateral paralysis of the arm, leg, and face
- Contralateral sensory deficits of the arm, leg, and face
- If the dominant hemisphere is involved: aphasia
- If the nondominant hemisphere is involved: apraxia, agnosia, unilateral neglect
- Homonymous hemianopia

**MIDDLE CEREBRAL ARTERY**

- Drowsiness, stupor, coma
- Contralateral hemiplegia of the arm and face
- Contralateral sensory deficits of the arm and face
- Global aphasia (if dominant hemisphere involved)
- Homonymous hemianopia

**ANTERIOR CEREBRAL ARTERY**

- Contralateral weakness or paralysis of the foot and leg
- Contralateral sensory loss of the toes, foot, and leg
- Loss of ability to make decisions or act voluntarily
- Urinary incontinence

**VERTEBRAL ARTERY**

- Pain in face, nose, or eye
- Numbness and weakness of the face on involved side
- Problems with gait
- Dysphagia
- Dysarthria

---

Manifestations are always sudden in onset, focal, and usually one sided. The most common manifestation is weakness involving the face and arm, and sometimes the leg. Other common manifestations are numbness on one side, loss of vision in one eye or to the side, speech difficulties, and difficulties with balance. The various deficits associated with involvement of a specific cerebral artery are collectively referred to as stroke syndromes, although the deficits often overlap, as shown in the box above.

Typical manifestations and complications include motor deficits, elimination disorders, sensory-perceptual deficits, language disorders, and behavioral changes. These may be transient or permanent, depending on the degree of ischemia and necrosis as well as time of treatment. As a result of the neurologic deficits, the client with a stroke has manifestations that involve many different body systems (see the box on page 1310).

## Motor Deficits

Body movement results from a complex interaction between the brain, spinal cord, and peripheral nerves. The motor areas of the cerebral cortex, the basal ganglia, and the cerebellum initiate voluntary movement by sending messages to the spinal cord, which then transmits the messages to the peripheral nerves. A stroke may interrupt the central nervous system component of this relay system and produce effects in the contralateral side ranging from mild weakness to severe limitation of any kind of movement.

## Manifestations and Complications of Stroke by Body System

**INTEGUMENT**

- Decubitus (pressure) ulcers

**NEUROLOGIC**

- Hyperthermia
- Neglect syndrome
- Seizures
- Agnosias
- Communication deficits
  a. Expressive aphasia
  b. Receptive aphasia
  c. Global aphasia
  d. Agraphia
- Visual deficits
  a. Homonymous hemianopia
  b. Diplopia
  c. Decreased acuity
- Cognitive changes
  a. Memory loss
  b. Short attention span
  c. Distractibility
  d. Poor judgment
  e. Poor problem-solving ability
  f. Disorientation
- Behavioral changes
  a. Emotional lability
  b. Loss of social inhibitions
  c. Fear
  d. Hostility

  e. Anger
  f. Depression
- Increased intracranial pressure
- Alterations in consciousness
- Sensory loss (touch, pain, heat, cold, pressure)

**RESPIRATORY**

- Respiratory center damage
- Airway obstruction
- Decreased ability to cough

**GASTROINTESTINAL**

- Dysphagia
- Constipation
- Stool impaction

**GENITOURINARY**

- Incontinence
- Frequency
- Urgency
- Urinary retention
- Renal calculi

**MUSCULOSKELETAL**

- Hemiplegia
- Contractures
- Bony ankylosis
- Disuse atrophy
- Dysarthria

---

Depending on the area of the brain involved, strokes may cause weakness, paralysis, and/or spasticity. The deficits include:

- **Hemiplegia:** paralysis of the left or right half of the body (see Figure 41–1 ■).

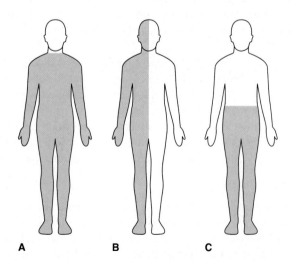

**Figure 41–1** ■ Types of paralysis. *A,* Tetraplegia is complete or partial paralysis of the upper extremities and complete paralysis of the lower part of the body. *B,* Hemiplegia is paralysis of one-half of the body when it is divided along the median sagittal plane. *C,* Paraplegia is paralysis of the lower part of the body.

- **Hemiparesis:** weakness of the left or right half of the body.
- **Flaccidity:** absence of muscle tone (hypotonia).
- **Spasticity:** increased muscle tone (hypertonia), usually with some degree of weakness. The flexor muscles are usually more strongly affected in the upper extremities and the extensor muscles are more strongly affected in the lower extremities.

When the corticospinal tract is involved, the affected arm and leg almost always are initially flaccid and then become spastic within 6 to 8 weeks. Spasticity often causes characteristic body positioning: adduction of the shoulder, pronation of the forearm, flexion of the fingers, and extension of the hip and knee. There is often foot drop, outward rotation of the leg, and dependent edema in the involved extremities.

The motor deficits may result in altered mobility, further impairing body function. The complications of immobility involve multiple body systems and include orthostatic hypotension, increased thrombus formation, decreased cardiac output, impaired respiratory function, osteoporosis, formation of renal calculi, contractures, and decubitus ulcer formation.

### Elimination Disorders

Disorders of bladder and bowel elimination are common. A stroke may cause partial loss of the sensations that trigger bladder elimination, resulting in urinary frequency, urgency, or incontinence. Control of urination may be altered as a result of cognitive deficits. Changes in bowel elimination are common; they result from changes in level of consciousness, immobility, and dehydration (Hickey, 2003).

## Sensory-Perceptual Deficits

A stroke may involve pathologic changes in neurologic pathways that alter the ability to integrate, interpret, and attend to sensory data. The client may experience deficits in vision, hearing, equilibrium, taste, and sense of smell. The ability to perceive vibration, pain, warmth, cold, and pressure may be impaired, as may proprioception (the body's sense of its position). The loss of these sensory abilities increases the risk for injury. Deficits may include:

- **Hemianopia:** the loss of half of the visual field of one or both eyes; when the same half is missing in each eye, the condition is called *homonymous hemianopia* (Figure 41–2 ■).
- **Agnosia:** the inability to recognize one or more subjects that were previously familiar; agnosia may be visual, tactile, or auditory.
- **Apraxia:** the inability to carry out some motor pattern (e.g., drawing a figure, getting dressed) even when strength and coordination are adequate.

Another form of sensory-perceptual deficit is the **neglect syndrome** (or unilateral neglect), in which the client has a disorder of attention. In this syndrome, the person cannot integrate and use perceptions from the affected side of the body or from the environment on the affected side, and ignores that part. In severe cases, the client may even deny the paralysis. This deficit is more common following a stroke of the right hemisphere where damage to the parietal lobe (a center for mediation of directed attention) results in perceptual deficits.

## Communication Disorders

Communication is a complex process, involving motor functions, speech, language, memory, reasoning, and emotions.

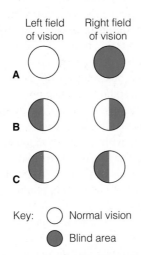

Key:   ○ Normal vision
        ● Blind area

**Figure 41–2 ■** Abnormal visual fields. *A,* Normal left field of vision with loss of vision in right field. *B,* Loss of vision in temporal half of both fields (bitemporal hemianopia). *C,* Loss of vision in nasal field of right eye and temporal field of left eye (homonymous hemianopia).

Communication problems are usually the result of a stroke affecting the dominant hemisphere. The left hemisphere is dominant in about 95% of right-handed people and 70% of left-handed people (Porth, 2002).

Many different impairments may occur, and most are partial. Disorders of communication affect both speech (the mechanical act of articulating language through the spoken word) and language (the vocal or written formulation of ideas to communicate thoughts and feelings). Language involves oral and written expression and auditory and reading comprehension. Among these disorders are:

- **Aphasia:** the inability to use or understand language; aphasia may be expressive, receptive, or mixed (global).
- Expressive aphasia: a motor speech problem in which one can understand what is being said but can respond verbally only in short phrases; also called *Broca's aphasia.*
- Receptive aphasia: a sensory speech problem in which one cannot understand the spoken (and often written) word. Speech may be fluent but with inappropriate content; also called *Wernicke's aphasia.*
- Mixed or global aphasia: language dysfunction in both understanding and expression.
- Dysarthria: any disturbance in muscular control of speech.

## Cognitive and Behavioral Changes

A change in consciousness, ranging from mild confusion to coma, is a common manifestation of a stroke. It may result from tissue damage following ischemia or hemorrhage involving either the carotid or vertebral arteries. Altered consciousness may also be the result of cerebral edema or increased intracranial pressure.

Behavioral changes include emotional lability (in which the client may laugh or cry inappropriately), loss of self-control (manifested by behavior such as swearing or refusing to wear clothing), and decreased tolerance for stress (resulting in anger or depression). Intellectual changes may include memory loss, decreased attention span, poor judgment, and an inability to think abstractly.

## COLLABORATIVE CARE

The client with a stroke may receive medical and/or surgical treatment. The focus in the acute care phase is on diagnosing the type and cause of the stroke, supporting cerebral circulation, and controlling or preventing further deficits.

### Diagnostic Tests

Diagnostic tests may be ordered to detect increased risk for a stroke or to identify pathophysiologic changes after a stroke has occurred.

- *Computed tomography (CT)* without contrast is the first imaging technique used to demonstrate the presence of hemorrhage, tumors, aneurysm, ischemia, edema, and tissue necrosis. A CT scan can also demonstrate a shift in intracranial contents and is useful in distinguishing the type of stroke (e.g., a hemorrhagic stroke results in an increase in density).

Nursing interventions for the client having a CT scan of the head are described in the box below.

- *Arteriography* of cerebral vessels is performed to demonstrate abnormal vessel structures, vasospasm, loss of vessel wall integrity, and stenosis of the carotid arteries.
- *Transcranial ultrasound Doppler (TCD)* studies are used to evaluate the velocity of the blood flow through the intracranial arteries and provide information about partial or complete occlusion.
- *Magnetic resonance imaging (MRI) test* may be conducted to detect shifting of brain tissues as a result of hemorrhage or edema. A *magnetic resonance angiography (MRA)* may be performed to detect occlusive disease of the large cerebral vessels.
- *Positron emission tomography (PET)* and *single-photon emission computed tomography (SPECT)* are used to examine cerebral blood flow distribution and metabolic activity of the brain. Both tests use very short-lived radionuclides that emit radioactive energy as they move through the circulation. PET allows the identification of the location and size of the stroke; SPECT provides information about the metabolism of and blood flow through the brain tissue affected by the stroke.

## Nursing Implications for Diagnostic Tests

### Computed Tomography (CT) of the Head

#### Preparation of Client
- Ensure a signed consent form.
- Check hospital policy on withholding food and fluids. Clients are usually on NPO status (except for the medications ordered as part of the test) for 8 hours before the test if it is done in the morning. If the test is done in the afternoon, the client may have a liquid breakfast.
- Give medications up to 2 hours before test.
- Assess for possible reaction to iodine dye (by asking about allergy to seafood). Document any allergy and inform the physician and radiology department.
- Remove metal hairpins, clips, and earrings.

#### Client and Family Teaching
- (*If applicable*) Do not drink or eat anything before the test except for the ordered medications.
- You may be given an intravenous infusion. When the contrast dye is injected, you may feel warm and have a metallic taste in the mouth.
- The exam lasts from 30 to 90 minutes.
- Your head will be positioned in a cradle, and a wide rubber strap will be applied snugly across the forehead during the test (to keep your head immobilized).
- The CT scanner is circular with a round opening. You are strapped to a special table, and the scanner revolves around the body part to be examined. The scanner makes a clicking noise.
- The test is painless.
- Someone is always immediately available during the test.

- *Lumbar puncture* may be performed to obtain cerebrospinal fluid for examination if there is no danger of increased intracranial pressure. (Removal of cerebrospinal fluid when intracranial pressure is increased can result in herniation of the brainstem.) A thrombotic stroke may elevate cerebrospinal fluid pressure; after a hemorrhagic stroke frank blood may be seen in the cerebrospinal fluid. Nursing interventions for the client having a lumbar puncture are described in the Nursing Implications box on the next page.

## Medications

Medications are administered to prevent a stroke in clients with TIAs or a previous stroke, and to treat the client during the acute phase of a stroke.

### Prevention

Antiplatelet agents are often used to treat clients with TIAs or who have had a previous stroke. Platelets are concentrated in high blood flow arteries, they adhere to endothelial tissue damaged by atherosclerosis and occlude the vessel. The drugs used to prevent clot formation and blood vessel occlusion include aspirin, clopidogrel (Plavix), dipyridamole (Persantine), pentoxifylline (Trental), and ticlopidine (Ticlid).

Daily low-dose aspirin reduces TIA occurrence and stroke risk by interfering with platelet aggregation. Ticlopidine (Ticlid) is a platelet-aggregation inhibitor that has shown reduction in thrombotic stroke risk.

### Acute Stroke

Pharmacologic agents are used to treat the client during the acute phase of an ischemic stroke to prevent further thrombosis formation, increase cerebral blood flow, and protect cerebral neurons. The type of medication used varies according to the type of stroke.

Anticoagulant drug therapy (discussed in Chapter 33) is often ordered for thrombotic stroke during the stroke-in-evolution phase but is contraindicated in completed stroke because it may increase the risk of cerebral hemorrhage. Anticoagulants are never administered to a client with a hemorrhagic stroke. Anticoagulants do not dissolve an existing clot but prevent further extension of the clot and formation of new clots. Sodium heparin may be given subcutaneously or by continuous IV drip, or warfarin sodium (Coumadin) may be given orally.

Thrombolytic therapy, using a tissue plasminogen activator such as recombinant altephase (Activase rt-pa), sometimes given concurrently with an anticoagulant, is used to treat thrombotic stroke. The drug converts plasminogen to plasmin, resulting in fibrinolysis of the clot. To be effective, it must be given within 3 hours of the onset of manifestations (Tierney et al., 2001).

Antithrombotic drugs, which inhibit the platelet phase of clot formation, have been used as a preventive measure for clients at risk for embolic and thrombotic CVA. Both aspirin and dipyridamole have been used for this purpose. These drugs are sometimes also used in combination with other drugs during acute treatment. Antiplatelet agents are contraindicated in clients with a hemorrhagic stroke.

## Nursing Implications for Diagnostic Tests

### Lumbar Puncture

#### Preparation of the Client

- Ensure a signed consent form (this consent may be obtained as part of the general consent given on admission to the hospital or agency).
- Ask the client to empty the bladder before the procedure begins.
- Help the client to assume a lateral recumbent position near the side of the bed. The client should assume the fetal position (knees flexed toward the head, head bent toward the chest), with the hands clasped around the knees.

#### Client and Family Teaching

- A local anesthetic is injected into the skin over the area of the needle insertion. This medication may cause a burning sensation.
- A long, thin needle is inserted into the lower back below the level of the spinal cord. Cerebrospinal fluid is withdrawn.
- The cerebrospinal fluid pressure is measured with a calibrated tube called a manometer.
- There may be slight pain down one leg during the procedure.
- It is important to remain still during the procedure.
- A small dressing is used to cover the place where the needle was inserted.

- After the procedure, remain flat in bed for the number of hours prescribed by the physician (this ranges from 4 to 24 hours). The nurses will take your vital signs and look under the small dressing at regular intervals.
- Drink fluids so that your body can replace the fluid that was withdrawn.
- If you have a headache or backache, ask for medications for pain.
- Notify your health care provider if you notice increased pain or drainage from the area where the procedure was done.

#### Postprocedure Nursing Care

- Take and record vital signs as indicated by agency standards.
- Monitor neurologic status at least every 4 hours for 24 hours following the procedure.
- Monitor the puncture site for leakage of cerebrospinal fluid or hematoma formation.
- Ensure that the client voids within 8 hours of the procedure.
- Encourage increased intake of fluids (up to 3000 mL in 24 hours).
- Administer analgesics as prescribed for pain.

---

Calcium channel blockers, such as nimodipine (Nimotop), are under investigation and have been used in clinical trials to reduce ischemic deficits and death from stroke. They block glutamate, an excitatory neurotransmitter, to reduce the sensitivity of neurons to ischemia.

Corticosteriods, such as prednisone or dexamethasone have been used to treat cerebral edema, but the results are not always positive. If the client has increased intracranial pressure, hyperosmolar solutions (such as mannitol) or diuretics (such as furosemide) may be administered. Anticonvulsants, such as phenytoin (Dilantin), and barbiturates may be prescribed if increased intracranial pressure causes seizures.

## Treatments

The treatments used in the medical management of a stroke include surgery, physical therapy, occupational therapy, and speech therapy.

### Surgery

Surgery may be performed to prevent the occurrence of a stroke or to restore blood flow when a stroke has already occurred. In people who have had TIAs or are in danger of having another stroke, a carotid endarterectomy at the carotid artery bifurcation may be performed to remove atherosclerotic plaque (Figure 41–3 ■). Nursing care for the client in the initial postoperative period following a carotid endarterectomy is described in the box on page 1314.

When an occluded or stenotic vessel is not directly accessible, an extracranial-intracranial bypass may be performed. Bypass of the internal carotid, middle cerebral, or vertebral arter-

ies may be required. The indications for the bypass are symptoms of ischemia caused by TIAs or a mild completed stroke. The procedure reestablishes blood flow to the affected area of the brain.

### Physical/Occupational/Speech Therapy

Physical therapy may help prevent contractures and improve muscle strength and coordination. Occupational therapy provides assistive devices and a plan for regaining lost motor skills that greatly improve quality of life after a stroke. In addition, the client with a communication disorder requires speech therapy.

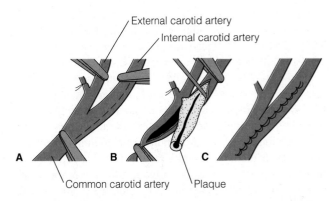

**Figure 41–3** ■ Carotid endarterectomy. *A,* The occluded area is clamped off and an incision is made in the artery. *B,* Plaque is removed from the inner layer of the artery. *C,* To restore blood flow through the artery, the artery is sutured, or a graft is completed.

## NURSING CARE OF THE CLIENT HAVING A CAROTID ENDARTERECTOMY

### POSTOPERATIVE CARE

- Position on the unoperated side and either maintain a flat position or elevate the head of the bed 30 degrees as prescribed. Maintain head and neck alignment and avoid rotating, flexing, or hyperextending head. *Pressure on the wound is undesirable. Elevating the head decreases edema in the operative site. Maintaining head and neck alignment prevents additional tension or pressure on the operative side.*
- Support the head when changing position. Teach to support the head with the hands when able to move about. *Supporting the head helps prevent stress on the operative site (which may cause bleeding and hematoma formation); it also helps reduce stress on the suture line.*
- Perform focused assessments to monitor for complications:
  a. *Hemorrhage.* Assess the dressing and the area under the neck and shoulders for drainage. Assess for increased pulse and decreased blood pressure. *The most common cause of respiratory problems is pressure on the trachea from a hematoma formation.*
  b. *Respiratory distress.* Assess respiratory rate, rhythm, depth, and effort. Observe for restlessness. Keep a tracheostomy tray at the bedside. *Respiratory distress may result from edema and hematoma formation, which may compress the trachea.*
  c. *Cranial nerve impairment.* Observe and record any facial drooping, tongue deviation, hoarseness, dysphagia, or loss of facial sensation. *Cranial nerves may be stretched during surgery, leading to temporary deficits in cranial nerve function.*
  d. *Hypertension* or *hypotension.* Take and record blood pressure at least hourly. Report any changes immediately and implement orders for medications to treat hypertension or hypotension. *About one-half of all clients having a carotid endarterectomy develop unstable blood pressure related to surgical denervation of the carotid sinus. Uncontrolled hypertension may precipitate a CVA. The most common problem is hypotension, possibly related to stimulation of the carotid body baroreceptors, which are exposed during surgery. Hypotension may result in myocardial ischemia.*

## NURSING CARE

**MediaLink** | **HEMORRHAGIC STROKE CARE PLAN**

Even though many people who have a stroke have full recovery, a substantial number are left with disabilities that affect their physical, emotional, interpersonal, and family status. The required nursing care is often complex and multidimensional, requiring consideration of continuity of care for clients in acute care settings, long-term care settings, rehabilitation centers, and the home.

Nurses caring for clients who have had a stroke require knowledge and skill to meet client needs during both the acute and the rehabilitative phases of care. The client often has multiple losses: loss of mobility, ability to provide self-care, communications, concept of self, and interpersonal or intimate relationships with others. Holistic, individualized nursing care is essential in all settings and focuses on promoting the achievement of maximum potential and quality of life.

The client's family is often faced with many changes. The young to middle-aged adult with a family member who has had a stroke may be faced with economic difficulties and social isolation. The middle-aged adult family member may become the caretaker for an older parent, in essence switching roles with the parent. An older adult may not be able to care for a spouse and may have to accept nursing home placement. In addition, the older adult who has no family may have to struggle alone to regain the ability to function independently. Although not all of these problems are amenable to nursing solutions, the nurse is most often the health care provider who assesses and identifies the needs of each individual and provides information and referrals to clients and families to help meet those needs.

Because a stroke has the potential to cause many different health problems, a wide variety of nursing diagnoses may be appropriate. It is important to remember that each person will be affected differently, depending on the degree of ischemia and the area of the brain involved. Nursing diagnoses discussed in this section focus on problems with cerebral tissue perfusion (specific to nursing care during the acute phase), physical mobility, self-care, communication, sensory-perceptual deficits, bowel and urine elimination, and swallowing (specific to prevention of complications and rehabilitation). See the Manifestations box on page 1310 for more information.

### Health Promotion

Health promotion activities focus on stroke prevention, especially for those people with known risk factors. It is important to discuss the importance of stopping smoking and drug use with clients of all ages. Maintaining a normal weight through diet and exercise can help reduce obesity, which increases the risk of hypertension and Type 2 diabetes mellitus (both in turn increase the risk of a stroke). Cholesterol levels should be screened regularly to monitor for hyperlipidemia. Regular health care to monitor for and treat cardiovascular disorders and to detect and treat infections such as infective endocarditis are important. It is also important to increase public awareness of the signs of a TIA or stroke and of the need to call 911 or to seek care immediately if the following warning signs or symptoms occur.

- Sudden weakness or numbness of the face, arm, or leg, especially on one side of the body
- Sudden confusion, difficulty speaking, or difficulty understanding speech
- Sudden trouble walking, dizziness, loss of coordination
- Sudden difficulty with vision in one or both eyes
- Sudden severe headache without a cause

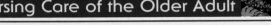

## Nursing Care of the Older Adult

### VARIATIONS IN ASSESSMENT FINDINGS—CVA

- Response to questions is often slower.
- Sensations, reflexes, and motor coordination are decreased.
- Alternating movements may be difficult.
- Gait may be slower and more deliberate.
- Motor strength is often decreased.
- Vision, taste, and sense of smell are often decreased.

## Assessment

The following data are collected through the health history and physical examination (see Chapter 40). Further focused assessments are described with the following nursing interventions. When assessing the older client, be aware of normal changes with aging, outlined in the box above.

- Health history: risk factors, drug use (medications and illegal), smoking history, when symptoms began, severity of symptoms, presence of incontinence, level of consciousness, family support system
- Physical assessment: motor strength, coordination, communication, cranial nerves

## Nursing Diagnoses and Interventions

The acute phase of a stroke is most often the time from admission to the hospital until the client is stabilized: usually 24 to 72 hours after admission (Hickey, 2003). Depending on the severity of the stroke, the client may be admitted to the intensive care unit. Regardless of the hospital setting, the nurse provides interventions to maintain body functions and prevent complications.

### Ineffective Tissue Perfusion (Cerebral)

The initial assessment and care of the client admitted for intensive care focuses on identifying changes that may indicate altered cerebral perfusion. The client's airway, breathing, circulation, and neurologic status are monitored and interventions are provided to maintain cerebral perfusion.

- Monitor respiratory status and airway patency. Auscultate pulmonary sounds and monitor respiratory rate and results of studies of arterial blood gases.
- Suction as necessary, using care to suction no longer than 10 to 15 seconds at any one time, and using sterile technique.
- Place in a side-lying position.
- Administer oxygen as prescribed.

*The client is often unconscious and breathing may be impaired. Suctioning removes secretions that not only obstruct airflow but also pose the risk for aspiration and pneumonia. Suctioning for longer than 15 seconds at a time may increase intracranial pressure (Hickey, 2003). Respiratory complications develop rapidly, as manifested by crackles and wheezes, rapid respirations, and respiratory acidosis. The administration of oxygen decreases the risk for hypoxia and hypercapnia, which can increase cerebral ischemia and intracranial pressure.*

**PRACTICE ALERT** *Positioning the client on the side allows secretions to drain out of the mouth, helping to prevent aspiration.* ■

- Monitor neurologic status.
- Assess mental status and level of consciousness: restlessness, drowsiness, lethargy, inability to follow commands, unresponsiveness.
- Monitor strength and reflexes, and assess for pain, headache, decreased muscle strength, sluggish pupillary reflexes, absent gag or swallowing reflexes, hemiplegia, Babinski's sign, and decerebrate or decorticate posturing. *Frequent monitoring of neurologic status is necessary to detect changes. Alterations in mental status, level of consciousness, movement, strength, and reflexes indicate increased intracranial pressure, the major cause of death in the acute phase of a stroke.*
- Continuously monitor cardiac status, observing for dysrhythmias. *A stroke may cause cardiac dysrhythmias, including bradycardia, PVCs, tachycardia, and AV block. Characteristic ECG changes include a shortened PR interval, peaked T waves, and a depressed ST segment.*
- Monitor body temperature. *Hyperthermia may develop if the hypothalamus is affected.*
- Maintain accurate intake and output records; measure urinary output via a Foley catheter. *A stroke may damage the pituitary gland, resulting in diabetes insipidus and the possibility of dehydration from greatly increased urinary output.*

**PRACTICE ALERT** *Diabetes insipidus is indicated by a large output of dilute urine; dehydration is indicated by scanty amounts of dark, concentrated urine.* ■

- Monitor seizures. Pad the side rails, and administer prescribed anticonvulsants. *Seizures may be the result of cerebral tissue damage or increased intracranial pressure. Padded side rails prevent injury if a seizure occurs. Anticonvulsants prevent or treat seizures.*

### Impaired Physical Mobility

The broad goals of care for clients with impaired mobility are to maintain and improve functional abilities (by maintaining normal function and alignment, preventing edema of extremities, and reducing spasticity) and to prevent complications.

- Encourage active ROM exercises for unaffected extremities and perform passive ROM exercises for affected extremities every 4 hours during day and evening shifts and once during the night shift. Support the joint during passive ROM exercises. *Active ROM exercises maintain or improve muscle strength and endurance, and help to maintain cardiopulmonary function. Passive ROM exercises do not strengthen muscles but do help maintain joint flexibility.*

**PRACTICE ALERT** *Both active and passive exercises increase venous return, decreasing the risk of thrombophlebitis.* ■

- Ensure safety when eating.
  - Position in upright sitting position with neck slightly flexed.
  - Order puréed or soft food.
  - Feed or teach client to eat by putting food behind the front teeth on the unaffected side of mouth and tilting the head slightly backward. Teach to swallow one bite at a time.

**PRACTICE ALERT** *After eating, check the mouth for "pocketing" of food, especially in the affected cheek.* ■

- Have suction equipment available at the bedside in case of choking or aspiration.
  *Sitting upright with the head and neck first slightly flexed and then tilted back helps the client swallow. The client can usually swallow puréed or soft foods more easily than liquid or solid foods. Using the unaffected side of the mouth helps prevent food from collecting in the mouth and makes swallowing safer; in addition, food is less likely to fall out of the mouth.*
- Minimize distractions and, if necessary, give step-by-step instructions for eating. *Distractions increase the risk of aspiration. Complex activities are easier to perform when broken down into small steps.*

## Using NANDA, NIC, AND NOC

Chart 41–1 shows links between NANDA nursing diagnoses, NIC, and NOC when caring for the client with a stroke.

## Home Care

Throughout the rehabilitation process, it is important to encourage self-care as much as possible but also to involve family members in the plan of care. Stress that ADLs may take twice as long as they did before the stroke. Emphasize that physical function may continue to improve for up to 3 months, and speech may continue to improve for even longer. Address the following topics in preparing the client and family for home care.

- Physical care, medications, physical therapy
- Realistic expectations
- Time off for the caregiver, respite care services
- Distributors for equipment and supplies
- Home environment conducive to using equipment (e.g., a wheel chair or walker)
- Home and equipment modifications (e.g., a raised toilet seat, grab bars in the bathroom, a bath chair, a vise lid opener, a long-handled shoehorn)
- Home health services
- Community resources, such as Meals-on-Wheels, senior centers, eldercare, large-print telephone dials, stroke clubs, Life-line (emergency alerting systems through a local hospital or agency).
- Helpful organizational resources:
  - American Heart Association
  - National Stroke Association
  - Stroke Clubs International
  - The National Institute of Neurological Disorders and Stroke

## CHART 41–1  NANDA, NIC, AND NOC LINKAGES

### The Client with a CVA

| NURSING DIAGNOSES | NURSING INTERVENTIONS | NURSING OUTCOMES |
|---|---|---|
| • Altered Cerebral Tissue Perfusion | • Acid-Base Management<br>• Cerebral Perfusion | • Electrolyte and Acid-Base Balance<br>• Circulation Status<br>• Cognitive Ability<br>• Neurologic Status |
| • Unilateral Neglect Management | • Unilateral Neglect<br>• Body Positioning: Self-Initiated | • Body Image |
| • Dressing/Grooming Self-Care Deficit | • Dressing<br>• Hair Care | • Self-Care: Dressing<br>• Self-Care: Grooming |
| • Powerlessness | • Self-Esteem Enhancement<br>• Self-Responsibility Enhancement | • Health Beliefs: Perceived Control<br>• Participation: Health Care Decisions |

*Note. Data from Nursing Outcomes Classification (NOC) by M. Johnson & M. Maas (Eds.), 1997, St. Louis: Mosby; Nursing Diagnoses: Definitions & Classification 2001–2002 by North American Nursing Diagnosis Association, 2001, Philadelphia: NANDA; Nursing Interventions Classification (NIC) by J.C. McCloskey & G. M. Bulechek (Eds.), 2000, St. Louis: Mosby. Reprinted by permission.*

MediaLink | STROKE RESOURCES

## Nursing Care Plan
## A Client with a Stroke

Orville Boren is a 68-year-old African American who had a stroke due to right cerebral thrombosis 1 week ago. He is a history instructor at the local community college. His hobbies are wood carving and gardening. Mr. Boren is also an active member of his church. For the past 2 years, Mr. Boren has been taking medication for hypertension, but his wife Emily reports that he often forgets to take it and that his blood pressure was high at his last physical examination. Mrs. Boren tells the staff that she has never had to worry about her husband's health before and that she wants to learn everything she can to care for him at home. However, she says that her husband was always the one to make the decisions and pay the bills. Mrs. Boren adds that all the children, grandchildren, neighbors, and family pastor want to see Mr. Boren back at home as soon as possible.

### ASSESSMENT

Carol Merck, RN, the nurse assigned to Mr. Boren, completes a health history and physical assessment, with Mrs. Boren providing information for the history. Mrs. Boren reports that her husband did have several spells of dizziness and blurred vision the week before his stroke, but they lasted only a few minutes and he believed them to be due to "old age and working out in the sun." On the morning of admission, Mr. Boren woke up and could not move his left arm or leg; he also could not speak sensibly. Mrs. Boren called 911, and an ambulance took her husband to the hospital.

Physical assessment findings include the following: Mr. Boren is drowsy but responds to verbal stimuli. Although he does not respond verbally, he can nod his head to indicate "yes" when asked questions. Flaccid paralysis is present in his left arm and left leg, with no response noted to touch in those extremities (he is left-handed). Visual fields are decreased in a pattern consistent with homonymous hemianopia. A CT scan, negative on admission, is repeated on the third day after admission and confirms the medical diagnosis of a right-brain stroke due to a thrombus of the middle cerebral artery.

Mr. Boren's medical treatment includes heparin sodium administered by continuous intravenous drip, with clotting studies to be performed every 4 hours and the dose adjusted accordingly.

### DIAGNOSES

- *Feeding self-care deficit* related to loss of the ability to use the left hand and arm
- *Impaired physical mobility* related to neurologic deficits causing left hemiplegia
- *Risk for impaired skin integrity* related to inability to change position
- *Sensory/perceptual alterations: visual* related to changes in visual fields
- *Impaired verbal communication* related to cerebral injury

### EXPECTED OUTCOMES

- Learn to use his right hand to feed himself.
- Participate in exercises necessary to maintain muscle strength and tone.
- Maintain skin integrity.
- Indicate understanding that visual fields may improve in a few weeks.
- Practice and implement speech therapy activities while at the same time using alternative methods of communication.

### PLANNING AND IMPLEMENTATION

- Arrange mealtimes so that he is sitting up by the window in a clean and private environment.
- Provide adaptive devices (silverware with thick handles and nonslip plates).
- Encourage Mrs. Boren to visit at mealtimes, to assist with meals, and periodically to bring a favorite food from home.
- Provide passive ROM exercises for his left arm and leg; schedule active ROM exercises for his right extremities as well as quadriceps and gluteal sets every 4 hours during waking hours.
- Keep his skin clean and dry at all times.
- Establish and maintain a regular schedule for turning when he is in bed.
- Place objects (e.g., call bell, tissues) on unaffected side and approach him from that side.
- Support attempts to communicate verbally; when he is not understood, he prefers to use a large marker and tablet.

### EVALUATION

Mr. Boren is discharged to his home after being in the hospital for 10 days. During the first 2 months after discharge, Martha Grimes, RN, the home health nurse, visits Mr. and Mrs. Boren at home. At the end of 2 months, Mr. Boren is using his right hand to feed himself. He has regained partial use of his left arm and leg and is using a walker to move around the house and yard; he is even able to work in his flower garden. His skin has remained intact, and his vision is back to normal. He is slowly relearning speech; this has been the most difficult change for him to accept. Once he writes on his tablet, "I think God has forgotten me."

### Critical Thinking in the Nursing Process

1. Hypertension is sometimes referred to as "the silent killer." Provide justifications for this statement.
2. The functional changes Mr. Boren has experienced may make a return to teaching difficult. What other uses of his knowledge and abilities might you suggest?
3. What would be your reply if, after you had completed passive ROM on Mr. Boren's left arm, he wrote: "I just ignore that part of my body—it doesn't work anyway"?

See Evaluating your Response in Appendix C.

# THE CLIENT WITH AN INTRACRANIAL ANEURYSM

An **intracranial aneurysm** is a saccular outpouching of a cerebral artery that occurs at the site of a weakness in the vessel wall. The weakness may be the result of atherosclerosis, a congenital defect, trauma to the head, aging, or hypertension. A ruptured cerebral aneurysm is the most common cause of a hemorrhagic stroke.

## INCIDENCE AND PREVALENCE

Approximately 5 million North Americans have intracranial aneurysms; most go through life without any manifestations of bleeding. However, it is estimated that 30,000 people will have a rupture of an intracranial aneurysm each year, and two-thirds of the survivors will have serious disabilities. Intracranial aneurysms are most common in adults age 30 to 60 (Hickey, 2003; Porth, 2002).

The exact etiology is unknown, but theories of cause include (1) a developmental defect in the vessel wall and (2) degeneration or fragility of the vessel wall due to conditions such as hypertension, atherosclerosis, connective tissue disease, or abnormal blood flow. Hypertension and cigarette smoking may be predisposing factors.

## PATHOPHYSIOLOGY

Intracranial aneurysms tend to occur at the bifurcations and branches of the carotid arteries and the vertebrobasilar arteries at the circle of Willis, with most aneurysms (85%) located anteriorly. They range in size from smaller than 15 mm to larger than 50 mm. Intracranial aneurysms tend to enlarge with time, making the vessel wall thin and increasing the probability of rupture.

There are several different types of intracranial aneurysms: A *berry aneurysm* is probably the result of a congenital abnormality of the tunica media of the artery. The aneurysm usually ruptures without warning. A *saccular aneurysm* is any aneurysm with a saccular outpouching, which distends only a small portion of the vessel wall. This type of aneurysm is often caused by trauma. In a *fusiform aneurysm,* the entire circumference of a blood vessel swells to form an elongated tube. Most aneurysms of this type occur as a result of the changes of arteriosclerosis. Fusiform aneurysms act as space-occupying lesions. In a *dissecting aneurysm,* the tunica intima pulls away from the tunica media of the artery, and blood is forced between the two layers. It may result from atherosclerosis, inflammation, or trauma.

Intracranial aneurysms typically rupture from the dome rather than the base, forcing blood into the subarachnoid space at the base of the brain. The aneurysm may also rupture and force blood into brain tissue, the ventricles, or the subdural space. This discussion focuses on intracranial hemorrhages due to rupture of a cerebral aneurysm. See Chapter 42 for further discussion of types of intracranial hemorrhage.

## MANIFESTATIONS AND COMPLICATIONS

An intracranial aneurysm is usually asymptomatic until it ruptures, although very large aneurysms may cause headache and/or neurologic deficits due to pressure on adjacent intracranial structures. Small leakages of blood may occur periodically, causing headache, nausea, vomiting, and pain in the neck and back. The client may also have prodromal manifestations before the rupture occurs, such as headache, eye pain, visual deficits, and a dilated pupil.

The manifestations of a ruptured intracranial aneurysm (and subsequent subarachnoid hemorrhage) include a sudden, explosive headache; loss of consciousness; nausea and vomiting; a stiff neck and photophobia (due to meningeal irritation); cranial nerve deficits; stroke syndrome manifestations; and pituitary malfunctions (that result primarily from changes in ADH secretion).

The severity of the rupture is often inferred from the manifestations of the subarachnoid hemorrhage. In one system, severity ranges from grade I, in which the client has no symptoms or a slight headache with some stiffness of the neck, to grade V, in which the client is in a deep coma with decerebrate posturing.

Fibrin and platelets seal off the bleeding point, but the escaped blood forms a clot that irritates the brain tissue. The resulting inflammatory response causes cerebral edema, and both the edema and the hemorrhage increase intracranial pressure (Hickey, 2003). Bleeding into the subarachnoid space causes meningeal irritation. Hypothalamic dysfunction and seizures are also potential complications. The major complications of a ruptured intracranial aneurysm are rebleeding, vasospasm, and hydrocephalus.

### Rebleeding

The greatest risk for rebleeding is within the first day after the initial rupture, and again in 7 to 10 days (when the initial clot breaks down). Rebleeding is manifested by a sudden severe headache, nausea and vomiting, decreasing levels of consciousness, and new neurologic deficits (Hickey, 2003). The mortality from rebleeding is as high as from the initial rupture.

### Vasospasm

Cerebral vasospasm is a common but dangerous complication that occurs between 3 and 10 days after a subarachnoid hemorrhage. It is associated with a large number of deaths and disability. A cerebral vasospasm narrows the lumen of one or more cerebral vessels, causing ischemia and infarction of tissue supplied by the affected vessels. The actual cause is unknown, but it occurs in blood vessels surrounded by thick blood clots, suggesting that some substance in the clot initiates the spasm. The manifestations vary according to the degree of spasm and the area of brain affected. Regional alterations may cause focal deficits (such as hemiplegia), whereas global alterations cause loss of consciousness.

### Hydrocephalus

**Hydrocephalus,** an abnormal accumulation of cerebrospinal fluid (CSF) within the cranial vault and dilation of the ventricles, is a potential complication of a ruptured intracranial aneurysm. Hydrocephalus is thought to be the result of obstruction of reabsorption of CSF through the arachnoid villi. The obstruction is caused by an increased protein content of the CSF because of lysis of blood in the subarachnoid space (Porth, 2002). The accumulation of cerebrospinal fluid increases intracranial pressure. Initial manifestations of hydrocephalus are typically nonspecific but commonly include decreasing levels of consciousness.

## COLLABORATIVE CARE

The care of the client with a ruptured intracranial aneurysm includes determining the location of the aneurysm, treating the manifestations of the hemorrhage, and preventing rebleeding and vasospasm. Surgery is the treatment of choice to repair the bleeding artery.

### Diagnostic Tests

The following diagnostic tests may be conducted to identify the site and extent of a ruptured intracranial aneurysm, as well as rebleeding.

- *CT scan* of the brain demonstrates blood in the subarachnoid space in most clients within the first 24 to 48 hours after rupture.
- *Lumbar puncture* may be performed to withdraw cerebrospinal fluid for analysis. The presence of blood in the cerebrospinal fluid confirms a subarachnoid hemorrhage. However, this procedure poses a risk of rebleeding and brain herniation (Porth, 2002).
- *Bilateral carotid* and *vertebral cerebral angiography* may be conducted to determine the site and size of an aneurysm. A contrast medium (if used) is injected into an artery, and X-ray films are taken to visualize the cerebral vessels. This diagnostic test is not conducted unless the client's condition is stable enough for surgery.

### Medications

If surgery is not possible because of the client's condition, medications may be used to reduce the risk of rebleeding and vasospasm until surgery is feasible.

Aminocaproic acid (Amicar, Epsikapron) is a fibrinolysis inhibitor used to treat excessive bleeding in acute, life-threatening situations. It prevents the lysis of any blood clot that has formed near the site of a rupture. This drug is used in the first 2 weeks after aneurysm rupture (or until the client has surgery) to reduce the risk of rebleeding. The drug is administered intravenously the first week and orally thereafter. Potential complications include pulmonary embolism, venous thrombosis, and focal ischemic neurologic deficits.

Calcium channel blockers, such as nimodipine (Nimotop), are used to improve neurologic deficits due to vasospasm following subarachnoid hemorrhage from ruptured intracranial aneurysms. The drug is administered orally for 3 weeks after the hemorrhage. It has been found to reduce the incidence of ischemic deficits from arterial spasm without side effects (Tierney et al., 2001).

Other medications that may be prescribed include:

- Anticonvulsants, such as phenytoin (Dilantin), to prevent seizures if the client has increased intracranial pressure.
- Stool softeners, such as docusate, to prevent constipation and straining with a bowel movement (which increases intracranial pressure and blood pressure). These, in turn, may cause rebleeding.
- Analgesics (e.g., acetaminophen or codeine) for headache.

### Surgery

Surgery for the treatment of intracranial aneurysm is done either to prevent rupture or to isolate the vessel to prevent further bleeding. Clients with good neurologic status may have surgery soon after the rupture. In clients with significant neurologic deficits, surgery may be delayed until they are more stable and less at risk for vasospasm.

There are several different types of surgery to repair a ruptured intracranial aneurysm or to prevent the rupture of an existing large aneurysm. The skull is opened (craniotomy), and the aneurysm is located. The neck of the aneurysm may be clipped with a metal clip (preventing the entry of blood into the aneurysm), or the involved artery may be clipped both proximally and distally to the aneurysm to isolate the affected area. Endovascular Gudlielmi detachable coils (GDCs) are used to treat aneurysms with narrow necks. The coil is inserted into the dome of the aneurysm and an electric current is passed through the coil to cause coagulation. The procedure, performed by a neuroradiologist, may be conducted either under general or local anesthesia (Bucher & Melander, 1999).

## NURSING CARE

### Nursing Diagnoses and Interventions

Nursing care is planned and implemented for the client with a ruptured intracranial aneurysm to prevent rebleeding as well as to meet needs resulting from neurologic deficits. Other appropriate nursing diagnoses and interventions are described earlier in the chapter in the discussion of nursing care for the client with a stroke.

### Ineffective Tissue Perfusion (Cerebral)

This discussion focuses on the care of the client immediately after the intracranial aneurysm ruptures. The expected outcome of care is preventing rebleeding and improving cerebral tissue perfusion.

- Institute aneurysm precautions to prevent rebleeding, as follows:
  - Keep the client in a private, quiet, darkened room. Disconnect or remove the telephone. Avoid using bright overhead lights. *A quiet environment helps prevent an increase in blood pressure, which could precipitate rebleeding. The client may experience photophobia (abnormal sensitivity to light) if hemorrhage has damaged the oculomotor nerve.*

- Elevate the head of the bed 30 to 45 degrees; follow prescribed activity orders (usually complete bed rest, but in some cases bathroom privileges may be approved). *Elevating the head of the bed promotes venous return from the brain and thus decreases intracranial pressure. Decreasing activity reduces the likelihood of increases in blood pressure.*
- Limit visitors to two family members at any one time, and limit the duration of visits. Monitor client response to visitors and decrease interactions if the client becomes agitated or upset. *Psychologic stress may increase blood pressure and the risk of rebleeding; however, social isolation may increase anxiety and stress. Each client (and family) must be individually evaluated.*
- Allow reading, watching television (if available), or listening to the radio (if available) to promote relaxation. *Although these passive activities were previously contraindicated for the client on aneurysm precautions, current therapy is based on the belief that these activities promote relaxation and help control blood pressure.*
- Prevent constipation and straining to have a bowel movement. Administer stool softeners as prescribed. Collaborate with the client and physician about use of a bedside commode or the bathroom. Do not administer enemas. *The client is at risk for constipation as a result of decreased mobility and the administration of narcotics (such as codeine) for headache. When straining to have a bowel movement, the client uses the Valsalva maneuver, which increases intracranial pressure and may precipitate rebleeding.*

**PRACTICE ALERT** *Maintaining a daily stool chart is an important assessment in preventing constipation.* ∎

- If the client is alert, and depending on physician preferences, allow to feed self and provide own personal care. *In many instances, self-care causes less anxiety and stress than care provided by the nurse. The extent of care provided varies according to client condition and physician preferences.*
- Monitor vital signs and neurologic status as indicated by client condition (frequency of assessments may range from every 15 minutes to every 4 hours). *Vital signs and neurologic assessments provide ongoing data for evaluation of changes indicative of increasing intracranial pressure and decreasing neurologic function. Report any change immediately to the physician.*

**PRACTICE ALERT** *A rising blood pressure and falling pulse rate are manifestations of increased intracranial pressure.* ∎

- Maintain seizure precautions: Have suction equipment and an oropharyngeal tube at the bedside, maintain the bed in the low position, and keep the side rails padded and raised. *Applying suction and inserting an oropharyngeal airway may be necessary to maintain an open airway in case of*

seizure. *A lowered bed and padded, raised side rails prevent injury if a seizure occurs.*
- Avoid positioning and activities that increase intracranial pressure such as coughing, sneezing, vomiting, sharply flexing the neck, blowing the nose, enemas, moving self up in bed, or cigarette smoking. *These measures help to prevent increasing intracranial pressure and rebleeding.*

## THE CLIENT WITH AN ARTERIOVENOUS MALFORMATION

An **arteriovenous (AV) malformation** is a congenital intracranial lesion, formed by a tangled collection of dilated arteries and veins, that allows blood to flow directly from the arterial into the venous system, bypassing the normal capillary network. Most AV malformations (90%) are located in the cerebral hemispheres; the remainder are found in the cerebellum and brainstem.

Rupture of vessels in the malformations account for 2% of all strokes. Clients with this condition develop manifestations before 40 years of age; it affects men and women equally (Porth, 2002). The manifestations are the result of spontaneous bleeding from the lesion into the subarachnoid space or brain tissue.

### PATHOPHYSIOLOGY

AV malformations displace rather than encompass normal brain tissue (Hickey, 2003). The pathophysiologic effects of an AV malformation are the result of the shunting of blood from the arterial to the venous system and of altered perfusion of cerebral tissue near the malformation. The shunting of arterial blood directly into the venous system within the malformation transfers the higher arterial pressure directly into the lower-pressure venous system. This increased pressure is likely to cause spontaneous bleeding or progressive expansion and rupture of a blood vessel.

Altered cerebral perfusion results when blood flow through a large, high-flow malformation is diverted from the normal cerebral circulation, causing tissue ischemia of the area surrounding the malformation. This is sometimes called a vascular "steal" phenomenon.

AV malformations range in size from very small to very large. Large malformations are usually initially manifested by seizure activity. In contrast, the manifestations of a small malformation are more often due to a hemorrhage that causes neurologic deficits. In both instances, the client may have recurrent headaches that do not respond to treatment.

### COLLABORATIVE CARE

AV malformations are diagnosed with the same diagnostic tests (CT scan, MRI, angiography) used to diagnose an intracranial aneurysm.

If the malformation is accessible, the ideal treatment is excision of the malformation and removal of any hematoma.

Large malformations may be treated by embolization. In this procedure, substances such as Gelfoam or metallic pellets are introduced into the involved area of the cerebral circulation, where they form emboli and gradually obstruct blood flow in the malformation. Inaccessible malformations are also treated with radiation therapy or laser therapy, to coagulate blood in the malformation and thicken its vascular elements, eventually obstructing it. When the malformation is excised or obstructed, blood flow is no longer shunted, and cerebral perfusion improves.

## NURSING CARE

Nursing care depends on the condition of the malformation. If hemorrhage has not occurred, teach the client to avoid activities that raise blood pressure or could cause injury. The client is usually given medications to control blood pressure and prevent seizures.

If the malformation ruptures and causes an intracranial hemorrhage, nursing care is the same as for any client who has had a hemorrhagic stroke (discussed earlier in this chapter).

# SPINAL CORD DISORDERS

## THE CLIENT WITH A SPINAL CORD INJURY

Nursing care of clients with disorders of the spinal cord takes place from the acute management phase through ongoing rehabilitation in a variety of settings. Although priorities of care may change depending on the client and setting, care focuses on maximizing function to preserve quality of life. The nurse provides independent care and also collaborates with other health care professionals to meet this goal.

## INCIDENCE AND PREVALENCE

A **spinal cord injury (SCI)** is usually due to trauma. There are an estimated 250,000 to 400,000 people with SCIs living in the United States. Although SCIs occur in people of all ages, they are most often seen in young adults age 16 to 30. The majority of the injuries are due to motor vehicle accidents; other causes include falls, violence, and sports injuries (with the majority from diving). Approximately 8000 people have a SCI each year, with the greatest risk for injury being in the summer (National Spinal Cord Injury Association, 1998; Porth, 2002).

The major causes of SCI are concussion, contusion, laceration, transection, hemorrhage, and damage to blood vessels that supply the spinal cord. If vertebrae are fractured and ligaments are torn, bony fragments can damage the cord and make the spinal column unstable. Injury to blood vessels supplying the cord can cause permanent damage. The injury is identified by vertebral level. For example, a C6 spinal cord injury is at the sixth cervical vertebra.

### Risk Factors

The three major risk factors for SCIs are age, gender, and alcohol or drug abuse. Young men are more prone to take risks than women. Older adults are more likely to have a cord injury from even minor trauma as a result of age-related vertebral degeneration. Motor vehicle crashes while under the influence of alcohol or drugs are a major source of trauma to people of all ages.

## OVERVIEW OF THE NORMAL SPINAL CORD

The spinal cord runs through the vertebral canal of the vertebral column from the foramen magnum to the L1 or L2 level. The cord provides a two-way pathway for the conduction of impulses and information to and from the brain and the body, serves as a major reflex center, and (through its attached spinal nerves) is involved in the sensory and motor innervation of the entire body below the head.

The cord consists of an outer region of white matter and an inner region of gray matter. The gray matter comprises the central canal of the cord, the posterior horns, the anterior horns, and the lateral horns. It is divided into a sensory half (dorsally) and a motor half (ventrally) and innervates somatic and visceral regions of the body. The white matter consists of tracts or pathways that convey information. The ascending (sensory) pathways carry information about proprioception, fine touch, discrimination, pain, temperature, deep pressure, and touch. The descending (motor) pathways carry information about movement. The pyramidal tracts control skilled voluntary movements (such as writing). The extrapyramidal tracts (all tracts other than the pyramidal tracts) bring about all other body movements. See Chapter 40 ⊙ for further information.

## PATHOPHYSIOLOGY

The primary injury causes microscopic hemorrhages in the gray matter of the cord and edema of the white matter of the cord. These initial pathologic changes are followed by the secondary injury, with mechanisms that increase the area of injury. The hemorrhages extend, eventually involving the entire gray matter. Microcirculation to the cord is impaired by edema and hemorrhage. The injured tissue releases norepinephrine, serotonin, dopamine, and histamine; these vasoactive substances cause vasospasm and further decrease microcirculation. As a result, vascular perfusion and oxygen tension of the affected area is decreased, which leads to ischemia.

When ischemia is prolonged, necrosis of both gray and white matter begins within a few hours, and within 24 hours the function of nerves passing through the injured area is lost. Although circulation returns to the white matter of the cord in about 24 hours, decreased circulation in the gray matter

MediaLink | SPINAL CORD INJURY CASE STUDY

continues. Because edema extends the level of injury for two cord segments above and below the affected level, the extent of injury cannot be determined for up to 1 week.

Tissue repair occurs over a period of 3 to 4 weeks. Phagocytes enter the area in 36 to 48 hours after the initial injury. Neurons degenerate and are removed by microphages in the first 10 days after the injury. Red blood cells disintegrate, and the hemorrhages are reabsorbed. Eventually the area of injury is replaced by acellular collagenous tissue, and the meninges thicken.

## Forces Resulting in SCI

SCIs are the result of the application of excessive force to the spinal column. The most common cause of abnormal spinal column movements are acceleration and deceleration (forces that are applied to the body, for example, in automobile crashes and falls). *Acceleration* occurs when external force is applied in a rear-end collision; the upper torso and head are forced backward and then forward. *Deceleration* occurs in a head-on collision; the external force is applied from the front. The head and body move forward until they meet a stationary object and then are forced backward. The following forces and movements (Figure 41–5 ■) may cause a variety of spinal cord injuries, with the extent of injury depending on the amount and direction of motion, and the rate of application of force.

- *Hyperflexion,* or forcible forward bending, may compress vertebral bodies and disrupt ligaments and intervertebral disks.
- *Hyperextension,* or forcible backward bending, often disrupts ligaments and causes vertebral fractures. A whiplash injury is a less severe form of hyperextension, with injury to soft tissues but no vertebral or spinal cord damage.
- *Axial loading,* a form of compression, is the application of vertical force to the spinal column (for instance, by falling and landing on the feet or buttocks or by diving into shallow water).
- *Excessive rotation,* in which the head is excessively turned, may tear ligaments, fracture articular surfaces, and cause compression fractures.

The alteration of the spinal cord and soft tissues caused by these abnormal movements is called **deformation.** In addition, the spinal cord may be penetrated by bullets and other foreign objects (e.g., sharp objects used as weapons, shrapnel from explosions). Penetrating injuries may cause vertebral fractures, tear ligaments and muscles, or cut through a part or all of the spinal cord. Complete severing of the cord is rare.

## Sites of Pathology

Injuries occur most often in the lumbar and cervical regions. The most frequent sites of injury of the cord are at the first, second, and fourth to sixth cervical vertebrae (C1, C2, C4 to C6);

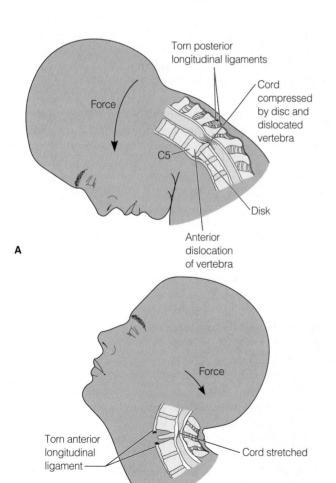

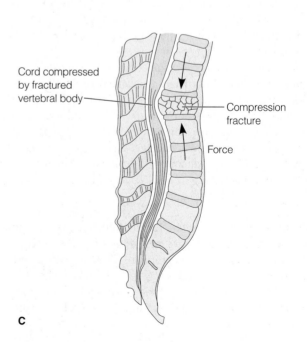

**Figure 41–5 ■** Spinal cord injury mechanisms. *A,* Hyperflexion. *B,* Hyperextension. *C,* Axial loading, a form of compression.

and the eleventh thoracic to second lumbar vertebrae (T11 to L2). Because the cervical spine has a wider range of movement than the rest of the spine, the cervical portion is more likely to be affected by externally applied forces. In addition, the cord fills most of the vertebral canal in the cervical and lumbar regions and thus is more easily injured. Damage to the vertebrae and ligaments causes the spinal column to become unstable, increasing the possibility of compression or stretching of the spinal cord with any further movement.

## Classification of SCI

SCIs are classified according to systems, for instance (1) as complete or incomplete cord injury, (2) by cause of injury, and (3) by level of injury. In clinical practice, these classifications often overlap. In a *complete SCI,* the motor and sensory neural pathways are completely interrupted (transected), resulting in total loss of motor and sensory function below the level of the injury. In an *incomplete SCI,* the motor and sensory pathways are only partially interrupted, with variable loss of function below the level of injury. Incomplete spinal cord injuries are further classified into syndromes as outlined in Table 41–1. The alterations in function that occur as the result of a spinal cord injury vary greatly depending on the amount of tissue damage and the level of injury.

## MANIFESTATIONS AND COMPLICATIONS

The spinal cord, the vertebrae, the intervertebral disks, the spinal nerves, the ligaments, and the surrounding soft-tissue structures are in such close anatomic proximity that any condition or injury affecting one structure may well affect any one or all of the other structures. The conditions with the most critical effects are disorders affecting the spinal cord. Disorders and injuries of the spinal cord have the potential to affect movement, perception, sensation, sexual function, and elimination. Manifestations and complications of SCI by body system are listed in the box below.

### Manifestations and Complications of Spinal Cord Injury by Body System

**Integument**
- Decubitus (pressure) ulcers

**Neurologic**
- Pain
- Areflexia
- Hypotonia
- Autonomic dysreflexia

**Cardiovascular**
- Spinal shock
- Paroxysmal hypertension
- Orthostatic hypotension
- Cardiac dysrhythmias
- Decreased venous return
- Hypercalcemia

**Respiratory**
- Limited chest expansion
- Decreased cough reflex
- Decreased vital capacity

**Gastrointestinal**
- Stress ulcers
- Paralytic ileus
- Stool impaction
- Stool incontinence

**Genitourinary**
- Urinary retention
- Urinary incontinence
- Neurogenic bladder
- Impotence
- Testicular atrophy
- Inability to ejaculate
- Decreased vaginal lubrication

**Musculoskeletal**
- Joint contractures
- Bone demineralization
- Osteoporosis
- Muscle spasms
- Muscle atrophy
- Pathologic fractures
- Paraplegia
- Tetraplegia

## TABLE 41-1   Incomplete Spinal Cord Injury Syndromes

| Type | Cause | Location | Deficits |
|---|---|---|---|
| Central syndrome | Cord transection Hyperextension | Cervical | Spastic paralysis of the upper extremities Variable paralysis of the lower extremities Variable effects on the bowel, the bladder, and sexual function |
| Anterior syndrome | Damage to the anterior spinal artery Infarction of the anterior spinal artery Hyperflexion | Anterior two-thirds of the cord | Paralysis below the level of injury Loss of temperature and pain sensation below the level of injury |
| Posterior syndrome | Vertebral dislocation Herniated disk Compression | Nerve roots | Weakness in isolated muscle groups Tingling, pain Decreased or absent reflexes in the involved area Bowel or bladder dysfunction |
| Brown-Séquard syndrome | Penetrating trauma | Hemisection of the anterior and posterior cord | Paralysis below the level of injury on the ipsilateral (same) side of the body Contralateral loss of temperature and pain sensation below the level of injury Ipsilateral loss of proprioception below the level of injury |
| Horner's syndrome | Incomplete cord transection | Cervical sympathetic nerves | Ipsilateral ptosis of the eyelid, constricted pupil, and facial anhidrosis (inability to perspire) |

## Spinal Shock

**Spinal shock** is the temporary loss of reflex function (called **areflexia**) below the level of injury. This response begins immediately after complete transection of the spinal cord, when connections between the brain and the spinal cord are interrupted and the cord does not function at all. The response also occurs (although in varying degrees) after partial transection as well as after spinal cord contusions, compression, and ischemia.

Normal activity of the spinal cord is dependent on constant impulses from the higher centers of the brain. When damage from an injury stops these impulses, spinal shock follows. There is loss of motor function, tendon reflexes, and autonomic function. Of particular concern is the effect on pulse and blood pressure; the parasympathetic system dominates in spinal shock, causing bradycardia and hypotension.

Spinal shock may begin within 1 hour of the injury. The condition may last from a few minutes to several months (although it usually lasts from 1 to 6 weeks), and then reflex activity returns. Spinal shock ends slowly, with the gradual reappearance of reflexes, hyperreflexia (increased reflex responses), muscle spasticity, and reflex bladder emptying.

The manifestations of acute spinal shock (which vary in degree) include the following:

- Bradycardia
- Hypotension
- Flaccid paralysis of skeletal muscles
- Loss of sensations of pain, touch, temperature, and pressure
- Absence of visceral and somatic sensations
- Bowel and bladder dysfunction
- Loss of the ability to perspire

A person with a cervical cord injury may also have neurogenic shock, resulting in cardiovascular changes. These changes are due to the inability of higher centers in the brainstem to modulate reflexes. As a result, vascular beds dilate, and the cardiac accelerator reflex is suppressed. The client experiences orthostatic hypotension and bradycardia. Other symptoms may include respiratory insufficiency due to loss of innervation of the diaphragm in C1 to C4 injuries, hypothermia, paralytic ileus, urinary retention, and oliguria.

Both bradycardia and hypotension may persist even after the spinal shock resolves. In addition to losing sympathetic control of the heart rate, the client with a high-level SCI experiences decreased peripheral resistance and loss of muscle activity. These changes result in sluggish blood flow and decreased venous return, increasing the risk for thrombophlebitis.

## Upper and Lower Motor Neuron Deficits

Injuries to the spinal cord are often classified as either *upper motor neuron lesions* or *lower motor neuron lesions*. Motor neurons are functional units that carry motor impulses. The upper motor neurons (located in the cerebral cortex, thalamus, brainstem, and corticospinal and corticobulbar tracts) are responsible for voluntary movement. When these motor pathways are interrupted, the client experiences spastic paralysis and hyperreflexia and may be unable to carry out skilled movement.

Lower motor neurons (located in the anterior horn of the spinal cord, the motor nuclei of the brainstem, and the axons that reach the motor end plate of skeletal muscles) are responsible for innervation and contraction of skeletal muscles. Interruption of lower motor neurons results in muscle flaccidity and extensive muscle atrophy, with loss of both voluntary and involuntary movement. If only some of the motor neurons supplying a muscle are affected, the client experiences partial paralysis (paresis); if all motor neurons to a muscle are affected, the client experiences complete paralysis. Hyporeflexia is also present.

## Paraplegia and Tetraplegia

Two common neurologic deficits resulting from an SCI are paraplegia and tetraplegia (see Figure 41–1). **Paraplegia** is paralysis of the lower portion of the body, sometimes involving the lower trunk. Paraplegia occurs when the thoracic, lumbar, and sacral portions of the spinal cord are injured, causing loss or impairment of sensory and/or motor function. **Tetraplegia,** formerly called quadriplegia, occurs when cervical segments of the cord are injured, impairing function of the arms, trunk, legs, and pelvic organs.

## Autonomic Dysreflexia

**Autonomic dysreflexia** (also called *autonomic hyperreflexia*) is an exaggerated sympathetic response that occurs in clients with SCIs at or above the T6 level. This response, which is seen only after recovery from spinal shock, occurs as a result of a lack of control of the autonomic nervous system by higher centers. When stimuli (such as a full bladder) are unable to ascend the cord, mass reflex stimulation of the sympathetic nerves below the level of the injured cord area occurs, triggering massive vasoconstriction. In response, the vagus nerve causes bradycardia and vasodilation above the level of injury. If untreated, autonomic dysreflexia can cause seizures, a stroke, or a myocardial infarction (Hickey, 2003). The complications of untreated dysreflexia are potentially fatal.

Autonomic dysreflexia is triggered by stimuli that would normally cause abdominal discomfort (a full bladder is the most common cause), by stimulation of pain receptors, and by visceral contractions (Porth, 2002). Causes include fecal impaction, bladder infections or stones, acute abdominal disorders, intrauterine contractions, ejaculation, and stimulation from pressure ulcers or ingrown toenails.

The manifestations of this condition include pounding headache; bradycardia; hypertension (with readings as high as 300/160); flushed, warm skin with profuse sweating above the lesion and pale, cold, and dry skin below it; and anxiety (Porth, 2002). Dysreflexia is a neurologic emergency and requires immediate treatment.

## COLLABORATIVE CARE

The client with an acute SCI requires emergency assessment and care and medications; sometimes the client also requires immobilization and surgery. The client is first assessed and stabilized at the scene of the accident, initially treated in the emergency room, and then admitted to the hospital intensive care unit.

## Emergency Care at the Scene

The danger of death from SCI is greatest when there is damage to or transection of the upper cervical region. When the injury is at the C1 to C4 level, respiratory paralysis is common, and the client who survives requires ventilator assistance to breathe. Injuries below C4 may increase the risk of respiratory failure if edema ascends the cord. It is of critical importance not to complicate the initial injury by allowing the fractured vertebrae to damage the cord further during transport to the hospital. Although at one time injuries to the high cervical cord were almost always fatal, advances in trauma care have greatly improved the survival rate.

All people who have sustained trauma to the head or spine, or who are unconscious, should be treated as though they have a spinal cord injury. Prehospital management includes rapid assessment of the ABCs (airway, breathing, circulation), immobilizing and stabilizing the head and neck, removing the person from the site of injury, stabilizing other life-threatening injuries, and rapidly transporting the person to the appropriate facility. Guidelines for emergency care are as follows:

- Avoid flexing, extending, or rotating the neck.
- Immobilize the neck, using rolled towels or blankets, or apply a cervical collar before moving the client onto a backboard.
- Secure the head by placing a belt or tape across the forehead and securing it to the stretcher.
- Maintain the client in the supine position.
- Transfer directly from the stretcher with backboard still in place to the type of bed that will be used in the hospital.

## Emergency Department Management

Assessment findings at the scene of the accident or in the emergency room vary according to the level of injury. The following findings indicate cervical injury.

- Paralysis or weakness of extremities
- Respiratory distress manifested by changes in arterial blood gas studies, cyanosis, flaring of the nostrils, use of accessory muscles of respiration, and restlessness
- Pulse rate below 60 and systolic BP below 80
- Decreased peristalsis

This finding indicates thoracic and lumbar injury:

- Paralysis or weakness of extremities

These findings indicate acute spinal shock:

- Loss of skin sensation
- Flaccid paralysis, areflexia
- Absent bowel sounds
- Bladder distention
- Decreasing blood pressure
- Absence of the cremasteric reflex in males (retraction of the left or right testicle in response to stimulation of the skin of, respectively, the inner left or right thigh)

The client in the emergency department with a suspected or identified SCI is also treated for respiratory problems, par-alytic ileus, atonic bladder, and cardiovascular alterations. Respiratory distress in the client with a cervical-level injury is treated by placing the client on a ventilator. Oxygen is administered to the client with a thoracic-level injury. Paralytic ileus (obstruction of the intestines due to lack of peristalsis) is common in clients with a spinal cord injury and is treated by the insertion of a nasogastric tube with connection to suction. To prevent overdistention of an atonic bladder, an indwelling catheter is inserted and connected to dependent drainage. Cardiovascular status is assessed on a continuous basis by inserting invasive monitoring devices, such as a Swan-Ganz catheter, and attaching the client to a cardiac monitor.

High-dose steroid protocol using methylprednisolone (Medrol) must be immediately implemented on admission to the emergency room. Clinical research indicates that the use of this adrenocorticosteroid is effective in preventing secondary spinal cord damage from edema and ischemia. The medication must be administered intravenously within 8 hours of the injury to be effective in preventing secondary damage. A loading dose is administered initially and a maintenance dose is continued for 23 hours.

## Diagnostic Tests

Diagnostic tests are ordered to identify the level and extent of injury, and to detect any complications.

- *X-ray films* of the cervical spine are taken immediately after admission to establish the level of injury and extent of vertebral injury. Thoracic and lumbar spine X-rays are taken at the same time if possible.
- *CT scan* or *MRI* illustrates changes in the vertebrae, spinal cord, and tissues around the cord.
- *Arterial blood gases* are measured to establish a baseline or to identify problems due to respiratory insufficiency.
- *Somatosensory evoked potential (SEP) studies* may be done to locate the level of spinal cord injury. In these tests, peripheral nerves are stimulated and response times measured.

## Medications

The pharmacologic treatment of the client with SCI is symptomatic. It is directed primarily toward decreasing edema from the injury, treating hypotension and bradycardia, and treating spasticity.

- Corticosteroids, discussed earlier in this section, may be used to decrease or control edema of the cord.
- Vasopressors are used in the immediate critical care phase to treat bradycardia or hypotension due to spinal and neurogenic shock. Examples of drugs are dopamine (Intropin) to treat hypotension in neurogenic shock and dobutamine (Dobutrex) to support cardiac function. Atropine should be available at the bedside to treat bradycardia.
- Antispasmodics are used to treat spasticity in clients with spinal cord injury. Both baclofen (Lioresal) and diazepam (Valium) may be used. A discussion of nursing implications of treatment with antispasmodics is found in the Medication Administration box on page 1328.

## Medication Administration

### Antispasmodics in Spinal Cord Injury

Baclofen (Lioresal)
Chlorzoxazone (Paraflex)
Cyclobenzaprine hydrochloride (Flexeril)
Diazepam (Valium)
Orphenadrine citrate (Norflex)

These drugs depress the central nervous system and inhibit the transmission of impulses from the spinal cord to skeletal muscle. They are used to control muscle spasm and pain associated with acute or chronic musculoskeletal conditions. They are not always effective in controlling spasticity resulting from cerebral or spinal cord conditions.

### Nursing Responsibilities

- Assess the client's spasticity and involuntary movements to obtain baseline data for comparison of results of therapy.

- Do not expect therapy to have effects for 1 week.
- Administer oral medications with food to decrease gastrointestinal symptoms.

### Client and Family Teaching

- These drugs may cause drowsiness, diplopia, and impotence.
- Take your medications with meals to decrease gastric irritation.
- Physical improvement may take several weeks.
- Report slurred speech, drooling, or inability to carry out normal functions to the physician.
- Do not stop taking the medication without consulting your health care provider.

---

- Analgesics such as nonsteroidal anti-inflammatory agents and tricylic antidepressants such as amitriptyline (Elavil) and imipramine (Tofranil) are administered to reduce pain.
- Histamine $H_2$ antagonists (e.g., ranitidine [Zantac]) are often administered to prevent stress-related gastric ulcers, a common complication in SCI.
- Anticoagulants (heparin or warfarin) may be given to prevent thrombophlebitis.
- Stool softeners may be administered as part of a bowel training program.

## Treatments

The treatments used in the management of an SCI include surgery, stabilization, and immobilization.

### Surgery

Early surgical treatment may be necessary if there is evidence of compression of the spinal cord by bone fragments or a hematoma. Surgery may also be done to stabilize and support the spine. However, many clients are treated with stabilization devices and do not require surgery. Surgeries that may be performed include a decompression laminectomy, a spinal fusion, and insertion of metal rods. Surgeries of the spine are discussed later in the chapter.

### Stabilization and Immobilization

The client with an SCI as a result of one or more dislocations or fractures of the cervical vertebrae may be immobilized by being placed in some type of traction or external fixation device to stabilize the vertebral column and prevent any further damage. Traction may also be used to stabilize the spinal column for clients who are not yet in a condition to have surgery or who have severe bleeding and edema of the injured cord. The physician applies the traction or fixation device; the nurse is responsible for assessments and interventions following the application.

Although used less frequently today, various devices provide cervical traction. Gardner-Wells tongs may be used (Figure 41–6 ■). In this type of traction, the physician applies

pins to the skull, approximately 1 cm above each ear, and weights are attached to the device.

The halo external fixation device is often used to provide stabilization if there is no significant involvement of the ligaments (Figure 41–7 ■). It is most often used to provide stability for fractures of the cervical and high thoracic vertebrae without cord damage. This device allows greater mobility, self-care, and participation in rehabilitation programs. The device is secured with four pins inserted into the skull, two in the frontal bone and two in the occipital bone. The halo ring is then attached to a rigid plastic vest lined with sheepskin. Nursing interventions for the client using a halo fixation device are described in the Nursing Care box on page 1329.

## NURSING CARE

Both during the acute phase and the rehabilitative phase, the client with a SCI has complex needs that involve all members of the health care team. Because these injuries are more common in younger clients, consideration of life-long effects on both the client and the family is essential. The nurse coordi-

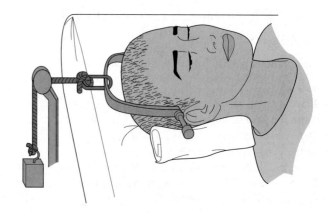

**Figure 41–6 ■** Cervical traction may be applied by several methods, including Gardner-Wells tongs.

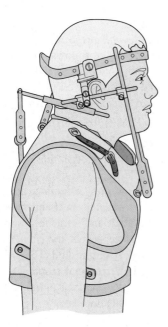

**Figure 41–7 ■** The halo external fixation device.

nates client care and develops and implements a care plan that is individualized to each client and family. The focus of the plan is to prevent the secondary complications of immobility and altered body functions, to promote self-care, and to educate the client and family.

## Health Promotion

Health promotion for SCI primarily involves preventing injuries. Nurses can provide valuable information in the community and in the workplace to prevent SCI. Programs that focus on wearing seat belts and using approved infant seats and child booster chairs in automobiles can do much to help decrease the number of SCIs each year. Educational programs

that promote workplace safety and farm safety should include information to prevent falls and how to use heavy equipment safely.

## Assessment

The following data are collected through the health history and physical examination (see Chapter 40). Further focused assessments are described with nursing interventions in the next section.

- Health history: time, location, and type of accident; location, duration, quality, and intensity of pain; dyspnea; sensation; paresthesia
- Physical examination: vital signs, motor strength, movement, spinal reflexes, bowel sounds, bladder distention

## Nursing Diagnoses and Interventions

Because an SCI has many possible effects, many nursing diagnoses may be appropriate. Nursing diagnoses discussed in this section focus on problems with physical mobility, gas exchange, dysreflexia, bowel and bladder elimination, sexual dysfunction, and self-esteem.

## Impaired Physical Mobility

After the initial period of spinal shock and areflexia, the client regains spinal reflex activity and muscle tone that is not under the control of higher centers. Clients with injuries above the level of T12 experience involuntary spastic movements of skeletal muscles. These movements reach a peak about 2 years after the injury and then gradually subside (Porth, 2002). Spasms impair the ability to carry out the activities of daily life and work. In addition, the paraplegia or tetraplegia increases the potential for impaired skin integrity, thrombophlebitis, and contractures.

The goals of care for clients with impaired mobility due to a spinal cord injury are to reduce the effects of spasticity and to

---

## NURSING CARE OF THE CLIENT IN HALO FIXATION

### NURSING RESPONSIBILITIES

- Maintain integrity of the halo external fixation device.
  a. Inspect pins and traction bars for tightness; report loosened pins to physician.
  b. Tape the appropriate wrench to the head of the bed for emergency intervention.
  c. Never use the halo ring to lift or reposition the client.
  *Loosening of the apparatus poses the risk of further damage to the cord. It is the responsibility of the nurse to maintain the integrity of the apparatus and the safety of the client.*
- Assess muscle function and skin sensation every 2 hours in the acute phase and every 4 hours thereafter.
  a. Assess motor function on a scale of 0 to 5, with 0 being no evidence of muscle contraction and 5 being normal muscle strength with full range of motion.
  b. Assess sensation by comparing touch and pain, moving from impaired to normal areas, and testing both the right and left sides of the body.

*Monitoring muscle function and skin sensation allows early identification of potential neurologic deficits.*
- Monitor pin sites each shift and follow hospital policy for pin care. Here are some general guidelines.
  a. Assess pin sites for redness, edema, and drainage.
  b. Depending on policy, clean each pin site with a sterile applicator dipped in hydrogen peroxide, apply a topical antibiotic, and cover with sterile 2-inch split gauze squares.
*Organisms can enter the body through the pin-insertion site; assessments and care are provided to detect signs of and prevent infection.*
- Maintain skin integrity.
  a. Turn the immobile client every 2 hours.
  b. Inspect the skin around edges of the vest every 4 hours.
  c. Change the sheepskin liner when it is soiled and at least once each week.

*These interventions prevent skin injury and irritation.*

prevent complications involving the skin, the cardiovascular system, and joint function.

- Perform passive ROM exercises for all extremities at least twice a day. Identify stimuli that cause spastic movements and either avoid the stimuli (such as certain exercises) or teach the client to expect the movements. *ROM exercises help prevent contractures and stretch spastic muscles, promoting rehabilitation.*
- Maintain skin integrity by turning every 2 hours, assessing pressure points at least once each shift, and using a special bed if necessary. The client may be placed on a regular or special bed, such as a kinetic bed. *Immobility compresses soft tissues and promotes the development of decubitus ulcers. The lack of sensory warning mechanisms and of voluntary motor control of skin dermatomes further increases the risk for altered skin integrity. Special beds allow movement or turning while keeping the spinal column in alignment.*
- Assess the lower extremities each shift for symptoms of thrombophlebitis. Observe for redness and for increased heat every shift; measure thigh and calf circumference daily. If antiembolic stockings (TEDs) are ordered, remove for 30 to 60 minutes each shift. Assess for skin impairment and provide skin care while TEDs are removed. *Clients with neurologic deficits are at high risk for deep vein thrombosis as a result of immobility, vasomotor dysfunction, and decreased venous return with venous stasis. Antiembolic stockings help to prevent the pooling of blood in the lower extremities and increase venous return, lessening the risk for venous stasis and thrombus formation.*

**PRACTICE ALERT** *Removing TED stockings each shift not only promotes healthy skin but also lets the nurse assess skin integrity.* ■

## Impaired Gas Exchange

Injuries at the level of T1 to T7 leave the phrenic nerve intact, but the innervation of intercostal muscles is affected, compromising respiratory function. In addition, because the abdominal muscles are paralyzed, the client cannot expel secretions by coughing. (Clients with cord injuries at C3 or above have paralysis of the respiratory muscles and cannot breathe without a ventilator.)

- Monitor vital capacity and respiratory effectiveness, assessing for tachycardia, restlessness, $Pao_2$ less than 60 mmHg, $Paco_2$ greater than 50 mmHg, and vital capacity less than 1L. *Clients with cervical cord injuries frequently require ventilatory support because of reduced vital capacity and inability to expel secretions by coughing.*

**PRACTICE ALERT** *Changes in arterial blood gases and vital capacity signal respiratory insufficiency.* ■

- Monitor for signs of ascending edema of the spinal cord, including difficulty in swallowing or coughing, respiratory stridor, use of accessory muscles of respiration, bradycardia,

and increased motor and sensory loss. *Hemorrhage and edema can further impair respiratory function.*

- Help the client to cough, as follows: Place the hand between the umbilicus and xiphoid process and push in and up as the client exhales and coughs. *The client who is unable to cough effectively and has decreased ventilatory capacity may develop atelectasis, pneumonia, and respiratory failure.*

## Ineffective Breathing Patterns

Respiratory function is impaired in the client with SCI in the cervical and thoracic levels if the diaphragm (innervated at C3 to C5), the intercostal muscles (innervated at T1 to T7), and the abdominal muscles are affected. In clients with injury at higher levels, assisted ventilation and a tracheostomy are necessary; when the injury is at lower levels, the client's ability to take a deep breath and cough is diminished. The goal of nursing interventions is to maintain normal respiratory rate (12 to 20 breaths per minute) and to prevent pulmonary complications such as atelectasis and pneumonia.

- Assess respiratory rate, rhythm, and depth every 4 hours (or more frequently if needed). Auscultate breath sounds as a part of respiratory assessment. *Injury to the cord in the cervical or thoracic regions can decrease respiratory function and increase the risk for respiratory problems.*

**PRACTICE ALERT** *Auscultate the lungs for crackles and wheezes.* ■

- Monitor results of oxygen saturation and arterial blood gas studies. *ABG studies provide information about gas exchange; decreasing Ph, oxygen, and oxygen saturation levels, and increasing carbon dioxide levels signal respiratory acidosis.*
- Help the client turn, cough, and deep breathe at least every 2 hours. Use assisted coughing as necessary. *Paralysis of intercostal or abdominal muscles decreases the ability to expel secretions by coughing; retained secretions increase the risk for pneumonia. The inability to breathe deeply may result in atelectasis.*
- Increase fluids given by mouth to 3000 mL per day (if oral intake is approved), according to client preference for type of liquids and predicated on the client's ability to swallow. *Increased fluid intake thins secretions, which can more easily be expelled and expectorated.*

## Dysreflexia

Autonomic dysreflexia is an emergency that requires immediate assessment and intervention to prevent complications of extremely high blood pressure (loss of consciousness, convulsions, and even death).

- Elevate the head of the client's bed and remove TEDs. *These measures increase pooling of blood in the lower extremities and decrease venous return, thus decreasing blood pressure.*
- Assess blood pressure every 2 to 3 minutes while at the same time assessing for stimuli that initiated the response (such as a full bladder, impacted stool, or skin pressure). *The most serious danger in dysreflexia is elevated blood pressure, which could precipitate a CVA, myocardial in-*

*farction, dysrhythmias, or seizures. If the client has a Foley catheter, ensure that there are no kinks in the tubing. If the client does not have a Foley catheter, drain the bladder with a straight catheter. If symptoms persist, assess for a fecal impaction. If an impaction is present, insert Nupercaine cream into the anus, wait 10 minutes, and manually remove the impaction.*

**PRACTICE ALERT** *Blood pressure readings may be as high as 300/160.* ■

- If blood pressure remains dangerously elevated, the physician may prescribe intravenous administration of diazoxide (Hyperstat). Other medications that may be used include nifedipine (Procardia) and hydralazine (Apresoline). *Diazoxide is an antihypertensive drug used in emergency situations to lower blood pressure in adults with dangerously high readings. Nifedipine and hydralazine are peripheral vasodilators that are administered to decrease the elevated blood pressure.*

### Altered Urinary Elimination and Constipation

Depending on the level of the injury, the client with a SCI may have alterations in bowel and bladder function. Clients with injuries to the cord at or above the S2 to S4 levels will have a neurogenic bladder, with deficits in control of micturition. Voluntary and involuntary bowel control is affected in the

client with a lower motor neuron injury. Both bowel and bladder retraining are possible; if not, some form of assisted elimination is necessary. Although an indwelling catheter may be used in the acute phase of care, the goal is to reestablish a catheter-free state.

- Monitor for manifestations of a full bladder. *Overdistention stretches the bladder and can lead to backflow of urine into the ureters and kidney; stasis of urine in an incompletely emptied bladder increases the risk for infection.*

**PRACTICE ALERT** *A distended bladder can be palpated over the lower abdomen above the symphysis pubis.* ■

- Teach client to use trigger voiding techniques prior to straight catheterization. These techniques include stroking the inner thigh, pulling the pubic hair, tapping on the abdomen over the bladder, and (in females) pouring warm water over the vulva. *These trigger voiding techniques stimulate parasympathetic nerve fibers to cause reflex activity and may facilitate voiding.*
- Teach self-catheterization to clients who will be able to carry out the procedure alone or with minimal assistance (Procedure 41–1). *Straight catheterization at regular intervals is part of bladder training because periodic distention and relaxation of the muscles of the bladder promote reflex bladder activity. In addition, self-care fosters independence.*

---

**Procedure 41–1** | **Client Self-Catheterization**

Self-catheterization on an intermittent basis (usually a part of self-care at home) is a clean rather than a sterile procedure. The hands should be washed before and after the procedure, and the urinary meatus should be cleaned by washing with soap and water.

### FEMALE SELF-CATHETERIZATION

- Attempt to void. If urine is not of sufficient quantity (at least 100 mL) or if you cannot void at all, do self-catheterization. *A large amount of residual urine means that more frequent catheterizations (every 4 to 6 hours) are necessary.*
- While sitting on the wheelchair or the commode, locate the urethra. Visualize the urethra by looking in a mirror, or palpate the urethra with a fingertip. *Visualization or palpation of the meatus is necessary for proper catheter insertion.*
- Lubricate the meatus with a water-soluble lubricant. *Lubrication facilitates the insertion of the catheter and reduces trauma to tissues.*

- Take a deep breath and insert the catheter tip 2 to 3 inches or until urine flows. *The catheter enters the bladder more easily when the sphincter is relaxed. The deep breath relaxes the sphincter. The female urethra is 1½ to 2½ inches long.*
- Hold the catheter securely and allow urine to drain until the flow stops. *Withdrawing and reinserting the catheter increase the risk of infection.*
- Withdraw the catheter and wash it with soap and water. Store the catheter in a clean container. *The catheter can be reused until it is too soft or too hard to be directed into and through the urinary meatus. Clean rather than sterile technique is usually used for self-catheterization at home.*

### MALE SELF-CATHETERIZATION

- Attempt to void. If urine is not of sufficient quantity (e.g., less than 100 mL) or if you cannot void at all, do self-catheterization. *A large amount of residual urine means that more frequent catheterizations (every 4 to 6 hours) are necessary.*

- Sit either on the commode or in the wheelchair. Hold the penis with slight upward tension and extend it to its full length. *Extending the penis straightens the urethra.*
- Lubricate the catheter from the tip to about 6 inches downward. *Lubrication is especially important for male catheterization because of the length of the urethra.*
- Take a deep breath and insert the catheter 6 to 7 inches or until urine flows. *The catheter enters the bladder more easily when the sphincter is relaxed. The deep breath relaxes the sphincter. The male urethra is about 6 inches long.*
- Hold the catheter securely and allow urine to drain until flow has stopped. *Withdrawing and reinserting the catheter increase the risk of infection.*
- Withdraw the catheter and wash it with soap and water. Store the catheter in a clean container. *The catheter can be reused until it is too soft or too hard to be directed into and through the urethra. Clean rather than sterile technique is usually used for self-catheterization at home.*

- Monitor residual urine throughout the bladder retraining program. *A residual urine amount of less than 80 mL after a triggered voiding is considered satisfactory.*
- Institute a bowel retraining program as follows:
  - Assess usual patterns of bowel elimination to establish best times for individualized program.
  - Maintain a high-fluid, high-fiber diet.
  - Use stool softeners as prescribed; rectal suppositories and enemas may be used 30 minutes after meals to stimulate stronger peristalsis and facilitate evacuation.
  - Maintain upright position if at all possible and ensure privacy.
  - If client is unable to evacuate, digital stimulation or manual removal on a regular basis may be the most effective long-term management.

  *A bowel retraining program to regulate the bowel through reflex activity may be instituted in clients with upper motor neuron injuries. The client with a lower motor neuron injury loses the defecation reflex, and bowel retraining is more difficult (if not impossible).*

## Sexual Dysfunction

Sexual intercourse is often still possible for the client with an SCI. In men, the general rule is that the higher the level of injury the greater the potential to have reflexogenic erections, although ejaculation or orgasm may not occur, and fertility is usually lower. However, ejaculation may be stimulated and the sperm used to inseminate the client's partner, so that fatherhood is a possibility. Men who have sacral-level injuries do not have reflexogenic erections but may have psychogenic erections. They are also more likely to remain fertile.

Women with SCI generally do not have sensation during sexual intercourse, but pregnancy is possible. However, pregnant women with an SCI are at increased risk for autonomic dysreflexia during labor and delivery. Birth control options should be discussed prior to discharge from the acute care setting.

A client with an SCI may be deeply concerned about alterations in sexual function. These concerns may lead to lowered self-esteem, altered self-image, or changes in feelings about being an attractive and desirable person. Assess concerns and provide a climate that is receptive to discussion about sexuality. Examples of objectives for sexual counseling for the client with an SCI are that the client will understand how the injury has altered sexual functioning, be aware of alternative ways of achieving sexual pleasure, and have a positive self-concept and body image.

- Include data about sexuality when obtaining the nursing history and database. *Sexuality is a private matter for most people, and the client may not discuss it unless the nurse introduces the topic.*
- Provide accurate information about the effect of the SCI on sexual function. *Accurate information gives the client a realistic picture of how the injury will affect sexuality.*
- Initiate a discussion with the client and partner of alternative means of gaining sexual satisfaction; these include the use of vibrators, and oral-genital and manual stimulation. *Alternatives to intercourse can meet sexual needs and help maintain the relationship with a significant other.*
- Refer for sexual counseling, if appropriate, or to local support groups where questions can be answered by others with similar concerns. *Knowing that others have had similar experiences can decrease social isolation and provide a means of learning alternative methods of sexual functioning.*

## Low Self-Esteem

An SCI is often the result of sudden trauma. Within moments, a formerly independent, fully functioning individual is suddenly unable to move and faces enormous adjustments in social, economic, and personal roles and relationships. Body image, self-esteem, and role performance are all affected by the damage. As a result, the client often demonstrates behaviors that may be difficult for the nurse to handle: depression, denial, and anger are often seen in the period immediately after the injury. In addition to these responses, the young adult client may act out by making sexually overt statements.

- Encourage talking about all aspects of physical function and care. *Talking provides a safe outlet for fears and frustrations and also increases self-awareness. Acceptance of self facilitates rehabilitation.*
- Encourage self-care and independent decision making. *Participating in self-care can promote positive coping; making decisions decreases feelings of powerlessness.*
- Help identify strategies to increase independence in desired roles; include both short- and long-term goals. Discuss assistive devices (such as hand-operated automobiles). *Identifying strategies to increase independence in the future fosters a positive self-concept and motivates the client to achieve rehabilitation goals.*
- Include family members and important others in discussions. *The realization that others do care and will continue to provide support is important in fostering positive self-regard.*
- Refer the client and family to support groups or for psychologic counseling. *Adjustment to change is more likely when the client and family seek peer and professional assistance.*

## Using NANDA, NIC, and NOC

Chart 41–2 shows links between NANDA nursing diagnoses, NIC, and NOC when caring for the client with an SCI.

## Home Care

Rehabilitation of the client with an SCI is an ongoing process that moves from intensive care through intermediate care to rehabilitation and then home care. Nursing interventions are necessary at all points in the process to prevent the complications of altered physical mobility and body functions, and to teach the client and family measures that promote independence in self-care.

Discharge planning should be addressed even in the initial plan of care while the client is in the critical care setting. Advance planning ensures continuity of care when the client leaves the hospital setting.

## CHART 41–2  NANDA, NIC, AND NOC LINKAGES

### The Client with a SCI

| NURSING DIAGNOSES | NURSING INTERVENTIONS | NURSING OUTCOMES |
|---|---|---|
| • Risk for Impaired Skin Integrity | • Pressure Management<br>• Pressure Ulcer Prevention | • Risk Control<br>• Tissue Perfusion: Peripheral<br>• Immobility Consequences: Physiological |
| • Risk for Injury | • Malignant Hyperthermia<br>• Surveillance: Safety<br>• Neurologic Monitoring | • Symptom Control Behavior |
| • Self-Care Deficit | • Bathing<br>• Dressing<br>• Feeding<br>• Bowel Management | • Self-Care: Bathing<br>• Self-Care: Dressing<br>• Self-Care: Eating<br>• Self-Care: Toileting |
| • Self-Esteem Disturbance<br>• Impaired Home Maintenance | • Self-Esteem Enhancement<br>• Home Maintenance Assistance<br>• Environmental Management | • Self-Esteem<br>• Mobility Level<br>• Self-Care: Instrumental Activities<br>of Daily Living |

*Note. Data from* Nursing Outcomes Classification (NOC) *by M. Johnson & M. Maas (Eds.), 1997, St. Louis: Mosby;* Nursing Diagnoses: Definitions & Classification 2001–2002 *by North American Nursing Diagnosis Association, 2001, Philadelphia: NANDA;* Nursing Interventions Classification (NIC) *by J.C. McCloskey & G. M. Bulechek (Eds.), 2000, St. Louis: Mosby. Reprinted by permission.*

The following should be included in teaching the client and family about care at home.

- Self-care activities (ADLs, exercises, bowel and bladder programs, skin care)
- Mobility (use of assistive devices: wheelchair, crutches, special automobiles)
- Preparation of the home environment
  - If the client is in a wheelchair, will steps, stairs, doors, or carpeted floors present physical barriers?
  - If a special bed is necessary, have arrangements been made, and is it in the home?
- Psychologic support
- Independent activities

- Community resources, such as Life-line (emergency alerting systems through a local hospital or agency), support groups, career centers for job retraining, counseling
- Coping skills for client and caregiver
- Referral to a home health agency and physical therapist for the client who is returning home
- Helpful resources:
  - The National Spinal Cord Injury Association
  - American Paralysis Association
  - Christopher Reeve Paralysis Foundation
  - Paralyzed Veterans of America
  - Canadian Paraplegic Association
  - Australian Quadriplegic Association

## THE CLIENT WITH A HERNIATED INTERVERTEBRAL DISK

A **herniated intervertebral disk,** also called a **ruptured disk,** herniated nucleus pulposus, or a slipped disk, is a rupture of the cartilage surrounding the intervertebral disk with protrusion of the nucleus pulposus (Figure 41–8 ■). Perhaps few neuro-orthopedic disorders are as challenging as those involving the intervertebral disks. Clients with herniation (rupture) of a disk have not only excruciating pain but also limited mobility. These problems may in turn cause alterations in role function, coping, and the ability to perform activities of daily living.

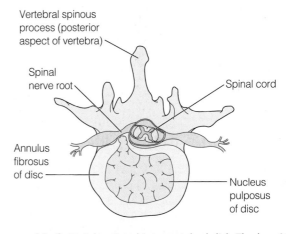

**Figure 41–8 ■** A herniated intervertebral disk. The herniated nucleus pulposus is applying pressure against the nerve root.

## Nursing Care Plan
## A Client with a SCI

Jim Valdez, a 19-year-old college sophomore, is admitted to the hospital by ambulance following an automobile accident. His family (father, mother, and sister) live 100 miles away and cannot visit often, although they are very concerned. On admission to the hospital, a CT scan of the spine shows a fracture and partial laceration of the cord at the C7 level. Mr. Valdez is in halo traction. One night, he tells the nurse, "I wish I had just died when I got hurt. I don't think I can stand to live like this."

### ASSESSMENT

When Mr. Valdez is admitted to the intensive care unit, he has flaccid paralysis involving all extremities. He has no sensation below the clavicle or in portions of his arms and legs. His bladder is distended and bowel sounds are absent. Other assessment findings include BP 90/56, P 50, T 97°F (36.1°C), arterial blood gases Ph 7.4, Pao$_2$ 96, Paco$_2$ 37, Sao$_2$ 96%. Oxygen per nasal cannula is given at 2 L/min, and halo traction is applied. A Foley catheter is inserted into his bladder, and a nasogastric tube is inserted into his stomach and attached to low-pressure continuous suction.

After 7 days, Mr. Valdez is moved from the intensive care unit to the neurosurgical unit for continuing care and planning for transfer to a rehabilitation hospital in his home town. His vital signs have stabilized and are normal for his age; respirations and oxygenation are normal. Other neurologic assessments remain the same.

### DIAGNOSES

- *Impaired physical mobility* related to paralysis of lower and upper extremities secondary to C7 injury
- *Bowel incontinence* related to lack of voluntary sphincter control secondary to C7 injury
- *Grieving* related to loss of the use of his arms and legs and the effect of that loss on finishing school and getting a job

### EXPECTED OUTCOMES

- Be actively involved in exercise programs.
- Have a soft, formed stool every second or third day.
- Verbally express his grief to parents and staff.

### PLANNING AND IMPLEMENTATION

- Conduct passive exercises on all extremities four times a day.
- Provide progressive mobilization by initially raising the head of the bed 90 degrees (repeat two to three times during the first

day of movement); if blood pressure remains normal, dangle for 5 minutes before transferring him to a chair.
- His usual time for a bowel movement is after breakfast; schedule retraining program for that time.
- Encourage a diet high in fiber and fluids. Likes whole-wheat bread, orange juice, and cola; does not like water.
- Promote grief work by providing time to express feelings. Explain to the family that his denial and anger are part of the grieving process.
- Determine food likes and dislikes and order preferred foods from the menu. Encourage his friends to bring in his favorite foods periodically.
- Take and record weight every third day, using the bed scales.

### EVALUATION

By the time Mr. Valdez is transferred to the rehabilitation hospital he is looking forward to learning how to use special equipment and getting his own motorized wheelchair. He is able to sit up in a chair without dizziness or hypotension. The use of ordered stool softeners combined with a high-fiber diet and fluid intake of 2000 to 3000 mL per day has maintained bowel elimination. Mr. Valdez and his parents have spent 3 hours talking about their feelings related to the accident and the future. Although the discussion is emotionally difficult, all three say they now feel much better. Mr. Valdez still has episodes of angry outbursts and tears, but he is more optimistic about what can be done and believes he can finish college. He selects foods from the menu each day and eats most of his meals, but he especially enjoys the times his friends bring in pizza or hamburgers.

### Critical Thinking in the Nursing Process

1. Considering Mr. Valdez's age and developmental level, do you think his emotional responses to his injury were appropriate?
2. Issues of sexuality are obviously important for the client with a spinal cord injury. How would you approach Mr. Valdez about this topic?
3. What would be your response as a male or female nurse if Mr. Valdez would allow only male nurses to provide care?
4. Outline a teaching program to help Mr. Valdez meet long-term urinary elimination needs.

See Evaluating your Response in Appendix C.

## INCIDENCE AND PREVALENCE

A herniated intervertebral disk may occur at any adult age. However, it is more common as people enter middle age and age-related changes occur. The nucleus pulposus loses fluid content, and the disks are less able to absorb shocks. The disks become smaller and slip out of place more easily. Aging causes degeneration in the annulus fibrosus and the posterior longitu-

dinal ligaments, and the vertebrae and disks are less able to respond to movement and are more easily injured.

Herniated intervertebral disks are more common in men than women. Most clients are between the ages of 30 and 50. The majority of herniated disks occur in the lumbar region (L4 or L5 to S1); when disks herniate in the cervical region, they most commonly do so at C6 to C7. Multiple herniations are not common, occurring in only about 10% of all clients (Hickey, 2003).

## PATHOPHYSIOLOGY

The intervertebral disks, located between the vertebral bodies, are made of an inner nucleus pulposus and an outer collar (the annulus fibrosus). The disks allow the spine to absorb compression by acting as shock absorbers. A herniated intervertebral disk occurs when the nucleus pulposus protrudes through a weakened or torn annulus fibrosus of an intervertebral disk. This protrusion may occur anywhere along the vertebral column, but herniation of thoracic disks is uncommon. The protrusion may occur spontaneously or as a result of trauma, with trauma (such as lifting heavy objects or falling) causing about half of all cases. Rupture of the disk allows herniation of the nucleus pulposus in a posterolateral direction, with compression of the associated nerve root. The resulting pressure on adjacent spinal nerves causes characteristic manifestations, which vary with the location and the amount of protruding disk material (see the box on this page). Occasionally the herniation is central rather than posterolateral, with pressure on the spinal cord.

The herniation may be abrupt or gradual. Lifting incorrectly or suddenly twisting the spine can cause rupture with immediate intense pain and muscle spasms. Gradual herniation is the result of degenerative changes, osteoarthritis, or ankylosis spondylitis. Clients with a gradual herniation have a slow onset of pain and neurologic deficits.

## Lumbar Disk Manifestations

The classic manifestation of a ruptured lumbar disk is recurrent episodes of pain in the lower back. The pain typically radiates across the buttock and down the posterior leg, although it may be experienced only in the leg. **Sciatica** is a term used to describe lumbar back pain that radiates down the posterior leg to the ankle and is increased by sneezing or coughing (the result of pressure on nerve roots L4, L5, S1, S2, or S3, which give rise to the sciatic nerve). Sciatica may be elicited by straight-leg raising: The client feels pain when lifting one leg while dorsiflexing the foot of that leg. Sciatica pain varies in intensity, ranging from mildly uncomfortable to excruciating. It is aggravated by a variety of positions and activities, including sitting, straining, coughing, sneezing, climbing stairs, walking, and riding in a car.

Other manifestations include postural deformity, motor deficits, sensory deficits, and changes in reflexes. In about 60% of clients with ruptured lumbar disks, the normal lumbar lordosis is absent. When standing, the client typically has a slight forward tilt to the trunk, scoliosis of the lumbar spine, slight flexion of the hip and knee on the affected side, and paravertebral muscle spasms (Hickey, 2003). Motor deficits include weakness and in some clients problems with sexual function and urinary elimination. Sensory deficits include paresthesias and numbness. Knee and ankle reflexes are decreased or absent.

## Cervical Disk Manifestations

Cervical disks that herniate laterally cause pain in the shoulder, neck, and arm. Other manifestations of lateral cervical hernia-

---

### Manifestations of a Ruptured Intervertebral Disk

#### L4 TO L5 LEVEL (AFFECTS FIFTH LUMBAR NERVE ROOT)

- Pain in hip, lower back, posterolateral thigh, anterior leg, dorsal surface of foot, great toe
- Muscle spasms
- Paresthesia over lateral leg and web of great toe
- Footdrop (rare)
- Decreased or absent ankle reflex
- Cauda equina syndrome (with complete nerve root compression): bowel and bladder incontinence, paralysis of lower extremities

#### L5 TO S1 LEVEL (AFFECTS FIRST SACRAL NERVE ROOT)

- Pain in midgluteal region, posterior thigh, calf to heel, plantar surface of the foot to the fourth and fifth toes
- Paresthesias in posterior calf and lateral heel, foot, and toes
- Difficulty walking on toes

#### C5 TO C6 LEVEL (AFFECTS SIXTH CERVICAL NERVE ROOT)

- Pain in neck, shoulder, anterior upper arm, radial area of forearm, thumb
- Paresthesia of forearm, thumb, forefinger and lateral arm
- Decreased biceps and supinator reflex
- Triceps reflex normal to hyperactive

---

tion include paresthesias, muscle spasms and stiff neck, and decreased or absent arm reflexes. Central cervical herniations result in mild, intermittent pain; however, the client may also experience lower extremity weakness, unsteady gait, muscle spasms, urinary elimination problems, altered sexual function, and hyperactive lower extremity reflexes.

## COLLABORATIVE CARE

Considerations for the client with a ruptured intervertebral disk include identifying the location of herniation and determining whether conservative treatment or surgery is indicated. Nursing care is directed toward preparing clients for diagnostic tests and providing teaching and care for the client who has either medical or surgical interventions.

### Diagnostic Tests

Diagnostic tests are ordered to differentiate the cause of back pain; for example, back and leg pain is also caused by spinal tumors, degenerative processes, or abdominal disease. Assessing pain is an important part of diagnosis.

- *Flat-plate X-ray films* may be taken of the lumbosacral or cervical area to identify skeletal deformities and narrowing of the disk spaces.
- *CT scans* are used to identify disk rupture or protrusion and may provide definitive diagnosis. However, if the client has

had previous back surgery or if more than one disk is involved, a CT scan may not clearly identify the ruptured disk.

- *MRI* is used to image the vertebral elements, thecal sac, disks, cerebrospinal fluid, nerve roots, and spinal cord. This noninvasive examination is increasingly being used to provide initial diagnosis.
- *Myelography* with contrast medium illustrates areas of herniation but does not provide the detail found with CT or MRI. However, myelography is diagnostic in 80% to 90% of all cases and is used both to rule out tumors and locate the herniation.

A myelogram is a radiologic examination of the subarachnoid space of the spinal canal, using a contrast agent. A myelogram is performed to visualize the lumbar, thoracic, or cervical area, or the whole spinal axis. It is used in the diagnosis of a spinal cord tumor, a herniated intervertebral disk, or a ruptured disk. Any obstruction of the flow of the contrast medium can be seen on X-ray film.

To perform a myelogram, a lumbar puncture is performed and about 10 mL of cerebrospinal fluid (CSF) is removed. A water-based contrast medium such as iopamidol (Isovue) is injected into the subarachnoid space. When the medium is injected, it diffuses up through the CSF and penetrates the nerve root sleeves, nerve rootlets, and narrow areas of the subarachnoid space. The head of the X-ray table is kept elevated at 30 degrees and the client is kept quiet to prevent rapid upward dispersion. If the contrast medium entered the cranial vault, it could cause seizures. The contrast medium is absorbed through the bloodstream and eliminated by the kidneys. Nursing implications for the care of a client having a myelogram are outlined in the box below.

- *Electromyography (EMG),* which measures electrical activity of skeletal muscles at rest and during voluntary contraction, may be conducted to identify specific muscles affected by the pressure of the herniation on the nerve roots.

## Medications

The client with a ruptured intervertebral disk is treated with medications to relieve pain and reduce swelling and muscle spasms. Pain is usually managed with nonsteroidal anti-inflammatory drugs (see Chapter 4). ⊂⊃ Muscle spasms are treated with muscle relaxants.

## Treatment

A ruptured intervertebral disk may be treated conservatively or with surgery.

### Conservative Treatment

A ruptured intervertebral disk is usually managed conservatively with bed rest and medication unless the client is experiencing severe neurologic deficits. The goals of treatment are

## Nursing Implications for Diagnostic Tests

### Myelography

#### Preparation of the Client

Ensure a signed informed consent.

- The meal prior to the procedure is usually omitted.
- The client should be well hydrated.
- Administer enemas or laxatives as ordered to ensure visualization of lumbar spine.
- Administer prescribed pretest medications, such as a sedative or diazepam (Valium).

#### Client and Family Teaching

- Remain NPO several hours before the test.
- The examination lasts about 1 hour.
- The position used to perform the examination will depend on the physician. You may have to lie on your stomach, sit and lean forward, or sit with the knees to the chest.
- A strap may be used to prevent falls, and the table will be tilted during the examination.
- A lumbar puncture ("spinal tap") is performed to inject the dye. A local anesthetic is used where the needle will be inserted. There may be a feeling of pressure during needle insertion. The needle is inserted below the level of the spinal cord.
- Tell the physician if you experience pain.
- It is important to stay in bed with the head of the bed elevated for at least 6 to 12 hours (the length of time will depend on physician preference and hospital policy).
- The nurse will check your blood pressure, pulse, and respirations. The nurse will also check your ability to feel and move at least every 4 hours (or more often) after the examination.

#### Postexamination Nursing Care

- Take and record vital signs and assess neurologic status as prescribed (and at least every 4 hours) for 24 hours postexamination. Record and report any changes.
- Assess the site of the lumbar puncture for leakage of cerebrospinal fluid or bleeding every 4 hours. Notify the physician of leakage or bleeding.
- Encourage increased intake of oral fluids to replace that withdrawn during the examination. (This may also help decrease a postmyelogram headache).
- Make sure that the client voids within 8 hours after the examination. If policy permits, allow male clients to stand at the bedside, or clients of either gender to use the bathroom. Notify the physician if the client has not voided within 8 hours.
- Administer analgesics as prescribed for postexamination pain, headache, or muscle spasms.
- Keep the client's head elevated at least 30 degrees (in bed or in a chair) for 12 hours, or as ordered.
- Resume diet if there is no nausea or vomiting.
- Force oral fluids to 2400 to 3000 mL in 24 hours, beginning immediately after the procedure.
- Administer prescribed medications for nausea.
- Do not give any phenothiazine derivatives for 48 hours (to reduce the possibility of seizures).

pain relief and healing of the involved disk by fibrosis. Conservative treatment is usually prescribed for 2 to 6 weeks. After that time, surgery may be considered. The treatment regimen depends on the severity of the manifestations but usually includes one or more of the following (Hickey, 2003):

- Decreasing activity level
- Avoiding flexion of the spine (e.g., do not lift, bend, or twist)
- Wearing a support garment, such as a corset or cervical collar
- Following a prescribed exercise program
- Using a firm mattress
- Taking prescribed medications for pain, inflammation, and muscle spasms

Some clients achieve pain relief with transcutaneous electrical stimulation (TENS) or transcutaneous neural stimulation (TNS). Another pain relief intervention is bed rest. It is important that the client use a firm mattress. The client should lie so that the pull on the affected nerve is reduced. Clients with lumbar involvement should usually flex the knees and elevate the head of the bed to about 30 degrees. After 4 days or less of bed rest, the client may begin walking and an exercise program designed by the physical therapist. This program includes teaching proper body mechanics and positioning, exercises to strengthen the back and decrease muscle spasms, massage, and the application of heat. Most clients report a good recovery after conservative management.

Medications used to treat back pain include nonnarcotic analgesics, anti-inflammatory drugs such as the nonsteroidal agents (NSAIDs), muscle relaxants, and sedative-tranquilizers.

## Surgery

Surgery is indicated for clients who do not respond to conservative management or have serious neurologic deficits. Several surgical interventions are used to treat a ruptured intervertebral disk. The type of surgery chosen depends on the location of the disk and the stability of the spinal column.

- A **laminectomy,** the type of surgery most often performed, is the removal of a part of the vertebral lamina. The surgery is done to relieve pressure on the nerves. It is often combined with removal of the protruding nucleus pulposus (*nuclectomy*). Nursing care for the client having a laminectomy is discussed in the box below. A *diskectomy* is the removal of the nucleus pulposus of an intervertebral disk. Diskectomy may be performed alone or along with a laminectomy.
- **Spinal fusion** is the insertion of a wedge-shaped piece of bone or bone chips between the vertebrae to stabilize them. The bone is usually taken from a client donor site, such as the iliac crest. A spinal fusion may also be performed through a spinal implant with a device called a BAK (a hollow titanium cylinder with holes) which is packed with grafted bone from a donor site and placed in the space where a disk is removed. Although not appropriate for all clients requiring a spinal fusion, this does require a short hospital stay and convalescence.
- *Foraminotomy* is an enlargement of the opening between the disk and the facet joint to remove bony overgrowth compressing the nerve. The location and size of the incision vary according to the surgeon's preference and the location and

## NURSING CARE OF THE CLIENT HAVING A POSTERIOR LAMINECTOMY

### PREOPERATIVE TEACHING

- Demonstrate and ask the client to practice logrolling; explain that it will be done by the nurses for the first day or two, and then the client can do it alone. *To ensure healing, the spinal column must remain in alignment when turning and moving.*
- Explain the importance of taking pain medications regularly and of asking for them before the pain is severe. Include information about the possibility of the pain being much the same after surgery. *Pain is easier to control if medications are taken before the pain is severe. Pain may be the same following surgery for a herniated intervertebral disk because edema due to surgery irritates and compresses the nerve roots.*
- Demonstrate the use of a fracture bedpan and ask the client to practice its use. *The client usually must remain flat in bed for a period of time following surgery. A fracture bedpan is more comfortable for clients who must lie flat.*
- Explain that the client may need to eat while lying flat. *This position prevents flexion of the spine.*
- Demonstrate and ask the client to practice deep breathing, the use of the incentive spirometer, and leg exercises. Ask the client to demonstrate these skills. *These measures prevent respiratory and circulatory complications.*

### POSTOPERATIVE CARE

- Maintain the client in a position that minimizes stress on the surgical wound. For clients with cervical laminectomy:
  a. Elevate the head of the bed slightly.
  b. Position a small pillow under the neck.
  c. Maintain the position of the cervical collar.

  For clients with lumbar laminectomy:
  a. Keep the bed flat or elevate the head of the bed slightly.
  b. Place a small pillow under the head.
  c. Place a small pillow under the knees, or use a pillow to support the upper leg when the client lies on one side.

  *These positions minimize stress on the surgical wound and suture line. A cervical collar provides stability and prevents flexing or twisting the neck.*
- Turn the client every 2 hours, using the logrolling technique. Teach the client not to use the side rails to change position. Maintain proper body alignment in all positions. *The client's body is turned as a single unit (usually with a turning sheet) to avoid movement of the operative area. Pulling on the side rails puts stress on the operative area and may also cause misalignment of the vertebral column.*

(continued on page 1338)

## NURSING CARE OF THE CLIENT HAVING A POSTERIOR LAMINECTOMY *(continued)*

### POSTOPERATIVE CARE *(continued)*

- Monitor the client for signs of nerve root compression.
  a. Cervical laminectomy: Assess hand grips and arm strength, ability to move the fingers, and ability to detect touch.
  b. Lumbar laminectomy: Assess leg strength, ability to wiggle the toes, and ability to detect touch.
  Compare bilateral findings. Report muscle weakness or sensory impairment to the physician immediately. *Loss of motor and sensory function may indicate nerve root compression.*
- Assess for hematoma formation as manifested by severe incisional pain that is not relieved by analgesics and decreased motor function. Report these findings to the surgeon immediately. *A hematoma may form at the surgical site. If untreated, it may cause irreversible neurologic deficits, including paraplegia and bowel/bladder dysfunctions (Hickey, 2003).*
- Assess for leakage of cerebrospinal fluid. Assess the dressing for increased moisture. Check the sheets for wetness when the client is lying supine; check for clear liquid running down the back when the client is sitting or standing. Gently palpate the sides of the wound to detect a bulge. Use a Dextrostrix strip to assess any leakage for the presence of glucose, a positive indicator of cerebrospinal fluid. *Although uncommon, leakage of cerebrospinal fluid greatly increases the risk for infection of the wound and of the meninges.*
- Assess for nerve root injury. Assess the client's ability to dorsiflex the foot (lumbar laminectomy) and the client's grip strength (cervical laminectomy). Assess the client who has had a cervical laminectomy for hoarseness. Report hoarseness to the physician and further assess the client's ability to swallow. *Nerve root compression may cause permanent damage, resulting in footdrop (in lumbar laminectomy clients) and hand weakness (in cervical laminectomy clients). Damage to the laryngeal nerve may cause permanent hoarseness. Impaired ability to swallow puts the client at risk for aspiration.*
- Assess for urinary retention. The client should void within 8 hours after surgery. If the physician allows, let males stand to void. Compare intake and output for each 8-hour period. *All clients who have received a general anesthetic are at risk for urinary retention. The client who has had a lumbar laminectomy*

may have even more difficulty voiding as a result of stimulation of sympathetic nerves during surgery.
- Assess for pain using a scale from 0 (no pain) to 10 (severe pain). Administer prescribed analgesics on a regular basis, or teach client to use PCA analgesia, if prescribed. Discuss client concerns about pain that is unrelieved by surgery. *Compression of the nerve root over time results in edema and inflammation. Because of surgery-induced edema, the client is likely to experience either the same pain or perhaps more severe pain in the period immediately after surgery. This pain usually persists for several weeks after surgery. In addition, many clients who have had a lumbar laminectomy have muscle spasms in the lower back, abdomen, and thighs for the first few days after surgery.*
- Assess for infection by taking and recording vital signs at least every 4 hours; report increased body temperature. Assess the wound and dressing for signs of infection: increased redness, drainage, pain, and pus. Use sterile technique to change dressings. *The surgical client is always at risk for infection; the client with a laminectomy is also at risk for arachnoiditis. This inflammation of the arachnoid layer of the spinal meninges results from wound infection or contamination during surgery and may cause the formation of painful adhesions.*
- Encourage deep breathing and the use of the incentive spirometer every 2 hours; coughing may be discouraged. *Anesthesia and immobility depress respiratory function. Coughing may be discouraged because it can disrupt healing tissues, especially in clients having a cervical laminectomy.*
- Increase mobility as prescribed. (The time frame for ambulation is prescribed by the physician; the routine here is representative.) Clients often sit on the side of the bed and dangle their legs the evening after surgery or the first day thereafter. Many clients ambulate the first or second postoperative day. To help the client out of bed, first elevate the head of the bed. Then bring the client's legs over the side of the bed at the same time that the upper body moves into the upright position. Clients should not ambulate without assistance until they are no longer dizzy or weak. *Early ambulation increases respiratory and circulatory function and decreases the risk of thrombophlebitis of the lower extremities. The vertebral column should remain in alignment while the client sits and stands. Safety must be considered throughout care.*

---

size of the ruptured disk. The posterior approach is taken for lumbar surgery. Either the posterior or the anterior approach may be taken for cervical disks.
- A *microdiskectomy,* in which microsurgical techniques are used, is performed through a very small incision. This type of surgery decreases the possibility of trauma to surrounding structures during surgery and allows early postoperative mobility and a short hospital stay.

## NURSING CARE

Nursing care for the client with a ruptured intervertebral disk may be provided through information in community and work settings, during conservative treatment, and during pre- and

postoperative treatment. The pain of the ruptured disk is often discouraging and debilitating, and may well affect the client's ability to work.

### Prevention

Proper body mechanics may help prevent the occurrence of a ruptured intervertebral disk. Teaching the proper method of lifting and moving heavy objects should begin when children enter school. This information should also be given to all workers who have lifting as part of their responsibilities; including nurses. The guidelines for proper body mechanics are as follows:

- Begin activities by spreading the feet apart to broaden the base of support.

- Use large muscles of the arms to lift and the legs to push when lifting.
- Work as closely as possible to the object that is to be lifted or moved.
- Slide, roll, push, or pull an object rather than lift it.
- When lifting, bend the knees and lift up over your center of gravity.

## Assessment

The following data are collected through the heath history and physical examination (see Chapter 40).

- Health history: type of employment, risk factors, pain (location, duration, intensity)
- Physical examination: muscle strength and coordination, sensation, reflexes

## Nursing Diagnosis and Interventions

Nursing care for clients with a herniated intervertebral disk focuses largely on pain management, both during conservative management and after surgery.

### Acute Pain

Clients with a ruptured intervertebral disk experience acute back and leg pain. Acute pain may be related to preoperative muscle spasms or nerve root compression. After surgery, the client may have pain at the site of the incision and in the surgical area.

- Encourage discussion of pain. Assess the degree of pain and identify contributing and relieving factors. *Pain is a subjective experience. The nurse needs to assess it thoroughly before initiating interventions.*
- Maintain bed rest as prescribed. Teach the client how to logroll (to turn the body without bending the spine) when changing positions. *Restricting activity and proper positioning may prevent muscle spasms.*
- Use a firm mattress or place a board under the mattress. *A firm bed supports the spinal column and muscles.*
- Teach the client to avoid turning or twisting the spinal column and to assume positions that decrease stress on the vertebral column (e.g., when in the supine position, flex the hips slightly). A small pillow may be placed under the knees (for clients with a herniated lumbar disk) or under the neck (for clients with a herniated cervical disk). *Correct body positions can decrease intradisk pressure.*
- Provide analgesic medications around the clock. *Intense pain can increase muscle spasms; maintaining serum levels of analgesics often prevents severe pain.*

**PRACTICE ALERT** *It is important to maintain a constant level of pain relief. Health care providers have the responsibility of relieving pain with adequate medications.* ■

### Chronic Pain

The client with a ruptured intervertebral disk often has pain for an extended period of time. Despite conservative treatment or previous surgery, pain may be ongoing or intermittent. If previous surgery has not relieved the pain, the client may be depressed or angry. Caring for a client with chronic pain is frustrating, and the client is often regarded as difficult.

- Treat the client's reports of pain with respect. *The client is the person experiencing the pain and is thus the expert about it.*
- Do not refer to the client as being addicted to pain medication. *All types of pain medications may be used legitimately to manage pain.*

**PRACTICE ALERT** *Although the client may develop tolerance to a narcotic analgesic, tolerance does not imply addiction.* ■

- Monitor the client carefully for any changes in condition. *Significant changes in the client's condition may go unrecognized when pain is present for a prolonged period of time.*
- Maintain written plans of care for pain management that are individualized and ensure continuity of care. *When the client makes several visits (for instance, to an emergency department or a pain clinic), written records help caregivers determine what is effective in managing pain and what is not.*
- Teach the client alternative methods of pain management. *Consider the client's coping style when recommending methods. Clients who have a passive coping style are often better able to manage pain by depending on others, taking medications, and resting. Clients with an active coping style are probably better able to manage pain by learning self-management methods, taking part in activities, and staying busy.*
- Develop effective methods of improving rest and sleep. Problems with rest and sleep make pain management more difficult. *Sleeping poorly at night contributes to decreased motivation, confused thinking, depression, and muscle aches.*
- Refer the client to a physical therapist for an exercise program, if appropriate. *The client needs to know exactly what exercises to do, how many repetitions are recommended, for how long, and how often. The client should not exercise to the point of causing increased pain.*
- Assess the need for referrals (and make them if necessary) for the client who is depressed or anxious. *Anxiety and depression often are a part of long-term chronic pain, making pain management more difficult. Suggest that referrals for help with the frustration (rather than "depression") may make a significant difference in the client's ability to manage pain.*

### Constipation

The client with a ruptured intervertebral disk often has problems with constipation because of reduced mobility and bed rest. Nursing interventions to alleviate and prevent constipation are important because straining to have a bowel movement can increase intradisk pressure, thus increasing pain.

- Assess the client's usual bowel routine, including diet, fluid intake, and the use of laxatives or enemas. *Effective interventions are based on individualized needs.*

---

**PRACTICE ALERT** *People who have used laxatives or enemas for long periods of time may be dependent on those methods of having a bowel movement.* ■

---

- Encourage a fluid intake of 2500 to 3000 mL per day unless contraindicated by the presence of renal or cardiac disease. *Adequate fluid intake facilitates the passage of feces.*
- Increase fiber and bulk in the diet. If the client is unable to tolerate increased fiber, consult with the physician about the use of stool softeners or bulk-forming agents. *Bulk and fiber promote regularity by retaining water in the large intestine.*

## Home Care

It is the nurse's responsibility to teach the client and family about chronic pain control, including specific interventions to alleviate pain. The nurse's role may be that of advocate and creative problem solver (see the Meeting Individualized Needs box on page 1341 for specific teaching topics). The following topics should be addressed:

- Often the goal is to control pain so that the client can perform normal activities of daily living, rather than to reach a pain-free state.
- Nonpharmacologic methods of pain management include relaxation techniques, guided imagery, distraction, hypnosis, and music. Joining a support group may be an effective intervention in coping with and managing pain.
- Clients may be referred to a physical therapist for education about body mechanics and back-strengthening exercises. Nurses should have the client demonstrate the exercises as a way of reinforcing teaching.

---

# Nursing Care Plan
## A Client with a Ruptured Intervertebral Disk

Maree Ivans is a 50-year-old lawyer who lives in Montana. She sustains ruptured intervertebral disks at C5 and C6 when she is thrown over the handlebars of her bicycle while mountain biking. Mrs. Ivans is the mother of two young adults; her husband operates a small business.

### ASSESSMENT

Immediately after the accident, Mrs. Ivans is taken to the nearest hospital by ambulance and evaluated by a neurosurgeon. Diagnostic tests include a CT scan, an MRI study, and X-ray films of the cervical vertebrae. The results demonstrate damaged ligaments and herniation of the C7 disk. Mrs. Ivans is sent home wearing a cervical collar to stabilize the area and is instructed to limit activity. Twisting or turning the neck is prohibited. After 2 weeks at home, Mrs. Ivans complains of having no appetite, being unable to sleep at night, and having acute pain in the neck and shoulders. She also has numbness and tingling in several fingers of her left (dominant) hand. A major concern is whether she will be able to return to work and resume her usual activities. A cervical laminectomy with spinal fusion is being discussed.

### DIAGNOSES

- *Acute pain* related to edema and muscle spasms
- *Impaired mobility* related to altered comfort
- *Disturbed sleep pattern* related to pain with movement
- *Risk for compromised family coping* related to altered lifestyle and lack of knowledge about the injury

### EXPECTED OUTCOMES

- State that her pain is decreased to the point of tolerance.
- Experience restful sleep as evidenced by statements of increased energy.
- Collaborate with her husband in discussing the injury and planning how best to meet household needs.

### PLANNING AND IMPLEMENTATION

- Take prescribed analgesics around the clock (when awake) to manage pain. Take prescribed muscle relaxants to control muscle spasms.
- Keep the cervical collar on at all times. Do not lift objects or bend or twist the neck.
- Follow a regular bedtime routine, sleeping on a firm mattress with a small pillow under the neck if desired.
- Drink six to eight full glasses of water each day.
- Increase fiber and bulk in the diet.

### EVALUATION

Following the acute care period, Mrs. Ivans's physical symptoms have decreased. She is able to manage her pain with oral analgesics and is sleeping better at night. She has begun a program of physical therapy and has continued to wear the cervical collar. After 2 months, Mrs. Ivans is so much improved that she begins to work half days. Her family has taken over cooking and cleaning responsibilities, and they remain sup ortive and understanding.

### Critical Thinking in the Nursing Process

1. Discuss the rationale for taking Mrs. Ivans to the hospital by ambulance after the bicycle accident.
2. Mrs. Ivans has grown children and a husband who provided help and support. How might the teaching you provide differ if the client who sustained this injury were a young single mother of two small children?
3. Design a teaching plan for Mrs. Ivans for the diagnosis, *Dressing/grooming self-care deficit*.

See Evaluating your Response in Appendix C.

## Meeting Individualized Needs

### TEACHING THE CLIENT WITH A RUPTURED INTERVERTEBRAL DISK

- Sleep on a firm mattress; use a bedboard if necessary.
- When lying in the supine position, flex the knees to approximately a 45-degree angle with a small pillow and use a small pillow under the head.
- Avoid any activities that flex the spine, such as bending or lifting, and do not twist the back.
- Follow your diet to maintain body weight or to lose weight if needed.
- Follow the prescribed exercise program.
  a. Lie flat on your back on the floor. Tighten your abdominal and buttock muscles and tilt your pelvis forward so that your lower back is flat on the floor (this is called a *pelvic tilt*). Hold the position for 3 seconds and repeat for prescribed number of times.
  b. Lying on the back on a firm surface, press the feet to the floor, tighten the abdominal muscles, and lift the upper half of the body off the floor. Hold the position for 3 seconds, and repeat as prescribed.
  c. Lying on your back on a firm surface, bring your knees up to the chest. Put your hands around your knees and raise the buttocks off the floor. Repeat as prescribed.
  d. Sit upright on the floor or a firm surface. Keep one leg straight and bend the other knee. Reach for the toes of the straightened leg. Switch legs. Repeat as prescribed.
  e. Stand upright. Squat down, flexing the hips and knees. Straighten your back. Stand upright by straightening the knees. Repeat as prescribed.
- Wear flat-heeled shoes that provide good support.
- Use proper lifting techniques. For instance, squat and use your thigh muscles to lift an object from the floor, and spread your feet to get a wide base of support when you lift while you are standing.

## THE CLIENT WITH A SPINAL CORD TUMOR

**Spinal cord tumors** may be benign or malignant, primary or metastatic. They may arise at any level of the spinal column. Of all spinal cord tumors, 50% are thoracic, 30% are cervical, and 20% are lumbosacral. They constitute about 0.5% to 1% of all tumors (Hickey, 2003). Tumors of the spinal cord are seen equally in men and in women, and they most often occur between the ages of 20 and 60. They are rarely seen in the older adult.

### CLASSIFICATION

Spinal cord tumors are classified by anatomic location as either intramedullary or extramedullary tumors. Intramedullary tumors, which make up about 10% of spinal tumors, arise from within the neural tissues of the spinal cord; those that occur include astrocytomas, ependymomas, glioblastomas, and medulloblastomas (Tierney et al., 2001). Extramedullary tumors arise from tissues outside the spinal cord, with commonly occurring tumors including neurofibromas, meningiomas, sarcomas, chordomas, and vascular tumors.

Extramedullary tumors are further categorized as intradural (arising from the nerve roots or meninges within the subarachnoid space) or extradural (arising from epidural tissue or the vertebrae outside the dura).

Tumors of the spinal cord are also classified as either primary or secondary (metastatic). Primary tumors, arising from the epidural vessels, spinal meninges, or glial cells, have an unknown cause. Secondary tumors are metastatic in origin, most commonly the result of malignancies of the lung, breast, prostate, gastrointestinal tract, or uterus.

### PATHOPHYSIOLOGY

Depending on their anatomic location, spinal cord tumors result in pathologic changes as a result of compression, invasion, or ischemia secondary to arterial or venous obstruction. Extramedullary tumors (whether benign or malignant) alter normal function through compression of the spinal cord, with destruction of white matter and eventual filling of the space around the spinal cord. Cord compression interferes with normal blood flow and membrane potentials, altering afferent and efferent motor, sensory, and reflex impulses. Compression of the spinal cord also causes edema, which can ascend the cord and cause further neurologic deficits. Intramedullary tumors both compress and invade. As the tumor grows within the cord, the cord also enlarges and thus distorts the white matter.

### MANIFESTATIONS

The manifestations of a spinal cord tumor depend on the anatomic location, level of occurrence, type of tumor, and spinal nerves involved. General manifestations of a spinal cord tumor include pain, motor and sensory deficits, changes in bowel and/or bladder elimination, and changes in sexual function. Pain is discussed here; specific manifestations by anatomic level are outlined in the box on page 1342.

Pain is often the first manifestation of a spinal cord tumor. It is caused by compression of the spinal cord, tension on the spinal nerves, or tumor attachment to the proximal dura (the covering of the spinal cord). The pain may be either localized or radicular. Localized pain is felt when pressure is applied over the spinous process of the involved area; this type of pain often accompanies metastatic tumors involving the vertebrae. Radicular pain is felt along the course of a nerve as a result of compression, irritation, or tension of a nerve root. The pain is often made worse by any activity that causes intraspinal pressure, such as sneezing or coughing.

Motor manifestations resulting from a spinal cord tumor include paresis and paralysis below the level of the tumor, spasticity, and hyperactive reflexes. The Babinski reflex may be positive. These deficits are the result of involvement of the corticospinal tracts.

## Manifestations of Spinal Cord Tumors

### CERVICAL CORD TUMORS

- Ipsilateral arm motor involvement, followed by ipsilateral and contralateral leg involvement, followed by contralateral arm involvement
- Paresis of the arms and legs
- Stiffness of the neck
- Paraplegia
- Pain in the shoulders and arms
- Hyperactive reflexes

### THORACIC CORD TUMORS

- Paresis and spasticity of one leg, followed by paresis and spasticity of the other leg
- Pain in the back and chest
- Positive Babinski reflex
- Bowel and bladder dysfunction
- Sexual dysfunction

### LUMBOSACRAL CORD TUMORS

- Paresis and spasticity of one leg, followed by paresis and spasticity of the other leg
- Pain in the lower back, radiating to the legs and perineal area
- Loss of sensation in the legs
- Bowel and bladder dysfunction
- Sexual dysfunction
- Decreased or absent ankle and knee reflexes

Many different sensory manifestations may occur, depending on the location and level of the tumor. Lateral tumor growth and compression affect the lateral spinothalamic tracts, causing pain, numbness, tingling, and coldness. If the tumor involves the posterior columns, the senses of vibration and proprioception of body parts are affected.

Bladder and bowel elimination and sexual function are often affected. Bowel elimination deficits include constipation that may progress to paralytic ileus. Initial bladder elimination deficits include frequency, urgency, and difficulty in voiding. The deficits may progress to urinary retention and a neurogenic bladder. In addition, the male client may be impotent.

*Syringomyelia* is a complication of some spinal cord tumors. In this condition, a fluid-filled cystic cavity forms in the central intramedullary gray matter. This syndrome causes pain, motor weakness, and spasticity.

## COLLABORATIVE CARE

The medical management of the client with a spinal cord tumor focuses first on diagnosis. Treatment depends on the type of tumor, its location, and the client's condition.

## Diagnostic Tests

The client with a spinal cord tumor undergoes many of the same diagnostic tests as does the client with a ruptured intervertebral disk. The following tests are often used to identify the tumor:

- *Flat-plate X-ray film* of the spine illustrates bony changes, such as erosion of the vertebral pedicles. Destruction of bone is usually the result of metastatic tumors.
- *CT scan* or *MRI* is used to visualize the tumor and may also demonstrate the site of cord compression.
- *Myelogram* may demonstrate complete blockage of cerebrospinal fluid circulation at the level of the tumor.
- *Lumbar puncture* may be performed to obtain cerebrospinal fluid for analysis. The cerebrospinal fluid in the client with a spinal cord tumor is commonly xanthochromic (having a yellow color), has increased protein, has few to no cells, and clots immediately (this cluster of findings is called Froin's syndrome).

## Medications

The client with a spinal cord tumor is given medications to relieve pain and control edema. If the pain is severe and the result of a metastatic tumor, an epidural catheter may be inserted for narcotic analgesic administration. Pain management for clients with a spinal cord tumor is provided by narcotic analgesics (see Chapter 4).

Steroids, such as dexamethasone (Decadron), are administered to control edema of the cord. The steroids are given in high doses for 3 days and then are rapidly tapered off (Tierney et al., 2001).

## Treatments

The treatments for spinal cord tumors include surgery and radiation therapy.

### Surgery

Intramedullary and intradural tumors are surgically excised when possible. Advances in microsurgical techniques and laser surgery have increased the possibility of tumor excision. Metastatic tumors may be partially excised to reduce cord compression; rapidly growing metastatic lesions may require surgical decompression to preserve motor, bowel, or bladder function.

The surgical excision is made through a laminectomy. The client with a tumor involving more than two vertebrae often has a spinal fusion and may also have rods inserted to stabilize the spinal column.

### Radiation Therapy

Radiation therapy is used to treat metastatic spinal cord tumors for several different reasons. It may be used on an emergency basis to treat the client with rapidly progressing neurologic deficits. It may be used to reduce pain. Radiation may also be used following surgical excision of as much tumor mass as possible.

Radiation of the spinal cord may cause the development of radiation-induced myelopathy. This complication of radiation exposure occurs over time, with manifestations of a *Brown-Séquard syndrome* developing 12 to 15 months after therapy. The manifestations may progress to paraplegia, sensory loss, and loss of bowel and bladder control (Hickey, 2003).

## NURSING CARE

Nursing care for the client with a spinal cord tumor is individualized in accordance with the type of tumor and the type of treatment. The client with a benign tumor that is removed by surgery has different health care needs than the client with a metastatic tumor, even though they may have similar neurologic deficits. The client with a spinal cord tumor (regardless of type) requires nursing care to monitor for neurologic changes, to provide pain management, and to manage motor and sensory deficits in order to preserve quality of life.

The assessments and nursing interventions for the client with a spinal cord tumor are similar to those described for the client with SCI or who is undergoing surgery for a ruptured intervertebral disk. The following nursing diagnoses may be appropriate for the client with a spinal cord tumor.

- *Anxiety* related to a diagnosis of malignant spinal cord tumor
- *Risk for constipation* related to the effects of spinal cord compression
- *Impaired physical mobility* related to weakness of lower extremities
- *Acute pain* related to compression of spinal nerve roots
- *Sexual dysfunction* related to effects of spinal cord compression
- *Urinary retention* related to the effects of spinal cord compression

Following surgical treatment, the client may be transferred to a rehabilitation center or may go home for the recovery period. Referrals for home care, occupational therapy, and physical therapy often help the client regain functional abilities. Teach family members how to move the client in the bed and from the bed to a chair. Also teach them how to provide physical care, care for any appliances (such as an indwelling catheter), and prevent or treat constipation.

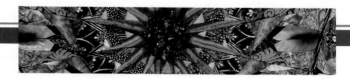

## EXPLORE MediaLink

NCLEX review questions, case studies, care plan activities, MediaLink applications, and other interactive resources for this chapter can be found on the Companion Website at www.prenhall.com/lemone.

Click on Chapter 41 to select the activities for this chapter. For animations, video clips, more NCLEX review questions, and an audio glossary, access the Student CD-ROM accompanying this textbook.

## TEST YOURSELF

1. Which of the following manifestations would alert you to the possibility that your client has had a TIA?

   a. Sudden severe pain over the left eye
   b. Numbness and tingling in the corner of the mouth
   c. Complete paralysis of the right arm and leg
   d. Loss of sensation and reflexes in both legs

2. What is the rationale for administration of a tissue plasminogen activator within the first 3 hours of a thrombotic stroke?

   a. To reduce the risk of vasospasm
   b. To decrease the risk of infection
   c. To increase platelet aggregation
   d. To cause fibrinolysis of the clot

3. Oxygen is often administered to the client who has had a stroke. Preventing hypoxia and hypercapnia through this treatment will lessen the risk of which complication?

   a. Fluid accumulation in the lungs

   b. Pulmonary emboli
   c. Increased intracranial pressure
   d. Rebleeding

4. What is the primary pathophysiologic process of spinal shock?

   a. Temporary loss of reflex function below the level of injury
   b. Loss of control of cardiovascular mechanisms
   c. Exaggerated sympathetic response
   d. Damage to the lower motor neurons

5. Your client has manifestations of autonomic dysreflexia. Which of these assessments would indicate a possible cause for this condition?

   a. Extreme hypertension
   b. Kinked catheter tubing
   c. Respiratory wheezes and stridor
   d. Skin breakdown over the coccyx

See Test Yourself answers in Appendix C.

# BIBLIOGRAPHY

Breteton, L., & Nolan, M. (2000). "You do know he's had a stroke, don't you?" Preparation for family care-giving: The neglected dimension. *Journal of Clinical Nursing, 9*(4), 498–506.

Bucher, L. & Melander, S. (1999). *Critical Care Nursing.* Philadelphia Saunders.

Buckley, D., & Guanci, M. (1999). Spinal cord trauma. *Nursing Clinics of North America, 34*(3), 661–687.

Chotikul, L. (2000). Spinal implants. *RN, 63*(5), 28–31.

Christensen, J., Cook, E., & Martin, B. (1997). Identifying denial in stroke patients. *Clinical Nursing Research, 6*(1), 105–118.

Davies, S. (1999). Dysphagia in acute strokes. *Nursing Standard, 13*(30), 49–55.

DeLisa, J., & Kirshblum, S. (1997). A review: Frustrations and needs in clinical care of spinal cord injury patients. *Journal of Spinal Cord Medicine, 20*(4), 384–390.

Duncan, P., & Lai, S. (1997). Stroke recovery. *Topics in Stroke Rehabilitation, 4*(3), 51–58.

Garner, C. (1999). Cancer-related spinal cord compression. *American Journal of Nursing, 99*(7), 34–35.

Gendreau-Webb, R. (2001). Action stat: Ischemic stroke. *Nursing, 31*(11), 120.

Gerhart, K., Charlifue, S., Weitzenkamp, D., Menter, R., & Whiteneck, G. (1997). Aging with spinal cord injury. *American Rehabilitation, 23*(1), 19–25.

Harding-Okimoto, M. (1997). Pressure ulcers, self-concept and body image in spinal cord injury patients. *SCI Nursing, 14*(4), 111–117.

Hayn, M., & Fisher, T. (1997). Stroke rehabilitation: Salvaging ability after the storm. *Nursing97, 27*(3), 40–46, 48.

Hickey, J. (2003). *The clinical practice of neurological and neurosurgical nursing* (4th ed.). Philadelphia: Lippincott.

Hock, N. (1999). Brain attack: The stroke continuum. *Nursing Clinics of North America, 34*(3), 689–723.

Huston, C. (1998). Cervical spine injury. *American Journal of Nursing, 98*(6), 33.

Identification and nursing management of dysphagia in adults with neurological impairment. *Best Practice, 4*(2), 1–6.

John, C. (1997). Time is of the essence. . . "Brain attack: Treating acute ischemic CVA." *Nursing97, 27*(6), 9–10.

Johnson, M., & Maas, M. (Eds.). (1997). *Iowa outcome project: Nursing outcomes classification (NOC).* St. Louis: Mosby.

Krause, J. (1998). Skin sores after spinal cord injury: Relationship to life adjustment. *Spinal Cord, 36*(1), 51–56.

LaFavor, K., & Ang, R. (1997). Managing autonomic dysreflexia through the use of clinical practice guidelines. *SCI Nursing, 14*(3), 83–86.

McAweeney, M., Tate, D., & McAweeney, W. (1997). Psychosocial interventions in the rehabilitation of people with spinal cord injury: A comprehensive methodologic inquiry. *SCI Psychosocial Process, 10*(2), 58–66.

McCloskey, J., & Bulechek, G. (Eds.). (2000). *Iowa intervention project: Nursing interventions classification (NIC)* (3rd ed.). St. Louis: Mosby.

McColl, M., Walker, J., Stirling, P., Wilkins, R., & Corey, P. (1997). Expectations of life and health among spinal cord injured adults. *Spinal Cord, 35*(12), 818–828.

McHale, J., Phipps, M., Horvath, K., & Schmelz, J. (1998). Expert nursing knowledge in the care of patients at risk of impaired swallowing. *Image: Journal of Nursing Scholarship, 30*(2), 137–141.

Mower, D. (1997). Brain attack: Treating acute ischemic CVA. *Nursing97, 27*(3), 34–39, 47–48.

National Spinal Cord Injury Association (1998). *Spinal cord injury statistics.* Available www.eskimo.com/~jlubin/disabled/nscia/fact02.html

Perry, L. (2001). Screening swallowing function of patients with acute stroke. Part 2. Detailed evaluation of the tool used by nurses. *Journal of Clinical Nursing, 10*(4), 474–481.

Petterson, M. (1997). Thrombolytic therapy in stroke management. *Critical Care Nurse, 17*(5), 88–93.

Porth, C. ( 2002). *Pathophysiology: Concepts of altered health states* (6th ed.). Philadelphia: Lippincott.

Routh, J. (1997). Consumer's perspective: Dressing and undressing following a stroke. *Topics in Stroke Rehabilitation, 4*(2), 94–98.

Sander, R. (1998). Stroke: The hidden problems. *Elderly Care, 10*(1), 27–32.

Shannon, M., Wilson, B., & Stang, C. (2002). *Health professionals drug guide 2002.* Upper Saddle River, NJ: Prentice Hall.

Sipski, M. (1997). Sexuality and spinal cord injury: Where we are and where we are going. *American Rehabilitation, 23*(1), 26–28.

Thompson, J., McFarland, G., Hirsch, J., & Tucker, S. (2002). *Mosby's clinical nursing* (5th ed.). St. Louis: Mosby.

Tierney, L., McPhee, S., & Papadakis, M. (Eds.). (2001). *Current medical diagnosis & treatment.* Stamford, CT: Appleton & Lange.

Westergren, A., Ohlsson, O., & Halberg, I. (2001). Eating difficulties, complications, and nursing interventions during a period of three months after a stroke. *Journal of Advanced Nursing, 35*(3), 416–426.

Whipple, B., & Komisarck, B. (1997). Sexuality and women with complete spinal cord injury. *Spinal Cord, 35*(3), 136–138.

# Nursing Care of Clients with Intracranial Disorders

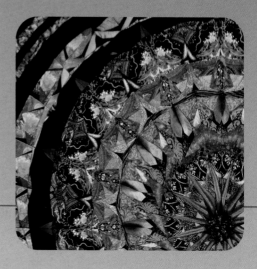

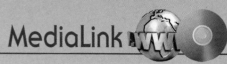

## www.prenhall.com/lemone

Additional resources for this chapter can be found on the Student CD-ROM accompanying this textbook, and on the Companion Website at www. prenhall.com/lemone. Click on Chapter 42 to select the activities for this chapter.

**CD-ROM**
- Audio Glossary
- NCLEX Review

*Animation*
- Coup-Contrecoup Injury

**Companion Website**
- More NCLEX Review
- Care Plan Activity
    Subdural Hematoma
- MediaLink Application
    Meningitis Prevention

## LEARNING OUTCOMES

After completing this chapter, you will be able to:

- Apply knowledge of normal anatomy, physiology, and assessments when providing nursing care for clients with intracranial disorders (see Chapter 40).

- Explain the pathophysiology, manifestations, collaborative care, and nursing care of altered level of consciousness and increased intracranial pressure.

- Describe the pathophysiology and manifestations of seizures, headaches, traumatic brain injury, intracranial infections, and brain tumors.

- Identify diagnostic tests used to identify and manage intracranial disorders.

- Discuss nursing implications for medications used to treat intracranial disorders.

- Explain collaborative care for clients with intracranial disorders.

- Describe nursing interventions in the preoperative and postoperative care of the client having intracranial surgery.

- Use the nursing process as a framework for providing individualized care to clients with intracranial disorders.

The client with an intracranial disorder presents a unique challenge to the nurse. Problems the client experiences in the acute stage of the disorder are often a prelude to long-term problems requiring ongoing management. These long-term problems range from alterations in the body's basic functioning to dysfunctions in the complex processes of the human mind. Systemic problems may accompany or develop secondary to an intracranial disorder. Intracranial disorders may affect the client's quality of life and that of the client's family. This chapter first discusses altered level of consciousness and increased intracranial pressure, followed by intracranial disorders that may manifest these and other health problems. Information specific to the client with a stroke is in Chapter 41.

# ALTERED CEREBRAL FUNCTION

The manifestations of altered cerebral function occur as a result of illness or injury. Assessment of the patterns of those manifestations helps determine the extent of the cerebral dysfunction and improvement or deterioration of cerebral function. Except in the case of direct damage to the brainstem and **reticular activating system (RAS),** brain function deterioration usually follows a predictable rostral to caudal progression, that is, a pattern in which higher levels of function are impaired initially, progressing to impairment of more primitive functions. Altered level of consciousness and behavior changes are early manifestations of the deterioration of the function of the cerebral hemispheres. Structures in the midbrain and brainstem are affected sequentially, with characteristic changes in level of consciousness; patterns of respiration, pupillary and oculomotor responses; and motor function (Porth, 2002). Manifestations of progressive deterioration of cerebral function are outlined in Table 42–1.

| TABLE 42–1 | Progression of Deteriorating Brain Function | | | |
|---|---|---|---|---|
| Level of Consciousness | Pupillary Response | Oculomotor Responses | Motor Responses | Breathing |
| Alert; oriented to time, place, and person | Brisk and equal; pupils regular | Eyes move as head turns Caloric testing (ear irrigation) produces nystagmus | Purposeful movement; responds to commands | Regular pattern with normal rate and depth |
| Responds to verbal stimuli; decreased concentration; agitation, confusion, lethargy; disoriented | Small and reactive | Roving eye movements; doll's eyes positive, with gaze fixed straight ahead; eye deviation away from cold caloric stimulus and toward warm stimulus | Purposeful movement in response to pain stimulus | Yawning, sighing respirations |
| Requires continuous stimulation to rouse | | | Decorticate posturing with upper extremity flexion | Cheyne-Stokes respirations with crescendo-decrescendo pattern in rate and depth followed by period of apnea |
| Reflexive positioning to pain stimulus | Pupils fixed (nonreactive) in midposition | Caloric testing produces nystagmus | Decerebrate posturing with adduction and rigid extension of upper and lower extremities | Central neurogenic hyperventilation with rapid, regular, and deep respirations; apneustic breathing with prolonged inspiration and pauses at full inspiration and following expiration |
| No response to stimuli | Pupils fixed in midposition | No spontaneous eye movement or nystagmus | Extension of upper extremities with flexion of lower extremities; flaccidity | Cluster or ataxic breathing with irregular pattern and depth of respirations; gasping respirations or apnea |

# THE CLIENT WITH ALTERED LEVEL OF CONSCIOUSNESS

**Consciousness** is a condition in which the person is aware of self and environment and is able to respond appropriately to stimuli. Full consciousness requires both normal arousal and full cognition.

- *Arousal,* or alertness, depends on the RAS, a diffuse system of neurons in the thalamus and upper brainstem.
- *Cognition* is a complex process involving all mental activities controlled by the cerebral hemispheres, including thought processes, memory, perception, problem solving, and emotion.

These two components of consciousness depend on the normal physiologic function of and connection between the arousal mechanisms of the reticular formation and the cognitive functions of the cerebral hemispheres. Because arousal and cognition are independent components of consciousness, each can act separately on stimuli. For example, the RAS reacts to the discomfort caused by a full bladder by waking the person in the middle of the night. Once awake, however, the frontal cortex alerts the person that the bladder is full and prompts the person to go to the bathroom and empty it.

The physiologic seat of consciousness, the reticular formation, is a mass of nerve cells and fibers that make up the core of the brainstem, extending from the medulla to the midbrain. The axons of reticular neurons are exceptionally long and branch outward to cells in the hypothalamus, thalamus, cerebellum, and spinal cord. A system of reticular neurons within the RAS passes steady streams of impulses through thalamic relays in order to stimulate the cerebral cortex into wakefulness. The body's sensory tracts interact with RAS neurons; this interrelationship helps control the strength of the RAS's rousing effect on the cerebrum.

Conditions that affect either the RAS or the function of the cerebral hemispheres can interfere with the normal level of consciousness. Terms describing altered level of consciousness (LOC) are listed and defined in Table 42–2. Nurses should remember that consciousness is a dynamic state: A client may pass from full consciousness to coma within hours or experience a slow diminishment of consciousness that does not become evident for weeks or months. The nurse can help provide effective care for a client with an altered level of consciousness by looking beyond the diagnostic labels of consciousness and accurately assessing the client's behavior and response to stimuli.

## PATHOPHYSIOLOGY

Level of consciousness may be altered by processes that affect the arousal functions of the brainstem, the cognitive functions of the cerebral hemispheres, or both. The major causes are (1) lesions or injuries that affect the cerebral hemispheres directly and widely or that compress or destroy the neurons of the RAS and (2) metabolic disorders.

| TABLE 42–2 | Terms Used to Describe Level of Consciousness |
| --- | --- |
| **Term** | **Characteristics of Client** |
| Full consciousness | Alert; oriented to time, place, and person; comprehends spoken and written words |
| Confusion | Unable to think rapidly and clearly; easily bewildered, with poor memory and short attention span; misinterprets stimuli; judgment is impaired |
| Disorientation | Not aware of or not oriented to time, place, or person |
| Obtundation | Lethargic, somnolent; responsive to verbal or tactile stimuli but quickly drifts back to sleep |
| Stupor | Generally unresponsive; may be briefly aroused by vigorous, repeated, or painful stimuli; may shrink away from or grab at the source of stimuli |
| Semicomatose | Does not move spontaneously; unresponsive to stimuli, although vigorous or painful stimuli may result in stirring, moaning, or withdrawal from the stimuli, without actual arousal |
| Coma | Unarousable; will not stir or moan in response to any stimulus; may exhibit nonpurposeful response (slight movement) of area stimulated but makes no attempt to withdraw |
| Deep coma | Completely unarousable and unresponsive to any kind of stimulus, including pain; absence of brainstem reflexes, corneal, pupillary, and pharyngeal reflexes and tendon and plantar reflexes |

## Arousal

Damage to the RAS impairs the person's ability to maintain wakefulness and arousal. Stroke is the most common cause of RAS destruction. Other causes include demyelinating diseases such as multiple sclerosis, tumors, abscesses, and head injury. Function of the RAS may be suppressed by compression of the brainstem, which produces edema and ischemia. Pressure and compression of the brainstem may be due to tumors, increased intracranial pressure, hematomas or hemorrhage, or aneurysm (McCance & Huether, 2002). Although it is possible to assess level of consciousness or arousal in the client with RAS damage, the impairment in arousal may make it impossible to assess cognitive function.

The function of the brain, especially the cerebral hemispheres, depends on continuous blood flow with unimpeded supplies of oxygen and glucose. Processes that disrupt this flow of blood and nutrients may cause widespread damage to the cerebral hemispheres, impairing arousal and cognition. Bilateral hemispheric lesions, such as global ischemia, or metabolic disorders, such as hypoglycemia, are the most common causes of altered LOC related to cerebral dysfunction of the hemispheres. Localized masses, such as a hematoma or cerebral edema that displace normal structures and cause direct or indirect pressure on the opposite hemisphere or brainstem can also affect LOC. The client who has widespread damage to the cerebral hemispheres but an intact RAS has sleep-wake cycles and may rouse in response to stimuli; the client cannot be said to be alert, however, because cognition is impaired.

Both localized neurologic processes and systemic disorders can alter LOC. Processes occurring within the brain, which may directly destroy or compress neurologic structures, include the following:

- Increased intracranial pressure
- Stroke
- Hematoma
- Intracranial hemorrhage
- Tumors
- Infections
- Demyelinating disorders

Any systemic condition that affects the delivery of blood, oxygen, and glucose to the brain or alters cell membranes may also alter LOC. If cerebral blood flow is impaired or the client becomes hypoxic or hypoglycemic, cerebral metabolism is impaired and level of consciousness declines rapidly. Clients at particular risk include those with poorly controlled diabetes and those with cardiac or respiratory failure.

Other metabolic alterations that can affect LOC include fluid and electrolyte imbalances, such as hyponatremia or hyperosmolality, and acid-base alterations, such as hypercapnia (an elevated arterial carbon dioxide level). Accumulated waste products and toxins from liver or renal failure can affect neuronal and neurotransmitter function, altering LOC. Drugs that depress the central nervous system (e.g., alcohol, analgesics, anesthetics) suppress metabolic and membrane activities in the RAS and cerebral hemispheres, thereby affecting LOC.

Seizure activity, abnormal electrical discharges from a local area of the brain or from the entire brain, commonly affects LOC. It appears that the spontaneous, disordered discharge of activity that occurs during a seizure exhausts energy metabolites or produces locally toxic molecules, altering LOC for a time after the seizure. Consciousness returns when the metabolic balance of the neurons is restored.

As the impairment of brain function progresses, more stimuli are required to elicit a response from the client. Initially, the client may rouse to verbal stimuli and respond appropriately to questions, remaining oriented to time, place, and person. With deterioration of neurologic function, the client becomes more difficult to rouse and may become agitated and confused when awakened. Orientation to time is lost initially, followed by orientation to place and then to person. Continuous stimulation or vigorous shaking is required to maintain wakefulness as LOC decreases. Eventually, the client does not respond, even with deep painful stimuli.

## Patterns of Breathing

Progressive impairment of neural function also causes predictable changes in breathing patterns as respiratory centers are affected. In normal respirations, a rhythmic pattern is maintained by neural centers in the pons and medulla that respond to changes in arterial levels of oxygen ($PaO_2$) and carbon dioxide ($PaCO_2$). When there is damage to the RAS or cerebral hemispheres, neural control of these centers is lost, and lower brainstem centers regulate breathing patterns by responding only to changes in $PaCO_2$, resulting in irregular respiratory patterns. As outlined in Table 42–1 and illustrated in Table 42–3, progressive deterioration in brain function is accompanied by decreasing LOC and changes in breathing patterns. The type of respirations, by area of cerebral damage, are as follows (Porth, 2002):

- *Diencephalon:* Cheyne-Stokes respirations
- *Midbrain:* neurogenic hyperventilation (may exceed 40 per minute), the result of uninhibited stimulation of the respiratory centers
- *Pons:* apneustic respirations, characterized by sighing on midinspiration or prolonged inhalation and exhalation; results from excessive stimulation of the respiratory centers
- *Medulla:* ataxic/apneic respirations (totally uncoordinated and irregular), probably as a result of the loss of responsiveness to $CO_2$

## Pupillary and Oculomotor Responses

The brainstem areas that control arousal are adjacent to areas that control the pupils. A predictable progression of pupillary

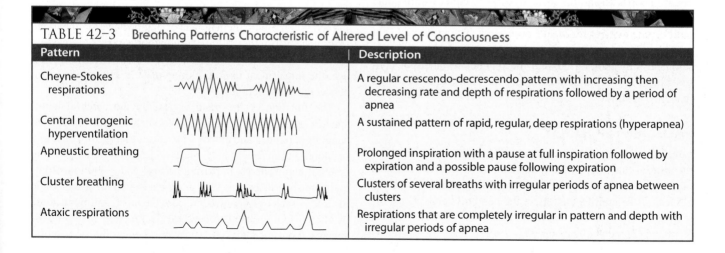

| TABLE 42–3 Breathing Patterns Characteristic of Altered Level of Consciousness | | |
| --- | --- | --- |
| **Pattern** | | **Description** |
| Cheyne-Stokes respirations | | A regular crescendo-decrescendo pattern with increasing then decreasing rate and depth of respirations followed by a period of apnea |
| Central neurogenic hyperventilation | | A sustained pattern of rapid, regular, deep respirations (hyperapnea) |
| Apneustic breathing | | Prolonged inspiration with a pause at full inspiration followed by expiration and a possible pause following expiration |
| Cluster breathing | | Clusters of several breaths with irregular periods of apnea between clusters |
| Ataxic respirations | | Respirations that are completely irregular in pattern and depth with irregular periods of apnea |

and oculomotor responses occurs as level of consciousness deteriorates toward coma (see Table 42–1). If the lesion or process affecting neurologic function is localized, effects may initially be seen in the *ipsilateral pupil* (the pupil on the same side as the lesion). With generalized or systemic processes, pupils are affected equally. If the pupils are small and equally reactive, metabolic processes affecting LOC may be present. With compression of cranial nerve III at the midbrain, the pupils may become oval or eccentric (off center). As the level of functional impairment progresses, the pupils become fixed (unresponsive to light) and, eventually, dilated.

In deteriorating LOC and coma, spontaneous eye movement is lost and reflexive ocular movements are altered. Normally, both eyes move simultaneously in the same direction; injury to the cranial nerve nuclei in the midbrain and pons can impair normal movement. **Doll's eye movements** are reflexive movements of the eyes in the opposite direction of head rotation; they are an indicator of brainstem function (Figure 42–1 ■). As a result of the oculocephalic reflex, the eyes move upward with passive flexion of the neck and downward with passive neck extension. As brainstem function deteriorates, this reflex is lost. The eyes fail to turn together and, eventually, remain fixed in the midposition as the head is turned.

Instilling cold water into the ear canal (cold caloric testing) tests the oculovestibular response. Normally, this stimulus causes **nystagmus** (lateral tonic deviation of the eyes) toward the stimulus. This reflex is also lost as brain function deteriorates.

## Motor Responses

The level of brain dysfunction and the side of the brain affected may be assessed by motor responses. These responses are the most accurate identifier of changes in mental status. In altered LOC, motor responses to stimuli range from an appropriate response to a command (e.g., "squeeze my hand" or "push my hands away with your feet") to flaccidity (see Table 42–1). Initially, the client may be able to move purposefully away from a noxious stimulus, for example, to brush the examiner's hand away from the face. As function declines, movements become more generalized (withdrawal, grimacing) and less purposeful.

Reflexive motor responses may occur, including *decorticate* posturing with flexion of the upper extremities accompanied by extension of the lower extremities. With further decline, *decerebrate* posturing is seen, with adduction and rigid extension of the upper and lower extremities. Without intervention, the client eventually becomes flaccid, with little or no motor response to stimuli.

## COMA STATES AND BRAIN DEATH

Possible outcomes of altered LOC and coma include full recovery with no long-term residual effects, recovery with residual damage (such as learning deficits, emotional difficulties, or impaired judgment), or more severe consequences such as persistent vegetative state (cerebral death) or brain death.

### Irreversible Coma

**Irreversible coma (persistent vegetative state)** is a permanent condition of complete unawareness of self and the environment, resulting from death of the cerebral hemispheres with continued function of the brainstem and cerebellum. While the homeostatic regulatory functions of the brain continue, the ability to respond meaningfully to the environment is lost.

The client in vegetative state has sleep-wake cycles and retains the ability to chew, swallow, and cough but cannot interact with the environment. When awake, the client's eyes may wander back and forth across the room, but they cannot track an object or person. In a **minimally conscious state,** the client is aware of the environment and can follow simple commands, manipulate objects, gesture or verbalize to indicate "yes/no" responses, and make meaningful movements (such as blinking or smiling) in response to a stimulus (McCance & Huether, 2002). Vegetative state is usually the result of severe head injury or global anoxia. With appropriate supportive care, the client may remain in this state for 2 to 5 years.

### Locked-In Syndrome

**Locked-in syndrome** is distinctly different from vegetative state, in that the client is alert and fully aware of the environment and has intact cognitive abilities, but is unable to

**Head in neutral position**

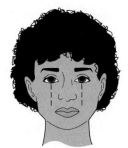

Eyes midline

**Head rotated to client's left**

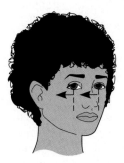

Doll's eyes present:
Eyes move right in
relation to head.

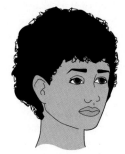

Doll's eyes absent:
Eyes do not move
in relation to head.
Direction of vision follows
head to left.

**Figure 42–1** ■ Doll's eye movements characteristic of altered level of consciousness.

communicate through speech or movement because of blocked efferent pathways from the brain. Motor paralysis affects all voluntary muscles, although the upper cranial nerves (I through IV) may remain intact, allowing the client to communicate through eye movements and blinking. In essence, the client is "locked" inside a paralyzed body in which he or she remains fully conscious of self and environment. Infarction or hemorrhage of the pons that disrupts outgoing nerve tracts but spares the RAS is the usual cause of locked-in syndrome. This condition may also result when the corticospinal tracts between the midbrain and pons are interrupted. Disorders of the lower motor neurons or muscles, such as acute polyneuritis, myasthenia gravis, or amyotrophic lateral sclerosis (ALS), may also paralyze motor responses, leading to locked-in syndrome.

## Brain Death

**Brain death** is the cessation and irreversibility of all brain functions, including the brainstem. Although the exact criteria for establishing brain death may vary somewhat from state to state, it is generally agreed that brain death has occurred when there is no evidence of cerebral or brainstem function for an extended period (usually 6 to 24 hours) in a client who has a normal body temperature and is not affected by a depressant drug or alcohol poisoning. Generally recognized criteria are:

- Unresponsive coma with absent motor and reflex movements.
- No spontaneous respiration (apnea).
- Pupils fixed (unresponsive to light) and dilated.
- Absent ocular responses to head turning and caloric stimulation.
- Flat EEG and no cerebral blood circulation present on angiography (if performed).
- Persistence of these manifestations for 30 minutes to 1 hour and for 6 hours after onset of coma and apnea.

Apnea in the comatose client is determined by the apnea test. The ventilator is removed while maintaining oxygenation by tracheal cannula and allowing the $Pco_2$ to increase to 60 mmHg or higher. This level of carbon dioxide is high enough to stimulate respiration if the brainstem is functional. The electroencephalogram (EEG) may be used to establish the absence of brain activity when brain death is suspected. A flat (isoelectric) EEG over a period of 6 to 12 hours in a client who is not hypothermic or under the influence of drugs that depress the central nervous system is generally accepted as an indicator of brain death (McCance & Huether, 2002).

## PROGNOSIS

The prognosis for clients with altered levels of consciousness and coma varies according to the underlying cause and pathologic process. Age and general medical condition also play a role in determining outcome. Young adults may fully recover following deep coma from head injury, drug overdose, or other cause. Recovery of consciousness within 2 weeks is associated with a favorable outcome. In general, the prognosis is poor for clients who lack pupillary reaction or reflex eye movements 6 hours after the onset of coma.

## COLLABORATIVE CARE

Management of the client with an altered LOC or coma must begin immediately. The focus of management is to identify the underlying cause, preserve function, and prevent deterioration if possible. Airway and breathing must be maintained during the initial acute stage until the diagnosis and prognosis can be established. Intravenous fluids are used to support circulation and to correct fluid, electrolyte, and acid-base imbalances. Treatment protocols to reduce increased intracranial pressure or control seizure activity (discussed later in this chapter) may be initiated. Changes in LOC associated with craniocerebral trauma, such as hematomas, often require immediate surgical intervention.

### Diagnostic Tests

Although the client's history and physical examination findings often indicate the cause of alterations in LOC, several diagnostic tests may be useful in establishing the diagnosis. The following tests may be ordered to evaluate for possible metabolic, toxic, or drug-induced disorders.

- *Blood glucose* is measured immediately when coma is of unknown origin and hypoglycemia is suspected or possible. The brain contains minimal stores of glucose and is dependent on a continuous supply for metabolism. When the blood glucose falls to less than 40 to 50 mg/dL, cerebral function declines rapidly. The client with type 1 diabetes is at particular risk for hypoglycemia-induced coma.
- *Serum electrolytes*—sodium, potassium, bicarbonate, chloride, and calcium in particular—are measured to assess for metabolic disturbances and guide intravenous therapy. Hyponatremia, in which serum sodium levels are below 115 mEq/L (normal level: 135 to 145 mEq/L), is associated with coma and convulsions, especially if it develops rapidly.
- *Serum osmolality* is evaluated. Both hyperosmolar and hypoosmolar states may be associated with coma. Hyperosmolality (above 320 mOsm/kg $H_2O$) causes cellular dehydration of brain tissue as fluid is drawn into the vascular system by osmosis. Hypo-osmolality (less than 250 mOsm/kg $H_2O$), by contrast, leads to cerebral edema and swelling, impairing consciousness.
- *ABGs* are drawn to evaluate arterial oxygen and carbon dioxide levels as well as acid-base balance. Hypoxemia is a frequent cause of altered LOC; increased levels of carbon dioxide are also toxic to the brain and can induce coma, particularly when the onset of hypercapnia is acute.
- *Serum creatinine* and *BUN* are measured to evaluate renal function.
- *Liver function tests,* including bilirubin, AST, ALT, LDH, serum albumin, and serum ammonia levels, are determined to evaluate hepatic function. High ammonia levels seen in hepatic failure interfere with cerebral metabolism and neurotransmitters, affecting level of consciousness.
- *Toxicology screening* of blood and urine is done to determine if altered LOC is the result of acute drug or alcohol toxicity. Serum alcohol levels are measured and the blood is assessed

for the presence of substances such as barbiturates, carbon monoxide, or lead.

- *CBC with differential* is done to assess for possible anemia or infectious causes of coma.
- *CT* and *MRI scanning* are done to detect neurologic damage due to hemorrhage, tumor, cyst, edema, myocardial infarction, or brain atrophy. These tests may also identify displacement of brain structures by large or expanding lesions. It is important to remember, however, that not all lesions or causes of altered LOC can be determined by CT scan or MRI.
- *EEG* is used to evaluate the electrical activity of the brain. The EEG is particularly valuable in identifying unrecognized seizure activity as a cause of altered LOC and is also useful in identifying certain infectious and metabolic causes of altered LOC. A normal EEG in an unresponsive client may identify locked-in syndrome. In addition to the baseline EEG, evoked responses may also be determined. The EEG is monitored as an auditory tone or other sensory stimulus is provided to assess the brain's responsiveness.
- *Radioisotope brain scan* is performed to identify abnormal lesions in the brain and evaluate cerebral blood flow.
- *Cerebral angiography* allows radiographic visualization of the cerebral vascular system. A radiopaque dye is injected into the carotid or vertebral arteries, followed by fluoroscopic and serial X-ray evaluation of the cerebral circulation. This exam can identify lesions such as aneurysms, occluded vessels, or tumors, and may also be used to determine cessation of cerebral blood flow and brain death.
- *Transcranial Doppler studies* use an ultrasound velocity detector that records sound waves reflected from RBCs in blood vessels to assess cerebral blood flow.
- *Lumbar puncture with CSF analysis* is performed when infection and possible meningitis are suspected as a cause of altered LOC.

## Medications

Medications are used to support homeostasis and normal function for the client with altered LOC, as well as to treat specific underlying disorders. An intravenous catheter is inserted, and fluid balance is maintained using isotonic or slightly hypertonic solutions, such as normal saline or lactated Ringer's solution. The client's response to fluid administration is monitored carefully for evidence of increased cerebral edema.

If hypoglycemia is present, 50% glucose is administered intravenously to restore cerebral metabolism rapidly. Conversely, insulin is administered to the client with hyperglycemia to reduce the blood glucose level and thus the serum osmolality. With narcotic overdose, naloxone is administered. Naloxone is a narcotic antagonist that competes for narcotic receptor sites, effectively blocking the depressant effect of the narcotic. Thiamine may be administered with glucose, particularly if the client is malnourished or known to abuse alcohol, to prevent exacerbation of Wernicke's encephalopathy, a hemorrhagic encephalopathy due to thiamine deficiency and associated with chronic alcoholism (Tierney et al., 2001).

Any underlying fluid and electrolyte imbalance is corrected by administering medications or appropriate electrolytes. For the client who is hyponatremic and has a low serum osmolality, furosemide (Lasix) or an osmotic diuretic such as mannitol may be administered to promote water excretion. Appropriate antibiotics are administered intravenously to the client with suspected or confirmed meningitis.

## Surgery

Although surgery is not indicated for most clients with altered LOC, it may be necessary if the cause of coma is a tumor, hemorrhage, or hematoma. Surgical intervention is discussed later in this chapter, in the section on brain tumors. When there is a risk of increased intracranial pressure, the client is monitored continuously. These measures are discussed in the section on increased intracranial pressure.

## Other Therapeutic Measures

Support of the airway and respirations is vital in the client with an altered LOC. The client who is drowsy but rousable may need little more than an oral pharyngeal airway. With more severe alterations in consciousness, the client may need endotracheal intubation to maintain airway patency, particularly if the cough and gag reflexes are absent. Mechanical ventilation is indicated when hypoventilation or apnea is present. Unless a do-not-resuscitate (DNR) order is in effect, mechanical ventilation should be initiated even if it has not been established that the disorder is reversible; without ventilatory support, cerebral anoxia develops rapidly, and brain death may ensue. ABGs are monitored frequently to determine the adequacy of ventilation. Hyperventilation may be used to reduce $PCO_2$ and promote cerebral vasoconstriction to reduce cerebral edema.

In clients with long-term alterations in consciousness, such as vegetative state or locked-in syndrome, measures to maintain nutritional status are initiated. Enteral feedings with a gastrostomy tube are preferred if the client is unable to take enough food by mouth without aspirating. In some cases, parenteral nutrition may be used.

# NURSING CARE

## Nursing Diagnoses and Interventions

Nursing care of the client with an altered LOC is planned and implemented for a variety of responses. Nursing diagnoses and interventions discussed in this section are directed toward the unconscious client and focus on problems with airway maintenance, skin integrity, contractures, and nutrition.

### Ineffective Airway Clearance

Ineffective airway clearance related to loss of the cough reflex and the inability to expectorate is a major problem for the unconscious client. The cough reflex may be absent or impaired when conditions that produce coma depress the function of the medullary centers.

- Assess ability to clear secretions. Monitor breath sounds, rate and depth of respirations, dyspnea, pulse oximeter, and the presence of cyanosis. *The client's ability to clear secretions serves as the initial assessment base for developing further interventions.*

- In unconscious clients or those without an intact cough reflex, maintain an open airway by periodic suctioning, limiting the time of suctioning to 10 to 15 seconds or less. *Periodic suctioning may be necessary to clear the airway of mucus, blood, or other drainage. Suctioning for more than 15 seconds in the client with increased intracranial pressure may cause hypercapnia, which in turn vasodilates cerebral vessels, increases cerebral blood volume, and increases intracranial pressure.*

**PRACTICE ALERT** *If the client has a basilar skull fracture or cerebral spinal fluid draining from the ears or nose, never suction nasally.* ■

- Turn from side to side every 2 hours, and maintain a side-lying position with the head of the bed elevated approximately 30 degrees. Do not position the unconscious client on the back. *Turning the client from side to side facilitates respirations, prevents the tongue from obstructing the airway, and helps prevent pooling of secretions in one area of the lungs (thus decreasing the risk of pneumonia).*
- If the client has a tracheostomy, provide tracheostomy care every 4 hours and suction when secretions are present (see Chapter 35 ⟨∞⟩ ), *to maintain an open airway.*

### Risk for Aspiration

The unconscious client with a depressed or absent gag and swallowing reflex is at high risk for aspiration. Drainage, mucus, or blood may obstruct the airway and interfere with oxygenation. Pooling of aspiration secretions in the lungs also increases the risk of pneumonia.

- Assess swallowing and gag reflexes every shift as appropriate to the client's level of consciousness. *Deepening levels of unconsciousness may cause a loss in swallow and gag reflexes.*
- Monitor for and report manifestations of aspiration: crackles and wheezes, dullness to percussion over an area of the lungs, dyspnea, tachypnea, cyanosis. *Early recognition facilitates prompt intervention.*
- Provide interventions to prevent aspiration:
  - Maintain NPO status.
  - Place in the side-lying position.
  - Provide oral hygiene and suctioning as needed.

*The side-lying position allows secretions to drain from the mouth rather than into the pharynx. Oral hygiene and suctioning remove secretions that might otherwise be aspirated.*

**PRACTICE ALERT** *Never give unconscious clients oral food and fluids because of the risk of aspiration.* ■

- Monitor the results of arterial blood gas analysis and pulse oximetry. Maintain records of trends. *Arterial blood gases and pulse oximetry directly measure the oxygen content of blood and are good indicators of the lungs' ability to oxygenate the blood.*

### Risk for Impaired Skin Integrity

The unconscious client is at risk for impaired skin integrity as a result of immobility and the inability to provide self-care. On average, healthy people change positions during sleep every 11 minutes; the unconscious client often cannot maintain the movement needed to prevent pressure on the skin, especially over bony prominences. As a result, the skin and subcutaneous tissues may become ischemic and prone to develop pressure ulcers. Perspiration and incontinence of urine and stool may exacerbate the problem. Nursing interventions are directed to maintaining the integrity not only of the skin, but also of the lips and mucous membranes.

- Assess skin every shift, especially over bony prominences and around genitals and buttocks. The large surface area of the skin bears weight and is in constant contact with the surface of the bed. *The skin, subcutaneous tissue, and muscles, especially those tissues over bony prominences, undergo constant pressure. This impairs normal capillary blood flow, which interferes with the exchange of nutrients and waste products. Tissue ischemia and necrosis may result and lead to the development of pressure ulcers.*
- Provide proper positioning. Reposition bed-ridden clients at least every 2 hours if this is consistent with the overall treatment goals. Keep the head of the bed elevated no higher than 30 degrees. Provide special pads and mattresses that distribute weight more evenly (e.g., silicone-filled pads, egg-crate cushions, turning frames, flotation pads). Lift the client instead of dragging the client across the sheet. *When the head of the bed is elevated above 30 degrees, the client's torso tends to slide down toward the foot of the bed. Friction and perspiration cause the skin and superficial fascia to remain fixed against the bed linens while the deep fascia and skeleton slide downward. When a person is pulled rather than lifted, the skin remains fixed to the sheet while the fascia and muscles are pulled upward. These sheering forces promote tissue breakdown.*
- Provide interventions to prevent breakdown of the skin and mucous membranes:
  - Keep bed linens clean, dry, and wrinkle free.
  - Provide daily bath with mild soap.
  - Cleanse the skin after urine and fecal soiling with a mild cleansing agent.
  - Provide oral care and lubricate the lips every 2 to 4 hours.
  - Maintain accurate intake and output records.
  - Keep the cornea moist by instilling methyl cellulose solution (0.5% to 1%) and apply protective eye shields or close the eyelids with adhesive strips if the corneal reflex is absent.

*Keeping linens clean, dry, and wrinkle free decreases the risk of injury from the shearing force of bed rest and protects against environmental factors that cause drying. Adequate hydration of the stratum corneum appears to protect the skin against mechanical insult. Preventing dehydration maintains circulation and decreases the concentration of urine, thereby minimizing skin irritation in people who are incontinent. Proper eye care prevents corneal abrasion and irritation.*

## Impaired Physical Mobility

Clients who are unconscious are unable to maintain normal musculoskeletal movement and are at high risk for contractures related to decreased movement. Because the flexor and adductor muscles are stronger than the extensors and abductors, flexor and adductor contractures develop quickly without preventive measures. Passive ROM exercises must be performed routinely to maintain muscle tone and function, to prevent additional disability, and to help restore impaired motor function.

- Maintain extremities in functional positions by providing proper support devices. Remove support devices every 4 hours for skin care and passive ROM exercises. Provide pillows for the axillary region; rolled washcloths may be placed in elevated hands; use splints to prevent plantar flexion (foot-drop). *Pillows in the axillary region help prevent adduction of the shoulder. Rolled washcloths help decrease edema and flexion contracture of the fingers. Splints are useful in preventing plantar flexion. Remove these support devices every 4 hours to increase circulation to the area.*
- Perform passive ROM exercises (unless contraindicated, as for the client with increased intracranial pressure) at least four times a day, keeping the following principles in mind:
  - Place one hand above the joint being exercised. The other hand gently moves the joint through its normal range of motion.
  - Move the body part to the point of resistance, and stop. *Placing one hand above the joint provides support against gravity and prevents unwanted movement. ROM exercises help prevent contractures by stretching muscles and tendons and maintaining joint mobility.*

## Risk for Imbalanced Nutrition: Less Than Body Requirements

The unconscious client is at risk for an alteration in nutrition related to a reduced or complete inability to eat. This is especially true for the client who is unconscious as the result of an infection or trauma, both of which increase metabolic requirements.

- Monitor nutritional status through daily weights (on bed scales) and laboratory data. *For accuracy, weigh the client at the same time each day, using the same scales. Ensure that the client wears the same clothing. Changes in laboratory data with decreased nutrition include a decrease in the levels of serum albumin and serum transferrin.*
- Assess the need for alternative methods of nutritional support (tube feeding or total parenteral nutrition) through collaboration with dietitian. *Clients unable to take oral food require parenteral nutrition or liquid feedings through a nasogastric, gastrostomy, or jejunostomy tube. Needs for protein, calories, zinc, and vitamin C increase during wound healing.*

## Support of the Family

Family members of a client with an altered level of consciousness are often very anxious. It is difficult for the family to deal with the client's uncertain prognosis. They may experience various conflicting emotions, such as guilt and anger. Reinforce information provided by the physician, and encourage the family to talk to the client as though he or she were able to understand. Explain that this communication may initially seem awkward, but in time it will feel appropriate. Evaluate the family's readiness to receive explanations regarding the client's treatment and care. The presence of many tubes (e.g., intravenous line, catheter, ventilator) may be overwhelming to the family. They may misperceive the seriousness of the situation if a thorough explanation is not given. Include the family in the client's care as much as they wish to be involved.

Allow significant others to stay with the client when possible. Reinforce the need for family members to care for themselves by encouraging adequate meals and rest. Offer to contact support services, such as friends, neighbors, and social services that the hospital may provide. Ask family members to leave a telephone number where they can be reached, and assure them that they will be called if any significant changes occur. Encourage family members to call if they have questions or concerns.

# THE CLIENT WITH INCREASED INTRACRANIAL PRESSURE

**Intracranial pressure (ICP)** is the pressure within the cranial cavity, usually measured as the pressure within the lateral ventricles (Porth, 2002). Transient increases in ICP occur with normal activities such as coughing, sneezing, straining, or bending forward. These transient increases are not harmful; however, sustained increases in intracranial pressure can result in significant tissue ischemia and damage to delicate neural tissue. Cerebral edema is the most frequent cause of sustained increases in ICP. Other causes include head trauma, tumors, abscesses, stroke, inflammation, and hemorrhage.

## OVERVIEW OF NORMAL INTRACEREBRAL BLOOD FLOW AND PERFUSION

In the adult, the rigid cranial cavity created by the skull is normally filled to capacity with three essentially noncompressible elements: the brain (80%), cerebrospinal fluid (10%), and blood (10%). A state of dynamic equilibrium exists; if the volume of any of the three components increases, the volume of the others must decrease to maintain normal pressures within the cranial cavity. This is known as the *Monro-Kellie hypothesis.* The normal intracranial pressure is 5 to 15 mmHg (measured intracranially with a pressure transducer while the client is lying with the head elevated 30 degrees) or 60 to 180 cm $H_2O$ (measured with a water manometer while the client is lying in a lateral recumbent position) (McCance & Huether, 2002).

Cerebral blood flow and perfusion are important concepts for understanding the development and effects of increased intracranial pressure. Whereas blood and CSF contribute an equal percentage to normal intracranial volume, vascular factors account for twice the amount of increase in ICP that CSF does. The brain requires a constant supply of oxygen and glucose to meet its metabolic demands; 15% to 20% of the resting cardiac output goes to the brain to meet its metabolic needs. Interruption of the cerebral blood flow leads to ischemia and disruption of the cerebral metabolism. Cerebral hemodynamics include the following:

- Cerebral blood volume is the amount of blood in the intracranial vault at any one time. Normally about 10%, most is in the venous system, and is determined by autoregulatory mechanism.
- Cerebral blood flow is normally maintained at about 750 mL/min, a rate that matches or exceeds local metabolic needs of the brain. Cerebral blood flow is regulated through vasoconstriction or vasodilation of the cerebral vessels in response to changes in arterial oxygen and carbon dioxide concentrations.
- Cerebral perfusion pressure (CPP) is the pressure required to perfuse brain cells. It is the difference between the mean arterial pressure (MAP) and the ICP. Normal cerebral perfusion pressure is 80 to 100 mmHg. CPP must be at least 50 mmHg to provide minimal blood flow to the brain.

*Autoregulation* is a compensatory mechanism in which cerebral arterioles change diameter to maintain cerebral blood flow when ICP increases. The two forms of autoregulation are pressure autoregulation and chemical or metabolic autoregulation.

In pressure autoregulation, stretch receptors within small blood vessels of the brain cause smooth muscle of the arterioles to contract. Increased arterial pressure stimulates these receptors, leading to vasoconstriction; when arterial pressure is low, stimulation of these receptors decreases, causing relaxation and vasodilation.

Chemical, or metabolic, autoregulation works in much the same way as pressure autoregulation. In this case, the stimulus is a buildup of metabolic by-products of cell metabolism, including lactic acid, pyruvic acid, carbonic acid, and carbon dioxide. Carbon dioxide and increased hydrogen ion concentration are potent cerebral vasodilators that may act locally or systemically to increase cerebral blood flow. Conversely, a fall in $PaCO_2$ causes cerebral vasoconstriction. Arterial oxygen tension ($PaO_2$) also affects cerebral blood flow, although it is a less powerful mechanism than that exerted by carbon dioxide and hydrogen ions.

## PATHOPHYSIOLOGY AND MANIFESTATIONS OF INCREASED ICP

Increased ICP (also labeled **intracranial hypertension**) may result from an increase in intracranial contents from a space-occupying lesion, cerebral edema (swelling), excess cerebrospinal fluid, or intracranial hemorrhage. Displacement of some CSF to the spinal subarachnoid space and increased CSF absorption are early compensatory mechanisms. The low-pressure venous system is also compressed, and cerebral arteries constrict to reduce blood flow. Brain tissue's ability to accommodate change is relatively restricted (Porth, 2002). The relationship between the volume of the intracranial components and intracranial pressure is known as *compliance.* When the capacity to compensate for increased intracranial pressure

is exceeded, *increased intracranial pressure (hypertension)* develops. Intracranial hypertension is a sustained state of increased ICP and is potentially life-threatening.

Autoregulatory mechanisms have a limited ability to maintain cerebral blood flow. When autoregulation fails, cerebrovascular tone is reduced and cerebral blood flow becomes dependent on changes in blood pressure. Autoregulation may be lost either locally or globally because of several factors, including increasing intracranial pressure, local or diffuse cerebral tissue ischemia or inflammation, prolonged hypotension, and hypercapnia or hypoxia.

With loss of autoregulation, intracranial pressure continues to rise and cerebral perfusion falls. Cerebral tissue becomes ischemic, and manifestations of cellular hypoxia appear. Because the neurons of the cerebral cortex are most sensitive to oxygen deficit, changes in cortical function are the earliest manifestations of increasing ICP (Porth, 2002). Behavior and personality changes occur; the client may become irritable and agitated. Memory and judgment are impaired, and speech pattern changes may be noted. The client's LOC decreases. As cerebral hypertension and hypoxia progress, the LOC continues to decrease in a predictable pattern to coma and unresponsiveness.

Pressure on the pyramidal tract often causes weakness (hemiparesis) on the contralateral side early in increased ICP. As ICP continues to increase, hemiplegia and abnormal motor responses, such as decorticate or decerebrate posturing (see Chapter 40), develop.

Altered vision is an early manifestation of increased ICP; it is caused by pressure on the visual pathways and cranial nerves. Blurred vision, decreased visual acuity, and diplopia are common. Pupillary and oculomotor responses are affected as well. Because the cause of increased ICP is often localized at first, pupillary changes, including gradual dilation and sluggish response to light, may initially be limited to the ipsilateral side.

Additional manifestations of increased ICP include headache, particularly on rising, that worsens with position changes. Headache is more common with slowly developing increased ICP and occurs because of pressure on pain-sensitive structures, such as the middle meningeal arteries, the venous sinuses, and the dura at the base of the skull. Papilledema (edema and swelling of the optic disk) may be noted on fundoscopic examination. Vomiting, often projectile and occurring without warning, may develop.

Ischemia of the vasomotor center in the brainstem triggers the CNS ischemic response, a late sign of increased ICP. Neuronal ischemia in the vasomotor center causes a marked increase in the mean arterial pressure (MAP), with a significant increase in systolic blood pressure and increased pulse pressure. The increased MAP causes reflexive slowing of the cardiac rate. This trio of manifestations (increased MAP, increased pulse pressure, and bradycardia) is known as *Cushing's response (or triad),* and represents the brainstem's final effort to maintain cerebral perfusion (Porth, 2002). The respiratory pattern also changes, often in the predictable progression outlined in Table 42–1. Although the temperature is usually normal in early stages, as ICP continues to increase, hypothalamic function is impaired and the temperature may rise dramatically.

## Manifestations of Increased Intracranial Pressure

- Decreased level of consciousness. *Early:* Confusion, restlessness, lethargy; disorientation, first to time, then to place and person. *Late:* Comatose with no response to painful stimuli.
- Pupillary dysfunction. Sluggish response to light progressing to fixed pupils; with a localized process, pupillary dysfunction is first noted on the ipsilateral side.
- Oculomotor dysfunction. Inability to move eye(s) upward; ptosis (drooping) of the eyelid.
- Visual abnormalities. Decreased visual acuity, blurred vision, diplopia.
- Papilledema. May be late sign.
- Motor impairment. *Early:* Hemiparesis or hemiplegia of the contralateral side. *Late:* Abnormal responses such as decorticate or decerebrate positioning; flaccidity.
- Headache. Uncommon but may occur with processes that slowly increase ICP; worse on rising in the morning and with position changes.
- Projectile vomiting without nausea.
- Cushing's response. Increased systolic blood pressure, widening pulse pressure, bradycardia.
- Respirations. Altered respiratory pattern related to level of brain dysfunction.
- Temperature. May be significantly elevated as compensatory mechanisms fail.

The manifestations of increased ICP are listed in the box above.

## Cerebral Edema

**Cerebral edema** is an increase in the volume of brain tissue due to abnormal accumulation of fluid. Cerebral edema is often associated with increased intracranial pressure; it may occur as a local process in the area of a tumor or injury, or it may affect the entire brain. Three types of cerebral edema have been identified and are described as follows (Porth, 2002). The client with intracranial hypertension may have more than one type.

- *Vasogenic edema,* an increase in the capillary permeability of cerebral vessels, occurs with impairment of the blood-brain barrier, allowing diffusion of water and protein into the interstitial spaces of the brain's white matter. A variety of pathologies, such as ischemia, hemorrhage, brain tumors and injuries, and infections (such as meningitis), may cause the increase in capillary permeability. The site of the brain injury, the level of increase in capillary permeability, and the client's systemic blood pressure influence the rate and extent of the edema's spread. Vasogenic edema is manifested by focal neurologic deficits, altered levels of consciousness, and severe intracranial hypertension.
- *Cytotoxic edema,* an increase of fluid in the intracellular space (primarily in the gray matter), involves changes in the functional or structural integrity of cell membranes due to pathologies such as water intoxication or severe ischemia, intracranial hypoxia, acidosis, and brain trauma. With abnormally low cerebral perfusion, oxygen and nutrients are depleted, intracranial cells switch to anaerobic metabolism, and

the sodium-potassium pump in the cell walls is impaired. Sodium diffuses into the cells, pulling fluid after it. The cells swell, and intracranial pressure rises. Accumulated metabolic waste products, such as lactic acid, contribute to a rapid deterioration of cell function. Cytotoxic edema is a slowly progressive process that results in altered consciousness. The edema may be so severe that it causes cerebral infarction with brain tissue necrosis.
- *Interstitial cerebral edema* involves movement of CSF across the ventricular wall, resulting in water and sodium in the periventricular white space. This type is seen more often in pathologies that obstruct CSF flow through the ventricles, such as hydrocephalus or purulent meningitis.

Cerebral edema tends to be proportional to the extent of the pathology precipitating it. Brain function is not disrupted by cerebral edema unless the edema causes an increase in ICP. When it does, a vicious cycle can ensue: Cerebral edema increases ICP, which in turn decreases cerebral blood flow. Brain tissue becomes hypoxic and ischemic, increasing toxic metabolic by-products, hydrogen ion concentration, and carbon dioxide levels in the tissue. Autoregulatory mechanisms cause vasodilation and increase cerebral blood flow, further increasing cerebral edema and intracranial pressure. Without effective intervention, the client's condition can deteriorate rapidly; intracranial pressure increases to the point where brain structures herniate.

## Hydrocephalus

**Hydrocephalus** is an increase in volume of CSF within the ventricular system, which becomes dilated. Hydrocephalus may increase ICP when it develops acutely. Hydrocephalus occurs when the production of CSF exceeds its absorption. It is generally classified as either noncommunicating or communicating hydrocephalus. *Noncommunicating hydrocephalus* occurs when CSF drainage from the ventricular system is obstructed. It may develop when a mass or tumor, inflammation or hemorrhage, or congenital malformation obstructs the ventricular system. *Communicating hydrocephalus* is a condition in which CSF is not effectively reabsorbed through the arachnoid villi. It may occur secondarily to subarachnoid hemorrhage or scarring from infection. In *normal pressure hydrocephalus,* seen most often in adults age 60 or older, ventricular enlargement causes cerebral tissue compression but the CSF pressure on lumbar puncture is normal. This condition may follow cerebral trauma or surgery, or the cause may not be known. Manifestations of hydrocephalus depend on the rate of its development. They may be mild and insidious in onset, presenting as progressive cognitive dysfunctions, gait disruptions, and urinary incontinence. If the process causing hydrocephalus is an acute one, the manifestations are those of increased ICP.

## Brain Herniation

If increased ICP is not treated, cerebral tissue is displaced toward a more compliant area. This can result in **brain herniation,** the displacement of brain tissue from its normal compartment under dural folds of the falx cerebri or through the tentorial notch or incisura of the tentorium cerebelli (Porth,

2002). Herniation of the cerebellum through the tentorium exerts pressure on the brainstem, with subsequent herniation through the foramen magnum. This is a lethal complication of increased ICP because it puts pressure on the vital centers of the medulla.

Brain herniation syndromes are generally categorized as supratentorial or infratentorial, depending on their location above or below the tentorium cerebelli (Figure 42–2 ■). Supratentorial herniation syndromes include cingulate herniation, central or transtentorial herniation, and uncal or lateral transtentorial herniation.

- *Cingulate herniation* (Figure 42–2A) occurs when the cingulate gyrus is displaced under the falx cerebri. Local blood supply and cerebral tissue are compressed, resulting in ischemia and further increases in intracranial pressure.
- *Central or transtentorial* herniation is the downward displacement of brain structures, including the cerebral hemispheres, basal ganglia, diencephalon, and midbrain through the tentorial incisura (Figure 42–2B). The client's neurologic signs may deteriorate rapidly, with decreased LOC progressing to coma, Cheyne-Stokes respirations progressing to central neurogenic hyperventilation, and pupils progressing from small and reactive to midsize and fixed. The client may demonstrate abnormal motor responses with unilateral decorticate posturing.
- *Uncal or lateral transtentorial* herniation occurs when a lateral mass displaces cerebral tissue centrally, forcing the medial aspect of the temporal lobe under the edge of the tentorial incisura (Figure 42–2C). The oculomotor nerve (cranial nerve III) often becomes trapped between the uncus and the tentorium, causing ipsilateral pupillary dilation. Other manifestations include alterations in LOC, motor deficits (which

may occur on the same side as the herniation because of compression of the cerebral peduncle on the opposite side), decreased sensation, respiratory changes, abnormal positioning, and eventual respiratory arrest.

- *Infratentorial herniation* results from increased pressure within the infratentorial compartment. Herniation may occur either upward, with structures displaced through the tentorial incisura, or downward, with displacement through the foramen magnum (Figure 42–2D). Downward displacement compresses the medulla, including its centers for controlling vital functions. Manifestations associated with medullary compression include coma, altered respiratory patterns, fixed pupils, and decorticate or decerebrate posturing. Respiratory or cardiac arrest may occur.

## COLLABORATIVE CARE

Care of the client with increased ICP is directed toward identifying and treating the underlying cause of the disorder, and controlling ICP to prevent herniation syndrome. Increased ICP is a medical emergency, and there is little time to complete lengthy diagnostic tests. The diagnosis must be made on the basis of observation and neurologic assessment; even subtle changes may be clinically significant.

### Diagnostic Tests

Diagnostic tests focus on identifying the presence of increased ICP and its underlying cause. A CT scan or MRI is generally the initial test. These tests are used to identify the possible causes of increased ICP (such as space-occupying lesions or hydrocephalus) and to evaluate therapeutic options. In general, a lumbar puncture is not performed when increased ICP is suspected because the sudden release of the pressure in the skull may cause cerebral herniation.

In addition to the diagnostic tests listed in the previous section for altered LOC, the following specific tests are ordered and their results closely monitored.

- *Serum osmolality* is an indicator of hydration status in the client with increased ICP. The test measures the number of dissolved particles (electrolytes, urea, glucose) in the serum. The normal range for the adult is 280 to 300 mOsm/kg $H_2O$. In addition to the restriction of fluids in the client with increased ICP, serum osmolality is maintained at a slightly elevated level (325 mOsm/kg $H_2O$) to draw excess intracellular fluid into the vascular system.
- *ABGs* are monitored frequently to assess pH and levels of oxygen and carbon dioxide. Hydrogen ions and carbon dioxide are both potent vasodilators; hypoxemia also causes vasodilation, although to a lesser degree.

### Medications

Medications play an important role in the management of increased ICP. Diuretics, particularly osmotic diuretics, are commonly used to reduce ICP and are the mainstays of pharmacologic treatment.

Osmotic diuretics work by increasing the osmolarity of the blood, thereby drawing water out of edematous brain tissue and

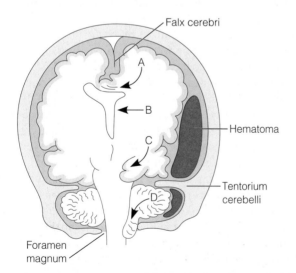

**Figure 42–2** ■ Forms of brain herniation due to intracranial hypertension. *A,* Cingulate herniation occurs when the cingulate gyrus is compressed under the falx cerebri. *B,* Central herniation occurs when a centrally located lesion compresses central and midbrain structures. *C,* Lateral herniation occurs when a lesion at the side of the brain compresses the uncus or hippocampal gyrus. *D,* Infratentorial herniation occurs when the cerebellar tonsils are forced downward, compressing the medulla and top of the spinal cord.

into the vascular system for elimination via the kidneys. The effects of these drugs vary with the type of injury. Regardless of the agent used, the optimal dose is the lowest that reduces ICP. Mannitol is the most commonly employed osmotic diuretic. Glucose, urea, and glycerol are other osmotic diuretics that may be used. Urine output by Foley catheter is monitored. Electrolyte levels are carefully assessed and potassium is replaced as indicated.

Loop diuretics, such as furosemide (Lasix) (the drug of choice) and ethacrynic acid (Edecrin), may be prescribed for some clients with increased ICP. These diuretics act on the renal tubule and are extremely effective in promoting diuresis. Additionally, loop diuretics may be used to manage the rebound effect that may occur with mannitol administration.

Antipyretics, such as acetaminophen, are used alone or in combination with a hypothermia blanket to treat hyperthermia.

Hyperthermia increases the cerebral metabolic rate and exacerbates an existing increase in ICP. Anticonvulsants are often required to manage seizure activity associated with brain injury and increased ICP. Gastrointestinal prophylaxis with histamine $H_2$ antagonists or sucralfate (Carafate) is often used, as clients with ICP are at increased risk for the development of stress ulcers.

To treat clients with severe, persistent intracranial hypertension that does not respond to other therapy, barbiturates may be used to induce coma. The mechanism of action of this controversial therapy is unclear, but it is thought to reduce metabolic demands in the injured brain. Because neurologic signs are masked, close monitoring of the client in induced coma is vital.

Nursing implications for these medications are described in the box below.

## Medication Administration

### Increased Intracranial Pressure

#### OSMOTIC DIURETICS

Mannitol (Osmitrol)
Urea
Glucose

Osmotic diuretics (hyperosmotic agents) draw fluid out of brain cells by increasing the osmolality of the blood. The effects of these drugs vary with the type of injury. Mannitol therapy is often initiated if the client's ICP has exceeded 15 to 20 mmHg for at least 10 minutes. Both intravenous bolus and continuous infusion techniques are used. Repeated use of mannitol can lead to continual elevations in serum osmolality, with attendant risk of seizures and serious fluid and electrolyte imbalance. Urea is seldom administered intravenously because a severe local reaction may result if leakage occurs at the injection site. Mannitol and urea are used cautiously if renal disease is present.

**Note:** Because the client with increased intracranial pressure often has an altered level of consciousness, client and family teaching is not discussed in this box.

#### Nursing Responsibilities
- Monitor vital signs, urinary output, central venous pressure (CVP), and pulmonary artery pressures (PAP) before and every hour throughout administration.
- Assess client for manifestations of dehydration.
- Assess client for muscle weakness, numbness, tingling, paresthesia, confusion, and excessive thirst.
- Assess client for pulmonary edema while administering the medication.
- Monitor neurologic status and intracranial pressure readings.
- Monitor renal function and serum electrolytes throughout therapy.
- Do not administer the medication if crystals are present in solution. Administer with an in-line filter. Observe infusion site frequently for infiltration.
- Do not administer mannitol solution with blood.
- Do not discontinue medication abruptly. Rebound migraine headaches may occur.

#### LOOP DIURETICS

Furosemide (Lasix)
Ethacrynic acid (Edecrin)

Loop diuretics such as furosemide and ethacrynic acid inhibit sodium and chloride reabsorption at the ascending loop of Henle. They cause a reduction in the rate of CSF production, thus reducing the ICP.

#### Nursing Responsibilities
- Monitor vital signs and electrolyte values closely.
- Assess fluid status throughout therapy.
- Monitor blood pressure and pulse before and during administration.
- Monitor renal laboratory studies closely.
- Use infusion pump to ensure accurate dosage.

#### INTRAVENOUS FLUIDS

Keeping the client moderately dehydrated to maintain serum osmolality can be effective in reducing cerebral edema. When giving intravenous fluids, closely monitor the osmolality of the solutions; if clients with increased ICP are given hypo-osmolar solutions, increased cerebral edema can occur. Preferred solutions include 0.45% to 0.9% sodium chloride solutions.

#### Nursing Responsibilities
- Monitor fluid status closely.
- Monitor neurologic status closely.
- Avoid administering hypo-osmolar solutions, such as 5% dextrose in water.
- Half-strength normal saline (0.45% sodium chloride) is considered a suitable fluid for a client who has increased intracranial pressure.
- Take care not to restrict fluids excessively in clients receiving dehydrating agents (such as osmotic or loop diuretics).

#### OTHER PHARMACOLOGIC INTERVENTIONS FOR ICP
- Antipyretics, such as acetaminophen, are used to reduce hyperthermia, thereby decreasing the high cerebral metabolism that contributes to ICP.
- Antiulcer drugs, such as histamine $H_2$ antagonists (for example, ranitidine [Zantac]) or sucralfate (Carafate), are used in clients with ICP to decrease the development of stress ulcers.
- Antihypertensive agents, such as beta-adrenergic blocking agents, may be used if the mean arterial pressure is high.
- Vasopressors may be used if the mean arterial pressure is low.
- Anticonvulsants may be given to prevent or treat seizures.

Intravenous fluids are usually necessary to maintain the client's fluid and electrolyte balance as well as vascular volume. If the client's blood pressure is unstable, vasoactive medications may be administered to maintain the MAP in a range that supports cerebral perfusion while minimizing increases in ICP. When enteral feeding is not possible, total parenteral nutrition may be administered.

## Treatments

### Surgery

Clients with increased ICP may undergo various intracranial surgical techniques to treat the underlying cause (see the discussion in the later section on brain tumors). In addition, infarcted or necrotic tissue may be resected to reduce brain mass. A drainage catheter or shunt may be inserted laterally via a burr hole into a ventricle to drain excess cerebrospinal fluid and reduce hydrocephalus. The removal of even a small amount of CSF may dramatically reduce ICP and restore cerebral perfusion pressure.

### ICP Monitoring

Intracranial pressure monitors facilitate continual assessment of ICP and are more precise than often vague clinical manifestations. With these devices, the effects of medical therapy and nursing interventions on ICP can also be monitored. In addition, cerebral perfusion pressure (the difference between MAP and ICP) can be readily calculated, allowing more precise manipulation of therapeutic measures to maintain cerebral perfusion and thereby prevent ischemia. The criteria for ICP monitoring depends on the client, but in general, clients who are comatose and have a Glasgow Coma Score of 8 or less should be monitored.

Basic monitoring systems include an intraventricular catheter, subarachnoid bolt or screw, and epidural probe (Figure 42–3 ■). Intraventricular fluid-filled catheters are placed in the anterior horn of the lateral ventricle (most often in the right side). They can both drain CSF and measure ICP. The ICP value is measured deep in the brain and is considered the most reflective of the whole brain pressure. Subarachnoid devices are placed in the subarachnoid space. Epidural catheters are usually fiberoptic pressure transducers; they do not penetrate the dura and are considered relatively noninvasive. A fiberoptic transducer-tipped catheter can be placed in the epidural, subdural, or l parenchymal space, with ICP values considered very accurate. Subarachnoid, epidural, or fiberoptic monitoring devices can drain CSF. The choice of monitor depends on both the suspected disorder and the physician's preference. Once the intracranial sensor is implanted, it is con-

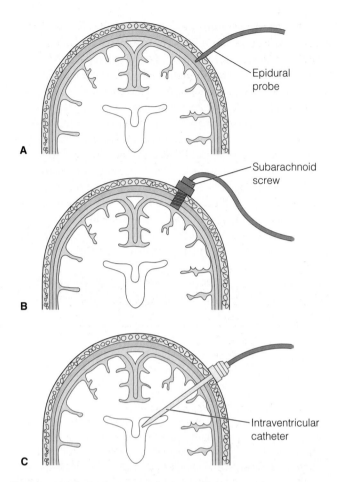

**Figure 42–3 ■** Types of intracranial pressure monitoring. *A*, Epidural probe. *B*, Subarachnoid screw. *C*, Intraventricular catheter.

nected to a transducer that converts the impulses to a signal that the recording device can translate into an oscilloscope tracing, digital value, or graphic recording. Factors that increase the risk for infection during ICP monitoring are listed in Box 42–1.

### Mechanical Ventilation

Clients who require intubation for airway management are placed on a ventilator. Mechanical ventilation may be used to maintain partial pressure of oxygen and carbon dioxide, thus preventing hypoxemia and hypercapnia, both of which can increase intracranial pressure (Hilton, 2001). It is important to maintain adequate oxygenation with a partial pressure of arterial oxygen at about 100 mmHg and a partial pressure of arterial

| BOX 42–1 ■ Risk Factors for Infection with Intracranial Pressure Monitoring | |
|---|---|
| **Factor** | **Rationale** |
| Intraventricular catheter | Is more invasive than other monitoring devices |
| Open head trauma or neurosurgery | Disrupts protective skin and skeletal barriers |
| Intracranial hemorrhage | Necessitates frequent flushing of catheter to maintain patency |
| Older adult | Tends to have impaired immune defenses |
| Monitoring for more than 3 to 5 days; or open system or frequent irrigation | Offers increased opportunity for pathogens to enter and grow |

carbon dioxide of about 35 mmHg (Bucher & Melander, 1999). The client with increased ICP and signs of impending herniation may be judiciously hyperventilated to cause cerebral vasoconstriction; however, this also increases cerebral ischemia.

## NURSING CARE

The nursing care of clients with increased ICP involves identifying those at risk and managing factors known to increase intracranial pressure. A major focus is protecting the client from sudden increases in ICP or a decrease in cerebral blood flow.

### Nursing Diagnoses and Interventions

Nursing interventions include performing neurologic assessments, maintaining the patency of the airway, ensuring adequate ventilation, positioning and moving, instituting seizure precautions, and monitoring fluids and electrolytes. Additionally, both client and family need emotional support during this period. The client with increased ICP has varied responses to actual or potential changes in physiologic processes (see the box below).

### Ineffective Tissue Perfusion: Cerebral

A number of disorders may lead to increased ICP, including cerebral edema, hydrocephalus, space-occupying lesions and hemorrhage, herniation syndromes, and changes in carbon dioxide concentrations. Increasing intracranial pressure alters cerebral perfusion and oxygenation of brain cells. The client with increased ICP requires intensive care, and often needs ventilator assistance.

- Assess for and report any of the manifestations of increasing ICP every 1 to 2 hours and as necessary. Assessment areas include level of consciousness, behavior, motor/sensory functions, pupillary size and reaction to light, and vital signs, including temperature. Look for trends, because vital signs alone do not correlate well with early deterioration. *Assessment of neurologic status establishes the client's clinical condition and provides a baseline to measure changes. Sudden changes in neurologic signs often indicate deterioration. An elevated temperature with increased oxygen consumption further increases intracranial pressure. Pupillary responses mirror the status of the midbrain and pons. Pressure on the brainstem may compromise the function of cranial nerves IX and X and protective mechanisms, such as the gag and cough reflexes.*

**PRACTICE ALERT**  *Often, the earliest manifestations of a change in intracranial pressure are alterations in the level of consciousness and breathing patterns.* ∎

- For the client on a ventilator: Maintain patency of the airway; preoxygenate with 100% oxygen before suctioning; limit suctioning to 10 seconds; suction gently. *Preoxygenation helps maintain oxygen levels during suctioning. Suctioning stimulates the cough reflex and Valsalva maneuver. Correct suctioning minimizes the risk of hypoxemia.*
- Monitor arterial blood gases (ABGs). *ABGs provide a reliable indicator of oxygen and carbon dioxide levels. If oxygen concentration is low, oxygen may be given or increased.*

## Nursing Research

### Evidence-Based Practice for Clients with Increased Intracranial Pressure

Nursing diagnoses are made based on the presence of defining characteristics. This study (Wall et al., 1995) was conducted to identify defining characteristics and risk factors for the nursing diagnoses of *Increased intracranial pressure* and *High risk for increased intracranial pressure*. Although this diagnosis is not listed in the NANDA taxonomy, the authors believe it should be. A national sample of nurses who care for clients with neurologic impairments were surveyed, and a number of defining characteristics were validated. The researchers concluded that the defining characteristics and risk factors identified in the literature represent these diagnoses well, although additional characteristics may be present in the clinical setting. Further clinical studies are recommended, with differentiation of characteristics specific to various settings and specialty areas.

The authors of this study believe that findings can assist nurses to identify relevant defining characteristics and risk factors, make a diagnosis, and implement appropriate interventions. Findings can also be helpful to students in learning critical thinking and diagnostic reasoning skills.

### IMPLICATIONS FOR NURSING

It is very important that nursing interventions be knowledge based. Studies such as this are important in defining the language of nursing and in facilitating the classification of nursing language. To provide safe and knowledgeable care, nurses must make accurate assessments, recognize and differentiate characteristics that support specific diagnoses, provide interventions, and evaluate outcomes of care.

### Critical Thinking in Client Care

1. Do you believe that increased intracranial pressure is a human response to an actual or a potential health problem? Can nurses select the interventions to treat this problem? Why or why not?
2. Provide a rationale for nursing assessment and monitoring of each of the following manifestations (defining characteristics) of increased intracranial pressure:
   a. Eye opening, motor and verbal responses
   b. Vital signs
   c. Pupillary responses
   d. Vomiting
   e. Headache
   f. Level of consciousness
3. Describe the rationale for administering intravenous fluids by an infusion pump to the client with a severe head injury.

- Elevate head of the bed to 30 degrees or keep flat, as prescribed; maintain the alignment of the head and neck to avoid hyperextension or exaggerated neck flexion; avoid prone position. *Keeping the head of the bed elevated facilitates venous drainage from the cerebrum. Obstruction of jugular veins can impede venous drainage from the brain (Sullivan, 2000).*
- Assess for bladder distention and bowel constipation. Administer stool softeners and use the Credé technique to empty the bladder. If the Credé technique is not effective, evaluate the pros and cons of urinary catheterization if the bladder remains distended. *Constipation and bladder distention increase intrathoracic or intra-abdominal pressure and place the client at risk for impaired venous drainage from the brain.*
- Assist in moving up in bed. Do not ask to push with heels or arms or push against a footboard. Avoid a footboard and restraints. *Moving up in bed requires pushing. Helping the client move prevents initiation of the Valsalva maneuver, which increases intracranial pressure.*
- Plan nursing care so that activities are not clustered together; avoid turning the client, getting the client on the bedpan, or suctioning within the same time period. Schedule nursing care to provide rest periods between procedures. *Multiple procedures, including certain nursing care activities, can increase ICP. Constant stimulation tends to increase ICP. Individualized nursing care ensures optimal spacing of activities and rest.*
- Provide a quiet environment, limiting noxious stimuli. Avoid jarring the bed. Try to limit situations that cause emotional upset; maintain a calm, reassuring manner; caution family members to refrain from unpleasant conversations or that may be emotionally stimulating to the client. *Noxious stimuli and emotional upsets cause an elevation in ICP.*
- Maintain fluid limitations, if prescribed. *Restricting fluids helps decrease cerebral edema by reducing total body water.*

### Risk for Infection

Although any client with an open head wound is at risk for infection, the interventions discussed here are for the client with an intracranial monitoring device. Most clinical units have written protocols for managing these systems. The following nursing actions serve only as a general guide.

- Keep dressings over the catheter dry, and change dressings on a prescribed basis (usually every 24 to 48 hours). *Wet dressings are conducive to bacterial growth.*
- Monitor the insertion site for leaking CSF, drainage, or infection. Monitor for manifestations of infection, including changes in vital signs, chills, increased WBC counts, and positive cultures of drainage. *Close monitoring helps detect the earliest signs of infection and helps prevent major complications. Fever is usually considered the key assessment. However, fever in a client with a neurologic disorder may be due to damage to the hypothalamus. Headache, generalized muscle aches, shivering, and chills may also be seen in the client with infection.*
- Use strict aseptic technique when in contact with the device. Check drainage system for loose connections. *The use of aseptic technique and monitoring drainage systems for loose connections helps prevent nosocomial infections. Most nosocomial infections are transmitted by health care workers who fail to wash their hands properly, to change gloves between clients, or to follow aseptic technique protocols. Invasive procedures provide an excellent opportunity for microbes to enter the body.*

### Client and Family Teaching

Teach the client at risk for increased ICP (and able to follow instructions) to avoid coughing, blowing the nose, straining to have a bowel movement, pushing against the bed rails, or performing isometric (muscle contracting) exercises. Advise the client to maintain head and neck alignment when turning in bed and to take rest periods.

Encourage the family to talk to the client, but maintain a quiet environment with a minimum of stimuli. Inform family members that upsetting the client may increase intracranial pressure and that they should avoid discussions that may distress the client. For clients unable to make decisions about treatment and to sign informed consent, the family must carry out these functions.

## THE CLIENT WITH A HEADACHE

**Headache** is pain within the cranial vault. Headache is one of the most common symptoms people experience, although its cause is frequently unknown. Headaches may occur as a result of benign or pathologic conditions, intracranial or extracranial conditions, diseases of other body systems, stress, musculoskeletal tension, or a combination of these factors.

Most headaches are mild, transient, and relieved by a mild analgesic. However, some headaches are chronic, intense, and recurrent. Manifestations of headache vary according to the cause, type, and precipitating symptoms.

## PATHOPHYSIOLOGY AND MANIFESTATIONS

Selected structures within the cranial vault are sensitive to pain. Pain-sensitive structures include supporting structures, such as the skin, muscles, and periosteum; the nasal cavities and sinuses; portions of the meninges, cranial nerves II, III, IV, V, VI, IX, and X; and cerebral vessels, including extracranial arteries and the venous sinuses. Most facial and scalp structures are sensitive to pain. Stretching (traction), inflammation, pressure compression, and dilation of the pain-sensitive structures of the cranial vault, scalp, and face can produce a headache. The most common types of headaches are tension, migraine, and cluster headaches (Table 42–4).

### Tension Headache

**Tension headache,** the most common type of headache, is characterized by bilateral pain, with a sensation of a band of tightness or pressure around the head. Sharply localized painful

## TABLE 42-4  Comparison of Migraine, Cluster, and Tension Headaches

| Type | Risk Factors | Frequency and Duration | Description | Prodromal and Associated Manifestations |
|------|--------------|------------------------|-------------|------------------------------------------|
| Migraine | Female<br>Family history of migraine headache.<br>Age not a risk factor. | Episodic:<br>• Tends to occur with stress and crisis.<br>• Often correlates with menstrual cycle.<br>• Can last hours to days. | Slow onset; pain becomes more severe, involving one side of head more than other. | Prodromal manifestations: visual defects, confusion, paresthesias.<br>Associated manifestations: nausea, vomiting, chills, fatigue, irritability, sweating. |
| Cluster | Male<br>Use of alcohol or nitrates.<br>May begin in early childhood. | Episodes are clustered together in rapid succession for a few days or weeks with remissions that last for months.<br>Can last a few minutes to a few hours. | May begin in infraorbital region and spread to head and neck; throbbing, deep pain, often unilateral. | Prodromal manifestations: uncommon.<br>Associated manifestations: flushing, tearing of eyes, nasal congestion, sweating and swelling of temporal vessels. |
| Tension | Related to tension and anxiety.<br>No family history.<br>Often begins in adolescence. | Episodic:<br>• Varies with amount of stress.<br>• Duration also varies; can be constant. | Tight, pressing, viselike; may involve neck and shoulders. | Prodromal manifestations: uncommon.<br>Associated manifestations: sustained contraction of neck muscles. |

spots (trigger points) may be present. The onset is gradual, and the intensity, frequency, and duration of the attack vary greatly. This type of headache is caused by sustained contraction of the muscles of the head and neck. It is often precipitated by stressful situations and anxiety. Secondary causes include disorders of the eyes, ears, sinuses, or cervical vertebrae. Abnormal posture associated with occupations that require bending over a desk (e.g., office workers, students) often precipitates tension-type headache. Additionally, slouching while reading or watching television can lead to muscle contraction. Most headaches are tension-type headaches.

## Migraine Headache

**Migraine headache** is a recurring vascular headache often initiated by a triggering event and usually accompanied by a neurologic dysfunction. It affects as many as 23 million people in the United States (5 million men and 18 million women) (Lin, 2001). It is more common between the ages of 25 to 55 years. There is often a positive family history. Headaches classified as migraines may differ in intensity, duration, and frequency. The exact causes of migraine are not fully understood, but they are believed to be the result of abnormalities in cerebrovascular blood flow, a reduction in brain and electrical activity, or increased release of sensory substances such as serotonin, norepinephrine, substance P, nitric oxide, and glutamate (McCance & Huether, 2002).

The classic migraine headache has several stages, including the aura stage, the headache stage (or period of throbbing), and the postheadache stage.

• The **aura** stage is characterized by sensory manifestations, usually visual disturbances such as bright spots or flashing lights zig-zagging across the visual fields. This stage lasts from 5 to 60 minutes. Less common sensory symptoms include numbness or tingling of the face or hand, paresis of an arm or leg, mild aphasia, confusion, drowsiness, and lack of coordination. Additionally, some clients experience a premonition the day prior to an attack. They may feel nervous or have other mood changes. The aura period corresponds with the initial physiologic change of vasoconstriction.

• The headache stage is characterized by vasodilation, a decline in serotonin levels, and the onset of throbbing headache. It appears that the pain is related to increased vessel permeability and polypeptide exudation by perivascular nerve endings rather than the vasodilation itself. Cerebral arteries are dilated and distended, with walls that are edematous and rigid. Beginning unilaterally, the headache eventually may involve both sides as it increases in intensity during the next several hours. Nausea and vomiting often occur. The client may be acutely ill and is often extremely irritable. The sensory organs often become hypersensitive, and the client withdraws from sound and light. The scalp is tender. The headache may last from several hours to a day or two.

• During the postheadache phase, the headache area is sensitive to touch, and a deep aching is present. The client is exhausted. Vessel size and serotonin levels return to normal.

A variety of factors are believed to trigger the onset of a migraine headache. Rapid changes in blood glucose levels, stress, emotional excitement, fatigue, hormonal changes due to menstruation, stimuli such as bright lights, and food high in tyramine or other vasoactive substances (e.g., aged cheese, nuts, chocolate, and alcoholic beverages) have been associated with migraine attacks. Hypertension and febrile states may make the disorder worse.

Another type of migraine headache is called a *migraine without aura*. This type is the most common and is associated with hereditary factors. The aura stage is absent; clients are aware only that a headache is eminent. The headache develops gradually, lasting hours to days, and may occur during periods of premenstrual tension and fluid retention. Chills, nausea and vomiting, fatigue, and nasal congestion are often present.

## Cluster Headache

The **cluster headache** is predominantly experienced by middle-aged men. The physiologic mechanism underlying cluster headaches is not well understood, but involves a vascular disorder, a disturbance of serotonergic mechanisms, a sympathetic defect, or dysregulation of the hypothalamus.

Although the headache may occur at any time, it typically begins 2 to 3 hours after falling asleep, awakens the person, and then lasts for less than 2 hours. Prodromal signs are absent. Intense unilateral pain around or behind one eye wakes the client. The pain is accompanied by rhinorrhea, lacrimation, flushing, sweating, facial edema, and possible miosis or ptosis on the affected side. Headaches last 30 minutes to a few hours and abate abruptly.

The attacks tend to occur frequently, in clusters of 1 to 8 daily, for weeks or a few months. The headaches often occur in the spring and fall and then disappear for an extended period. The same side of the head is involved in each cluster of attacks. Attacks may be triggered by drinking alcohol or eating specific foods, or there may be no known precipitating event.

## COLLABORATIVE CARE

Identifying the underlying cause(s) of the headache is the initial focus of collaborative care. If the underlying cause is treatable, the headache will often decrease or disappear. An accurate diagnosis of the type of headache is key to the treatment.

Therapeutic management for migraine headache includes a combination of client teaching, medications, and measures to control contributing factors. Dietary changes such as eliminating caffeine, cured meats, monosodium glutamate (MSG), and foods containing tyramine (red wine, aged cheese, and others) may be necessary. Stress management or biofeedback are also part of the overall strategy. Treatment protocols for cluster headache include eliminating aggravating factors (e.g., consumption of alcohol) and using medications and oxygen inhalation. The management of tension headaches is directed toward reducing the client's level of stress and relieving pain with ice and aspirin or NSAIDs.

## Diagnostic Tests

Diagnosis and treatment are based on history, the identification of triggering or precipitating events, and the type of headache. A thorough history and physical examination are integral parts of the assessment. Neurodiagnostic testing may be done to rule out a structural disease process. Testing may

include a brain scan, MRI, X-ray studies of the skull and cervical spine, EEG, or lumbar puncture for CSF if inflammation is suspected. Serum metabolic screens and hypersensitivity testing also may be performed if systemic problems are suspected.

## Medications

Pharmacologic management depends on the type of headache. The goals of treatment are to reduce the frequency and severity of headaches and to limit or relieve a headache that is beginning or in progress.

The management of migraine headache includes administering medications to prevent pain (prophylactic therapy) as well as drugs to stop (or abort) a headache in progress. The client with frequent migraine headaches is a candidate for prophylactic therapy. Drugs used to reduce the frequency and severity of migraine follow:

- Methysergide maleate (Sansert) is a serotonin antagonist that competitively blocks serotonin receptors in the CNS and is also a potent vasoconstrictor.
- Propranolol hydrochloride (Inderal) is a beta blocker that prevents dilation of vessels in the pia mater and inhibits serotonin uptake.
- Verapamil (Isoptin) is a calcium channel blocker that is thought to prevent migraine by controlling cerebral vasospasms.

When the manifestations of migraine are recognized early, several medications may be used to abort or limit the severity and duration of the headache. Ergotamine tartrate (Cafergot) is a complex drug that reduces extracranial blood flow, decreases the amplitude of cranial artery pulsation, and decreases basilar artery hyperperfusion. Administered at the onset of an attack, ergotamine controls up to 70% of acute attacks. Sumatriptan (Imitrex) is available in oral, nasal spray, or subcutaneous injection forms. It binds with serotonin$_1$ receptors and is rapidly effective. Zolmitriptan (Zomig), a selective serotonin$_1$ receptor agonist, is administered orally and is effective in the treatment of acute headache. Once a migraine is in progress, a narcotic analgesic such as codeine or meperidine (Demerol) may be required. Antiemetics may be prescribed to control nausea and vomiting.

Many of the same medications used for migraine also prevent or treat cluster headache. Because the onset of cluster headaches is abrupt, abortive therapy is not possible. Medications such as ergotamine tartrate may be given in suppository form at bedtime to prevent headache during the episodic attacks. Clients may find that inhaling 100% oxygen at 7 L/min for 15 minutes at the onset of an attack relieves their headache (Tierney et al., 2001).

Nonnarcotic analgesics such as aspirin or acetaminophen may relieve tension headaches. Additionally, tranquilizers such as diazepam may reduce muscle tension.

Nursing implications for drugs commonly prescribed for headaches are described in the Medication Administration box on pages 1363–1364.

# Medication Administration

## Headaches

### BETA BLOCKERS

> Propanolol hydrochloride (Inderal)
> Nadolol (Corgard)
> Atenolol (Tenormin)
> Timolol maleate (Blocadren)

Beta blockers are effective in the prophylactic treatment of headache. They act by combining with beta-adrenergic receptors to block the response to sympathetic nerve impulses, circulating catecholamines, or adrenergic drugs.

#### Nursing Responsibilities

- Before beginning therapy, determine pulse and blood pressure in both arms with client lying, sitting, and standing.
- Assess baseline and monitor serum glucose level, CBC, electrolytes, and liver and renal function studies.
- Note any history of diabetes or impaired renal function.
- Note the rate and quality of respirations; drugs in this category may cause dyspnea and bronchospasm.
- Administer the drug with meals to prevent gastrointestinal disturbances.
- Be alert that beta blockers cause bradycardia and the heart rate may not rise in response to stress, such as exercise or fever. Notify the primary health care provider if pulse falls below 50 or if blood pressure changes significantly.
- Teach the client or family member how to take a pulse and blood pressure reading.

#### Client and Family Teaching

- Take the medication with meals to provide a coating for the gastrointestinal tract and prevent gastrointestinal disturbances.
- Return for blood work as prescribed.
- Take the last dose of the day at bedtime.
- Rise from a sitting or lying position to a standing position slowly to avoid dizziness and falls.
- Take pulse and blood pressure each day and maintain a record of readings.
- Avoid excessive intake of alcohol, coffee, tea, or cola. Consult with the health care provider before taking any over-the-counter medications.
- Report any cough, nasal stuffiness, or feelings of depression to the health care provider.

### TRICYCLIC ANTIDEPRESSANTS

> Imipramine hydrochloride (Tofranil)
> Amitriptyline hydrochloride (Elavil)

The tricyclic antidepressants have been successful in the prophylaxis of cluster and migraine headaches. Although the exact mechanism is not known, they do prevent the reuptake of norepinephrine or serotonin, or both. They are chemically related to the phenothiazines, and as such they exhibit many of the same pharmacologic effects (e.g., anticholinergic, antiserotonin, sedative, antihistaminic, and hypotensive effects).

#### Nursing Responsibilities

- Assess baseline CBC and liver function studies, heart sounds, and neurologic status before initiating prescribed therapy.

#### Client and Family Teaching

- Make position changes slowly.
- Chew sugarless gum to relieve dry mouth.
- Do not abruptly quit taking the medication.

### ERGOT ALKALOID DERIVATIVES

Methysergide maleate (Sansert)

Methysergide is an ergot alkaloid derivative structurally related to LSD. It acts by stimulating smooth muscle, leading to vasoconstriction. It is thought that methysergide prevents headaches by blocking the effects of serotonin, a powerful vasodilator believed to play a role in vascular headaches. It also inhibits the release of histamine from mast cells and prevents the release of serotonin from platelets.

#### Nursing Responsibilities

- Note any history of renal or hepatic disease.
- Assess baseline eosinophil and neutrophil counts before beginning therapy.
- Administer the drug with meals or milk to minimize gastrointestinal irritation due to increased hydrochloric acid production.
- Assess for renal, central nervous system, and cardiovascular complications.
- Drug dosage should be gradually reduced over 2 to 3 weeks to prevent rebound headaches. A drug-free interval of 3 to 4 weeks is required with each 6-month course of therapy to prevent complications.
- Monitor for signs of ergotism, such as coldness or numbness of the fingers and toes, nausea, vomiting, headache, muscle pain, and weakness. Vasoconstriction may further impair peripheral circulation and increase blood pressure.

#### Client and Family Teaching

- Take the medication with meals or milk to minimize gastrointestinal upset.
- Report to the primary care provider nervousness, weakness, rashes, hair loss, or swelling of the extremities.
- Weigh daily and report any unusual weight gain to the primary care provider.
- Return to the primary care provider for a checkup at least every 6 months or as instructed. Do not take the drug on a regular basis for longer than 6 months, but do not abruptly stop taking it.
- Return for follow-up blood work as ordered.

### SEROTONIN SELECTIVE AGONIST

> Sumatriptan succinate injection (Imitrex)
> Zolmitriptan (Zomig)
> Rizatriptan Benzoate (Maxalt)

Binds to vascular receptors to vasoconstrict cranial blood vessels and relieve migraine headache.

#### Nursing Responsibilities

- Assess for history of peripheral vascular disease, renal or hepatic problems, and pregnancy.
- Evaluate relief of migraine headache, and assess for side effects of photophobia, sound sensitivity, and nausea and vomiting.

(continued on page 1364)

## Medication Administration

### Headaches (continued)

#### Client and Family Teaching

- Do not use more than two injections in a 24-hour period, and allow at least 1 hour between injections.
- Use the autoinjector to administer the medication, and follow instructions for proper method of giving the injection and disposing of the syringe.
- Report wheezing, heart palpitations, skin rash, swelling of the eyelids or face, or chest pain to the health care provider immediately.

#### CALCIUM CHANNEL BLOCKERS

> Verapamil (Isoptin)
> Nifedipine (Procardia)

The calcium channel blockers may have value in controlling cerebral vasospasms by two mechanisms: inhibiting the influx of calcium into the cerebral artery and interfering with the destruction of erythrocytes and aggregation of platelets.

#### Nursing Responsibilities

- These drugs cause peripheral vasodilation. Therefore, monitor blood pressure and pulse during the initial administration of the drug. Any excessive hypotensive response and tachycardia may precipitate angina. Request written parameters for safe drug administration.
- Monitor intake and output and daily weights. Assess for manifestations of congestive heart failure: weight gain, peripheral edema, dyspnea, rales, and jugular vein distention.
- Teach client and family members how to take pulse and blood pressure readings.

#### Client and Family Teaching

- Take the medication with meals to reduce gastrointestinal irritation.
- Take pulse and blood pressure before taking medications each day at the same time, and follow instructions regarding when to withhold medication and when to contact the provider. Keep a record of pulse and blood pressure readings.
- Report any side effects, such as dizziness, vertigo, unusual flushing, facial, warmth, or headaches, to the primary care provider.
- Report immediately any swelling of the hands or feet, pronounced dizziness, or chest pain accompanied by sweating, shortness of breath, or severe headaches.

#### NONSTEROIDAL ANTI-INFLAMMATORY DRUG (NSAID): SALICYLATE

Acetylsalicylic acid (Ecotrin, Bufferin)

Acetylsalicylic acid, or aspirin, is a nonnarcotic analgesic, antipyretic, anti-inflammatory agent used to relieve headache pain.

#### Nursing Responsibilities

- Determine the type and pattern of pain. If aspirin was used in the past for pain control, note its effectiveness.
- Note any history of peptic ulcers or other conditions that may suggest potential problems with the use of salicylates.
- Assess clients receiving anticoagulant therapy for bruises, bleeding of the mucous membranes, or blood in the urine or stool.

#### Client and Family Teaching

- Take aspirin after meals or before meals with an antacid and a full glass of water to minimize gastric irritation.
- Report ringing in the ears, unusual bleeding of gums, bruising, or black tarry stools to the primary health care provider.
- Monitor blood glucose levels carefully (if you have diabetes), and report hypoglycemia if it occurs.

#### ERGOTAMINE

> Caffeine-ergotamine tartrate combination (Cafergot)
> Ergotamine tartrate (Gynergen)

Ergot alkaloids vasoconstrict the cerebral blood vessels, decreasing the amplitude of the pulsations of the cranial arteries. The major use of ergot alkaloids is the treatment of migraine headaches. Cafergot has the same actions as Gynergen, in addition, the caffeine it contains provides a vasoconstrictive action, enhancing the effects of ergotamine.

#### Nursing Responsibilities

- Because the drug accumulates in the body and is eliminated slowly, ergotamine poisoning may occur. Sepsis, renal and vascular disease, heavy smoking, malnutrition, pregnancy, contraceptive hormones, and fever can increase the risk of ergotamine poisoning.
- These drugs are contraindicated in clients with diabetes mellitus, sepsis, hepatic or renal disease, peripheral and coronary artery disease, hypertension, and pregnancy.

#### Client and Family Teaching

- Take the drug immediately at onset of headache.
- Report the following to your health care provider: pain in the leg muscles, weakness, and coldness or numbness of fingers or toes.
- A dose of Cafergot taken late in the day may prevent sleep because of the effects of caffeine.

## Complementary Therapies

The following complementary therapies are used to relieve the pain of headaches.

- Intake of vitamin D, elemental calcium, riboflavin (vitamin B), and magnesium
- Acupuncture
- Relaxation, guided imagery, massage
- Regular exercise
- Magnetic field therapy
- Herbal therapy
- Osteopathic manipulation

## NURSING CARE

### Health Promotion

Teach clients with tension headaches relaxation techniques, such as massage and biofeedback. Counseling for chronic anxiety may also be helpful. Triggers for migraine or cluster headache should be identified and, if possible, eliminated. For example, avoiding physical and emotional stress, having regular and consistent sleep patterns, eating meals regularly, and avoiding specific foods or alcohol can be incorporated into daily life and are helpful.

## Assessment

Collect the following data through the health history and physical examination.

- Health history: history of intracerebral trauma, tumor, or infection; detailed history and description of headache characteristics; family history; triggering factors; effects of recurring headaches on lifestyle, ADLs, and role performance
- Physical assessment: skin (diaphoresis, pallor, flushing), eyes (sensitivity to light, tearing), muscle strength and movement

## Nursing Diagnoses and Interventions

The primary response of the client requiring nursing interventions is acute pain. Develop nursing interventions to help the client identify strategies for controlling the pain and discomfort of the headache.

### Acute Pain

Headaches originate from both intracranial and extracranial sources and range in severity from benign, transient discomfort to severe, incapacitating pain. Interventions focus on teaching the client self-care measures to control or relieve the pain, and reducing any associated problems, such as nausea and vomiting or anxiety.

- Teach to maintain a diary of headaches, including duration, onset, location, relation to menstruation or food intake, and related manifestations such as factors that relieve or intensify the pain. *A thorough assessment of the headache is essential for both the client and the health care provider to identify the circumstances and patterns of headache occurrence.*
- Ask the client to rate the pain or discomfort on a scale of 0 to 10 (with 10 being the worst pain). *Using a scale to rate the pain provides an objective measure of the client's subjective experience of the pain or discomfort. The scale can also be used to evaluate the effectiveness of pain relief measures.*
- Teach to minimize light, noise, and activity and rest in a quiet, nonstimulating environment when experiencing a headache. *Manipulating the environment helps reduce noxious stimuli that may increase pain.*
- Teach to use noninvasive and nonpharmacologic pain relief measures such as deep breathing or relaxation to facilitate self-management of pain (see Chapter 4). *Alternative strategies to control pain can help reduce tension and may help to increase the client's sense of control over the pain.*
- If appropriate, teach to apply cold compresses or dry heat to the head and neck. *The application of cold can cause vasoconstriction, which helps reduce pain in vascular headaches. Application of heat can reduce muscle tension and improve circulation.*

- Teach to follow good nutrition guidelines, get regular exercise and sleep, and minimize stress. *Headaches are more likely to occur when ill, tired, or under stress.*

## Home Care

In addition to implementing comfort measures, client education has a high priority. Develop a teaching plan to help the client learn how to limit attacks (e.g., by avoiding precipitating factors) and reduce the effects of the headache. Provide specific information about prescribed medications. Referrals for methods of stress reduction may be necessary for clients with long-term or migraine headaches.

# THE CLIENT WITH A SEIZURE DISORDER

**Seizures** are "paroxysmal motor, sensory, or cognitive manifestations of spontaneous, abnormally synchronous discharges of collections of neurons in the cerebral cortex" (Porth, 2002, p. 1189). This abnormal neuronal activity, which may involve all or part of the brain, disturbs skeletal motor function, sensation, autonomic function of the viscera, behavior, or consciousness. The term **epilepsy** is used to denote any disorder characterized by recurrent seizures. Epilepsy is categorized as a paroxysmal disorder because its manifestations are discontinuous; that is, minutes, days, weeks, or even years may elapse between seizures.

## INCIDENCE AND PREVALENCE

Epilepsy and seizures affect approximately 2.3 million Americans, costing an estimated $12.5 billion in medical expenses and lost or reduced earnings. About 10% of Americans will experience a seizure. People of all ages are affected, but particularly children and the elderly. The incidence of epilepsy is increasing. Researchers have suggested that the increase may be due to technologic advances in obstetric and pediatric care that allow extremely high-risk neonates to survive and to other technologic advances that have improved survival rates after craniocerebral trauma.

Isolated seizure episodes may occur in otherwise healthy people for a variety of reasons, including an acute febrile state, infection, metabolic or endocrine disorder (such as hypoglycemia), or exposure to toxins. Epilepsy may be idiopathic (that is, it may have no identifiable cause), or it may be secondary to birth injury, infection, vascular abnormalities, trauma, or tumors. Older adults may experience seizures as a result of vascular diseases (the most common cause in adults over 60) and degenerative disorders such as Alzheimer's disease.

## PATHOPHYSIOLOGY AND MANIFESTATIONS

Normally, when the mind is actively working, electrical activity in the brain is unsynchronized; when the mind is at rest, electrical activity is mildly synchronized. It is believed that most seizures arise from a few unstable, hypersensitive, and hyperreactive neurons in the brain. During a seizure, these neurons produce a rhythmic and repetitive hypersynchronous

## Nursing Care Plan
## A Client with a Migraine Headache

Betty Friedman is a 25-year-old grade-school teacher. Her friends and the other teachers regard Ms. Friedman as an enthusiastic person who sets high standards for herself and strives for perfection. During the spring semester, Ms. Friedman begins to miss work and sometimes appears very nervous. One day, another teacher notices Ms. Friedman running down the hall and into the restroom; the teacher finds Ms. Friedman vomiting. As she washes up, Ms. Friedman tells the other teacher that she has been having headaches since she began menstruating, but that they have never been as intense and frequent as during this past year. They even wake her from her sleep. Ms. Friedman agrees to see the nurse practitioner, Jane Schickadanz, at the school clinic for evaluation.

### ASSESSMENT

During her health history, Ms. Friedman relates that each month before her menstrual cycle she becomes nervous and sees flashing lights. She also has difficulty expressing herself and thinking clearly. The next day she develops a "sick headache." She states that the headache can last 1 to 2 days and that afterwards she cannot brush her hair because her scalp hurts. Ms. Friedman attributes these symptoms to PMS and adds that she thinks she is allergic to cheese and nuts because she gets very sick after eating them. After assessment, and in consultation with the physician, Ms. Schickadanz diagnoses Ms. Friedman's problem as a migraine with aura headache. Sumatriptan succinate (Imitrex) injections are prescribed.

### DIAGNOSES

- *Acute pain* related to vasodilation of cerebral vessels and a decreased serotonin level
- *Deficient knowledge* pain management
- *Altered role performance* related to pain

### EXPECTED OUTCOMES

- Experience reduced frequency and duration of pain.
- Identify the available resources for helping with self-management of pain.

### PLANNING AND IMPLEMENTATION

- Ask to keep a diary of her headaches for the next month, noting times of their occurrence, location and duration of pain, and factors that trigger the onset, such as her menstrual period or certain foods.
- Teach techniques for administering the subcutaneous injection and for disposing of the syringe and guidelines for administration. Teach to take the medication at the first awareness of an impending attack.
- Suggest an appointment with a counselor to learn methods of relaxation and stress relief.
- Request dietary referral for elimination of foods that might precipitate headaches.

### EVALUATION

Four weeks after beginning medication therapy with Imitrex and relaxation techniques, Ms. Friedman has noted a decrease in the intensity of the headaches. She reports that the medication has stopped the headaches, which, she has noted, tend to occur more frequently immediately before her menstrual period. She is walking for 30 minutes each day and has made changes in her usual diet. Ms. Friedman states, "I feel good about going to work with my kids at school and knowing I can control my pain."

### Critical Thinking in the Nursing Process

1. List the questions you would include in a health history that would identify stressors consistent with migraine headaches.
2. Develop a teaching plan for Ms. Friedman that includes methods of reducing fluid retention before her menstrual period, as well as a suggested diet based on the food guide pyramid.
3. Design a plan of care for Ms. Friedman for the nursing diagnosis, *Disturbed sleep pattern*.

See Evaluating Your Response in Appendix C.

---

discharge. Although the exact initiating factor for seizure activity has not been identified, several theories have been proposed (Porth, 2002):

- Alterations in the permeability of, or ion distribution across, cell membranes
- Alterations in the excitability of neurons resulting from glial scarring or decreased inhibition of activity in the cerebral cortex or thalamic region
- Imbalances of excitatory and inhibitory neurotransmitters such as acetylcholine (ACh) or gamma aminobutyric acid (GABA)

All people have a seizure threshold; when this threshold is exceeded, a seizure may result. In some people, the seizure threshold may be abnormally low, increasing their risk for seizure activity; in other people pathologic processes may alter the seizure threshold (Porth, 2002). The neurons that initiate seizure activity are called the *epileptogenic focus*. Abnormal neuronal activity may remain localized, causing a partial or focal seizure, or it may spread to involve the entire brain, causing generalized seizure activity. Seizures may also be provoked or unprovoked. *Unprovoked (primary* or *idiopathic) seizures* have no identifiable cause, with multiple episodes diagnosed as a seizure disorder or epilepsy. *Provoked (secondary) seizure* etiologies include febrile seizures in children, toxemia of pregnancy, rapid withdrawal from alcohol or barbiturates, systemic metabolic conditions (such as hypoglycemia, hypoxia, uremia, and electrolyte imbalances), and pathologies of the brain (such as meningitis, cerebral bleeding, or cerebral edema).

Metabolic needs of the brain increase dramatically during seizure activity. The demand for adenosine triphosphate (ATP), the energy source of the brain, increases by approximately 250%. Consequently, the demand for glucose and oxygen (which are needed to produce ATP) increases, and oxygen consumption increases by about 60%. To supply this increased oxygen need and remove carbon dioxide and other metabolic by-products, cerebral blood flow increases to about 2.5 times that of the normal rate. As long as oxygenation, blood glucose levels, and cardiac function remain normal, cerebral blood flow can respond to this increased metabolic demand of the brain. If cerebral blood flow cannot meet these needs, however, cellular exhaustion and cellular destruction may result.

Although seizures may be categorized in several different ways, the classification developed by the International League Against Epilepsy is the most useful clinically (Tierney et al., 2001). Seizures are divided into those that affect only part of the brain (partial seizures) and those that are generalized.

## Partial Seizures

**Partial seizures** involve the activation of only a restricted part of one cerebral hemisphere. A partial seizure accompanied by no alteration in consciousness is called a *simple partial seizure;* one in which consciousness is impaired is called a *complex partial seizure.*

The manifestations of simple partial seizures depend on the involved area of the brain. Manifestations may include alterations in motor function, sensory signs, or autonomic or psychic symptoms. Typically, the motor portion of the cortex is affected, causing recurrent muscle contractions of a contralateral part of the body, such as a finger or hand, or the face. This motor activity may stay confined to one area or spread sequentially to adjacent parts, a phenomenon known as a *Jacksonian march* or *Jacksonian seizure.* Manifestations of a simple partial seizure involving the sensory portion of the brain may include abnormal sensations or hallucinations. Disruptions in the function of the autonomic nervous system, with resulting tachycardia, flushing, hypotension, and hypertension, or psychic manifestations, such as a sense of déjà vu or inappropriate fear or anger, may also be experienced during a simple partial seizure.

During a complex partial seizure, consciousness is impaired and the client may engage in repetitive, nonpurposeful activity, such as lip smacking, aimless walking, or picking at clothing. These behaviors are known as *automatisms.* During the seizure, the client loses conscious contact with the environment; amnesia is common after the seizure, and several hours may elapse before the client regains full consciousness. Complex partial seizures usually originate in the temporal lobe and may be preceded by an aura, such as an unusual smell, a sense of déjà vu, or a sudden intense emotion.

## Generalized Seizures

**Generalized seizures** involve both hemispheres of the brain as well as deeper brain structures, such as the thalamus, basal ganglia, and upper brainstem. Consciousness is always impaired with generalized seizures. Absence and tonic-clonic seizures are the common forms of generalized seizure activity; they occur more frequently (especially in children) than partial seizures.

### Absence Seizures

**Absence (petit mal) seizures** are characterized by a sudden brief cessation of all motor activity accompanied by a blank stare and unresponsiveness. Absence seizures are more common in children than in adults. The seizure typically lasts only 5 to 10 seconds, although some may last for 30 seconds or more. Movements such as eyelid fluttering or automatisms such as lip smacking may occur during an absence seizure. Seizure activity may vary from occasional episodes to several hundred per day.

### Tonic-Clonic Seizures

**Tonic-clonic seizures** are the most common type of seizure activity in adults. This type of seizure activity follows a typical pattern. An aura may precede generalized seizure activity. The aura may be a vague sense of uneasiness or an abnormal sensation (such as a smell of burning rubber or seeing bright light). Often, however, the seizure occurs without warning.

The seizure begins with a sudden loss of consciousness and sharp tonic muscle contractions (the *tonic phase* of the seizure). With the muscle contraction, air is forced out of the lungs, and the client may cry out. Postural control is lost, and the client falls to the floor in the opisthotonic posture (Figure 42–4A■). Muscles are rigid, with the arms and legs extended and the jaw clenched. Urinary incontinence is common; bowel incontinence may also occur. Breathing ceases and cyanosis develops during the tonic phase of a seizure. The pupils are fixed and dilated. The tonic phase lasts an average of 15 seconds, although it may persist for up to a minute.

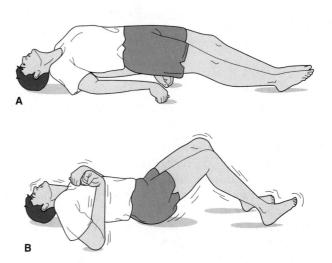

**Figure 42–4 ■** Tonic-clonic seizures in grand mal seizures. *A,* Tonic phase. *B,* Clonic phase.

The *clonic phase,* which follows the tonic phase, is characterized by alternating contraction and relaxation of the muscles in all the extremities along with hyperventilation (Figure 42–4B). The eyes roll back, and the client froths at the mouth. The clonic phase varies in duration and subsides gradually. The entire tonic-clonic portion of the seizure generally lasts no more than 60 to 90 seconds.

Following the clonic phase of seizure activity, the client remains unconscious and unresponsive to stimuli. This period is known as the *postictal period* or *phase.* The client is relaxed and breathes quietly. The client regains consciousness gradually and may be confused and disoriented on waking. Headache, muscle aches, and fatigue often follow the seizure, and the client many sleep for several hours. Amnesia of the seizure is usual; the client also may not recall events just prior to the seizure activity.

Because of the lack of warning with tonic-clonic seizures, the client may experience injury. Head injury, fractures, burns, or motor vehicle crashes may occur secondarily to seizure activity.

## Status Epilepticus

**Status epilepticus** can develop during seizure activity. In this case, the seizure activity becomes continuous, with only very short periods of calm between intense and persistent seizures. The repetitive seizures may be of any type, although they are usually generalized tonic-clonic (Porth, 2002). Repeated seizures have a cumulative effect, producing muscular contractions that can interfere with respirations. The client is in great danger of developing hypoxia, acidosis, hypoglycemia, hyperthermia, and exhaustion if the convulsive activity is not halted. Status epilepticus is considered a life-threatening medical emergency that requires immediate treatment

## COLLABORATIVE CARE

Initial treatment focuses on controlling the seizure; the long-term goal is to determine the cause and prevent future seizures. Collaborative care includes diagnostic testing, medications, and, in some cases, surgery.

## Diagnostic Tests

Diagnostic testing is performed to confirm the seizure diagnosis and to determine any treatable causes and precipitating factors. The tests include:

- *Complete neurologic exam* to determine the focal neurologic deficit or the focus or origin of seizure activity.
- *Electroencephalogram (EEG)* to help confirm the seizure diagnosis and localize any lesion(s). See the box on this page for the nursing implications of EEG.
- *Skull X-rays* to identify possible fractures, deformities in bony structures, or calcification.
- *MRI* or *CT scan* to determine the presence of a tumor, congenital lesions, edema, infarct, hemorrhage, arteriovenous malformation, or a structural deviation, such as ventricular enlargement.

## Nursing Implications for Diagnostic Tests

### Electroencephalogram (EEG)

An EEG is used to detect abnormal brain function. It provides a graphic record of the brain's electrical activity (brain waves) and is useful in evaluating seizure activity.

### Client Preparation

- Explain the procedure, emphasizing the importance of cooperation.
- Withhold fluids, foods, and medications (as prescribed) that may stimulate or depress brain waves. These include anticonvulsants, tranquilizers, depressants, and caffeine-containing foods (e.g., coffee, tea, colas, and chocolate). Medications are usually withheld for 24 to 48 hours before the test.
- Help the client wash the hair before the test.

### Client and Family Teaching

- The test takes about 1 hour.
- The test is painless and will be performed while sitting in a comfortable chair or lying on a stretcher.
- The electrodes are applied to the scalp with a thick paste.
- During the test, you will first be asked to breathe in and out deeply for a few minutes. Then, you will close your eyes while a light is flashed on them and, finally, you will lie quietly with your eyes closed.
- After the test, the nurse will help you wash the paste out of your hair.

- *Lumbar puncture* to determine the presence of infection (meningitis) or elevated protein levels in the CSF.
- *Blood studies* to assess blood count, electrolytes, blood urea, and blood glucose.
- *Electrocardiogram (ECG)* to rule out underlying cardiac dysrhythmias.

## Medications

Anticonvulsant medications can reduce or control most seizure activity. These medications do not cure the disorder; they only manage its manifestations. Anticonvulsant medications generally act in one of two ways: by raising the seizure threshold or by limiting the spread of abnormal activity within the brain.

The goals of medications for epilepsy are to protect the client from harm and to reduce or prevent seizure activity without impairing cognitive function or producing undesirable side effects. Ideally, the lowest possible dose of a single medication that will control the client's seizures is prescribed; often, however, several medications must be tried before the most effective is identified, and a combination of drugs may be needed to manage the client's seizures. Therapy is individualized, based on the type of seizure activity and the client's response to the medication. Nursing implications for these drugs are described in the Medication Administration box on the page 1369; drug interactions are listed in Box 42–2. The success rate is higher in clients with partial and secondary tonic-clonic seizures when carbamazepine (Tegretol), phenytoin (Dilantin), or valproic acid (Depakote) is used. Another

## Medication Administration

### Seizures

#### ANTICONVULSANTS

Examples of anticonvulsants are:

Phenytoin (Dilantin)

Phenobarbital

Primidone (Mysoline)

Carbamazepine (Tegretol)

Valproic acid (Depakene)

Ethosuximide (Zarontin)

Clonazepam (Klonopin)

Gabapentin (Neurontin)

Lamotrigine (Lamictal)

Tiagabine HCL (Gabitril)

Anticonvulsant agents are used to control chronic seizures and involuntary muscle spasms or movements characteristic of certain neurologic diseases. These drugs act in the motor cortex of the brain to reduce the spread of electrical discharges from the rapidly firing epileptic foci in this area. These agents control seizures without impairing the normal functions of the CNS. Drugs effective against one type of seizure may not be effective against another; anticonvulsant therapy must be individualized.

#### Nursing Responsibilities

- Monitor blood pressure, pulse, and respirations.
- Note evidence of CNS side effects, such as blurred vision, dimmed vision, slurred speech, nystagmus, or confusion. Gingival hyperplasia may be noted in clients taking phenytoin.
- Recognize that if clients are to be on prolonged therapy, they may need a diet rich in vitamin D.
- Monitor the serum calcium level as ordered; phenytoin can contribute to demineralization of bone.
- When administering anticonvulsants intravenously, monitor closely for respiratory depression and cardiovascular collapse.

- Administer gabapentin 2 hours after antacids.
- Administer tiagabine HCL with food.

#### Client and Family Teaching

- Take the exact dosage prescribed. Do not increase, decrease, or discontinue the dosage without obtaining the primary care provider's approval; doing so may lead to convulsions.
- Avoid hazardous tasks until the drug has been regulated. Anticonvulsant drugs may at first decrease mental alertness and cause drowsiness, headache, dizziness, and incoordination of muscles. These effects are usually dose related and may disappear with a change of dosage or continued therapy.
- If you are taking phenytoin (Dilantin), maintain good oral hygiene: Use a soft toothbrush, massage the gums, and floss daily.
- It is very important to obtain liver function studies regularly as ordered by the primary care provider. This will help detect early signs of hepatitis and other liver problems. Report for all scheduled laboratory studies, including complete blood count, kidney and liver function studies, and drug levels.
- Carry identification indicating the type of seizures for which you are being treated.
- Do not take gabapentin 1 hour before or less than 2 hours after an antacid.
- If you are taking lamotrigine and develop a rash, tell your health care provider.
- Take Tiagabine HCL (Gabitril) with food.

---

medication approved for partial seizures is tiagabine (Gabitril), a GABA inhibitor. If the client has been seizure free for at least 3 years, withdrawal of medications may be considered, with the dose of one drug at a time reduced over weeks or months. There is no way of predicting which clients can remain seizure free without medication, but if seizures reoccur, the same medications usually provide good control.

Status epilepticus requires immediate intervention to preserve life. Establishing and maintaining the airway is a priority. A solution of 50% dextrose is administered intravenously to prevent hypoglycemia. Diazepam (Valium) or lorazepam (Ativan) is given intravenously, and the dose repeated in 10 minutes if necessary to stop seizure activity. Phenytoin (Dilantin) is also administered intravenously for longer-term control of seizures. Phenobarbital may also be administered to clients in status epilepticus.

### Treatments

#### Surgery

When all attempts to control the client's seizures fail, excision of the tissue involved in the seizure activity may be an effective and safe treatment alternative. An estimated 5% of clients with epilepsy may be candidates for surgery. The goal of surgery is to reduce the client's uncontrollable seizures.

To be selected as a candidate for surgery, the client must be highly motivated and psychologically prepared. A psychologic screening is required because the preoperative

| BOX 42–2 | ■ Drug Interactions with Anticonvulsants |
| --- | --- |

- *Valproic acid (Depakene) and phenobarbital.* Blood levels of phenobarbital may rise significantly when valproic acid is added to the client's medication regimen.
- *Phenobarbital and digoxin.* This combination may increase the metabolism of digoxin, resulting in decreased digoxin levels.
- *Phenobarbital and sodium warfarin (Coumadin).* Phenobarbital may decrease the absorption of sodium warfarin from the gastrointestinal tract and decrease the drug's anticoagulant response.
- *Disulfiram (Antabuse) and phenobarbital.* This combination may inhibit the metabolism of the anticonvulsant drug and increase the incidence of side effects associated with the anticonvulsant drug.
- *Carbamazepine and oral contraceptives.* Carbamazepine decreases the effectiveness of oral contraceptives.
- *Other drugs.* Other drugs reported to interact with anticonvulsant drugs include aspirin, certain antibiotics, isoniazid, acetazolamide (Diamox), antacids, folic acid, and narcotics.

preparation is extensive and time-consuming and because the surgery is long and requires that the client remain awake during surgery so that he or she can cooperate and respond to commands. The EEG is monitored during surgery to identify the epileptogenic focus and evaluate the effect of surgical intervention.

## NURSING CARE OF THE CLIENT WITH SEIZURES WHO IS HAVING SURGERY

### PREOPERATIVE CARE

- For most clients, anticonvulsant medications are withheld the morning or evening of the day before surgery. *Anticonvulsant medications may interfere with intraoperative EEG monitoring.*
- For clients with frequent and/or severe seizures, however, a partial dose of medication may be administered. *This prevents seizures or status epilepticus during surgery.*
- A low dose of analgesics is administered before surgery. *The client must remain awake throughout the lengthy procedure to respond to commands during EEG recording.*

### POSTOPERATIVE CARE

- Anticonvulsant medications are administered parenterally until the client can tolerate oral fluids; medications are then continued orally. *It is common for the client to have seizures in the early postoperative period.*
- Steroids are administered for the first 3 days after surgery and are tapered and then discontinued during the following week. *Steroids are given to decrease cerebral edema.*

General postoperative care for the client with intracranial surgery follows the nursing management guidelines outlined later in the chapter. Specific preoperative and postoperative care for a client with a seizure disorder is described in the box above.

Resective surgery, with removal of the epileptogenic focus, is an option that is still in its early stages. Candidates for this type of surgery include those who are unresponsive to medical management, who have a unilateral focus, and who have impaired quality of life from seizures. Resections of the temporal lobe are most commonly performed and are most effective for partial complex seizures.

### Vagal Nerve Stimulation

Vagal nerve stimulation is approved as a treatment for clients with partial-onset seizures who do not respond to drugs and are not candidates for surgery. The mechanism of action is unknown.

## NURSING CARE

### Health Promotion

Health promotion activities for the client with seizures focus on teaching to reduce the incidence of seizure activity and to promote safety. Stress the following:

- Know the importance of follow-up care, of keeping medical appointments, and of continuing to take anticonvulsant medications as prescribed even when no seizures are experienced.
- Review any state and local laws that apply to people with seizure disorders. Driving a motor vehicle is usually prohibited for 6 months to 2 years after a seizure episode. Usually, a driver's license can be reinstated or obtained after a seizure-free period and a letter from the nurse practitioner or physician.
- Teach client and family members measures to prevent injury at home:
  - Avoid smoking when alone or in bed.
  - Avoid alcohol.
  - Avoid becoming excessively tired.
  - Install grab bars in the shower and tub area.
  - Do not lock doors of the bedroom or bathroom.
  - Avoid an excessive intake of caffeine.

### Assessment

Collect the following data through the health history and physical examination.

- Health history: past seizures: age when the client's first seizure occurred, most recent seizure, factors precipitating a seizure, any warning signs (aura), prophylactic anticonvulsant therapy, and specific concerns the client may have about the seizures
- Physical assessment: important data used in determining an accurate diagnosis that describe manifestations obtained from nursing assessments before, during, and after a seizure (Table 42–5 lists nursing assessments with rationale.)

### Nursing Diagnoses and Interventions

Nursing care of clients with a seizure disorder focuses on providing care during and immediately after the seizure and on client teaching. The client with seizures has a wide variety of responses to actual or potential changes in health status; interventions discussed in this section focus on facilitating physical and psychologic comfort and safety.

### Risk for Ineffective Airway Clearance

During a seizure, the tongue may fall back and obstruct the airway, the gag reflex may be depressed, and secretions may pool at the back of the throat. These may put the client at risk for an obstructed airway. Most seizures occur in the home or community; also teach these interventions to the client's family.

- Provide interventions to maintain a patent airway:
  - Loosen clothing around the neck.
  - Turn on the side.
  - Do not force anything into the mouth.
  - If prescribed and available, administer oxygen by mask.
  *Although it was at one time believed that it was necessary to place a padded tongue blade in the client's mouth during a seizure, this is no longer recommended; an improperly placed tongue blade can obstruct the airway. Turning the client on the side allows secretions to drain from the mouth.*

## TABLE 42-5 Nursing Assessments Before, During, and After a Seizure

| Assessment | Rationale |
| --- | --- |
| What was the client's level of consciousness? If consciousness was lost, at what point? | Indicates area of brain involved and type of seizure. |
| What was the client doing just before the attack? | May suggest precipitating factors. |
| In what part of the body did the seizure start? | May indicate the site of seizure activity in the brain tissue; for example, if jerking movements were first observed in right hand, the seizure focus may be in left motor cortex in the area of the hand. |
| Was there an epileptic cry? | Usually indicates the tonic stage of a generalized tonic-clonic seizure. |
| Were any automatisms such as eyelid fluttering, chewing, lip smacking, or swallowing observed? | Often seen in complex, partial, and absence seizures. |
| How long did movements last? Did the location or character change (tonic to clonic)? Did movements involve both sides of the body or just one? | Indicates areas in which focal activity originated. |
| Did the head and/or eyes turn to one side and, if so, which side? | Helps localize the focus of the seizure. During the seizure, the head and eyes typically will turn away from the side of the epileptogenic focus. |
| Were there changes in pupillary reactions? | Indicates involvement of the autonomic nervous system. |
| If the client fell, was the head hit? | Skull X-ray studies may be needed to rule out subdural hematoma or fracture. |
| Was there foaming or frothing from the mouth? | Usually indicates a tonic-clonic seizure. |

- Teach family members or significant others how to care for the client during a seizure to prevent airway obstruction. *Family members are often the only people present to provide this emergency intervention.*

### Anxiety

The client with a seizure disorder is understandably anxious about the future, with questions about ability to go to school, work, have a family, and drive a car. Feelings of embarrassment about having a seizure in public and rejection by others are common and also increase the client's anxiety.

- Provide support by explaining that concerns are normal. *It is important to be sensitive to the effect of seizures on the client's self-concept and body image; alterations in these areas not only increase anxiety but also cause withdrawal from socialization with others. Demonstrating acceptance of the client's concerns allows further discussion.*
- Help identify safe leisure activities. *Worrying about being hurt if a seizure occurs may cause withdrawal from social activities that are pleasurable.*
- Provide information about sources and support groups. *Sharing information with other people with similar health problems allows for a more realistic viewpoint; accurate information can clear up misconceptions that cause anxiety.*
- Provide accurate information about hiring practices and legal limitations on driving or operating heavy or dangerous machinery. *Accurate information decreases anxiety about the unknown. The American Disabilities Act prohibits discrimination; however, there are legal limitations on driving until the person is proved free of seizures.*

### Using NANDA, NIC, and NOC

Chart 42-1 shows links between NANDA nursing diagnosis, NIC, and NOC when caring for the client with a seizure disorder.

### Home Care

Teaching follows a systematic assessment of the needs of both the client and family. Include family members so that they can learn seizure management, including the care and observations

## CHART 42-1 NANDA, NIC, AND NOC LINKAGES

### The Client with a Seizure Disorder

| NURSING DIAGNOSES | NURSING INTERVENTIONS | NURSING OUTCOMES |
| --- | --- | --- |
| • Risk for Aspiration<br>• Risk for Falls<br>• Anxiety | • Aspiration Precautions<br>• Fall Prevention<br>• Anxiety Reduction | • Neurological Status<br>• Safety Behavior: Fall Prevention<br>• Anxiety Control<br>• Acceptance: Health Status |

*Note. Data from Nursing Outcomes Classification (NOC) by M. Johnson & M. Maas (Eds.), 1997, St. Louis: Mosby; Nursing Diagnoses: Definitions & Classification 2001–2002 by North American Nursing Diagnosis Association, 2001, Philadelphia: NANDA; Nursing Interventions Classification (NIC) by J.C. McCloskey & G. M. Bulechek (Eds.), 2000, St. Louis: Mosby. Reprinted by permission.*

necessary before and during a seizure. Stress the importance of safety and keeping the airway patent.

Help both the client and family adjust to a diagnosis of epilepsy. Address the following topics.

- Misconceptions, common fears, and myths about epilepsy
- The importance of wearing a MedicAlert band or carrying a medical alert card at all times
- Avoiding alcoholic beverages and limiting coffee intake

- Taking showers versus tub baths, because of safety issues during a generalized seizure
- Factors that may trigger a seizure, such as abrupt withdrawal from medication, constipation, fatigue, excessive stress, fever, menstruation, sights and sounds such as television, flashing video, and computer screens
- Helpful resources:
  - American Epilepsy Society
  - Epilepsy Foundation

## Nursing Care Plan
## A Client with a Seizure Disorder

Janet Carlson is a 19-year-old college student who lives with her parents and one younger sister. Although Janet had seizures while she was in grade school, they have been controlled with medication. However, she had a tonic-clonic seizure yesterday and immediately made an appointment with her family physician. She is currently taking phenytoin (Dilantin) 300 mg/day as a maintenance medication to prevent seizures.

### ASSESSMENT
Evita Farias, RN, completes a health history for Ms. Carlson. During the history, she tells Ms. Farias that she has been under stress because of difficulties in completing her course requirements this semester. She has not been sleeping as many hours per night, and sometimes she forgets to take her medication. Janet's serum phenytoin level is 8 mg/mL. Therapeutic level is 10 to 20 mg/ml.

### DIAGNOSES
- *Risk for injury* related to recurrence of generalized tonic-clonic seizure activity and low serum phenytoin levels
- *Deficient knowledge* related to activities that may trigger seizure occurrence, the effect of stress on seizures, and medication information

### EXPECTED OUTCOMES
- Will verbalize precipitating and triggering factors related to the onset of seizures.
- Will verbalize the relationship between emotional and physical stress and seizures.
- Will verbalize the importance of taking anticonvulsant medications.

### PLANNING AND IMPLEMENTATION
- Teach client and her family the following:

- Current information about seizures
- Care during and after a seizure
- Medication protocols
- Factors and activities that can trigger seizures
- The importance of follow-up care
- Refer client and her family to a local epilepsy support group.
- Recommend that she purchase and wear a MedicAlert bracelet.

### EVALUATION
Ms. Carlson is instructed to continue taking Dilantin 300 mg/day. She states the importance of nutrition, rest, and measures to reduce stress. She also discusses the importance of maintaining the proper blood levels of her medication, stating that too little or too much of the medication could cause problems. Ms. Carlson recognizes that the seizure problems had recurred during a busy time in school during which she had forgotten to take her medication. She is now wearing a MedicAlert bracelet. Ms. Farias provides the Carlsons with the telephone number of the Epilepsy Foundation of America.

### Critical Thinking in the Nursing Process
1. If you were Ms. Carlson's nurse, would your teaching differ if she were living alone? If so, how?
2. Ms. Carlson tells you that although she knows she should not drive a car, she often drives her friend to work. How would you approach this problem?
3. Ms. Carlson states that "it's embarrassing to wear a MedicAlert bracelet." How would you respond, and what recommendation(s) would you make?

See Evaluating Your Response in Appendix C.

## TRAUMATIC BRAIN INJURY

**Traumatic brain injury (TBI)** is a leading cause of death and disability in the United States. The National Head Injury Foundation defines TBI as a traumatic insult to the brain capable of causing physical, intellectual, emotional, social, and vocational changes. A TBI may be classified as a *penetrating (open) head injury* (e.g., resulting from a knife, bullet, or baseball bat) or a *closed head injury* (a blunt injury to the brain that does not result in an open skull fracture).

## INCIDENCE AND PREVALENCE

The CDC estimates that each year 1 million people in the United States are treated and released from hospital emergency departments as a result of TBI: 230,000 people are hospitalized and survive: and 50,000 people die. Additionally, more than 80,000 are discharged with TBI-related injuries, and 5.3 million Americans are living today with a TBI-related disability.

## Risk Factors

Motor vehicle accidents (MVAs) are a major cause of TBI; elevated blood alcohol levels contribute significantly to the risk of MVA and subsequent injury. Other causes of head injury include falls, sports injuries, occupational injuries, assaults, and gunshot wounds. Adults age 15 to 30 are at the greatest risk, with the male to female ratio of 3:1 (McCance & Huether, 2002). Other risk factors include being over the age of 75 and living in a high-crime area.

## MECHANISMS OF CRANIOCEREBRAL TRAUMA

Specific damage following craniocerebral injuries is related to the mechanism of the injury (how it occurs), the nature of the injury (type), and the location of the injury (where it occurs).

Injuries to the head can occur through several mechanisms:

- *Acceleration injury* is sustained when the head is struck by a moving object, such as a swinging bat.
- *Deceleration injury* occurs when the head hits a stationary object, such as a concrete wall.
- *Acceleration-deceleration injury* (also called a *coup-contrecoup phenomenon*) occurs when the head hits an object and the brain "rebounds" within the skull (Figure 42–5 ■). The brain is injured at the point of impact (the coup) and on the opposite side of the impact (the countrecoup). Two or more areas of the brain can be injured as a result of this phenomenon.
- *Deformation injuries* are those in which the force deforms and disrupts the integrity of the impacted body part (e.g., skull fracture).
- Head injuries can also be classified as *blunt* or *penetrating*.

Types of craniocerebral trauma include injuries to the skull (including fractures), injuries to the brain (including concussion and contusion), and intracranial hemorrhage (including hematomas). Brain injury can result either from the direct effects of the trauma on brain tissue or from secondary responses to trauma, such as cerebral edema, hematoma, swelling, or increased intracranial pressure.

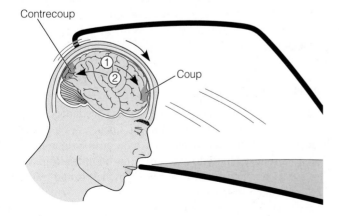

**Figure 42–5** ■ Coup-contrecoup head injury. Following the initial injury (coup), the brain rebounds within the skull and sustains additional injury (contrecoup) in the opposite part of the brain.

## THE CLIENT WITH A SKULL FRACTURE

A **skull fracture** is a break in the continuity of the skull. It may occur with or without damage to the brain; however, intracranial trauma often results from skull fractures. The considerable force of impact significantly increases the risk of underlying hematoma formation. Disruption of the skull can also cause cranial nerve injury, allow bacteria to enter the cranial vault, or allow CSF to leak out.

## PATHOPHYSIOLOGY AND MANIFESTATIONS

Skull fractures are classified as open or closed. In an open fracture, the dura is torn, and in a closed fracture, the dura is not torn. Skull fractures are further classified into one of four categories: linear, comminuted, depressed, or basilar (Table 42–6).

*Linear fractures* are the most common, accounting for 80% of all skull fractures. They typically extend from the point of impact toward the base of the skull. Although the risk of infection or CSF leakage is minimal with this type of fracture because the dura usually remains intact, subdural or epidural hematomas (a collection of blood) frequently underlie the fracture. A hematoma (discussed later in this chapter) places pressure on underlying brain tissue, increasing both intracranial pressure and the risk of brain damage.

*Comminuted* and *depressed skull fractures* increase the risk of direct damage to brain tissue from bruising (*contusion*) and bone fragments. However, the risk of secondary brain injury may be reduced in these fractures, because in breaking the bone, the traumatic impact energy is distributed and dissipated. If the skin overlying the fracture is lacerated or the dura is torn, the risk of infection is greater.

*Basilar skull fractures* involve the base of the skull and usually are extensions of adjacent fractures, although they may occur independently. Although most basilar skull fractures are uncomplicated, they may involve the sinuses of the frontal bone or the petrous portion of the temporal bone (middle ear).

MediaLink | COUP-CONTRECOUP INJURY ANIMATION

| TABLE 42–6 | Types of Skull Fractures |
| --- | --- |
| **Type** | **Description** |
| Linear (simple) | Simple, clean break in skull. Occurs with low-velocity injuries. |
| Comminuted | Bone is crushed into small, fragmented pieces. Usually seen with high-impact injuries. |
| Depressed | Inward depression of bone fragments. Usually due to a powerful blow to the skull. The dura may or may not be intact. Bone fragments may penetrate into the brain tissue. |
| Basilar | Occurs at the base of the skull. May be linear, comminuted, or depressed. |

If the dura is disrupted, CSF may leak through the tear. Manifestations of CSF leakage may include **rhinorrhea** (CSF leakage through the nose) or **otorrhea** (CSF leakage from the ear). Basilar skull fractures can be difficult to identify on X-ray film, but they have certain common manifestations. For example, blood may be visible behind the tympanic membrane (*hemotympanum*), or ecchymosis may be noted over the mastoid process (known as *Battle's sign*). Bilateral periorbital ecchymosis ("raccoon eyes") is another possible manifestation. If CSF leakage is present, the risk of infection is high. Other complications of basilar skull fractures include injury to the internal carotid artery and compression of cranial nerve II, VI, or VII.

## COLLABORATIVE CARE

Treatment of a client with a skull fracture depends on the type and location of the fracture. Skull fracture may be only one of several head injuries.

A simple linear fracture generally requires bed rest and observation for underlying injury to brain tissue or hematoma formation. No specific treatment is required. Depressed skull fractures require surgical intervention, usually within 24 hours of the injury, to debride the wound completely and remove bone fragments, which may become embedded in brain tissue or cerebral blood vessels. If depressed deeply, the bone may be elevated. If cerebral edema is not present, a cranioplasty with insertion of acrylic bone may be performed. Basilar skull fractures do not require surgery unless CSF leakage persists. Regular neurologic assessments and observation for manifestations of meningitis are required for the hospitalized client. Antibiotics may be administered prophylactically.

## NURSING CARE

The client with a craniocerebral trauma may have a variety of responses and health care needs, depending on the location and extent of the trauma. Many of those problems with related nursing interventions are discussed in other sections of this chapter, including seizures, increased intracranial pressure, and bleeding within the brain.

### Nursing Diagnoses and Interventions

This section discusses the risk for infection, a problem common in the client with an open head wound from a skull fracture.

#### Risk for Infection

The client with a skull fracture is at high risk for infection related to possible access to the cranial contents through a tear in the dura. In an open, depressed fracture, the wound may be contaminated by dirt, hair, or other debris.

- Monitor for otorrhea or rhinorrhea. *Open fractures of the skull increase the possibility of leakage of CSF from the ears or nose.*
- Test drainage of clear fluid from ear and nose for glucose by using a glucose reagent strip, such as Dextrostix. *Clear*

*drainage that tests positive for glucose indicates leakage of CSF.*

- Observe blood-tinged fluid for "halo" sign. *CSF dries in concentric rings on gauze or tissues.*
- Keep the nasopharynx and the external ear clean. Place a piece of sterile cotton in the ear, or tape a sterile cotton pad loosely under the nose; change dressings when they become wet. *Wet dressings facilitate movement of organisms.*
- Instruct client not to blow nose, cough, or inhibit sneeze; sneeze through open mouth. *Blowing the nose and coughing increase ICP. Withholding a sneeze forces bacteria backward.*
- Use aseptic technique at all times when changing head dressings or ICP monitor dressings and insertion sites. *Using aseptic technique reduces the possibility of introducing infection.*

### Home Care

The client and family need to be informed about the degree of injury that has occurred with the skull fracture. The client with a linear fracture, who may not be hospitalized, will need teaching that focuses on the need to monitor progress closely. To prevent complications, advise the client and family to go to the emergency room if the client experiences any of the following:

- Growing drowsiness or confusion
- Difficulty waking (instruct a family member to wake the client every 2 hours during the first night home)
- Vomiting
- Blurred vision
- Slurred speech
- Prolonged headache
- Blood or clear fluid leaking from the ears or nose
- Weakness in an arm or leg
- Stiff neck
- Seizure

## THE CLIENT WITH A FOCAL OR DIFFUSE BRAIN INJURY

Even when the skull and other structures overlying the brain remain intact, a blow to the head can cause significant brain injury. Closed head injuries may result in either diffuse or focal damage to the brain. They range in severity from mild to severe.

### PATHOPHYSIOLOGY

Brain injury results from both primary and secondary mechanisms. Primary injury results from the impact. A blow to the head, even with no break in the skull, can cause serious and diffuse brain injury. Injury to axons disrupts oligodendroglia and direct mechanical disruption is caused by debris and leakage. The immediate vascular response to the injury results in increased capillary permeability to solutes.

Secondary injury is the progression of the initial injury resulting from events that affect perfusion and oxygenation of brain cells. These events include intracranial edema, hematoma, infection, hypoxia, or ischemia. Cerebral ischemia is the most common cause of secondary brain injury (Porth, 2002). Ischemia leads to cerebral hypoxia, with consequences of increased glial permeability to sodium (cyctotoxic edema), an influx of calcium with changes in electrophysiology and release of free fatty acids and lactic acidosis.

Acute brain injury affects all body systems as well as the central nervous system. Systemic effects of acute brain injury are listed in Box 42–3.

## Focal Brain Injuries

**Focal brain injuries** are specific, grossly observable brain lesions confined to one area of the brain. The force of the impact produces contusions from direct contact with the inside of the skull that in turn may cause epidural hemorrhage and subdural and intracerebral hematomas. The mechanisms of injury are coup and/or contrecoup damage of the brain at the point of the impact and the rebound effect. The damaged brain area is surrounded by edema, contributing to increased ICP. Infarction and necrosis, multiple hemorrhages, and edema are found within the contused areas. The maximum effects of the injury peak in 18 to 36 hours (McCance & Huether, 2002).

Intracranial hemorrhage can result directly from the trauma (e.g., beneath a fracture) or from shearing forces on cerebral arteries and veins that occur with acceleration-deceleration. Depending on the site and rate of bleeding, manifestations may appear immediately or may not become evident for hours or even weeks. Intracranial hemorrhages and the hematomas they cause place pressure on surrounding structures, causing manifestations of an expanding focal lesion. They also cause increased ICP, leading to altered levels of consciousness and potential herniation syndromes. Intracranial hematomas are classified by their location as

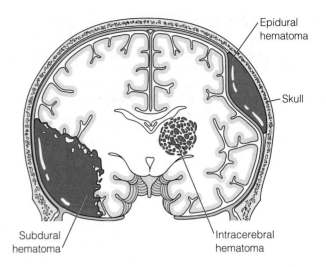

**Figure 42–6 ■** Three types of hematomas: epidural hematoma, subdural hematoma, and intracerebral hematoma.

epidural, subdural, or intracerebral. Table 42–7 compares the frequency, locations, common sites, precipitating factors, and clinical manifestations of intracranial hematomas; Figure 42–6 ■ illustrates their locations.

### Contusion

A **contusion** is a bruise of the surface of the brain, typically accompanied by small, diffuse venous hemorrhages. Both white and gray matter may have a bruised, discolored appearance. A decrease in pH, with accumulation of lactic acid and decreased oxygen consumption, may hinder cell function. Contusions (and other focal brain injuries) occur when the brain strikes the inner skull, often with a *coup* (point of impact) lesion and a *contrecoup* lesion on the opposite side of the brain. Contusions

| BOX 42–3 ■ Systemic Effects of Acute Brain Injury | |
|---|---|
| **Cause** | **Effect** |
| ■ Stimulation of the sympathetic nervous system, which stimulates the adrenal cortex and medulla to increase glucocorticoid and mineralocorticoid levels | ■ Increased metabolism of carbohydrates, fats, and proteins<br>■ Retention of sodium and water |
| ■ Stimulation of the sympathetic nervous system, increasing the serum catecholamine levels | ■ Hypertension<br>■ EEG changes<br>■ Dysrrhymias (bradycardia, sinus tachycardia) |
| ■ Altered release of ADH from the posterior pituitary | ■ Retention of water or diuresis and diabetes insipidus |
| ■ Neurogenic pulmonary dysfunction | ■ Abnormal respiratory patterns<br>■ Reduced residual capacity with retention of $CO_2$, vasodilation, and increased ICP<br>■ Pulmonary edema |
| ■ Stress response to trauma | ■ Hyperglycemia |
| ■ Increased platelet, plasma fibrinogen, and thromboplastin levels | ■ Decreased clotting and prothrombin times<br>■ Vascular occlusion<br>■ Disseminated intravascular coagulation<br>■ Anemia |
| ■ Immunosuppression | ■ Infection |
| ■ Decreased gastric motility and increased gastric acidity | ■ Gastritis<br>■ Gastric ulcers |

TABLE 42-7 Comparison of Intracranial Hematomas

| | Location/Common Site | Precipitating Factors | Manifestations |
| --- | --- | --- | --- |
| **Epidural Hematoma** 2% to 6% of all types of head injuries | Located in the space between the skull and the dura mater Common site: the temporal bone (over the middle meningeal artery) | Skull fractures Contusion | Momentary loss of consciousness followed by a lucid period lasting from a few hours to 1 to 2 days Rapid deterioration in level of consciousness (drowsiness to confusion to coma) Seizures Headache Hemiparesis (may be ipsilateral or contralateral) Fixed dilated ipsilateral pupil Rise in blood pressure with decreases in pulse and respirations indicates a rapidly increasing hematoma |
| **Subdural Hematoma** Approximately 29% of all types of head injuries | Located in the space below the dural surface (between the dura and arachnoid and pia mater layers of meninges) Common site: may occur any place in cranium | Closed head injury Acceleration-deceleration injury Cerebral atrophy (seen in older adults) Chronic alcoholism Use of anticoagulants Contusion | Acute: • Headache • Drowsiness • Agitation • Slowed thinking • Confusion Subacute: • Same as those of acute subdural hematoma but develop more slowly Chronic: • Manifestations may not appear until weeks to months after injury • Confusion, slowed thinking, drowsiness |
| **Intracerebral Hematoma** 14% to 15% of all types of head injuries | Located directly in the brain tissue Common sites: frontal or temporal region | Gunshot wounds Depressed bone fractures Stab injury Long history of systemic hypertension Contusions | Headache Deteriorating consciousness to deep coma Hemiplegia on contralateral side Dilated pupil on the side of the clot |

occur most frequently near bony prominences of the skull. Cerebral edema can follow contusion, resulting in increased ICP. Contusions; small, diffuse venous hemorrhages; and brain swelling are at their peak 12 to 24 hours after injury.

Manifestations of contusion depend on the size and location of the brain injury. An initial loss of consciousness occurs; level of consciousness may remain altered, and behavior changes such as combativeness may persist for an extended period. Full consciousness may be regained extremely slowly, and residual deficits may persist; in some clients, full level of consciousness never really returns. Focal effects of the contusion may cause loss of reflexes, hemiparesis (muscular weakness of one-half of the body), or abnormal posturing. Manifestations of increased ICP may occur if cerebral edema develops. Regaining full LOC may take an extended period of time and residual deficits may persist.

## Epidural Hematoma

An **epidural hematoma** (also called an extradural hematoma) develops in the potential space between the dura and the skull, which normally adhere to one another. As the blood collects, the expanding hematoma strips the dura away from the skull. Epidural hematomas affect young to middle-aged adults more frequently than older adults, because the dura becomes more tightly attached to the skull with aging.

Epidural hematomas usually result from a skull fracture, resulting in a torn artery, often the middle meningeal artery. Because epidural hematomas are arterial in origin, they tend to develop rapidly. The client may lose consciousness with the initial injury, and then have a brief lucid period before the level of consciousness rapidly declines from drowsiness to coma as the hematoma expands, stripping the dura away from the skull and placing pressure on brain tissue. Other manifestations include headache; vomiting; a fixed, dilated pupil on the same side (ipsilateral) as the hematoma; contralateral (opposite side) hemiparesis or hemiplegia; and possible seizures. Because epidural hematomas usually develop rapidly, timely intervention is vital to prevent significant increases in ICP and herniation.

## Subdural Hematoma

**Subdural hematomas,** in which a localized mass of blood collects between the dura mater and the arachnoid mater, are more common than epidural hematomas. Acute subdural hematomas are unusually located at the top of the head, and develop within 48 hours of the initial head injury. Chronic subdural hematomas develop over weeks or months. The chronic type is seen most often in the older adult and people who have some brain atrophy with subsequent enlarged epidural space. These hematomas are often venous in origin, although they may involve bleeding from small arteries as well. Subdural hematomas may form without direct trauma or contusion; acceleration-deceleration forces may tear the bridging veins that connect veins on the surface of the cerebral cortex to the dural sinuses. As blood collects, it places direct pressure on underlying brain tissue.

Acute subdural hematomas develop rapidly following head injury. Although a lucid period may occur, the client commonly develops drowsiness, confusion, and enlargement of the ipsilateral pupil within minutes or hours of the injury. If responsive, the client may complain of a unilateral headache. Hemiparesis and respiratory pattern changes may occur.

Chronic subdural hematomas are often associated with relatively minor trauma such as a fall. Weeks to months may elapse before manifestations of the hematoma occur; the initial trauma may have been forgotten. Chronic subdural hematomas may also occur spontaneously in the older adult or in clients with bleeding disorders. Manifestations of the hematoma develop slowly and may be mistaken for the onset of dementia in the older adult. Slowed thinking, confusion, drowsiness, or lethargy are common early manifestations. Other manifestations include headache, dilation and sluggishness of the ipsilateral pupil, and possible seizures.

### Intracerebral Hematoma

**Intracerebral hematomas** may be single or multiple, and are associated with contusions. They may occur in any location but usually are found in the frontal or temporal lobes. They may result from closed head trauma, particularly contusion or shearing of small blood vessels deep within the hemispheres. Intracerebral hematomas can also accompany other types of head trauma such as lacerations. Older adults are particularly vulnerable to intracerebral hemorrhage because cerebral blood vessels are more fragile and easily torn.

The manifestations of intracerebral hematoma vary according to the location of the hematoma. Headache may develop, along with decreasing level of consciousness, hemiplegia, and dilation of the ipsilateral pupil. The expanding clot increases intracranial pressure, and herniation may occur.

## Diffuse Brain Injury (DBI)

A **diffuse brain injury (DBI)** affects the entire brain and is caused by a shaking motion, with twisting movement (rotational acceleration) the primary mechanism of injury. Shearing stresses on brain tissue cause axonal damage from shearing, tearing, or stretching of nerve fibers. The most serious axonal injuries are located farthest from the brainstem, with the frontal and temporal axonal tracts being most vulnerable to injury. Physical deficits resulting from diffuse brain injuries include spastic paralysis, peripheral nerve injury, swallowing disorders, visual and hearing impairments, and taste and smell disorders. Damage decreases the speed of information processing and responding and disrupts attention, resulting in serious cognitive and affective impairments. Cognitive deficits that may result include disorientation and confusion, short attention span, problems with memory and learning, perceptual problems, and poor judgment. Possible behavioral deficits include agitation, impulsivity, depression, and social withdrawal.

Initially, the damage involves tearing of axons, blood vessels, and brain tissue (visible only by electron microscope). The number of damaged axons progressively increases, with pathology involving the nucleii and axons. The damaged axons, which resemble sausage links, regress into round balls called *retraction balls* (visible with light microscopy). After several weeks, the retraction balls are replaced by clusters of microglia. In the final phase, astrocytosis (equivalent to scarring) occurs at the site of axonal damage, accompanied by demyelination of long axon tracts.

The categories of DBI (McCance & Huether, 2002) include mild concussion, classic cerebral concussion, and diffuse axonal injury.

### Mild Concussion

**Mild concussion** involves temporary axonal disturbances. It is defined as a momentary interruption of brain function with or without loss of consciousness (Porth, 2002). A concussion may be associated with an immediate, brief loss of consciousness on impact. Altered consciousness may last only seconds or persist for several hours. Amnesia for events immediately preceding and following the injury (*retrograde* and *antegrade amnesia*) is common. Other manifestations of concussion include headache, drowsiness, confusion, dizziness, and visual disturbances such as diplopia or blurred vision (see the box below).

The grades of mild concussion, with manifestations, are as follows:

- Grade I: Momentary amnesia, confusion, and disorientation
- Grade II: Momentary confusion and retrograde amnesia that develops after 5 to 10 minutes
- Grade III: Confusion and retrograde amnesia that are present from impact

### Classic Cerebral Concussion (Grade IV)

A **classic cerebral concussion** involves diffuse cerebral disconnection from the brainstem RAS. An immediate loss of consciousness occurs, lasting less than 6 hours. Both retrograde and anterograde amnesia occur. Cerebral contusions may be present. In a severe concussion, a brief seizure and respiratory

---

## Manifestations of Concussion

- Immediate loss of consciousness (lasting usually no longer than 5 minutes)
- Amnesia for events surrounding injury
- Headache
- Drowsiness, confusion, dizziness
- Visual disturbances
- Possible brief seizure activity with transient apnea, bradycardia, pallor, and hypotension

### Postconcussion Syndrome

- Persistent headache
- Dizziness
- Irritability and insomnia
- Impaired memory and concentration, learning problems

arrest may occur; transient pallor, bradycardia, and hypotension may accompany loss of consciousness.

Following concussion, clients may develop **postconcussion syndrome** with persistent headache, dizziness, irritability, insomnia, impaired memory and concentration, and learning problems. Postconcussion syndrome may last for several weeks or, rarely, up to a year.

### Diffuse Axonal Injury

**Diffuse axonal injury (DAI)** is a brain injury in which a high-speed acceleration-deceleration injury, typically associated with motor vehicle crashes, causes widespread disruption of axons in the white matter. Focal lesions may be found in the corpus callosum, midbrain, and brainstem. An immediate loss of consciousness occurs. The prognosis is poor; most clients with severe DAI either die or remain in persistent vegetative state.

DAI may range from mild to severe. In mild DAI, coma lasts 6 to 24 hours, and cognitive, psychologic, and sensorimotor deficits may persist. In moderate DAI, injury and impairment is spread throughout the cererbral cortex and diencephalon. There is axonal tearing, coma lasting more than 24 hours, and often incomplete recovery. In severe DAI, axonal injury occurs in both cerebral hemispheres, the diencephalon, and the brainstem. Immediate autonomic dysfunction occurs, and increased ICP is manifested in 4 to 6 days. Profound cognitive and sensorimotor deficits occur, involving movement, verbal and written communication, ability to learn and reason, and ability to modulate behavior.

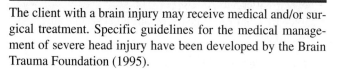

## COLLABORATIVE CARE

The client with a brain injury may receive medical and/or surgical treatment. Specific guidelines for the medical management of severe head injury have been developed by the Brain Trauma Foundation (1995).

### Concussion

Following a concussion, the client may be observed for 1 to 2 hours in the emergency department, and then discharged home with instructions for further observation to detect manifestations of secondary injury. If the loss of consciousness extended more than 2 minutes, the client may be admitted to the hospital for observation.

### Acute TBI

Recognition and management of acute TBI with transport to an ED is essential to client outcomes. Morbidity and mortality increase with hypotension (systolic pressure less than 90 mmHg) and hypoxia (PaO$_2$ less than 60 mmHg) (Bucher & Melander, 1999). Assessment of the client's airway, breathing, and circulation (ABCs), with management of dysfunction, is necessary to decrease the secondary effects of the brain injury. An intracranial pressure monitor probe may be inserted to assess ICP and monitor therapy to reduce cerebral edema and maintain cerebral perfusion. Osmotic diuretics such as mannitol also may be administered to reduce cerebral edema.

### Diagnostic Tests

Diagnostic testing may be done to monitor hemodynamic status and detect conditions that may contribute to cerebral edema.

- *Skull X-rays* detect skull fractures and assess penetrating objects.
- *ABGs* are analyzed, with particular attention to oxygen and carbon dioxide levels. Adequate oxygenation is vital to maintain cerebral metabolism; carbon dioxide is a potent vasodilator, and increased levels may contribute to cerebral edema and increased ICP.
- *Blood count, serum glucose and electrolyte levels,* and *serum osmolarity* are assessed to monitor for infection or conditions that can affect cerebral blood flow or metabolism.
- *CT scan* or *MRI* is ordered to detect contusions and lesions associated with diffuse axonal injury. CT scan shows normal findings in concussion but characteristic lesions with contusion and DAI.
- Other diagnostic tests may include an *EEG* and possibly a *lumbar puncture* to assess for bleeding.

### Treatments

#### Management of Increased ICP

Increased ICP is managed (as described in a previous section) to reestablish equilibrium of the intracranial contents and prevent secondary brain damage. Treatments include airway management, hyperventilation (used if signs of herniation appear), fluid resuscitation, positioning, temperature regulation, and medications. Medications other than those previously discussed include a category of drugs called neuroprotectants. These drugs are used to treat or alter some of the pathologic pathways that occur in ischemia, and must be administered within a short time of the injury to be effective. Classifications of the drugs include lipid peroxidase inhibitors, free radical scavengers, receptor antagonists, calcium channel blockers, and gangliosides (Bucher & Melander, 1999).

#### Surgery

Small subdural hematomas can frequently be reabsorbed and may be treated conservatively, with close observation and supportive care. However, the treatment of choice for epidural hematomas and large acute subdural hematomas is surgical evacuation of the clot. This can often be performed through *burr holes* made into the skull (Figure 42–7 ■). In an epidural hematoma, the bleeding vessel can also be ligated during this procedure, preventing further bleeding. Rebleeding may occur following evacuation of an acute subdural hematoma in older adults and clients with chronic alcoholism. A craniotomy is necessary to evacuate chronic subdural hematomas because the hematoma tends to solidify, making it difficult or impossible to remove through burr holes. Surgery is less successful in treating intracerebral hematomas because of widespread tissue damage. Supportive care to manage intracranial pressure and prevent complications is provided.

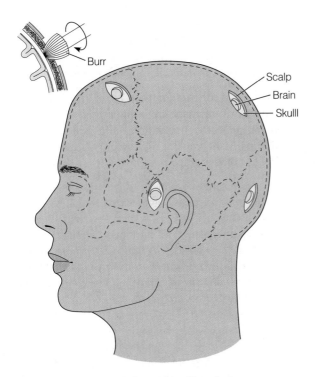

**Figure 42–7** ■ Possible locations of burr holes.

# NURSING CARE

## Health Promotion

The best way to treat any injury is to prevent it from happening. Public education must continue to stress the importance of safe driving, the dangers of driving under the influence of alcohol or drugs, and the necessity of wearing seat belts. Legislation has mandated such motor vehicle changes as seat belts, child safety seats, and airbags. Other behaviors that can reduce the morbidity and mortality associated with TBI are wearing bicycle and motorcycle helmets, learning and following gun safety rules, promoting farm safety, and teaching older adults about safety (such as preventing falls) in the home.

## Assessment

Collect the following data through the health history and physical examination (see Chapter 40). When assessing the older adult, be aware of normal changes with aging, described in Box 42–4.

- Health history: A history of the injury is helpful in understanding the nature of the craniocerebral trauma; knowledge about loss of consciousness assists the nurse in planning care
- Physical examination: neurologic assessment, including pupils, LOC, Glasgow Coma Scale, brainstem reflexes (cornea, cough, gag, extraocular movements), vital signs; skull and face (deformity, lacerations, bruising, bleeding); movement of extremities

## Nursing Diagnoses and Interventions

Nursing care of the client in the acute care phase initially focuses on maintaining an effective airway and breathing pattern. Nursing care is also directed toward continuous assessment and monitoring of neurologic function as well as other body systems. This close monitoring provides early recognition and treatment of problems and complications, and initiation of aggressive forms of therapy that may be needed.

Many nursing diagnoses associated with traumatic brain injury correspond with those outlined previously in the sections on the client with altered level of consciousness and increased intracranial pressure. Specific nursing diagnoses discussed in this section focus on problems with decreased intracranial adaptive capacity, airway clearance, and breathing patterns.

### Decreased Intracranial Adaptive Capacity

The client with a traumatic brain injury has or is at high risk for increased ICP. As the mechanisms that normally compensate for changes in intracranial pressure are compromised, intracranial pressure increases in disproportional response to a variety of stimuli. (See the discussion earlier in the chapter for other nursing diagnoses and interventions for the client with increased ICP).

- Monitor for manifestations of increased ICP, including eye opening response, motor response, and verbal response. *These responses evaluate the ability to integrate commands with conscious and involuntary movement.*
- Monitor for changes in vital signs: bradycardia or tachycardia, varying breathing patterns, hypertension, and/or widening pulse pressure. *Vital signs vary depending on the site of impairment. Cushing's triad (bradycardia, increased systolic blood pressure, and increased pulse pressure) indicates brainstem ischemia leading to cerebral herniation.*
- Assess for vomiting, headache, lethargy, restlessness, purposeless movements, and changes in mentation. *These manifestations may be early indicators of intracranial pressure changes.*
- Monitor temperature and initiate hypothermia treatment as prescribed. *Impaired hypothalmic function can interfere with temperature regulation. Hyperthermia may increase ICP.*
- Monitor fluid status: Regularly compare intake and output, review serum osmolality, and use infusion pump to administer IV fluids (if prescribed). *Osmotic diuretics, if used to treat cerebral edema, may cause hypotension and decreased cardiac output.*

**PRACTICE ALERT** *Overhydration from rapid infusion of IV fluids may cause or further increase increased ICP.* ■

## Ineffective Airway Clearance

The primary objective in the care of any trauma client is maintaining a patent airway to prevent hypoxia. However, in the initial acute care phase, the risk of cervical vertebral fractures and spinal cord injury may complicate the process of establishing a patent airway. In addition, other multisystem injuries may complicate the interpretation of vital signs. In general, all unconscious people with a head injury should be intubated with an endotracheal tube to prevent aspiration. Clients with head trauma may also require a tracheostomy to provide an airway and be placed on a ventilator.

- Assess neurologic manifestations on a regular schedule. *Changes in neurologic manifestations may indicate increased ICP, with the risk of further depression of the respiratory system and respiratory arrest.*
- Maintain head and neck in neutral alignment, immobilized until injury is determined. *Head rotation and neck flexion are associated with increased ICP, decreased jugular venous outflow, and localized changes in cerebral blood flow (Sullivan, 2000). Immobilization prevents spinal cord injury in suspected or actual fractures of the cervical spine; spinal cord injury at this level would further impair respiratory function.*
- Clear the nose and mouth of mucus and blood. *This ensures patency of the upper airway.*

- Suction the airway as needed, limiting suctioning time to no more than 10 seconds at one time. Do not suction the nasal passages until a dural tear has been ruled out. *Suctioning is usually necessary to maintain a patent airway.*

## Ineffective Breathing Pattern

The client with a traumatic brain injury and hematoma is at high risk for ineffective breathing pattern related to increased ICP. If ICP increases dramatically, tentorial herniation may occur, leading to sudden respiratory arrest.

- Monitor the respiratory pattern for rate, depth, and rhythm every 2 hours if the client is not on a ventilator. Assess breath sounds, presence of cyanosis, restlessness, and use of accessory respiratory muscles. Monitor pulse oximetry and blood gas levels. *Head injuries may cause alterations in respirations. An increased respiratory rate may indicate hypoxia. A decrease in respiratory rate may be the result of depression of the medullary respiratory center.*

**PRACTICE ALERT** *In general, an initial increase in intracranial pressure causes respirations to slow; as the pressure continues to increase, respirations become rapid.* ■

- Monitor ICP readings. *Continuous measurement of ICP is used to diagnose and monitor increased intracranial pressure. As ICP increases, herniation may occur, leading to respiratory arrest and death.*
- If the client is not intubated, prepare for oxygen administration and/or tracheal intubation if respiratory distress occurs. *Supplying oxygen prevents hypoxia until a hematoma can be evacuated, relieving pressure on the respiratory center.*
- Prepare for cranial surgery if deteriorating respiratory pattern and neurologic changes are noted. *Surgical intervention usually consists of placing several burr holes in the skull or performing a craniotomy to remove the hematoma. (Intracranial surgery is discussed later in the chapter.) However, the cerebral edema and increased intracranial pressure may cause death even if surgery is performed.*

## Using NANDA, NIC, and NOC

Chart 42–2 shows links between NANDA nursing diagnoses, NIC, and NOC when caring for the client with an acute brain injury.

## Home Care

### Concussion

Inform the client and family that a postconcussion syndrome sometimes occurs. If the client experiences persistent headaches and dizziness, is uncharacteristically emotional, seems overly tired, or has difficulty paying attention or remembering, the health care provider should be notified. Explain that these manifestations may persist for some time. Rehabilitation may help the client compensate for memory impairment and attention deficits.

## CHART 42-2  NANDA, NIC, AND NOC LINKAGES

### The Client with an Acute Brain Injury

| NURSING DIAGNOSES | NURSING INTERVENTIONS | NURSING OUTCOMES |
|---|---|---|
| • Acute Confusion | • Delirium Management<br>• Surveillance: Safety | • Cognitive Ability<br>• Neurological Status: Consciousness<br>• Memory |
| • Risk for Aspiration | • Aspiration Precautions<br>• Vomiting Management | • Neurological Status |
| • Hyperthermia | • Temperature Regulation | • Thermoregulation |
| • Impaired Memory | • Memory Training | • Memory |
| • Disturbed Sensory Perception | • Cerebral Perfusion Promotion<br>• Environmental Management<br>• Cerebral Edema Management<br>• ICP Monitoring | • Cognitive Ability<br>• Neurological Status |

*Note. Data from Nursing Outcomes Classification (NOC) by M. Johnson & M. Maas (Eds.), 1997, St. Louis: Mosby; Nursing Diagnoses: Definitions & Classification 2001–2002 by North American Nursing Diagnosis Association, 2001, Philadelphia: NANDA; Nursing Interventions Classification (NIC) by J.C. McCloskey & G. M. Bulechek (Eds.), 2000, St. Louis: Mosby. Reprinted by permission.*

## Acute Brain Injury

Clients who survive an acute brain injury will require long-term physical care and rehabilitation. Although recovery is highly individualized, many clients who regain consciousness require life-long care; others remain in a coma or vegetative state. The family often expects the client to recover fully after the coma subsides, and they need information about the real possibility of residual deficits in self-care, emotional responses, cognition, communication, and movement. Topics that should be addressed for home care include:

• The need to encourage self-care and independence as much as possible.

• Positioning, movement, and skin care to prevent contractures and pressure ulcers.
• Safety issues.
• Equipment needs, such as a wheelchair and hospital bed.
• Vocational counseling and services.
• Referral to community resources and support groups.
• Helpful resources:
  • National Head Injury Foundation
  • Brain Trauma Foundation
  • International Center for Individuals with Disabilities

## Nursing Care Plan

### A Client with a Subdural Hematoma

Wong Lee is a 50-year-old tug boat mechanic who is married and has three sons. Although Mr. Lee has been through rehabilitation twice for alcoholism, he has not been able to quit drinking. His physician has explained the physical consequences and the possible interaction between alcohol and the anticoagulant Mr. Lee is taking for chronic atrial fibrillation. While attending a family reunion, during which he eats a large meal and drinks several beers, Mr. Lee joins a game of softball. Mrs. Lee is concerned that Mr. Lee has consumed too much alcohol to play ball in the heat, but Mr. Lee is adamant and states that he wants to pitch. During the end of the second inning, the batter hits a ball that strikes Mr. Lee in the head. Mr. Lee stumbles and drops to the ground, holding his head. He does not lose consciousness and gets up on his own. His sons and wife try to persuade him to go to the hospital, but Mr. Lee insists he feels fine.

Two weeks later, after an evening of consuming several mixed drinks, Mr. Lee develops a headache. He attributes the headache to a hangover, but instead of improving the next day, the headache becomes steadily worse. He becomes confused and disoriented. His wife, concerned that his drinking is increasing again, calls the physician, who admits Mr. Lee to the detoxification center at the local hospital. A CT scan is performed. The diagnosis of a subdural hematoma is made, and Mr. Lee is transferred to the neurosurgical unit.

### ASSESSMENT

When Saundra Knight, the nurse on the neurosurgical unit, enters the room, she notices that Mr. Lee is sitting in bed, laughing and giddy. As she begins to talk to Mr. Lee, he states, "Don't ask me anything—I can't think. My headache is getting worse." Over the next few hours, the giddiness subsides, and Mr. Lee becomes drowsy. Ms. Knight reports a Glasgow Coma Scale score of 11. An

*(continued on page 1382)*

## Nursing Care Plan

## A Client with a Subdural Hematoma *(continued)*

ICP monitor is inserted and reveals increased intracranial pressure. Mr. Lee is scheduled to have burr holes and hematoma evacuation that afternoon.

### DIAGNOSES

- *Risk for ineffective breathing pattern* related to pressure on respiratory center by intracranial hematoma
- *Ineffective cerebral tissue perfusion* related to increased intracranial pressure secondary to cerebral edema

### EXPECTED OUTCOMES

- Maintain a respiratory rate and rhythm within normal limits.
- Maintain adequate cerebral perfusion, as evidenced by stable vital signs, stable neurologic status, and no decrease in level of consciousness.

### PLANNING AND IMPLEMENTATION

- Perform neurologic assessment every 2 hours or as needed.
- Monitor vital signs every 2 hours or as needed.
- Explain to the family the procedure for intracranial surgery.

### EVALUATION

The first day postoperatively, Mr. Lee begins breathing on his own without ventilatory support. His respiratory rate and rhythm are within normal limits, with no signs of abnormal breath sounds. The ICP monitor readings are appropriate, and Mr. Lee shows significant improvement in level of consciousness, with a Glasgow Coma Scale score of 15. Mr. Lee continues to improve and is discharged to home 5 days after surgery.

### Critical Thinking in the Nursing Process

1. Describe the similarities and differences between Mr. Lee's disorder and the manifestations of other types of intracranial hematomas.
2. Mr. Lee kept trying to pull out his ICP line. You know he should not be restrained, because pulling against restraints increases restlessness and increases intracranial pressure. What would you do?
3. Write a care plan for Mr. Lee for the nursing diagnosis, *Acute confusion*.

See Evaluating Your Response in Appendix C.

## THE CLIENT WITH A CENTRAL NERVOUS SYSTEM INFECTION

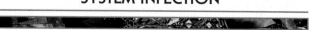

The central nervous system (CNS), including the meninges, neural tissues, and blood vessels, may be directly affected by bacteria, viruses, fungi, protozoans, and rickettsiae. The CNS may also be affected by toxins from bacterial infections. The major CNS infections include meningitis, encephalitis, and brain abscesses.

## INCIDENCE AND PREVALENCE

The most common infection of the meninges is bacterial meningitis. The mortality rate is 25% in adults. Brain abscess occur 2 times more often in men than in women, with the median age for abscess formation 30 to 40 years (McCance & Huether, 2002). Meningococcal meningitis may occur in epidemics among people who are in close contact with one another, such as military recruits and students living in dormitories. Pneumococcal meningitis, in contrast, primarily affects the very young and very old.

The incidence of pathogenic infections of the CNS increases with the onset of AIDS. Clients who are HIV positive may have CNS infections caused by toxoplasmosis, cryptococcus, tuberculosis, herpes simplex, cytomegalovirus, or a polyoma virus (resulting in progressive multifocal leukoencephalopathy).

## Risk Factors

Those at highest risk are the young, frail older adults, those with debilitating diseases, and the immunosuppressed (such as clients having radiation therapy or chemotherapy treatments).

Other risk factors are having AIDS, having an infection elsewhere in the body, and having a skull fracture or invasive neurosurgery (King, 1999).

## PATHOPHYSIOLOGY AND MANIFESTATIONS

When pathogens enter the CNS and the meninges, an inflammatory process results. The pathology of CNS infections includes the invading pathogens, the subsequent inflammation, and the increase in intracranial pressure that may result from the inflammatory processes. Both the pathogenic damage and the increased ICP may result in brain damage and life-threatening complications.

### Meningitis

**Meningitis** is an inflammation of the pia mater, the arachnoid, and the subarachnoid space. Inflammation spreads rapidly throughout the CNS because of the circulation of CSF around the brain and spinal cord. Infection is the usual cause of meningitis, although chemical meningitis may also occur (Porth, 2002). Meningitis may be acute or chronic, and it may be bacterial, viral, fungal, or parasitic in origin.

In meningitis, the infecting organisms usually reach the CNS in one of two ways: by direct extension, such as can occur after cranial trauma or invasive procedures (e.g., ICP monitoring devices or neurosurgery); or through the bloodstream secondary to another infection in the body.

The organism responsible for meningitis must overcome nonspecific and specific host defense mechanisms to invade and replicate in the CSF. These defenses include the skin barrier, the blood-brain barrier, the nonspecific inflammatory response, and the immune response. Host response to the particular pathogen is responsible for the manifestations of clinical meningitis. The organisms that initiate the host response in meningitis demonstrate an affinity for the nervous system. They colonize and invade the nasopharyngeal mucosa, survive intravascularly, and penetrate the CNS if the blood-brain barrier is damaged, as can happen during surgery, the inflammatory response, or cerebral edema.

Infection of the CSF and meninges causes an inflammatory response in the pia, arachnoid, and CSF. Because the meninges and subarachnoid space are continuous around the brain, spinal cord, and optic nerves, the infection and inflammatory response is always cerebrospinal, involving both the brain and the spinal cord. Inflamed blood vessels in the area leak fluids as cell permeability increases. Purulent exudate infiltrates cranial nerve sheaths and blocks the choriod plexus and subarachnoid villi. Increased ICP occurs as brain tissue responds to the pathogen. With an increase in ICP, cerebral perfusion decreases and cerebral autoregulation is lost.

### Bacterial Meningitis

The causative organisms of bacterial meningitis include *Neisseria meningitis,* meningococcus, *Streptococcus pneumoniae, Haemophilus influenzae,* and *E. coli.* Risk factors include head trauma with a basilar skull fracture, otitis media, sinusitis, neurosurgery, systemic sepsis, or immunocompromise (Porth, 2002).

Once the pathogen enters the central nervous system, it or its toxic products (free radicals) initiate an inflammatory response in the meninges, CSF, and ventricles. Meningeal vessels become engorged, and their permeability increases. Phagocytic white blood cells migrate into the subarachnoid space, forming a purulent exudate that thickens and clouds the CSF and interferes with its flow. Rapid exudate formation causes further inflammation and edema of meningeal cells. Blood vessel engorgement, exudate formation, impaired CSF flow, and cellular edema cause the intracranial pressure to increase.

The client with bacterial meningitis typically presents with fever and chills, headache, back and abdominal pain, and nausea and vomiting. (The older adult may not have a high fever, but may rather exhibit confusion). Meningeal irritation causes *nuchal rigidity,* with a very stiff neck and positive Brudzinski's sign (flexion of the neck that causes the hip and knee to flex) and positive Kernig's sign (inability to extend the knee while the hip is flexed at a 90-degree angle). Photophobia is present; the client may also experience diplopia. With meningococcal meningitis, a rapidly spreading petechial rash involving the skin and mucous membranes may be noted. The client may also have increased ICP, manifested by decreased LOC, seizures, changes in vital signs and respiratory pattern, and papilledema. The manifestations of bacterial meningitis are listed in the box in the following column.

Complications of bacterial meningitis include arthritis, cranial nerve damage, and hydrocephalus. Cranial nerve VIII, the auditory nerve, is frequently affected, with resulting nerve deafness. Thrombophlebitis may develop in cerebral vessels, with infarction of surrounding tissues (Porth, 2002).

## Manifestations of Bacterial Meningitis

- Restlessness, agitation, and irritability
- Severe headache
- Signs of meningeal irritation:
  a. Nuchal rigidity (stiff neck)
  b. Positive Brudzinski's sign
  c. Positive Kernig's sign
- Chills and high fever
- Confusion, altered LOC
- Photophobia (aversion to light), diplopia
- Seizures
- Signs of increased ICP (widened pulse pressure and bradycardia, respiratory irregularity, decreased LOC, headache, and vomiting)
- Petechial rash (in meningococcal meningitis)

### Viral Meningitis

Acute viral meningitis, also called aseptic meningitis, is a less severe disease than bacterial meningitis. It can be caused by numerous viruses, such as herpes simplex, herpes zoster, Epstein-Barr virus, or cytomegalovirus (CMV). Viral meningitis most often appears after a case of mumps. Although viral infection also triggers the inflammatory response, the course of the disease is benign and of short duration. Recovery is uneventful.

The manifestations of viral meningitis are similar to those of bacterial meningitis, although usually milder. The client may have a mild flulike illness prior to the onset of meningitis. Headache is intense and is accompanied by malaise, nausea, vomiting, and lethargy. Photophobia may be present. The client generally remains oriented, although possibly drowsy. Temperature is mildly elevated. Neck stiffness, positive Brudzinski's sign, and positive Kernig's sign are usually present.

## Encephalitis

**Encephalitis** is an acute inflammation of the parenchyma of the brain or spinal cord. It is almost always caused by a virus, but it may also be caused by bacteria, fungi, and other organisms. Other less common causes include ingested lead; postvaccination encephalitis (from vaccines for measles, mumps, and rabies), and HIV (Porth, 2002). See Table 42–8 for a list of the most common causes of encephalitis.

### Viral Encephalitis

Viruses depend on living tissue for reproduction and become highly destructive when they invade brain tissue. The inflammatory response extends over the cerebral cortex, the white matter, and the meninges, with degeneration of the neurons. The pathology of encephalitis includes local necrotizing hemorrhage, which ultimately becomes generalized, with prominent edema. There is progressive degeneration of nerve cell bodies. The inflammatory response in encephalitis does not cause exudate formation as it does in meningitis. Certain viruses show a propensity for specific areas of the brain (e.g., herpes simplex virus involves frontal and temporal lobes). The

## TABLE 42-8   Causes of Encephalitis

| Cause | Comments |
|---|---|
| Arboviruses | Transmitted by bites from ticks and mosquitoes. <br> Bites from ticks occur more frequently in spring. <br> Bites from mosquitoes occur in middle to late summer. <br> Most common types are St. Louis and eastern and western equine encephalitis. <br> May destroy major parts of the lobe or hemisphere. <br> Two-thirds of clients who develop eastern equine encephalitis either die or develop severe residual disabilities (e.g., seizures, blindness, deafness, speech disorders, or mental retardation). <br> The incubation is 5 to 15 days. <br> Mortality rates associated with arboviruses are higher than those associated with enteroviruses. |
| Enteroviruses, such as echovirus, coxsackievirus, poliovirus, paramyxovirus (the virus that causes mumps), and varicella-zoster (the virus that causes chickenpox) | Infection occurs more frequently in summer (except infection by the mumps virus, which occurs more frequently in early winter). <br> Some degree of protection can be afforded by immunization against measles, mumps, and poliomyelitis. <br> Mortality rates are lower than those associated with herpes simplex type 1 virus. |
| Herpes simplex type 1 virus | Most common nonepidemic encephalitis in North America. <br> Can occur any time of year and throughout the world. <br> Has an affinity for the inferomedial portions of the frontal and temporal lobes. <br> Prognosis is grave but not hopeless: Mortality rate can be as high as 40%, and client may die within 2 weeks. |
| Amebic meningoencephalitis due to infection by *Naegleria* and *Acanthamoeba* protozoa | Both protozoa are found in warm fresh water. <br> Enter the nasal mucosa of people swimming in ponds or lakes. <br> May also be found in soil and decaying vegetation. <br> Incidence of infection is increasing in North America. |
| Exogenous poisoning | May occur after ingestion of lead or arsenic or inhalation of carbon monoxide. |

virus gains access to the CNS via the bloodstream or along peripheral or cranial nerves, or it may already be present in the meninges in the client with meningitis.

The manifestations of viral encephalitis vary, depending on the organism and area of the brain affected. Usual manifestations are similar to those of meningitis, including fever, headache, seizures, stiff neck, and altered LOC. The client may be disoriented, agitated and restless, or lethargic and drowsy. As the disease progresses, the LOC deteriorates, and the client may become comatose.

### Arbovirus Encephalitis

The arboviruses are arthropod (mosquito or tick) borne agents that infect humans. They include many different types, including Western equine encephalitis, St. Louis encephalitis, and Rift Valley fever. Adults are most often infected with St. Louis encephalitis, with older adults affected more often. The arthropods may live in small mammals and birds, or may be carried by horses and deer. The newest arboviral encephalitis in the United States is West Nile encephalitis, first identified in 1999. Bird infections began in New York and are spreading across the continent.

The arthropod-borne agents cause widespread degeneration of nerve cells, and edema and necrosis with or without hemorrhage occur. Increased ICP may develop. Manifestations include fever, malaise, sore throat, nausea and vomiting, stiff neck, tremors, paralysis of extremities, exaggerated deep tendon reflexes, seizures, and altered level of consciousness.

## Brain Abscess

A **brain abscess** is an infection with a collection of purulent material within the brain tissue. Approximately 80% are found in the cerebrum and 20% are cerebellar.

The causes of a brain abscess include open trauma and neurosurgery; infections of the mastoid, middle ear, nasal cavity, or nasal sinuses; metastatic spread from distant foci (such as heart, lungs, skin, abscessed teeth, and dirty needles); and arising from other associated areas of infection. The immunocompromised are at increased risk for abscesses. The most common pathogens causing the abscess are streptococci, staphylococci, and bacteroids. Yeast and fungi may also cause brain abscess.

A brain abscess results from the presence of microorganisms in the brain tissue. If the abscess is encapsulated, it has the ability to enlarge and, therefore, behave as a space-occupying lesion within the cranium. This predisposes the client not only to the systemic effects of the inflammatory process but also to the serious consequences of increased intracranial pressure. Occasionally, the abscess does not become encapsulated; instead, it spreads through the brain tissue to the subarachnoid space and ventricular system.

Initially, the client exhibits the general symptoms associated with an acute infectious process, such as chills, fever, malaise, and anorexia. Because brain abscess generally forms after infection, the client may consider these signs to be an exacerbation of that illness. The client may experience seizures, altered level of consciousness, and manifestations of increased ICP. As the abscess enlarges, specific symptoms are related to location; for example the client with a frontal lobe abscess may have contralateral hemiparesis, expressive aphasia, focal seizures, and frontal headache.

## COLLABORATIVE CARE

Bacterial meningitis is a medical emergency that, if not treated immediately, can be fatal within days. Successful management depends on rapid diagnosis and aggressive treatment to eradicate the infecting organism and support vital functions. The client may be placed in strict or respiratory isolation until the organism has been identified, depending on hospital policy. Universal precautions apply to CSF as well as blood.

Treatment for viral meningitis focuses on managing client symptoms and is supportive. Antipyretics and analgesics may provide relief. Antibiotic therapy is not indicated, and isolation precautions are not required.

Treatment of the client with a brain abscess focuses on prompt initiation of antibiotic therapy. Other manifestations are treated symptomatically, as with the client diagnosed with meningitis or encephalitis. If pharmacologic management is not effective, the abscess may be drained or, if it is encapsulated, removed.

### Diagnostic Tests

The diagnosis of meningitis is based on manifestations and diagnostic tests results. The following diagnostic tests may be ordered.

- *Lumbar puncture* with examination of the CSF is the definitive diagnostic measure for bacterial meningitis. Data that indicate bacterial meningitis include turbid, cloudy fluid; a markedly increased white blood cell count and protein content; and a decreased glucose content. The opening pressure on the lumbar puncture is elevated. In contrast, CSF analysis in the client with encephalitis may have a normal CSF analysis and pressure or may have some lymphocytes. The client with a brain abscess will have a markedly elevated pressure with elevated protein content and elevated WBC count. Glucose content is normal. (As a lumbar puncture in the presence of a space-occupying lesion can result in brain herniation and death, a CT scan is performed first if neurologic findings support such a lesion.)
- *Gram stain* and *culture of the CSF* are performed. Gram stain is used to determine if a bacterial infection is present. Cultures are used to determine the specific agent; no bacteria are cultured from the CSF in viral meningitis. Culture results take several days.
- *Counterimmunoelectrophoresis (CIE)* is a laboratory test that may be ordered to determine the presence of viruses or protozoa.
- *Polymerase chain reaction techniques* may be used to detect viral DNA or RNA in spinal fluid. This test is especially sensitive to herpes simplex.
- *MRI* can detect focal edema and hemorrhage in encephalitis.
- *CT scan* will show an area of increased contrast surrounding a low-density core with brain abscess.

## Medications

### Meningitis

Immediate intravenous administration of a broad-spectrum antibiotic that crosses the blood-brain barrier into the subarachnoid space is instituted in cases of bacterial meningitis. Once culture reports identify the causative organism, drug therapy is continued from 7 to 21 days, using the most effective drug or drugs specific to that bacterium. The cephalosporin antibiotics are preferred. A major concern in the treatment of CNS infections is penicillin-resistant streptococci. Recommendations for treatment are for a broad-spectrum cephalosporin, such as rifampin (Rifadin), cefotaxime (Claforam), or vancomycin (Vancocin). However, as the bacteria are killed, the toxins they release increase production of inflammatory cytokines, which are potentially lethal. Steroids such as dexamethasone (Decadron) are often give with the antibiotics to suppress inflammation. The CDC recommends that the client remain on isolation for 24 hours after the start of antibiotic therapy.

### Encephalitis

Treatment for encephalitis consists of administering specific medications and preventing complications. Fungal meningitis is treated with antifungal agents, such as amphotericin-B (Amphotec), flucytosine (Ancobon), and fluconazole (Diflucan). Viral encephalitis is treated with intravenous acyclovir (Zoviran) or vidarabine (Vira-A).

### Brain Abscess

Antibiotic therapy is the primary treatment for brain abscess. A combination of broad-spectrum antibiotics is used if the infecting organism is unknown.

An intraventricular method of medication administration uses an Ommaya reservoir that has been surgically implanted into a lateral ventricle of the brain (Figure 42–8 ■). This device

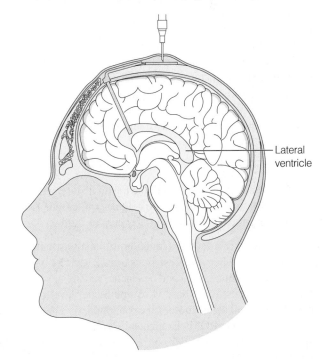

Lateral ventricle

**Figure 42–8** ■ Ommaya reservoir for medication administration.

is used to enhance CSF absorption of antibiotics and to maintain treatment over an extended period of time.

Anticonvulsant medications such as phenytoin (Dilantin) are often prescribed to prevent or control seizure activity. Antipyretic and analgesic medications may provide symptomatic relief; however, analgesics that have a depressant effect on the CNS (such as opiates) are avoided to prevent masking of early manifestations of deteriorating LOC. The client initially may require antiemetics to control nausea and vomiting. Fluid and electrolyte status is maintained through intravenous fluid replacement until the client is able to resume oral intake.

## Surgery

Surgical drainage of an encapsulated abscess may be necessary. The decision to perform surgery is based on the client's general condition, the stage of abscess development, and the site of the abscess.

## NURSING CARE

Central nervous system infections are serious illnesses, with potentially life-threatening effects and complications. Nursing assessments and interventions are critical in identifying changes in the client's neurologic status and preventing complications from increased ICP.

## Health Promotion

The following help to prevent central nervous system infections.

- Vaccinations for meningococcal, pneumococcal, and hemophilic meningitis
- Administration of prophylactic rifampin (Rifadin) for people exposed to meningococcal meningitis
- Mosquito control with repellants, insecticides, and protective clothing
- Destruction of the insect larvae and elimination of breeding places, such as pools of stagnant water
- Vaccination against Japanese B encephalitis (recommended for summer travelers to rural East Asia)
- Prompt diagnosis and treatment of infections of the head, neck, and respiratory system
- Careful asepsis for care of any client with an open head injury or postoperative neurosurgery

## Assessment

Collect the following data through the health history and physical examination (see Chapter 40). Further focused assessments are described with nursing interventions below.

- Health history: risk factors (concurrent infections, other illnesses, travel), when manifestations began, severity of manifestations, current nausea and headache, seizures
- Physical examination: Glasgow Coma Scale, level of consciousness, vital signs, motor function, pupillary check, cranial nerves, neck ROM, Brudzinski's sign, Kernig's sign, skin (rash, petechiae, purpura), muscle movement and strength, speech

## Nursing Diagnoses and Interventions

In planning and implementing nursing care for the client with a CNS infection, the prognosis may depend on the supportive care given. The client is often very ill, and the combination of fever, dehydration, and cerebral edema may predispose the client to seizures. Airway obstruction, respiratory arrest, or cardiac dysrhythmias may occur. Nursing diagnoses and interventions previously discussed for the client with an altered LOC, increased ICP, and seizures are also appropriate for the client with a CNS infection. Nursing interventions in this section focus on altered protection and risk for fluid volume deficit.

### Ineffective Protection

Clients with CNS infections are less able to protect themselves against insults from both internal and external sources. The effects of the inflammation and resulting pathophysiologic processes may include pain, fever, altered LOC, seizures, increased ICP, and cranial nerve dysfunction. In addition, pathophysiologic effects on the brain from toxins or thrombosis of a cerebral vessel may lead to permanent neurologic deficits, such as loss of motor function or dementia.

- Assess neurologic status on a regular basis. *Many complications are evidenced by changes in neurologic manifestations.*
- Assess vital signs, including temperature, on a regular basis. *The client often has a high temperature throughout the illness, ranging from 101°F (38°C) to 105°F (40.5°C).*

**PRACTICE ALERT** *Hyperthermia may result from increased intracranial pressure, while an increased temperature can also increase ICP.* ■

- Monitor levels of consciousness. Assess levels of orientation, memory, attention span, and response to stimuli. *Early in the infection, the client often has problems with memory and orientation. There may be problems with following commands, restlessness, irritability, and combativeness. As the illness progresses, the level of consciousness decreases to lethargy and finally into deep coma.*
- Assess for manifestations of seizure activity, and institute seizure precautions:
  - Monitor twitching of hands or face and tonic-clonic movements.
  - Have an oral airway and suction equipment readily available.
  - Pad side rails, maintain bed in low position, and keep side rails up.
  *Irritation of the cerebral cortex secondary to meningeal inflammation may cause seizures. Careful monitoring and seizure precautions are necessary to prevent injury.*
- Assess for manifestations of cranial nerve damage; monitor extraocular movements, facial movement, dizziness, ability to hear, double vision, drooping upper eyelids (*ptosis*), and pupillary changes. *Cranial nerve dysfunction may result from inflammation or vascular changes in the brain.*

- Assess for manifestations of increased intracranial pressure: decreased pulse, increased blood pressure, widening pulse pressure, respiratory changes, and vomiting. *Increased intracranial pressure results from infectious or inflammatory exudate, cerebral edema, and hydrocephalus.*
- Administer prescribed medications and maintain prescribed fluid restrictions. *Diuretics are often prescribed to prevent increases in ICP, anticonvulsants are prescribed to prevent or control seizures, and antibiotics are prescribed to eradicate the bacteria. Fluids may be restricted to help prevent increased ICP.*

### Risk for Deficient Fluid Volume

The client is at risk for fluid volume deficit related to increased metabolic rate, diaphoresis, and fluid restrictions.

- Assess for presence, or worsening, of fluid volume deficit.
  - Measure and compare intake and output every 2 to 4 hours.
  - Monitor daily body weights.
  - Monitor skin turgor.
  - Monitor condition of mucous membranes.
  - Monitor urine amount, color, and odor.
  - Monitor BUN:creatinine ratio.

  *The elastic property of the skin depends partially on interstitial fluid volume. If there is a fluid volume deficit, skin flattens more slowly after a pinch is released. Mucous membranes are dry. In fluid volume deficit, urine output is decreased, urine is dark in color and concentrated with a strong odor, and urine specific gravity is greater than 1.020, and BUN will rise out of proportion to serum creatinine.*

---

**PRACTICE ALERT** *An acute weight loss of 1 lb represents a fluid loss of approximately 500 mL.* ■

- When administering fluids, either orally or parenterally, consider concurrent illnesses. For example, clients with increased intracranial pressure or renal failure require complex management. See Chapter 5 🔗 for a further discussion of fluid volume deficit.

## Using NANDA, NIC and NOC

Chart 42–3 shows links between NANDA nursing diagnoses, NIC, and NOC when caring for the client with a CNS infection.

## Home Care

The importance of preventive measures, such as recognizing predisposing conditions, is a major focus for client education. People who have had close contact with the client with meningitis should be assessed for fever, headache, or neck stiffness. Some physicians believe that those closest to the client are candidates for antimicrobial prophylaxis. Also address the following topics.

- The need to report any signs or symptoms of ear infection, sore throat, or upper respiratory infection
- The names and purposes of all medications that may be prescribed
- The importance of taking all medication until completely gone, because some clients may think it is acceptable to stop the medication as soon as they feel better

---

## CHART 42–3 NANDA, NIC, AND NOC LINKAGES

### The Client with a CNS Infection

| NURSING DIAGNOSES | NURSING INTERVENTIONS | NURSING OUTCOMES |
|---|---|---|
| • Risk for Imbalanced Body Temperature | • Temperature Regulation<br>• Vital Signs Monitoring<br>• Cerebral Edema Management | • Infection Status |
| • Acute Confusion | • Delirium Management<br>• Surveillance: Safety | • Cognitive Ability<br>• Neurological Status: Consciousness<br>• Memory |
| • Self-Care Deficit | • Self-Care Assistance | • Self-Care: ADLs<br>• Self-Care: Bathing<br>• Self-Care: Hygiene<br>• Self-Care: Eating<br>• Self-Care: Toileting |

*Note.* Data from *Nursing Outcomes Classification (NOC) by M. Johnson & M. Maas (Eds.), 1997, St. Louis: Mosby; Nursing Diagnoses: Definitions & Classification 2001–2002 by North American Nursing Diagnosis Association, 2001, Philadelphia: NANDA; Nursing Interventions Classification (NIC) by J.C. McCloskey & G. M. Bulechek (Eds.), 2000, St. Louis: Mosby.* Reprinted by permission.

## Nursing Care Plan
## A Client with Bacterial Meningitis

Monty Cook is a 22-year-old musician who plays in a local rock band. He is unmarried and lives with his parents. He is known by everyone in the community as a quiet, low-key, easygoing person and an excellent guitar player. During a performance 2 days ago, he had difficulty playing his guitar, complaining of bright stage lights blazing in his eyes. When he tried to keep his head down to prevent the lights from hurting his eyes, he noticed his neck was very stiff. After the performance, one of the newest members of the band remarked that it certainly was not their best performance. Monty responded angrily that maybe the new members of the group needed more practice. Then he stomped out and went home to bed.

He wakes at 4:00 A.M. with a severe headache, sweating, and chills; his temperature is 102°F, and he cannot bend his neck without severe pain. His mother recognizes that he is agitated and irritable, which is uncharacteristic. Frightened, she rushes him to the hospital emergency room. A lumbar puncture performed in the emergency room reveals turbid, cloudy fluid, a markedly increased white blood cell count, and protein with a decreased glucose content. Bacterial meningitis is the medical diagnosis. Mr. Cook is admitted to the hospital for treatment and care.

### ASSESSMENT
When the nurse, Aisha Aldi, enters Mr. Cook's isolation room, she sees him thrashing about in the bed, talking incoherently, and becoming more agitated. On assessment, Ms. Aldi notes dry mucous membranes, cracked lips, and small petechiae over the upper torso and abdomen. Mr. Cook's temperature is 104°F. Kernig's sign is positive. Intravenous broad-spectrum antibiotics are prescribed and initiated. After the first 2 hours on duty, Ms. Aldi notes a decrease in Mr. Cook's level of consciousness.

### DIAGNOSES
- *Hyperthermia* related to infection and abnormal temperature regulation by hypothalamus
- *Disturbed thought processes* related to intracranial infection
- *Ineffective protection* related to progression of illness

### EXPECTED OUTCOMES
- Have a decrease in body temperature.
- Become less restless and agitated.
- Remain free of injury.

### PLANNING AND IMPLEMENTATION
- Monitor vital signs every 2 hours.
- Provide sponge baths if temperature continues to rise.
- Provide a quiet, nonstimulating environment with the shades drawn.
- Provide oral care every 4 hours.
- Measure and compare intake and output every 2 hours.
- Perform neurologic assessments every 2 to 4 hours.
- Monitor for and report seizure activity and decreasing level of consciousness.
- Keep bed in low position with side rails elevated.
- Administer prescribed intravenous antibiotics.

### EVALUATION
After 4 days of antibiotic therapy, Mr. Cook's temperature has returned to near normal. Ms. Aldi notes that he has begun opening his eyes and visually tracking her as she moves about the room. Mr. Cook responds to a request to squeeze Ms. Aldi's fingers and after several hours asks her what had happened. On day 5, Mr. Cook states that he feels better and his headache is gone. He asks for sips of juice and begins urinating regularly. Seven days after admission, Mr. Cook is discharged and is able to go home with his mother. He has some weakness in his legs, but otherwise has no evidence of neurologic deficits.

### Critical Thinking in the Nursing Process
1. What strategies should the nurse use to decrease the environmental stimuli for Mr. Cook, and what is the rationale for doing these?
2. If you were caring for Mr. Cook in the initial phase of the illness and he became combative, what would you do?
3. Develop a plan of care for Mr. Cook for the nursing diagnosis, *Acute pain*. Consider the effect of narcotics on respiratory function in designing the plan.

See Evaluating Your Response in Appendix C.

## THE CLIENT WITH A BRAIN TUMOR

**Brain tumors** are growths within the cranium, including tumors in brain tissue, meninges, pituitary gland, or blood vessels. Brain tumors may be benign or malignant, primary or metastatic, and intracerebral or extracerebral. Regardless of type or location, brain tumors are potentially lethal as they grow within a closed cranial vault and displace or impinge on CNS structures.

## INCIDENCE AND PREVALENCE

An estimated 17,000 new cases of malignant brain tumors are diagnosed in the United States each year (American Cancer Society, 2001). In addition, more than 100,000 people die each year from metastatic brain tumors (Porth, 2002). Although brain tumors can occur in any age group, the highest incidence is among young children and among adults ages 50 to 70. In the adult population, the most common tumor is glioblastoma multiforme, followed by meningioma and cytoma. Glioblastomas represent more than 50% of all primary intracranial lesions.

The cause of many brain tumors is unknown. Although a number of chemical and viral agents can cause brain tumors in laboratory animals, there is no evidence that these agents cause tumors in humans. Other factors associated with brain tumors include heredity, cranial irradiation, and exposure to some chemicals (Porth, 2002).

## TABLE 42-9  Classification of Brain Tumors

| Tumor Type | Tumor | Characteristics |
|---|---|---|
| **Primary Tumors**<br>Intracerebral tumors<br>Account for 40% to 50% of all brain tumors<br>Originates from neuroglia and invades brain tissue<br>Most common type of brain tumor | *Glioma*<br>• Astrocytoma<br><br>• Glioblastoma multiforme<br>• Ependymoma<br><br><br>• Oligodendroglioma<br><br>• Astroblastoma | <br>Most common glioma<br>Graded I to IV according to degree of cell differentiation<br>Most malignant form<br>Fast growing<br>Tumor that develops from lining of ventricles<br>Graded I to IV according to degree of cell differentiation<br>Slow growing<br>Rare, slow growing<br>May be encapsulated<br>Benign |
| Extracerebral tumors<br>Tumors arising from the supporting structures of the nervous system<br>Account for 10% to 15% of all brain tumors | Medulloblastoma<br><br><br>Meningioma<br><br><br>Acoustic neuroma | Fast growing and malignant<br>Occurs primarily in children; can occur in adults<br>Found in cerebellum<br>Slow growing<br>Develops in meninges (especially dura)<br>Firm and encapsulated<br>Slow growing<br>Benign<br>Originates from Schwann cells of the cranial nerve XIII<br>May also affect cranial nerves V, VII, IX, and X<br>Also called neurofibromatosis<br>Genetic origin due to autosomal dominant mendelian trait<br>Firm, encapsulated lesions attached to nerve |
| Congenital (developmental) tumors<br>Account for 4% to 8% of all brain tumors | Hemangioblastoma<br><br>Craniopharyngioma | Vascular tumor<br>Slow growing<br>Originates from Rathke's pouch<br>Solid or cystic tumor<br>Compresses pituitary gland<br>Presses on the third ventricle and may cause blockage of cerebrospinal fluid (CSF) |
| Pituitary adenomas<br>Slow growing<br>Account for 8% to 12% of all brain tumors | Chromophobic<br><br>Eosinophilic<br>Basophilic | Account for 90% of pituitary tumors<br>Nonsecreting tumor<br>Secreting tumors that produce growth hormone<br>Secreting tumors that produce adrenocorticotropic hormone<br>Fast growing |
| **Secondary Tumors**<br>Metastatic brain tumors<br>    Slow-growing tumors that arise from other parts of the body<br>Account for 10% of all brain tumors<br>Tumors of the lung, breast, lower gastrointestinal tract, pancreas, kidney, skin | | <br><br><br><br><br>Usually well differentiated from the brain |

## PATHOPHYSIOLOGY AND MANIFESTATIONS

Brain tumors may be classified as benign or malignant, based on the tissue type and characteristics of the cells. The use of the term *benign* may be misleading. A tumor that is benign by histologic examination but is surgically inaccessible may continue to expand, increasing intracranial pressure and causing neurologic deficits, herniation, and finally death. In discussions of brain tumors, the term *malignant* is used to describe the lack of cell differentiation, the invasive nature of the tumor, and its ability to metastasize.

Brain tumors also may be classified as primary or metastatic, depending on their origin (Table 42–9). Primary tumors of CNS tissue arise from the cells and structures that are found within the brain, for example, neurons and neuroglia. The primary intracranial tumors that originate in the skull cavity but not from brain tissue itself arise from the supporting structures; including the meninges, pituitary gland, and pineal gland. Primary brain tumors rarely metastasize outside the central nervous system. Metastatic brain tumors originate from structures outside the brain, such as the breasts, lungs, and prostate gland.

Focal disturbances take place when there is compression of brain tissue and infiltration or direct invasion of brain parenchyma with destruction of neural tissue. As the tumor grows, edema develops in adjacent tissues. The mechanism is not completely understood, but it is thought that an osmotic gradient causes the tumor to absorb fluid. Some tumors may cause hemorrhage. Venous obstruction and edema due to breakdown of the blood-brain barrier increase intracranial volume and intracranial pressure. Obstruction of the circulation of CSF from the lateral ventricles to the subarachnoid space causes hydrocephalus.

An estimated 25% of people with cancer develop brain metastasis. Metastatic brain tumors present in the same way as primary brain tumors, with increased ICP, and focal and/or diffuse cerebral dysfunction. The most common source of intracranial metastasis is cancer of the lung. Other common primary sites are the breast, kidney, and gastrointestinal tract. The metastasis reaches the brain through the circulation. In more than 75% of cases, the tumors are multiple and are scattered through the cerebellum and cerebrum (McCance & Huether, 2002).

Multiple manifestations can develop as a result of the growth of the tumor, while others are related to the location of the lesion (see the box below). Some of the more common manifestations include changes in cognition or consciousness, headache that is usually worse in the morning, seizures, and vomiting. Compression of brain tissue and the invasion of the brain tumor into the cerebral tissue may lead to changes typi-

cally seen with cerebral edema and increased ICP. Cerebral blood supply may diminish as the tumor compresses blood vessels. Shifts in brain tissue can occur, leading to brain herniation syndromes and, if untreated, death.

## COLLABORATIVE CARE

Treatment for a brain tumor may involve chemotherapy, radiation therapy, surgery, or any combination of these. Several variables are considered when selecting the appropriate treatment modality: the size and location of the tumor, the type of tumor, related symptoms (such as neurologic deficits), and the client's overall condition.

### Diagnostic Tests

The following diagnostic tests may be ordered.

- *CT scan* or *MRI* with gadolinium enhancement can locate the tumor and define its size, shape, extent to which normal anatomy is distorted, and the degree of any associated cerebral edema.
- *Arteriography* may show stretching or displacement of cerebral vessels by the tumor, as well as the presence of tumor vascularity.
- *EEG* provides information about cerebral function, may demonstrate focal or diffuse changes, and is useful if seizures are present.
- *Endocrine studies* are conducted if a pituitary tumor is suspected.

### Medications

The choice of drug for treatment is based on the type of tumor, its location, and the client's response to therapy. The use of chemotherapy to treat brain tumors is still emerging. An intraventricular method of medication administration uses an Ommaya reservoir that has been surgically implanted into a lateral ventricle of the brain (see Figure 42–8). Other medications that may be prescribed include corticosteroids and anticonvulsants.

### Treatments

#### Surgery

Surgery is used to remove tumors, to reduce the size of the tumor, or for symptom relief (*palliation*). The type of procedure, the surgical approach, and the timing of surgery (emergency versus planned procedure) influence the overall nursing management of the client having intracranial surgery.

Some of the more common intracranial neurosurgical procedures follow:

- **Burr hole.** A hole made in the skull with a special drill. The hole may facilitate the evacuation of an extracerebral clot, or a series of holes may be made in preparation of craniotomy (see Figure 42–7).
- **Craniotomy.** A surgical opening into the cranial cavity (Figure 42–9 ■). For a craniotomy, a series of burr holes are made. The bone between the holes is then cut with a special

## Manifestations of Brain Tumors

### FRONTAL LOBE TUMORS

- Inappropriate behavior
- Personality changes
- Inability to concentrate
- Impaired judgment
- Recent memory loss
- Headache
- Expressive aphasia
- Motor dysfunctions

### PARIETAL LOBE TUMORS

- Sensory deficits: paresthesia, loss of two-point discrimination, visual field deficits

### TEMPORAL LOBE TUMORS

- Psychomotor seizures

### OCCIPITAL LOBE TUMORS

- Visual disturbances

### CEREBELLUM TUMORS

- Disturbances in coordination and equilibrium

### PITUITARY TUMORS

- Endocrine dysfunction
- Visual deficits
- Headache

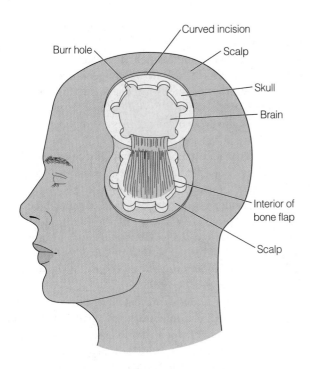

**Figure 42–9** ■ In a craniotomy, a portion of the skull and overlying scalp is removed to allow access to the brain.

saw called a craniotome. The tumor is excised, and the bone flap is turned down. A craniotomy may also be performed to repair defects associated with traumatic head injuries or to repair a cerebral aneurysm.

A *supratentorial craniotomy* refers to surgery above the tentorium. It provides access to the frontal, temporal, parietal, and occipital lobes. The incision for this procedure is usually within the hairline over the area involved.

An *infratentorial craniotomy* refers to surgery below the tentorium. Access is provided to lesions in the cerebellum and the brainstem. The incision is made at the nape of the neck, around the occipital lobe.

- **Craniectomy.** An excision of a portion of the skull and complete removal of the bone flap. This procedure may be done to provide decompression after cerebral edema. Pressure on the brain structures is lessened by providing space for expansion.
- **Cranioplasty.** Plastic repair to the skull in which synthetic material is inserted to replace the cranial bone that was removed. This procedure may be performed after a large craniectomy. The plastic repair restores the contour and integrity of the cranium.

### Radiation Therapy

Radiation therapy may be administered alone or as adjunctive therapy with surgery. Radiation is often the treatment of choice for surgically inaccessible tumors; it may also be used to decrease the size of a tumor prior to surgery. Tumors that were not completely excised by surgery may also be treated with radiation.

### Specialty Procedures

Technologic advances—including the development of special instruments, the use of stereotaxic techniques for localizing a specific target, and the use of the laser beam—have greatly advanced neurosurgical practice. Microsurgery involves an operating microscope with microinstruments and supportive illumination equipment. With stereotaxic techniques, the client is positioned to allow location of discrete areas of the brain that control specific functions and exact locations of deep brain lesions. The use of a laser beam for excision of a tumor results in less damage to surrounding tissue and less postoperative swelling. The gamma knife, which is not actually a knife but a gamma unit, consists of a heavily shielded helmet containing 201 sources of cobalt-60, which is capable of destroying deep and otherwise inaccessible lesions in a single treatment session.

## NURSING CARE

The nursing care of the client with a brain tumor includes support during the diagnostic period and specific management as directed by the selected treatment. The foundation for care is data from the health history and physical assessment, which includes identifying neurologic deficits. This information directs planning and implementing care. Many of the alterations in health commonly experienced by the client with a brain tumor have been discussed throughout this chapter, including altered level of consciousness, increased intracranial pressure, and seizures. The client will require intensive care in the immediate postoperative period.

### Nursing Diagnoses and Interventions

This section of the chapter focuses on nursing interventions for the client who has intracranial surgery. The nursing diagnoses discussed are anxiety, risk for infection, ineffective protection, acute pain, and disturbed self-esteem.

### Anxiety

The diagnosis of a brain tumor brings anxiety and feelings of uncertainty about the future. Both the client and family members are likely to be apprehensive and require education and emotional support.

- Assist through routine medical procedures, including blood work and radiologic studies. *Baseline laboratory and radiologic studies are needed to ensure that the client has no other preexisting medical condition. Explaining the procedures and assisting the client through this process helps decrease anxiety.*
- Reinforce, clarify, and repeat information. *Both client and family may have limited understanding of the scheduled diagnostic tests, procedures, and treatment modalities. The client may be confused or have altered thought processes as a result of the tumor. Information may need to be repeated or reexplained.*

- Encourage client and family to verbalize feelings, questions, and fears; provide realistic information appropriate to their level of understanding. *Verbalization helps reduce anxiety and fear.*
- Review client and family strengths and effective coping skills. *Personal strengths, support systems, and coping skills can aid in the development of appropriate strategies to reduce anxiety.*
- Arrange for a member of the clergy to visit if desired. *Faith in a higher being is often a strong source of strength and support.*
- Provide preoperative teaching, including the following information.
  - Type of anesthesia and surgery
  - Time surgery will begin and expected length of procedure and recovery room stay
  - Where the client will be taken after surgery (CCU, ICU) (If possible, show the client and family the CCU or ICU and introduce them to the nurse who will be in charge of care after the surgery.)
  - Where family can wait during and following surgery
  - Appearance of the client after surgery, which may include swollen, bruised eyelids and other facial features; a large dressing covering the head; and a tracheostomy or endotracheal tube
  - Behavior of the client after surgery, which will differ depending on the site of surgery, although cognitive and behavioral changes are common
  
  *Information about what to expect reduces anxiety.*
- Allow time for client and family to be together. *Clients and families need quiet time together to support each other and prepare emotionally for surgery.*

## Risk for Infection

The client who has had intracranial surgery is at risk for infection from multiple invasive lines, the scalp wound, and the risk of introduction of bacteria into the operative area. The nurse provides interventions to monitor for and prevent infection.

- Assess for leakage of CSF:
  - Presence of glucose in clear drainage from ears, nose, or wound
  - Complaints of "something dripping down the back of the throat"
  - Constant swallowing
  
  *These manifestations indicate an opening in the dura, which provides an avenue for an ascending infection.*
- Provide interventions to prevent contamination of area leaking CSF:
  - If leaking from the nose: Keep head of bed elevated 20 degrees unless contraindicated; do not suction nasally; do not clean nose; tell client not to put finger in nose; do not insert packing.
  - If leaking from the ear: Position client on side of leakage unless contraindicated; do not clean ear; tell client not to put finger in ear; do not insert packing.
  - Place a sterile dressing over the area of drainage and change as soon as it becomes damp.
  
  *Leakage of CSF indicates a break in the dura and increases the risk of an ascending infection. Surgery may be necessary*

*to repair the break; however, the leak usually heals spontaneously in about 1 week.*
- Monitor and report manifestations of infection:
  - Take and record temperature on a regular basis.
  - Assess IV insertion sites for redness, swelling, drainage, and pain.
  - Assess scalp wound for redness, swelling, bulging, drainage, and pain.
  - Assess for manifestations of meningitis: fever and chills, increasing headache, neck stiffness, positive Kernig's or Brudzinski's sign, photophobia.
  - Monitor laboratory reports for increased white blood cell count.
  
  *Intact skin is the first line of defense against infection. Any break in the skin increases the risk of infection. Intracranial surgery increases the risk of meningitis, with infectious agents ascending into the brain.*
- Implement interventions to prevent infection:
  - Use strict aseptic technique when changing dressings and when caring for wound drains and ICP monitor lines.
  - Keep the client's hands away from drains and dressings; use mitten restraints if necessary.
  - Administer prescribed antibiotics.
  
  *Sterile technique decreases the risk of introducing infection into a wound. Antibiotics are usually prescribed prophylactically to prevent infection.*

## Ineffective Protection

The client who has intracranial surgery does not have normal human defenses against changes in intracranial pressure and is also at risk from cerebral edema and a shift of intracerebral contents. In addition, the surgery may cause cerebral bleeding or hematoma formation.

- Monitor for manifestations of increased intracranial pressure:
  - Restlessness, agitation, and decreasing level of consciousness
  - Headache
  - Vomiting
  - Seizures
  - Decreasing sensory and motor function
  - Changes in pupil size and reaction
  - Changes in vital signs: altered respiratory rate or depth, increasing pulse pressure, decreasing pulse rate, increasing blood pressure
  - Abnormal posturing
  
  *Increasing intracranial pressure is manifested by alterations in the functions and centers controlled by the brain.*
- Implement interventions to decrease the risk of increased intracranial pressure:
  - Elevate the head of the bed 15 to 30 degrees as prescribed (unless contraindicated).
  - Avoid neck flexion or rotation; keep head in midline position unless a large bone flap or mass was removed; then position the client on unoperated side to decrease venous congestion in the operative area.
  - Do not take rectal temperatures.

- Avoid clustering activities that increase intracranial pressure: suctioning, turning, bathing.
- Administer medications to prevent vomiting.
- Do not suction for more than 10 seconds at one time.
- Teach the client (if possible) to avoid coughing, sneezing, and straining to have a bowel movement.
- Maintain fluid restrictions as prescribed.
- For internal shunts: Avoid pressure on the shunt, reservoir, or tubing. Pump the shunt as prescribed.
- For external shunts: Avoid kinks in tubing, and maintain the drainage collecting device and client's head at the prescribed levels.

*Keeping the head of the bed slightly elevated facilitates venous drainage from the brain. Neck flexion or rotation disrupts circulation to and from the brain. Rectal stimulation, suctioning, turning, bathing, coughing, sneezing, and straining to have a bowel movement all initiate Valsalva's maneuver, which constricts the jugular veins and impairs venous return from the brain. Fluid restriction may be prescribed to dehydrate the client slightly and lessen ICP.*

- Maintain (as much as possible) a quiet, calm, softly lighted environment. Avoid excessive sensory stimulation. *These interventions promote rest and decrease stimulation, thereby reducing ICP.*
- Implement interventions to prevent seizures or, if they occur, to prevent injury to the client:
  - Pad side rails of the bed.
  - Place bed in lowest position, and keep side rails up.
  - Carry out interventions to prevent and treat increased intracranial pressure.
  - Have an oral airway and suction equipment immediately available.
  - Administer prescribed anticonvulsants.
  - If a seizure occurs: Maintain a patent airway; do not restrain client; do not force anything into the client's mouth; provide physical and emotional support.

*These interventions promote safety and help prevent injury. Anticonvulsants are often prescribed prophylactically to prevent seizures after intracranial surgery.*

- Carefully monitor hydration status. Compare trends in intake and output, laboratory results of serum osmolality, and urine specific gravity and osmolality. *Changes in fluid balance and osmolality may result from excess intravenous fluids, osmotic diuretics, surgically induced diabetes insipidus or syndrome of inappropriate antidiuretic hormone secretion, fever, diarrhea, tube feedings, or hyperglycemia.*

## Acute Pain

The client who has intracranial surgery has pain, manifested as a headache, as a result of either compression or displacement of brain tissue or from increased intracranial pressure. A headache may also be a manifestation of meningitis.

- Assess the location, duration, and intensity of the pain, using a scale from 0 (no pain) to 10 (worst pain) in the client who can verbally communicate. *The client is the best source of information about pain.*

- Implement interventions to reduce the pain:
  - Raise the head of the bed slightly.
  - Reduce noise and bright lights in the room.
  - If allowed, loosen head dressing.
  - Administer narcotic analgesics with caution.

*Nonpharmacologic measures may be used to reduce increased intracranial pressure and headache.*

**PRACTICE ALERT** *Narcotic analgesics mask changes in eye signs and depress respirations.* ■

## Disturbed Self-Esteem

The client who has intracranial surgery has many alterations that affect self-esteem and body image. Physical changes include a loss of hair on the scalp, swelling and bruising in the eyelids and face, and perhaps an indentation in the skull. The client is no longer independent in self-care, but must depend on others to meet basic needs. There are often long-term neurologic deficits, affecting areas such as speech, vision, and motor abilities, which require changes in roles and relationships.

- Assess for verbal and nonverbal manifestations of negative self-esteem:
  - Denial of changes
  - Preoccupation with changes
  - Refusal to look in the mirror
  - Withdrawal from family and friends
  - Expressions of grief and loss (see Chapter 11) ⬛⬛

*Low self-esteem can be initiated by stressful situations and changes in body image.*

- Provide interventions to improve self-concept:
  - Limit negative self-assessment.
  - Help focus on positive areas of life.
  - Help identify sources of support and strength.
  - Help identify and use helpful coping methods.
  - Encourage significant others to visit.
  - Encourage independence in self-care.

*Self-esteem is derived from one's own perceptions of competence and from the responses of others. When one's self-concept and self-ideal are congruent, self-esteem is enhanced.*

## Home Care

The effect of the possible outcomes following the surgery produces fear in both client and family, interfering with their ability to retain information. Also, the client may have cognitive or neurologic deficits that interfere with learning. Family members also must be assessed for their ability to cope with the stress of the surgery. Information may have to be repeated several times.

Clients and their families who have experienced intracranial surgery require emotional support. The process of recovery is often extended and may involve adaptation to change in body image and management of any motor or sensory deficits. The family should be involved in the care of the client. If family members are willing, they may begin to assist with ADLs while the client is in the hospital, such as assisting with personal hygiene and meals. Clients should also be encouraged to

## Nursing Care Plan
## A Client with a Brain Tumor

Claire Lange is a 44-year-old television announcer. During one night's broadcast, she confuses several major news items so badly that her co-anchor tries to correct her. Ms. Lange responds angrily that she does not need any help and then rises and storms off the set. As she leaves the camera area, she limps noticeably and appears to drag her left leg. The show's producer asks her what is wrong; she screams that nothing is wrong—she simply has another headache. He follows her to her dressing room and inquires about her headaches. She tells him that they come and go but have been getting worse lately. He then asks her if she has injured her left leg; she responds that the leg was weak because she was tired. As the producer leaves the dressing room, Ms. Lange begins to shake and collapses on the floor. The producer recognizes that she is having a seizure and calls for an ambulance.

Ms. Lange is admitted to the neurology floor of the local hospital for evaluation. A CT scan, MRI study, and EEG are completed and identify an intracranial mass. A biopsy of the mass is positive for malignant cells. A glioma in the frontal lobe is identified, and surgery is scheduled for that week.

### ASSESSMENT

When Clara Rosetti, RN, enters Ms. Lange's room, she sees Ms. Lange looking at her shoulder-length hair in the mirror. Ms. Lange tells Ms. Rosetti that she has never in her life worn her hair any shorter, and "Now you're going to cut it all off!" She paces the room and makes the statement, "I guess the hair isn't really important if I survive this situation." She also says that she has a headache.

### DIAGNOSES

- *Acute pain* (headache) related to tumor and increase in intracranial pressure
- *Disturbed body image* related to upcoming hair loss and cranial incision
- *Anxiety* related to unknown future following surgery

### EXPECTED OUTCOMES

- Verbalize the causes of pain.
- Verbalize an understanding of the changes in body appearance that are associated with the scheduled intracranial surgery (e.g., shaving of the head prior to surgery, cranial incision, facial swelling postoperatively).

- Identify measures that will help minimize the effect of the hair loss.
- Verbalize a reduction in anxiety.

### PLANNING AND IMPLEMENTATION

- Assess level of discomfort using a rating scale of 0 to 10.
- Provide a quiet, nonstimulating environment.
- Position the client for comfort, keeping the head of the bed elevated to promote venous drainage.
- Assess level of consciousness for potential increases in ICP.
- Encourage to verbalize feelings about the surgery.
- Suggest measures that may help minimize the hair loss, such as the use of turbans, scarves, hats, and wigs.
- Suggest relaxation techniques to decrease anxiety.

### EVALUATION

By the time of surgery, Ms. Lange has recognized the relationship between the brain tumor and the headache. She states that lying in a flat position and coughing increase the headache. The head of the bed is kept at a 30- to 45-degree angle. Daily activities are spaced to provide periods of rest. Ms. Lange demonstrates no significant changes in level of consciousness. She has talked about the effect of the hair loss and her television responsibilities. Ms. Lange has learned that the hair preparation would be done in surgery and that the hair would be saved for her. She states she has already consulted her hair stylist and that "scarves and turbans are on the way."

### Critical Thinking in the Nursing Process

1. Outline interventions to decrease intracranial pressure both before and after surgery.
2. When making your initial assessments on the morning of surgery, you find that Ms. Lange has a decreased pulse and increased blood pressure. She tells you her headache is worse and suddenly vomits. What do you do now?
3. Ms. Lange asks you to be sure that she has absolutely no visitors after surgery, because she knows how ugly she will look. How would you respond?
4. Design a plan of care for Ms. Lange for the nursing diagnosis, *Powerlessness*.

See Evaluating Your Response in Appendix C.

---

take an active role in their own care. Discharge planning includes a discussion of the following topics: medication information; wound care; the use of wigs, turbans, hats, or colorful scarves; and the importance of follow-up visits. In addition, emphasize the importance of reporting manifestations such as stiff neck, increasing headache, elevated temperature, new motor or sensory deficits, vision changes, or seizures.

Provide information about the overall treatment plan, management of deficits and/or disabilities, and future needs. Specific teaching topics are as follows:

- Safety measures for motor deficits, sensory deficits, lack of coordination, seizures, and cognitive deficits
- Comfort measures for nausea, vomiting, and pain
- Measures for communication if aphasia is present
- Measures to improve vision if visual deficits are present
- How to buy wigs and hairpieces
- Referrals to support groups and community resources
- Helpful resources:
  - American Cancer Society
  - American Brain Tumor Association
  - National Brain Tumor Foundation

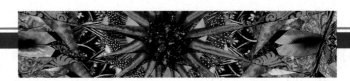

 # EXPLORE MediaLink

NCLEX review questions, case studies, care plan activities, MediaLink applications, and other interactive resources for this chapter can be found on the Companion Website at www.prenhall.com/lemone.

Click on Chapter 42 to select the activities for this chapter. For animations, video clips, more NCLEX review questions, and an audio glossary, access the Student CD-ROM accompanying this textbook.

## TEST YOURSELF

1. Which of the following pathophysiologic events results in irregular respiratory patterns as LOC decreases?

   a. Pressure on the meninges
   b. Reflexive motor responses
   c. Loss of the oculocephalic reflex
   d. Brainstem responds only to changes in $Paco_2$

2. The unconscious client has depressed or absent gag and swallowing reflexes. Which nursing diagnosis would be appropriate?

   a. *Decreased intracranial adaptive capacity*
   b. *Risk for aspiration*
   c. *Imbalanced nutrition: Less than body requirements*
   d. *Ineffective breathing pattern*

3. What is the rationale for the use of osmotic diuretics to treat increased ICP?

   a. Hyperthermia increases the cerebral metabolic rate and exacerbates increased ICP
   b. Increased blood osmolality draws edematous fluid into the vascular system

   c. Clients with ICP are at increased risk for gastrointestinal hemorrhage
   d. Brain injury and increased ICP often cause seizures

4. What manifestation is consistently assessed in clients with generalized seizures?

   a. Loss of consciousness
   b. Repetitive nonpurposeful activity
   c. Tonic movements
   d. Clonic movements

5. When assessing a client with a head injury, you test fluid dripping from one ear for glucose. What are you assessing for?

   a. Infection
   b. Blood
   c. CSF
   d. Serum

See Test Yourself answers in Appendix C.

## BIBLIOGRAPHY

American Cancer Society. (2001). *Cancer facts and figures–2001.* Atlanta: ACS.

Barker, E. (1998). The xenon CT: A new neuro tool. *RN, 61*(2), 22–25.

Brain Trauma Foundation and the Joint Section on Neurotrauma and Critical Care of the American Association of Neurological Surgeons and the Congress of Neurological Surgeons. (1995). *Guidelines for the management of severe head injury.* Park Ridge, IL: The Brain Trauma Foundation.

Bucher, L., & Melander, S. (1999). *Critical Care Nursing.* Philadelphia: Saunders

Chiocca, E. (1997). Action stat! Bacterial meningitis. *Nursing, 27*(9), 33.

Dodick, D. (1997). Headache as a symptom of ominous disease. . . what are the warning signals? *Postgraduate Medicine, 101*(5), 46–50, 55–56, 62.

Duff, D., & Wells, D. (1997). Postcomatose unawareness/vegetative state following severe brain injury: A content methodology. *Journal of Neuroscience Nursing, 29*(5), 305–307, 312–317.

Edmeads, J. (1997). Headaches in older people: How are they different in this age group? *Postgraduate Medicine, 101*(5), 91–94, 98, 100.

Fettes, I. (1997). Menstrual migraine: Methods of prevention and control. *Postgraduate Medicine, 101*(5), 67–70, 73–75, 77.

Hickey, J. (2003). *The clinical practice of neurological and neurosurgical nursing* ( 5th ed.). Philadelphia: Lippincott.

Hilton, G. (2001). Emergency: Acute head injury. *American Journal of Nursing, 101*(9), 51–52.

———.(1997). Seizure disorder in adults: Evaluation and management of new onset seizures. *Nurse Practitioner: American Journal of Primary Health Care, 22*(9), 42, 54, 49–50.

Horowitz, S., Passik, S., & Malkin, M. (1996). "In sickness and in health": A group intervention for spouses caring for patients with brain tumors. *Journal of Psychosocial Oncology, 14*(2), 43–56.

Johnson, M., & Maas, M. (Eds.). (1997). *Nursing outcomes classification (NOC).* St. Louis: Mosby.

Kee, J. (2001). *Handbook of laboratory and diagnostic tests* (4th ed.). Upper Saddle River, NJ: Prentice Hall.

Kidd, P., & Wagner, K. (2001). *High-acuity nursing* (3rd ed.). Upper Saddle River, NJ: Prentice Hall.

King, D. (1999). Central nervous system infections. Basic concepts. *Nursing Clinics of North America, 34*(3), 761–771.

Levitt, M., Lamb, S., & Voss, B. (1996). Brain tumor support group: Content themes and mechanisms of support. *Oncology Nursing Forum, 23*(8), 1247–1356.

Lin, Jong-mi. (2001). Overview of migraine. *Journal of Neuroscience Nursing, 33*(1), 6–13.

Liporace, J. (1997). Women's issues in epilepsy: Menses, childbearing and more. . . *Postgraduate Medicine, 102*(1), 123–124, 127–129, 133–135.

Long, L., & McAuley, J. (1996). Epilepsy: A review of seizure types, etiologies, diagnosis, treatment, and nursing implications. *Critical Care Nurse, 16*(4), 83–92.

Long, L., & Reeves, A. (1997). The practical aspects of epilepsy: Critical components of comprehensive patient care. *Journal of Neuroscience Nursing, 29(4)*, 249–254.

McCance, K., & Huether, S. (2002). *Pathophysiology: The biologic basis for disease in adults and children* (4th ed.). St. Louis: Mosby.

McCloskey, J., & Bulechek, G. (Eds.). (2000). *Nursing interventions classification (NIC)* (3rd ed.). St. Louis: Mosby.

McKenry, L., & Salerno, E. (1998). *Pharmacology in nursing* (20th ed.). St. Louis: Mosby.

McNair, N. (1999). Traumatic brain injury. *Nursing Clinics of North America, 34*(3), 637–659.

McNew, C., Hunt, S., & Warner, L. (1997). How to help your patient with epilepsy. *Nursing, 27*(9), 56–63.

Miller, L, & Chol, C. (1997). Meningitis in older patients: How to diagnose and treat a deadly infection. *Geriatrics, 52*(8), 43–44, 47–50, 55.

Myers, F. (2000). Meningitis: The fears, the facts. *RN, 63*(11), 53–57.

North American Nursing Diagnosis Association. (2001). *Nursing diagnoses: Definitions & classification 2001–2002.* Philadelphia: NANDA.

Porth, C. (2002). *Pathophysiology: Concepts of altered health states* (6th ed.). Philadelphia: Lippincott.

Schultz, R. (1997). Eggs and brains. . . the basics of head trauma. *Emergency Medical Services, 26*(4), 29–34, 75.

Shafer, P. (1999). Epilepsy and seizures. *Nursing Clinics of North America, 34*(3), 743–759.

Shannon, M., Wilson, B., & Stang, C. (2002). *Drug guide 2002.* Upper Saddle River, NJ: Prentice Hall.

Sullivan, J. (2000). Positioning of patients with severe traumatic brain injury: Research-based practice. *Journal of Neuroscience Nursing, 32*(4), 204–209.

Tierney, L., McPhee, S., & Papadakis, M. (Eds.). (2001). *Current medical diagnosis & treatment* (40th ed.). New York: McGraw-Hill.

Wall, B., Howard, J., & Perry-Phillips, J. (1995). Validation of two nursing diagnoses: Increased intracranial pressure and high risk for increased intracranial pressure. In M. Rantz & P. LeMone (Eds.). *Classification of nursing diagnoses: Proceedings of the 11th conference* (pp. 166–170). Glendate, CA: CINAHL.

Wright, M. (1999). Resuscitation of the multi-trauma patient with head injury. *AACN Clinical Issues, 10*(1), 32–45.

Yarbo, C., Frogge, M., Goodman, M., & Groen-wald, S. (Eds.). (2001). *Cancer nursing: Principles and practice* (5th ed.). Sudbury, MA: Jones & Bartlett.

### CHAPTER 43

# Nursing Care of Clients with Neurologic Disorders

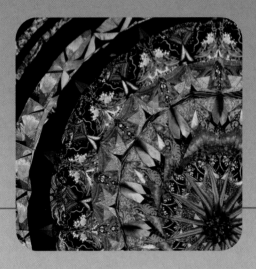

MediaLink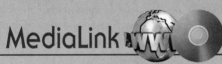

**www.prenhall.com/lemone**

Additional resources for this chapter can be found on the Student CD-ROM accompanying this textbook, and on the Companion Website at www. prenhall.com/lemone. Click on Chapter 43 to select the activities for this chapter.

**CD-ROM**
- Audio Glossary
- NCLEX Review

*Animations*
- Multiple Sclerosis
- Dopamine
- Levodopa

*Videos*
- Akinesia
- Bradykinesia

**Companion Website**
- More NCLEX Review
- Case Study
    Parkinson's Disease
- Care Plan Activity
    Guillain-Barré Syndrome
- MediaLink Application
    Alzheimer's Disease

## LEARNING OUTCOMES

After completing this chapter, you will be able to:

- Apply knowledge of normal anatomy, physiology, and assessments when providing nursing care for clients with neurologic disorders (see Chapter 40).

- Explain the pathophysiology of neurologic disorders.

- Identify diagnostic tests used to diagnose selected neurologic disorders.

- Discuss the nursing implications of medications used to treat clients experiencing neurologic disorders.

- Discuss collaborative care for clients with neurologic disorders.

- Provide appropriate nursing care to clients undergoing neurologic surgery.

- Use the nursing process as a framework for providing individualized care to clients with neurologic disorders.

This chapter discusses a variety of neurologic disorders. Included are degenerative disorders, peripheral nervous system disorders, and disorders caused by neurotoxins and viruses. For many of the disorders, nursing care is based on similar nursing diagnoses. To avoid repeating those diagnoses and interventions for each disorder, they have been divided among the nursing care discussions as appropriate.

# DEGENERATIVE NEUROLOGIC DISORDERS

Degenerative neurologic disorders can affect the central nervous system and the peripheral nerves. By progressively disrupting cognitive processes or motor functions, disorders such as multiple sclerosis, Alzheimer's disease, and Parkinson's disease strike at the core of an individual's sense of personal autonomy and well-being and can be psychologically and emotionally devastating to family members and caregivers.

Ongoing medical research into degenerative neurologic disorders offers an increasing measure of hope to clients and their families. The discovery of genetic or biochemical markers associated with some of these disorders is leading to the development of effective screening and diagnostic methods. In addition, new drugs may make it possible to halt the progression of the disorders in some clients, transforming the disorders into manageable conditions.

## THE CLIENT WITH ALZHEIMER'S DISEASE

**Alzheimer's disease (AD)** (also called *dementia of Alzheimer type [DAT]* or *senile disease complex*) is a form of dementia characterized by progressive, irreversible deterioration of general intellectual functioning. **Dementia** is defined by the World Health Organization as a chronic or progressive disease of the brain in which multiple cortical functions, calculation, learning capacity, language, and judgment are disturbed. Impairments of cognitive function are usually accompanied by deterioration in emotional control, social behavior, and motivation.

Memory loss is usually the first sign of Alzheimer's disease. Memory deficits are initially subtle and family members and friends may not suspect a problem until the disease progresses and symptoms become more noticeable. Family members may also deny the symptoms and hide deficits until the person exhibits unsafe or extremely unusual behavior. Progression of the disease varies, but the course is one of deteriorating cognition and judgment with eventual physical decline and total inability to perform ADLs. With the loss of the ability to perform even the most basic ADLs, the burden of meeting the client's needs shifts to the caregiver.

## INCIDENCE AND PREVALENCE

Alzheimer's disease is the most common degenerative neurologic illness and the most common cause of cognitive impairment (Porth, 2002). It accounts for about two-thirds of cases of dementia in America, affecting adults in middle to late life.

Scientists estimate that more than 4 million people have AD, and the number of people with AD doubles every 5 years beyond age 65.

## Risk Factors and Warning Signs

As one ages, the risk of developing AD increases. With numbers of older people increasing, this type of dementia is predicted to also increase. The risk factors for AD are older age, family history, and female gender. Warning signs are:

- Memory loss that affects job skills
- Difficulty performing familiar tasks
- Problems with language
- Disorientation to time and place
- Poor or decreased judgment
- Problems with abstract thinking
- Misplacing things
- Changes in mood or behavior
- Changes in personality
- Loss of initiative

Recognizing early symptoms is important, because the cause of dementia (such as from depression or hypothyroidism) may be reversible. Dementia from AD is not reversible. Treatment, however, can maximize quality of life and allow the affected person to plan for the future.

## PATHOPHYSIOLOGY

The exact cause of AD is unknown. Theories include loss of neurotransmitter stimulation by choline acetyltransferase, mutation for encoding amyloid precursor protein, and alteration in apolipoprotein E. Other possible causes are gene defects on chromosomes 14, 19, or 21, which may lead to clumping and precipitation of insoluble amyloid as plaques. The role of protein kinase C, the link between AD and aluminum, a viral cause, an autoimmune cause, and mitochondrial defects that alter cell metabolism and protein processing are being studied (McCance & Huether, 2002).

Two types of AD exist: *Familial AD* follows an inheritance pattern and *sporadic AD* has no obvious inheritance pattern. AD is further described as early onset (occurring in people younger than 65) and late onset (occurring in people age 65 and older). Early-onset AD usually affects people ages 30 to 60, is relatively rare, and often progresses more rapidly than late-onset AD.

Several structural and chemical changes in the brain occur with AD, especially in the hippocampus and the frontal and temporal lobes of the cerebral cortex. As AD destroys neurons in the hippocampus and related structures, short-term memory fails and the ability to perform easy and familiar tasks declines. The effect of AD on neurons in the cerebral cortex is loss of language skills and judgment. Emotional outbursts and behavior changes (such as wandering and agitation) begin to occur and become more frequent as the disease progresses. Eventually, other areas of the brain are affected; all affected areas begin to atrophy, and the person becomes totally helpless and unresponsive.

Characteristic findings in the brains of AD clients are loss of nerve cells and the presence of *neurofibrillary tangles* and *amyloid plaques* (Figure 43–1 ■). Neurofibrillary tangles result when a tau, a kind of protein in the neurons, becomes distorted and twisted. Tau normally holds together the microtubles, which guide nutrients and molecules to the end of the axon. In AD, tau changes and twists into pairs of filaments, which then join to form tangles. As tau no longer maintains the transport system, communication is lost between neurons. Death of neurons may follow, contributing to the development of dementia.

Groups of nerve cells (and especially the terminal axons) degenerate and clump around an amyloid core as plaque. They are found in the spaces between the neurons of the brain. These plaques, which develop first in areas used for memory and cognition, disrupt transmission of nerve impulses. The plaques

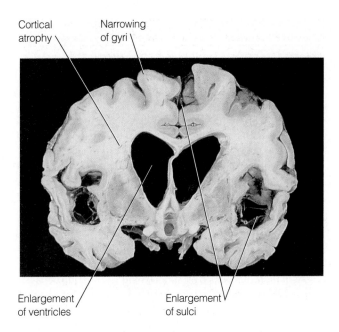

Figure 43–2 ■ Changes in neuroanatomy associated with Alzheimer's disease. Note areas of cortical atrophy, narrowing of the gyri, enlargement of sulci, and ventricular dilation.

consist primarily of insoluble deposits of beta-amyloid, a protein fragment from a larger protein called amyloid precursor protein (APP), mixed with other neurons and nonnerve cells. It is not yet known if plaque formation causes AD or if plaques are a by-product of the AD process.

Blood flow to the affected areas of the brain is decreased. The brain atrophies, and corresponding enlargement of ventricles and sulci is evident (Figure 43–2 ■). As AD progresses, more areas of the brain are affected, with symptoms correlating to those affected areas of the brain. For example, neuronal and neurotransmitter losses in the parietal lobe result in problems with perception and interpretation of environmental stimuli; deficits in the frontal lobe cause changes in personality and emotional lability.

## MANIFESTATIONS

Alzheimer's disease is classified into three stages based on the client's manifestations and abilities, as outlined in the Manifestations box on page 1400. It is important to note that the progression of AD varies for each individual and may not precisely follow the model.

### Stage I AD

In stage I, a client typically appears physically healthy and alert, and cognitive deficits can go undetected unless thorough and periodic evaluations are performed. Usually, family members are the first to notice lapses in memory, subtle changes in personality, or problems in doing simple calculations. AD clients and families may consciously or unconsciously compensate for cognitive deficits by adjusting schedules and routines. Clients may seem restless, forgetful, or uncoordinated.

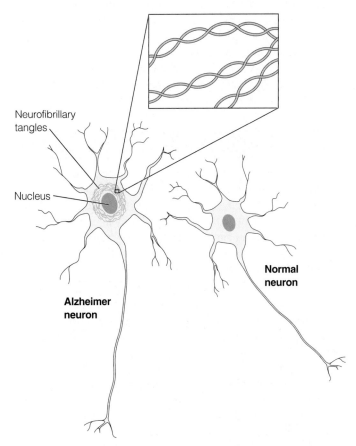

Figure 43–1 ■ Neuron with neurofibrillary tangles seen in Alzheimer's disease.

## Manifestations of Alzheimer's Disease

### STAGE I: APPROXIMATELY 2 TO 4 YEARS

• Short-term memory loss: Forgets location and names of objects and has difficulty learning new information; long-term memory is unaffected.
• Decreased attention span.
• Subtle personality changes: Lacks spontaneity; denial, irritability, and depression are possible.
• Mild cognitive deficits: Attempts to adjust to and cover up memory loss.
• Visuospatial deficits: Some problems with depth perception.

### STAGE II: APPROXIMATELY 2 TO 12 YEARS

• Impaired cognition: Obvious memory deficits and confusion; loss of abstract thinking; astereognosis and agraphia; inability to do math calculations; loss of ability to tell time and time disorientation, manifested as "sundowning"; wandering behavior.

• Personality changes: Becomes easily agitated and irritable; may have delusions or hallucinations.
• Visuospatial deficits: Is unable to dress self; has poor spatial orientation.
• Impaired motor skills: Paces and is restless at times; motor apraxia is evident when using familiar objects.
• Impaired judgment: Diminished social skills; inability to drive a car; inability to make decisions (e.g., choose clothing).

### STAGE III: APPROXIMATELY 2 TO 4 YEARS OR LONGER

• Cognitive abilities grossly decreased or absent: Is usually disoriented to time, place, and person.
• Communication skills usually absent: Is frequently mute.
• Motor skills grossly impaired or absent: Limb rigidity and posture flexion; bowel and bladder incontinence.

## Stage II AD

In stage II, memory deficits are more apparent, and the client is less able to behave spontaneously. Clients may wander and get lost, even in their own homes. Although progression of manifestations continues and orientation to place and time deteriorates, AD clients may still have periods of mental lucidity and engage in time-oriented conversations. Generally, however, clients become more confused and lose their sense of time, leading to changes in sleeping patterns, agitation, and stress. AD clients are less able to make even simple decisions and to adapt to environmental changes. Some AD clients develop severe attacks related to seemingly minor events; this reaction may result from a progressively lowered stress threshold. **Sundowning** is another behavioral change, characterized by increased agitation, time disorientation, and wandering behaviors during afternoon and evening hours; it is accelerated on overcast days.

Language deficits are common in stage II. They include *paraphasia* (using the wrong word), *echolalia* (repetition of words or phrases), and *scanning speech,* in which the client appears to search for words. Eventually, total *aphasia* (absence of speech) may occur. Frustration and depression are common among AD clients as the full extent and implications of the deficits become obvious.

The AD client slowly loses the ability to perform simple tasks required for hygiene or eating because sequencing of tasks is lost. For example, the client may open a can of soup but not remember to pour it into a pan to heat it. Instead, the client might place the can directly on the burner and leave the heat on high even after a smoke alarm sounds. The AD client may falsely interpret the smoke alarm as a telephone ringing, a tornado warning siren, or an ambulance siren. Thus, safety is a high priority for the client in stage II.

Sensorimotor deficits in stage II include *apraxia,* the inability to perform purposeful movements and use objects correctly; *astereognosis,* the inability to identify objects by touch; and *agraphia,* the inability to write. Problems related to malnutri-

tion and decreased fluid intake, such as anemia and constipation, may be evident. Sleep pattern disturbances are also common and are related to the loss of time orientation, sundowning phenomenon, and depression.

## Stage III AD

Stage III brings increasing dependence, with inability to communicate, loss of continence, and progressive loss of cognitive abilities. Common complications include pneumonia, dehydration, malnutrition, falls, depression, delusions, and paranoid reactions. The prognosis of a client with AD is poor, with an average life expectancy of 7 years from time of diagnosis. Death frequently occurs from pneumonia secondary to aspiration.

## COLLABORATIVE CARE

There is no cure for AD, and the main objective of care is to provide an environment that matches the client's functional abilities. Nurses, physicians, physical therapists, and social workers collaborate with the client's family to provide the least restrictive environment in which the client can safely function.

### Diagnostic Tests

Alzheimer's disease is diagnosed by ruling out causes for the client's manifestations. The only definitive method of diagnosis is postmortem examination of brain tissue. An extensive workup is especially important, because the dementia may be due to a reversible or treatable condition. For example, an older client's misuse of medications can lead to overdosing and resulting confusion. Other categories of conditions that may be considered and ruled out include depression, infection, hypothyroidism, dehydration, heart disease, stroke, and chronic obstructive respiratory disease.

The following diagnostic tests may be done.

• *EEG* may reveal a slowed pattern in the later stages of the disorder.

---

**Orientation to Time**
"What is the date?"

**Registration**
"Listen carefully. I am going to say three words. You say them back after I stop. Ready? Here they are …
HOUSE (pause), CAR (pause), LAKE (pause). Now repeat those words back to me."
[Repeat up to 5 times, but score only the first trial.]

**Naming**
"What is this?" [Point to a pencil or pen.]

**Reading**
"Please read this and do what it says." [Show examinee the words on the stimulus form.]
CLOSE YOUR EYES.

---

**Figure 43–3 ■** Mini Mental Status Examination Examples.

*Reproduced by special permission of the Publisher, Psychological Assessment Resources, Inc., 16204 North Florida Avenue, Lutz, Florida 33549, from the Mini Mental State Examination, by Marshal Folstein and Susan Folstein, Copyright 1975, 1998, 2001 by Mini Mental LLC, Inc. Further reproduction is prohibited without permission of PAR, Inc. The MMSE can be purchased form PAR, Inc. by calling (800) 331-8378 or (813) 968-3303.*

- *MRI* and *CT scan of the brain* demonstrates shrinkage of the hippocampus as well as changes in other parts of the brain.
- *Positron emission tomography (PET) scan* allows visualizing the activity and interactions of various parts of the brain as they are used during cognitive operations involving information processing.
- *Psychometric evaluation* using the Folstein Mini Mental Status Examination form (Figure 43–3 ■) or a similar instrument reflects the loss of memory and other cognitive skills over time.

Other tests may be performed, depending on the client's manifestations. For example, if the client has hypertension and memory changes, cerebral vascular studies are indicated to exclude multi-infarct dementia or other problems. Ruling out reversible dementia disorders requires evaluation of specific laboratory studies, such as thyroid function studies and measurement of electrolyte and vitamin levels.

Guidelines for the early recognition and assessment of AD have been established by the Agency for Healthcare Research and Quality. A diagnosis of Alzheimer's disease requires the presence of dementia, onset between age 40 and 90 years (most often after age 65), and absence of systemic or brain disorders that could cause mental changes.

## Medications

Cholinesterase inhibitors are used to treat mild to moderate dementia in AD. Tacrine hydrochloride (Cognex) was the first medication specifically approved for the treatment of AD. Donepezil hydrochloride (Aricept) is used to treat mild to moderate AD dementia with some success. Rivastigmine tartrate (Exelon) is also used to treat mild to moderate AD symptoms. It improves the ability to carry out ADLs, decreases agitation and delusions, and improves cognitive function. See the box below for information about medications used to treat AD.

---

## Medication Administration

### The Client with Alzheimer's Disease (AD)

**CHOLINERGIC (PARASYMPATHOMIMETICS); CHOLINESTERASE INHIBITORS**

Tacrine hydrochloride (Cognex)
Donepezil hydrochloride (Aricept)
Rivastigmine tartrate (Exelon)

In the early stages of AD, the pathologic changes in neurons result in a deficiency of acetylcholine (a key neurotransmitter involved in cognitive functioning). Cholinesterase inhibitors slow the breakdown of acetylcholine release by the remaining intact neurons. In addition, rivastigmine tartrate inhibits the $G_1$ form of acetyl-cholinesterase (found in higher levels in the brain of clients with AD), so less acetylcholine is degraded. The drugs are used to improve memory in mild to moderate AD dementia.

### Nursing Responsibilities
- Administer tacrine hydrochloride 1 hour before meals, if possible.
- Administer donepezil hydrochloride at bedtime.
- Administer rivastigmine tartrate (both capsules and liquid) with food. Liquid form may be administered undiluted or mixed with water, juice, or soda. Stir to completely dissolve.

- Monitor for jaundice, increased bilirubin levels, and other signs of liver involvement, such as rising serum aminotransferase (AST, ALT) levels. Therapy is usually decreased when the enzyme level exceeds 4 times normal limits and discontinued when the level reaches 5 times normal.
- Observe for gastrointestinal bleeding and gastric ulcer pain.
- Monitor for cholinergic-related problems: bladder outlet obstruction, seizures, and slowed cardiac rate.
- Assist with ambulation as dizziness is a common side effect.
- Monitor glycemic control in clients with diabetes.
- Assess for improvement in AD symptoms, especially in reasoning, memory, and ADLs.

### Client and Family Teaching
- Notify the physician promptly if jaundice, seizures, slowed heart rate, GI bleeding, or difficulty urinating occurs.
- Follow directions for times and instructions about administration of specific medication.
- Follow your health care provider's recommendation for periodic EEG, blood tests, and urine tests.
- These medications do not cure AD, and will at some point become ineffective as the disease progresses.

Depression often accompanies AD and is treated with the appropriate medication. Antihistamines and tricyclic antidepressants that have high anticholinergic activity are usually avoided because they can increase AD symptoms. Occasionally clients with AD require tranquilizers such as thioridazine (Mellaril) or haloperidol (Haldol) to manage severe agitation. Other therapies under study to prevent or delay the onset of AD include antioxidants such as vitamin E, anti-inflammatory agents, and estrogen replacement therapy in women.

## Complementary Therapy

The following types of complementary therapy may be used in treating the manifestations of AD.

- Massage, which decreases agitation
- Herbs
  - Ginko biloba, which is thought (among other actions) to improve cognition
  - Huperzine A, a traditional Chinese medicine, which acts as an acetylcholinesterase inhibitor
- Coenzyme Q10, an antioxidant that naturally occurs in the body
- Supplements, such as zinc, selenium, and evening primrose oil
- Therapies involving art, music, sound, and dance

## NURSING CARE

Clients with AD often require intensive, supportive nursing interventions directed at the physical and psychosocial responses to illness. Equally important, the nurse can facilitate the long-term support of these clients by providing teaching and referrals to follow-up care in the community.

## Health Promotion

Health promotion for the client with AD focuses on maintaining functional abilities and safety. If the client will be cared for at home, address safety considerations (see the box below)

as well as the caregivers' abilities to meet the client's basic needs, such as maintaining hygiene and other ADLs. Adapt nursing interventions and teaching to the client's stage of Alzheimer's disease.

## Assessment

Collect the following data through the health history and physical examination (see Chapter 40). Further focused assessments are described with nursing interventions below.

- Health history: family member/caregiver support, living arrangements, ability to carry out ADLs, drug use, work history (e.g., exposure to metals), previous history of multiple strokes, brain injury or brain infection, family history of dementia, sleep pattern, changes in cognition and memory, ability to communicate, changes in behavior
- Physical assessment: height/weight, orientation, abstract reasoning, mental status

## Nursing Diagnoses and Interventions

During the early stage of AD, nursing care focuses on helping the client make minor adaptations to his or her environment. As the client becomes progressively unable to manage self-care tasks, more adaptations are required. Equally important, the caregiver needs much support—both physical and psychosocial—as the client becomes increasingly dependent.

### Impaired Memory

Impaired memory is an appropriate nursing diagnosis in stage I AD. At this stage, techniques to help with the memory loss should be included in teaching for both the client and the caregiver.

- Suggest complementary therapies, such as meditation, massage, or exercise. *These activities can help reduce stress, which can aggravate memory loss.*
- Suggest using a calendar, keeping lists of reminders, or asking someone else to remind of appointments and events. *Written or verbal reminders are helpful if memory is impaired.*

## Meeting Individualized Needs: Safety Interventions for the Client with AD

### DECREASING THE RISK OF FALLS

- Assess usual environment for hazards, such as throw rugs, electrical cords, and slick floors.
- Observe areas of special concern, such as the bathroom, kitchen, and stairs, and modify as needed; for example, provide skidproof surfaces, and mark stairs to show depth.
- Evaluate muscle strength and gait; consult a physical therapist to plan exercises to increase strength and balance.
- Check shoes for fit and support.
- Inquire about alcohol use and medications that affect balance or cause mobility problems; for example, antihypertensive agents can cause dizziness with position changes.
- Use night-lights and increase daytime lighting in dark areas, such as hallways.
- Keep traffic areas free from clutter.

### DECREASING THE INJURIES RELATED TO COGNITIVE IMPAIRMENTS

- Secure items that may be mistakenly ingested, such as cleaning preparations and house plants.
- Modify potentially unsafe areas, such as unenclosed porches.
- Provide double lock systems to outside doors and doors to rooms that are off-limits.
- Protect from fire hazards; for example, make matches and cigarettes inaccessible.
- Fence the yard with a locked gate to prevent wandering.
- Modify the controls on the oven and stove.
- Adjust the water heater to a safe temperature.

### GENERAL SAFETY CONSIDERATIONS

- Plan a calling system for emergencies; have children call at about the same time every day as a check.
- Ensure that the cognitively impaired family member has no access to objects in the home such as knives and guns.

- Recommend using a medication box labeled with days and times. *A medication box is a good way to remember to take medications.*

**PRACTICE ALERT** *It may be necessary to teach the caregiver how to refill the medication box, or to stress the importance of spot-checking if the client fills it.* ■

- If safety is a concern (such as turning on the stove and forgetting it), suggest using alternatives such as a microwave. Program emergency numbers into the telephone. Ask client to consider a Life-line telephone program. *These measures can increase safety.*
- Suggest using cues, such as an alarm on a watch or a pocket computer, to trigger actions at designated times. *Cues are often helpful when memory loss is a problem.*

## Chronic Confusion

Clients with AD often have memory deficits that make functioning in a nonstructured environment difficult. Many of the nursing interventions for this diagnosis need to be modified over time as the client continues to lose cognitive function.

- Label rooms, drawers, and other items as needed. *Visual cues promote the highest possible degree of independence for the client.*
- Remove potential hazards (such as sharp knives or potentially harmful liquids or chemicals) from the environment. *Ensuring safety is a critical factor in providing care.*
- Keep environmental stimuli to a minimum: Decrease noise levels; speak in a calm, low voice; and take an unhurried approach. *Minimizing sensory input and maintaining a calm manner may decrease anxiety.*
- Begin each interaction by identifying self and calling client by name. See Box 43–1 for other communication techniques. *These techniques provide information for the client with memory loss.*
- Limit questions to those that require a simple yes or no response. *Questions need to be appropriate to the client's ability as decision making and verbal skills decline.*
- Orient to the environment, person, and time as able; place large, easy-to-read calendars and clocks in the client's line of vision. Make references to the season or day of the week when conversing with the client. *Orient the client according to his or her level of ability; orienting to precise time may not be possible in the later stages of AD.*
- Provide boundaries by placing red or yellow tape on the floor. *Boundaries help the client stay within safe areas.*

**PRACTICE ALERT** *Red and yellow are more easily seen by older adults.* ■

- Provide continuity in nursing staff. *This not only promotes consistency of care for the client but also allows the nurse to determine more accurately changes in the client's condition.*

---

**BOX 43–1 ■ Communication Techniques for the Client with AD**

- Face the client and talk directly to him or her; call the client by name.
- When first approaching the client, identify yourself.
- Use simple sentences and words with few syllables.
- Speak in a calm, low voice.
- Ask one question at a time. Use questions that require only a yes or no response.
- Keep nonverbal communication relaxed and parallel to the verbal communication.
- Avoid giving the impression of being in a hurry; try to have a relaxed approach.
- Observe for anxiety—wringing hands, pacing, darting eye movements—and alter your approach to decrease anxiety.
- Avoid arguing with clients; do not insist on orienting client to reality; the client's point of reference may not be based in reality.
- Give plenty of time for the client with AD to process what you are trying to say; do not expect clients to perform skills beyond their abilities.
- Repeat explanations in simple terms.

---

- Repeat explanations simply and as needed to decrease anxiety. *Loss of short-term memory leads to loss of a point of reference; eventually, AD clients think they are experiencing everything for the first time.*

## Anxiety

Managing the AD client's behaviors associated with anxiety, restlessness, and confusion is a major challenge confronting nurses and caregivers. Frequently, clients are relatively calm in the morning hours, only to experience increasing periods of agitation in the afternoon and evening hours. The AD client may even waken from the night's sleep with confusion, fearfulness, or panic attacks.

- Monitor for early behaviors of fatigue and agitation. *Early assessment of problems results in prompt intervention to promote rest or to remove the client from the situation causing anxiety.*
- Remove from situations that are causing increased anxiety, such as noisy activities involving large groups. *High-stimulus situations may increase anxious feelings and agitation.*
- Keep daily routine as consistent as possible. *Providing a structured day enhances feelings of familiarity and decreases stress.*
- Schedule rest periods or quiet times throughout the day. *Fatigue contributes to anxiety and lowers the stress threshold.*
- Provide quiet activities, such as listening to favorite music, in the afternoon or early evening. *Quiet activities may help decrease sundowning.*
- If confusion and agitation persist or escalate, assess for physical causes such as decreased oxygenation, infections, fatigue, constipation, and electrolyte imbalance. *Physical factors can increase agitation in clients with AD.*
- Use therapeutic touch or gentle hand massage. *These activities induce relaxation and have a calming effect.*

## Hopelessness

As the client and family recognize the impact of AD on their lives, they may feel a sense of hopelessness and powerlessness. They may not have the coping skills to deal effectively with the diagnosis and anticipated problems. The increasingly degenerative, irreversible nature of the disorder tends to diminish hope; only the ability to adapt to the many problems can restore it.

- Assess the client's and family's response to the diagnosis and understanding of AD; encourage expression of feelings. *Understanding the client/family's perspective enables the nurse to dispel myths about AD.*
- Provide realistic information about the disorder; provide information at the client/family's level of understanding. *Client and family may need to have separate sessions. Factual information provides a foundation for decision making.*
- Avoid criticizing or judging expressed feelings. *An environment accepting of the expression of real feelings promotes both further expression of feelings and willingness to discuss other issues.*
- Support positive family bonds and enhance communication among family members; promote mutual positive regard. *Strong family relationships can provide direction for living and convey a willingness to share the burden.*
- Encourage the client to make as many decisions as possible. *Self-determination enhances a feeling of control over a situation and may give a sense of hope.*
- Encourage the client and family to seek spiritual guidance that previously inspired hope. *The client's church is a legitimate support system. Belief in God can inspire hope beyond present circumstances.*

## Caregiver Role Strain

Most caregivers of clients with AD are spouses or other family members. Because AD is a chronic and eventually debilitating disorder, caregivers may feel overwhelmed by their responsibilities. The caregiving spouse faces not only the responsibility for the client's multiple physical demands but also economic and psychosocial stressors. An area that must be discussed is the ability and safety of the client in driving an automobile. Although is may be necessary, the loss of independence represented by the loss of the ability to drive may further trigger anxiety and anger. Fear of the future, loss of income, loss of companionship and a mate—combined with fatigue—make the caregiver vulnerable. Caregivers may become physically and mentally exhausted and socially isolated because of the overwhelming responsibilities of providing total care to the incapacitated family member.

- Teach the caregivers self-care techniques, such as taking rest periods and avoiding fatigue. *Fatigue adds to stress and potentially leads to poor decision making.*
- Have the caregivers list and regularly take part in physical activities they enjoy, such as walking or swimming. *Regular physical exercise decreases stress.*
- Refer the caregivers to local AD support groups. Suggest books pertinent to the subject. *Explicit suggestions in locating support systems and providing specific information promotes coping.*
- Refer the caregivers to Meals-on-Wheels, home health, respite care, and other community services. *Community agencies can relieve some of the daily care burdens, thus providing time for other activities. Programs that support caregivers have been shown to delay nursing home placement.*
- Ensure the family knows that hospice care is available during the end stages of AD. *Hospice services can support the family during this difficult time.*

## Using NANDA, NIC, and NOC

Chart 43–1 shows links between NANDA nursing diagnoses, NIC, and NOC when caring for the client with AD.

## Home Care

Teaching for clients and families centers initially on explaining the disorder and exploring available support systems. Anticipate the need to reexplain the disorder and its consequences, as clients and families may be in shock or denial during the initial period of the disease.

---

### CHART 43–1 NANDA, NIC, AND NOC LINKAGES

#### The Client with AD

| NURSING DIAGNOSES | NURSING INTERVENTIONS | NURSING OUTCOMES |
|---|---|---|
| • Chronic Confusion | • Dementia Management<br>• Anxiety Reduction<br>• Family Support<br>• Environmental Management: Safety | • Cognitive Orientation<br>• Distorted Thought Control<br>• Identity<br>• Safety Behavior |
| • Disturbed Sleep Pattern | • Sleep Enhancement<br>• Security Enhancement | • Sleep<br>• Anxiety Control<br>• Comfort Level |
| • Self-Care Deficit | • Self-Care Assistance | • Cognitive Ability<br>• Anxiety Control |

*Note. Data from Nursing Outcomes Classification (NOC) by M. Johnson & M. Maas (Eds.), 1997, St. Louis: Mosby; Nursing Diagnoses: Definitions & Classification 2001–2002 by North American Nursing Diagnosis Association, 2001, Philadelphia: NANDA; Nursing Interventions Classification (NIC) by J.C. McCloskey & G. M. Bulechek (Eds.), 2000, St. Louis: Mosby. Reprinted by permission.*

In addition to explaining the anticipated changes with AD, suggest practical solutions to identified problems. It is important to evaluate both the client and caregivers; interventions must be appropriate for the family's situation and resources. Maintaining the least restrictive environment that promotes safety for the client is a major goal of teaching. Using memory cues, such as labeling drawers to indicate the specific types of clothing and labeling rooms, can help orient the client and foster independence. Consistency in the environment and daily routine is an essential part of care. Emphasizing realistic expectations means adjusting care and communication techniques to the client's level of ability.

Address the following topics for home care of the client and for the caregiver.

- Support groups and peer counseling are helpful in handling caregiver stress.
- A person with AD who is confused or agitated is not comfortable and is usually frightened.

- Plan care that matches the person's level of coping, using a consistent routine.
- Provide regular rest periods to decrease the client's stress and fatigue (these do not increase nighttime wandering).
- Plan care for the caregiver. Periodic respite care during the initial stages, with plans for increasing assistance to meet the client's daily needs as the disease progresses, may be sufficient. Referrals to the appropriate agency for long-term care, including skilled nursing facilities, may be indicated. Family members may need help adjusting to the idea of extended care but may be relieved to relinquish the physical care needs.
- Suggest the following resources:
  - Alzheimer's Association
  - Alzheimer's Disease and Related Disorders Association
  - Alzheimer's Disease Education and Referral Center
  - National Institute of Neurological and Communicative Disorders and Stroke

## Nursing Care Plan
## A Client with AD

Arthur and Ruth Joste, both age 73, have been married for 47 years; he is a retired history teacher, and she has been a homemaker. They have four children; two live in the same town, and two live out of state. Arthur has noticed that he is having problems remembering friends' names and phone numbers; his wife has been asking him if he is driving in the correct direction when they go shopping.

Mrs. Joste has severe osteoarthritis and is unable to lift heavy objects or perform all but light housekeeping tasks. For about 18 months, Mrs. Joste has been aware of her husband's progressive cognitive decline, including forgetting current news from last night's newspaper; miscalculating checkbook balances; neglecting his hygiene needs; and confusing their children's and grandchildren's names. The Jostes are referred to a neurologist for evaluation.

### ASSESSMENT
Martha Spital, RN, assesses Mr. Joste at the neurologist's office. She notes that he is unable to recall his home address without prompting, to name the correct date (although he does know the day of the week), to subtract serial 7s more than twice, and to recall two of three objects. He is alert to his surroundings. Mr. Joste scores 21 of a possible 30 points on the Mini Mental Status Exam. Mrs. Joste states that the problems seem to be getting worse with time and that she has had to "cover up" mistakes for her husband. Mr. Joste seems easily agitated, and his wife reports that his sleep habits are "jumbled"; he has long periods of wakefulness in the nighttime hours.

Following a thorough evaluation and diagnostic testing to rule out other possible disorders, the neurologist tells the couple that Mr. Joste has probable dementia of the Alzheimer's type. Both have feared this diagnosis; they want to know how they can be sure that Mr. Joste has this disease and what they can do to prevent further decline. Both are obviously much saddened, and they verbalize their feelings of being overwhelmed. The Jostes intend to remain in their home "for as long as we can."

### DIAGNOSES
- *Chronic confusion* related to deterioration of brain function and dementia
- *Self-care deficits* related to forgetfulness and declining physical abilities
- *Risk for injury* related to decreased orientation
- *Disturbed sleep pattern* related to time disorientation
- *Caregiver role strain* (wife) related to need to care for self and husband

### EXPECTED OUTCOMES
- Remain free of injury.
- Navigate home environment with modifications as needed.
- Participate in grooming and hygiene activities with prompting and supervision.
- Obtain a minimum of 7 uninterrupted hours of sleep a night.
- Mrs. Joste will participate in a minimum of two out-of-home activities a week.

### PLANNING AND IMPLEMENTATION
The home health nurse, Erick Montane, RN, makes a home visit to evaluate the environment, assess available support, and determine needs. He meets two of the Jostes' children, Dawn and Jay, who live in the same community and are willing to participate as much as possible in providing care and modifying the home.

Mr. Montane discusses the importance of establishing and maintaining a consistent daily routine. He emphasizes the importance of matching activities to Mr. Joste's mental abilities to avoid frustration and increased agitation. Mr. Montane recommends labeling drawers with their contents, such as Mr. Joste's sock drawer. Labeling rooms may eventually be necessary.

Because his inability to comprehend and process information distresses and agitates Mr. Joste, Mr. Montane teaches the family to modify their communications to fit Mr. Joste's cognitive ability, such as using simple, direct statements and directions.

*(continued on page 1406)*

## Nursing Care Plan
## A Client with AD *(continued)*

Mr. Montane recommends that family members keep background noise to a minimum because this may be a source of confusion.

After touring the home, Mr. Montane makes the following recommendations about safety:

- Remove throw rugs from hallways, and tack down any remaining carpets.
- Secure the kitchen, bathroom, and workshop cabinets as well as the controls on the oven and stove.
- Modify the doors so that negotiating locks requires a two-step system of unlocking, such as with a deadbolt and a key.
- Provide extra lighting in dark areas, especially a night-light in the bathroom.

Mr. Montane explains that Mrs. Joste will need assistance with housekeeping as Mr. Joste continues to decline. Mr. Montane provides referrals to community services, including Meals-on-Wheels, which can supply a daily meal. He also suggests that the Jostes obtain the services of a home health aide to provide daily hygiene care. Most of the remaining home maintenance needs can be met with the children's help.

Mr. and Mrs. Joste and the two children attend the weekly local support group meetings for Alzheimer's disease and related disorders for approximately 3 months; thereafter, Mrs. Joste attends with her daughter.

### EVALUATION

Six months after the initial home visit and family planning session, Mr. Joste:

- Has not had a fall, burn, or other injury.
- Has periods of confusion when outside his home, but 90% of the time is oriented to place when at home.
- Has attended several support group meetings until 3 months ago. Currently, his wife attends weekly, and a daughter occa-sionally accompanies her. She has continued to participate in their church and maintains contact with a few friends. She is finding it harder to leave her husband unattended for even a few minutes.

- Is able to clean and dress himself with prompting; he is not able to choose his own clothing. If hygiene articles are "set up" (e.g., if the toothpaste is placed on the toothbrush), he remembers to perform the hygiene activity. The children have been replacing buttons and zippers with Velcro closures on his clothing.
- Sleeps an average of 6 hours a night with a 30-minute nap in the afternoon; this pattern is consistent with his previous sleep pattern.
- Has seemed to be more easily agitated for the past month. He wanders from room to room, apparently looking for something. These behaviors are worse in the evening and on cloudy days. Mrs. Joste acknowledges her progressive inability to care for her husband.

### Critical Thinking in the Nursing Process

1. Develop a tool to teach safety needs for the client and family with Alzheimer's disease.
2. List five interventions to decrease agitation in cognitively impaired older adults; give three additional examples of activities suited to an older adult with AD who has osteoarthritis.
3. You are caring for a client in Stage 2 Alzheimer's disease. She is 65 inches (165 cm) tall and weighs 132 lb (59.9 kg); she has lost 3 lb within the past month. The client has difficulty focusing on eating and is easily agitated. Describe your plan for ensuring that she takes in enough nutrition to meet her needs.

See Evaluating Your Response in Appendix C.

## THE CLIENT WITH MULTIPLE SCLEROSIS

**Multiple sclerosis (MS)** is a chronic demyelinating disease of the central nervous system, associated with an abnormal immune response to an environmental factor. The symptoms of MS vary according to the area of the nervous system affected. The initial onset may be followed by a total remission, making diagnosis difficult. In about 60% of clients, MS is characterized by periods of exacerbation, when symptoms are highly pronounced, followed by periods of remission. The end result, however, is progression of the disease with increasing loss of function.

### INCIDENCE AND PREVALENCE

Approximately 500,000 people in the United States have MS. Females are affected 2 times more often than males, and the incidence is highest in young adults (age 20 to 40). The disease occurs more commonly in temperate climates, including the northern United States. This association is established by approximately age 15, and moving to or from a temperate climate after that age does not change it.

The onset of MS is usually between 20 and 50 years of age, with a peak at age 30. MS is the most prevalent CNS demyelinating disorder, and is a leading cause of neurologic disability in young adults. Although all races are affected, MS is primarily a disease of Caucasians. Although a definite genetic factor has not been established, 15% of those with MS have a relative with the disease (McCance & Huether, 2002).

### PATHOPHYSIOLOGY

MS is believed to occur as a result of an autoimmune response to a prior viral infection in a genetically susceptible person. The infection, which is thought to occur early in life, activates T cells. T cells usually move in and out of the CNS across the blood-brain barrier, but for an unknown reason, they remain in the CNS in people with MS. The T cells facilitate infiltration by other leukocytes, and an inflammatory

| BOX 43–2 ■ | Classifications of Multiple Sclerosis |
|---|---|

**Relapsing-remitting:** The most common clinical course of MS, characterized by exacerbations (acute attacks) with either full recovery or partial recovery with disability.

**Primary progressive:** Steady worsening of disease from the onset with occasional minor recovery.

**Secondary progressive:** Begins as with relapsing-remitting, but the disease steadily becomes worse between exacerbations.

**Progressive-relapsing:** This rare form continues to progress from the onset but also has exacerbations.

process follows. Inflammation destroys myelin and oligodendrocytes (myelin-producing cells), leading to axon dysfunction. The myelin sheaths are fatty, segmented wrappings that normally protect and insulate nerve fibers and increase the speed of transmission of nerve impulses. In multiple sclerosis, these myelin sheaths of the white matter of the spinal cord, brain, and optic nerve are destroyed in patches, called plaques, along the axon (see *Pathophysiology Illustrated* on pages 1408–1409). The **demyelination** of nerve fibers slows and distorts the conduction of nerve impulses and sometimes results in the total absence of impulse transmission. The neurons usually affected by MS are located in the spinal cord, brainstem, cerebral and cerebellar areas, and the optic nerve.

Both plaques and diffuse lesions form as demyelinating lesions. Plaques typically are scattered through the white matter of the CNS, although they may extend into adjacent gray matter. Early manifestations are the result of inflammatory edema in and around the plaque and partial demyelination. These manifestations typically disappear within weeks after the initial episode. With progression of the disease, the demyelination and plaque formation result in scarring of glia (*gliosis*) and degeneration of axons. Continued loss of function leads to permanent disability, usually over about 20 years.

There are four classifications of MS: relapsing-remitting, primary progressive, secondary progressive, and progressive-relapsing (Box 43–2). Most individuals with MS present with the relapsing-remitting type.

Various stressors have been suggested as triggers for MS. These stressors include febrile states, pregnancy, extreme physical exertion, and fatigue. These precipitating factors can also cause a relapse of the manifestations during the course of the disease.

## MANIFESTATIONS

The manifestations of MS vary according to the areas destroyed by demyelination and the affected body system (see *Multisystems Effects of MS* on page 1410). Fatigue is one of the most disabling manifestations, and affects almost all clients with MS. The manifestations, categorized by the established syndromes of MS, include:

*Mixed or Generalized Type (50% of cases)*

- Manifestations include optic nerve involvement, with visual blurring, fogginess, or haziness; and impaired color perception. There is also decreased central visual acuity, area of diminished vision in the visual fields, acquired color vision deficit (especially to red and green), and an altered pupillary reaction to light.
- Brainstem lesions (cranial nerves III to XII) are noted, with nystagmus, dysarthria, deafness, vertigo, vomiting, tinnitus, facial weakness, and decreased sensation. Other manifestations include diplopia and eye pain, and cognitive dysfunctions involving concentration, short-term memory, word finding, and planning.
- Mood alterations are manifested as depression more often than euphoria.

*Spinal Type (25% of cases)*

- Weakness and/or numbness is noted in one or both extremities (most often the legs).
- Upper motor neuron involvement is manifested by stiffness, slowness, weakness (spastic paresis).
- Bladder dyfunctions include urgency, hesitancy, and incontinence.
- Bowel dysfunction is most often seen as constipation.
- Neurogenic impotence is noted.

*Cerebellar Type (5% of cases)*

- Client shows manifestations of nystagmus, ataxia, and hyptonia.

*Amaurotic Form (5% of cases)*

- Client develops blindness.

Short-lived attacks of neurologic deficits indicate the temporary appearance or worsening of manifestations. Conditions that cause short-lived attacks include (1) minor increases in body temperature or serum calcium concentrations (both increase the leakage of current through demyelinated neurons) and (2) functional demands that exceed conduction capacity. Paroxysmal attacks are sensory or motor manifestations that occur abruptly and last for only seconds or minutes; the manifestations are paresthesias, dysarthria and ataxia, and tonic head turning. Paroxysmal attacks, which may occur many times a day, result from the direct transmission of nerve impulses between adjacent demyelinated axons (McCance & Huether, 2002).

## COLLABORATIVE CARE

Management of the client with MS varies according to the severity of the manifestations. The focus is on retaining the optimal level of functioning possible, given the degree of disability. Rehabilitation—physical, occupational/vocational, and psychosocial—is a cornerstone of a team approach to treatment. During exacerbations, the focus of interventions shifts to controlling manifestations and quickly returning to remission.

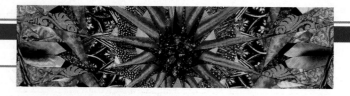

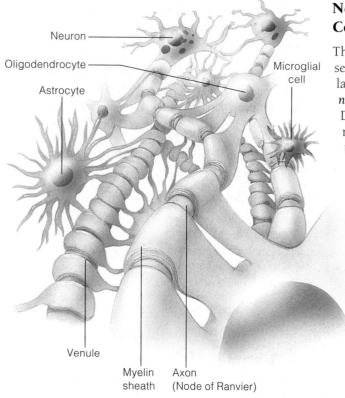

Neuron

Oligodendrocyte

Astrocyte

Microglial cell

Venule

Myelin sheath

Axon (Node of Ranvier)

## Normal Anatomy of the Central Nervous System

The central nervous system (CNS) is composed of several cell types arranged in a dense, interconnected lattice. The basic functional cell of the CNS is the *neuron*, which transmits electrochemical impulses. Dendrites, thin projections extending from the neuron body, receive impulses that are passed down the neuronal axon for transmission to other cells. Myelin, a lipid-protein substance, surrounds the axons, insulating them and speeding nerve impulse transmission.

Neurons are surrounded by a network of neuroglial cells:

- *Astrocytes* support neurons and connnect them to surrounding capillaries and venules.
- *Microglia* are motile phagocytic cells.
- *Oligodendrocytes* wrap concentric layers of myelin around nearby axons.

## Acute Attack

Multiple sclerosis (MS) is a demyelinating disease in which axonal myelin in the central nervous system is eroded, destroyed, and replaced by scar tissue.

An autoimmune process apparently triggered by genetic and environmental factors is believed to cause inflammation of venules in the CNS. This disrupts the blood–brain barrier, allowing lymphocytes to enter CNS tissue. These lymphocytes proliferate and produce IgG, an antibody that attacks and damages myelin and causes the release of inflammatory chemicals and edema. As the inflammation subsides, the myelin regenerates and manifestations of the disease subside.

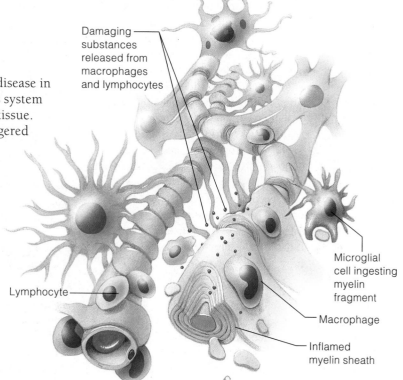

Damaging substances released from macrophages and lymphocytes

Lymphocyte

Microglial cell ingesting myelin fragment

Macrophage

Inflamed myelin sheath

## Chronic Lesion

After repeated inflammatory attacks, myelin is irreparably damaged. Segments of axons become totally demyelinated and may degenerate. Astrocytes proliferate in damaged regions of the CNS (a process call *gliosis*), forming plaques. The plaques are scattered throughout the CNS, appearing as gray or pinkish lesions. The relapsing-remitting character of MS and the scattered areas of damage within the CNS account for the variable nature of MS manifestations.

Damaged oligodendrocyte

Proliferating astrocytes

Demyelinated axon

## Abnormal Nerve Impulse Transmission

In an undamaged neuron, nerve impulses travel down the axon by "leaping" from one node of Ranvier to the next, thus greatly increasing the speed of impulse transmission. When nerve impulses travel down an axon damaged by MS, they are significantly slowed and weakened as they pass across the surface of demyelinated areas. Impulses may be blocked entirely when axons degenerate. The weakening or interruption of the transmission of nerve impulses and plaque formation within the CNS cause the manifestations of MS, including extremity weakness, paresthesias, visual disturbances, bladder dysfunction, and vertigo.

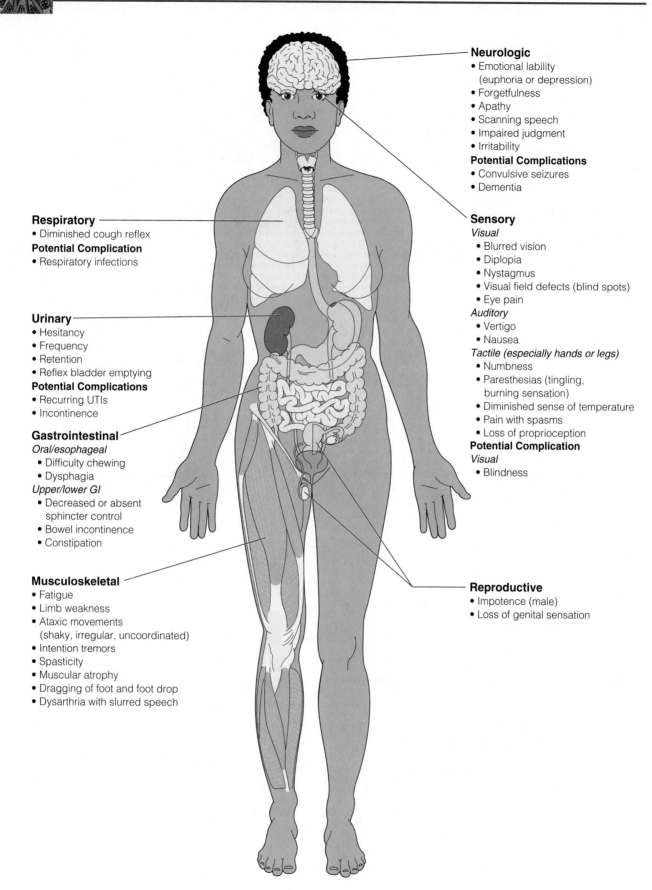

**Neurologic**
- Emotional lability
  (euphoria or depression)
- Forgetfulness
- Apathy
- Scanning speech
- Impaired judgment
- Irritability

**Potential Complications**
- Convulsive seizures
- Dementia

**Sensory**

*Visual*
- Blurred vision
- Diplopia
- Nystagmus
- Visual field defects (blind spots)
- Eye pain

*Auditory*
- Vertigo
- Nausea

*Tactile (especially hands or legs)*
- Numbness
- Paresthesias (tingling,
  burning sensation)
- Diminished sense of temperature
- Pain with spasms
- Loss of proprioception

**Potential Complication**

*Visual*
- Blindness

**Respiratory**
- Diminished cough reflex

**Potential Complication**
- Respiratory infections

**Urinary**
- Hesitancy
- Frequency
- Retention
- Reflex bladder emptying

**Potential Complications**
- Recurring UTIs
- Incontinence

**Gastrointestinal**

*Oral/esophageal*
- Difficulty chewing
- Dysphagia

*Upper/lower GI*
- Decreased or absent
  sphincter control
- Bowel incontinence
- Constipation

**Musculoskeletal**
- Fatigue
- Limb weakness
- Ataxic movements
  (shaky, irregular, uncoordinated)
- Intention tremors
- Spasticity
- Muscular atrophy
- Dragging of foot and foot drop
- Dysarthria with slurred speech

**Reproductive**
- Impotence (male)
- Loss of genital sensation

## Diagnostic Tests

Diagnosis of MS is challenging because the disease does not present uniformly. Initially, a thorough history and physical examination are completed, and their importance in establishing a diagnosis cannot be overemphasized. Diagnostic tests vary with the presenting complaints. MRI is the most definitive test available; however, it is one of several laboratory and diagnostic tests that may be performed when establishing the diagnosis.

- *Cerebral spinal fluid (CSF) analysis* reveals an increased number of T lymphocytes that are reactive with antigens, indicating the presence of an immune response in the client. Of MS patients, 80% have elevated levels of immunoglobulin G (IgG) in the CSF. IgG may not be increased during the initial period of the disease.
- *MRI studies* are performed. Cerebral MRI detects multifocal lesions in the white matter. Serial MRIs may be performed to chart the course of the disease. MRI of the spinal cord or optic nerves can detect lesions in these areas.
- *CT scan* of the brain shows atrophy and white matter lesions. In about 25% of clients with MS, enlarged ventricles are visible on CT.
- *Positron emission tomography (PET) scan* measures brain activity. In MS clients, the scan reveals areas with changes in glucose metabolism.

- *Evoked response testing* of visual, auditory, or somatosensory impulses may show delayed conduction.

## Medications

Medications slow the progression of MS and decrease the number of attacks. See the Medication Administration box on pages 1411–1412 for information about these medications.

The medications used during an exacerbation are aimed at decreasing inflammation to inhibit manifestations and induce remission. Frequently, a combination of adrenocorticotrophic hormone (ACTH) and glucocorticoids is used to decrease inflammation and suppress the immune system. Immunosuppressive agents, including azathioprine (Imuran) and cyclophosphamide (Cytoxan), are also used. Some centers administer cyclophosphamide monthly to prevent exacerbations.

Other medications treat the manifestations of MS, such as muscle spasms. Anticholinergics are sometimes administered for bladder spasticity; cholinergics are given if the client has a problem with urinary retention related to flaccid bladder.

## Treatments

Although medications are the primary method of controlling manifestations, other treatments include surgery, dietary management, and rehabilitative therapies.

---

# Medication Administration

## The Client with Multiple Sclerosis

### IMMUNOMODULATORS

Interferon beta-1a (Avonex)
Interferon beta-1b (Betaseron)
Glatiramer acetate (Copaxone, Copolymer-1)

Interferon beta-1a, interferon beta-1b, and glatiramer acetate are administered to clients with relapsing-remitting MS to prolong the time of onset to disability. Their use is based on the assumption that MS is an immunologically mediated disease. Interferon beta-1b produces a decrease in the MS lesions in some clients. Some clients, however, develop a decrease in the absolute neutrophil count and increases in the levels of liver enzymes. Anxiety, confusion, and depression with suicidal tendencies also have been reported. Other adverse reactions include pain, inflammation, hypersensitivity at the injection site, and generalized flulike manifestations. Some women experience menstrual disorders. Pregnant women should not take these medications.

### Nursing Responsibilities

- Assess baseline parameters to evaluate drug side effects: psychologic profile, liver function tests, and CBC with differential. Monitor CBC and liver function tests every 3 months or as prescribed.
- Assess injection site and report ulceration promptly (pain and redness are common reactions).
- Evaluate client's baseline neurologic, sensory, and motor function. Monitor changes in condition and function.
- Report if client is pregnant or breast-feeding.

### Client and Family Teaching

- This drug may cause depression and thoughts of suicide; report these feelings immediately to the physician.
- The medication is reconstituted and should be discarded if it becomes discolored or precipitates out. Administer the medication within 3 hours of reconstitution. Rotate injection sites, and avoid any areas that are red or show other skin reactions.
- Seek follow-up care to monitor neurologic changes, CBC, and liver function.
- Avoid prolonged exposure to sunlight.

### ADRENOCORTICOSTEROID THERAPY

Adrenocorticotropic hormone (ACTH) (Acthar)
Prednisone (Deltasone, Meticorten, Orasone)
Methylprednisolone (Medrol, Solu-Medrol)

Adrenocorticosteroids are used both to sustain a remission and to treat exacerbations of MS. ACTH is usually given to induce a remission; it is administered intravenously for 1 week and may be followed by oral prednisone therapy. Another protocol involves administering ACTH intravenously for 3 days followed by intramuscular injections every 12 hours for 1 week (Hickey, 2002). The drugs are given to suppress the immune system, implicated in the etiology of MS. If the drug is used long term, the usual steroid precautions are indicated, such as monitoring for

*(continued on page 1412)*

## Nursing Research

### Evidence-Based Practice to Improve Quality of Life in Clients with Multiple Sclerosis

Quality of life is a critical factor in living with chronic illnesses like multiple sclerosis. Regardless of health status or functional disabilities, quality of life is made up of the same factors and relationships important to healthy people. It is experienced when basic needs are met and opportunities are available to pursue and achieve life goals. Gulick (1997) conducted a study to investigate the extent to which demographic and self-reported health and role predicted quality of life in 153 people with multiple sclerosis.

Analysis of data resulted in the following findings specific to people with MS:

- Marriage, work, and health are major contributors to a positive outlook on life.
- Living with a spouse, followed by employment, were the most important demographic variables related to quality of life.
- Depression may result from anxieties about the loss of body function; loss of normal pleasures; and loss of social, business, and personal factors of life.
- Recreation and socialization are important correlates of quality of life.

### IMPLICATIONS FOR NURSING

Nurses can help clients with MS identify aspects of their health and roles/relationships that adversely and positively affect quality of life. By identifying strengths and weaknesses, nurses can provide interventions to enhance the client's quality of life. Those interventions would include sexuality counseling, provision of assistive devices to enable greater mobility, and referral to support groups.

### Critical Thinking in Client Care

1. In reflecting on the manifestations of multiple sclerosis, what factors can you identify as potential strengths and weaknesses for a client?
2. As a person with MS ages, disabilities often become more severe. How would you adapt teaching plans for home care for the following people?
   - A 29-year-old mother of two toddlers, diagnosed 1 year ago
   - A 45-year-old man who has worked in construction all his life
   - A 60-year-old woman who is a college professor

*adapting utensils and foods can ensure that nutritional needs are met.*

- Teach interventions related to altered bowel and bladder function: fluid intake of at least 2000 mL daily, bowel routine as indicated to prevent constipation, self-catheterization skills as necessary. *Maintaining optimal bowel and bladder function decreases the risk of urinary tract infection and bowel impaction.*

### Using NANDA, NIC, and NOC

Chart 43–2 Shows links between NANDA nursing diagnoses, NIC, and NOC when caring for the client with MS.

### Home Care

The nurse adapts teaching approaches based on the MS client's needs. The inconsistent and erratic nature of the disease can make teaching difficult. Initial teaching focuses on a

---

### CHART 43–2  NANDA, NIC, AND NOC LINKAGESS

#### The Client with MS

| NURSING DIAGNOSES | NURSING INTERVENTIONS | NURSING OUTCOMES |
|---|---|---|
| • Impaired Physical Mobility | • Energy Management<br>• Exercise Therapy: Ambulation<br>• Exercise Therapy: Joint Mobility | • Mobility Level<br>• Ambulation: Walking<br>• Joint Movement: Active |
| • Disturbed Sensory Perception: Visual | • Communication Enhancement<br>• Environment Management<br>• Eye Care | • Neurological Status |
| • Urinary Retention | • Urinary Catheterization<br>• Urinary Retention Care | • Urinary Elimination |
| • Sexual Dysfunction | • Sexual Counseling | • Self-Esteem |
| • Interrupted Family Processes | • Family Process Promotion<br>• Emotional Support<br>• Support System Enhancement | • Role Performance |

*Note. Data from Nursing Outcomes Classification (NOC) by M. Johnson & M. Maas (Eds.), 1997, St. Louis: Mosby; Nursing Diagnoses: Definitions & Classification 2001–2002 by North American Nursing Diagnosis Association, 2001, Philadelphia: NANDA; Nursing Interventions Classification (NIC) by J.C. McCloskey & G. M. Bulechek (Eds.), 2000, St. Louis: Mosby. Reprinted by permission.*

realistic explanation of MS. Referral to a support group early in the course of the disease also is indicated. Social support can make a positive difference in a client's ability to cope with MS. Address the following topics in preparing the client for home care.

- Various treatment options and their side effects
- Information about medications, particularly steroid use, and about possible interactions with prescription or over-the-counter medications

- Ongoing care from nurses, counselors, and physical, occupational, and speech therapists, as well as the physician and community health nurse.
- Helpful resources:
  - National Multiple Sclerosis Society
  - National Institute of Neurological and Communicative Disorders and Stroke

## Nursing Care Plan
## A Client with MS

George McMurphy, a 45-year-old from northern Minnesota, was diagnosed with MS approximately 5 years ago. He states that he probably had mild symptoms as long ago as 10 years. He works as a manager for a large grocery store chain near his home. He lives at home with his wife and two children, ages 12 and 15. Recently, Mr. McMurphy has had increasing problems with urinary incontinence, lack of energy, weakness, extreme fatigue, and altered mobility from spasticity in his leg muscles. He also has a fever, chest congestion, and a cough productive of green sputum. He is admitted to the hospital for evaluation and treatment of pneumonia and exacerbation of his MS.

### ASSESSMENT
Denise Miller, RN, primary care nurse, is assigned to care for Mr. McMurphy. His major complaint is the inability to "bring up all this sputum; I feel rotten from being so congested. I hate not being able to get to work and for my wife having to tend to my personal needs." Vital signs are as follows: BP 134/84, P 94, R 30, T 102°F (38.8°C). Mr. McMurphy is admitted for an acute exacerbation of the disorder, probably triggered by pneumonia. He will be treated with ACTH and intravenous antibiotics during this admission.

### DIAGNOSES
- *Ineffective airway clearance* related to lung infection and thick mucus
- *Activity intolerance* related to fatigue and spasticity
- *Self-care deficit: Toileting, feeding, and grooming* related to muscle weakness

### EXPECTED OUTCOMES
- Be able to clear airway.
- Have breath sounds clear to auscultation and pulse oximetry readings above 95%.
- Be able to ambulate using assistive devices, if needed.
- Perform self-care activities without becoming overly fatigued and tired.
- Verbalize methods to adapt daily routine to his level of tolerance.

### PLANNING AND IMPLEMENTATION
- Initiate pulmonary hygiene measures (e.g., incentive spirometry, turning, deep breathing and coughing, breathing exercises, and postural drainage) at least every 2 hours. Assess lung sounds, oxygen saturation, and ability to clear airway.

- Teach the importance of maintaining an oral fluid intake of at least 2000 mL per day to prevent tenacious sputum and to prevent urinary tract infections. Teach signs and symptoms of urinary and respiratory infections.
- Encourage participation in decision making about care.
- Assist with ADLs only as needed, based on level of fatigue and muscle weakness.
- Plan self-care activities so that they are performed during periods of peak level of energy; intersperse rest periods throughout the day.
- Refer to an MS support group.
- Refer to physical and occupational therapists for counseling regarding control of spasticity and possible splinting of spastic muscles.
- Consult a urologist for assessment of bladder incontinence; teach intermittent catheterization. Alternatively, the use of an external condom catheter may be indicated.

### EVALUATION
Mr. McMurphy is discharged 3 days following admission. He states that he feels stronger; on discharge, he has no problem clearing his airway. Although he continues to pace his activities to avoid fatigue, his muscle strength and "tiredness" have improved. He is able to complete ADLs unassisted.

Pulmonary function has returned to normal, prehospitalization levels: ABGs and pulse oximetry are within normal limits. Both Mr. McMurphy and his wife have listed several ways to modify their daily routine to allow more rest and decreased stress. Follow-up visits to his primary care physician have been arranged, and they have been provided with information about the local MS support group.

### Critical Thinking in the Nursing Process

1. Describe approaches the nurse could take to ensure that Mr. McMurphy does not exceed his activity tolerance.
2. Develop a teaching plan for Mr. McMurphy to help prevent future respiratory infections.
3. Develop a care plan for Mr. McMurphy for the nursing diagnosis, *Risk for injury* related to fatigue, muscle weakness, and spasticity.

See Evaluating Your Response in Appendix C.

# THE CLIENT WITH PARKINSON'S DISEASE

**Parkinson's disease (PD)** is a progressive, degenerative neurologic disease characterized by *tremor at rest* (resting or **nonintention tremor**), muscle rigidity, and *akinesia* (poverty of movement). People with PD are faced with multiple problems involving independence in ADLs, emotional well-being, financial security, and relationships with caregivers.

## INCIDENCE AND PREVALENCE

Parkinson's disease is one of the most common neurologic disorders affecting older adults, affecting up to 1 million people in the United States. Although it may occur in younger people, the onset of PD is most often after age 40, with the mean age being 60. Men are affected more than women.

Parkinson's-like manifestations, called *secondary parkinsonism,* may result from other disorders such as trauma, encephalitis, tumors, toxins, and drugs. Drug-induced parkinsonism, which is usually reversible, may occur in people taking neuroleptics, antiemetics, antihypertensives, and illegal designer drugs containing the chemical MPTP (McCance & Huether, 2002). Carbon monoxide or cyanide poisoning can also cause secondary parkinsonism. This discussion focuses on primary Parkinson's disease, the cause of which is unknown.

## PATHOPHYSIOLOGY

Coordinated, voluntary body movement is achieved through the actions of neurotransmitters in the basal ganglia of the brain. Some neurotransmitters facilitate the transmission of excitatory nerve impulses, while other neurotransmitters inhibit their transmission. Together, this system allows control of movement. A disturbed balance between excitatory and inhibitory neurotransmitters causes disorders of voluntary motor function.

In PD, neurons in the cerebral cortex atrophy and are lost, and the dopaminergic nigrostriatal (pigmented) pathway degenerates. Also, the number of specific dopamine receptors in the basal ganglia decreases. These pathologic processes cause a decrease in dopamine (a neurotransmitter that helps regulate nerve impulses involved in motor function). The usual balance of dopamine (an inhibitory neurotransmitter) and acetylcholine (an excitatory neurotransmitter) in the brain is disrupted, and dopamine no longer inhibits acetylcholine. The failure to inhibit acetylcholine is the underlying basis for the manifestations of the disorder. Parkinson's disease has five stages, outlined in Box 43–3.

## MANIFESTATIONS

Parkinson's disease begins with subtle symptoms. Clients complain of feeling tired and seem to move more slowly; a slight tremor may accompany the fatigue. In a small percentage of clients, dementia is the initial presenting symptom. The manifestations of PD are presented in the box on page 1417.

---

| BOX 43–3 | ■ Stages of Parkinson's Disease |
|---|---|

I  Unilateral involvement only, usually with minimal or no functional impairment.

II  Bilateral or midline involvement, without impairment of balance.

III  First sign of impaired righting reflexes, evidenced as unsteadiness as the client turns or demonstrated when the client is pushed from standing equilibrium with the feet together and eyes closed. Functionally, the client is somewhat restricted in activities but may have some employment potential, depending on the type of employment. Clients are physically capable of leading independent lives, and their disability is mild to moderate.

IV  Fully developed, severely disabling disease; the client is still able to walk and stand unassisted but is markedly incapacitated.

V  Client is confined to bed or wheelchair unless aided.

---

## Tremor at Rest

Tremor at rest is usually the first manifestation experienced, with upper extremities more often affected. Resting tremors of the hand show a "pill rolling" motion of the thumb and fingers (given this name as this is the way in which medicinal pills were formed in the early days of medicine). The tremor may be controlled with purposeful, voluntary movement, and is worsened by stress and anxiety. Clients have progressive impairment in performing skills that require dexterity and fine muscle control, such as writing and eating.

## Rigidity and Akinesia

Manifestations related to motor and postural effects include rigidity, akinesia, and uncoordinated movements. *Rigidity* (resulting from involuntary contraction of all skeletal muscles) makes both active and passive movement difficult. It is manifested as increased resistance to passive range of motions. Although the extremity moves, it does so in a jerky motion, called *cogwheel rigidity*. The first manifestation of rigidity may be muscle cramps in the toes or hands, but most often the client describes stiffness, heaviness, or aching in muscles.

*Akinesia* is the most common and crippling manifestation. All striated muscles are affected, including those that involve chewing, swallowing, and speaking. Slowed or delayed movements affect the eyes, mouth, and voice, causing a masklike face and softened or muffled voice. Disorders of swallowing result in problems with eating and with drooling. Clients have a staring gaze with minimal change in expression (Figure 43–4 ■). Akinetic movements include both hypokinesia and bradykinesia. *Hypokinesia* (decreased frequency or absence of associated movements) is one of the earliest manifestations. Clients describe being "frozen" in place as voluntary movement is lost, and they sit or lie in one position without movement for long periods of time. **Bradykinesia** (slow movement) is experienced as difficulty in starting, continuing, or coordinating movements. Both of these disorders

## Medication Adm[...]

**The Client with Parkins[...]**

### DOPAMINERGICS

Levodopa (Larodopa, Dopa[...]
Carbidopa-levodopa (Sine[...]
Amantadine (Symmetrel)

These drugs have their major [...]
disease, improving mobility w[...]
tremor. Levodopa is a metabo[...]
like dopamine, it can cross th[...]
converted to dopamine in the[...]
enzyme, and stimulates do[...]
dopamine/acetylcholine co[...]
decarboxylase from converti[...]
peripheral tissues; therefore,[...]
combination with levodopa. A[...]
sia and also elevates mood.

Levodopa is avoided in cli[...]
severe angina pectoris, transi[...]
The "on-off" phenomenon oc[...]
for several years; this phenc[...]
pected dyskinesias and lack o[...]

Common side effects are [...]
urine and sweat; dyskinesias, [...]
therapy; dysrhythmias; orthos[...]
reactions, such as hallucinati[...]
are particularly susceptible to [...]

### Nursing Responsibilitie[...]
- Establish the client's baselir[...]
  ADLs and administering th[...]
  and coordination.
- To avoid adverse reaction[...]
  status before initiating ther[...]
- Monitor medications kno[...]
  tions: anticholinergics, py[...]
  alter the effectiveness of [...]
  cause severe hypertensior[...]
  effects.
- Withhold levodopa for 8 h[...]
  to avoid potentiating the e[...]

### Client and Family Teac[...]
- Levodopa may not take eff[...]
- Do not alter dosages of me[...]
  tion may not result in bett[...]
  severe side effects.
- Your protein intake should[...]
  the day's meals. Avoid foo[...]
  beef, ham, avocado, beans,[...]
- Levodopa may cause a ch[...]
  less, however.
- To prevent side effects:
  - Prevent nausea by takin[...]
  - Change position slowly [...]
    and risk of falling.
  - Prevent constipation by [...]
    cising regularly.
- Notify practitioner if you be[...]
  tary movements or cardiac [...]

## Manifestations of Parkinson's Disease

### MANIFESTATIONS RELATED TO MOTOR DYSFUNCTION
- Nonintention tremor
- Bradykinesia or akinesia
  a. Slowed movements; inability to initiate voluntary movements
  b. Slowed speech, low amplitude
  c. Poor articulation
  d. Decreased eye movements (i.e., blinking)
  e. Masklike, expressionless face
- Rigidity
- Posture and gait disturbances
  a. Trunk tilted forward
  b. Shuffling gait, propulsive at times
  c. Retropulsion
- Complications: falls, fractures, impaired communication, social isolation

### MANIFESTATIONS RELATED TO AUTONOMIC SYSTEM DYSFUNCTION
- Skin problems
  a. Seborrhea
  b. Excess sweating on face and neck, absence of sweating of trunk and extremities
  c. Mottled skin
- Heat intolerance
- Postural hypotension
- Constipation
- Complications: skin breakdown, dizziness, falls, constipation

### MANIFESTATIONS RELATED TO COGNITIVE AND PSYCHOLOGIC DYSFUNCTION
- Dementia
  a. Memory loss
  b. Lack of insight and problem-solving ability
  c. Declining intellectual abilities
- Anxiety
- Depression
- Complications: loss of ability to function, social isolation

of movement are interspersed with freezing, which is brought about by turning, increasing the effort to move, or making visual or touch contacts.

### Abnormal Posture

The loss of normal postural reflexes results in postural abnormalities, including disorders of postural fixation, equilibrium, and righting. Involuntary flexion of the head and shoulders means the person with PD cannot maintain an upright position of the trunk when sitting or standing. This problem of postural fixation results in the characteristic stooped, leaning forward position. Disorders of equilibrium follow loss of postural fixation with an inability to make adjustments when leaning or falling. The client takes short, accelerated steps, also characteristic of PD, to try to maintain an upright position when walking.

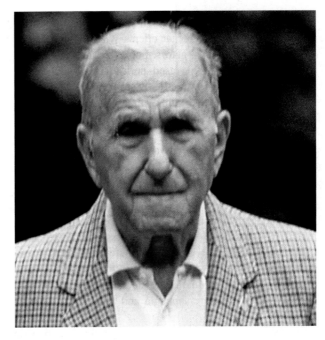

**Figure 43–4** ■ In Parkinson's disease, the client's face lacks expression or animation.

*Source: Yoav Levy/Phototake NYC.*

### Autonomic and Neuroendocrine Effects

Many manifestations result from the loss of functions controlled by the autonomic nervous system. Elimination problems include constipation and urinary hesitation or frequency. Clients may experience problems related to orthostatic hypotension, including dizziness with position change. Eczematous skin changes and seborrhea are related to the increase in sweat gland activity secondary to increased sebotropic hormone production.

### Mood and Cognition

Both depression and dementia are pathologies associated with PD. Depression occurs in half of all clients and a third have dementia. Dementia, resulting from loss of cholinergic cells, loss of neurons, senile plaques, neurofibrillary tangles, and amyloid changes in small blood vessels, is seen more often in clients over the age of 70. The client manifests confusion, disorientation, memory loss, distractibility, and changes in abstraction and judgment. *Bradyphrenia* may also occur, resulting in slow thinking and a decreased ability to form thoughts, plan, and decide.

### Sleep Disturbances

Clients with PD also have sleep disturbances, although they may experience decreased manifestations during sleep in the early stages. The ability to fall and stay sleep is affected by acetylcholine. Muscle rigidity may compromise sleep because of the inability to change position. This lack of muscle movement causes the client to awaken and consciously shift position.

MediaLink | AKINESIA/BRADYKINESIA VIDEOS

## Interrelated Effects

Some of the manifestations th
have multiple contributing fac
is common because of decre
creased peristalsis is not the o
(resulting in being unable to dr
etary changes from dysphagia
constipation.

The following complicatio
son's disease.

- Oculogyric crisis, in which t
  eral and upward gaze
- Paranoia and hallucinations,
- Impaired communication du
  writing, and expressiveness
- Falls from balance, posture,
- Infections, such as pneumor
- Malnutrition related to dys
  meals
- Altered sleep patterns due t
  effects (nightmares, dreams)
  gics (hyperreflexia, muscle
- Skin breakdown and pressur
  incontinence, malnutrition, a
- Depression and social isolat

## PROGNOSIS

Prognosis is poor, owing to th
ultimately affects multiple phy
tion. Psychosocial effects ar
family needs more support as t
Total disability is usually seer
The leading cause of death is

## COLLABORATIV

Diagnosis is based primarily c
cal examination, and is made
manifestations: tremor at rest,
tural instability. Intervention:
the disorder and include medic
to retain the optimal level of
proach is essential for these cl

## Diagnostic Tests

Diagnostic studies may su
Parkinson's disease; howeve
Parkinson's disease from otl
ever, PET scan will show dec
dopa. Tests are usually perfc
produce secondary parkinson
ordered.

- *Drug screens* determine the
  ins that cause secondary pa
  reserpine, or carbon monox

---

## Nursing Research

### Evidence-Based Practice for Preventing Falls in Clients with PD

Although clients with PD are at risk for and experience frequent falls, not much research has been done to identify the risk factors involved with this population. Gray and Hildebrand (2000) conducted this study to collect demographic, environmental, and medical history data. They also asked subjects to maintain a fall diary for a 3-month period. Of the 118 participants, 59% reported one or more falls (a total of 237 falls).

Analysis of data resulted in the following factors involved in an increased risk for falls in people with PD:

- Duration and severity of manifestations of PD, especially freezing, involuntary movements, and postural disorders that affected gait while walking (Clients with PD for more than 15 years were 5 times more likely to fall than those with PD for 5 years or less. Of subjects who reported episodes of freezing, 80% had falls.)
- Postural hypotension
- Using an aid to walk, such as a cane or walker
- Requiring help with ADLs
- Giving up usual activities
- Daily alcohol intake

### IMPLICATIONS FOR NURSING

Nurses play an important role in identifying clients with PD who are at risk for falls, and in teaching clients and caregivers how to prevent them. A fall risk assessment should be an integral part of the nursing assessment. Clients and caregivers can be alerted to factors that increase the risk, and take preventive measures to reduce injuries. For example, being aware of the fall risk with turning, standing, walking, and freezing can increase attention to safety measures. In addition, stress the risk of alcohol intake, as well as intake and timing of medications and avoiding changes in the client's environment.

### Critical Thinking in Client Care

1. How would interventions for the nursing diagnosis, *Risk for falls,* differ in a 60-year-old man who lives alone and an 88-year-old woman who is a resident in a nursing home?
2. Postural hypotension and lightheadedness may be side effects of medications for PD. Outline a teaching plan to decrease the risk for falls from these manifestations.
3. What factors would you include in a home assessment that would increase the client's risk for falls?

---

### Imbalanced Nutrition: Less Than Body Requirements

Tremors, altered gait, and impaired chewing and swallowing can cause nutritional problems in the client with PD. As the disorder progresses, interventions for ensuring optimal nutrition need to be adapted to the client's functional abilities. Assess the client's swallow reflex before starting any feeding program. During the initial stages of the disorder, some clients may have the nursing diagnosis, *Imbalanced nutrition: More than body requirements,* if kcal intake exceeds energy expenditure.

- Assess nutritional status and self-feeding abilities; consult with occupational or speech therapist, if needed. *An initial assessment of abilities ensures that interventions are personalized to the client's current functional abilities.*
- Teach caregivers how to prepare foods of proper consistency as determined by swallowing function. *The client may aspirate food that is too liquid.*
- Weigh weekly. *Early recognition of weight loss allows for intervention.*
- Teach eating methods to decrease tremors, such as holding a piece of bread in the hand that is not holding an eating utensil. *Nonintention tremor may be reduced through purposeful activity.*
- Encourage diet that is high in bulk and fluids. *Several anti-Parkinson's medications can cause constipation.*

### Disturbed Sleep Pattern

Rigidity and weakness can cause clients with Parkinson's disease to lose the ability to move and change positions during sleep. The resulting discomfort causes periods of wakefulness. Medications to treat Parkinson's disease contribute to sleep pattern disturbance; for example, levodopa can cause vivid dreams. Nurses can help accurately assess the sleep pattern disturbance and in planning interventions to improve or increase sleep time.

- Assess sleep pattern and existing conditions that may affect sleep, such as depression or pain. *Clients experiencing anxiety, depression, and dementia have a difficult time falling asleep and may wake up more at night.*

**PRACTICE ALERT** *Remember to assess pain status; lack of adequate pain control may interfere with sleep.* ∎

- Explain the disease process and the effects of decreased dopamine on the sleep-wake cycle. *Depending on the dosage, levodopa causes less REM sleep and deep sleep.*
- Review the client's medication. *Bromocriptine and levodopa, especially if used with an anticholinergic, can cause vivid dreams. Other medications (diuretics, theophylline, hypnotics) also may interfere with sleep.*
- Teach how to modify lifestyle activities that affect sleep:
  - Institute a routine of activities with limited rest periods during the day; avoid napping close to bedtime. Avoid strenuous exercise in the evening. *Daytime sleeping may contribute to decreased nighttime sleeping. Vigorous exercise just before bedtime may act as a stimulant.*
  - Incorporate diet modifications, such as limiting caffeine and alcohol intake. *Caffeine is a stimulant, and alcohol may cause early-morning awakenings, increased daytime sleepiness, and nightmares.*
  - Drink a glass of milk before bedtime. *Milk contains L-tryptophan, which produces sedative effects by shortening the time taken to fall asleep (sleep latency).*

## CHART 43–3  NANDA, NIC, AND NOC LINKAGES

### The Client with PD

| NURSING DIAGNOSES | NURSING INTERVENTIONS | NURSING OUTCOMES |
|---|---|---|
| • Impaired Physical Mobility | • Energy Management<br>• Exercise Therapy: Ambulation | • Mobility Level<br>• Ambulation: Walking |
| • Self-Care Deficits | • Bathing/Hygiene<br>• Dressing/Hair Care<br>• Feeding<br>• Toileting | • Self-Care: ADLs<br>• Self-Care: Bathing<br>• Self-Care: Dressing<br>• Self-Care: Feeding<br>• Self-Care: Toileting |
| • Constipation<br>• Imbalanced Nutrition: Risk for Less than Body Requirements | • Bowel Management<br>• Nutrition Management<br>• Swallowing Therapy<br>• Self-Care Assistance: Feeding | • Bowel Elimination<br>• Nutritional Status |

*Note. Data from* Nursing Outcomes Classification (NOC) *by M. Johnson & M. Maas (Eds.), 1997, St. Louis: Mosby;* Nursing Diagnoses: Definitions & Classification 2001–2002 *by North American Nursing Diagnosis Association, 2001, Philadelphia: NANDA;* Nursing Interventions Classification (NIC) *by J.C. McCloskey & G. M. Bulechek (Eds.), 2000, St. Louis: Mosby. Reprinted by permission.*

- Adapt the environment to aid in sleep (e.g., darken the room and decrease noises). *Reducing environmental stimuli decreases external sleep disturbances.*

## Using NANDA, NIC, and NOC

Chart 43–3 shows links between NANDA nursing diagnoses, NIC, and NOC when caring for the client with PD.

## Home Care

It is important for both the client and the family to maintain independence and self care as long as possible. To maintain function and quality of life, the following topics should be addressed.

- Realistic expectations
- Equipment suppliers
- Home environment conducive to using equipment
- Referrals to speech therapist, occupational therapist, physical therapist, dietitian
- Gait training and exercises for improving ambulation, speech, swallowing, and self-care
- Increased fluid intake of 3000 mL/day and increased fiber in every meal
- Stool softeners or laxatives as needed for bowel elimination
- Swallowing during eating and taking medications (Have suction equipment available and know the Heimlich maneuver if choking occurs.)
- Foods that can be easily swallowed (such as pureed or soft) and feed six small meals a day if possible
- Helpful resources:
  - American Parkinson's Disease Association
  - National Parkinson Foundation, Inc.
  - Parkinson's Disease Foundation
  - The National Institute of Neurological Disorders and Stroke

MediaLink | PARKINSON'S DISEASE RESOURCES

## Nursing Care Plan
## A Client with PD

Walter Avneil, age 78, was diagnosed with PD at age 64. His wife died 5 years ago and he has no other family living. Mr. Avneil worked for more than 40 years as a mechanic in a large factory. He is a resident of a long-term care facility. During his last clinic visit for a review of his medications, the following assessment was made.

### ASSESSMENT
Elderly white male with history of PD for the past 14 years. Skin oily and damp. Tremors in both hands and the lips. Gait is slow and shuffling, with a forward leaning posture. Speech slow and slurred. Face expressionless. Has lost 10 lb since last visit 3 months ago. Has been on levodopa with carbidopa since diagnosis. States major problems are "eating problems, bowel problems, walking problems."

### DIAGNOSIS
- *Constipation* related to lack of exercise, decreased food intake, and effects of medications
- *Impaired verbal communication* related to lip tremors, slow/slurred speech, and facial muscle involvement of PD
- *Imbalanced nutrition: Less than body requirements* related to difficulty swallowing and chewing
- *Impaired physical mobility* related to rigidity and bradykinesia

### EXPECTED OUTCOMES
- Have a soft stool at least every other day.
- Practice exercises provided by speech therapist twice a day.

*(continued on page 1424)*

## Nursing Care Plan
### A Client with PD (continued)

- Increase number of calories, fluids, and fiber in diet provided at long-term facility.
- Improve joint mobility and ability to ambulate.

### PLANNING AND IMPLEMENTATION

- Discuss problems with bowel elimination with staff at long-term facility; suggest increasing fluids to 3000 mL per day and also increasing fiber in the diet with oatmeal for breakfast, and more fruits and vegetables at meals.
- Encourage exercises provided by speech therapist to improve speech and swallowing. If these are not effective, make a referral for another evaluation.
- Discuss diet plan with dietitian at the long-term care facility, including consistency of foods and number of calories. Suggest dietitian be a part of swallowing evaluation by the speech therapist.
- Refer for physical therapy and occupational therapy for a program to improve gait and joint mobility, and to decrease risk of falling.

### EVALUATION

In a return visit 3 months later, Mr. Avneil reports that "my bowels are working better." He has gained 7 lb, and the staff report that this is related to multiple factors, including practicing his swallow-ing exercises, getting more exercise that stimulated his appetite, and changing his diet to six small meals a day of soft or pureed foods. The staff is offering him liquids at meals and snack times, and he usually drinks all they give him. His speech is not much improved. He posture and gait are somewhat better, and he is doing the exercises provided by the physical therapist and occupational therapist. Mr. Avneil's functional abilities have improved so much that the staff is considering training sessions specific to care of residents with PD.

### Critical Thinking in the Nursing Process

1. Although Mr. Avneil did not mention it, the staff reports that he is frustrated by not being able to dress himself. What suggestions could you make to facilitate his independence?
2. Mr. Avneil spends most of his time alone, although he enjoys the company of the other residents. List assessments and interventions you might provide to increase his diversional activity.
3. The loss of his wife and the debilitating effects of his disease increase Mr. Avneil's risk for chronic sorrow. What might you suggest the long-term staff do to reduce this risk?

See Evaluating Your Response in Appendix C.

## THE CLIENT WITH HUNTINGTON'S DISEASE

**Huntington's disease,** also called **chorea,** is a progressive, degenerative, inherited neurologic disease characterized by increasing dementia and chorea (jerky, rapid, involuntary movements). It is a single-gene autosomal-dominant inherited disease that causes localized death of neurons of the basal ganglia (Porth, 2002). The exact cause is unknown, but postmortem studies have demonstrated a decrease in gamma-aminobutyric acid (GABA), an inhibitory neurotransmitter in the basal ganglia. There is also a decrease in acetylcholine levels, suggesting that the manifestations are the result of an imbalance in dopamine and acetylcholine. Although carriers can be identified, there is no cure for the disease. Huntington's disease causes progressive chorea, speech problems, and dementia.

Because the client is usually asymptomatic until age 30 to 40, he or she may already have passed the gene to the next generation. The psychologic impact is devastating to clients and their families. The family not only experiences guilt from passing the disease from one generation to the next, but also is faced with the overwhelming long-term care needs of those affected. It is common for several family members to be afflicted with the disease.

### PATHOPHYSIOLOGY

Huntington's disease causes destruction of cells in the caudate nucleus and putamen areas of the basal ganglia. Other areas of the brain, such as the frontal lobes, may selectively atrophy. Several neurotransmitters and their receptors are decreased, including GABA and acetylcholine. The neurotransmitter dopamine is not affected in Huntington's disease, but the decrease in acetylcholine results in a relative excess of dopamine in the basal ganglia. Whereas in Parkinson's disease a deficit of dopamine causes slow movement or lack of movement, in Huntington's disease the opposite occurs: There is a relative excess of dopamine, causing excessive, uncontrolled movement.

### MANIFESTATIONS

Manifestations primarily involve abnormal movement and progressive dementia (see the box on page 1425). The progression and sequence of manifestations varies somewhat; however, initially the psychologic manifestations are more debilitating than the choreiform movements.

Early signs of personality change include severe depression, memory loss with decreased ability to concentrate, emotional lability, and impulsiveness. The client experiences frequent mood swings ranging from uncontrollable periods of anger to apathy. Eventually, signs of dementia, including disorientation, confusion, and lack of sense of time, become evident and interfere with self-care.

Motor symptoms usually parallel personality and mood changes. The motor symptoms worsen with environmental stimuli and emotional stress but are absent when the client is sleeping. Initially, movement problems are described as "fidgeting" or restlessness, followed by progressive worsening of

## Manifestations of Huntington's Disease

### MOTOR EFFECTS

**Early**

- Restlessness
- "Fidgety" feeling
- Minor gait changes—unsteady on feet
- Posture and positioning disturbances, frequent falls
- Inability to keep the tongue from protruding
- Slurred speech with poor articulation
- Complications: increasing problem with self-care activities, such as bathing, grooming, eating

**Late**

- Chorea—severely altered gait with irregular, uncontrollable movement; the distal extremity is most affected; shoulders shrug arrhythmically
- Facial grimacing—raising of eyebrows, uncontrollable protrusion of the tongue
- Dysphagia
- Unintelligible speech
- Impaired diaphragmatic movement
- Complications: immobility, aspiration, choking, and, eventually, total dependence, poor oxygenation, emaciation, and cachexia

### PSYCHOSOCIAL EFFECTS

**Early**

- Irritability
- Outbursts of rage alternating with euphoria
- Depression
- Complication: suicide

**Late**

- Decreasing memory
- Loss of cognitive skills
- Eventual dementia
- Complication: total dependence

abnormal movements. The choreiform movements, which begin in the face and arms and then involve the entire body, are manifested by facial grimaces, tongue protrusion, jerky movement of the distal arms or legs, and a rhythmic, lurching gait that almost resembles a dance. (The term *chorea* comes from *choreia*, the Greek word meaning "dance.") Gait changes cause uncoordinated movements and contribute to frequent falls.

The muscles of swallowing, chewing, and speaking are affected, leading to dysphagia and dysarthria and associated problems with communication and nutrition. The client's constant movement and difficulty in swallowing contribute to weight loss and eventual cachexia. Breathing is impaired because the diaphragm is unable to move effectively.

The manifestations slowly progress over approximately 15 to 20 years after initial symptoms appear. Prognosis is poor, with inevitable debilitation and total dependence. Death usually results from aspiration pneumonia or another infectious process.

## COLLABORATIVE CARE

There is no cure for Huntington's disease, and treatment addresses the disease's manifestations. Nurses provide care to clients with Huntington's disease in a variety of community settings. Initially, clients and families can manage care needs at home, but as the disease progresses, the client requires constant supervision, such as that provided in day care facilities. Eventually, skilled long-term care is needed. Clients who develop acute problems may be hospitalized until the crisis is managed. Because of the inevitable total multisystem debilitation of clients with Huntington's disease, nurses and other caregivers face many challenges.

### Diagnostic Tests

Genetic testing is the only test available to diagnose clients suspected of having Huntington's disease. Both blood and amniotic fluid may be tested for the presence of chromosome 4 using DNA analysis. The test can predict with 95% accuracy which offspring have the disease.

### Medications

The following medications are given for palliation of the symptoms of Huntington's disease.

- Antipsychotics, specifically phenothiazines and butyrophenones, are effective in Huntington's disease because they block dopamine receptors in the brain. The therapeutic goal is to restore the balance among the neurotransmitters.
- Antidepressants are prescribed in the early stage of the disease; however, medications are no substitute for intense follow-up counseling for clients and families.

## NURSING CARE

Nurses are faced with a multitude of challenges when caring for families who have Huntington's disease, including physiologic, psychosocial, and ethical problems. Physiologic problems are related to the progressive and eventually debilitating nature of the disease. Psychosocial concerns occur as a result of the client's personality and mental changes, the family's responsibility for providing care, and the guilt implicit in a genetically transmitted disease. Ethical difficulties relate to the genetic nature of the disease: DNA testing for the marker on chromosome 4 can determine whether the person is a carrier of the disease before he or she begins to exhibit manifestations. Children of people with Huntington's disease are thus faced with the choice of finding out whether they will eventually be affected. If they choose not to be tested, they may pass the disease on to yet another generation; and if a fetus is affected, they may face the decision of whether to undergo an abortion.

### Nursing Diagnoses and Interventions

Initially, much of the nursing care focuses on teaching about the disease, psychologic support, and genetic counseling. As manifestations become more severe, nursing considerations center on problems related not only to immobility and altered nutrition, but also to the increasing self-care deficits. Families and clients experiencing Huntington's disease face many psychosocial issues. Nurses must be prepared to listen actively as well as to provide comfort and encouragement throughout the lengthy illness. There are many possible nursing diagnoses for the client with Huntington's disease; this section focuses on nursing diagnoses related to aspiration, nutrition, skin integrity, and communication.

### Risk for Aspiration

Uncoordinated movements and swallowing and chewing problems put the client at high risk for aspiration.

- Maintain in an upright position while the client eats; support the head. *Proper positioning may prevent aspiration during mealtime.*
- Teach the Heimlich maneuver to caregivers and family members. *Aspiration is a real possibility; caregivers must be prepared to reestablish the client's airway.*
- Provide food that is thick enough to manage, such as thick soups, mashed potatoes, stews, or casseroles. *These foods are more readily tolerated and manipulated by the tongue than liquids.*
- Make sure food is swallowed before giving another spoonful of food. *The automatic phase of swallowing may be disrupted in the client with Huntington's disease; providing adequate time and smaller bites may improve the ability to manipulate foods.*
- Provide a calm, relaxing eating environment. *Stress worsens choreiform movements and inappropriate behaviors.*

### Imbalanced Nutrition:
### Less Than Body Requirements

Clients with Huntington's disease have unpredictable choreiform movements of the extremities and decreased ability to control muscles involved with chewing and swallowing. Families and caregivers are challenged to provide sufficient calories to maintain the client in positive nitrogen balance.

- Evaluate current weight and nutritional status, including serum albumin and transferrin levels. *Establishing a baseline is crucial for meeting individual caloric, protein, vitamin, and mineral needs.*
- Assess ability to swallow and manipulate eating utensils. *Aspiration is an ever-present danger that must be avoided; utensils may need to be adapted to client's abilities, if client is able to assist at all.*
- Continue feeding even if the client physically turns away from the meal. *Involuntary choreiform movements should not be interpreted as a refusal to eat.*
- Provide high-kcal, nutritious foods and sufficient snacks; request input from a dietitian. *The constant movement of Huntington's disease increases caloric requirements.*
- Avoid milk; provide frequent oral hygiene. *Milk tends to thicken secretions. Decreasing thick secretions may improve ability to swallow and enable the client to ingest more calories.*

### Impaired Skin Integrity

Skin integrity is only one component of the client's general need for protection and avoidance of injury. Several factors increase the risk for impaired skin integrity, including poor nutritional status, eventual total immobility, and incontinence.

- Evaluate the skin for actual and potential areas of breakdown. *Establishing a baseline is necessary to modify care and provide prophylactic protection of high-risk pressure areas.*
- Determine nutritional status, especially serum albumin level and vitamin, mineral, and kcal intake. *Optimal nutritional status and positive nitrogen balance help prevent skin breakdown and formation of pressure ulcers.*
- Turn and inspect the skin at least every 2 hours, giving special consideration to areas that are most prone to breakdown, such as heels and coccyx. *Pressure points are particularly susceptible to skin breakdown.*
- Provide ROM exercises on a regular schedule in the daytime. *Movement stimulates circulation, which provides oxygenation and allows nutrients to reach muscles and skin.*
- Keep the skin clean and dry; pay particular attention to the perineal area if incontinent. *Skin in close proximity to perineal area, such as the sacral area, is highly susceptible to breakdown due to exposure to wet, acidic urine and fecal material.*
- Place on an alternating-pressure mattress with foot board. *Decreasing pressure on bony prominences and preventing shearing forces serve to prevent skin breakdown.*
- Pad side rails and headrests of special chairs; have the client wear a football-type helmet. *The client's violent movements can cause trauma to the head and extremities.*

### Impaired Verbal Communication

The inability to control muscles related to speech, swallowing, and facial movement contributes to problems of verbal communication. Because Huntington's disease affects fine motor movement, especially the distal portion of the extremities, the hands are not effective in communication. As the disease progresses, mental abilities are also compromised, making both receptive and expressive communication impossible.

- Choose alternative methods of communication while the client is able to participate. *Anticipatory planning may facilitate communication and decrease anxiety.*
- Continue to incorporate therapeutic communication techniques, even though client is not responsive: maintain eye contact, use touch, and talk directly to the client rather than to others in the room. *These techniques enhance the individual's dignity and worth.*
- Seek input from family about client's usual preferences and how they are communicated; be alert for subtle cues. *Nonverbal communication techniques may be individualized and more readily recognized by the family member or caregiver that usually provides care.*
- Continue talking to the client, even though there is no apparent response. *Hearing may not be impaired, even though the client cannot speak.*

---

**BOX 43–4** ■ **Inheritance of an Autosomal Dominant Trait**

- The abnormal trait is dominant over the normal characteristics—in the case of Huntington's disease, neurologic functioning.
- People affected usually have at least one parent who also is affected.
- Each offspring has a 50% risk of being affected. In other words, transmission of the dominant trait is independent of number of children who may or may not already have the disease.
- Both sexes are equally affected because the inheritance is autosomal dominant, not X-linked.
- Children who are not affected will not genetically transmit the disease to their children.

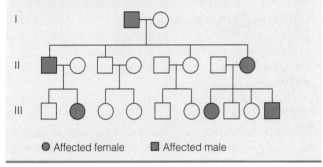

● Affected female ■ Affected male

## Home Care

Clients with Huntington's disease and their families know how devastating the illness is as they may have cared for a parent or other close family member who has suffered through the illness. Many families are overwhelmed with just the thought of the physical and psychosocial debilitation that the disease brings. Fear, anxiety, and hopelessness leading to depression are common reactions. Teaching ways to cope effectively with the psychosocial and physical changes is an integral part of the nurse's responsibilities. Referrals to appropriate agencies, such as the Huntington's Disease Foundation and local support groups or a psychologist, should be part of the nursing plan.

Another aspect of client teaching concerns the genetic transmission of Huntington's disease; refer clients and family members to a geneticist. Nurses are frequently involved with clarifying information, especially concerning the transmission, course of illness, and prognosis. A caring, sensitive approach is crucial. Information about transmission of an autosomal-dominant trait is presented in Box 43–4.

Nurses in the community are often the professionals with whom families have the most contact. Teaching family members ways to prevent injury from falls and methods to avoid malnutrition are part of holistic care. Measures to assist with incontinence are instituted when indicated.

## THE CLIENT WITH AMYOTROPHIC LATERAL SCLEROSIS

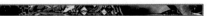

**Amyotrophic lateral sclerosis (ALS),** or **Lou Gehrig's disease,** is a progressive, degenerative neurologic disease characterized by weakness and wasting of the involved muscles, without any accompanying sensory or cognitive changes. The name is derived from the pathophysiologic processes of muscle atrophy (*amyotrophy*) resulting from lower motor neuron involvement and lateral sclerosis of the corticospinal tract in the lateral column of the spinal cord resulting from upper motor neuron involvement. Death results in 2 to 5 years after onset of the symptoms, usually due to respiratory failure.

ALS is the most common motor neuron disease in the United States, with approximately 5000 new cases diagnosed each year (McCance & Huether, 2002). There are several types, categorized as sporadic ALS (no family history of ALS) and familial ALS (a family history of ALS). Most people are between 40 and 60 years of age at diagnosis; the incidence is higher in men in the earlier ages but becomes equal with women after menopause. Classic ALS (Lou Gehrig's disease) occurs most often in the early 50s. There is a genetic factor involved, with familial ALS linked to chromosome 21 defects. Most of the physiologic problems a client with ALS encounters are related to swallowing and managing secretions, communication, and dysfunction of the muscles used in respiration.

## PATHOPHYSIOLOGY AND MANIFESTATIONS

ALS results from the degeneration and demyelination of motor neurons in the anterior horn of the spinal cord, brainstem, and cerebral cortex. ALS involves both upper and lower motor neurons. Death of the motor neurons results in axonal degeneration, demyelination, glial proliferation, and scarring along the corticospinal tract. In the early stages of the disease, surviving motor neurons sprout new branches to reinnervate affected muscle fibers, preserving muscle strength. However, when more than half of the lower motor neurons are affected, reinnervation fails and weakness is evidenced (Ross, 1999).

Although the pathogenesis of ALS is not clear, abnormal glutamate metabolism and hydrogen peroxide production are being studied. Echovirus RNA have also been isolated in spinal cord tissue in some clients with nonfamilial ALS (McCance & Huether, 2002). Environmental factors, excess intracellular calcium, and antibodies to calcium channels are also being researched.

The initial manifestations may relate to dysfunction of upper motor neurons, lower motor neurons, or both. Dysfunction of upper motor neurons (located in the cerebral cortex and conduct impulses within the central nervous system) results in spastic, weak muscles with increased deep-tendon reflexes. Dysfunction of lower motor neurons (which originate in the gray matter of the spinal cord or the brainstem cranial nerves and innervate skeletal muscles) results in muscle flaccidity, paresis (weakness), paralysis, and atrophy.

Weakness and paresis are common early complaints. The weakness may initially affect only one muscle group. Manifestations vary according to the particular muscle group involved; **fasciculations,** or focal twitching, of involved muscles are common in the early stage of the disorder. With the loss of muscle innervation, the muscles atrophy, and paralysis results. Clinically, the muscle mass decreases, and clients complain of progressive fatigue. Typically, the disease first affects the hands, then the shoulders, upper arms, and finally the legs.

Increasing brainstem involvement causes progressive atrophy of the tongue and facial muscles with eventual dysphagia and dysarthria. Emotional lability and loss of control occur, but dementia is not part of the pathologic progression of ALS. Vision, hearing, sensation, and cognitive ability usually remain intact. A summary of manifestations is presented in the box below.

About 50% of clients die within 2 to 5 years of diagnosis, but the course of the disease varies. Eventually, the client faces total debilitation and dependence. Death frequently results from aspiration pneumonia, another infectious process, or respiratory failure.

## COLLABORATIVE CARE

Because many treatable disorders may cause manifestations similar to those that appear in the initial stage of ALS, a thorough evaluation is required. Once ALS is diagnosed, the primary goal is to support the client and family in meeting physical and psychosocial needs, particularly as the disease progresses.

Medical and nursing care for clients with ALS is primarily supportive. Referral to community health nurses for home health management is indicated. Occupational, physical, speech, and respiratory therapy are major supportive and rehabilita-

## Manifestations of ALS

### MUSCULOSKELETAL SYSTEM

- Weakness and fatigue
- "Heaviness" of legs
- Fasciculations
- Uncoordinated movements, loss of fine motor control in hands
- Spasticity
- Paresis
- Hyperreflexia
- Atrophy
- Problems with articulation
- Complications: paralysis, loss of ability to perform ADLs, total immobility, aspiration, loss of verbal communication

### RESPIRATORY SYSTEM

- Dyspnea
- Difficulty clearing airway
- Complications: pneumonia, eventual respiratory failure

### NUTRITIONAL EFFECTS

- Difficulty chewing
- Dysphagia
- Complication: malnutrition

### EMOTIONAL EFFECTS

- Loss of control, lability
- Complication: depression

tive treatments. As the disorder progresses and swallowing becomes ineffective, a gastrostomy tube may be indicated to provide adequate nutritional intake. Ventilatory assistance should be discussed with clients before the need occurs.

## Diagnostic Tests

A number of disorders may mimic early ALS, including hyperthyroidism, hypoglycemia, compression of the spinal cord, toxic agents, infections, and neoplasms. In addition to diagnostic studies performed to rule out other suspected conditions, the following tests may be ordered.

- *EMG* is done to differentiate a neuropathy from a myopathy. Fibrillations of the muscle at rest supports the diagnosis of ALS.
- *Muscle biopsy* reflects tissue changes consistent with atrophy and loss of muscle fiber.
- *Serum creatine kinase (CK) enzyme levels* are usually elevated; however, this finding is not specific to ALS.
- *Pulmonary function studies* may be ordered if respiratory involvement is a factor.

## Medications

Riluzole (Rilutek), an antiglutamate, is the first medication developed to treat ALS. It inhibits the presynaptic release of glutamic acid in the CNS and protects neurons against the excitotoxicity of glutamic acid. This oral medication is administered without food at the same time each day. Clients are regularly monitored for liver function, blood count, blood chemistries, and alkaline phosphatase. They should be warned to report any febrile illness to their health care provider and to avoid alcohol.

## NURSING CARE

Nursing care focuses on current health problems and on anticipating future difficulties. As with other disorders causing incapacitation and dependence, individualized nursing goals and interventions relate to decreasing complications, especially those associated with loss of muscular function and immobility; promoting independence to the extent possible; initiating referrals, particularly to a support group for both client and family; and providing physical and psychosocial support as indicated.

Of special consideration is planning for the client's eventual inability to communicate. Because the client's eye muscles and movements remain intact, signals can be prearranged before the loss of speech.

### Nursing Diagnoses and Interventions

Two nursing diagnoses that frequently apply to clients with ALS are Risk for disuse syndrome and Ineffective breathing pattern.

#### Risk for Disuse Syndrome

Clients with ALS are at risk for developing problems associated with bed rest not only because they cannot move and reposition themselves but also because they frequently have altered nutritional and hydration status. Nursing interventions focus on

In myasthenia gr[...]
muscular junction re[...]
ber of acetylcholine r[...]
diminished acetylcho[...]
in the muscle's abilit[...]
of acetylcholine. A [...]
junction and one aff[...]
Figure 43–5 ■.

In about 75% of cl[...]
gland, which is usuall[...]
duce antibodies becau[...]
of tumors. It is belie[...]
toantigen that trigger[...]
gravis. The exact mec[...]
antibody production i[...]

Myasthenia gravis[...]
the thymus, thyroto[...]
arthritis, and lupus er[...]
nosed when a client [...]

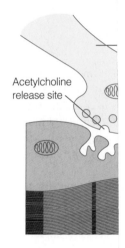

**A** Normal neuromus[...]

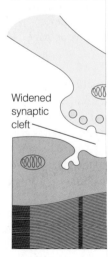

**B** Myasthenia gravis

**Figure 43–5** ■ *A, A[...]
showing the changes [...]
interfere with the transr[...]*

---

preventing skin breakdown and infections, such as urinary tract infections.

- Assess current condition for baseline parameters, particularly skin over bony prominences, lung sounds, and vital signs. *Understanding client's current condition allows accurate future assessment and realistic planning.*
- Assess skin; provide skin care, and obtain an alternating-pressure mattress. *Pressure points are at risk for breakdown; early detection is crucial to instituting appropriate care.*
- Institute active ROM exercises, as the client is able. Perform passive ROM exercises every 2 hours, when the client is turned. *Contractures can develop within a week because extensor muscles are weaker than flexor muscles.*
- Maintain positive nitrogen balance and hydration status: Monitor albumin levels, hemoglobin and hematocrit levels, and urine specific gravity. *Adequate protein is required to maintain osmotic pressure and prevent edema; positive nitrogen balance promotes optimal body functioning.*
- Monitor for manifestations of infection; for example, assess urine, especially if a urinary catheter is present. *Urinary catheters place clients at high risk for sepsis; bed rest places the client at greater risk for urinary stasis.*

**PRACTICE ALERT** *Urinary tract infection is indicated by cloudy, foul-smelling urine, pain on urination, fever, and general malaise.* ■

### Ineffective Breathing Pattern

As the muscle weakness of ALS continues, clients become less able to breathe. The respiratory muscles are affected, and clients eventually may require ventilatory assistance. The nurse must initiate measures to support the existing respiratory effort.

- Obtain a baseline assessment of breathing pattern, air movement, and oxygen saturation. *Assessments indicating the client's current condition provide data to plan individualized interventions.*
- Turn at least every 2 hours. *Movement enhances the ability to move pulmonary secretions and prevents stasis.*
- Elevate the head of the bed at least 30 degrees, suction as indicated, and provide oxygen. *This supports ventilation and enhances lung expansion as the client's condition changes.*
- Assess temperature and lung sounds routinely; obtain sputum culture as indicated. *Early detection of a possible infectious process leads to prompt treatment.*

**PRACTICE ALERT** *A pulmonary infection is indicated by respiratory difficulty, crackles and/or wheezes, cough productive of yellow or green sputum, fever, and malaise.* ■

### Home Care

Initial teaching centers on explaining the disease process, expected course, and prognosis. Referral to a social worker to determine home care needs and financial assistance is helpful.

---

Counseling and referrals to a community health nurse, dietitian, and physical, speech, and occupational therapists can help the family meet the client's changing needs and abilities. The need for realistic anticipation of needs cannot be overemphasized.

As the client becomes more debilitated, family members or other care providers focus on preventing complications. For example, family members need to know how to suction the client and perform the Heimlich maneuver to prevent aspiration. Teaching the family how to prevent problems related to immobility is a primary consideration for the nurse.

Another focus of teaching is basic care needs, such as care required to meet elimination needs. Teach families methods to establish a bowel routine, considerations related to a urinary catheter, and the need to promptly report manifestations of an infection.

Throughout the early stage and continued care of the client and family with ALS, much consideration is given to psychosocial concerns. Depression, anger, and denial may be initial reactions; refer the client and family to an ALS support group, social worker, psychologist, or psychiatrist as indicated.

## THE CLIENT WITH CREUTZFELDT-JAKOB DISEASE

**Creutzfeldt-Jakob disease (CJD, spongiform encephalopathy)** is a rapidly progressive, degenerative, neurologic disease that causes brain degeneration without inflammation. The disease is transmissible and progressively fatal. The causative agent is believed to be an abnormal form of a cellular glycoprotein known as the prion protein. Transmission of the agent is by direct contamination with infected neural tissue, such as during eye and brain surgery. The injection of contaminated human growth hormone from cadaveric pituitaries has also been implicated.

A new disease, called **new variant CJD (vCJD)** is also a rare, degenerative, fatal brain disorder, but is not the same as the classic form of CJD. New variant CJD, referred to as "mad-cow disease" is believed due to consumption of cattle products contaminated with bovine spongiform encephalopathy (BSE). This form primarily affects younger people. As the illness is fatal and is associated with infected cattle, severe restrictions have been placed on the importation of cattle, sheep, and goats; and on products from these animals from countries in which BSE is known to exist. To date, no case of this cattle disease has been detected in the United States, but it has been identified in England, France, Ireland, Italy, and Canada.

In the United States, the annual incidence of the classic form of CJD is estimated to be between 0.9 and 31.3 cases per million people. It primarily affects adults over the age of 50; men and women are affected equally. The peak age for onset is between the ages of 55 and 74. The disease occurs worldwide, but clusters occur in several areas, more often in England, Chile, and Italy.

## PATHOPHYSIOL(

Creutzfeldt-Jakob dise
the gray matter of the
volving the formation
produces severe deme
and characteristic chan
of brain tissue, the bra
tion of astrocytes (indi

The disease, which
agnosis, has characteri
is characterized by m
reflex, sleep disturbar
experiences rapid dete
age function. Tremors
Babinski reflex are oft
dementia in almost all
comatose and exhibit (

### COLLABOR/

The disease is diagno
tion, specific EEG cha
diagnosis of CJD can
tion. It is often diffi
Alzheimer's disease, e

There is no specifi
progression of CJD. (
disease's manifestation

### NURSING C

The nurse may ident
Jakob disease when cc

Many etiologic agents
system disorders. Au
mental toxins such as
cies can affect the peri

### THE CLIENT V

**Myasthenia gravis** is
acterized by fatigue an
Clients experience per
mild forms of the diso
to a few muscle group
become generalized
weakened.

### Manifestations of Myasthenia Gravis

**OCULAR AND FACIAL**

- Ptosis
- Diplopia
- Facial weakness
- Dysphagia
- Dysarthria
- Complications: difficulty closing eyes, aspiration, impaired communication and nutrition

**MUSCULOSKELETAL**

- Weakness and fatigue
- Decreased function of hands, arms, legs, and neck muscles
- Complications: inability to perform ADLs and self-care activities, complications related to immobility, myasthenic and cholinergic crises

**RESPIRATORY**

- Weakening of intercostal muscles
- Decrease in diaphragm movement
- Breathlessness and dyspnea
- Poor gas exchange
- Complications: decreasing ability to walk, eat, and perform other ADLs, pneumonia

**NUTRITIONAL**

- Inability to chew and swallow
- Decreasing ability to move tongue
- Impairment of fine motor movements: inability to feed self
- Complications: weight loss, dehydration, malnutrition, aspiration

impaired speech, and anxiety. **Cholinergic crisis** is the result of overdosage with anticholinesterase (cholinergic) medications used to treat myasthenia gravis. Gastrointestinal symptoms, severe muscle weakness, vertigo, and respiratory distress are signs of cholinergic crisis. Both types of crises are emergency, life-threatening situations; clients frequently require ventilatory assistance. Differentiation is based on the client's response to edrophonium chloride (Tensilon). In myasthenic crisis the test is positive, and in cholinergic crisis the test is negative (see the discussions following).

### COLLABORATIVE CARE

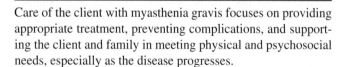

Care of the client with myasthenia gravis focuses on providing appropriate treatment, preventing complications, and supporting the client and family in meeting physical and psychosocial needs, especially as the disease progresses.

### Diagnostic Tests

Diagnostic tests are conducted following a thorough history and physical examination, with special attention to the facial, oculomotor, laryngeal, and respiratory muscles. Diagnostic tests include the following:

- *Tensilon test:* The client is injected with edrophonium chloride (Tensilon), a short-acting anticholinesterase. Clients

with myasthenia gravis show a significant improvement in muscle strength that lasts approximately 5 minutes. This test is also used to differentiate myasthenic crisis (caused by insufficient medication, so the client shows improvement with the drug) from cholinergic crisis (caused by overmedication, so the client does not show improvement).

- *EMG studies* demonstrate a reduced amplitude of the action potential in response to electrical stimulation when myasthenia gravis is present.
- *Antiacetylcholine receptor antibody serum levels* are increased in about 80% of clients with myasthenia gravis; this test is also useful in follow-up of effectiveness of therapy.
- *CT scan* of the chest may demonstrate abnormalities in the thymus.
- *Single-fiber electromyography* detects delayed or failed neuromuscular transmission in muscle fibers supplied by a single nerve fiber.
- *Repetitive 2- or 3-Hz stimulation* of motor nerves helps indicate a disturbance of neuromuscular transmission.
- *Serum assay* of circulating acetylcholine receptor antibodies, if increased, is diagnostic of myasthenia gravis with a sensitivity of 80% to 90% (Tierney et al., 2001).

### Medications

The primary group of medications used to treat myasthenia gravis is the anticholinesterases. These drugs act at the neuromuscular junction and allow acetylcholine to concentrate at the receptor sites, thus promoting muscle contraction. Pyridostigmine (Mestinon) is the most commonly used acetylcholinesterase inhibitor for myasthenia gravis. The client's decrease in symptoms guides dosage.

Immunosuppression with glucocorticoids, typically prednisone, is another pharmacologic therapy aimed at improving muscle strength. Clients must be aware of the need to stay on the drug at the prescribed dose to determine the least amount required for efficacy. If clients do not respond to prednisone alone, it may be combined with other immunosuppressive agents, such as cyclosporine or azathioprine (Imuran). Medications used to treat myasthenia gravis are discussed in the box on page 1433.

### Surgery

Approximately 75% of clients with myasthenia gravis have dysplasia of the thymus gland. Therefore, thymectomy is often recommended for clients younger than 60. The two surgical approaches used are the transcervical approach, which is considered less invasive, and the transternal approach. The latter approach allows a more extensive removal of the gland; however, it also poses more potential complications because it involves splitting the sternum.

Preoperatively, clients may be tapered from steroid therapy. Usually, pyridostigmine is administered to prevent muscular manifestations during the perioperative period. Postoperative nursing care focuses on preventing complications and controlling pain. Nursing implications for the client undergoing thymectomy are presented on page 1433. Remission is obtained in about 40% of clients but may take several years to achieve. Refer to Chapter 36 ⟳ for care of the client having

# Medication Administration

## The Client with Myasthenia Gravis

### ANTICHOLINESTERASES/CHOLINESTERASE INHIBITORS

> Neostigmine (Prostigmin)
> Ambenonium (Mytelase Caplets)
> Pyridostigmine (Mestinon, Regonol)
> For diagnosis: edrophonium chloride (Tensilon)

Cholinesterase inhibitors are used in myasthenia gravis to enhance the effects of acetylcholine at the remaining skeletal muscle receptors. Cholinesterase inhibitors do not cure or change the underlying pathophysiologic processes, but they can provide effective, lifelong improvement of symptoms. Because the cholinesterase inhibitors are nonselective, the neuromuscular, muscarinic, and ganglionic junctions are each affected.

Adjusting the dose to obtain maximum benefit with minimal side effects is a major consideration when administering cholinesterase inhibitors. Initially, small doses are given followed by incremental increases until optimal muscle strength is obtained. The dose may need to be adjusted when activities result in symptoms of undermedication, such as increased ptosis. Severe undermedication results in myasthenic crisis. Although a sustained release form of pyridostigmine is available for bedtime use, it should not be used during the day because of its inconsistent absorption.

When the client takes an overdose of anticholinesterase inhibitors, a cholinergic crisis occurs. Clients and family members must be taught the symptoms and actions to take in each crisis. The oral dose of neostigmine is approximately 30 times greater than parenteral doses.

Cholinesterase inhibitors should not be administered to clients experiencing obstruction of the intestinal or urinary tract. Caution is advised when administering these drugs to clients with asthma, hyperthyroidism, bradycardia, or peptic ulcer disease. Cholinesterase inhibitors can cross the placenta; reproductive counseling is indicated.

### Nursing Responsibilities

- Obtain a baseline assessment of muscle strength and abilities, concentrating on swallowing and ptosis.
- Administer the medication parenterally if the client has dysphagia.
- Check the dose of the medication carefully when changing from oral to parenteral routes.
- Evaluate the effectiveness of the medication and document the response, for example, time when fatigue occurs in relation to activities.
- Promptly recognize and respond to manifestations of excessive stimulation of muscarinic receptors: excess salivation, urinary urgency, bradycardia, gastrointestinal hypermotility, diaphoresis. Atropine can be administered to combat these manifestations. Respiratory depression and failure can occur and require mechanical ventilation.
- Have a muscarinic antagonist (e.g., physostigmine) readily available to treat poisoning.

### Client and Family Teaching

- Balancing symptom control with dosage is crucial; record time of dose and response in a journal. Note the time of day when fatigued and any adverse effects, such as excess salivation, sweating, slow heartbeat, and diarrhea.
- Take the medication about 30 minutes prior to meals to enhance swallowing and chewing.
- Report manifestations of myasthenic crisis immediately: severe muscle weakness, fast heartbeat, restlessness, difficulty breathing, increasing difficulty swallowing or speaking.
- Report slow heartbeat, increased salivation or sweating, and/or decreased blood pressure immediately:
- Review possible causes of myasthenic crisis: physical or emotional stress, infection, or reduction in the medication dosage.
- Wear or carry MedicAlert identification.

# NURSING CARE OF THE CLIENT HAVING A THYMECTOMY

## PREOPERATIVE CARE

- Reinforce the physician's explanation of the procedure, and prepare the client for chest tubes and tracheostomy. *Realistic preparation of what to expect postoperatively encourages compliance and allays anxiety.*
- Anticipate the need for alternative communication. *The client may have a tracheostomy; preoperative planning facilitates communication after surgery.*
- Allow sufficient time for questions. *Thymectomy is a major surgery requiring either a thoracotomy and sternal split or transcervical approach. The client is usually anxious, and adequate time must be allocated to preoperative instruction.*

## POSTOPERATIVE CARE

- Provide meticulous pulmonary hygiene: turning, deep breathing, and coughing at least every 2 hours; use an incentive spirometer. *Regardless of surgical approach, measures are aimed at preventing pulmonary complications of atelectasis and pneumonia.*
- Clients with a thoracotomy and sternal split procedure will require care of the anterior chest tube. Observe for complications; such as pneumothorax. *Air may enter the thoracic cavity—be alert for sudden chest pain and dyspnea, decreased breath sounds, and early signs of shock, such as restlessness.*
- Manage pain with scheduled analgesic therapy. *Maintaining a therapeutic blood level of analgesic provides better pain control than waiting until the client requests medication, as on a prn basis.*

a thoracotomy and chest tubes. A tracheostomy may be required when the diaphragm or intercostal muscles are involved.

## Plasmapheresis

Plasma exchange in myasthenia gravis may be used in conjunction with other therapies; for example, it may be performed prior to surgical intervention. The goal of therapy is to remove the antiacetylcholine receptor antibodies, thus improving severe muscle weakness, fatigue, and other symptoms. The procedure is frequently performed when respiratory muscle involvement is evident. See Figure 43–7 ■ and the box below for nursing care.

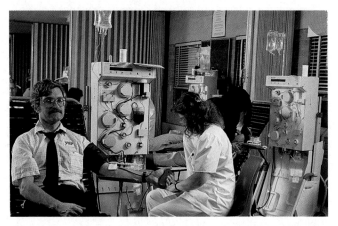

**Figure 43–7 ■** Plasmapheresis is a procedure used to separate the blood's cellular components from plasma. About 50 mL per minute is withdrawn to the centrifuge in the plasmapheresis machine. The plasma is replaced with donor plasma or colloids and returned to the client.

*Courtesy of Baxter Healthcare Corporation.*

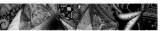

### BOX 43–5 ■ Client and Family Teaching: Myasthenia Gravis

- Schedule periods of rest and avoid stress; conserve energy when possible.
- Avoid cigarette smoke, alcohol, and beverages with quinine (e.g., tonic water).
- Take medications as prescribed. If manifestations change, consult the physician; the dose may need to be adjusted.
- Avoid extremes of temperature; an environment that is too hot or too cold may cause an exacerbation of myasthenia gravis.
- Avoid people with upper respiratory infections; infections can result in an exacerbation and extreme weakness.

## NURSING CARE

Because avoiding fatigue is a major part of teaching, it is important to incorporate interventions to enhance rest and conserve energy (see Box 43–5). Suggest sitting while preparing meals and while performing hygiene and grooming, for example. Anticipating problems, such as impaired communication, and developing alternative solutions can be helpful in promoting independence.

### Nursing Diagnoses and Interventions

Nursing care of clients with myasthenia gravis focuses not only on present problems but also on anticipated needs. Preventing myasthenic and cholinergic crises and providing psychologic support to clients and families are two important aspects of care. Individualized care depends on the specific therapy insti-

## NURSING CARE OF THE CLIENT TREATED WITH PLASMAPHERESIS

### PREPROCEDURE CARE

- Teach about the procedure and what to expect, including what the machine looks like, the need for arterial and venous insertion sites, and the length of time of the procedure (2 to 5 hours). *Giving information, answering questions, and addressing concerns decreases anxiety.*
- Check with physician about holding medications until after the procedure. *Medications may be removed from the body as an incidental part of the plasmapheresis process.*
- Assess vital signs and weight. *Baseline parameters are necessary to evaluate for fluid imbalances and response to therapy.*
- Assess CBC, platelet count, and clotting studies. *Clients undergoing plasmapheresis are at high risk for anemia and coagulation problems secondary to hemolysis of cells.*
- Check blood type and crossmatch for replacement blood products. *Hypersensitivity reactions can occur, and close monitoring is important.*

### CARE DURING THE PROCEDURE AND POSTPROCEDURE

- Observe for dizziness or hypotension. *Hypovolemia is a complication of plasma exchange, especially during the procedure when up to 15% of the client's blood volume is in the cell separator.*
- Apply pressure dressing to access site(s). *Direct pressure helps decrease or prevent bleeding.*
- Monitor for infection and bruises at the intravenous port site. *The site of vascular access is at risk for complications and must be routinely and carefully assessed for signs of infection and for bleeding or hematoma formation.*
- Monitor electrolytes and signs of electrolyte loss. Report imbalances, and replace electrolytes as ordered. Observe for circumoral tingling, Chvostek's and Trousseau's signs if calcium levels are low, and cardiac dysrhythmias and leg cramps if potassium levels are low. *Hypocalcemia and hypokalemia may occur. Hypocalcemia occurs because the anticoagulant citrate dextrose binds with calcium.*
- Reevaluate preprocedure laboratory data, especially CBC, platelet count, and clotting times. *The cell-separating process can damage cells; anticoagulation is part of the procedure.*

tuted. This section discusses the nursing diagnoses related to ineffective airway clearance and impaired swallowing; other nursing diagnoses that commonly apply, such as that related to fatigue, are addressed in other sections of this chapter.

## Ineffective Airway Clearance

The underlying causes for ineffective airway clearance for the person with myasthenia gravis include poor cough mechanism, decreased rib cage expansion, diminished diaphragm movement, and decreased expiratory effort. The following interventions require particular attention if the client undergoes a thymectomy.

- Assist with turning, deep breathing, and coughing at least every 2 hours. Teach proper coughing techniques; use an incentive spirometer every 2 hours while the client is awake. *Position changes promote lung expansion; coughing helps clear secretions from the tracheobronchial tree.*
- Place in a semi-Fowler's position. *This position expands the lungs and alleviates pressure from the diaphragm, especially important considerations if the client is obese.*
- Maintain hydration status and monitor for dehydration; use a humidifier as needed. If needed, teach family how to perform percussion, postural drainage, and suction. *Interventions to liquefy secretions, such as ensuring a daily fluid intake of up to 2500 mL (perhaps via feeding tube or parenteral route), help the client mobilize and expectorate sputum.*
- Assess lung sounds, the rate and character of respirations, and pulse oximetry readings at least every 4 hours or as indicated by client's condition. *Monitoring for hypoxia and worsening of client's ability to move air alerts the nurse to early signs of arteriovenous shunting.*

## Impaired Swallowing

Clients with myasthenia gravis have weakness of the laryngeal and pharyngeal muscles involved with swallowing. Alterations in swallowing place the client at risk for poor nutrition as well as for possible aspiration. Family members need to be included in teaching, particularly the person who prepares and assists with meals.

- Assess the ability to safely manage various consistencies of foods; consult with a speech pathologist for evaluation. *Dysphagic clients are at risk for aspiration; matching food consistency to the client's ability to swallow enhances safety.*
- Plan meals to promote medication effectiveness. *Pyridostigmine should be given 30 minutes before the meal to provide optimal muscle strength for swallowing and chewing.*
- Have the client eat slowly, using small bites of food. Schedule meals during periods when the client is adequately rested; develop a daily schedule incorporating rest periods. *Fatigue may add to dysphagia, putting the client at greater risk for aspiration.*
- If necessary, give cues while eating, such as: "Chew your food thoroughly; swallow." *Keeping client focused may enhance swallowing.*

- Teach caregivers the Heimlich maneuver and how to suction. *Knowing specific measures to take in case of aspiration decreases both the client's and family's anxiety and promotes confidence in managing potential problems.*

## Home Care

Teaching for the client and family with myasthenia gravis focuses on prevention and recognition of crisis situations, understanding the disorder, and methods for coping with both physical and psychosocial problems. Setting realistic goals with the client and family provides opportunities for self-assessment and promotes active participation in rehabilitation.
Address the following topics.

- The importance of maintaining consistency in medication dosage and management
- Realistic expectations
- Methods to avoid fatigue and undue stress; specific measures for avoiding upper respiratory infections and exposure to extreme heat or cold
- Birth control measures or referral for counseling (Pregnancy can exacerbate symptoms; also, medications used to control myasthenia gravis, such as neostigmine bromide (Prostigmin), cross the placenta.)
- Referral to support groups
- Helpful resources such as the Myasthenia Foundation

## THE CLIENT WITH GUILLAIN-BARRÉ SYNDROME

**Guillain-Barré syndrome (GBS)** is an acute inflammatory demyelinating disorder of the peripheral nervous system characterized by an acute onset of motor paralysis (usually ascending). The classification of Guillain-Barré subtypes includes acute inflammatory demyelinating polyradiculoneuropathy, acute axonal motor neuropathy, acute motor and sensory axonal neuropathy, and Miller-Fisher syndrome.

Guillain-Barré syndrome is one of the most common peripheral nervous system disorders. The cause is unknown, but precipitating events include a respiratory or gastrointestinal viral or bacterial infection 1 to 3 weeks prior to the onset of manifestations, surgery, viral immunizations, and other viral illnesses. In 60% of cases, *Campylobacter jejuni* is identified as the cause of the preceding infection. Approximately 80% to 90% of clients with GBS have a spontaneous recovery with little or no residual disabilities. However, the disease has a 4% to 6% mortality rate, and up to 10% of cases have permanent disabling weakness, imbalance, and sensory loss (McCance & Huether, 2002).

The disease is characterized by progressive ascending flaccid paralysis of the extremities, accompanied by paresthesias and numbness. About 20% of clients have respiratory involvement to the point that ventilatory assistance is required. GBS is often a medical emergency.

## Nursing Care Plan
## A Client with Myasthenia Gravis

Kirsten Avis, a 44-year-old homemaker and mother of two teenage sons, was diagnosed with myasthenia gravis 2 years ago. She takes an anticholinesterase medication, pyridostigmine (Mestinon), four times a day. Over the past month she has been experimenting with decreasing the dose of her pyridostigmine because she has "felt so good." She was prescribed 60 mg of pyridostigmine three times a day before meals and one-half of a long-acting 180 mg pyridostigmine tablet at night.

Three days ago, she began having chills and fever and her myasthenic symptoms became markedly worse. Mrs. Avis is easily fatigued and has been experiencing increasing weakness, bilateral ptosis, and mild dysphagia in the late afternoon and evenings.

### ASSESSMENT

Lela Silva, RN, is caring for Mrs. Avis. Physical examination of Mrs. Avis reveals severe muscle weakness bilaterally in her hands, arms, and thorax. Her voice is nasal, and she speaks slowly; the longer she speaks, the more difficult it becomes to understand her. She is anxious and dyspneic. Her complaints of weakness, dysphagia, dysarthria, problems with mobility, and ptosis are more pronounced later in the day. Vital signs are as follows: BP 138/88, P 88, R 28, T 102.4°F (39°C).

Some improvement in muscle weakness is noted following a restful night's sleep; however, the respiratory distress is more evident, and Mrs. Avis is increasingly restless. She is moved to the intensive care unit for advanced monitoring and possible ventilatory assistance. The medical diagnosis is myasthenic crisis secondary to pulmonary infection.

### DIAGNOSES

- *Impaired gas exchange* related to ineffective breathing pattern and muscle weakness
- *Risk for aspiration* related to difficulty swallowing
- *Fatigue* related to increased energy needs from muscular involvement

### EXPECTED OUTCOMES

- Pulse oximetry readings will be maintained at 92% or above.
- No aspiration will occur.
- Will verbalize decreasing fatigue when performing ADLs.
- Will state the correct method of medication dosing and demonstrate how she will maintain schedule.

### PLANNING AND IMPLEMENTATION

Mrs. Avis's manifestations improve following administration of edrophonium chloride (Tensilon) to verify myasthenic crisis. She is placed on oxygen by mask and suctioned as needed; equipment for possible intubation and ventilation is made readily available. She is placed in a semi-Fowler's position, and vital signs are assessed every 5 minutes during the acute exacerbation. The nurses in the intensive care unit remain in constant attendance throughout the crisis period and provide explanations to Mrs. Avis in an effort to decrease her stress and to avoid further severity of manifestations.

Three days after the crisis period, Mrs. Avis is moved to a progressive nursing care unit. Nurses follow up on teaching her the manifestations of both myasthenic and cholinergic crises. They discuss the need to wear MedicAlert identification and review medication administration techniques with Mrs. Avis. The nurses emphasize in particular that Mrs. Avis must not split time-released medications.

Within 5 days, Mrs. Avis's condition stabilizes, and her weakness decreases sufficiently to allow discharge home. Although her temperature has returned to normal and her respiratory status has improved, she still has a productive cough. Oral antibiotics are prescribed for 2 weeks, after which she will have a follow-up visit with her primary care provider. She is instructed to seek treatment promptly if respiratory symptoms or temperature indicate recurrence of infection.

### EVALUATION

Mrs. Avis is discharged without developing aspiration pneumonia or any symptoms of aspiration. Her airway was maintained throughout the myasthenic crisis, and her pulse oximetry readings remained above 92% once oxygen therapy was initiated. On discharge, pulse oximetry is above 95% without oxygen therapy. Mrs. Avis states that her fatigue and weakness have significantly improved.

Both Mrs. Avis and her husband are able to explain the difference between myasthenic and cholinergic crises and to identify methods to avoid both problems. Mrs. Avis correctly relates her proper medication regimen and makes an appointment for a follow-up visit with her physician.

### Critical Thinking in the Nursing Process

1. What is the rationale for administering Tensilon to evaluate a myasthenic crisis?
2. Develop a plan to teach Mrs. Avis how to avoid fatigue when preparing and eating meals.
3. Develop a nursing care plan for Mrs. Avis for the nursing diagnosis, *Ineffective role performance.*

See Evaluating Your Response in Appendix C.

| BOX 43–6 | ■ Stages of Guillain-Barré Syndrome |

## I. ACUTE STAGE

■ Characterized by severe and rapid weakness, especially, in the lower extremities; loss of muscle strength progressing to quadriplegia and respiratory failure; decreasing deep-tendon reflexes; decreasing vital capacity; paresthesias, numbness; pain, especially nocturnal; facial muscle involvement (inability to wrinkle forehead or change expressions).

■ Involvement of the autonomic nervous system manifested by bradycardia, sweating, fluctuating blood pressure, notably hypotension, which may last for 2 weeks.

## II. STABILIZING/PLATEAU STAGE

■ Occurs 2 to 3 weeks after initial onset.

■ Marks the end of changes in condition; characterized by a "leveling off" of symptoms.

■ Generally, the labile autonomic functions stabilize.

## III. RECOVERY STAGE

■ May take from several months to 2 years.

■ Marked by improvement in symptoms.

■ Generally, muscle strength and function return in descending order.

## PATHOPHYSIOLOGY AND MANIFESTATIONS

The primary pathophysiologic process in Guillain-Barré syndrome is the destruction of myelin sheaths covering the axons of peripheral nerves. The demyelination is thought to be the result of both a humoral- and cell-mediated immunologic response. The loss of myelin results in poor conduction of nerve impulses, causing sudden muscle weakness and loss of reflex response. Other manifestations occur when nerve conduction to various muscles is interrupted. The stages of Guillain-Barré syndrome and their usual manifestations are presented in Box 43–6.

Muscles, sensory nerves, and cranial nerves are commonly affected in clients with GBS. Most people experience symmetric muscle weakness, initially in the lower extremities. The weakness and sensory loss then ascends to the upper extremities, torso, and cranial nerves. Sensory involvement includes severe pain, paresthesia, and numbness. Cognition and level of consciousness are not affected. Facial nerve involvement results in the inability to change facial expressions and close the eyes. Muscles involved with chewing, swallowing, and speaking may be affected.

Paralysis of intercostal and diaphragmatic muscles may alter respiratory function. These clients require ventilatory assistance and supportive care. Involvement of the autonomic nervous system is characterized by fluctuating blood pressure, cardiac dysrhythmias and tachycardia, paralytic ileus, syndrome of inappropriate antidiuretic hormone (SIADH) secretion and urinary retention.

The weakness usually plateaus or improves by the fourth week. Strength then improves slowly over days or months.

Most affected individuals have full recovery. Women who have had Guillain-Barré syndrome are at increased risk for relapse in the first trimester of pregnancy.

## COLLABORATIVE CARE

Interventions during the acute phase (1 to 3 weeks) focus primarily on ensuring oxygenation via ventilatory assistance and preventing complications from immobility. Rehabilitation time to regain muscle strength and function varies; most people return to full presyndrome muscle function within 6 months to 2 years.

Care of the client with Guillain-Barré syndrome requires a team approach. From the initial acute phase through rehabilitation, many members of the health care team are involved. An accurate and rapid diagnosis is needed to ensure prompt supportive treatment, particularly if there is respiratory involvement combined with widespread paralysis.

### Diagnostic Tests

Diagnosis of Guillain-Barré syndrome is made after a thorough history and clinical examination. It must be differentiated from several disorders, among them influenza, heavy metal poisoning, Lyme disease, and cranial hemorrhage. Diagnosis is made based on manifestations, history of a recent viral infection, elevated CSF protein levels, and EMG studies. Although there is no specific test to diagnose this syndrome, several findings support and confirm the diagnosis.

• *CSF analysis* shows increased protein levels with a normal cell count. This elevation is caused by active demyelination.

• *EMG studies* reflect decreased nerve conduction with fibrillations during the severe stage of the syndrome.

• *Pulmonary function tests* and *ABGs* are performed when respiratory function is compromised. Abnormal results reflect the decreased ventilatory function.

### Medications

There are no medications available for the specific treatment of Guillain-Barré syndrome. Other medications may be prescribed to provide support or prophylaxis, or to combat concurrent problems; for example, antibiotics may be prescribed for urinary tract or respiratory infections. Morphine is commonly administered to control muscle pain. Anticoagulation therapy is usually instituted to prevent thromboembolic complications, such as deep-vein thrombosis and pulmonary embolism, which are associated with prolonged bed rest. If hypotension is a problem, vasopressors are prescribed.

### Treatments

#### Surgery

Tracheostomy is performed if respiratory failure occurs. Clients who need ventilatory support are usually able to be weaned after 2 to 3 weeks, but the time frame varies greatly. When the client's vital capacity reaches 8 to 10 mL/kg, he or she may be weaned from the ventilator (Hickey, 2002). Insertion of a temporary pacemaker may be indicated for bradycardia.

## Plasmapheresis

Plasma exchange has been beneficial, particularly when performed within the first 2 weeks of the syndrome's development. Antibodies are removed, and immunosuppressive agents are administered concurrently. Clients typically have five exchanges during an 8- to 10-day period (see the Nursing Care box on page 1434).

## Dietary Management

Nutritional support for the client who is immobilized for prolonged periods of time is crucial. Maintaining positive nitrogen balance, ensuring sufficient fluid intake and electrolyte balance, and ensuring recommended caloric intake are goals of therapy. When swallowing problems occur, total parenteral nutrition may be indicated if feeding via a nasogastric or gastrostomy tube is ineffective.

## Physical and Occupational Therapy

Long-term physical and occupational therapy is crucial to recovery. Clients with Guillain-Barré syndrome usually require prolonged rehabilitation care, which begins during the acute phase and focuses on preventing complications and limiting the effects of immobility. The severe muscle atrophy and loss of muscle tone require that clients relearn many functions and skills, such as walking. Compromise in respiratory function may delay physical rehabilitation; clients need positive reinforcement when they make even small gains in their progress. Continued attention to pain control is essential because paresthesia and pain can interfere with physical therapy.

## NURSING CARE

Many of the nursing interventions for clients with this syndrome involve assessing neurologic function, preventing problems of immobility, ensuring adequate hydration and nutrition, and promoting respiratory function. Anticipating needs of both the client and family is an important aspect of care. For example, developing an alternative method of communication before it is necessary may decrease anxiety. It is very important that nursing care focus on preventing complications that may be fatal by following a rigorous predetermined schedule for turning and pulmonary toilet, using strict aseptic technique, and providing continuous psychosocial support.

## Nursing Diagnoses and Interventions

Anxiety and powerlessness are major nursing considerations. The client is almost always admitted to the ICU for care, and is mentally alert but suddenly mute, ventilator dependent, and immobile. Refer to previous nursing care sections in this chapter for interventions related to anxiety, imbalanced nutrition, impaired swallowing, impaired verbal communication, and ineffective airway clearance. This section focuses on managing the nursing diagnoses related to pain and risk for impaired skin integrity.

### Acute Pain

Pain experienced with Guillain-Barré syndrome varies. Frequently, there is a "stocking-glove" pattern, with pain in the hands, feet, and legs. Pain and tenderness in muscles can be severe; interventions must be individualized to client needs. The intense pain combined with altered sensations leads to anxiety; nursing interventions can make a difference in breaking the cycle of increasing pain that leads to increased anxiety and in turn causes more pain.

- Listen to the description of pain; determine presence of triggers or a pattern. *Acknowledging the client's perception of pain is a basis for treatment; listening establishes trust.*
- Use a pain scale for determining extent of pain. *Consistent measurement is essential to evaluate degree of pain and effectiveness of intervention.*
- Use complementary therapies to help manage pain:
  - Application of heat/cold
  - Guided imagery
  - Relaxation techniques
  - Massage

  *Presenting options for managing pain gives the client control over the situation and helps reduce anxiety. Noninvasive interventions may augment the therapeutic benefit of medications.*
- Provide analgesics as indicated; administer on a regular schedule rather than waiting until pain becomes severe. *Anticipating and managing pain before it becomes severe decreases anxiety and averts the cycle of increased anxiety leading to increased pain.*
- Monitor for side effects of analgesics, particularly respiratory depression; assess respirations and lung sounds. Perform routine pulmonary hygiene measures and monitor for aspiration. *Clients with Guillain-Barré syndrome have a weakened thoracic musculature; frequent respiratory monitoring is indicated.*

### Risk for Impaired Skin Integrity

During the acute and plateau stages of Guillain-Barré syndrome, clients are at risk for problems related to immobility and malnutrition. Impaired skin integrity is one such problem. Preventing areas of skin breakdown is important. Prophylactic interventions will help ensure that ingested protein and calories are used to maintain ideal body weight and other body functions rather than to heal an avoidable problem. Implicit in the following interventions is maintenance of adequate nutrition.

- Inspect bony prominences and provide skin care at least every 2 hours. Reposition the client and clean, dry, and lubricate the skin as needed. *These activities stimulate circulation and ensure even distribution of body weight; baseline observations allow discovery of early signs of altered integrity.*
- Pad bony prominences, such as sacral area, heels, and elbows. *This decreases shearing tears on these pressure points.*
- Use an alternating-pressure mattress or water bed. *Relieving pressure stimulates circulation and promotes oxygenation of tissues.*
- Monitor for incontinence and provide thorough skin care following each episode of incontinence. *Urine is caustic to the skin, and the moisture promotes skin breakdown.*

## Home Care

Clients and family members are frequently stunned by the rapid deterioration of function and fear that the paralysis will be permanent. Regularly reinforce teaching because the client's high anxiety level may interfere with listening and understanding. When possible, include the client and family in decision making; for example, seek their input when planning a daily schedule of care that incorporates various therapies.

Referrals to appropriate therapists are a component of anticipating needs; speech, nutritional, occupational, and physical therapists are an integral part of rehabilitation. Another focus of care is teaching both the client and family; incorporate explanations for interventions aimed at promoting self-care. For further information, refer the client and family to the Guillain-Barré Syndrome Foundation, International.

Teaching the rationales for preventive measures reinforces the client's and family's understanding and may promote compliance during the lengthy rehabilitation. For example, because of autonomic nerve involvement, clients need to be monitored for cardiac dysrhythmias and taught to avoid changing position suddenly to prevent orthostatic hypotension.

# CRANIAL NERVE DISORDERS

Disorders of the cranial nerves may be caused by intracranial trauma or by pathologic processes. The pairs of cranial nerves, described in Chapter 40, are numbered in the order in which they arise in the brain and are named according to their anatomic characteristic or primary function. The most common cranial nerve disorders are those affecting the trigeminal (cranial nerve V) and the facial (cranial nerve VII) nerves. These disorders, discussed in the following sections, result primarily in pain or loss of sensory or motor function.

## THE CLIENT WITH TRIGEMINAL NEURALGIA

**Trigeminal neuralgia,** also called **tic douloureux,** is a chronic disease of the trigeminal cranial nerve (V) that causes severe facial pain. The trigeminal nerve has three divisions: the ophthalmic, the maxillary, and mandibular (Figure 43–8 ■). The ophthalmic division supplies the forehead, eyes, nose, temples, meninges, paranasal sinus, and part of the nasal mucosa. The maxillary division supplies the upper jaw, teeth, lip, cheeks, hard palate, maxillary sinus, and part of the nasal mucosa. The mandibular division supplies the lower jaw, teeth, lip, buccal mucosa, tongue, part of the external ear, and the meninges. Sensory fibers of the nerve conduct impulses for touch, pain, and temperature; motor fibers innervate the temporal and masseter muscles used for chewing and lateral movement of the jaw. The maxillary and mandibular divisions are the divisions of the trigeminal nerve affected in almost all cases of this disorder.

Trigeminal neuralgia occurs more commonly in middle and older adults and affects women more often than men. The actual cause is unknown; however, contributing factors include irritation from flulike illnesses, trauma or infection of the teeth or jaw, and pressure on the nerve by an aneurysm, a tumor, or arteriosclerotic changes of an artery close to the nerve (Hickey, 2002).

## PATHOPHYSIOLOGY AND MANIFESTATIONS

Trigeminal neuralgia is characterized by brief (lasting a few seconds to a few minutes), repetitive episodes of sudden severe facial pain. The pain may occur as often as hundreds of times a day to as infrequently as a few times a year. The unilateral pain is experienced over the surface of the skin. It most often begins near one side of the mouth and rises toward the ear, eye, or nostril on the same side of the face. Clients describe the pain as stabbing or lightning-like and often respond to the pain by wincing or grimacing.

Stimulating specific areas of the face, called *trigger zones,* may initiate the onset of pain. These trigger zones usually parallel the distribution of the nerve and typically follow a track leading from just over the eyebrow to the ridge of the cheekbone, along the nasolabial fold, around the corner of the mouth, and down the side of the chin. The episodes of pain are initiated by many factors, including light touch, eating, swallowing, talking, sneezing, shaving, chewing gum, brushing the teeth, or washing the face. Other factors that may trigger a pain episode include changes in temperature and exposure to wind. In an attempt to control the pain, clients may refuse to wash, shave, eat, or talk.

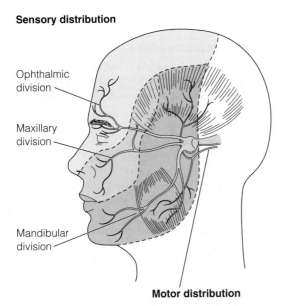

**Sensory distribution**

Ophthalmic division

Maxillary division

Mandibular division

**Motor distribution**

**Figure 43–8 ■** Sensory and motor distribution of the trigeminal nerve. The three sensory divisions are ophthalmic, maxillary, and mandibular.

The episodes of pain may recur for several weeks or months. The disease then spontaneously goes into remission, and the client is free of pain for periods lasting from days to years. As the client grows older, the remissions tend to become shorter, and a dull ache may be present between episodes of acute pain.

## COLLABORATIVE CARE

There are no specific diagnostic tests for trigeminal neuralgia. The disorder is diagnosed by the characteristic location and type of pain. The disorder is treated by pharmacologic or surgical interventions.

### Medications

The drug most useful in controlling the pain is the tricyclic anticonvulsant carbamazepine (Tegretol). If carbamazepine is ineffective, other medications such as the anticonvulsants phenytoin (Dilantin) or gabapentin (Neurontin), or the skeletal muscle relaxant baclofen (Lioresal) may be used. These drugs are administered to decrease paroxysmal afferent impulses and stop the pain. Drugs in this category may cause side effects of dizziness, nausea, and drowsiness. In addition, liver function, bone marrow function, and blood levels of the medications should be monitored on a regular basis.

### Surgery

If medications do not control the pain, surgical procedures may be performed, including various types of **rhizotomy**, the surgical severing of a nerve root. Closed surgical interventions by percutaneous rhizotomy involve inserting a needle through the cheek into the foramen ovale at the base of the brain and partially destroying the trigeminal nerve with glycerol (an alcohol), by radiofrequency-induced heat, or by balloon compression of the trigeminal ganglion. These procedures carry less risk and result in shorter hospital stays than do open procedures, but there is a possibility of recurrence of pain. Following surgery, the client may have some facial numbness, but there usually is no residual paralysis. The involved side of the face is insensitive to pain. The client will have some loss of facial sensation (e.g., to temperature and/or touch) and is at risk for loss of the corneal reflex. Closed procedures provide long-term pain relief and are well tolerated by the older adult. Nursing care of the client undergoing a percutaneous rhizotomy is presented in the box below.

It has been found that some structural abnormalities (such as an artery or vein compressing the nerve) may cause the neuralgia, and if so, decompression and separation of the blood vessel from the nerve root produces lasting relief of the pain (Tierney et al., 2001). The Jannetta procedure involves locating and lifting the involved vessel and placing a small piece of silicone sponge between the vessel and the nerve. Possible complications of the procedure include headache and facial pain.

## NURSING CARE

Nursing care for the client with trigeminal neuralgia involves teaching self-management at home after medical or surgical intervention. Primary client concerns are managing pain, maintaining nutrition, and preventing injury.

### Nursing Diagnoses and Interventions

Interventions for managing pain and improving nutritional intake are addressed here; teaching to prevent injury following surgery is discussed under client and family teaching.

#### Acute Pain

The client with trigeminal neuralgia has excruciating pain and often avoids ADLs and socializing with others in an attempt to prevent the onset of pain. Pain management is fully discussed in Chapter 4. ⬥⬥ Nursing interventions for pain in clients with this disorder focus on strategies for self-management.

## NURSING CARE OF THE CLIENT HAVING PERCUTANEOUS RHIZOTOMY

### POSTOPERATIVE CARE

- Follow routine postoperative interventions for clients having surgery (see Chapter 7). ⬥⬥
- Monitor cranial nerve function every 2 to 4 hours:
  a. Assess the corneal reflex by lightly touching the cornea with a wisp of cotton. If the reflex is intact, the client will blink. *Severing the ophthalmic division of the trigeminal nerve destroys the corneal reflex and leaves the cornea at risk for dryness and injury.*
  b. Assess the facial nerve by asking the client to blow out the cheeks, wrinkle the forehead, frown, wink, and close both eyes tightly. Test taste by placing bitter, salty, and sweet substances on the anterior portion of the tongue. *Facial weakness is evidenced by changes in movement in the involved side of the face. The facial nerve also innervates the anterior two-thirds of the tongue.*
  c. Assess the function of the oculomotor muscles by asking the client to follow your finger through the cardinal positions of vision (see Chapter 40). *The eyes should move together; alterations in movement indicate an abnormal response.*
  d. Assess the motor portion of the trigeminal nerve by asking the client to clench the teeth while you palpate the tightness of the contracted masseter and temporal muscles: *Loss of motor function is indicated by loss of bulk and tightness of these muscles.*
  e. Apply, as prescribed; an ice pack to the jaw on the operative site. *Cold decreases bleeding and swelling.*
  f. Teach the client to avoid rubbing the eye on the involved side. *Loss of the corneal reflex removes protection because the client no longer has the sensation of pain in the involved eye. Rubbing the eye could cause corneal abrasions.*

- Identify factors that trigger an attack, and discuss strategies to avoid these precipitating factors. *Most clients can clearly identify trigger zones and triggering factors. Identification is the first step in pain control.*
- Determine usual response to pain. *Sensitivity and reaction to pain are influenced by previous experiences with pain, age, gender, emotional factors, and cultural background.*
- Assess factors that affect the ability to influence pain tolerance, including the knowledge and cause of the pain, the meaning of the pain, the ability to control the pain, cultural background, and support systems. *Pain tolerance, which is the duration and intensity of pain a person is willing to endure, differs greatly among individuals and may also vary within particular clients in different situations.*
- Monitor the effects of the medication prescribed for the neuralgia. *If the prescribed medication does not provide relief, other medications or methods of treatment may be used to control the pain.*

### Risk for Altered Nutrition: Less Than Body Requirements

Clients often refuse to eat during periods of pain attacks, fearing that the movements of chewing may precipitate the pain. In addition, the chronic nature of the illness often causes depression, which may depress the appetite.

- Monitor dietary intake and weight at each visit, and ask the client to keep a weekly weight record. *Ongoing assessments are necessary for early detection of nutritional deficiencies.*
- Discuss the temperature and consistency of foods eaten, and suggest referral to a dietitian if necessary. *Hot or cold foods may trigger an attack; soft, warm, or cool foods are less likely to act as triggers.*
- Suggest chewing on the unaffected side of the mouth. *Chewing on the unaffected side is less likely to trigger an attack of pain and so facilitate food intake.*
- If unable to tolerate oral food, tube feedings may be necessary. *Adequate kcal and nutrients for metabolic processes are essential.*

### Home Care

The client with trigeminal neuralgia who is receiving medical treatment and providing self-care at home requires teaching about the disease process, the medication(s) being taken, and ways to reduce the incidence of attacks or pain. Diet teaching and assistance with self-management of pain are also important. For example, if the home setting is drafty and attacks of pain are triggered by wind blowing across the face, it may be necessary to encourage the client to put weather stripping around windows and doors. Family members are also included in teaching. To prevent injury to affected areas, the following topics should be addressed.

### Eye Care

- Do not rub the eyes; use artificial tears four times a day if the eyes are dry or irritated.
- Wear an eyepatch at night.
- Wear protective sunglasses or goggles when outside, when working in dusty areas, when mowing the lawn, and when using any type of spray material (e.g., hair spray, cleaning materials, paint, insecticides).
- Remember to blink frequently.
- Check your eyes for redness or swelling each day.
- Schedule regular eye examinations.

### Face and Mouth Care

- Chew on the unaffected side of the mouth.
- Avoid eating hot foods or drinking hot liquids.
- After every meal, brush your teeth and inspect the inside of your mouth for food that may collect between the gums and cheek.
- Have regular dental examinations; you will not be able to feel pain associated with gum infection or tooth decay.
- Use an electric razor to shave the face.
- Protect your face from very cold or windy conditions.

## THE CLIENT WITH BELL'S PALSY

**Bell's palsy,** also called *facial paralysis,* is a disorder of the seventh cranial (facial) nerve, characterized by unilateral paralysis of the facial muscles. The facial nerve is primarily a motor nerve that supplies all the muscles associated with expression on one side of the face. The sensory component innervates the anterior two-thirds of one side of the tongue.

This disorder can occur at any age but is seen most often in adults between 20 and 60. The incidence is equal in men and women. The exact cause of the disorder is unknown, although inflammation of the nerve and a relationship to the herpes simplex virus have been suggested (Tierney et al., 2001).

### PATHOPHYSIOLOGY AND MANIFESTATIONS

The onset of Bell's palsy is usually sudden and almost always involves one side of the face. Pain behind the ear or along the jaw may precede the paralysis. Manifestations of Bell's palsy are listed in the box below.

The client initially notices numbness or stiffness of one side of the face that distorts the appearance. As the disease progresses, the distortion becomes more obvious, and the face appears asymmetric. The facial paralysis causes the entire side of the face to droop, and the client cannot wrinkle the forehead, close the eye, or pucker the lips on the affected side. When the client attempts to smile, the lower facial muscles

### Manifestations of Bell's Palsy

- Paralysis of the facial muscles on one side of the face
- Paralysis of the upper eyelid with loss of the corneal reflex on the affected side
- Loss or impairment of taste over the anterior portion of the tongue on the affected side
- Increased tearing from the lacrimal gland on the affected side

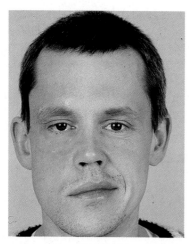

**Figure 43–9** ■ The client with Bell's palsy shows the typical drooping of one side of the face.

*Source: NIH/Phototake NYC.*

are pulled to the opposite side of the face. Some clients have only mild manifestations, whereas others have complete facial paralysis (Figure 43–9 ■). Clients often believe they have had a stroke.

Eighty percent of clients recover completely within a few weeks to a few months (and three-fourths recover without any treatment). Of those remaining, 15% recover some function but have some permanent facial paralysis; these clients are usually older, have diabetes mellitus, or have more severe manifestations, such as vertigo, a sensitivity to noise, and deep head pain.

## COLLABORATIVE CARE

There are no definitive laboratory or diagnostic tests for Bell's palsy, nor are there any specific treatments. The only medical treatment that influences outcome is the use of corticosteroids, but their use has also been questioned (Tierney et al., 2001). Care of the client with Bell's palsy is supportive, as described below.

## NURSING CARE

Although clients provide self-care at home, the nurse plays a key role in teaching the client and family about the disease and how to prevent injury and maintain nutrition. The client is often anxious about his or her appearance and may require counseling if any deficits in facial expression become permanent. The following topics should be addressed.

- Use artificial tears four times a day to lubricate the eye; wear an eye patch or tape the eye shut at night. Wear sunglasses or goggles when outside, when working in dusty conditions, and when using any type of spray.
- Massage combined with warm, moist heat often is effective in relieving the pain.
- A soft diet that does not require chewing and six small meals a day are helpful. Chew slowly on the unaffected side and avoid hot foods. Clean the mouth and carefully inspect the area between the gums and cheek for food after each meal.
- As function returns, practice wrinkling the forehead, closing the eyes, blowing air out of the puckered mouth, and whistling for 5 minutes three or four times a day.

# NEUROLOGIC DISORDERS RESULTING FROM VIRAL INFECTIONS AND NEUROTOXINS

A variety of disorders of the nervous system may have toxic or infectious causes. Although these disorders are not common, those included here require significant nursing care when they do occur.

## THE CLIENT WITH POSTPOLIOMYELITIS SYNDROME

**Postpoliomyelitis syndrome** is a complication of a previous infection by the poliomyelitis virus. This disease was epidemic in the 1940s and 1950s, but has largely been eradicated through immunization with oral live trivalent virus vaccine. However, it is thought that nearly 50% of the estimated 1.63 million people in the United States who had the disease are reexperiencing manifestations of the acute illness. These people have struggled for years to rehabilitate themselves and lead productive lives. Now, as they reach retirement age, they again experience symptoms which may be physically and psychologically incapacitating.

The poliomyelitis virus destroys some of the motor cells of the anterior horn cells of the spinal cord, causing neuromuscu-

lar effects that range from mild to severe flaccid paralysis and atrophy. The primary cause of death is respiratory arrest (Tierney et al., 2001).

Manifestations of motor neuron degeneration and weakness may emerge years after the initial infection. Most clients with postpoliomyelitis syndrome initially had a more severe case of polio and required hospitalization, contracted the disease after the age of 10, required ventilator assistance for respiration, and had paralysis in all four extremities. The incidence is slightly higher in women. As the population ages, it is projected that the number of older adults with postpoliomyelitis syndrome will increase.

## PATHOPHYSIOLOGY AND MANIFESTATIONS

The pathophysiologic process in postpoliomyelitis syndrome is not known. The manifestations include fatigue, muscle and joint weakness, loss of muscle mass, respiratory difficulties, and pain. These manifestations typically begin 25 to 35 years after the initial illness. The manifestations are most often seen in muscles affected by the initial infection, but new muscle groups may also be affected. In addition to neuromuscular manifestations, the client may experience cold intolerance, dizziness, headaches, urinary incontinence, and sleep disorders.

## COLLABORATIVE CARE

Postpoliomyelitis syndrome is diagnosed by a previous history of polio and the current manifestations. Diagnostic studies of nerve conduction, muscle strength, and pulmonary function determine current physical status. Treatment addresses the manifestations, and often involves physical therapy and pulmonary rehabilitation programs.

## NURSING CARE

The client with postpoliomyelitis syndrome faces the challenge of unexpected physical changes. Clients are often anxious about how others will react or what the future holds. Respiratory dysfunction may result in the need for oxygen. Muscular weakness and decreased pulmonary function may make walking difficult, if not impossible. Activities of daily living, independent self-care, and careers are threatened.

Many clients have not fully recovered psychologically from having polio and may respond to a recurrence of symptoms with denial and disbelief. Older clients may not know they had polio as children. Nurses are responsible for assessing and identifying the manifestations of postpoliomyelitis syndrome. It is essential to question middle to older adults about a past history of polio when conducting the health history and to ask specific questions about manifestations that the client may be experiencing.

### Home Care

The nurse individualizes teaching to meet the physical and psychosocial needs of the client and family. Provide candid explanations, and teach the client how to prevent fatigue, promote optimal respiratory function, meet self-care needs, modify ADLs, and maintain safety. Follow-up care with nurses, physicians, physical therapists, respiratory therapists, and counselors is indicated. Referral to a support group can make a positive difference in the client's and family's ability to cope with the disorder.

## THE CLIENT WITH RABIES

**Rabies** is a rhabdovirus infection of the central nervous system transmitted by infected saliva that enters the human body through a bite or an open wound. This is a critical illness that almost always causes death if untreated. The rabies virus is carried by both wild and domestic animals, including bats, skunks, foxes, raccoons, cats, and dogs. After an incubation period that may last from 10 days to many years (norm is 3 to 7 weeks), the virus travels to the brain of the infected animal via the nerves. It multiplies and migrates to the salivary glands.

## PATHOPHYSIOLOGY

The client with rabies usually has a history of an animal bite but may also become infected through an abrasion or open wound that is exposed to the infected saliva. The virus spreads from the wound to local muscle cells and then invades the peripheral nerves. It eventually travels to the central nervous system. The incubation period in humans varies according to the severity and location of the bite. For example, bites on the face may result in manifestations in 10 days to a few weeks, whereas bites on the lower extremities may incubate for as long as 1 year.

## MANIFESTATIONS

The manifestations occur in stages. During the initial, or prodromal, stage, the site of the wound is painful and then exhibits various paresthesias. The infected person is anxious, irritable, and depressed. General manifestations of infection (such as headache, loss of appetite, and sore throat) may appear. The person may also have increased sensitivity to light and sounds, and the skin is especially sensitive to changes in temperature.

The prodromal stage is followed by an excitement stage. The infected person has periods of excitement that alternate with periods of quiet. Attempts to drink cause such painful larynogospasms that the person refuses to drink (a phenomenon called hydrophobia). Large amounts of thick, tenacious mucus are present. The client experiences convulsions, muscle spasms, and periods of apnea. Death occurs approximately 7 days from the onset of manifestations and is usually due to respiratory failure.

## COLLABORATIVE CARE

Animals that bite are kept under observation, if possible, for 7 to 10 days to detect rabies manifestations. Sick animals should be euthanized and their brains examined for presence of the rabies virus, which is detected by fluorescent antibody testing. The blood of an infected person can also be tested with the same diagnostic study to demonstrate the presence of rabies antibodies.

## NURSING CARE

Nursing care for clients with rabies is provided in an intensive care unit, with the client in a quiet, darkened room to decrease stimulation as much as possible. The client requires interventions to maintain the airway, maintain oxygenation, and control seizures. Standard precautions are essential, because the rabies virus is present in the saliva of the client. If an open wound of a health care provider is contaminated with infected saliva, the provider must receive postexposure immunizations.

### Health Promotion

Client and family teaching focuses on the importance of immunizing pets, providing proper care of wounds, seeking immediate medical attention for animal bites, and obtaining treatment after any suspicious bite.

Because the untreated disease is almost always fatal, the best intervention is prevention. Preventive activities follow:

- Immunize household dogs and cats; immunize people who are exposed to animals.
- Local treatment of animal bites and scratches:
  - Carefully and thoroughly clean and flush wounds with soap and water to remove the saliva and dilute the viral exposure.
  - Immediately take the person with the bite for emergency treatment.
- Postexposure care:
  - Rabies immune globulin (RIG) is administered for passive immunization. Up to 50% of the globulin is infiltrated around the wound, and the rest is administered intramuscularly. At the same time, an inactivated human diploid cell vaccine (HDCV) is administered intramuscularly, with 1 mL given on the day of exposure and on days 3, 7, 14, and 28 after exposure (Tierney et al., 2001). Rabies immune globulin and rabies vaccine (HDCV) should never be given in the same syringe or at the same site. Local and mild systemic reactions include itching, tenderness, headaches, muscle aches, and nausea.
  - If RIG is not available, equine rabies antiserum may be administered after testing the client for horse serum sensitivity.

## THE CLIENT WITH TETANUS

**Tetanus,** more commonly called **lockjaw,** is a disorder of the nervous system caused by a neurotoxin elaborated by *Clostridium tetani.* This anaerobic bacillus lives in the soil. Spores of the bacillus enter the body through open wounds contaminated with dirt, street dust, or feces (animal or human). The wounds may result from scratches or abrasions, bee stings, abortions, surgery, trauma, burns, or intravenous drug use. Incidence is highest among people who have never been immunized, older adults whose immunity has been lost, and women. The majority of cases occur in people over age 50. Tetanus has a high mortality rate, with death occurring in over 40% of all cases. Contaminated lesions of the head and face are more dangerous than those in other parts of the body.

## PATHOPHYSIOLOGY

When the spores of *Clostridium tetani* enter the open wound, they germinate and produce a toxin called tetanospasmin. The incubation period averages 8 to 12 days but can range from 5 days to 15 weeks (Tierney et al., 2001). The toxins are absorbed by the peripheral nerves and carried to the spinal cord, where they block the action of inhibitory enzymes at spinal synapses and interfere with transmission of neuromuscular impulses. As a result, even minor stimuli cause uncontrolled muscle spasms.

## MANIFESTATIONS

The manifestations often begin with pain at the site of the infection. The infected person has stiffness of the jaw and neck and dysphagia. There is often profuse perspiration and drooling from increased salivation. As the infection progresses, the person experiences hyperreflexia, spasms of the jaw muscles (*trismus*) or facial muscles, and rigidity and spasms of the abdominal, neck, and back muscles. Generalized tonic seizures are caused by even minor stimuli, and the person assumes a typical opisthotonic position during the seizures: The head is retracted, the back is arched, and the feet are extended. The muscle spasms are painful. The person may be unable to breathe from spasms of the glottis and respiratory muscles. Despite these physical effects, the client has no change in mental status.

The complications of tetanus include urinary retention and airway obstruction from the spasms. Cardiac and respiratory failure are late, life-threatening complications.

## COLLABORATIVE CARE

There are no specific diagnostic tests for tetanus; diagnosis is based on manifestations. Tetanus is completely preventable by active immunization. Immunization for children includes tetanus toxoid, administered as part of the diphtheria-pertussis-tetanus (DPT) immunization series. In adults, immunization is obtained by administering tetanus toxoid as two doses 4 to 6 weeks apart, with a third dose in 6 to 12 months. All individuals should have a booster dose every 10 years throughout life or at the time of a major injury if the last booster dose was given more than 5 years prior to the injury.

If a wound is contaminated or if the person's immunization status is uncertain, passive immunization with tetanus immune globulin is administered. Active immunization with tetanus toxoid is begun at the same time. The wound is carefully and thoroughly debrided and antibiotics administered.

The client with tetanus requires intensive care in an area of minimal stimulation. Penicillin is administered to help destroy the toxin-producing organism. Muscle spasms and seizures are controlled by chlorpromazine (Thorazine) or diazepam (Valium), often combined with a sedative. Anticoagulants may be prescribed to prevent venous thrombosis. In severe cases, seizures and spasms are controlled with paralysis by a curare-like medication, and airway obstruction is managed by mechanical ventilation.

## NURSING CARE

Nursing care for the client with tetanus is intensive and focuses on assessments and interventions to promote safety, prevent injury, maintain nutrition, and maintain pulmonary and cardiovascular function. The client usually requires in-hospital care for 2 to 5 weeks. The nursing care plan commonly includes the following:

- Place in a quiet, darkened room to decrease stimuli that cause muscle spasms and seizures.

- Provide only necessary physical care, and do so during periods of maximal sedation to decrease tactile stimulation that causes muscle spasms.
- Maintain oxygenation through mechanical ventilator and frequent suctioning of secretions.
- Maintain intravenous access for the administration of fluids and medications.
- Administer prescribed antibiotics, anticonvulsants, and sedatives. In the case of cardiovascular complications, administer prescribed beta-adrenergic blocking agents such as propranolol (Inderal).
- Provide adequate nutrition through prescribed nutritional support, such as total parenteral nutrition.
- Monitor respiratory and cardiovascular status and provide immediate interventions for respiratory or cardiovascular failure.
- Monitor fluid and electrolyte status. Ensure adequate fluid intake to maintain hydration and urinary output.
- Monitor urinary output, which should be maintained at 1.5 to 2 L per day.
- Monitor for the hazards of immobility, including constipation, pneumonia, deep vein thrombosis, and pressure ulcers.

### Health Promotion

Tetanus is a preventable disorder, and nurses have a major role in promoting immunizations for all children and for educating adults about the need for booster doses. The older population is especially at risk for never having been immunized or for letting immunizations lapse. Information for this age group can be provided through activities such as community health fairs and programs at senior citizen groups.

It is also necessary to teach the proper care of wounds. All wounds, no matter how small, should be thoroughly washed with soap and water. All foreign material should be carefully flushed out or removed from a wound, and medical care should be sought for wounds that are more extensive or contaminated.

## THE CLIENT WITH BOTULISM

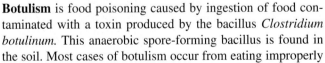

**Botulism** is food poisoning caused by ingestion of food contaminated with a toxin produced by the bacillus *Clostridium botulinum*. This anaerobic spore-forming bacillus is found in the soil. Most cases of botulism occur from eating improperly canned or cooked foods, especially home-canned vegetables and fruits, smoked meats, and vacuum-packed fish. The mortality rate is high if the disease is untreated.

## PATHOPHYSIOLOGY AND MANIFESTATIONS

The toxins liberated by *Clostridium botulinum* are absorbed by the gastrointestinal tract and bound to nerve tissues. They block the release of acetylcholine from nerve endings and thus cause respiratory paralysis due to paralysis of skeletal muscles. Manifestations usually appear 12 to 36 hours after ingestion of the contaminated food.

The manifestations of botulism usually begin with visual disturbances such as diplopia, loss of accommodation, and fixed, dilated pupils. Ptosis is often present. Gastrointestinal manifestations include nausea and vomiting, diarrhea, dysphagia, and dry mouth. Involvement of the larynx is manifested by dystonia (impaired muscle tone). Paralysis of all muscle groups progresses throughout the body, with respiratory paralysis causing death if the client is not placed on a mechanical ventilator. There is no effect on mental status.

## COLLABORATIVE CARE

Infection with the Clostridium toxin is verified by laboratory analysis of the serum and stool and of suspected food, if possible. If botulism is suspected, the state health department and the Centers for Disease Control and Prevention should be notified for assistance with laboratory assays and procuring botulism antitoxin. All people who may have eaten the contaminated food must be located and observed.

Any toxins in the gastrointestinal system are removed by cathartics, enemas, and gastric lavage. The client with respiratory paralysis is placed on a mechanical ventilator and may require a tracheostomy. Botulism antitoxin is administered to eradicate toxins in the circulation. Nutritional support is often provided with total parenteral nutrition. Intravenous fluids are administered to prevent dehydration and renal failure. If ventilation can be maintained, the client often recovers without further neurologic deficits.

## NURSING CARE

The client with botulism is hospitalized, and interventions focus on monitoring for respiratory failure and providing ventilatory assistance if necessary. Ongoing assessments are also made for manifestations of paralytic ileus and urinary retention. The client will be NPO until able to swallow and breathe; therefore, hydration and nutritional status are monitored. Teach the client and family that fatigue and weakness may persist for up to a year. During this time, the client may need to modify ADLs and take rest periods throughout the day.

### Health Promotion

Education of the public to prevent botulism is important. Address the following topics at health fairs and community programs and explain them to rural residents who do home canning.

- Home-canned foods must be processed in a pressure cooker rather than in boiling water because the organism is difficult to kill.
- Do not eat home-processed foods that have a change in color, are soft, contain gas bubbles, or have a bad odor.
- Always heat both home-processed and commercial foods at temperatures over 248° F (120 C) or boil for 10 minutes before tasting or eating them.
- Discard home-processed or commercially canned or bottled foods with defective seals.
- Discard commercially prepared canned foods that are damaged or have bulging sides or leaking contents.

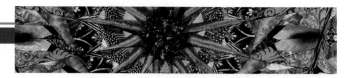

 EXPLORE MediaLink

NCLEX review questions, case studies, care plan activities, MediaLink applications, and other interactive resources for this chapter can be found on the Companion Website at www.prenhall.com/lemone.

Click on Chapter 43 to select the activities for this chapter. For animations, video clips, more NCLEX review questions, and an audio glossary, access the Student CD-ROM accompanying this textbook.

## TEST YOURSELF

1. What manifestation is usually the first indication of the onset of AD?

    a. Total inability to perform ADLs
    b. Sundowning
    c. Subtle memory deficits
    d. Inability to communicate

2. Which of the following nursing diagnoses is appropriate for clients with MS, regardless of type or severity?

    a. *Fatigue*
    b. *Risk for aspiration*
    c. *Acute pain*
    d. *Impaired gas exchange*

3. The manifestations of Parkinson's disease are the result of:

    a. Autoimmune responses to a viral infection
    b. The failure of dopamine to inhibit acetylcholine

    c. Effects of a neurotoxin
    d. A genetic defect

4. What drug classification is the medication used to treat ALS?

    a. Dopamine agonist
    b. Anticholinergic
    c. Antiinflammatory
    d. Antiglutamate

5. How can the nurse prevent tetanus?

    a. Teach safe food preparation techniques
    b. Promote immunizations for all children
    c. Demonstrate proper disposal of soiled dressings
    d. Promote immunization of household pets

See Test Yourself answers in Appendix C.

## BIBLIOGRAPHY

Alzheimer's Disease and Related Disorders Association, Inc. (2000). Available www.Alzheimers.org

Andresen, G. (1998). Dx dementia. But what kind? *RN, 61*(6), 26–29.

Baker, L. (1998). Sense making in multiple sclerosis: The information needs of people during an acute exacerbation. *Qualitative Health Research, 8*(1), 106–120.

Bell, V., & Troxel, D. (2001). Spirituality and the person with dementia–A view from the field. *Alzheimer's Care Quarterly, 2*(2), 31–45.

Boyden, K. (2000). The pathophysiology of demyelination and the ionic basis of nerve conduction in multiple sclerosis: An overview. *Journal of Neuroscience Nursing, 32*(1), 49–53, 60.

Center for Disease Control. (2001). *Bovine spongiform encephalopathy and Creutzfeldt-Jakob disease.* Available www.cdc.gov/ncidod/diseases

Charles, T., & Swash, M. (2001). Amyotrophic lateral sclerosis: Current understanding. *Journal of Neuroscience Nursing, 33*(5), 245–253.

Costa, M. (1998). Trigeminal neuralgia. *American Journal of Nursing, 98*(6), 42–43.

Dewing, J. (2001). Care for older people with a dementia in acute hospital settings. *Nursing Older People, 13*(3), 18–20.

Epps, C. (2001). Recognizing pain in the institutionalized elder with dementia. *Geriatric Nursing, 22*(2), 71–79.

Fontaine, K. (2000). *Healing practices: Alternative therapies for nursing.* Upper Saddle River, NJ: Prentice Hall.

Fowler, S. (1997). Hope and a health-promoting lifestyle in persons with Parkinson's disease. *Journal of Neuroscience Nursing, 29*(2), 111–116.

Gerdner, L., & Hall. G. (2001). Chronic confusion. In M. Maas, K. Buckwalter, M. Hardy, T. Tripp-Reimer, M. Titler, & J. Specht (Eds.), *Nursing care of older adults: Diagnoses, outcomes, & interventions* (pp. 421–441). St. Louis: Mosby.

Gray, P., & Hildebrand, K. (2000). Fall risk factors in Parkinson's disease. *Journal of Neuroscience Nursing, 32*(4), 222–228.

Greenway, M., & Walker, A. (1998). Home health: Helping caregivers cope with Alzheimer's disease. *Nursing98, 28*(2), 32hh 1–2, 4–6.

Gulick, E. (1997). Correlates of quality of life among persons with multiple sclerosis. *Nursing Research, 46*(6), 305–311.

Herndon, C., Young, K., Herndon, A., & Dole, E. (2000). Parkinson's disease revisited. *Journal of Neuroscience Nursing, 32*(4), 216–221.

Hickey, J. (2002). *The clinical practice of neurological and neurosurgical nursing* (5th ed.). Philadelphia: Lippincott.

Johnson, M., & Maas, M. (Eds.). (1997). *Nursing outcomes classification (NOC).* St. Louis: Mosby.

Kee, J. (1998). *Handbook of laboratory and diagnostic tests with nursing implications* (4th ed.). Upper Saddle River, NJ: Prentice Hall.

Lisak, D. (2001). Overview of symptomatic management of multiple sclerosis. *Journal of Neuroscience Nursing, 33*(5), 224–230.

McCance, K., & Huether, S. (2002). *Pathophysiology: The biologic basis for disease in adults and children.* St. Louis: Mosby.

McCloskey, J., & Bulechek, G. (Eds.). (2000). *Nursing interventions classification (NIC)* (3rd ed.). St. Louis: Mosby.

McKenry, L., & Salerno, E. (1998). *Pharmacology in nursing* (20th ed.). St. Louis: Mosby.

McMahon-Parkes, K., & Cornock, M. (1997). Guillain-Barré syndrome: Biological basis, treatment and care. *Intensive & Critical Care Nursing, 13*(1), 42–48.

Mini-mental state exam. (1975). *J Psychiatric Research, 12,* 189–198. Oxford: Elsevier Science.

National Parkinson Foundation, Inc. (2001). New approaches for treating tremor. Available www.Parkinson.org/treatment.htm

North American Nursing Diagnosis Association. (2001). *Nursing diagnoses: Definitions & classification 2001–2002*. Philadelphia: NANDA.

O'Donnell, L. (1997). Immune-mediated neurological diseases. Management of myasthenia gravis—An overview. *Journal of Care Management, 3*(6 Disease Management Digest), 4–5, 17–18.

Porth, C. (2002). *Pathophysiology: Concepts of altered health states* (6th ed.). Philadelphia: Lippincott.

Ross, A. (1999). Neurologic degenerative disorders. *Nursing Clinics of North America, 34*(3), 725–742.

Schutte, D., Williams, J., Schutte, B., & Maas, M. (1998). Alzheimer's disease genetics: Practice and education implications for special care unit nurses. *Journal of Gerontological Nursing, 24*(1), 40–48, 58–64.

Segatore, M. (1998). Managing the surgical orthopaedic patient with Parkinson's disease. *Orthopaedic Nursing, 17*(1), 13–22.

Shannon, M., Wilson, B., & Stang, C. (2002). *Health professional's drug guide 2002*. Upper Saddle River, NJ: Prentice Hall.

Spratto, G., & Woods, A. (1998). *Delmar's therapeutic class drug guide for nurses 1998*. Albany, NY: Delmar.

Tierney, L., McPhee, S., & Papadakis, M. (Eds.). (2001). *Current medical diagnosis & treatment* (40th ed.). Stamford, CT: Appleton & Lange.

Worsham, T. (2000). Easing the course of Guilllain-Barre syndrome. *RN, 63*(3), 46–50.

Zaveruha, A., Bishop, D., St. Clair, A., & Moreau, K. (1997). Rabies update for nurse practitioners. *Clinical Excellence for Nurse Practitioners, 1*(6), 367–375.

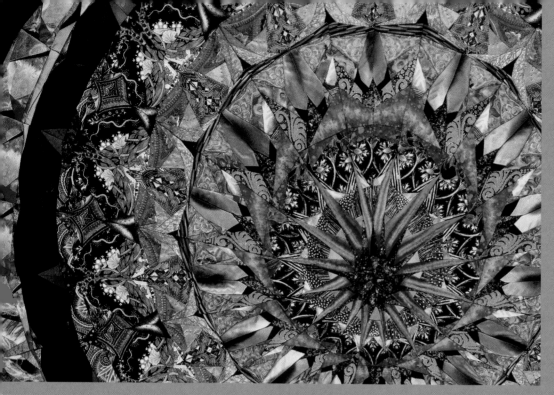

# RESPONSES TO ALTERED VISUAL AND AUDITORY FUNCTION

### CHAPTER 44

# Assessing Clients with Eye and Ear Disorders

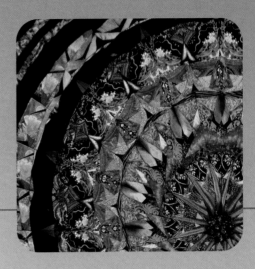

## LEARNING OUTCOMES

After completing this chapter, you will be able to:

- Review the anatomy and physiology of the eye and the ear.

- Explain the physiologic processes involved in vision, hearing, and equilibrium.

- Identify specific topics for consideration during a health history interview of the client with health problems of the eye or ear.

- Describe techniques for assessing the structure and function of the eye and ear.

- Identify abnormal findings that may indicate impairment in the function of the eye and the ear.

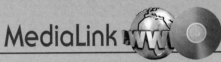

## MediaLink

### www.prenhall.com/lemone

Additional resources for this chapter can be found on the Student CD-ROM accompanying this textbook, and on the Companion Website at www.prenhall.com/lemone. Click on Chapter 44 to select the activities for this chapter.

**CD-ROM**
- Audio Glossary
- NCLEX Review

*Animations*
- Ear Anatomy
- Eye Anatomy

**Companion Website**
- More NCLEX Review
- Functional Health Pattern Assessment
- Case Study
    Otitis Media

Vision and hearing allow us to experience the world in which we live. The eyes and ears provide pathways for visual and auditory stimuli to reach the brain. In addition, specialized structures within the ear help maintain position sense and equilibrium. Deficits in vision and hearing may limit self-care, mobility, independence, communication, and relationships with others

## REVIEW OF ANATOMY AND PHYSIOLOGY
### The Eye and Vision

The eyes are complex structures, containing 70% of the sensory receptors of the body. Each eye is a sphere measuring about 1 inch (2.5 cm) in diameter, surrounded and protected by a bony orbit and cushions of fat. The primary functions of the eye are to encode the patterns of light from the environment through photoreceptors and to carry the coded information from the eyes to the brain. The brain gives meaning to the coded information, allowing us to make sense of what we see. Both extraocular and intraocular structures are considered parts of the eye.

#### Extraocular Structures
Although the extraocular structures of the eye are outside the eyeball, they are vital to its protection. These structures are the eyebrows, eyelids, eyelashes, conjunctiva, lacrimal apparatus, and extrinsic eye muscles (Figure 44–1 ■).

The eyebrows shade the eyes and keep perspiration away from them. The eyelids are thin, loose folds of skin covering the anterior eye. They protect the eye from foreign bodies, regulate the entry of light into the eye, and distribute tears by blinking. The eyelashes are short hairs that project from the top and bottom borders of the eyelids. An unexpected touch to the eyelashes initiates the blinking reflex to protect the eyes from foreign objects.

The conjunctiva is a thin, transparent membrane that lines the inner surfaces of the eyelids and also folds over the anterior surface of the eyeball. The palpebral conjunctiva lines the upper and lower eyelids, whereas the bulbar conjunctiva loosely covers the anterior sclera (the white part of the eye). The conjunctiva is a mucous membrane that lubricates the eyes. The lacrimal apparatus is composed of the lacrimal gland, the puncta, the lacrimal sac, and the nasolacrimal duct. Together, these structures secrete, distribute, and drain tears to cleanse and moisten the eye's surface.

The six extrinsic eye muscles control movement of the eye, allowing it to follow a moving object and move precisely. The muscles also help maintain the shape of the eyeball. The cranial nerves control the extrinsic muscles (Figure 44–2 ■).

#### Intraocular Structures
The intraocular structures transmit visual images and maintain homeostasis of the inner eye. Those in the anterior portion of each eyeball are the sclera and the cornea (forming the outermost coat of the eye, called the fibrous tunic), the iris, the pupil, and the anterior cavity (Figure 44–3 ■).

The white sclera lines the outside of the eyeball, and protects and gives shape to the eyeball. The sclera gives way to the cornea over the iris and pupil. The cornea is transparent, avascular, and sensitive to touch. The cornea forms a window that allows light to enter the eye and is a part of its light-bending apparatus. When the cornea is touched, the eyelids blink (the *corneal reflex*) and tears are secreted.

The iris is a disc of muscle tissue surrounding the pupil and lying between the cornea and the lens. The iris gives the eye its color and regulates light entry by controlling the size of the pupil. The pupil is the dark center of the eye through which light enters. The pupil constricts when bright light enters the eye and when it is used for near vision; it dilates when light conditions are dim and when the eye is used for far vision. In response to intense light, the pupil constricts rapidly in the pupillary light reflex.

The anterior cavity is made of the anterior chamber (the space between the cornea and the iris) and the posterior chamber (the space between the iris and the lens). The anterior cavity is filled with a clear fluid, the aqueous humor. Aqueous humor is con-

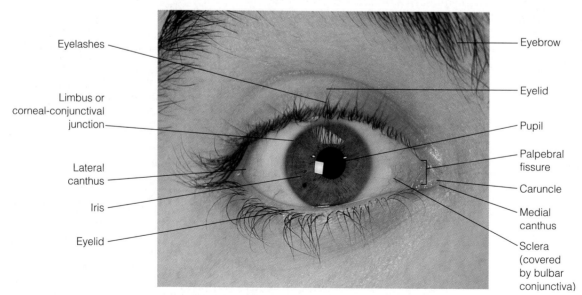

**Figure 44–1 ■** Accessory and external structures of the eye.

*Source: Todd Buck*

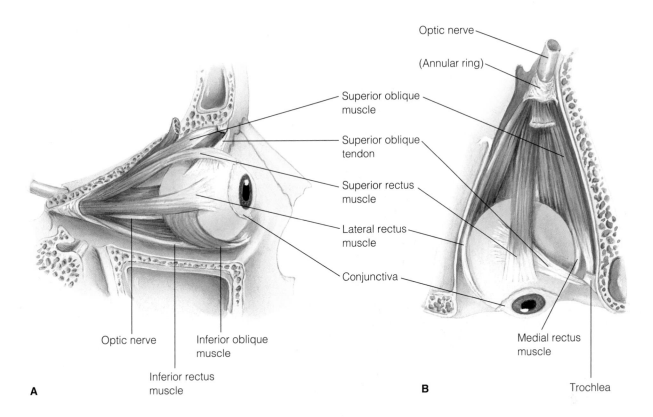

| Name | Controlling cranial nerve | Action |
|---|---|---|
| Lateral rectus | VI (abducens) | Moves eye laterally |
| Medial rectus | III (oculomotor) | Moves eye medially |
| Superior rectus | III (oculomotor) | Elevates eye or rolls it superiorly |
| Inferior rectus | III (oculomotor) | Depresses eye or rolls it inferiorly |
| Inferior oblique | III (oculomotor) | Elevates eye and turns it laterally |
| Superior oblique | IV (trochlear) | Depresses eye and turns it laterally |

**Figure 44–2** ■ Extraocular muscles. *A,* Lateral view of the right eye. *B,* Superior view of the right eye. *C,* Innervation of the extraocular muscles by the cranial nerves.

stantly formed and drained to maintain a relatively constant pressure of from 15 to 20 mmHg in the eye. The canal of Schlemm, a network of channels that circles the eye in the angle at the junction of the sclera and the cornea, is the drainage system for fluid moving between the anterior and posterior chambers. Aqueous humor provides nutrients and oxygen to the cornea and the lens.

The intraocular structures that lie in the internal chamber of the eye are the posterior cavity and vitreous humor, the lens, the ciliary body, the uvea, and the retina.

The posterior cavity lies behind the lens. It is filled with a clear gelatinous substance, the vitreous humor, which supports the posterior surface of the lens, maintains the position of the retina, and transmits light. The lens is a biconvex, avascular, transparent structure located directly behind the pupil. It can change shape to focus and refract light onto the retina.

The uvea, also called the vascular tunic, is the middle layer of the eyeball. This pigmented layer has three components: the iris, ciliary body, and choroid. The ciliary body encircles the lens, and along with the iris, regulates the amount of light reaching the retina by controlling the shape of the lens. Most of the uvea is made up of the choroid, which is pigmented and vascular. Blood vessels of the choroid nourish the layers of the eyeball. Its pigmented areas absorb light, preventing it from scattering within the eyeball.

The retina is the innermost lining of the eyeball. It has an outer pigmented layer and an inner neural layer. The outer layer, next to the choroid, serves as the link between visual stimuli and the brain. The transparent inner layer is made up of millions of light receptors in structures called rods and cones. Rods enable vision in dim light as well as peripheral

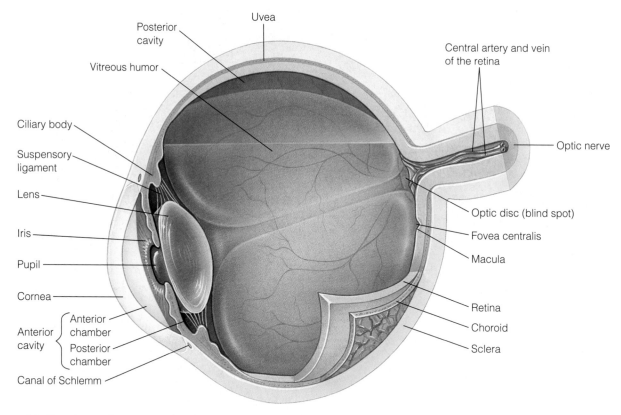

**Figure 44–3** ■ Internal structures of the eye.

vision. Cones enable vision in bright light and the perception of color. The optic disc, a cream-colored round or oval area within the retina, is the point at which the optic nerve enters the eye. The slight depression in the center of the optic disc is often called the physiologic cup. Located laterally to the optic disc is the macula, a darker area with no visible blood vessels. The macula contains primarily cones. The fovea centralis is a slight depression in the center of the macula that contains only cones and is a main receptor of detailed color vision.

## The Visual Pathway

The optic nerves are cranial nerves formed of the axons of ganglion cells. The two optic nerves meet at the optic chiasma, just anterior to the pituitary gland in the brain. At the optic chiasma, axons from the medial half of each retina cross to the opposite side to form pairs of axons from each eye. These pairs continue as the left and right optic tracts (Figure 44–4 ■). The crossing of the axons results in each optic tract carrying information from both eyes. The left optic tract carries visual information from the lateral half of the retina of the left eye and the medial

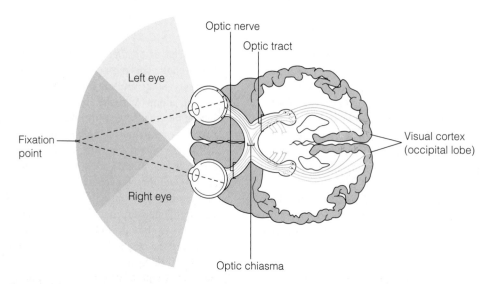

**Figure 44–4** ■ The visual fields of the eye, and the visual pathways to the brain.

half of the retina of the right eye, whereas the right optic tract carries visual information from the lateral half of the retina of the right eye and the medial half of the retina of the left eye.

The ganglion cell axons in the optic tracts travel to the thalamus and create synapses with neurons, forming pathways called optic radiations. The optic radiations terminate in the visual cortex of the occipital lobe. Here the nerve impulses that originated in the retina are interpreted.

The visual fields of each eye overlap considerably, and each eye sees a slightly different view. Because of this overlap and the crossing of the axons, information from both eyes reaches each side of the visual cortex, which then fuses the information into one image. This fusion of images accounts for the ability to perceive depth; however, depth perception depends on visual input from two eyes that both focus well.

## Refraction

Refraction is the bending of light rays as they pass from one medium to another medium of different optical density. As light rays pass through the eye, they are refracted at several points: as they enter the cornea, as they leave the cornea and enter the aqueous humor, as they enter the lens, and as they leave the lens and enter the vitreous humor. At the lens, the light is bent so that it converges at a single point on the retina. This focusing of the image is called accommodation. Because the lens is convex, the image projected onto the retina (the real image) is upside down and reversed from left to right. This real image is coded as electric signals that are sent to the brain. The brain decodes the image so that the person perceives it as it occurs in space.

The eyes are best adapted to see distant objects. Both eyes fix on the same distant image and do not require any change in accommodation. For people with *emmetropic* (normal) vision, the distance from the viewed object at which the eyes require no accommodation is 20 ft (6 m). This point is called the far point of vision. To focus for near vision, the eyes must instantly accommodate the lens, constrict the pupils, and converge the eyeballs. Accommodation is accomplished by contraction of the ciliary muscles. This contraction reduces the tension on the lens capsule so that it bulges outward to increase the curvature. This change in shape also achieves a shorter focal length, another requirement for focusing close images on the retina. The closest point on which a person can focus is called the near point of vision; in young adults with normal vision this is usually 8 to 10 inches (20 to 25 cm). Pupillary constriction helps eliminate most of the divergent light rays and sharpens focus. Convergence (the medial rotation of the eyeballs so that each is directed toward the viewed object) allows the focusing of the image on the retinal fovea of each eye.

## ASSESSING THE EYE

Data about the function of the eyes and vision are gathered both during the health assessment interview to collect subjective data and the physical assessment to collect objective data.

## Health Assessment Interview

This section provides guidelines for collecting subjective data about the functions of the eye and ear through a health assessment interview.

A health assessment interview to determine problems with the eyes and vision may be part of a health screening, may focus on a chief complaint (such as blurred vision or an eye infection), or may be part of a total health assessment. If the client has a health problem involving one or both eyes, analyze its onset, characteristics and course, severity, precipitating and relieving factors, and any associated symptoms, noting the timing and circumstances. For example, you may ask the client:

- Describe the type of pain you experience in your eyes. When did it begin? How long does it last?
- Have you noticed rings of color around streetlights at night?
- When did you first notice having difficulty reading the paper?

Throughout the interview, be alert to nonverbal behaviors (such as squinting or abnormal eye movements) that suggest problems with eye function. Explore problems such as watery, irritated eyes or changes in vision. Assess the client's use of corrective eyewear and care of eyeglasses or contact lenses. If the client uses eye medications, ask about the type and purpose as well as the frequency and duration of use. When taking the history, find out about eye trauma, surgery, or infections, as well as the date and results of the last eye examination. In addition, ask the client about a medical history of diabetes, hypertension, thyroid disorders, glaucoma, cataracts, and eye infections. Include questions about a family history of nearsightedness or farsightedness, cancer of the retina, color blindness, and any other eye or vision disorders.

Collect information about environmental or work exposure to irritating chemicals, participation in sports or hobbies that pose the risk of eye injury, and the use of protective eyewear during dangerous activities.

Further interview questions and leading statements, categorized by functional health patterns, can be found on the Companion Website.

## Physical Assessment of the Eye and Vision

Physical assessment of the eyes and of visual acuity may be performed as part of a total assessment or separately for clients with known or suspected problems of the eyes. The eyes and vision are primarily assessed through inspection of external structures and assessment of visual fields and visual acuity, extraocular muscle function, and internal structures. Palpation (e.g., of a blocked lacrimal duct) may be used if a problem is identified. Prior to the examination, collect all necessary equipment—visual acuity charts, an opaque eye cover, a pen, a penlight, a cotton-tipped applicator, and an ophthalmoscope—and explain the techniques to the client to decrease anxiety. The client may sit or stand during the assessment.

## Assessing Visual Fields

Visual fields are tested to assess the functioning of the macula and peripheral vision. The visual fields of the examiner (which must be normal to perform this assessment) are used as the standard. To measure visual fields, sit directly opposite the client at a distance of 18 to 24 inches. Ask the client to cover one eye with the opaque cover while you cover your own eye opposite to the client (for example, if the client covers the right eye, you cover your left eye). Ask the client to look directly at you. Move the penlight from the periphery toward the center from right to left, above and below, and from the middle of each of these directions. Both you and the client should see the penlight enter the field of vision at the same time.

### Vision Assessment with Abnormal Findings (✓)

Visual acuity is assessed with the Snellen chart or the E chart for testing distance vision and the Rosenbaum chart for testing near vision. The Snellen chart contains rows of letters in various sizes, with standardized numbers at the end of each row. The number at the end of the row indicates the visual acuity of a client who can read the row at a distance of 20 feet. (If the client is unable to read or does not read English, you can use the E chart to test visual acuity.) The top number at the end of the row is always 20, representing the distance between the client and the chart. The bottom number is the distance (in feet) at which a person with normal vision can read the line. A person with normal vision can read the row marked 20/20. To conduct the assessment, ask the person to stand 20 feet from the chart in a well-lit area. Ask the client to cover one eye with an opaque cover (Figure 44–5 ■). Then ask the client to read each row of letters, moving from largest letters to the smallest ones that the client can see. Measure visual acuity in the other eye in the same way, and then assess visual acuity while the client has both eyes uncovered. You may test the client who wears corrective lenses with and without the lenses.

The Rosenbaum chart is held at a distance of from 12 to 14 inches from the eyes, with visual acuity measured in the same manner as with the Snellen chart (Figure 44–6 ■). A gross estimate of near vision may also be assessed by asking the person to read from a magazine or newspaper.

- Assess distant vision, using the Snellen or E chart.
  - ✓ Changes in distant vision are most commonly the result of **myopia** (nearsightedness). For example, a reading of 20/100 indicates impaired distance vision. A person has to stand 20 feet from the chart to read a line that a person with normal vision could read 100 feet from the chart.

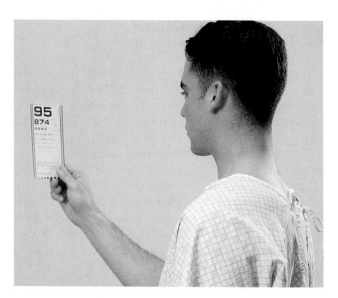

**Figure 44–6** ■ Testing near vision using Rosenbaum eye chart.

- Assess near vision, using a Rosenbaum chart or a card with newsprint held 12 to 14 inches from the client's eyes.
  - ✓ Changes in near vision, especially in clients over 45, can indicate **presbyopia,** impaired near vision resulting from a loss of elasticity of the lens related to aging. In younger clients, this condition is referred to as **hyperopia** (farsightedness).

### Eye Movement and Alignment Assessment with Abnormal Findings (✓)

- Assess the cardinal fields of vision to gain information about extraocular eye movements. Ask the client to follow a pen or your finger while keeping the head stationary. Move the pen or your finger through the six fields one at a time, returning to the central starting point before proceeding to the next field (Figure 44–7 ■). The eyes should move through each field without involuntary movements.
- The cover-uncover test is a test for strabismus, a weakening of a muscle that causes one eye to deviate from the other when the person is focusing on an object. To conduct the test, hold a pen or your finger about 1 foot from the eyes and ask the person to focus on that object. Cover one of the client's eyes and note any movement in the uncovered eye; as you remove the cover, assess for movement in the eye that was just uncovered. Repeat the procedure with the other eye.
- Assess convergence. Ask the client to follow an object as you move it toward the client's eyes; normally both eyes converge toward the center.
  - ✓ Failure of the eyes to converge equally on an approaching object may indicate a neuromuscular disorder or improper eye alignment.
- Assess extraocular movements.
  - ✓ Failure of one or both eyes to follow the object in any given direction may indicate extraocular muscle weakness or cranial nerve dysfunction.
  - ✓ An involuntary rhythmic movement of the eyes, nystagmus, is associated with neurologic disorders and the use of some medications.

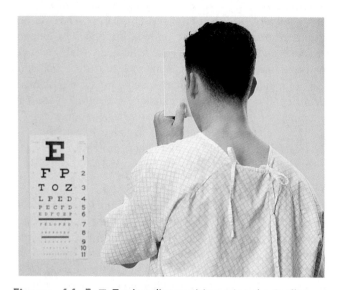

**Figure 44–5** ■ Testing distant vision using the Snellen eye chart.

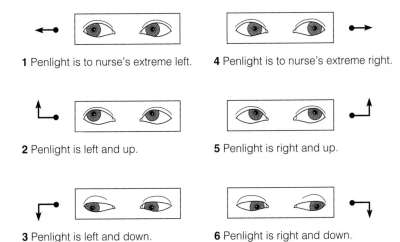

**1** Penlight is to nurse's extreme left.

**4** Penlight is to nurse's extreme right.

**2** Penlight is left and up.

**5** Penlight is right and up.

**3** Penlight is left and down.

**6** Penlight is right and down.

**Figure 44–7** ■ The six cardinal fields of vision.

• Assess the corneal light reflex. Direct a light source onto the bridge of the nose from 12 to 15 inches. Observe for equal reflection of the light from each eye.
  ✓ Reflections of the light from different sites on the eyes reveal improper alignment.

## Pupillary Assessment with Abnormal Findings (✓)

• Observe pupil size and equality.
  ✓ Pupils that are unequal in size may indicate a severe neurologic problem, such as increased intracranial pressure.
• Assess direct and consensual pupil response. Ask the client to look straight ahead. Shine a light obliquely into one eye at a time. Observe for constriction of the pupil in the illuminated eye. Test both eyes. To test consensual pupil response, again shine a light obliquely into one eye at a time as the client looks straight ahead. Observe constriction of the pupil in the opposite eye.
  ✓ Failure of the pupils to respond to light may indicate degeneration of the retina or destruction of the optic nerve.
  ✓ A client who has one dilated and unresponsive pupil may have paralysis of the oculomotor nerve.
  ✓ Some eye medications may cause unequal dilation, constriction, or inequality of pupil size. Morphine and similar drugs may cause small, unresponsive pupils, and anticholinergic drugs such as atropine may cause dilated, unresponsive pupils.
• Test for accommodation. Hold an object at a distance of a few feet from the client. The pupils should dilate. Ask the client to follow the object as you bring it to within a few inches of the client's nose. The pupils should constrict and converge as they change focus to follow the object.
  ✓ Failure of accommodation along with lack of pupil response to light may signal a neurologic problem.
  ✓ Lack of response to light with appropriate response to accommodation is often seen in clients with diabetes.

## External Eye Assessment with Abnormal Findings (✓)

• Inspect the eyelids.
  ✓ Unusual redness or discharge may indicate an inflammatory state due to trauma, allergies, or infection.

✓ Drooping of one eyelid, called **ptosis,** may be the result of a stroke, indicate a neuromuscular disorder, or be congenital (Figure 44–8 ■).
✓ Unusual widening of the lids may be due to **exophthalmos,** protrusion of the eyeball due to an increase in intraocular volume. Exophthalmos is often associated with hyperthyroid conditions (see Chapter 17).
✓ Yellow plaques noted most often on the lid margins are referred to as *xanthelasma* and may indicate high lipid levels.
✓ An acute localized inflammation of a hair follicle is known as a hordeolum (sty) and is generally caused by staphylococcal organisms (Figure 44–9 ■).

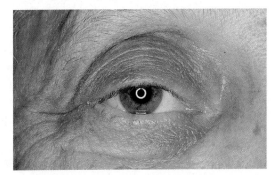

**Figure 44–8** ■ Ptosis.

*Source: Leonard Lessen/Peter Arnold, Inc.*

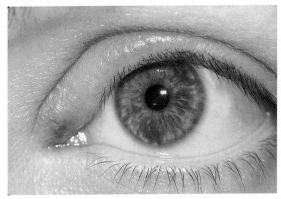

**Figure 44–9** ■ Hordeolum.

*Source: Science Photo Library/Photo Researchers, Inc.*

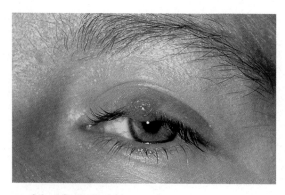

**Figure 44–10 ■** Chalazion.

*Source: Custom Medical Stock Photo, Inc.*

✓ A chalazion is an infection or retention cyst of the meibomian glands (Figure 44–10 ■). The swelling is firm and not painful.
- Inspect the puncta.
  ✓ Unusual redness or discharge from the puncta may indicate an inflammation due to trauma, infection, or allergies.
- Inspect the bulbar and palpebral conjunctiva.
  ✓ Increased erythema or the presence of exudate may indicate acute conjunctivitis.
  ✓ A cobblestone appearance is often associated with allergies.
  ✓ A fold in the conjunctiva, called a *pterygium,* may be seen as a clouded area that extends over the cornea. This is an abnormal growth of the bulbar conjunctiva, usually seen on the nasal side of the cornea. It may interfere with vision if it covers the pupil.
- Inspect the sclera.
  ✓ Unusual redness may indicate an inflammatory state as a result of trauma, allergies, or infection.
  ✓ Yellow discoloration of the sclera may be seen in conditions involving the liver, such as hepatitis.
  ✓ Bright red areas in the sclera are often subconjunctival hemorrhages and may indicate trauma or bleeding disorders. They may also occur spontaneously.
- Inspect the cornea.
  ✓ Dullness, opacities, or irregularities of the cornea may be abnormal.
  ✓ *Corneal arcus* is a thin, grayish white arc seen toward the edge of the cornea. It is normal in older clients.
- Assess corneal sensitivity. Lightly touch a wisp of cotton to the client's cornea. This action should cause a blink reflex.
  ✓ Failure of the blink reflex may indicate a neurologic disorder.
- Inspect the iris.
  ✓ Lack of clarity of the iris may indicate a cloudiness of the cornea.
  ✓ Constriction of the pupil accompanied by pain and circumcorneal redness indicates acute iritis.

### Internal Eye Assessment with Abnormal Findings (✓)

Assess internal structures of the eye by using the ophthalmoscope, an instrument that allows visualization of the lens, the vitreous humor, and the retina. Box 44–1 provides guidelines for using the ophthalmoscope.

- Inspect for the red reflex.
  ✓ Absence of a red reflex often indicates improper position of the ophthalmoscope, but also may indicate total opacity of the pupil by a cataract or a hemorrhage into the vitreous humor.
- Inspect the lens and vitreous body.
  ✓ A *cataract* is an opacity of the lens, often seen as a dark shadow on ophthalmoscopic examination. It may be due to aging, trauma, diabetes, or a congenital defect.
- Inspect the retina.
  ✓ Areas of hemorrhage, exudate, and white patches may be a result of diabetes or long-standing hypertension.
- Inspect the optic disc.
  ✓ Loss of definition of the optic disc, as well as an increase in the size of the physiologic cup, results from papilledema from increased intracranial pressure.
- Inspect the blood vessels of the retina.
  ✓ Glaucoma often results in displacement of blood vessels from the center of the optic disc due to increased intraocular pressure.
  ✓ Hypertension may cause an apparent narrowing of the vein where an arteriole crosses over.
  ✓ Engorged veins may occur with diabetes, atherosclerosis, and blood disorders.
- Inspect the retinal background.
  ✓ Variations in color or a pale color overall may indicate disease.
- Inspect the macula.
  ✓ Absence of the fovea centralis is common in older clients. It may indicate macular degeneration, a common cause of loss of central vision.
- Palpate over the lacrimal glands, puncta, and nasolacrimal duct.
  ✓ Tenderness over any of these areas or drainage from the puncta may indicate an infectious process. (Wear gloves if you see any drainage.)
  ✓ Excessive tearing may indicate a blockage of the nasolacrimal duct.

## REVIEW OF ANATOMY AND PHYSIOLOGY
### The Ear and Hearing

As a sensory organ, the ear has two primary functions, hearing and maintaining equilibrium. Anatomically, the ear is divided into three areas: the external ear, the middle ear, and the inner ear (Figure 44–11 ■). Each area has a unique function. All three are involved in hearing, but only the inner ear is involved in equilibrium.

### The External Ear

The external ear consists of the auricle (or pinna), the external auditory canal, and the tympanic membrane.

The auricles are elastic cartilage covered with thin skin. They contain sebaceous and sweat glands and sometimes hair.

## BOX 44–1   ■  Guidelines for Using the Ophthalmoscope

The ophthalmoscope has a head and a handle. (See the figure below.) The head contains a focus wheel (also called a lens selector dial) located on the side, lenses of varying magnification, and an opening through which the eye structures are visualized. The focus wheel adjusts the lens refraction, which is measured in diopters. The diopter measurements range from 0 to +40 when the lens is rotated clockwise, and from 0 to −25 when the lens is rotated counterclockwise. By moving the focus wheel, the examiner can converge or diverge light rays to visualize the retina.

The handle usually contains batteries that can be plugged into a wall socket for recharging.

Before the examination, explain the procedure to the client. Assemble the ophthalmoscope. Wash your hands and wear disposable gloves if the client has any drainage from the eyes. Darken the room (to allow the pupils of the client to dilate), and ask the client to look straight ahead, focusing on a fixed point such as an object on the wall. Hold the ophthalmoscope in one hand, resting the index finger on the focus wheel (see the figure at right).

1. Turn on the ophthalmoscope light, and set focus wheel to 0 diopters. Hold the ophthalmoscope in your right hand with your index finger on the focus wheel. Standing in front of the client, position yourself at a 15-degree angle to the client's line of vision.

2. Hold the opening of the ophthalmoscope up to your right eye and direct the light toward the client's right eye from a distance of about 12 inches.

3. As the beam of light falls on the client's pupil, observe for the red reflex, which appears as a sharply outlined orange glow from within the pupil. This glow is the reflection of the light from the retina.

4. Move closer to the client, turning the focus wheel clockwise toward the positive numbers as needed to maintain clear focus.

5. Examine the lens and the vitreous body, both of which should be clear.

6. Gradually rotate the focus wheel counterclockwise toward the negative numbers as needed, focusing on a structure of the retina (such as the disc or a blood vessel). Turn the focus wheel until the image is clear. Examine the structures of the retina as follows:

   a. The optic disc (see the accompanying figure). Assess for size, shape, color, distinct margins, and the physiologic cup. The disc is round to slightly oval and about 1.5 mm in diameter. It has a yellow to pink color that is lighter than the retina itself. The margins should be sharp and clear. The physiologic cup is a small depression that occupies about one-third of the optic disc, lying temporal to the center of the disc.

   b. The vessels of the retina. Assess for color, arteriolar light reflex, ratio of arterioles to veins, and arteriovenous crossings. The arterioles are red, brighter than the veins, and about one-fourth smaller. The arterioles normally have a

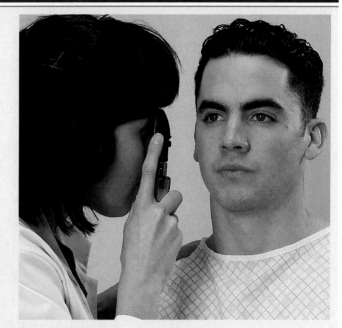

Technique for holding an ophthalmoscope.

narrow light reflex from the center of each vessel; veins do not have this light reflex. The ratio of arterioles to veins is usually 2:3 or 4:5. The vessels normally cross and become smaller toward the periphery.

   c. The retinal background. Assess color and changes in color. The retina is normally reddish orange and regular in color.

   d. The macula. Assess size and color. To assess the macula, ask the client to look directly into the ophthalmoscope light. The macula is temporal to the optic disc, appears slightly darker than the retina, and has no visible vessels. The fovea centralis may be seen as a bright spot of light. Because looking directly into the light causes some discomfort, conduct this portion of the examination last. The macula is often difficult to visualize.

7. Using the same technique, examine the left eye.

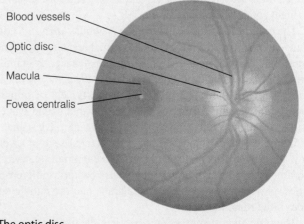

Blood vessels

Optic disc

Macula

Fovea centralis

The optic disc.

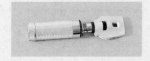

An ophthalmoscope.

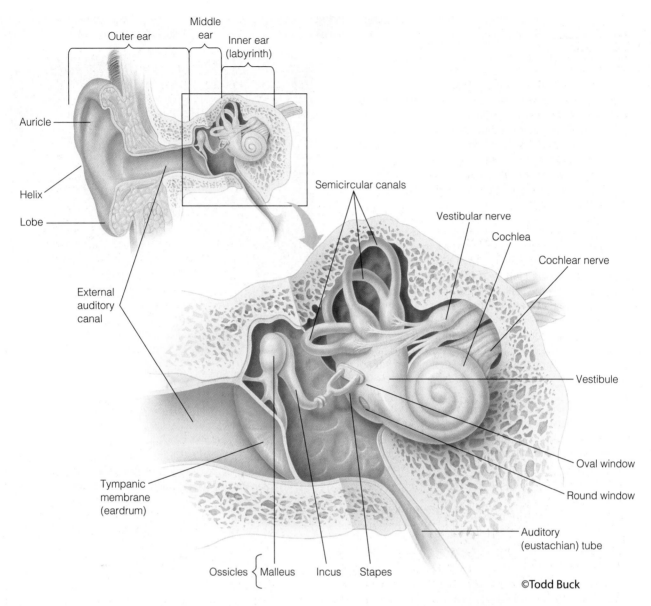

**Figure 44–11** ■ Structures of the external ear, middle ear, and inner ear.

©Todd Buck

Each auricle has a rim (the *helix*) and a lobe. The auricle serves to direct sound waves into the ear.

The external auditory canal, which is about 1 inch (2.5 cm) long, extends from the auricle to the tympanic membrane. The canal is lined with skin that contains hair, sebaceous glands, and ceruminous glands. The external auditory canal serves as a resonator for the range of sound waves typical of human speech and actually increases the pressure that sound waves in this frequency range place on the tympanic. The canal's ceruminous glands (modified apocrine glands) secrete a yellow to brown waxy substance called **cerumen** (earwax). Cerumen traps foreign bodies; it also has bacteriostatic properties, protecting the tympanic membrane and the middle ear from infections.

The tympanic membrane lies between the external ear and the middle ear. It is a thin, semitransparent, fibrous structure covered with skin on the external side and mucosa on the inner side. The membrane vibrates as sound waves strike it; these vibrations are transferred as sound waves to the middle ear.

## The Middle Ear

The middle ear is an air-filled cavity in the temporal bone. The middle ear contains three auditory ossicles: the malleus, the incus, and the stapes. These bones extend across the middle ear. The medial side of the middle ear is a bony wall containing two membrane-covered openings, the oval window and the round window. The posterior wall of the middle ear contains the mastoid antrum. This cavity communicates with the mastoid sinuses, which help the middle ear adjust to changes in pressure. It also opens into the eustachian tube, which connects with the nasopharynx. The eustachian tube helps to equalize the air pressure in the middle ear by opening briefly in response to differences between middle ear pressure and atmospheric pressure. This action also ensures that vibrations of the tympanic membrane remain adequate. The mucous membrane lining the middle ear is continuous with the mucous membranes lining the throat.

The malleus attaches to the tympanic membrane and articulates with the incus, which in turn articulates with the stapes. The stapes fits into the oval window. When the tympanic membrane vibrates, the vibrations are conducted across the middle ear to the oval window by the ossicles. The vibrations then set in motion the fluids of the inner ear, which in turn stimulate the hearing receptors. Two small muscles attached to the ossicles contract reflexively in response to sudden loud noises, thus decreasing the vibrations and protecting the inner ear.

### The Inner Ear

The inner ear, also called the labyrinth, is a maze of bony chambers located deep within the temporal bone, just behind the eye socket. The labyrinth is further divided into two parts: the bony labyrinth, a system of open channels that houses the second part, the membranous labyrinth. The bony labyrinth is filled with a fluid similar to cerebrospinal fluid called perilymph, which bathes the membranous labyrinth. Within the chambers of the membranous labyrinth is a fluid called endolymph.

The bony labyrinth has three regions: the vestibule, the semicircular canals, and the cochlea. The vestibule is the central portion of the inner ear, one side of which is a bony wall containing the oval window. Two sacs within the vestibule (the saccule and the utricle) join the vestibule with the cochlea and the semicircular canals. The saccule and the utricle contain receptors for equilibrium that respond to changes in gravity and changes in position of the head. The three semicircular canals each project into a different plane (anterior, posterior, and lateral). Each canal contains a semicircular duct that communicates with the utricle of the vestibule. Each duct has an enlarged area at one end containing an equilibrium receptor that responds to angular movements of the head.

The cochlea is a tiny bony chamber that houses the organ of Corti, the receptor organ for hearing. The organ of Corti is a series of sensory hair cells, arranged in a single row of inner hair cells and three rows of outer hair cells. The hair cells are innervated by sensory fibers from cranial nerve VIII. The organ of Corti is supported in the cochlea by the flexible basilar membrane, which has fibers of varying lengths that respond to different sound wave frequencies.

### Sound Conduction

Hearing is the perception and interpretation of sound. Sound is produced when the molecules of a medium are compressed, resulting in a pressure disturbance evidenced as a sound wave. The intensity or loudness of sound is determined by the amplitude (height) of the sound wave, with greater amplitudes causing louder sounds. The frequency of the sound wave in vibrations per second determines the pitch or tone of the sound, with higher frequencies resulting in higher sounds. The human ear is most sensitive to sound waves with frequencies between 1000 and 4000 cycles per second, but can detect sound waves with frequencies between 20 and 20,000 cycles per second.

Sound waves enter the external auditory canal and cause the tympanic membrane to vibrate at the same frequency. The ossicles not only transmit the motion of the tympanic membrane to the oval window but also amplify the energy of the sound wave. As the stapes moves against the oval window, the perilymph in the vestibule is set in motion. The increased pressure of the perilymph is transmitted to fibers of the basilar membrane and then to the organ of Corti (directly above the basilar membrane). The up-and-down movements of the fibers of the basilar membrane pull the hair cells in the organ of Corti, which in turn generates action potentials that are transmitted to cranial nerve VIII and then to the brain for interpretation.

Several brainstem auditory nuclei transmit impulses to the cerebral cortex. Fibers from each ear cross, with each auditory cortex receiving impulses from both ears. Auditory processing is so finely tuned that a wide variety of sounds of different pitch and loudness can be heard at any one time. In addition, the source of the sound can be localized.

### Maintenance of Equilibrium

The inner ear also provides information about the position of the head. This information is used to coordinate body movements so that equilibrium and balance are maintained. The types of equilibrium are static balance (affected by changes in the position of the head) and dynamic balance (affected by the movement of the head).

Receptors called maculae in the utricle and the saccule of the vestibule detect changes in the position of the head. Maculae are groups of hair cells; these cells have protrusions covered with a gelatinous substance. Embedded in this gelatinous substance are tiny particles of calcium carbonate called otoliths (ear stones), which make the gelatin heavier than the endolymph that fills the membranous labyrinth. As a result, when the head is in the upright position, gravity causes the gelatinous substance to bear down on the hair cells. When the position of the head changes, the force on the hair cells also changes, bending them and altering the pattern of stimulation of the neurons. Thus, a different pattern of nerve impulses is transmitted to the brain, where stimulation of the motor centers initiates actions that coordinate various body movements according to the position of the head.

The receptor for dynamic equilibrium is in the crista, a crest in the membrane lining the ampulla of each semicircular canal. The cristae are stimulated by rotatory head movement (acceleration and deceleration) as a result of changes in the flow of endolymph and of movement of hair cells in the maculae. The direction of endolymph and hair cell movement is always opposite to the motion of the body.

## ASSESSING THE EAR

Data about the function of the ears and hearing are gathered both during the health assessment interview to collect subjective data and the physical assessment to collect objective data.

### Health Assessment Interview

The health history assessment to collect subjective data about the ears and hearing may be part of a health screening, may focus on a chief complaint (such as hearing problems or pain in the ear), or may be part of a total health assessment. If the

## BOX 44–2 ■ Guidelines for Using the Otoscope

The otoscope has a handle that contains batteries for the light and various specula that fit onto the handle. (See the accompanying figure.) This instrument is used to inspect the auditory canal and the tympanic membrane. A pneumatic otoscope is used to determine the mobility of the tympanic membrane. A pneumatic otoscope has an attached rubber bulb that can be squeezed to inject air into the auditory canal, causing a normal tympanic membrane to move in and out.

Before the examination, explain the procedure to the client. Assemble the otoscope, using the largest speculum that will fit into the client's auditory canal without discomfort. Wash your hands; wear disposable gloves if the client has any drainage from the ears. Turn on the otoscope light. Ask the client to tip the head slightly toward the shoulder opposite the ear being examined. When the client is in this position, the auditory canal is aligned with the speculum.

1. Hold the handle of the otoscope in your dominant hand. If the client is restless, hold the otoscope handle upward, resting the hand against the client's head. If the client is cooperative, hold the handle downward.
2. For adult clients, grasp the superior portion of the auricle and pull up, out, and back to straighten the auditory canal. (See the accompanying figure.)
3. Insert the speculum into the ear and advance it gently. Assess the walls of the auditory canal while advancing the speculum, inspecting for color, obstructions, hair growth, and cerumen. Old cerumen is very dark and may obstruct visualization of part or all of the tympanic membrane.
4. Move the otoscope so that you can see the tympanic membrane. You may need to realign the auditory canal by gently continuing to pull up and back on the auricle. A normal membrane is semitransparent, allowing visualization of a portion of the auditory ossicles. The concave nature of the tympanic membrane and its oblique position in the auditory canal account for the triangular light reflex (cone of light) seen on otoscopic examination.
5. Note the color and surface of the membrane. The normal tympanic membrane is pearly gray, shiny, and semitransparent. The surface should be continuous, intact, and either flat or concave.
6. Identify the landmarks of the tympanic membrane (see the accompanying figure):
   a. The cone of light, located over the anteroinferior quadrant.
   b. The malleus, pars tensa, annulus, pars flaccida, and malleolar folds.
7. Assess movement of the tympanic membrane. If the auditory tube is patent, the membrane moves in and out when air is injected (or when the client performs the Valsalva maneuver).
8. Gently withdraw the speculum. If the speculum is soiled with drainage or cerumen, use a clean speculum for the other ear.
9. Using the same technique, examine the other ear.

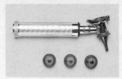

An otoscope.

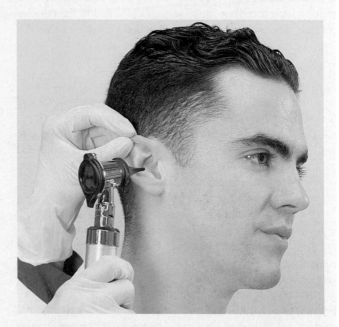

Technique for using an otoscope.

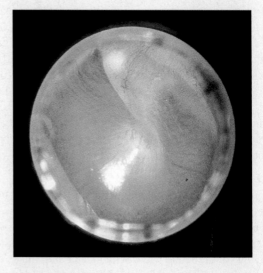

Structures of the tympanic membrane visible through the otoscope.

client has a problem involving one or both ears, analyze its onset, characteristics and course, severity, precipitating and relieving factors, and any associated symptoms, noting the timing and circumstances. For example, you may ask the following questions.

- Have you noticed any difficulty hearing high-pitched sounds, low-pitched sounds, or both?
- When did you first notice the ringing in your ears?
- Is your workplace very noisy? If so, do you wear protective ear equipment at work?

Throughout the examination, be alert to nonverbal behaviors (such as inappropriate answers or requests to repeat statements) that suggest problems with ear function. Explore changes in hearing, ringing in the ears (*tinnitus*), ear pain, drainage from the ears, or the use of hearing aids. When taking the history, ask about trauma, surgery, or infections of the ear as well as the date of the last ear examination. In addition, ask the client about a medical history of infectious diseases, such as meningitis or mumps, as well as the use of medications that may affect hearing. Because ear problems tend to run in families, ask about a family history of hearing loss, ear problems, or diseases that could result in such problems. If the client has a hearing aid, ascertain the type and assess measures for its care.

Specific questions and leading statements, categorized by functional health patterns, can be found on the Companion Website.

## Physical Assessment of the Ear and Hearing

Physical assessment of the ear and hearing may be performed as part of a total health assessment or separately for clients with known or suspected problems with the ears. The ears and hearing are assessed primarily through inspection of external structures, the external auditory canal, and the tympanic membrane. Hearing acuity is assessed by voice tests and tuning fork tests. The external structures may be palpated.

Equipment includes an otoscope and a tuning fork. The client should be sitting, and the examiner's head should be level with the head of the client. Prior to the assessment, collect all necessary equipment and explain the techniques to the client to decrease anxiety.

The auditory canal and tympanic membrane are inspected with the otoscope. Guidelines for use of the otoscope are listed on the previous page in Box 44–2.

### Hearing Assessment with Abnormal Findings (✓)

Tuning forks are used to determine whether a hearing loss is conductive or perceptive (sensorineural) (Figure 44–12 ■).

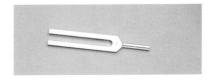

**Figure 44–12** ■ A tuning fork.

Hold the tuning fork at the base and make it ring softly by stroking the prongs or by lightly tapping them on the heel of the opposite hand. The vibrating tuning fork emits sound waves of a particular frequency, measured in Hertz (Hz). Tuning forks with a frequency of 512 to 1024 Hz are preferred for auditory evaluation, because that range corresponds to the range of normal speech.

- Perform the **Weber test.** Place the base of a vibrating tuning fork on the midline vertex of the client's head (Figure 44–13 ■). Ask whether the client hears the sound equally in both ears or better in one than the other. Sound is normally heard equally in both ears.
  ✓ Sound heard in, or lateralized to, one ear indicates either a conductive loss in that ear or a sensorineural loss in the other ear. Conductive losses may be due to a buildup of cerumen, an infection such as otitis media, or perforation of the eardrum.
- Perform the **Rinne test.** Place the base of a vibrating tuning fork on the client's mastoid bone. Ask the client to indicate when the sound is no longer heard. When the client does so, quickly reposition the tuning fork in front of the client's ear close to the ear canal. Ask whether the client can hear the sound. If the client says yes, ask the client to indicate when the sound is no longer heard. The client with no conductive hearing loss will hear the sound twice as long by air conduction as by bone conduction (Figure 44–14 ■).
  ✓ Bone conduction is greater than air conduction in the ear with a conductive loss. The normal pattern is AC>BC (air conduction greater than bone conduction).
- Perform the **whisper test.** Ask the client to occlude one ear with a finger. Stand 1 to 2 feet away from the client, on the

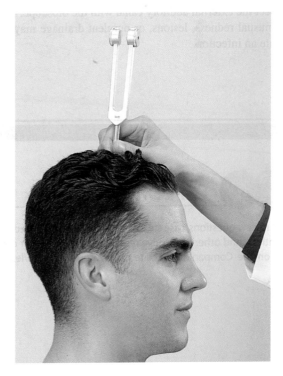

**Figure 44–13** ■ Performing the Weber test.

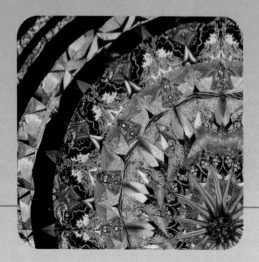

### CHAPTER 45

# Nursing Care of Clients with Eye and Ear Disorders

## MediaLink

### www.prenhall.com/lemone

Additional resources for this chapter can be found on the Student CD-ROM accompanying this textbook, and on the Companion Website at www. prenhall.com/lemone. Click on Chapter 45 to select the activities for this chapter.

**CD-ROM**
- Audio Glossary
- NCLEX Review

**Animations**
- Ear Abnormalities
- Middle Ear Dynamics
- Pilocarpine

**Companion Website**
- More NCLEX Review
- Case Study
  Retinal Detachment
- Care Plan Activity
  Hearing Aid

## LEARNING OUTCOMES

After completing this chapter, you will be able to:

- Use knowledge of normal anatomy and physiology of the eye and ear and assessments to provide care for clients with disorders of the eyes and ears (see Chapter 44).

- Describe the pathophysiology of commonly occurring disorders of the eyes and ears, relating their manifestations to the pathophysiologic process.

- Identify diagnostic tests used to diagnose eye and ear disorders.

- Discuss the nursing implications for medications prescribed for clients with eye and ear disorders.

- Provide appropriate care for the client having eye or ear surgery.

- Use the nursing process as a framework for providing care to clients with impaired vision or hearing.

Vision and hearing provide the primary means of input for much of what we know about the world. The ability to receive and organize information orients us to our surroundings. These senses allow us to communicate easily, gain access to information, and derive pleasure from the sights and sounds of the world around us.

This chapter discusses conditions affecting vision and hearing as the result of eye and ear disorders. Nursing care focuses on clients with vision and hearing deficits that can result from the disorders presented.

# EYE DISORDERS

Any portion of the eye and its protective structures may be affected by an acute or chronic condition. Disorders and diseases of the outer, visible portion of the eye often cause discomfort and may have cosmetic effects. The effect on vision can often be prevented or reversed with proper treatment of the disorder. The client who has had eye surgery or minor trauma may have either temporary or permanent visual impairment. Disorders affecting the internal structures or the function of the eye are more likely to have adverse effects on vision. Although these disorders often cannot be prevented or cured, some can be controlled and vision corrected to normal or near normal. Although many eye disorders do not pose a threat to vision, the client may perceive a threat and therefore feel anxiety.

## THE CLIENT WITH AGE-RELATED CHANGES IN VISION

Not all conditions affecting the eye are pathologic; some are associated with normal aging (See Figures 45–1 ■ and 45–2 ■). The pupil decreases in size and does not dilate readily, reducing the amount of light that reaches the retina. Night vision is affected, and increased light intensity is necessary for reading and handwork. The lens becomes less elastic, making it increasingly difficult to focus for near vision. Clients notice that "their arms have become too short" to read the newspaper comfortably. With aging, the lens discolors and opacifies, causing it to absorb more of the short wavelengths of light, resulting in a decrease in color perception. This change affects the green, blue, and violet hues in particular. Clients may tend to choose brighter colors of clothing and decor as color perception changes.

Other effects of aging on the eye include changes in the vitreous humor, atrophy of the choroid, thinning of the retina, and degenerative changes in the optic nerve (Hazzard et al., 1998). Depth perception and the ability to see lines of demarcation (e.g., the edges of steps or a change in direction of walls) diminish with age.

As the aging client loses subcutaneous tissue, the eyes may recess into the eye sockets, creating tissue folds on the upper lids. These structural changes, along with a decrease in eye mobility, can limit the older adult's vision upward and to the sides. Nurses can help the client by placing signs at eye level, not above. Checking for low-hanging objects that the client may not see can prevent head injuries.

Changes of the eye and vision commonly associated with the aging process are summarized in Table 45–1.

## THE CLIENT WITH AN INFECTIOUS OR INFLAMMATORY EYE DISORDER

The extraocular structures—the eyelids, eyelashes, and conjunctiva in particular—are vulnerable to inflammation and infection because of their constant exposure to the environment. When inflamed, these normally protective structures may perform their functions less effectively and may cause discomfort and changes in the client's appearance. The corneal reflex and tears (which contain antibodies and lysozyme, an antibacterial enzyme) protect the eye against most hazards. As tear production decreases with aging, the risk of infection increases.

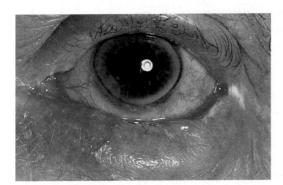

**Figure 45–1** ■ Entropion.

*Source: Science Photo Library/Photo Researchers, Inc.*

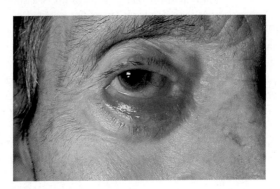

**Figure 45–2** ■ Ectropion.

*Source: Science Photo Library/Photo Researchers, Inc.*

| TABLE 45–1    Age-Related Changes in the Eye and Vision | | |
|---|---|---|
| **Physiologic Change** | **Conditions** | **Effect on Vision** |
| Changes that lead to altered protection of the eye | • Senile entropion: Inversion of the lid margins<br>• Senile ectropion: Eversion of the eyelid margin<br>• Decreased corneal sensitivity<br><br>• Decreased tear secretion | • Lashes may cause corneal irritation and damage<br>• Conjunctival exposure and possible inflammation<br>• Increased potential for damage due to foreign body or trauma<br>• Increased potential for infection or damage due to environmental pollution |
| Changes that affect vision | • Flattening of the cornea<br><br>• Pupillary constriction<br><br><br><br>• Decreased lens elasticity and increased lens density<br><br><br><br><br><br><br><br>• Loss of sensory cells at the periphery of the retina | • Reduced refractory power and decreased visual acuity<br>• Reduction in the amount of light reaching the retina to approximately one-third of previous amount (in younger years)<br>• Decreased visual acuity, affecting close vision especially<br>• Increased problems with glare (scattering of light rays)<br>• Decreased color perception, especially in blue, green, and violet spectra<br>• Decreased visual fields (peripheral vision) |
| Mechanical changes that may affect vision | • Senile enophthalmos: Sinking in of the eyes giving a "hollow-eyed" appearance<br>• Decreased eye motility | • May limit peripheral vision in all directions: to the sides, upward, and downward<br>• Increased difficulty with looking upward and convergence |
| Cosmetic changes | • Yellowing of the sclera due to fatty deposits<br>• Arcus senilis: Formation of a grayish yellow ring at the corneal margin | • None<br>• None |

# PATHOPHYSIOLOGY AND MANIFESTATIONS
## Eyelid Infections and Inflammations

The most common disorder affecting the eyelids is **marginal blepharitis,** an inflammation of the glands and lash follicles on the margins of the eyelids. This inflammatory disorder can be caused by a staphylococcal infection or it may be seborrheic in origin; commonly, both types are present. Seborrheic blepharitis is usually associated with seborrhea (dandruff) of the scalp or eyebrows. Irritation, burning, and itching of eyelid margins are common manifestations of blepharitis. The eye appears red-rimmed with mucous discharge, and there is crusting or scaling of lid margins. Lid margins may ulcerate, resulting in a loss of eyelashes.

Infection of one or more of the sebaceous glands of the eyelid may cause a **hordeolum (sty).** Hordeolum is a staphylococcal abscess that may occur on either the external or internal margin of the lid (see Figure 44–9). An external hordeolum is characterized initially by acute pain at the lid margin and redness. A small tender raised area is visible. The client may also experience photophobia, tearing, and the sensation of a foreign body in the affected eye. Internal hordeola are seen on the conjunctival side of the lid and may have more severe manifestations.

Chronic inflammation of a meibomian gland may lead to formation of a **chalazion,** a granulomatous cyst or nodule of the lid (see Figure 44–10). It presents as a hard swelling on the lid, and surrounding conjunctival tissue is reddened. Chalazion may also follow a hordeolum that was inadequately treated. Unlike a hordeolum, a chalazion is painless. It may slowly increase in size and eventually require removal, but most resolve within several months.

## Conjunctivitis

The conjunctiva lines the inner lid and covers the outer portion of the eye to the margin of the cornea. **Conjunctivitis,** inflammation of the conjunctiva, is the most common eye disease and most often results from bacterial or viral infections. These infections are usually transmitted to the eye by direct contact (e.g., hands, tissues, towels). Allergens, chemical irritants, and exposure to radiant energy such as ultraviolet light from the sun or tanning devices can also lead to this common condition. Its severity can range from mild irritation with redness and tearing to conjunctival edema, hemorrhage, or a severe necrotizing process with tissue destruction.

### Acute Conjunctivitis

Infectious conjunctivitis may be bacterial, viral, or fungal in origin. Bacterial conjunctivitis, also known as "pink eye," is highly contagious, and often is caused by *Staphylococcus* and *Haemophilus.* Adenovirus infection is the leading cause of conjunctivitis in adults. Systemic infections that may affect the eyes include herpes simplex and other viral infections. Contact with genital secretions infected with Gonococcus can cause gonococcal conjunctivitis, a medical emergency that can lead to corneal perforation.

Redness and itching of the affected eye are common manifestations of acute conjunctivitis (Figure 45–3 ■). The client may also complain of a scratchy, burning, or gritty sensation. Pain is not common; however, photophobia may occur. Tearing

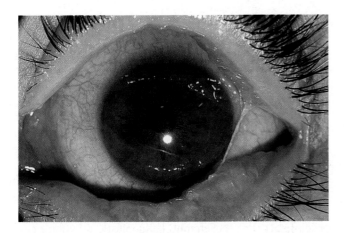

**Figure 45–3** ■ The appearance of an eye with conjunctivitis.

*Source: Buddy Crofton/Medical Images, Inc.*

and discharge accompany the inflammatory process. The discharge may be watery, purulent, or mucoid, depending on the cause of conjunctivitis. The client may have associated manifestations such as pharyngitis, fever, malaise, and swollen preauricular lymph nodes.

## Trachoma

**Trachoma,** a chronic conjunctivitis caused by *Chlamydia trachomatis,* is a significant preventable cause of blindness worldwide that remains endemic in sub-Saharan Africa, the Middle East, and parts of Asia. In the United States, it can be found in Native Americans of the Southwest, but less frequently. Trachoma is contagious, transmitted primarily by close personal contact (eye-to-eye, hand-to-eye) or by fomites such as towels, handkerchiefs, and flies. Certain forms of trachoma are transmitted during delivery when the newborn is exposed to contaminated genital secretions of the mother (Braunwald et al, 2001).

Early manifestations of trachoma include redness, eyelid edema, tearing, and photophobia. Small conjunctival follicles develop on the upper lids. The inflammation also causes superficial corneal vascularization and infiltration with granulation tissue. Scarring of the conjunctival lining of the lid causes entropion (see Figure 45–1). The lashes then abrade the cornea, eventually causing ulceration and scarring. The scarred cornea is opaque, resulting in loss of vision.

## Corneal Infections and Inflammations

The clear cornea allows light rays to enter the eye and transmits images onto the retina. It helps to focus light on the retina and protects the internal eye structures. The cornea has three major layers: the outermost epithelium, which consists of five or six layers of cells that are constantly being renewed; the stroma, which makes up 90% of corneal tissue; and the single-cell thickness endothelium adjacent to the aqueous humor of the anterior chamber. The cornea is avascular tissue; the central cornea is dependent on atmospheric oxygen to meet its metabolic needs. Because there is no blood supply, immune defenses have difficulty fending off infections of the cornea.

Corneal scarring or ulceration are two major causes of blindness worldwide.

### Keratitis

**Keratitis** is an inflammation of the cornea and may be caused by many of the microorganisms that cause conjunctivitis. Other causes include hypersensitivity reactions, ischemia, tearing defects, trauma, and interrupted sensory innervation of the cornea (Porth, 2002). Keratitis is described as either ulcerative or nonulcerative. Ulcerative keratitis causes inflammation and ulceration of the cornea, resulting in altered visual acuity. Inflammation that involves only the epithelial layer of the cornea is nonulcerative and does not destroy the cornea or visual acuity. When the inflammatory process involves both the conjunctiva and the cornea, the term *keratoconjunctivitis* may be used.

### Corneal Ulcer

A **corneal ulcer,** local necrosis of the cornea, may be caused by infection, exposure trauma, or the misuse of contact lenses. A frequent cause is bacterial infection following trauma or contact lens overuse. Herpes viruses, including herpes simplex and herpes zoster, are a leading cause of ulcerative corneal disease. Corneal ulcers may also complicate bacterial conjunctivitis, trachoma, gonorrhea, and other acute infections. Clients who are immunosuppressed because of disease or drug therapy are at particular risk for developing corneal ulcers due to infection.

In corneal ulceration, a portion of the epithelium and/or stroma is destroyed. Ulcers may be superficial or deep, penetrating underlying layers and posing a risk of perforation. Fibrous tissue may form during healing, resulting in scarring and opacity of the cornea. Perforation can lead to infection of deeper eye structures or extrusion of eye contents. Partial or total vision loss may result.

When the cornea becomes inflamed, the client commonly experiences tearing, discomfort ranging from a gritty sensation in the eye to severe pain, decreased visual acuity, and blepharospasm (spasm of the eyelid and inability to open the eye). A discharge may be present, especially if the conjunctiva is also inflamed. Corneal ulceration may be visible on direct examination.

## Uveitis and Iritis

The middle vascular layer of the eye, including the choroid, the ciliary body, and the iris, is known as the uvea and uveal tract. **Uveitis** is inflammation of all or part of this vascular layer. **Iritis,** inflammation of the iris only, occurs more commonly than uveitis.

Uveitis is usually a disease limited to the eye; it may be idiopathic or caused by an autoimmune process, infection, parasitic disease, or trauma. Approximately 40% of cases can be linked to a systemic disease, often an arthritic or autoimmune disorder such as ankylosing spondylitis, Reiter's syndrome, rheumatoid arthritis, or sarcoidosis (see Chapter 39). Uveitis has also been linked with tuberculosis and syphilis.

Manifestations of uveitis include pupillary constriction and erythema around the limbus. The client may complain of severe eye pain and photophobia, as well as blurred vision.

## COLLABORATIVE CARE

Management of the client with an infectious or inflammatory eye disorder is directed toward establishing an accurate diagnosis and prompt treatment to reduce the risk of permanent vision deficit.

The history and physical assessment are key in diagnosing these disorders. The diagnosis can often be made based on clinical manifestations without using any diagnostic procedures. Accurate diagnosis of conjunctivitis is especially important, because other potentially vision-threatening conditions, such as acute uveitis or acute angle-closure glaucoma, can also cause a red eye. Although many eye disorders can be treated in an outpatient clinic, the client with a severe corneal infection or ulcer may require hospitalization. Corneal ulcers are medical emergencies, requiring prompt referral to an ophthalmologist for treatment. Pressure dressings may be applied to both eyes for comfort and to reduce the risk of perforation and loss of eye contents.

### Diagnostic Tests

The following tests may be ordered to identify the cause and extent of eye infections or inflammations.

- *Fluorescein stain* with slit lamp examination allows visualization of any corneal ulcerations or abrasions, which appear green with staining.
- *Conjunctival or ulcer scrapings* are examined microscopically or cultured to identify the organisms.

Additional laboratory testing such as blood counts or antibody titers may be used to identify any underlying infectious or autoimmune processes.

### Medication

Infectious processes involving the lids, conjunctiva, or cornea are treated with antibiotic or antiviral therapy as appropriate. Topical anti-infectives applied as either eye drops or ointment may include erythromycin, gentamicin, penicillin, bacitracin, sulfacetamide sodium, amphotericin B, or idoxuridine. For severe infections, central ulcers, or cellulitis, anti-infectives may be administered by subconjunctival injection and/or systemic intravenous infusion.

Antihistamines are used to minimize symptoms of conjunctivitis when an allergic response underlies the inflammatory process. Corticosteroids may be prescribed for keratitis related to systemic inflammatory disorders or trauma; however, it is important to avoid their use with local infections to avoid suppressing the immune and inflammatory responses. Immunosuppressive therapy with azathioprine (Imuran) or cyclosporine (Sandimmune) may be used to suppress the inflammatory response in clients with severe uveitis. Atropine may also be prescribed for the client with associated inflammation of the iris. The client may require analgesics such as acetaminophen and/or codeine for pain management.

### Corneal Transplant

Once the cornea has become scarred and opaque, no treatment can restore its clarity. The first successful corneal transplant (or *keratoplasty*), replacement of diseased cornea by healthy corneal tissue from a donor, was performed in 1906. Current corneal transplant procedures have a success rate of approximately 90%.

Corneas are harvested from the cadavers of uninfected adults who were under the age of 65 and who died as a result of acute trauma or illness. After harvesting, the cornea can be stored in a tissue-culture medium for up to 4 weeks before being used as a graft. Corneal transplantation is usually an elective surgery, although emergency transplantation may be required for perforation of the cornea.

Corneal transplant may be either lamellar or penetrating. In a lamellar keratoplasty, the superficial layer of cornea is removed and replaced with a graft. The anterior chamber remains intact. In a penetrating keratoplasty, a button or full thickness of cornea is removed and replaced by donor tissue (Figure 45–4 ■). The graft is then sutured in place using suture finer than human hair and a continuous or interrupted stitch. Because the cornea is avascular, these sutures remain in place for up to a year to ensure healing.

Most corneal transplants are performed on an outpatient basis, and clients do not generally require hospitalization. The eye is patched for 24 hours following surgery. Narcotic analgesia may be required initially, because the cornea is extremely sensitive. Corticosteroid eye drops are ordered to reduce the in-

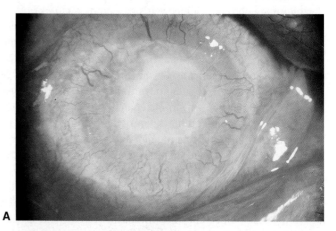

A

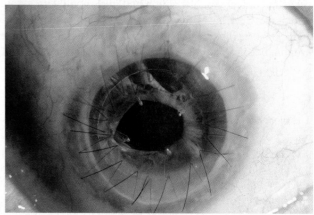

B

**Figure 45–4** ■ Corneal transplant. *A,* The diseased, opaque cornea. *B,* The diseased cornea is removed and a corneal graft is sutured in place using material finer than a human hair.

*Source: Custom Medical Stock Photo, Inc.*

flammatory response to surgery, preventing edema of the graft. Antibiotic drops may also be prescribed to prevent infection.

The risk of transplant rejection is low in this procedure. Because the cornea is avascular, there is little exposure of the transplanted corneal tissue to the host's immune defenses (Porth,

2002). When rejection does occur, it occurs within 3 weeks of the transplant, beginning with inflammation at the edge of the grafted tissue and spreading to involve the entire graft.

See the box below for nursing care of the client undergoing eye surgery.

## NURSING CARE OF THE CLIENT HAVING EYE SURGERY

### PREOPERATIVE CARE

- Review Chapter 7 ⊝ for routine preoperative care.
- Assess the visual acuity of the client's nonoperative eye prior to surgery. *The client with limited visual acuity in the nonoperative eye may need additional assistance and attention in the postoperatively to ensure safety and maintain ADLs.*
- Assess the client's support systems and the possible effect of impaired vision on lifestyle and ability to perform ADLs in the postoperative period. *Vision in the operative eye may be impaired during the postoperative period, limiting the client's depth perception and mobility. Safety measures such as installing handrails and removing throw rugs in the client's home are often useful, especially if the client has limited vision in the unaffected eye.*
- Teach the client measures to prevent eye injury postoperatively. The client should avoid vomiting, straining at stool, coughing, sneezing, lifting more than 5 lb, and bending over at the waist. *These activities increase intraocular pressure temporarily and may be associated with postoperative complications.*
- Remove all eye makeup and contact lenses or glasses prior to surgery. Store them in a safe place. Have glasses readily available for the client on return from surgery. *Maintaining visual acuity in the unaffected eye helps reduce the client's fear and maintain safety.*
- Administer preoperative medications and eye drops or ointments as prescribed. *Mydriatic (pupil-dilating) or cycloplegic (ciliary-paralytic) drops and drops to lower intraocular pressure may be prescribed preoperatively. Preanesthetic medications may also be ordered.*

### POSTOPERATIVE CARE

- Review Chapter 7 for routine postoperative care.
- Monitor status of the eye dressing following surgery. *Assess dressings for the presence of bleeding or drainage from the eye, as either could indicate a surgical complication.*
- Maintain the eye patch or eye shield in place. *The eye patch or shield helps prevent inadvertent injury to the operative site.*
- Place the client in a semi-Fowler's or Fowler's position, having the client lie on the unaffected side. *These positions reduce intraocular pressure in the affected eye.*
- After surgery for a detached retina, the client is positioned so that the detachment is dependent or inferior. For example, if the outer portion of the left retina is detached, the client is positioned on the left side. *Positioning so that the detachment is inferior maintains pressure on that area of the retina, improving its contact with the choroid.*
- Assess the client, and medicate or assist to avoid vomiting, coughing, sneezing, or straining as needed. *These activities increase intraocular pressure.*
- Assess comfort and medicate as necessary for complaints of an aching or scratchy sensation in affected eye. Immediately report any complaint of sudden, sharp eye pain to the physician. *An*

*abrupt increase in or onset of eye pain may indicate hemorrhage or other ocular emergency requiring immediate intervention to preserve sight.*
- Assess for potential surgical complications:
  a. Pain in or drainage from the affected eye
  b. Hemorrhage with blood in the anterior chamber of the eye
  c. Flashes of light, floaters, or the sensation of a curtain being drawn over the eye (indicators of retinal detachment)
  d. Cloudy appearance to the cornea (corneal edema)
  *Evidence of any of the above manifestations or unusual complaints by the client should be reported to the physician at once. Early intervention is often necessary to preserve sight.*
- Approach the client on the unaffected side. *This approach facilitates eye contact and communication.*
- Place all personal articles and the call bell within easy reach. *These measures prevent stretching and straining by the client.*
- Assist with ambulation and personal care activities as needed. *Assistance may be necessary to maintain safety.*
- Administer antibiotic, anti-inflammatory, and other systemic and eye medications as prescribed. *Medications are prescribed postoperatively to prevent infection or inflammation of the operative site, maintain pupil constriction, and control intraocular pressure.*
- Administer antiemetic medication as needed. *It is important to prevent vomiting to maintain normal intraocular pressures.*

### Client and Family Teaching
- Teach the client and family about home care.
  a. The proper way to instill eye drops
  b. The name, dosage, schedule, duration, purpose, and side effects of postoperative medications
  c. The proper use of the eye patch and eye shield
  d. The need to avoid scratching, rubbing, touching, or squeezing the affected eye
  e. Measures to avoid constipation and straining, and activity limitations
  f. Symptoms that should be reported to the physician, including eye pain or pressure, redness or cloudiness, drainage, decreased vision, floaters or flashes of light, or halos around bright objects
  g. The need to wear sunglasses with side shields when outdoors. *Photophobia is common after eye surgery.*
- Remind the client that vision may not stabilize for several weeks following eye surgery. New corrective lenses, if necessary, are not prescribed until vision has stabilized. The client should make and keep recommended follow-up appointments with the physician. *Clients may be alarmed that vision seems worse after surgery than before and need reassurance that visual acuity usually improves with time and healing of the affected eye.*
- Provide referral to a community home health agency for assistance with home care after discharge as needed.

## Complementary Therapies

Careful cleansing of the lid margins using a "no-tears" baby shampoo is often recommended for marginal blepharitis. Soaking the lids with warm saline compresses prior to cleansing facilitates the removal of crusts and exudate in blepharitis or conjunctivitis. Frequent eye irrigations may be ordered to remove the copious purulent discharge associated with conjunctivitis. Local heat applications may be used to treat hordeolum or chalazion; excision and drainage may be required if this is not effective.

## NURSING CARE

The nursing role in management of clients with infections and inflammatory eye disorders may involve direct care, but more often focuses on prevention and providing education. Nurses working in clinics and outpatient surgical settings care for clients undergoing corneal transplant.

## Health Promotion

Education is a vital strategy for preventing infectious and inflammatory eye disorders. Teach all clients about proper eye care, including the importance of not sharing towels and makeup and avoiding rubbing or scratching the eyes as well as preventing trauma and infection. Emphasize the importance of not using old eye makeup, which can cause eye infections. Teach contact lens users appropriate care and cleaning techniques. Stress the importance of periodic removal of lenses, even extended-wear lenses. In general, lenses should be removed at night, even though manufacturers may claim it is safe to wear them while sleeping. Emphasize the need to follow cleaning instructions precisely to avoid bacterial contamination of lenses and possible corneal infection. If the client experiences a corneal abrasion or keratitis, instruct the client to avoid wearing contact lenses until the cornea has healed completely.

## Assessment

Collect the following data through health history and physical examination (see Chapter 44). Additional focused assessments are described with the interventions below. When assessing an older client, be aware of normal changes associated with aging (see Table 45–1).

- Health history: risk factors; presence of redness, discomfort, tearing, photophobia, edema, and drainage; symptom onset
- Physical assessment: visual acuity; inspect eyelids, conjunctiva, sclera, and cornea; extraocular movements

## Nursing Diagnoses and Interventions

Nursing care focuses primarily on preventing complications from the underlying infectious or inflammatory eye disorder. The priority nursing diagnoses include risk of altered vision, pain, and risk for injury.

### Risk for Disturbed Sensory Perception: Visual

Disorders affecting the conjunctiva or cornea may disrupt the integrity or clarity of these structures. Because the cornea plays a vital role in focusing light on the retina, corneal damage can affect vision, impairing visual acuity and even causing legal blindness.

- Assess vision with and without corrective lenses. *Assessment provides a baseline to evaluate possible changes in vision resulting from the inflammatory disorder or therapy.*
- Instruct about thorough handwashing before inserting or removing contact lenses or instilling any eye medications. Teach to avoid touching or rubbing the eyes. Instruct to use a new, clean cotton-tipped swab or cotton ball for cleaning each eye. *Handwashing is the single most important measure to prevent transmission of infection to the eye. Touching or rubbing the eyes increases the risk of infection and corneal trauma. Using a new swab or cotton ball prevents cross-contamination between eyes.*
- Emphasize the importance of proper care of contact lenses specific to the type of lens used. *Clients who wear hard contact lenses must remove them daily, because the central cornea needs exposure to atmospheric oxygen. Although soft and extended-wear lenses allow the cornea to "breathe," improper cleaning carries a major risk for infection.*
- Teach the importance of using eye protection when engaging in potentially dangerous activities. *Trauma increases the risk of infection and scarring of the cornea.*

**PRACTICE ALERT** *Suspect corneal perforation with complaints of sudden, severe eye pain and photophobia.* ∎

- If corneal perforation is suspected, place in the supine position, close the eye, and cover it with a dry, sterile dressing. Notify the physician immediately. *Corneal perforation may occur without warning in clients with corneal ulcers and places the client at risk for loss of eye contents. Emergency measures are taken to reduce intraocular pressure and maintain eye integrity to preserve vision.*

### Acute Pain

The cornea of the eye is extremely sensitive. Corneal disorders frequently cause significant pain. Pain, in turn, increases the client's stress response and interferes with rest, potentially impairing healing.

- Assess pain, using verbal and nonverbal cues. *Pain is a subjective experience and can be evaluated only by the client's response and in terms of its effect on the client.*
- Administer prescribed analgesia routinely in the first 12 to 24 hours after corneal surgery. *Routine administration of analgesics prevents pain from reaching a level of severity at which it becomes difficult to relieve.*
- Patch both eyes if necessary. *Patching both eyes reduces eye movement and irritation of the affected eye.*

- Teach to apply warm compresses to reduce inflammation and pain. *Warm compresses for 15 minutes, three to four times a day, promote comfort for clients with keratitis or corneal injury.*
- Instruct to use dark sunglasses with appropriate UV protection when out of doors, even on cloudy days. *True photophobia, often associated with corneal disorders, causes eye pain with increased light intensity.*
- Teach to instill prescribed eyedrops as ordered. *Prescribed medications may reduce inflammation and eliminate infection, reducing discomfort.*

### Risk for Injury

The client who has undergone corneal transplantation has an increased risk for injury for several reasons. The eye on which surgery was performed is patched for 24 hours after surgery, changing the client's depth perception and increasing the risk for falls. Increased intraocular pressure or trauma to the eye may damage the graft, resulting in graft rejection.

- Instruct to call for help before getting up or ambulating after surgery. Ensure access to the call light. *It may take time for the client to adjust to changes in depth perception caused by the eye patch. Assistance helps prevent falls that may not only injure the client but also traumatize the operative site.*

> **PRACTICE ALERT** *Administer prescribed antiemetics and stool softeners postoperatively to prevent vomiting and straining at stool, activities that increase intraocular pressure, damaging suture lines.* ∎

- Encourage to deep breathe and use the incentive spirometer to promote lung expansion. *These important postoperative measures help prevent pulmonary complications. Coughing is avoided because it increases intraocular pressure.*
- Teach how to apply an eye shield at night after the eye patch is removed. *An eye shield may be recommended at night to prevent inadvertent rubbing or trauma to the eye during sleep.*
- Instruct not to rub or scratch the eye. *Rubbing or scratching may disrupt suture lines or damage the grafted tissue.*
- Reinforce the importance of using eye protection during hazardous activities. *Following a corneal transplant, the client has the same risk of eye injury as other people who perform hazardous activities.*

### Using NANDA, NIC, and NOC

Chart 45–1 shows links between NANDA nursing diagnoses, NIC, and NOC when caring for the client with infectious or inflammatory eye conditions.

### Home Care

Following medical treatment for infectious or inflammatory eye conditions, teach clients to manage these conditions at home. Emphasize to the family ways to prevent transmission of infection. If the client is unable to administer eye medications or to perform other eye care techniques, involve the family in the teaching session. The following topics should be included.

- Safety and medical asepsis when cleansing the eye
- Instillation of prescribed eye drops and ointments
- Application of an eye patch and where to obtain supplies
- Avoidance of activities such as excessive reading while eye inflamed
- Follow-up appointments after corneal transplant surgery
- Signs of graft rejection
- Avoidance of activities that increase intraocular pressure such as straining, coughing, sneezing, bending over, lifting heavy objects
- Helpful resources:
  - National Eye Institute
  - Lighthouse National Center for Vision and Aging

## THE CLIENT WITH EYE TRAUMA

Over 2 million eye injuries occur each year. Many eye injuries are minor, but without timely and appropriate intervention, even a minor injury can threaten vision. For this reason, all eye injuries should be considered medical emergencies requiring immediate evaluation and intervention.

## PATHOPHYSIOLOGY AND MANIFESTATIONS

Any part of the eye, especially the exposed parts, may be affected by trauma. Foreign bodies, abrasions, and lacerations are the most common types of eye injury. Traumatic injury may also be due to a burn, penetrating objects, or blunt force.

### CHART 45–1 NANDA, NIC, AND NOC LINKAGES

#### The Client with an Infectious or Inflammatory Eye Disorder

| NURSING DIAGNOSES | NURSING INTERVENTIONS | NURSING OUTCOMES |
|---|---|---|
| • Disturbed Sensory Perception<br>• Ineffective Health Maintenance | • Surveillance: Safety<br>• Health Education | • Vision Compensation Behavior<br>• Health-Promoting Behavior |

*Note. Data from Nursing Outcomes Classification (NOC) by M. Johnson & M. Maas (Eds.), 1997, St. Louis: Mosby; Nursing Diagnoses: Definitions & Classification 2001–2002 by North American Nursing Diagnosis Association, 2001, Philadelphia: NANDA; Nursing Interventions Classification (NIC) by J.C. McCloskey & G. M. Bulechek (Eds.), 2000, St. Louis: Mosby. Reprinted by permission.*

**Corn**

Disrupt
a corne
sion in
such as
and che

Supe
general
phobia
stroma
increase

**Burns**

The out
by heat
most co
eye. An
drain cle
often im
stances
chemica
sive dan
ally caus

Explo
thermal
corneal
pending
be know
arc burn,

In add
a caustic
of eye p
Burns ma
eye may
is redder
larly with
hazy, and

**Penetr**

Perforatic
flakes or
grinding,
eye. Gun
trate the e
taneously
or small r
ily appare
the layers
resulting
contents (

Penetr
swelling o
that comn
wound to
tissue for
or comple
of eye con

# THE CLIENT WITH REFRACTIVE ERRORS

Refractive errors are the most common problem affecting visual acuity; they result from an alteration in the shape of the eyeball, an abnormal curvature of the cornea, or a change in the lens focusing power. People with **emmetropia** see near and far objects clearly because light rays focus directly on the retina. In **myopia** (nearsightedness) the eyeball is elongated, causing the image to focus in front of the retina instead of on it. Objects in close range are seen clearly and those at a distant are blurred. The eyeball is short in **hyperopia** (farsightedness), causing the image to focus behind the retina. People with this condition see objects clearer at a distance than those close to them.

With age, the elasticity of the lens decreases, leading to loss of accommodation; the resultant condition is **presbyopia.** The client cannot see close objects without reading glasses. **Astigmatism** develops with abnormal curvature of the cornea or eyeball, causing the image to focus at multiple points on the retina.

Eye glasses or contact lenses provide nonsurgical correction of refractive errors. Corrections can be combined for several errors such as myopia and astigmatism. Newer surgical techniques such as laser in situ keratomileusis (LASIK) reshape the cornea to correct refractive errors. It is performed in an outpatient surgery center. Operative risks are for postoperative infection and corneal scarring; in addition, the limitations of the correction are discussed with the client. Postoperatively the nurse administers antibiotics and analgesics and prepares the client for self-care at home.

# THE CLIENT WITH CATARACTS

A **cataract** is an opacification (clouding) of the lens of the eye. This opacification can significantly interfere with light transmission to the retina and the ability to perceive images clearly.

## PATHOPHYSIOLOGY

Cataracts are a common and significant cause of visual deficits in the elderly. It is estimated that 50% to 70% of people over the age of 65 have some degree of cataract formation; however, only a small percentage of those have impaired vision as a result of the cataract. This population accounts for more than 1.35 million cataract surgeries in the United States yearly (Porth, 2002).

The majority of cataracts are senile cataracts, formed as a result of the normal aging process. As the lens ages, its fibers and proteins change and degenerate, losing clarity. This process generally begins at the periphery of the lens, gradually spreading to involve the central portion. As the cataract continues to develop, the entire lens may become opaque. When only a portion of the lens is affected, the cataract is called immature. A mature cataract is opacity of the entire lens.

Several risk factors for senile cataracts have been identified. Long-term exposure to sunlight (UV-B rays) contributes; cigarette smoking and heavy alcohol consumption are associated with earlier cataract development. Although senile cataracts are by far the most common, cataracts also may be congenital or acquired in origin. Eye trauma, including injury to the lens capsule by a foreign body, blunt trauma, or exposure to heat or radiation, can precipitate cataract formation. Other factors implicated include inflammation of the eye and some systemic diseases. Diabetes mellitus is associated with earlier development of cataracts, especially when the blood glucose level is not carefully controlled at normal or near normal levels. Certain drugs such as corticosteroids, chlorpromazine (Thorazine), and busulfan (Myleran), when taken systemically, may also prompt the formation of cataracts.

## MANIFESTATIONS

Cataracts tend to occur bilaterally unless related to eye trauma. Fortunately, their development is usually not symmetric, and one cataract generally matures more rapidly than the other. As a cataract matures and interferes with light transmission through the lens, the client experiences decreased visual acuity, affecting both close and distance vision. Light rays are scattered as they pass through the lens, causing the client to complain of glare. Because of the increased glare, the client also has difficulty adjusting between light and dark environments. The client also describes an inability to distinguish between color hues. In the client with a mature cataract, the pupil may appear cloudy gray or white rather than black.

# COLLABORATIVE CARE

The diagnosis of a cataract is made based on the history and eye examination with the Snellen vision test. Ophthalmoscopic examination confirms the diagnosis by identifying the location and extent of a cataract. As the cataract matures, ophthalmoscopy reveals a dark area instead of the red reflex. Surgical removal is the only treatment used at this time for cataracts; no medical treatment is available to prevent or treat them. If the client presents with bilateral cataracts, surgery is only performed on one eye at a time. If an intraocular lens (an artificial lens to replace the diseased lens of the eye) is to be implanted during surgery, the corneal curvature and anteroposterior diameter of the eye are measured prior to surgery to determine the lens power needed for the intraocular lens implant.

Surgical removal of the cataract and lens is indicated when the cataract has developed to the point that vision and activities of daily living are affected. A mature cataract may also be removed when it causes a secondary condition such as glaucoma or uveitis.

Cataract surgery is usually done on an outpatient basis, using local anesthesia. If general anesthesia is required, the client may be hospitalized overnight. Using an operating microscope, the surgeon makes a small incision at the edge of the cornea and extracts the lens using either forceps or a supercooled probe (cryoextraction), or emulsification and aspiration. In the latter technique, ultrasound vibrations are used to break the lens material into fragments (phacoemulsification), which are then suctioned out of the eye.

The entire lens and its surrounding capsule may be removed in a procedure called intracapsular extraction (Figure 45–5A ■). Extracapsular extraction is the most common procedure presently used to treat cataracts. It involves removal of the nucleus and cortex of the lens, leaving the posterior capsule intact (Figure 45–5B). The remaining capsule supports the lens implant and protects the retina. An additional advantage to extracapsular lens removal is the smaller incision required.

After removal of the lens, the eye can no longer focus light on the retina, and vision is seriously affected. Usually a polymethylmethacrylate (PMMA or Plexiglas) intraocular lens is implanted at the time of surgery to provide for light refraction and restore visual acuity. This implant rapidly restores binocular vision and depth perception. An anterior chamber lens implant is used following intracapsular lens removal. In an anterior chamber implant, the lens is lodged in the anterior chamber of the eye, resting over the pupil. In a posterior implant, the lens is positioned in the posterior capsule to restore vision following an extracapsular lens extraction. The posterior chamber lens is positioned behind the iris and stabilized by the remaining posterior capsule.

For some clients, convex corrective glasses or contact lenses may be used instead of intraocular lens implants to correct vision after cataract removal. Although contact lenses can provide excellent vision correction following cataract surgery, they may be difficult for some clients to adapt to or manipulate. The client with a preexisting refractive error may continue to require corrective lenses and often needs a prescriptive change after surgery.

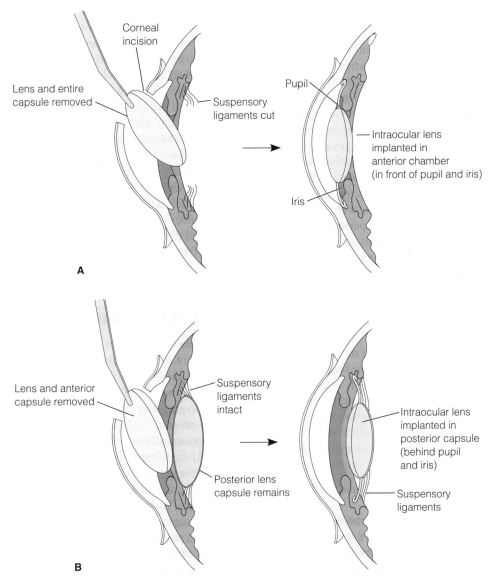

**Figure 45–5** ■ Cataract removal with intraocular lens implant. *A,* Intracapsular cataract extraction with removal of the entire lens and capsule. The intraocular lens is implanted in the eye's anterior chamber. *B,* Extracapsular cataract extraction with removal of the lens and anterior capsule, leaving the posterior capsule intact. The intraocular lens is implanted within posterior capsule.

TABLE 45-2    A Comparison of Open-Angle and Angle-Closure Glaucoma

| | Open-Angle Glaucoma | Angle-Closure Glaucoma |
|---|---|---|
| Incidence | • Common<br>• Accounts for 90% of all cases of glaucoma | • Uncommon |
| Risk Factors | • Over age 35<br>• Genetic link<br>• African American ancestry | • Narrow anterior chamber angle<br>• Aging<br>• Asian ancestry |
| Pathophysiology | • Impaired aqueous outflow through the canal of Schlemm<br>• Cause unknown<br>• Gradual, consistent increase in intraocular pressure<br>• Usually bilateral | • Pupil dilation or lens accommodation causes already narrowed angle to close, blocking aqueous outflow<br>• Rapid rise in intraocular pressure<br>• Usually unilateral |
| Manifestations | • No initial manifestations<br>• Frequent lens changes in glasses<br>• Impaired dark adaptation<br>• Halos around lights<br>• Gradual reduction of visual fields with preservation of central vision until late in the disease<br>• Mild to severe increased intraocular pressure | • Abrupt onset of eye pain, headache<br>• Decreased visual acuity<br>• Nausea and vomiting<br>• Reddened conjunctiva<br>• Cloudy cornea<br>• Fixed pupil<br>• Rapid, significant increase in intraocular pressure |
| Management | • Topical medications such as miotics, betablockers, prostaglandin analogues<br>• Carbonic anhydrase inhibitors<br>• Laser trabeculoplasty, trabeculectomy | • Topical miotics or betablockers<br>• Systemic osmotic agents, carbonic anhydrase inhibitors<br>• Laser iridotomy or peripheral iridectomy |

## Angle-Closure Glaucoma

Acute angle-closure (also called narrow-angle or closed-angle) glaucoma is the other, less common form of primary glaucoma in adults. It accounts for approximately 5% to 10% of all cases of glaucoma (Porth, 2002).

Approximately 1% of people over the age of 35 have narrowed anterior chamber angles; the incidence is higher in older adults and in people of Asian ancestry. Narrowing of the anterior chamber angle occurs because of corneal flattening or bulging of the iris into the anterior chamber. When the lens thickens during accommodation or the iris thickens during pupil dilation, this angle can close completely. Closure of the angle blocks the outflow of aqueous humor through the trabecular meshwork and canal of Schlemm, and the intraocular pressure rises abruptly (Figure 45-7B). This abrupt increase in intraocular pressure damages the neurons of the retina and the optic nerve, leading to a rapid and permanent loss of vision if not treated promptly.

Episodes of angle-closure glaucoma are typically unilateral. However, in clients who have had angle-closure glaucoma of one eye, the other eye is at increased risk in the future.

Because of the effect of pupil dilation on aqueous outflow in angle-closure glaucoma, episodes often occur in association with darkness, emotional upset, or other factors that cause the pupil to dilate. Clients may have intermittent episodes lasting several hours before having a more typical prolonged attack of angle-closure glaucoma. For clients with a history of the condition, it is vital to avoid medications such as atropine and other anticholinergics, which have a mydriatic or pupil-dilating effect.

### Manifestations

Symptoms such as severe eye and face pain, general malaise, nausea and vomiting, seeing colored halos around lights, and an abrupt decrease in visual acuity are associated with acute episodes of angle-closure glaucoma. The conjunctiva of the affected eye may be reddened and the cornea clouded with corneal edema. The pupil may be fixed (nonreactive to light) at midpoint.

## COLLABORATIVE CARE

Although glaucoma cannot be predicted, prevented, or cured, in most cases it can be controlled and vision preserved if diagnosed early. Because the most prevalent type of glaucoma, open-angle, has few symptoms, routine eye examinations are recommended for early detection. Measurement of intraocular pressure, fundoscopy to assess the optic disk, and visual field testing are used for diagnosis and monitoring of treatment effectiveness.

### Diagnostic Tests

The following diagnostic studies are used to detect and evaluate for the presence, severity, type, and effects of glaucoma.

• *Tonometry* indirectly measures intraocular pressure. Either contact or noncontact tonometry may be used. In contact tonometry, the eye is anesthetized, and the force needed to produce an indentation in the cornea is measured using a Schiötz tonometer (Figure 45-8 ■) or a Goldmann applanation tonometer. Noncontact tonometry measures the time required to flatten the cornea with a puff of air to determine the

M

Th

CA

Th
are
lar
giv

N
•

•

as n
cho
the

Su

Sur
clos
glat

vol
teri
filtr

a g
arou
the
wor
bec
pati

mai
teri
rem
nel
jun
und
tem
gen

coa
usi
tior
pro
ocu
of a
aqu

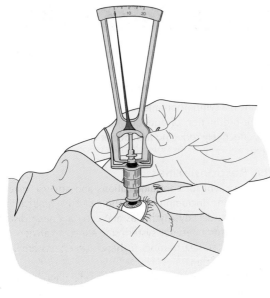

**Figure 45–8** ■ The Schiötz tonometer for measuring intraocular pressure.

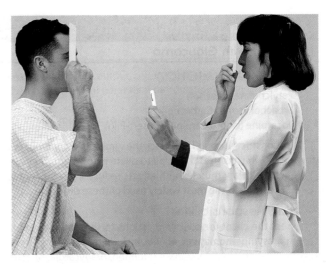

**Figure 45–9** ■ Visual field testing. Peripheral vision or visual fields are assessed by testing the client's ability to detect an object brought into the line of vision from the periphery. The client's peripheral vision is compared to the nurse examiner's. Each eye is tested separately.

intraocular pressure. No anesthesia is needed. Routine tonometry screening is recommended for all people over the age of 60. A single elevated pressure reading does not warrant a diagnosis of glaucoma; variations in intraocular pressure occur throughout the day.

• *Fundoscopy* identifies pallor and an increase in the size and depth of the optic cup on the optic disk. These changes are significant for diagnosing glaucoma.
• *Gonioscopy* uses a goniscope to measure the depth of the anterior chamber. This test differentiates open-angle from angle-closure glaucoma.
• *Visual field testing* (Figure 45–9 ■) identifies the degree of central visual field narrowing and peripheral vision loss. The client with glaucoma may retain 20/20 central vision even though there is severe peripheral vision loss.

## Medications

Although medications cannot cure glaucoma, many clients with open-angle glaucoma can control intraocular pressure and preserve vision indefinitely with medications. Medications are used alone or in combination with the timing and dosage individually determined by pressure measurements. The primary pharmacologic agents used to treat glaucoma are the cholinergics (miotics), adrenergics (mydriatics), beta-adrenergic blocking agents, carbonic anhydrase inhibitors, and prostaglandin analogs.

Cholinergics or miotics (pilocarpine, carbachol) cause contraction of the sphincter of the iris, constricting the pupil, and contraction of the ciliary muscle that promotes accommodation for near vision. The net effect is to facilitate aqueous humor outflow by increasing drainage through the trabecular meshwork in open-angle glaucoma. In angle-closure glaucoma, pupillary constriction flattens the iris, opening the angle and the canal of Schlemm. Miotics are administered topically as

drops, with the dose and frequency dependent on the preparation prescribed and the client response.

The adrenergic agonists epinephrine and dipivefrin may be prescribed along with miotics to counteract the effect of the miotic on accommodation. Epinephrine decreases the production of aqueous humor by the ciliary body, further reducing the intraocular pressure.

Timolol (Timoptic) is a beta-adrenergic blocking agent that also acts to decrease the production of aqueous humor in the ciliary body. Beta-adrenergic blockers have a longer duration of activity than the miotics, allowing fewer doses per day. When administering beta blockers or teaching a client about their use, it is important to remember that ophthalmic preparations can produce the systemic effects of other beta blockers, including bronchospasm, bradycardia, and heart failure.

Dorzolamide (Trusopt), a carbonic anhydrase inhibitor, decreases the production of aqueous humor and reduces intraocular pressure. It is used with other drugs to control pressures and in clients for whom beta blockers are contraindicated because of heart failure or reactive airway disease. Acetazolamide (Diamox), a systemic carbonic anhydrase inhibitor, also may be used for some clients.

Prostaglandin analogs such as latanoprost (Xalatan) are a newer class of ophthalmics prescribed to increase aqueous outflow. They are similar to beta blockers in their longer duration of action, thus requiring only a daily dose.

Nursing implications for the medications used to control chronic glaucoma are outlined in the Medication Administration box on pages 1480–1481.

In acute angle-closure glaucoma, diuretics may be administered intravenously to achieve a rapid decrease in intraocular pressure prior to surgical intervention. Both the carbonic anhydrase inhibitor acetazolamide and osmotic diuretics, such

Americans and Asians. All people over the age of 40 are encouraged to receive an eye examination every 2 to 4 years, including tonometry screening. Those with a predominant family history should be evaluated more frequently, every 1 to 2 years. After the age of 65, yearly ophthalmologic examinations are recommended.

## Assessment

Collect the following data through a health history and physical examination (see Chapter 44).

- Health history: family history; presence of altered vision, halos, and excessive tearing; sudden, severe eye pain; use of corrective lenses
- Physical examination: distant and near vision, peripheral fields, retina for optic nerve cupping

## Nursing Diagnoses and Interventions

Nursing care planning focuses on problems associated with the temporary or permanent visual impairment, the resultant increased risk for injury, and the psychosocial problems of anxiety and coping.

### Risk for Disturbed Sensory Perception: Visual

Whether glaucoma and resulting impaired vision is the client's primary problem or a preexisting condition in a client with another disorder, it must be a primary consideration in nursing care planning.

- Address by name and identify yourself with each interaction. Orient to time, place, person, and situation as indicated. State the purpose of your visit. *The client with impaired vision must rely on input from the other senses. A lack of visual cues increases the importance of verbal ones. For example, the visually impaired client cannot see the nurse checking an intravenous infusion and needs a verbal explanation of who is in the room and why. When the client's normal daily routine is disrupted by illness or hospitalization, additional sensory input such as a radio, television, and explanations of the routine and activities are useful to maintain the client's orientation.*
- Provide any visual aids that are routinely used. Keep them close, making sure that the client knows where they are and can reach them easily. *Easy access encourages the client to use these items and enhances the ability to provide self-care.*
- Orient to the environment. Explain the location of the call bell, personal items, and the furniture in the room. If able, tour client's room, including the bathroom and sink. *Visually impaired clients are usually very capable of providing self-care in a known environment.*
- Provide other tools or items that can help compensate for diminished vision:
  a. Bright, nonglare lighting
  b. Books, magazines, and instructions in large print
  c. Books on tape
  d. Telephones with oversize pushbuttons
  e. A clock with numbers and hands that can be felt

- Assist with meals by:
  a. Reading menu selections and marking choices.
  b. Describing the position of foods on a meal tray according to the clock system, for example, "On the plate, the peas are at 9 o'clock, the mashed potatoes at 1 o'clock, and the chicken breast at 6 o'clock. The milk glass is at 2 o'clock on the tray above the plate, and coffee is at 11 o'clock."
  c. Placing the utensils in a readily accessible position.
  d. Removing lids from containers, buttering the bread, and cutting meat, as needed.
  e. If the visual impairment is new or temporary, the client may need feeding or continued assistance during the meal.
  *Providing assistance during eating is important to maintain the client's nutritional status. The client may be ashamed of needing help or embarrassed to request it and may respond by not eating or by claiming not to be hungry.*
- Assist with mobility and ambulation as needed:
  a. Have the client hold your arm or elbow, and walk slightly ahead as a guide. Do not hold the client's arm or elbow.
  b. Describe the surroundings and progress as you proceed. Warn in advance of potential hazards, turns, and steps.
  c. Teach to feel the chair, bed, or commode with the hands and the back of the legs before sitting.
  *These measures help ensure the client's safety while providing for mobility and helping prevent complications associated with immobility.*
- If the vision loss is unilateral and recent, provide instructions related to unilateral vision loss and change in depth perception:
  a. Caution about the loss of depth perception and teach safety precautions, such as reaching slowly for objects and using visual cues as to distance, especially when driving.
  b. Teach to scan, turning the head fully toward the affected side to identify potential hazards and looking up and down to compensate for the loss of depth perception.
  *The client with a unilateral vision loss is often unaware of its effect on peripheral vision and depth perception.*

### Risk for Injury

Whether the client is experiencing a sudden loss of vision due to acute angle-closure glaucoma or significant visual impairment due to inadequately managed chronic glaucoma, both are at an increased risk for injury. Clients who have had surgical interventions for glaucoma are at even greater risk.

- Assess ability to perform activities of daily living. *Clients may be reluctant to request assistance, believing that they should be able to perform these familiar tasks. Careful assessment and provision of needed assistance help prevent injury and maintain the client's self-esteem.*

**PRACTICE ALERT** *Keep traffic area free of clutter to reduce the risk for injury in visually impaired clients.* ■

- Notify housekeeping and place a sign on the client's door to alert all personnel not to change the arrangement of the client's room. *The visually impaired client is at high risk for falling when in an unfamiliar environment. It is important to maintain a safe, familiar room when the client is hospitalized.*
- Raise two or three side rails on the client's bed. *Raised rails remind clients to ask for assistance before ambulating in an unfamiliar environment.*
- Discuss possible adaptations in the home to help the client remain as independent as possible and prevent falls or other injuries. *Often minor changes in the home environment, such as removing scatter rugs and small items of furniture, allow the client to navigate safely in this already familiar environment.*

### Anxiety

The actual or potential loss of sight threatens the client's self-concept, role functioning, patterns of interaction, and, potentially, environment. The visually impaired client who functions well in a familiar environment will feel anxious in the unfamiliar setting of a hospital or care facility.

- Assess for verbal and nonverbal indications of level of anxiety and for normal coping mechanisms. Repeated expressions of concern or denial that the vision change will affect the client's life indicate anxiety. Nonverbal indicators include tension, difficulty concentrating or thinking, restlessness, poor eye contact, and changes in vocalization (rapid speech, voice quivering). Physical indicators include tachycardia, dilated pupils, cool and clammy skin, and tremors. *The client may not recognize this feeling as anxiety. Identifying and acknowledging the anxiety state can help the client recognize and deal with it.*
- Encourage to verbalize fears, anger, and feelings of anxiety. *Verbalizing helps externalize the anxiety and allows fears to be addressed.*
- Discuss perception of the eye condition and its effects on lifestyle and roles. *Discussion provides an opportunity to correct misperceptions and introduce alternative activities and assistive devices for the visually impaired.*
- Introduce yourself when entering the room, explain all procedures fully before and as they are being performed, and use touch to convey proximity and caring. *The visually impaired client must rely on the other senses to make up for the loss of sight. Because the client cannot see what you are doing, complete explanations of even simple tasks such as refilling a water glass help to relieve anxiety.*
- Identify coping strategies that have been useful in the past and to adapt these strategies to the present situation. *Previously successful coping strategies may be employed to increase the client's sense of control.*

## Using NANDA, NIC and NOC Linkages

Chart 45–2 shows links between NANDA nursing diagnoses, NIC, and NOC when caring for the client with glaucoma.

## Home Care

Clients with glaucoma require teaching about lifetime strategies for managing their chronic disorder at home. They need to understand the importance of lifetime therapy to control the disease and prevent blindness. If a permanent visual impairment has resulted, the client needs information on achieving the maximum possible independence while maintaining safety. The following topics should be discussed with the client and family:

- Prescribed medications including proper way to instill drops
- Importance of not taking certain prescription and over-the-counter medications without consulting a physician
- Periodic eye examinations with intraocular pressure measurement
- Risks, warning signs, and management of acute angle-closure glaucoma
- Possible surgical options
- Community resources, such as Visually Impaired Society, local library, and transportation services
- Helpful resources:
  - National Glaucoma Foundation
  - Young and Under Pressure Glaucoma Foundation
  - Glaucoma Research Foundation
  - Prevention of Blindness Society

MediaLink | GLAUCOMA RESOURCES

---

### CHART 45–2   NANDA, NIC, AND NOC LINKAGES

#### The Client with Glaucoma

| NURSING DIAGNOSES | NURSING INTERVENTIONS | NURSING OUTCOMES |
| --- | --- | --- |
| • Disturbed Sensory Perception | • Eye Care<br>• Coping Enhancement<br>• Coping | • Symptom Control<br>• Sensory Function: Vision |
| • Anxiety | • Anxiety Reduction | • Anxiety Control |

*Note. Data from Nursing Outcomes Classification (NOC) by M. Johnson & M. Maas (Eds.), 1997, St. Louis: Mosby; Nursing Diagnoses: Definitions & Classification 2001–2002 by North American Nursing Diagnosis Association, 2001, Philadelphia: NANDA; Nursing Interventions Classification (NIC) by J.C. McCloskey & G. M. Bulechek (Eds.), 2000, St. Louis: Mosby. Reprinted by permission.*

## Nursing Care Plan
## A Client with Glaucoma and Cataracts

Lila Rainey is an 80-year-old widow who lives alone in the house she and her late husband built 50 years ago. She has worn glasses for nearsightedness since she was a young girl. She was diagnosed 4 years ago with chronic open-angle glaucoma, for which she takes timolol maleate (Timoptic) 0.5%. Recently she has noticed difficulty reading and watching television despite a new lens prescription. She has stopped driving at night because the glare of oncoming headlights makes it difficult for her to see. Mrs. Rainey's ophthalmologist has told her that she has cataracts but that they do not need to come out until they bother her. Although her glaucoma is still controlled with timolol maleate 0.5%, one drop in each eye twice a day, her intraocular pressure measurements have been gradually increasing. Mrs. Rainey has taken 325 mg of aspirin daily since a TIA 8 years ago. She is being admitted to the outpatient surgery unit for a cataract removal and intraocular lens implant in her right eye.

### ASSESSMENT

Mrs. Rainey is admitted to the eye surgery unit by Susan Schafer, RN. In her assessment, Ms. Schafer finds Mrs. Rainey to be alert and oriented, though apprehensive about her upcoming surgery. Assessment findings include BP 134/72, P 86, R 18. Mrs. Rainey's neurologic, respiratory, cardiovascular, and abdominal assessments are essentially normal. Her pupils are round and equal, and react briskly to light and accommodation. Her conjunctivae are pink; sclera and corneas, clear. Using the ophthalmoscope, Ms. Schafer notes that the red reflex in Mrs. Rainey's right eye is diminished. Ophthalmic examination shows visual acuity of 20/150 OD (right eye) and 20/50 OS (left eye) with corrective lenses. Her intraocular pressures are 21 mmHg OD and 17 mmHg OS. On fundoscopic exam, no disease of the blood vessels, retina, macula, or disc is found. Ms. Schafer reviews the operative procedure with Mrs. Rainey, answering her questions and telling her what to expect after surgery. Following preoperative protocols, Mrs. Rainey is prepared and transported to surgery.

### DIAGNOSIS

- *Disturbed sensory perception: Visual* related to myopia and lens extraction
- *Anxiety* related to anticipated surgery
- *Deficient knowledge:* lack of information regarding postoperative care
- *Impaired home maintenance* related to activity restrictions and impaired vision

### EXPECTED OUTCOMES

- Regain sufficient visual acuity to maintain ADLs, including reading and watching television for enjoyment.
- Demonstrate a reduced level of anxiety.
- Demonstrate the procedure for instilling eye drops postoperatively.

- Demonstrate knowledge of the home care she will require after surgery, signs of complications, and actions to take if complications occur.
- Use appropriate resources to assist with home maintenance until vision stabilizes and activity restrictions are lifted.

### PLANNING AND IMPLEMENTATION

- Provide a safe environment, placing the call light and personal care items within easy reach.
- Encourage Mrs. Rainey to express her fears about surgery and its potential effect on vision.
- Explain all procedures related to surgery and recovery.
- Instruct her to avoid shutting the eyelids tightly, sneezing, coughing, laughing, bending over, lifting, or straining to have a bowel movement. Teach her to wear glasses during the day and an eye shield at night to prevent injury to the surgical site.
- Explain and demonstrate the procedure for administering eye drops.
- Provide verbal and written instructions about postoperative care, including a schedule of follow-up examinations, potential complications, and actions to take in response.
- Refer Mrs. Rainey to a discharge planner or social worker to help establish a plan for home maintenance.

### EVALUATION

Mrs. Rainey is discharged the morning after her surgery. She is visibly relieved when the eye patch is removed because her vision in the operated eye is better than before surgery, even without her glasses. She is able to relate the recommended activity restrictions. Mrs. Rainey administers her own eye drops before discharge and relates an understanding of the prescribed postoperative care and safety precautions. Mrs. Rainey's daughter plans to visit her mother two to three times a week to help with laundry and vacuuming until Mrs. Rainey is able to resume all her household activities. Mrs. Rainey says that she won't "be so scared when I need my other eye done." She understands the chronic nature of her glaucoma and says that her vision is too important for her to neglect her timolol drops and routine eye exams.

### Critical Thinking in the Nursing Process

1. Why did it become more difficult to control Mrs. Rainey's intraocular pressure as her cataract matured?
2. Identify medications that are commonly prescribed following cataract surgery. What are the risks of interactions between these medications and Mrs. Rainey's timolol drops?
3. Develop a care plan for the nursing diagnosis, *Self-care deficit: Dressing/grooming,* related to visual impairment and restricted bending.

See Evaluating Your Response in Appendix C.

## THE CLIENT WITH A RETINAL DETACHMENT

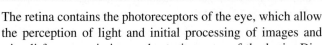

The retina contains the photoreceptors of the eye, which allow the perception of light and initial processing of images and stimuli for transmission to the optic center of the brain. Disruption of this neural layer of the eye by trauma or disease interferes with light perception and image transmission, potentially resulting in blindness.

Both primary eye conditions and systemic diseases can affect the retina and interfere with vision. Retinal tears or detachments can occur either spontaneously or as a result of trauma.

## PATHOPHYSIOLOGY AND MANIFESTATIONS

Separation of the retina or sensory portion of the eye from the choroid, the pigmented vascular layer, is known as a **retinal detachment.** Although retinal detachment may be precipitated by trauma, it usually occurs spontaneously. The vitreous humor normally adheres to the retina at the optic disk, the macula, and the periphery of the eye. With aging, the vitreous humor shrinks and may pull the retina away from the choroid. Aging therefore is a common risk factor, as are myopia and aphakia, absence of the lens (e.g., following lens removal for cataracts) (Porth, 2002; Tierney et al., 2001).

The retina may actually tear and fold back on itself, or the retina may remain intact but no longer adhere to the choroid (Figure 45–10 ■). A break or tear in the retina allows fluid from the vitreous cavity to enter the defect. This, along with fluid that escapes from choroid vessels, the pull of gravity, and traction exerted by the vitreous humor, separates the retina from the choroid. The detached area may rapidly increase in size, increasing loss of vision. Unless contact between the retina and choroid is reestablished, the neurons of the retina become ishemic and die, causing permanent vision loss. For this reason, retinal detachment is a true medical emergency, requiring prompt ophthalmologic referral and treatment.

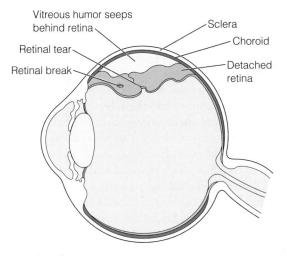

**Figure 45–10** ■ Retinal detachment.

### Manifestations of Retinal Detachment

- Floaters: irregular, dark lines or spots in the field of vision
- Flashes of light
- Blurred vision
- Progressive deterioration of vision
- Sensation of a curtain or veil being drawn across the field of vision
- If the macula is involved, loss of central vision

When the retina detaches, the client experiences floaters, or "spots," and lines or flashes of light in the visual field. Often the client describes the sensation of having a curtain drawn across the vision, much like a curtain being drawn over a window. The area of the visual field affected is directly related to the area of detachment. For example, because light rays cross as they pass through the lens, a retinal tear in the superior portion of the eye results in a deficit in the lower part of the visual field. The client feels no pain, and the eye appears normal to visual inspection. Common manifestations of retinal detachment are listed in the box above.

## COLLABORATIVE CARE

The manifestations and examination of the ocular fundus by ophthalmoscopy establish the diagnosis of retinal detachment. Early diagnosis and intervention are vital. If the condition is left untreated, the detached portion will become necrotic because of separation from the vascular supply of the choroid. The result is permanent blindness in that portion of the eye. If an ophthalmologist is not readily available, the client's head is positioned so that gravity pulls the detached portion of the retina into closer contact with the choroid.

Interventions are directed toward bringing the retina and choroid back into contact and reestablishing the blood and nutrient supply to the retina. Either cryotherapy, using a supercooled probe, or laser photocoagulation may be used to create an area of inflammation and adhesion to "weld" the layers together.

A surgical procedure called *scleral buckling* also may be used. In this procedure, an indentation or fold is created in the sclera, bringing the choroid into contact with the retina. Contact is maintained with a local implant on the sclera or an encircling strap or "buckle." Air may also be injected into the vitreous cavity, a procedure called pneumatic retinopexy. The client is positioned so that the air bubble pushes the detached portion of the retina into contact with the choroid.

With a retinal tear, it may be necessary to use surgical instruments to manipulate the detached section of retina into place. Air or a liquid is then injected into the vitreous to maintain retinal contact with the choroid, or laser therapy used to create a bond.

MediaLink | RETINAL DETACHMENT CASE STUDY

## NURSING CARE

The nursing focus for the client with a detached retina is on early identification and treatment. Because early intervention is vital to preserve the client's sight, nurses must recognize early manifestations of retinal detachment and intervene appropriately to obtain definitive treatment for the client. Retinal detachment can be successfully treated on an outpatient basis, often in an ophthalmologist's office. For these clients, the nursing focus is on education.

### Ineffective Tissue Perfusion: Retinal

Restoring contact between the retina and choroid is a priority of nursing and medical care for the client with retinal detachment. Vitreous humor may leak through a retinal tear, and fluid exudate may collect behind the tear, causing further retinal detachment. If the macula is detached, central vision is lost, and the client's prognosis for full vision restoration is poorer.

**PRACTICE ALERT** *Carefully assess anyone who complains of a sudden rapid loss of vision because these are often medical emergencies.* ■

- Assess for other manifestations of eye disease. *Retinal detachment is painless and has no outward manifestations. The client with a red eye or cloudy cornea may be experiencing acute angle-closure glaucoma rather than retinal detachment.*
- Notify physician and the ophthalmologist immediately. *Immediate medical intervention is required in clients with retinal detachment to preserve vision.*
- Position so the area of detachment is inferior. For instance, for a superior temporal retinal detachment of the right eye (with corresponding vision loss in the inferior medial visual field of that eye), place supine with the head turned to the right. *Correct positioning allows the contents of the posterior portion of the eye to place pressure on the detached area, bringing the retina in closer contact with the choroid.*

### Anxiety

The client with retinal detachment has a rapid decline in vision in the affected eye, often occurring spontaneously and without pain. Unless the client has had previous episodes, he or she usually does not know what is causing the problem. Anxiety and fear of complete vision loss are common, expected reactions.

- Maintain a calm, confident attitude while carrying out priority interventions. *Administering care in a calm although urgent manner helps reassure the client that the problem is treatable and that appropriate measures are being taken.*
- Reassure that most retinal detachments are successfully treated, usually on an outpatient basis. *Reassurance can help allay the client's fear of permanent vision loss.*
- For spontaneous detachments, assure that he or she did not cause the detachment to occur. *The client may believe that the detachment is related to a specific activity and feel guilty for "causing" this loss of vision.*

- Explain all procedures fully, including the reason for positioning. *Explanations facilitate the client's understanding and help relieve anxiety in unfamiliar settings.*
- Allow supportive family members or friends to remain with the client as much as possible. *Additional support helps lower the client's anxiety level.*

## Home Care

Teaching the client undergoing surgical repair of retinal detachment is similar to that for clients experiencing other types of eye surgery (see page 1469). If the retina remains detached, the client needs instructions about the change in peripheral vision or other visual fields and changes in depth perception.

Discuss the following topics with the client and family to prepare for home care:

- Limitations on positioning the head following pneumatic retinopexy
- Activity restrictions such as no bending or straining at stool
- Use of eye shield
- Early manifestations and the importance of seeking immediate treatment
- Follow-up treatment with the ophthalmologist

## THE CLIENT WITH MACULAR DEGENERATION

The leading cause of blindness in people over the age of 65 is **macular degeneration** (Quillen, 1999). The macula is the area of the retina that receives light from the center of the visual field and that has the greatest visual acuity. Factors associated with macular degeneration include aging, smoking, hypertension, and hypercholesterolemia. The destructive changes in the macula occur most often as a response to the aging process. It affects males and females equally and is seen more frequently in people of European ancestry.

Age-related macular degeneration is thought to result from gradual failure of the outer pigmented layer of the retina (the retinal layer adjacent to the choroid), which removes cellular waste products and keeps the retina attached to the choroid. This failure causes photoreceptor (sensory) cells to be lost at an increasing rate. In addition, waste and toxins from cell breakdown further damage the cells of the outer pigmented retinal layer. Serous fluid may enter the subretinal space, leading to retinal detachments and depriving sensory cells of oxygen and nutrients, increasing cell death. The process is typically bilateral and slowly progressive.

Two forms of macular degeneration exist. *Atrophic degeneration* (dry) causes gradual and progressive vision loss because of atrophy and degeneration of the outer pigmented retinal layer. Vision loss is more rapid and severe in *exudative degeneration;* this form accounts for 90% of people who are legally blind because of macular degeneration. In exudative degeneration (wet), a proliferation of new blood vessels (neovascularization) form in the subretinal space. These vessels leak serous fluid or blood into the retina, separating the pigmented retina from the choroid or separating the neurosensory retina (innermost layer) from the pigmented retina (Tierney et al., 2001).

When the macula is damaged, central vision becomes blurred and distorted, but peripheral vision remains intact. Distortion of vision in one eye is a common initial manifestation; straight lines appear wavy or distorted (Figure 45–11A ■). With the loss of central vision, activities that require close central vision, such as reading and sewing, are particularly affected (Figure 45–11B).

There is currently no effective treatment for atrophic macular degeneration. Laser photocoagulation may slow the exudative form if performed early in the course of the disease to seal leaking capillaries and stop exudation. Large-print books and magazines, the use of a magnifying glass, and high-intensity lighting can help the client to cope with the reduced vision of macular degeneration.

Nurses should be alert for clients demonstrating new and rapid onset manifestations of macular degeneration and promptly refer these clients for ophthalmologic evaluation. Early intervention may preserve a greater degree of vision and slow the progress of the disease. For clients with slowly progressive manifestations, the nursing focus is on helping the client and family members adapt to the gradual decline in vision by recommending visual aids and other coping strategies. Client education materials should be in a large-print format.

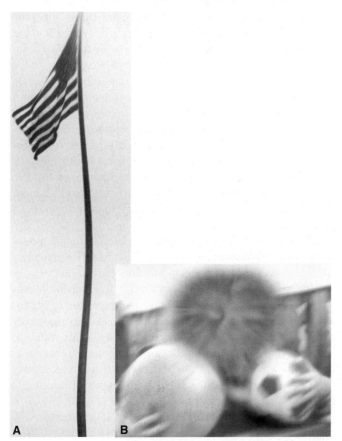

**Figure 45–11 ■** *A,* The visual distortion of straight lines typical of early macular degeneration. *B,* Loss of central vision with advanced macular degeneration.

*Courtesy of Prevent Blindness America (A); the National Eye Institute, National Institutes of Health (B).*

## THE CLIENT WITH RETINITIS PIGMENTOSA

**Retinitis pigmentosa** is a hereditary degenerative disease characterized by retinal atrophy and loss of retinal function progressing from the periphery to the central region of the retina. It is inherited as an autosomal dominant, autosomal recessive, or X-linked trait and may be associated with other genetic defects (Braunwald et al, 2001; Porth, 2002).

In retinitis pigmentosa, the genetic defect appears to cause production of an unstable form of rhodopsin, the receptor protein of rod cells in the retina. Rod cells degenerate, initially at the periphery of the retina. The areas of degeneration and cell death slowly expand, causing vision to narrow. Central vision is finally lost as well.

The initial manifestation of retinitis pigmentosa, difficulty with night vision, is often noted during childhood. As the disease progresses, there is slow loss of visual fields, photophobia, and disrupted color vision. The progression to tunnel vision and blindness is gradual; the client may be totally blind by age 40.

Currently, there is no effective treatment for retinitis pigmentosa. Research into the role that defective rhodopsin plays in the disease holds future promise for the development of therapy that may at least slow its progress.

Clients with retinitis pigmentosa may benefit from low-vision aids, much like those for the client with macular degeneration. Additionally, information about the disease and its progress is vital so the client can plan for the eventual total loss of sight. Clients with retinitis pigmentosa should be referred for genetic counseling prior to starting a family to determine the risk of transmitting the disease to their children.

## THE CLIENT WITH DIABETIC RETINOPATHY

In the United States, **diabetic retinopathy** is the leading cause of new blindness in people age 20 to 74. While approximately 85% of diabetics will develop retinopathy, the majority will not become blind (Braunwald et al, 2001). Diabetic retinopathy is a vascular disorder affecting the capillaries of the retina. The capillaries become sclerotic and lose their ability to transport sufficient oxygen and nutrients to the retina. Retinopathy is seen in both type 1 and type 2 diabetes. In the diabetic, the extent of retinopathy is reflective of the length of time the client has had the disease and the degree of control that has been maintained. Nursing care of the client with diabetes is discussed in Chapter 18. ⊂⊃

Diabetic retinopathy has two major forms: *nonproliferative* or background retinopathy and *proliferative* retinopathy. Nonproliferative retinopathy is typically the initial form seen. The venous capillaries of the eye dilate and develop microaneurysms that may then leak, causing retinal edema, or they may rupture, causing small hemorrhages into the retina. On ophthalmoscopic examination, yellow exudates, cotton-wool patches indicative of retinal ischemia, and red-dot hemorrhages

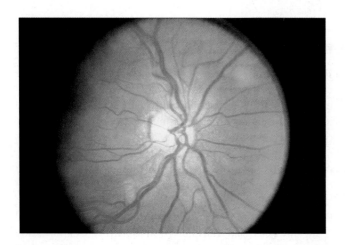

**Figure 45–12** ■ Appearance of the ocular fundus in diabetic retinopathy.

*Courtesy of the National Eye Institute, National Institutes of Health.*

are observed (Figure 45–12 ■). When the peripheral retina is involved, the client may experience few symptoms other than light glare. Edema of the macula or a large hemorrhage may cause vision loss.

Diabetic retinopathy may progress to the proliferative form. This disease is marked by large areas of retinal ischemia and the formation of new blood vessels (neovascularization) spreading over the inner surface of the retina and into the vitreous body. These vessels are fine and fragile, making them permeable and easily ruptured. Blood and blood protein leakage contribute to retinal edema, and hemorrhage into the vitreous body may occur. The vessels gradually become fibrous and firmly attached to the vitreous body, increasing the risk of retinal detachment.

Clients with diabetes should be examined yearly by an ophthalmologist. The development of any new visual manifestations is an additional indication for prompt ophthalmologic examination and possibly retinal angiography.

Laser photocoagulation is used to treat both the nonproliferative and proliferative forms of diabetic retinopathy. Leaking microaneurysms are sealed and proliferating vessels destroyed, reducing the risk of hemorrhage, retinal edema, and retinal detachment. This treatment also slows the progress of aneurysms and new vessel formation; however, it does not cure the disorder. Clients with severe proliferative retinopathy may undergo vitrectomy to remove vitreous hemorrhage or treat associated retinal detachments (Tierney et al., 2001).

As with many other eye disorders, the nursing care focus for diabetic retinopathy is primarily educational. The newly diagnosed diabetic client needs to understand the importance of regular eye examinations beginning approximately 5 years after the onset of type 1 diabetes and at the time of onset of type 2 diabetes. Changes of diabetic retinopathy may already be present when type 2 is diagnosed.

Teach the client to report promptly any new visual manifestation, including blurred vision; black spots (floaters), cobwebs, or flashing lights in the visual field; or a sudden loss of vision in one or both eyes. Emphasize to the client that careful blood glucose control may help prevent diabetic retinopathy

from developing; it may also slow its progress. The client's blood pressure should also be maintained within normal limits to prevent further damage to retinal vessels. Although diabetic retinopathy cannot be halted or cured, its progress can be slowed with aggressive management. Much of the burden for this management falls on the client, increasing the importance of good teaching.

## THE CLIENT WITH HIV INFECTION

More than 50% of people infected with the human immunodeficiency virus (HIV) develop an infectious or noninfectious ocular condition, generally as a late manifestation of the disease (Braunwald et al., 2001).

HIV retinopathy, manifested as cotton-wool spots around the optic nerve, is the most common noninfectious ophthalmic lesion in AIDS. Cotton-wool spots indicate areas of retinal ischemia. Microaneurysms and dot-, blot-, or flame-shaped hemorrhages may also be seen in HIV retinopathy.

Neoplasms common in the client with AIDS can also affect the eye. Kaposi's sarcoma may affect the external surface or anterior segment of the eye or the eyelids. Kaposi's lesions vary in color (red, brown, or purple) and in size, shape, and location. Conjunctival lesions resemble a benign subconjunctival hemorrhage. Kaposi's lesions of the lid may cause **ptosis** (drooping of the lid) and abnormal lid function. Vision or eye position and movement may be affected by the tumor or by the effect of increased intracranial pressure on the cranial nerves.

The most serious and frequent opportunistic eye infection associated with HIV infection is cytomegalovirus (CMV) retinitis. CMV retinitis develops in 10% to 15% of people with AIDS, generally when CD4 cell counts drop below 50 mL. Initially unilateral, CMV retinitis commonly progresses to become bilateral because of the systemic nature of the infection. CMV invades the retina of the eye directly, producing exudate and cotton-wool spots, hemorrhage, cell death, and necrosis. Visual field deficits develop and can progress to eventual blindness.

Corneal ulcers from opportunistic bacterial, fungal, protozoal, or viral infections are also associated with HIV infection. Toxoplasmic and fungal retinal infections may occur.

The client with an HIV-associated ocular condition may complain of a change in visual acuity, blurring, floaters, or gaps in the field of vision. Extensive retinal damage may cause retinal detachment and symptoms of flashing lights, multiple floaters, and a loss of vision. Because the observed changes in the retina are nonspecific, it is important for the examining physician to know that the client is HIV positive in order to make an accurate diagnosis.

In addition to the general treatment of HIV infection with retroviral medications such as zidovudine (AZT) and didanosine (ddI), specific therapies may be directed toward the ocular manifestations of the disease. CMV retinitis is commonly treated with the antivirals ganciclovir (Cytovene) and foscarnet sodium (Foscavir).

**Procedure 45-1**

# Removing and Reinserting a Prosthetic Eye

## SUPPLIES

- Gloves
- Clean basin or plastic denture cup
- Sterile normal saline or soap and water for cleaning the prosthesis
- Gauze squares or cotton cloth for cleaning the socket
- A bulb syringe for irrigation if necessary

## BEFORE THE PROCEDURE

Most clients who have an artificial eye provide self-care and require little assistance. However, it may be necessary for the nurse to remove an eye prosthesis from the unconscious or debilitated client. Explain the procedure to the client and provide for privacy.

## PROCEDURE

- Follow standard precautions.
- Wash the hands and put on clean exam gloves.
- To remove the prosthesis, either

- Pull down the lower lid and gently exert outward and upward pressure on the lower edge of the prosthesis. This pressure usually causes the prosthesis to slip out.
- Pull down the lower lid and apply a moistened suction cup to the prosthesis by squeezing the device. Twist gently to remove the prosthesis from the socket.
- Wash the prosthesis using mild soap and water or normal saline. Rinse thoroughly. Do not use abrasives or chemicals for cleaning.
- If the prosthesis is not immediately replaced in the eye socket, store it in a clearly labeled plastic container lined with a soft cloth or gauze squares. Avoid scratching or damaging the prosthesis. Store it in a safe place to prevent loss.
- If irrigation of the eye socket is ordered, have the client lean over a sink or basin if possible, or position on the affected side with a clean emesis basin to hold the irrigant as it flows out of the socket.

Gently hold the lids open and irrigate the socket using a bulb syringe and clean warm water.
- Reinsert the prosthesis.
  a. Moisten the prosthesis with warm normal saline or water.
  b. Gently hold the lids open, inserting the upper edge of the prosthesis under the upper lid first, then the lower edge under the lower lid using slight pressure.
  c. If a suction device is used, attach it to the cleaned prosthesis over the pupil. Holding the lids open, insert the prosthesis using the above procedure, then remove the suction cup by squeezing it gently and exerting slight pressure on the edge of the cup with the lower lid.

## AFTER THE PROCEDURE

Ensure that the client is comfortable. Chart the procedure and any abnormal findings, such as drainage or inflammation.

---

Although treatment of ocular Kaposi's sarcoma is usually not indicated, conjunctival lesions may be excised for comfort or cosmetic reasons. Lid lesions may be treated with radiation or intralesional chemotherapy.

## THE CLIENT WITH AN ENUCLEATION

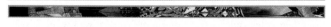

Occasionally surgical removal of an eye is necessary because of trauma, infection, glaucoma, intractable pain, or malignancy. This procedure is known as **enucleation.**

Enucleation is performed under local or general anesthesia. After the globe is removed, the conjunctiva and eye muscles are sutured to a round implant inserted into the orbit to maintain its shape. A pressure dressing is left in place for 24 to 48 hours. The client is permitted out of bed on the day of surgery. Hemorrhage and infection are the most commonly seen complications.

Postoperative nursing care includes teaching, psychologic support, and observation for potential complications. The client may be instructed to apply warm compresses and instill antibiotic ointment or drops postoperatively.

Within 1 week, a temporary prosthesis called a conformer is fitted into the empty socket. The permanent prosthesis is individually designed to closely resemble the client's other eye. The prosthesis can be fitted 1 to 2 months after surgery. Often it is difficult to discern which eye is functional and which is

the prosthesis. Procedure 45–1 outlines the proper way to remove and reinsert an eye prosthesis when the client is unable to do so.

## THE CLIENT WHO IS BLIND

Visual impairment exists on a continuum from blindness to decreased visual acuity that can be corrected with refractive lenses to normal or near normal. The legal definition of blindness is visual acuity no better than 20/200 in the better eye with optimal correction, or a visual field of less than 20 degrees (compared to the normal of 180 degrees). Total blindness usually indicates that the client has no light perception at all. In practical terms, a person with a visual deficit sufficient to need assistive devices or aid from other people for normal activities of daily living is considered blind.

Ten to 12 million people in the United States have a visual impairment that cannot be corrected. More than 500,000 Americans are legally blind. Worldwide, between 40 and 50 million people have visual impairment significant enough to be considered blind.

The major worldwide causes of blindness are as follows:

1. Cataracts
2. Trachoma
3. Glaucoma

4. Onchocerciasis (river blindness), a parasitic infection transmitted by flies that causes opacification of the cornea, inflammation of the iris and choroid (uveitis), and eventual destruction of vision
5. Nutritional deficiencies including xerophthalmia and keratomalacia due to vitamin A deficiency
6. Trauma

## PATHOPHYSIOLOGY

Although approximately two-thirds of all cases of blindness worldwide are either preventable or curable, it continues to be prevalent because of lack of access to care, fear of surgery or other treatment, poor sanitation and nutrition, and ignorance of need. In the United States, sanitation measures, better access to health care, and a higher level of nutrition have reduced the threat of infectious disorders to vision. However, glaucoma and cataracts remain significant causes of blindness. Other major causes of blindness in the United States include retinal diseases such as diabetic retinopathy, macular degeneration, and congenital disorders.

## NURSING CARE

Blind people need to cope not only with the loss of a significant sense but often also with societal attitudes that make them feel inferior, helpless, and inadequate. The idea of losing the sense of vision is uniformly feared, leaving sighted people unable to understand the magnitude and impact of the loss in those who have experienced it. Because of this fear and confusion, sighted people are unsure of what the blind expect from them.

The adjustment of the person who is born blind and raised to become an independent member of society differs from that of the person who has been sighted and becomes blind. The person who has been blind from birth has developed numerous adaptive strategies that the newly blind person has yet to learn.

Although adaptation may be easier for the client who has experienced a gradual loss of vision than for someone with an abrupt loss, both must grieve the lost sense. The blind client needs to grieve the lost body part as well as the loss of mobility, self-sufficiency, perhaps economic security, and, to a certain extent, contact with reality as it has been perceived. The client's self-concept and self-esteem are threatened. Anger, denial, remorse, and self-pity are not uncommon in the initial period following loss of sight. Interpersonal relationships and roles are affected. Communication patterns change with the loss of the ability to perceive many nonverbal cues. Expressions of sexuality may be impaired.

Acceptance of the change from sighted to blind is characterized by releasing the hope that vision will be regained. Self-esteem increases as the client attempts and masters activities of self-sufficiency such as completing ADLs, cooking, and becoming mobile outside the known home environment.

Health professionals often confuse the role of the blind person with the role of the client, seeing the person as helpless, dependent, and lacking in personal identity and control. Although nurses need to take blindness into account in planning care and maintaining client safety, it is vital to give the blind client the same respect and decision-making power that all clients deserve. Nurses who have dealt with their own emotions and responses to vision loss are better prepared to help the client adapt.

Nurses can foster independence in the hospitalized client with a significant vision deficit by doing the following:

- Orient to the environment verbally and physically. Describe the client's room using a central point such as the bed. Lead the client around the room, identifying chairs, sink, bathroom, and other landmarks. Be sure that only the client moves objects such as chairs, personal items, and clothing. Leave doors either fully open or closed as the client wishes, but, to preserve the client's safety, do not leave doors partially open. Keep the room and hallways where the client will be ambulating free of clutter.
- Use verbal communication freely. Describe activities going on around the client. Introduce yourself as you enter the room and let the client know when you are leaving.
- Provide other sensory stimuli such as radio and television as desired by the client.
- Orient to food trays by using the face of a clock to describe the position of food items on the plate and tray (unless the client has always been blind and cannot visualize a clock face).
- When assisting with ambulation, allow to hold your arm as you walk slightly ahead. Do not hold the client's arm. Verbally describe the environment, such as, "There will be two steps up 5 feet ahead."
- Do not hesitate to ask what assistance the client desires.

For the client with a new loss of sight, refer to available services. Counseling can help the client cope with and eventually adapt to the loss of sight. People who are blind are eligible for mobility training, assistance with relearning self-care activities, education in the use of braille to communicate, and vocational and other forms of rehabilitation. Local, state, and national agencies such as the American Foundation for the Blind, National Braille Association, and National Federation for the Blind coordinate services for the blind. Many assistive devices are available, including guide or pilot dogs, computer services, talking books and tape players, and low-vision aids.

Although each client with a significant vision deficit has individualized needs, the following nursing diagnoses may be appropriate for the blind client.

- *Disturbed sensory perception: Visual* related to trauma or disease process
- *Bathing/hygiene, dressing/grooming, feeding self-care deficit* related to impaired vision
- *Deficient knowledge* related to lack of information about available resources
- *Hopelessness* related to loss of vision
- *Grieving* related to loss of a body part
- *Risk for situational low self-esteem* related to significant change in body image

# EAR DISORDERS

For a person to hear, sound waves must enter the external auditory meatus and travel through the ear canal to vibrate the tympanic membrane and bony structures of the middle ear, which in turn activate the receptors of the cochlea. Trauma or disease involving any portion of this pathway can affect hearing. **Tinnitus,** the perception of sound such as ringing, buzzing, or roaring in the ears, is another potential result of problems affecting the auditory system.

Disorders of the external ear, including the auricle, auditory meatus, and ear canal, can affect the conduction of sound waves and hearing. Obstruction of the external auditory canal or damage to the tympanic membrane, which separates the outer from the middle ear, may lead to conductive hearing loss. Infection or inflammation, trauma, and obstruction of the ear canal with cerumen (wax) or a foreign body are the most common conditions affecting the external ear.

Disorders of the middle ear may be either acute or chronic. Unless these disorders are treated promptly and effectively, damage and scarring of middle ear structures can result in a permanent conductive hearing loss. Infectious or inflammatory disorders such as otitis media and mastoiditis are the most common conditions affecting the middle ear. Otosclerosis, a genetic condition, may also affect the structures of the middle ear.

## THE CLIENT WITH EXTERNAL OTITIS

**External otitis** is inflammation of the ear canal. Commonly known as *swimmer's ear,* it is most prevalent in people who spend significant time in the water. Competitive athletes, including swimmers, divers, and surfers, are particularly prone to external otitis. Wearing a hearing aid or ear plugs, which hold moisture in the ear canal, is an additional risk factor. Although *Pseudomonas aeruginosa* or other bacterial infection is the most common cause, external otitis may also be due to fungal infection, mechanical trauma (such as cleaning the ear with hair pins), or a local hypersensitivity reaction.

## PATHOPHYSIOLOGY AND MANIFESTATIONS

Disruption of the normal environment within the external auditory canal typically precedes the inflammatory process. Retained moisture, cleaning, or drying of the ear canal remove the protective layer of cerumen, an acidic, water-repellent substance with antimicrobial properties. Its removal leaves the skin of the ear canal vulnerable to invasion and infection. For surfers, the presence of *exostoses,* bony growths in the ear canals resulting from prolonged exposure to cold, predisposes to impaction and retained moisture within the canal.

The client with external otitis often complains of a feeling of fullness in the ear. Ear pain typically is present and may be severe. The pain of otitis externa can be differentiated from that associated with otitis media by manipulation of the auricle. In external otitis, this maneuver increases the pain, whereas the client with otitis media experiences no change in pain perception. Odorless watery or purulent drainage may be present. The ear canal appears inflamed and edematous on examination.

## COLLABORATIVE CARE

Management of the client with an external ear disorder focuses on restoring the normal balance of the external ear and canal and teaching the client how to prevent future problems.

For otitis externa, the following steps are recommended in treatment.

- Thorough cleansing of the ear canal, particularly if drainage or debris is present
- Treatment of the infection with local antibiotics; if cellulitis is present, systemic antibiotics may be necessary
- Medication to relieve the pain and itching
- Teaching on the prevention of future episodes of swimmer's ear

A topical antibiotic is often prescribed for the treatment of otitis externa. A topical corticosteroid may be ordered in combination with the antibiotic to provide immediate relief of the pain, swelling, and itching. Polymyxin B-neomycin-hydrocortisone (Cortisporin Otic) is a typical combination preparation used to treat external otitis; these antibiotics are effective against *Pseudomonas.* It is important to identify known sensitivity to any of the drugs in this preparation prior to initiating therapy. Clients who are sensitive to neomycin may develop dermatitis, in which case the drug must be stopped. Other preparations such as 1% tolnaftate solution (Tinactin) may be prescribed for a fungal infection of the ear canal.

## NURSING CARE

External otitis can cause severe pain and discomfort. Although the disorder is rarely serious enough to require hospitalization, the nurse teaches the client about the disorder, comfort measures, and prevention of future episodes.

### Impaired Tissue Integrity

External otitis may result from attempts to clean the ear canal with a toothpick, cotton-tipped applicator, or other implement that damages the skin, allowing an infectious organism to invade the tissue. Even if the canal is not damaged by attempts to clean it, the cleaning process often interrupts normal mechanisms, causing cerumen and debris to collect in the canal. This collected debris, in turn, tends to trap water within the canal, causing maceration of the skin.

- Inform that ear canals rarely need cleansing beyond washing of the external meatus with soap and water. Teach clients of all ages not to clean ear canals with any implement. *"Cleaning" increases the risk of tissue damage and impairs the normal mechanism that clears the canal of accumulated cerumen and debris.*

- Teach client (and, if necessary, a family member) how to instill prescribed ear drops:
  a. Wash the hands.
  b. Warm the medication briefly by holding the container in the hand or placing it in a pocket for approximately 5 minutes before instilling the drops. *Warming the medication promotes comfort.*
  c. Lie on the unaffected side; if sitting, tilt the head toward the unaffected side. *This position allows gravity to assist in moving the medication to the inner portion of the ear canal.*
  d. Partially fill the ear dropper with medication.
  e. Using the nondominant hand, straighten the ear canal by pulling the pinna of the ear up and back. *Straightening helps the medication travel along the length of the canal.*
  f. Administer the prescribed number of drops into the ear canal. *It is important that the full amount of prescribed medication be administered to penetrate the length of the canal and achieve full effectiveness.*
  g. Remain in the side-lying position for approximately 5 minutes after the instillation of drops. *This position allows the medication to penetrate into deeper portions of the canal and prevents it from running out when the head is moved upright.*
  h. Loosely place a small piece of cotton in the auditory meatus for 15 to 20 minutes. *The cotton helps keep the medication in the canal.*
- Teach to avoid getting water in the affected ear until it is fully healed. Cotton balls may be used while showering to prevent water from entering the ear canal. The client should refrain from water sports and activities until approved by the primary care provider. *Retained moisture in the ear canal can further impair skin integrity, increasing inflammation.*

## Home Care

The client is ultimately responsible for carrying out the prescribed treatment regimen in external otitis and for implementing measures to prevent future episodes. Teaching is vital. Provide verbal and written instructions on use of the prescribed medications. Teach the client care measures to prevent recurrent episodes especially important in swimmers, divers, and surfers (Box 45–1).

Cellulitis of the surrounding tissue is a possible complication of external otitis. Instruct the client to report to the primary care provider any increase in pain, swelling, or redness of surrounding tissues; fever; or other manifestations of infection such as malaise or increased fatigue.

## THE CLIENT WITH IMPACTED CERUMEN AND FOREIGN BODIES

The external auditory canal can be obstructed by cerumen or foreign bodies. The curved shape and narrow lumen of the canal make it particularly vulnerable to obstruction.

---

**BOX 45–1** ■ **Teaching to Prevent External Otitis**

- Stay out of the water until the acute inflammatory process is completely resolved. Ideally, allow 7 to 10 days before resuming water activities.
- Take precautions to keep the ear canal dry while in the water.
  a. Use silicone earplugs, which can keep water out of the ear without reducing hearing significantly.
  b. Wear a tight-fitting swim cap or wet suit hood, especially in cold ocean water. Although these do not prevent water from entering the ear, they protect the ear from the cold and possibly slow the formation of bony growths in the ears. They also protect the ear from sand and other water debris.
- Immediately after swimming, dry the ear canal. Allow water to drain by tilting the head and jumping to shake water out of the ear. Dry the outer ear with a towel, then use a hair dryer on the lowest setting several inches from the ear to dry the canal.
- Do not insert cotton swabs or other objects into the ear canal to dry it. This removes the protective layer of cerumen and may damage the skin of the canal, increasing the risk of bacterial infection. In addition, if debris such as sand is present, the swab may actually push debris further into the canal, forming an impacted mass.
- Use a drying agent in the ear canal after swimming. A 2% acetic acid solution or 2% boric acid in ethyl alcohol is effective in drying the canal and restoring its normal acidic environment.
- If it is necessary to remove impacted debris from the ear canal, irrigate the ear with warm tap water. A bulb syringe available over the counter or a 20 mL syringe attached to a short Teflon intravenous catheter (with the needle removed) is effective. With the head tilted toward the affected side, direct a stream of warm water toward the upper wall of the ear canal, allowing the water to run out into a bowl or sink. Repeated instillations may be necessary to break up and flush out impacted wax and debris.

---

As cerumen dries, it moves down and out of the ear canal. In some individuals it tends to accumulate, narrowing the canal. Aging is a risk factor for cerumen impaction, because less is produced and it is harder and drier. The accumulation of cerumen is often aggravated by attempting to remove it using cotton-tipped swabs or hairpins, which pack it more deeply into the ear canal. A study of cerumen impaction, common ear-cleaning practices, and hearing acuity in older adults is summarized in the Nursing Research box on page 1493.

A variety of objects become foreign bodies in the ear canal. In adults, implements used to clean the ear canal may break and become lodged. Insects also may enter the ear canal and be unable to exit.

When the ear canal becomes occluded with either cerumen or a foreign body, the client experiences a conductive hearing loss in the affected ear. Manifestations include a sensation of fullness, along with tinnitus and coughing due to stimulation of the vagal nerve. The foreign body or impacted cerumen may be

## Nursing Research

### Evidence-Based Practice for Ear-Cleaning and Hearing Loss

A descriptive study of the incidence of cerumen impaction, ear-cleaning practices, and hearing loss in three groups of adults over the age of 60 included people living independently and participating in senior citizen center activities, and clients in personal care homes and nursing homes (Ney, 1993). The researchers found that individuals living independently had significantly fewer cerumen impactions than those in the other groups. This finding may reflect the higher level of activity of the independent adults, facilitating the natural drainage of cerumen from the ear canal, or better hygiene practices of that group. Approximately one-third of the subjects inserted an object (usually a cotton-tipped applicator) into the ear canal for the purpose of cleaning on a regular or periodic basis.

Some degree of hearing deficit was demonstrated in two-thirds of the subjects, with 18% of the population unable to hear any tone presented. Loss at the highest frequency was the most common deficit noted.

### IMPLICATIONS FOR NURSING

This study demonstrates the potential role nurses can play in identifying hearing deficits, preventing further conductive deficit from impacted cerumen, and teaching clients about appropriate ear-hygiene measures.

The higher incidence of impacted cerumen in residents of personal care homes and nursing homes demonstrates the need for routine assessment of the ear canal and cleaning as necessary. Clients who routinely clean the ear canals using an object such as a cotton-tipped swab, hairpin, paper clip, or nail need to be taught alternative methods. Several subjects in this study used alcohol or hydrogen peroxide to soften cerumen; only one used a commercial product specifically for that purpose. Nurses can have a positive impact by increasing awareness of acceptable alternatives.

### Critical Thinking in Client Care

1. Why is the resident of a personal care home or nursing home at higher risk for developing a cerumen impaction?
2. How can nurses in these settings prevent cerumen from accumulating to this degree?
3. How can the nurse in a long-term care setting screen the hearing of the residents to identify possible deficits?

---

visualized on otoscopy. Impacted cerumen appears as a yellow, brown, or black mass in the canal.

Treatment focuses on clearing the canal. If there is no evidence of tympanic membrane perforation, irrigation of the canal is often the initial therapy.

Impacted wax, objects, or insects may require physical removal using an ear curet, forceps, or right-angle hook inserted via an otoscope and ear speculum. Mineral oil or topical lidocaine drops are used to immobilize or kill insects prior to their removal from the ear. When an organic foreign body such as a bean or an insect is suspected, water should not be instilled into the ear canal, because it may cause the object to swell, making its removal more difficult. Smooth, round objects present the biggest challenge to remove from the ear canal. Suction applied using a piece of soft intravenous tubing may be effective.

Nurses are often involved in identifying and relieving obstructions of the ear canal, especially in outpatient and community settings. Any client with evidence of a new conductive hearing loss or complaints of discomfort and fullness in one ear should be evaluated for possible obstruction. Inability to visualize the tympanic membrane or observation of a dark, shiny mass obstructing the canal may indicate a need for an irrigation or other procedure to clear the canal. It is important to determine that the tympanic membrane is intact before irrigating; assessment by a physician or advanced practitioner may be necessary if a ruptured membrane is suspected.

Because obstruction of the ear canal with cerumen or a foreign body is generally preventable, teaching is a key component of nursing care. Clients need to know appropriate care measures for the external ear. Although the ear canal rarely needs cleaning, the client prone to cerumen impaction needs teaching about the use of mineral oil or commercial products to soften wax and of irrigation to remove it. All clients should un-

derstand the importance of not inserting anything smaller than a finger wrapped with a washcloth into the ear canal to avoid trauma to the canal or eardrum. Stress the risk of impacting cerumen against the tympanic membrane when using cotton-tipped swabs to clean the ear canal. Additionally, the swab may break and lodge in the canal. If ear drops have been prescribed, teach the client and a family member how to instill them.

## THE CLIENT WITH OTITIS MEDIA

**Otitis media,** inflammation or infection of the middle ear, primarily affects infants and young children but may also occur in adults. The tympanic membrane, which separates the middle ear from the external auditory canal, protects the middle ear from the external environment. The auditory (eustachian) tube connects the middle ear with the nasopharynx to help equalize the pressure in the middle ear with the atmospheric pressure. Unfortunately, this connecting tube also provides a route by which infectious organisms enter the middle ear from the nose and throat, causing otitis media, the most common disease of the middle ear.

## PATHOPHYSIOLOGY AND MANIFESTATIONS

There are two primary forms of otitis media: (1) serous and (2) acute or suppurative. Both forms are associated with upper respiratory infection and auditory tube dysfunction. The auditory tube is narrow and flat, normally opening only during yawning and swallowing. Allergies or upper respiratory tract infections can cause edema of the tube lining, impairing its function. Air within the middle ear is trapped and gradually absorbed, creating negative pressure in this space.

## Serous Otitis Media

Serous otitis media occurs when the auditory tube is obstructed for a prolonged time, impairing equalization of air pressure in the middle ear. Air within the middle ear space is gradually absorbed; the tube obstruction prevents more air from entering the middle ear. The resulting negative pressure in the middle ear causes sterile serous fluid to move from the capillaries into the space, forming a sterile effusion of the middle ear.

Upper respiratory infection or allergies such as hay fever predispose the client to serous otitis media. Clients with narrowed or edematous auditory tubes may also be subject to barotrauma or barotitis media. In these clients, the middle ear cannot adapt to rapid changes in barometric pressure as occur during air travel or underwater diving. Barotrauma tends to occur during descent in an airplane, because negative pressure within the middle ear causes the auditory tube to collapse and lock. However, underwater diving places even greater stress on the auditory tube and middle ear (Tierney et al., 2001).

Typical manifestations of serous otitis media include decreased hearing in the affected ear and complaints of "snapping" or "popping" in the ear. On examination, the tympanic membrane demonstrates decreased mobility and may appear retracted or bulging. Fluid or air bubbles are often visible behind the drum. Severe pressure differences as occur with barotrauma may cause acute pain, hemorrhage into the middle ear, rupture of the tympanic membrane, or even rupture of the round window with sensory hearing loss and severe **vertigo** (a sensation of whirling or rotation). *Hemotympanum*, bleeding into or behind the tympanic membrane, may be observed on otoscopic examination.

## Acute Otitis Media

The auditory tube also provides a route for the entry of pathogens into the normally sterile middle ear, resulting in acute or suppurative otitis media. Acute otitis media typically follows an upper respiratory infection. Edema of the auditory tube impairs drainage of the middle ear, causing mucus and serous fluid to accumulate. This fluid is an excellent environment for the growth of bacteria, which may enter from the oronasopharynx via the auditory tube. Although a viral upper respiratory infection may predispose the client to a middle ear infection, the bacteria *Streptococcus pneumoniae*, *Haemophilus influenzae*, and *Streptococcus pyogenes* account for most cases of otitis media in adults. Invasion and colonization of the middle ear by bacteria and the resultant migration of white blood cells cause pus formation. Accumulated pus can increase middle ear pressure sufficiently to rupture the tympanic membrane. The bacterial infection may also migrate internally, causing mastoiditis, brain abscess, or bacterial meningitis. A more common complication of otitis media is a persistent conductive hearing loss, which typically resolves when the middle ear effusion clears.

The client with acute otitis media experiences mild to severe pain in the affected ear. The client's temperature is often elevated. Diminished hearing, dizziness, vertigo, and tinnitus are

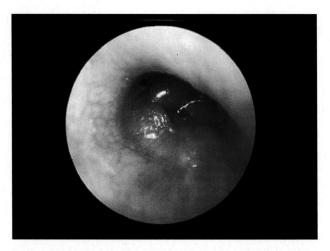

**Figure 45–13** ■ A red, bulging tympanic membrane of otitis media.

*Source: Janet Hayes/Medical Images, Inc.*

common associated complaints. Pus within the mastoid air cells often causes mastoid tenderness in acute otitis media. On otoscopic examination, the tympanic membrane appears red and inflamed or dull and bulging (Figure 45–13 ■). Decreased movement of the membrane is demonstrated by tympanometry or air insufflation. Spontaneous rupture of the tympanic membrane releases a purulent discharge. **Myringotomy** (an incision of the tympanic membrane) may be performed to relieve the pressure.

## COLLABORATIVE CARE

The diagnosis of otitis media is usually based on the history and the physical examination. The tympanic membrane may be visualized with a pneumatic otoscope that allows a puff of air to be instilled into the ear canal so that the examiner can evaluate the mobility of the tympanic membrane. Generally, the tympanic membrane moves slightly when air is instilled or the client performs the Valsalva maneuver. Less movement is seen in clients with auditory tube dysfunction and acute otitis media with effusion.

### Diagnostic Tests

- *Impedance audiometry*, also known as tympanometry, is an accurate diagnostic test for otitis media with effusion. In this test, an audiometer with a sealed probe tip is used to deliver a continuous tone to the tympanic membrane. The instrument also records the energy reflected from the surface of the tympanic membrane, allowing measurement of the compliance of the tympanic membrane and middle ear system. With middle ear effusion, compliance is reduced.
- A *CBC* may be performed to assess for an elevated WBC indicative of acute bacterial infection. If the tympanic membrane has ruptured or a tympanocentesis or myringotomy is performed, drainage is cultured to determine the infecting organism.

## Medications

Auditory tube dysfunction and serous otitis media are treated with decongestants and autoinflation of the middle ear. Decongestants are used to reduce the mucosal edema of the auditory tube and improve its patency. They may be administered either systemically or by intranasal spray. Although controversial, a short course of oral corticosteroids may be prescribed for clients with serous otitis media. (Refer to Chapter 17 ⟠ for further discussion of these medications.)

The client with auditory tube dysfunction may be taught to autoinflate the middle ear by performing the Valsalva maneuver or by forcefully exhaling against closed nostrils. Additionally, the client is advised to avoid air travel and underwater diving.

Acute otitis media is treated with antibiotic therapy, especially amoxicillin, trimethoprim-sulfamethoxazole, cefaclor, or azithromycin for 5 to 10 days. This course of treatment is long enough to ensure eradication of the infective organism; yet, short enough to reduce the incidence of bacterial resistance. (See Chapter 8 ⟠ for further discussion of antibiotics). Symptomatic relief may be provided by analgesics, antipyretics, antihistamines, and local application of heat.

## Surgery

A myringotomy or tympanocentesis may be performed to relieve excess pressure in the middle ear and prevent spontaneous rupture of the eardrum. To perform a tympanocentesis, the physician inserts a 20-gauge spinal needle through the inferior portion of the tympanic membrane, allowing aspiration of fluid and pus from the middle ear to relieve pressure and, if necessary, obtain a specimen for culture. *Myringotomy,* or surgical drainage of the middle ear, may be performed to relieve severe pain or when complications of acute otitis media, such as mastoiditis, are present. As soon as the pressure is released, pain subsides and hearing improves.

Clients who do not respond to antibiotic therapy may require myringotomy with insertion of ventilation (tympanostomy) tubes. Small tubes are inserted into the inferior portion of the tympanic membrane, providing for ventilation and drainage of the middle ear during healing. The tube is eventually extruded from the ear, and the tympanic membrane heals. While the tube is in place, it is important to avoid getting any water in the ear canal because it may then enter the middle ear space.

## NURSING CARE

Clients with otitis media are commonly treated in outpatient and community settings. The nursing role is primarily one of support and education.

## Health Promotion

Health promotion for otitis media focuses on educating clients about the importance of seeking medical care for prolonged, severe ear pain with or without drainage combined with an up-

per respiratory tract infection. Untreated or repeated attacks of otitis media can progress to a chronic form of otitis media, acute mastoiditis, or eardrum perforation.

## Assessment

Collect assessment data through a health history and physical examination (see Chapter 44).

- Health history: recent upper respiratory infection, presence of pain in affected ear, sense of fullness or pressure in the ear, change in hearing
- Physical examination: hearing test, inspect tympanic membrane

## Nursing Diagnosis and Interventions

Pain can be a significant problem for clients with otitis media, as can the risk of damage to delicate tissues of the middle ear by the infectious and inflammatory processes.

### Pain

Tissue edema, effusion of the middle ear, and the inflammatory response can affect the pain-sensitive tissues of the middle ear in otitis media, causing acute discomfort. This discomfort is increased by pressure changes, such as those that occur during air travel or underwater diving.

- Assess pain for severity, quality, and location. *A thorough assessment is important to determine the source of the pain. The pain of otitis media, unlike that of external otitis, is not aggravated by movement of the external ear.*
- Encourage the use of mild analgesics such as aspirin or acetaminophen every 4 hours as needed to relieve pain and fever. *These nonprescription medications are effective in reducing the perception of pain. Aspirin also has anti-inflammatory properties that may help relieve the inflammation of the ear.*
- Advise to apply heat to the affected side unless contraindicated. *Heat dilates blood vessels, promoting the reabsorption of fluid and reducing swelling.*
- Instruct to avoid air travel, rapid changes in elevation, or diving. *A rapid change in barometric pressure can increase the client's pain significantly.*
- Instruct to report promptly an abrupt relief of pain to the primary care provider. *Pain that subsides abruptly may indicate spontaneous perforation of the tympanic membrane with relief of pressure within the middle ear.*

### Home Care

The client who has otitis media needs teaching about the disorder, its causes and prevention, and any specific treatment recommended or prescribed. Discuss the following topics with the client and family.

- Antibiotic therapy and potential side effects
- Importance of completing all ordered doses
- Follow-up examinations in 2 to 4 weeks
- Avoid swimming, diving, or submerging the head while bathing if ventilation tubes are in place

If surgical intervention is necessary, teach the client and family members about the surgery and postoperative care. Provide instruction about any special postoperative precautions, such as avoiding water in the ear canals or avoiding sudden changes in air pressure.

## THE CLIENT WITH ACUTE MASTOIDITIS

The mastoid process is a portion of the temporal bone of the skull lying adjacent to the middle ear. It is full of air cavities called mastoid air cells or mastoid sinuses. The infection of acute otitis media always extends into the mastoid air cells; effective treatment of acute otitis media eliminates the infection from the mastoid cells as well. When treatment is ineffective, pus remains in the mastoid air cells, and acute **mastoiditis,** bacterial infection of the mastoid process, may develop.

## PATHOPHYSIOLOGY AND MANIFESTATIONS

In acute mastoiditis, the bony septa between mastoid air cells are destroyed and cells coalesce to form large spaces. Portions of the mastoid process are eroded. With chronic infection, an abscess may form, or bony sclerosis of the mastoid may result. Acute mastoiditis increases the risk of meningitis because only a very thin bony plate separates mastoid air cells from the brain. Fortunately, this complication is rare since the advent of effective antibiotic therapy for treating otitis media.

Manifestations of acute mastoiditis usually develop approximately 2 to 3 weeks after an episode of acute otitis media and include recurrent earache and hearing loss on the affected side. The pain is persistent and throbbing; tenderness is present over the mastoid process (behind the ear). It may also be red and inflamed. Swelling of the process can cause the auricle of the ear to protrude more than normal. Fever may be accompanied by tinnitus and headache. Profuse drainage from the affected ear may be noted.

## COLLABORATIVE CARE

In addition to the manifestations of acute mastoiditis, loss of septa between mastoid air cells may be noted on radiologic examination. Acute mastoiditis is treated aggressively with antibiotic therapy. Intravenous ticarcillin-clavulanate (Timentin) and gentamicin may be used initially, with therapy tailored to the specific organism once culture results are obtained. Antibiotics are continued for at least 14 days. Infections that do not respond to medical therapy or that pose a high risk of spreading to the brain may necessitate **mastoidectomy,** surgical removal of the infected mastoid air cells, bone, and pus, and inspection of the underlying dura for possible abscess. The extent of tissue destruction determines the extent of surgery required. In a modified mastoidectomy, as much tissue is preserved as possible to avoid disruption of hearing. A radical mastoidectomy involves removal of middle ear structures including the incus and malleus as well as the diseased portions of the mastoid process. Unless reconstruction is performed at the time of

surgery, this surgery results in conductive hearing loss. **Tympanoplasty,** surgical reconstruction of the middle ear, can restore or preserve hearing.

## NURSING CARE

Prevention is the primary focus of collaborative and nursing care related to mastoiditis. Adequate, effective antibiotic treatment of acute otitis media prevents mastoiditis in nearly all instances.

Following surgical intervention, carefully assess the wound and drainage for evidence of infection or other complications. The client's hearing may be temporarily or permanently affected, depending on the extent of the surgery. If the client has impaired hearing in the unaffected ear as well, develop a means of communication with the client prior to surgery. If the hearing is preserved in the unaffected ear, position the client with that ear toward the door. Speak slowly and clearly; do not shout or speak unusually loudly. Be sure that family and staff know about the client's hearing loss and use appropriate communication techniques. Assist the client with ambulation initially, because dizziness and vertigo are not unusual following surgery. Nursing care of the client having ear surgery is discussed in the box on page 1497.

### Home Care

When teaching about acute mastoiditis, stress the importance of complying with the prescribed antibiotic therapy and recommendations for follow-up. Instruct the client and family to report any adverse reactions to the primary care provider so that therapy can be adjusted. Teach the client and family how to change the surgical dressing using aseptic technique. Provide referrals to appropriate community agencies for the client with a new hearing loss resulting from mastoiditis or its treatment.

## THE CLIENT WITH CHRONIC OTITIS MEDIA

**Chronic otitis media** involves permanent perforation of the tympanic membrane, with or without recurrent pus formation and often accompanied by changes in the mucosa and bony structures (ossicles) of the middle ear. Chronic otitis media is usually a consequence of recurrent acute otitis media and auditory tube dysfunction, but may also result from trauma or other diseases.

Marginal perforations, which usually occur in the posterior-superior portion of the tympanic membrane, are associated with more complications than central perforations. With marginal perforations, squamous epithelium may migrate from the ear canal into the middle ear, where it begins to desquamate and accumulate, forming a *cholesteatoma* (a cyst or mass filled with epithelial cell debris). Its incidence is highest in young adults. The desquamating epithelium continues to accumulate and remains infected, producing collagenases (enzymes) that destroy adjacent bone. The inflammatory process compromises

# NURSING CARE OF THE CLIENT HAVING EAR SURGERY

## PREOPERATIVE CARE

- Review Chapter 7 ⊚ for routine preoperative care.
- Assess the client's hearing or verify documentation of preoperative hearing assessment. *These data are important in evaluating the results of the surgical procedure.*
- Agree on a means of communication to be used after surgery. *Hearing may be impaired after surgery.*
- Explain that blowing of the nose, coughing, and sneezing are restricted to prevent pressure changes in the middle ear and potential disruption of the surgical site. If the client needs to cough or sneeze, leaving the mouth open minimizes pressure changes in the middle ear. *Providing teaching and the opportunity to practice before surgery promotes the client's cooperation in the postoperative period.*

## POSTOPERATIVE CARE

- Review Chapter 7 for routine postoperative care.
- Assess the client for bleeding or drainage from the affected ear. *Infection and hemorrhage are possible complications.*
- Administer antiemetics as ordered to prevent vomiting. *Vomiting may increase the pressure in the middle ear, disrupting the surgical site.*
- Elevate the head of bed and have the client lie on the unaffected side. *This position minimizes the pressure in the middle ear.*
- Assess for vertigo or dizziness, especially with ambulation or movement in bed. Avoid unnecessary movements such as turning. Take measures to ensure safety when the client gets up and ambulates. *Surgery on the ear may disrupt the client's equilibrium, increasing the risk of falling.*
- Assess the client's hearing postoperatively. Stand on the client's unaffected side to communicate and use other meas-

ures such as written messages as needed for effective communication with the hearing-impaired client. Reassure the client that decreased hearing acuity immediately after surgery is expected. *Hearing improvement, if an expected result of the ear surgery, typically does not occur until ear plugs are removed, and edema and drainage at the operative site have resolved. If no reconstruction of the middle ear is done or the cochlea is involved, permanent hearing loss in the affected ear may be an expected result.*
- Remind client to avoid coughing, sneezing, or blowing the nose. *These increase pressure in the middle ear.*

### Client and Family Teaching

- Provide instructions for home care.
  a. To prevent contamination of the ear canal, avoid showers, shampooing, and immersing the head until the physician says you can do so.
  b. Keep the outer ear plug clean and dry, changing it as needed. Do not remove inner ear dressing until the physician so orders.
  c. Avoid blowing the nose; if you need to cough or sneeze, keep the mouth open.
  d. Do not swim or dive without physician approval. Check with the physician regarding air travel.
  e. Meclizine hydrochloride (Antivert) or other antiemetic/antihistamine medication may be necessary for up to 1 month following surgery.
  f. Fever, bleeding, increased drainage, increased dizziness, or decreased hearing after discharge may indicate a complication. Notify the physician if any of these occur.

---

blood supply to the stapes, causing its destruction and conductive hearing loss. Cholesteatomas are benign and slow-growing tumors, which can enlarge to fill the entire middle ear. Untreated, the cholesteatoma can progressively destroy the ossicles and erode into the inner ear, causing profound hearing loss.

Systemic antibiotics are prescribed for exacerbations of purulent otitis media. Tympanic membrane perforation is repaired with a tympanoplasty to restore sound conduction and the integrity of the middle ear. A cholesteatoma may require radical mastoidectomy to remove the tympanic membrane, ossicles, and tumor. The mastoid air cells and middle ear are converted into an open cavity, which can be inspected and cleaned as necessary.

As with other complications of acute otitis media, a priority of nursing care is prevention of chronic otitis media and cholesteatoma. Clients with chronic otitis media need to understand various treatment options and their risks and benefits, as well as the long-term risk of not treating a perforated tympanic membrane. They are also taught how to instill ear drops, to clean the external auditory meatus, and to not irrigate the ear when the tympanic membrane is perforated or if they think it might be.

If surgical treatment of chronic otitis media will affect the client's hearing, include this information in preoperative teaching. Teach the client and family how to use alternative means of communication if this will be necessary postoperatively. When an assistive device is ordered, teach the client and a family member about its use.

## THE CLIENT WITH OTOSCLEROSIS

**Otosclerosis** is a common cause of conductive hearing loss. Abnormal bone formation in the osseous labyrinth of the temporal bone causes the footplate of the stapes to become fixed or immobile in the oval window. The result is a conductive hearing loss.

Otosclerosis is a hereditary disorder with an autosomal dominant pattern of inheritance. It occurs most commonly in Caucasians and in females. The progressive hearing loss typically begins in adolescence or early adulthood and seems to be accelerated by pregnancy. Although both ears are affected, the rate of hearing loss is asymmetric. Because bone conduction of sound is retained, the client may be able to use the telephone but have difficulty conversing in person. Tinnitus may also be associated with otosclerosis.

On examination, a reddish or pinkish-orange tympanic membrane may be noted because of increased vascularity of the middle ear. The Rinne test (see Chapter 44) shows bone sound conduction to be equal to or greater than air conduction, an abnormal finding.

Clients with otosclerosis may choose conservative treatment, relying on a hearing aid to improve their ability to hear and interact with others. Sodium fluoride may be prescribed to slow bone resorption and overgrowth. Surgical treatment involves a stapedectomy and middle ear reconstruction or a stapedotomy. A *stapedectomy* is a microsurgical technique for removing the diseased stapes. A metallic prosthesis is then inserted, with one end connected to the incus and the other inserted into the oval window. *Stapedotomy* involves creation of a small hole in the footplate of the stapes and insertion of a wire or platinum ribbon prosthesis. An argon, KTP, or $CO_2$ laser may be used for surgery. Surgery usually restores hearing for the client with otosclerosis.

Education and referral of the client to appropriate community agencies are important nursing care priorities for the client with otosclerosis. For the client who chooses surgical treatment, nursing care is similar to that for other clients undergoing ear surgery. The following nursing diagnoses may be appropriate:

- *Risk for injury* related to hearing loss or postoperative vertigo
- *Disturbed sensory perception: Auditory* related to bony sclerosis of the stapes
- *Impaired verbal communication* related to hearing loss
- *Anxiety* related to concern about transmission of genetic disorder to children

## THE CLIENT WITH AN INNER EAR DISORDER

Disorders affecting the inner ear are much less common than disorders of the outer or middle ear. Inner ear disorders affect equilibrium and may also affect sensorineural hearing, the perception of sound. Labyrinthitis and Meniere's disease are the most common diseases of the inner ear. Vertigo may be a disorder of the inner ear itself or a manifestation of other disorders.

## PATHOPHYSIOLOGY AND MANIFESTATIONS

The inner ear (also called the labyrinth) contains the cochlea and the semicircular canals. The hair cells and neurons that allow sound perception and transmission to the auditory center of the brain are in the cochlea. The semicircular canals filled with endolymph are the primary organs involved in maintaining equilibrium. Disruption of this portion of the ear by an inflammatory process or excess endolymph not only affects balance but may also result in permanent hearing loss.

## Labyrinthitis

**Labyrinthitis,** also called otitis interna, is an inflammation of the inner ear. It is an uncommon disorder, because the bony protection of the membranous labyrinth makes it difficult for organisms to enter the inner ear. However, bacteria, viruses, and other organisms may enter and infect the inner ear through the oval window during acute otitis media, through the cochlear aqueduct during meningitis, or through the blood. Viral labyrinthitis is suspected when the client has a sudden onset of symptoms after an upper respiratory infection or when there is no evidence of concurrent otitis media.

Inflammation of the labyrinth typically causes vertigo, sensorineural hearing deficit, and **nystagmus** (rapid involuntary eye movements).

Vertigo, a sensation of motion when there is none, or an exaggerated sense of motion in response to movement, is the hallmark manifestation of inner ear disorders. The vertigo of labyrinthitis is severe and often accompanied by nausea and vomiting. Any movement can aggravate the vertigo, and falling is a significant risk if the client attempts to stand. Vertigo lasts days to weeks in labyrinthitis, making client education a vital component of care.

Hearing loss in the ear affected by labyrinthitis may be temporary or permanent. If inflammation destroys tissue of the membranous labyrinth, the hearing loss may be complete and permanent.

The involuntary rhythmic eye movements of nystagmus may not be present in all clients with labyrinthitis. When present, the eye movement is typically horizontal. Applying positive or negative pressure to the tympanic membrane of the affected ear may stimulate nystagmus, as will caloric testing (irrigating the ear canal with warm or cool water). Although nystagmus may also be a symptom of brainstem or cerebellar dysfunction, vertigo and hearing loss are not typically associated with those disorders.

## Meniere's Disease

**Meniere's disease,** also known as endolymphatic hydrops, is a chronic disorder of unknown cause characterized by recurrent attacks of vertigo with tinnitus and a progressive unilateral hearing loss. This disorder affects men and women equally, with adults between the ages of 35 and 60 at highest risk.

The cause of Meniere's disease is unclear. It is brought about by an overaccumulation of endolymph, the fluid in the membranous labyrinth of the inner ear. The excess fluid is thought to be caused by impaired reabsorption of endolymph in the endolymph duct or sac (Porth, 2002). The lymphatic channels dilate in response, resulting in labyrinthine dysfunction. Autonomic nervous system control of labyrinthine circulation may be impaired, or damage to the inner ear from severe otitis media or a head injury can precipitate Meniere's disease. A family history of the disease increases risk, suggesting a possible genetic link in some clients. In many clients, however, it is idiopathic, thought to be precipitated by a viral injury to the fluid transport system of the inner ear. Immune dysfunction also may contribute.

The onset of Meniere's disease may be gradual or sudden. It is characterized by recurrent attacks of vertigo, gradual loss of hearing, and tinnitus. Attacks may be preceded by a feeling of fullness in the ears, and a roaring or ringing sensation. The sensorineural hearing loss and tinnitus are usually unilateral but can become bilateral. Attacks of severe rotary vertigo occur abruptly and often unpredictably, lasting from minutes to hours. An attack may be linked to increased sodium intake, stress, allergies, vasoconstriction, or premenstrual fluid retention. As the disease continues, hearing loss progresses and the vertigo can be severe enough to cause immobility, nausea, and vomiting. Attacks are often accompanied by hypotension, sweating, and nystagmus.

## Vertigo

Normally, the integration of input from the labyrinths, eyes, muscles, joints, and neural centers maintains balance and posture. This input and integration can be affected by disorders of the labyrinth, vestibular nerve or nuclei, eyes, cerebellum, brainstem, or cerebral cortex, causing vertigo. Vertigo is a disorder of equilibrium. The sensation of whirling, rotation, or movement is described as either subjective or objective.

Clients with subjective vertigo report the sensation of being in motion in a stable environment. This is not always a sense of spinning; the client may have a sense of tumbling or falling forward or backward. The sensation is reversed in objective vertigo; clients report a sensation of stability in a moving environment. This motion may be perceived as the room spinning around the client or the ground rocking beneath the client's feet. Dizziness, which may be mistaken for vertigo, is a sensation of unsteadiness, lack of balance, lightheadedness, or movement within the head. The person who is dizzy does not have the rotational sensation felt with vertigo.

Vertigo may be disabling, resulting in falls, injury, and difficulty walking. Attacks of vertigo are often accompanied by nausea and vomiting, nystagmus, and autonomic symptoms such as pallor, sweating, hypotension, and salivation.

## COLLABORATIVE CARE

The manifestations associated with inner ear disorders are similar, making testing necessary to establish a diagnosis. Once the diagnosis is determined, collaborative care is directed toward managing symptoms and preventing permanent hearing loss.

The following diagnostic studies may be ordered.

- *Electronystagmography* evaluates the vestibulo-ocular reflex by identifying eye movements (nystagmus) in response to caloric testing. Water is instilled directly into the ear canal so that it contacts the tympanic membrane while eye motion is recorded. In clients with impaired vestibular function, the normal nystagmus response is blunted or absent. This portion of the test is contraindicated in clients who have a perforated tympanic membrane.
- *Rinne* and *Weber tests* of hearing (see Chapter 44) show decreased air and bone conduction on the affected side if a sensorineural hearing loss is present. In Meniere's disease,

audiology shows sensorineural hearing loss involving the low tones.

- *X-rays* and *CT scans* of the petrous bones are used to evaluate the internal auditory canal. In clients with Meniere's disease, the vestibular aqueducts may be shorter and straighter than normal.
- *Glycerol test* is conducted by giving the client oral glycerol to decrease fluid pressure in the inner ear. An acute temporary hearing improvement is considered diagnostic for Meniere's disease.

Once the diagnosis is established, specific treatments can be ordered. Clients with labyrinthitis or an acute attack of Meniere's disease may require hospitalization to manage the vertigo and its effects. Atropine is used to decrease the parasympathetic nervous system response. A central nervous system depressant such as diazepam (Valium) or lorazepam (Ativan) may be an alternative to atropine. Parenteral droperidol (Inapsine) provides both a sedative and antiemetic effect, making it a useful drug for acute attacks. Antivertigo/antiemetic medications such as meclizine (Antivert), prochlorperazine (Compazine), or hydroxyzine hydrochloride (Vistaril) are prescribed to reduce the whirling sensation and nausea. If the nausea and vomiting are severe, intravenous fluids may be necessary to maintain fluid and electrolyte balance. Bed rest in a quiet, darkened room with minimal sensory stimuli and minimal movement provides the most comfort for the client.

Large doses of antibiotics, often administered intravenously, are prescribed for labyrinthitis when the cause is thought to be bacterial. No specific therapy is indicated for viral labyrinthitis.

Management of the client between acute attacks of Meniere's disease is directed at preventing future attacks and preserving hearing. A low-sodium diet and an oral diuretic such as furosemide (Lasix) or hydrochlorothiazide/triamterene (Dyazide) help maintain a lower labyrinthine pressure. The Furstenberg diet, a salt-free neutral ash diet, may be prescribed if moderate sodium restriction is ineffective in controlling attacks. Clients should avoid tobacco, which causes vasoconstriction and can precipitate an attack, along with alcohol and caffeine.

When medical interventions are ineffective in controlling episodes of vertigo in Meniere's disease, surgical intervention may be necessary. Surgical *endolymphatic decompression* relieves the excess pressure in the labyrinth; a shunt is then inserted between the membranous labyrinth and the subarachnoid space to drain excess fluid away from the labyrinths and maintain lower pressure. This procedure preserves hearing for the majority of the clients. Vertigo is relieved in approximately 70% of clients, but the sensations of fullness and tinnitus remain for about 50% of people after the surgery.

Destruction of a portion of the acoustic nerve is an alternative to shunting procedures. In a *vestibular neurectomy*, the portion of the cranial nerve VIII controlling balance and sensations of vertigo is severed. This procedure relieves vertigo for up to 90% of clients. Although there is a risk of damage to the cochlear portion of the nerve and resultant hearing loss, for most clients hearing loss stabilizes after neurectomy, even improving for some.

The surgery of last resort for Meniere's disease is a **labyrinthectomy.** The labyrinth is completely removed, destroying cochlear function. This procedure is used only when hearing loss is nearly complete and vertigo is persistent. Although labyrinthectomy relieves vertigo in nearly all cases, the client may remain unsteady and have continued problems with balance.

After surgery on the inner ear, the client is positioned to minimize ear pressure and vertigo. The client's movement is restricted, and assistance is provided when the client gets up. Antiemetics and antivertigo medications are used to manage the symptoms resulting from disruption of the inner ear. Complications include infection and leakage of cerebral spinal fluid.

## NURSING CARE

The client with an inner ear disorder has multiple nursing care needs related to the manifestations of the disorder.

### Health Promotion

Health promotion focuses on identifying clients with potential inner ear disorders. Persistent episodes of dizziness, ringing in the ears, balance problems, or loss of hearing should be reported to a health care provider. Clients diagnosed early may have a lower risk for injury and can be taught strategies for maintaining as near normal as possible their work and social life.

### Assessment

Collect the following data for the client with potential inner ear disorders through a health history and physical examination. Assess the older client further for other medical causes of imbalance and dizziness. Neurologic dysfunction, musculoskeletal and cardiovascular disorders, and endocrine problems often contribute to the older client's unsteadiness.

- Health history: medication use; presence of vertigo, nystagmus, nausea and vomiting, and hearing loss; balance problems; frequency and duration of symptoms
- Physical examination: hearing, tinnitus, balance

### Nursing Diagnoses and Interventions

The risk for trauma in clients with inner ear disorders is great. Attacks of vertigo may occur without warning and can be so severe that the client is unable to remain upright. If frequent attacks are accompanied by vertigo, the client's nutrition may be compromised. Constant or intermittent tinnitus can interfere with sleep and rest. Finally, because nearly all inner ear disorders are associated with some degree of hearing loss, which may be progressive, the client has significant psychosocial needs.

### Risk for Trauma

Because of the unpredictable nature of attacks, the client with vertigo due to an inner ear disorder needs to learn strategies for dealing with an acute episode. Because vertigo tends to be chronic except in acute viral labyrinthitis, the emphasis is on helping the client develop strategies to reduce the frequency of attacks and the risk of injury.

- Monitor for vertigo, nystagmus, nausea, vomiting, and hearing loss. *Monitoring is important to determine the severity of impairment, the duration of attacks, and the client's ability to predict an impending attack.*

**PRACTICE ALERT** *During an acute attack of vertigo, keep on bed rest with the side rails raised and the call light readily accessible.* ■

- Instruct to not get up without assistance during episodes of vertigo. *During attacks of vertigo, assistance reduces the risk of falling.*
- Teach to avoid sudden head movements or position changes. *Sudden movement may precipitate an attack of vertigo.*
- Administer prescribed medications as ordered, including antiemetics, diuretics, and sedatives. *These medications may reduce the frequency, severity, and duration of vertigo attacks.*
- Instruct that when sensing an impending attack it is best to respond by taking the prescribed medication and lying down in a quiet, darkened room. *These measures help protect the client from injury and may shorten the duration and reduce the severity of the attack.*
- Advise to pull to the side of the road and wait for the symptoms to subside if an attack occurs while the client is driving. *Perception and judgment necessary for safe driving may be impaired during an acute attack; pulling off the road is vital to protect the safety of the client and others.*
- Discuss the effect of unilateral hearing loss on the ability to identify the direction from which sounds come. To ensure safety, encourage the client to use other senses (e.g., when crossing the street). *Just as depth perception changes when vision is lost in one eye, sound perception and differentiation of direction change when hearing is lost unilaterally.*

### Sleep Pattern Disturbance

The tinnitus often associated with inner ear disorders may be loud and continuous, interfering with the client's ability to concentrate, relax, and sleep. It may be perceived as a continuous high-pitched whine, buzzing, ringing, or humming sound. In some clients, it may have a pulsatile quality.

- Refer for a complete hearing and ear examination if one has not been done. *Although most tinnitus is associated with hearing loss, often due to noise exposure, it may also be associated with treatable conditions such as impacted cerumen, hypertension, cerebrovascular disorders, and other conditions.*
- Discuss options for masking tinnitus to promote concentration and sleep.
  a. Ambient noise from a radio or sound system
  b. Masking device or white-noise machine
  c. Hearing aid that produces a tone to mask the tinnitus
  d. Hearing aid that amplifies ambient sound

## CHART 45–3  NANDA, NIC, AND NOC LINKAGES

### The Client with Inner Ear Disorders

| NURSING DIAGNOSES | NURSING INTERVENTIONS | NURSING OUTCOMES |
| --- | --- | --- |
| • Disturbed Sensory Perception: Auditory | • Communication Enhancement: Hearing Deficit | • Hearing Compensation Behavior<br>• Risk Control: Hearing Impairment |
| • Risk for Trauma | • Environmental Management: Safety | • Safety Behavior: Fall Prevention |
| • Disturbed Sleep Pattern | • Sleep Enhancement | • Sleep |

*Note. Data from* Nursing Outcomes Classification (NOC) *by M. Johnson & M. Maas (Eds.), 1997, St. Louis: Mosby;* Nursing Diagnoses: Definitions & Classification 2001–2002 *by North American Nursing Diagnosis Association, 2001, Philadelphia: NANDA;* Nursing Interventions Classification (NIC) *by J.C. McCloskey & G. M. Bulechek (Eds.), 2000, St. Louis: Mosby. Reprinted by permission.*

*These techniques or devices help mask the subjective perception of tinnitus, allowing the client to focus on something other than the sound.*

- Discuss the possible risks and benefits of medications to treat tinnitus. *Many medications have been used to treat tinnitus; oral antidepressants such as nortriptyline (Aventyl, Pamelor) taken at bedtime have been shown to be most effective.*

## Using NANDA, NIC, and NOC

Chart 45–3 shows links between NANDA nursing diagnoses, NIC, and NOC when caring for the client with an inner ear disorder.

## Home Care

Because disorders of the inner ear disrupt balance, safety is a primary focus of teaching. The nurse assists the client to identify possible hazards in the home environment. Discuss the following points during the teaching session.

- Change positions slowly, especially when ambulating.
- Turn the whole body rather than just the head.
- Sit down immediately with the onset of vertigo and lie down if possible.
- Take prescribed antiemetic and antivertigo medications.
- Wear MedicAlert identification.
- If appropriate, discuss the surgical procedure, the immediate postoperative period, and the long-term effects of the surgery.
- Discuss alternative communication techniques as needed.
- Suggest the following resources.
  - Better Hearing Institute
  - Self-Help for Hard of Hearing People

## THE CLIENT WITH AN ACOUSTIC NEUROMA

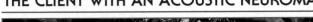

An **acoustic neuroma** or **schwannoma** is a benign tumor of cranial nerve VIII. It typically occurs in adults between the ages of 40 and 50. Acoustic neuromas are common and account for 7% to 8% of intracranial tumors (Way & Doherty, 2003).

These tumors usually occur in the internal auditory meatus, compressing the auditory nerve where it exits the skull to the inner ear. Both the vestibular and cochlear branches are af-

fected; however, the tumor arises from the vestibular division of the auditory nerve twice as often. If allowed to grow, the tumor eventually destroys the labyrinth, including the cochlea and vestibular apparatus. As the tumor expands, it erodes the wall of the internal auditory meatus. The tumor may eventually impinge on the inferior cerebellar artery, which provides blood to the lateral pons and medulla, the brainstem, and the cerebellum. An obstructive hydrocephalus can also occur. Cranial nerves VII (facial) and V (trigeminal) are often affected by the expanding tumor; the tumor frequently wraps around the facial nerve.

Early manifestations of an acoustic neuroma are those associated with disorders of the inner ear: tinnitus, unilateral hearing loss, and nystagmus. Dizziness or vertigo may occur. As the tumor expands and occupies increasing amounts of space in the closed cranium, the client experiences neurologic signs related to the area of the brain affected.

The presence of the tumor can generally be identified on CT or MRI scans. X-ray films of the petrous pyramid of the temporal bone may show erosion caused by the tumor.

The treatment of choice for an acoustic neuroma is surgical excision. In surgery, every effort is made to preserve this nerve and its function as well as other cranial nerves that may be affected. Small tumors of the vestibular division of the acoustic nerve may be excised using microsurgical techniques; hearing can often be preserved. A translabyrinthine approach provides good access to the tumor and allows the facial nerve to be preserved. However, this approach destroys hearing in the affected ear, and it is usually used only when the tumor is large or little effective hearing remains in the affected ear. Larger tumors require craniotomy for removal; facial nerve paralysis is a common result of surgery.

Postoperative nursing care focuses on preserving cerebral function. Position the client to minimize cerebral edema and monitor frequently for signs of increased intracranial pressure. Because the gag reflex may be affected, assess the client carefully before food and fluids are allowed by mouth. Speech therapy is often prescribed for the client after surgery. Because deficits may not resolve for a long time after surgery, education and support are vital components of nursing care for the client. (See Chapter 40 ⊙⊙ for care of the client undergoing craniotomy).

## THE CLIENT WITH A HEARING LOSS

Approximately 10 million adults in the United States are hearing impaired. The problem of hearing loss is particularly significant in older adults, affecting an estimated 24% of people between the ages of 65 and 74, and up to 39% of those over age 75. As many as 70% of nursing home residents have impaired hearing. Hearing loss is more prevalent in lower socioeconomic groups of older adults (Hazzard et al., 1998).

Lesions in the outer ear, middle ear, inner ear, or central auditory pathways can result in hearing loss. The process of aging also can affect the structures of the ear and hearing. Hearing loss is classified as conductive, sensorineural, or mixed, depending on what portion of the auditory system is affected. Profound deafness is often a congenital condition.

Clients with a hearing loss, whether conductive or sensorineural, may display signs that caregivers can recognize. The voice volume of the hearing-impaired client frequently increases, and the client positions the head with the better ear toward the speaker. The client frequently may ask people to repeat what they have said or respond inappropriately to questions or statements. A question may elicit a blank look if the client has not heard or understood its content.

## PATHOPHYSIOLOGY AND MANIFESTATIONS

Hearing loss impairs the ability to communicate in a world filled with sound and hearing individuals. A hearing deficit can be partial or total, congenital or acquired. It may affect one or both ears. In some types of hearing loss, the ability to perceive sound at specific frequencies is lost. In others, hearing is diminished across all frequencies.

### Conductive Hearing Loss

Anything that disrupts the transmission of sound from the external auditory meatus to the inner ear results in a conductive hearing loss. The most common cause of conductive hearing loss is obstruction of the external ear canal. Impacted cerumen, edema of the canal lining, stenosis, and neoplasms all may lead to canal obstruction. Other etiologic factors for conductive loss include a perforated tympanic membrane, disruption or fixation of the ossicles of the middle ear, fluid, scarring, or tumors of the middle ear.

With conductive hearing loss, there is an equal loss of hearing at all sound frequencies. If the level of sound is greater than the threshold for hearing, speech discrimination is good. Because of this, the client with a conductive hearing loss benefits from amplification by a hearing aid.

### Sensorineural Hearing Loss

Disorders that affect the inner ear, the auditory nerve, or the auditory pathways of the brain may lead to a sensorineural hearing loss. In this type of hearing loss, sound waves are effectively transmitted to the inner ear. In the inner ear, however, lost or damaged receptor cells, changes in the cochlear apparatus, or auditory nerve abnormalities decrease or distort the ability to receive and interpret stimuli.

A significant cause of sensorineural hearing deficit is damage to the hair cells of the organ of Corti. In the United States, noise exposure is the major cause. Exposure to a high level of noise (e.g., standing close to the stage or speakers at a rock concert) on an intermittent or continuing basis damages the hair and supporting cells of the organ of Corti. Ototoxic drugs also damage the hair cells; when combined with high noise levels, the damage is greater and resultant hearing loss more profound. Ototoxic drugs include aspirin, furosemide (Lasix), aminoglycosides, vancomycin (Vancocin), antimalarial drugs, and chemotherapy such as cisplatin (Platinol). Other potential causes of sensory hearing loss include prenatal exposure to rubella, viral infections, meningitis, trauma, Meniere's disease, and aging.

Tumors such as acoustic neuromas, vascular disorders, demyelinating or degenerative diseases, infections (bacterial meningitis in particular), or trauma may affect the central auditory pathways and produce a neural hearing loss.

Sensorineural hearing losses typically affect the perception of high-frequency tones more than of low-frequency tones. This loss makes speech discrimination difficult, especially in a noisy environment. Hearing aids are often not useful, because they amplify both speech and background noise. The increased sound intensity may actually cause discomfort for the client.

### Presbycusis

With aging, the hair cells of the cochlea degenerate, producing a progressive sensorineural hearing loss. In presbycusis, hearing acuity begins to decrease in early adulthood and progresses as long as the individual lives. Higher pitched tones and conversational speech are lost initially. Hearing aids and other amplification devices are useful for most clients with presbycusis.

Because the hearing loss of presbycusis is gradual, the client and family may not realize the extent of the deficit. The hearing-impaired individual may be described as unsociable or paranoid. The family may worry that the person is becoming increasingly forgetful, absent minded, or perhaps "senile." Depression, confusion, inattentiveness, tension, and negativism have been noted in hearing-impaired older adults. Functional problems such as poor general health, reduced mobility, and impaired interpersonal communication are also associated with hearing loss. Caregivers need to be alert for signs of impaired hearing such as cupping an ear, difficulty understanding verbal communication when the person cannot see the speaker's face, difficulty following conversation in a large group, and withdrawal from social activities.

### Tinnitus

Tinnitus is the perception of sound or noise in the ears without stimulus from the environment. The sound may be steady, intermittent, or pulsatile and is often described as a buzzing, roaring, or ringing.

Tinnitus is usually associated with hearing loss (conductive or sensorineural); however, the mechanism producing the sound is poorly understood. It is often an early symptom of noise-induced hearing damage and drug-related ototoxicity. Tinnitus is especially associated with salicylate, quinine, or quinidine toxicity. Other etiologic conditions include obstruction of the auditory meatus, presbycusis, inflammations and infections of the middle or inner ear, otosclerosis, and Meniere's disease. Most tinnitus, however, is chronic and has no pathologic importance.

Tinnitus that is intermittent or slight enough to be masked by environmental sounds is often well tolerated. When it is loud, continuous, and not responsive to treatment, tinnitus can be a significant stressor. It can interfere with activities of daily living, sleep, and rest.

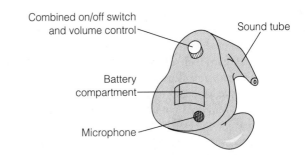

**Figure 45–14** ■ An in-ear hearing aid.

## COLLABORATIVE CARE

The best treatment for hearing loss is prevention. Clients need to know the potential for hearing damage and how to prevent it. Awareness of the effects of noise exposure, especially when combined with the ototoxic effects of aspirin or other drugs, is important to prevent sensorineural hearing loss.

### Diagnostic Tests

Hearing evaluation includes gross tests of hearing (such as the whisper test), the Rinne and Weber tests, and audiometry.

- *Rinne and Weber tests* compare air and bone sound conduction. When bone conduction of sound is better than air conduction, the hearing deficit is a conductive loss. The Rinne test can identify even mild conductive hearing losses. If both air and bone conduction are impaired, a sensorineural loss is indicated. (See Chapter 44.)
- *Audiometry* identifies the type and pattern of hearing loss. Specific sound frequencies are presented to each ear by either air or bone conduction.
- *Speech audiometry* identifies the intensity at which speech can be recognized and interpreted.
- *Tympanometry* is an indirect measurement of the compliance and impedance of the middle ear to sound transmission. The external auditory meatus is subjected to neutral, positive, and negative air pressure while the resultant sound energy flow is monitored.

### Amplification

A hearing aid or other amplification device can help many clients with hearing deficits. These assistive devices do nothing to prevent, minimize, or treat the hearing loss itself, but they amplify the sound presented to the hearing apparatus of the ear. Amplification may bring the level of sound above the hearing threshold for the client, allowing more accurate perception and interpretation of its meaning. For the client with distorted sound perception, the hearing aid may be less helpful, because it simply amplifies the distorted sound.

Unfortunately, less than one-fifth of older clients with a hearing deficit have a hearing aid. Denial of the deficit, other health problems, poor visual acuity, decreased manual dexterity, and cost all contribute to this low usage. Hearing aids must

be individually prescribed by an audiologist. Proper design, proper fit, and regular maintenance are necessary for their effectiveness.

Hearing aids are available in a variety of styles, each with advantages and disadvantages. The newest and least noticeable style fits entirely in the ear canal. This small and unobtrusive device allows use of the telephone and can be worn during exercise. Because of its small size, the client must have good manual dexterity to insert it, clean it, and change the batteries. For this reason, older clients or clients with impaired dexterity may be unable to use it.

The in-ear style of aid fits into the external ear and is more visible than the in-canal aid (Figure 45–14 ■). Its larger size makes manipulation somewhat easier, although it still may be difficult for less dextrous individuals. A greater degree of amplification is possible with the in-ear aid. Many have a toggle switch for telephone usage. With both the in-canal and in-ear style, cleaning is important. Small portals may become plugged with cerumen, interfering with sound transmission.

The behind-ear hearing aid allows finer adjustment of the level of amplification and is easier for the client to manipulate (Figure 45–15 ■). For the client who wears glasses, this style can be modified, with all components fitting into the temple of the eyeglasses.

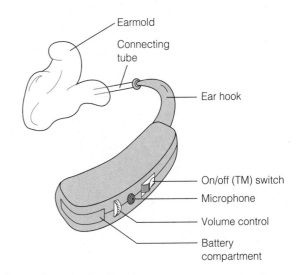

**Figure 45–15** ■ A behind-ear hearing aid.

Clients with profound hearing loss may require a body hearing aid. The microphone and amplifier of this aid are contained in a pocket-sized case that the client clips on to clothing, slips into a pocket, or carries in a harness. The receiver is attached by a cord to the case and clips onto the ear mold, which delivers the sound to the ear canal.

For the client who does not have a hearing aid, an *assistive listening device,* or "pocket talker," with a microphone and "Walkman" type earpieces, is useful. Pocket talkers are available over the counter or through an audiologist and are relatively inexpensive. The earpiece requires no special fitting, and the external microphone allows the client to focus on the desired sound rather than simply amplifying all sounds. Assistive listening devices may also be used in conjunction with a hearing aid.

Clients with tinnitus may find a white-noise masking device helpful to promote concentration and rest. These devices conduct a pleasant sound to the affected ear, allowing the client to block out the abnormal sound.

## Surgery

Reconstructive surgeries of the middle ear, such as a stapedectomy or tympanoplasty, may be useful for the client with a conductive hearing loss. Stapedectomy is the removal and replacement of the stapes. This procedure is used for clients with a conductive hearing loss related to otosclerosis.

In a tympanoplasty, the structures of the middle ear are reconstructed to improve conductive hearing deficits. Chronic otitis media with necrosis and scarring of the middle ear is a common indication for this type of surgery.

For the client with a sensorineural hearing loss, a cochlear implant may be the only hope for restoring sound perception. Two types of cochlear implant are available. The first uses an electrode implanted in the cochlea to stimulate remaining, intact, excitable auditory neurons (Figure 45–16 ■). A small

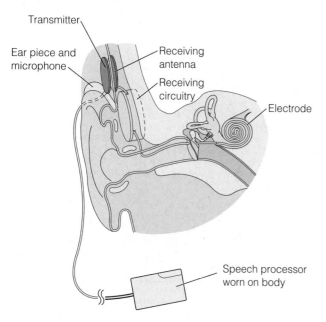

Transmitter

Ear piece and microphone

Receiving antenna

Receiving circuitry

Electrode

Speech processor worn on body

**Figure 45–16** ■ A cochlear implant for sensorineural hearing loss.

processor carried outside the body receives sound through a microphone and sends a signal to a transmitter mounted behind the ear. The transmitter then sends the signal to a receiver implanted under the skin, which in turn transmits it to the electrode implanted in the cochlea.

The second type of cochlear implant is used when no excitable auditory nerve fibers are available. The external microphone-transmitter sends the signal to an implanted receiver, which transmits the stimulus via an electrode implanted in the brainstem over the cochlear nucleus.

Cochlear prostheses provide the client with the perception of sound but not normal hearing. The client is able to recognize warning sounds such as automobiles, sirens, telephones, and doors opening or closing. They also receive stimuli to alert them to incoming communication so they can focus on the person speaking. Many clients can learn to interpret the perceived sounds as words, especially with newer implant devices.

## NURSING CARE

In planning and implementing nursing care for the client with a hearing deficit, the nurse needs to consider the type and extent of hearing loss, the client's adaptation to the loss, and the availability of assistive hearing devices and the client's ability and willingness to use them.

### Health Promotion

Health care personnel can be instrumental in preventing hearing loss through education. It is important to promote environmental noise control and the use of ear protection. The Occupational Safety and Health Administration (OSHA) requires ear protection for work environments that consistently exceed 85 decibels. Teaching for primary prevention focuses on the following:

- Care of the ears and ear canals, including cleaning and treatment of infection
- No placing of any hard objects into the ear canal
- Use of plugs to protect the ears during swimming or diving
- Protecting the hearing by avoiding intermittent or frequent exposure to loud noise
- Monitoring for side effects with ototoxic medications
- Hearing evaluation when hearing difficulty is present

### Assessment

Collect the following data through a health history and physical examination (see Chapter 44).

- Health history: ototoxic medication use; presence of upper respiratory tract infection, previous bacterial or viral infections; high noise level exposure; presence of vertigo, tinnitus, unsteadiness, or imbalance
- Physical examination: external ear, tympanic membrane; hearing, cranial nerve

## Nursing Diagnoses and Interventions

This section focuses on the problems of having a hearing deficit, impaired communication, and social isolation for the client who is hearing impaired.

### Disturbed Sensory Perception: Auditory

Whether the client's hearing deficit is partial or total, impaired sound perception is the primary problem. The client needs to understand what causes the deficit and what to expect for the future. Nursing interventions focus on maximizing available hearing and preventing further deterioration to the extent possible.

- Encourage to talk about the loss of hearing and its effect on activities of daily living. *Hearing loss affects each individual in a different way. The client may be denying the extent of the deficit or grieving the loss. Listening to the client and providing support encourage the client to develop coping strategies.*
- Provide information about the type of hearing loss. Refer to an audiologist for evaluation of the hearing loss and possible exploration of amplification devices. *With improved understanding of the deficit, the client can plan ways to compensate.*
- Replace batteries in hearing aids regularly and as needed. *Hearing aid batteries last approximately 1 week. If a battery is old or has been improperly stored, the life may be reduced further.*
- If the hearing aid has a toggle switch for microphone/telephone, be sure it is in the appropriate position. *This ensures proper amplification with the hearing aid.*

**PRACTICE ALERT** *Check hearing aids for patency, cleaning out cerumen as necessary.* ∎

### Impaired Verbal Communication

A hearing deficit impairs the client's ability to receive and interpret verbal communication. A hearing loss affects the client's ability to follow conversations, use the telephone, and enjoy television or other forms of entertainment.

- Wave the hand or tap the shoulder before beginning to speak.
- When speaking, face the client and keep the hands away from the face.
- Keep your face in full light.
- Reduce the noise in the environment before speaking.
- Use a low voice pitch with normal loudness.
- Use short sentences and pause at the end of each sentence.
- Speak at a normal rate, and do not overarticulate.
- Use facial expressions or gestures.
- Provide a magic slate for written communication.

This prepares the client to receive incoming communication. Hearing-impaired individuals often lip-read, making good visibility of the speaker's face necessary. Excessive environmental noise interferes with the ability to perceive the message. Higher tones are typically lost with presbycusis and other types of hearing loss. Using short sentences and pausing give the client time to interpret the message. Overarticulating

makes it more difficult to follow the flow and to lip-read. Nonverbal cues and written messages enhance the client's understanding.

- Be sure hearing aid is properly placed, is turned on, and has fresh batteries. *The client may not be aware that the hearing aid is not functioning well.*
- Do not place intravenous catheters in the dominant hand. *The client may need to use that hand to write.*
- Rephrase sentences when there is difficulty understanding. *Hearing losses may affect different sound tones, making some words more difficult to comprehend. Using alternative words and phrases may increase the client's ability to perceive the message.*
- Repeat important information. *The nurse makes sure that the client understands the information.*
- Inform other staff about the client's hearing deficit and effective strategies for communication. *Consistent use of effective strategies for communication decreases the client's frustration.*

### Social Isolation

The client with impaired hearing often becomes socially isolated. This isolation may be self-imposed because of the client's difficulty in communicating, especially in a group. Often, however, the isolation comes about gradually and without intention. The client finds social settings such as family dinners or community gatherings increasingly difficult. Friends and family become frustrated trying to communicate with the hearing-impaired person, and invitations to participate in social activities dwindle.

- Identify the extent and cause of the social isolation. Help to differentiate the reality of the isolation and its cause from the client's perception of isolation. *Hearing-impaired clients may be unaware that they are isolated. Identifying factors that contribute to the isolation may provide the impetus the client needs to remedy the hearing loss. Clients may also experience paranoid thinking as a result of the impaired communication and believe that friends and family have purposely begun to avoid interactions.*
- Encourage to interact with friends and family on a one-to-one basis in quiet settings. *Clients with impaired hearing are more successful in understanding conversations that take place in small groups and quiet settings.*
- Treat with dignity and remind friends and family that a hearing deficit does not mean loss of mental faculties. *Inappropriate responses due to a hearing deficit can cause others to perceive the client as "stupid" or demented.*
- Involve in activities that do not require acute hearing, such as checkers and chess. *The client has an opportunity to interact socially without the stress of straining to hear.*
- Obtain a pocket talker or encourage the client and family to do so.
- Refer the client to an audiologist for evaluation and possible hearing-aid fitting.
- Refer to resources such as support groups and senior citizen centers. *These groups provide new social outlets.*

---

### CHART 45–4 NANDA, NIC, AND NOC LINKAGES

**The Client with a Hearing Loss**

| NURSING DIAGNOSES | NURSING INTERVENTIONS | NURSING OUTCOMES |
|---|---|---|
| • Impaired Verbal Communication<br><br>• Social Isolation | • Communication Enhancement: Hearing Deficit<br>• Social Enhancement | • Communication: Receptive Ability<br><br>• Loneliness<br>• Social Involvement<br>• Well-Being |

*Note. Data from Nursing Outcomes Classification (NOC) by M. Johnson & M. Maas (Eds.), 1997, St. Louis: Mosby; Nursing Diagnoses: Definitions & Classification 2001–2002 by North American Nursing Diagnosis Association, 2001, Philadelphia: NANDA; Nursing Interventions Classification (NIC) by J.C. McCloskey & G. M. Bulechek (Eds.), 2000, St. Louis: Mosby. Reprinted by permission.*

---

## Using NANDA, NIC, and NOC

Chart 45–4 shows links between NANDA nursing diagnoses, NIC, and NOC when caring for the client with a hearing loss.

## Home Care

For the client with a permanent hearing loss, teaching relates to managing the deficit and developing coping strategies. The nurse can refer the client to an audiologist to evaluate the usefulness of a hearing aid. In addition, discuss the following topics as appropriate for each client.

• Use, care, and maintenance of a hearing aid

• Strategies for coping with the hearing deficit
• Voicing a preference for individual visits and small group interactions rather than large social functions
• Helpful resources include the following:
  • American Deafness and Rehabilitation Association
  • International Hearing Dog, Inc.
  • National Association for the Deaf
  • National Institute on Deafness and Other Communication Disorders
  • Self-Help for Hard of Hearing People

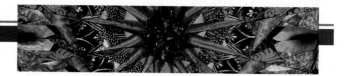

 **EXPLORE MediaLink**

NCLEX review questions, case studies, care plan activities, MediaLink applications, and other interactive resources for this chapter can be found on the Companion Website at www.prenhall.com/lemone.

Click on Chapter 45 to select the activities for this chapter. For animations, video clips, more NCLEX review questions, and an audio glossary, access the Student CD-ROM accompanying this textbook.

---

## TEST YOURSELF

1. A client complains of decreasing peripheral vision and halos around lights. These manifestations are characteristic of:
   a. Retinal detachment
   b. Open-angle glaucoma
   c. Cataract
   d. Macular degeneration

2. A client with Meniere's disease experiences frequent attacks of vertigo and tinnitus. Of the following teaching points, which one has the highest priority for this client?
   a. Provide instruction about a low-sodium diet
   b. Encourage the client to stop smoking

   c. Instruct the client about antiemetic medications
   d. Teach the client to sit down immediately during an attack

3. A patient with glaucoma also has a history of bradycardia. Which medication should the nurse discuss with the physician before administering it?
   a. Pilocarpine (Isopto Carpine)
   b. Acetazolamide (Diamox)
   c. Timolol (Timoptic)
   d. Epinephrine (Epitrate)

4. During the first 24 hours after eye surgery, what is the rationale for placing the client in a semi-Fowler's position on the unaffected side?

   a. To reduce intraocular pressure in the affected eye
   b. To prevent hemorrhage in the affected eye
   c. To prevent accidental scratching of the cornea
   d. To increase retinal contact with the choroid

5. The nurse should suspect a potential hearing impairment when a client demonstrates which one of the following manifestations:

   a. Speaks in soft tones
   b. Complains of persistent ear ringing
   c. Asks for questions to be repeated
   d. Socially withdraws from group interactions

See Test Yourself answers in Appendix C.

## BIBLIOGRAPHY

Ackley, B. J., & Ladwig, G. B. (2002). *Nursing diagnosis handbook: A guide to planning care* (5th ed.). St. Louis: Mosby.

Andreoli, T. E., Bennett, J. C., Carpenter, C. C. J., & Plum, F. (1997). *Cecil essentials of medicine* (4th ed.). Philadelphia: W. B. Saunders Company.

Barnes, G. (1997). The suitability of cataract patients for day surgery. *Professional Nurse, 12*(4), 264–268.

Braunwald, E., Fauci, A. S., Kasper, D. L., Hauser, S. L., Longo, D. L, & Jameson, J. L. (2001). *Harrison's principles of internal medicine* (15th ed.). New York: McGraw-Hill.

Bullock, B. A. & Henze, R. L. (2000). *Focus on pathophysiology*. Philadelphia: Lippincott.

Coleman, A. L. (1999, November, 20). Glaucoma. *The Lancet, 354*, 1803–1810.

Copstead, L. E. & Banasik, J. L. (2000). *Pathophysiology biological and behavioral perspectives* (2nd ed.). Philadelphia: W. B. Saunders.

Demers, K. (2001). Hearing screening. *Journal of Gerontological Nursing, 27*(11), 8–9.

Duffield, P. (1997). Primary care diagnosis of acute closed-angle glaucoma. A case report. *Advance for Nurse Practitioners, 5*(11), 67.

Elfervig, L. S. (1998). Age-related macular degeneration. *Nurse Practitioner Forum, 9*(1), 4–6.

Eliopoulos, C. (2001). *Gerontological nursing* (5th ed.). Philadelphia: Lippincott.

Galant, J. J. (1997). Differential diagnosis of decreased vision: A case study. *Journal of the American Academy of Nurse Practitioners, 9*(9), 421–425.

Hazzard, W. R., Blass, J. P., Ettinger, W. H., Jr., Halter, J. B., Ouslader, J. G. (Eds.). (1998).

*Principles of geriatric medicine and gerontology* (4th ed.). New York: McGraw-Hill.

Ho-Shing, D. (2000). Treating glaucoma with drainage and pericardial grafts. *AORN, 71*(6), 1237–1251.

Johnson, M., & Maas, M. (Eds.). (2000). *Nursing outcomes classification (NOC)*. St. Louis: Mosby.

Jupiter, T., & Spivey, V. (1997). Perception of hearing loss and hearing handicap on hearing aid use by nursing home residents. *Geriatric Nursing, 18*(5), 201–207.

Kupecz, D. (2001). Keeping up with recent ophthalmic drug approvals. *The Nurse Practitioner, 26*(4), 61–62, 64, 67.

McCloskey, J. C., & Bulechek, G. M. (Eds.). (2000). *Nursing interventions classification (NIC)* (3rd ed.). St. Louis: Mosby.

National Institutes of Health, National Eye Institute. (2001). National Eye Institute low vision resource list. Available www.nei.nih.gov/health/lowvision/resources.htm

_____ . (2001). National Eye Institute statement on detection of glaucoma. Available www.nei.nih.gov/nehep/statements.htm

_____ . (2001). National Eye Institute statement on vision screening in adults. Available www.nei.nih.gov/news/statements/visions_task.htm

Ney, D. F. (1993, March/April). Cerumen impaction, ear hygiene practices, and hearing acuity. *Geriatric Nursing, 14*, 70–73.

Norwood-Chapman, L., & Burchfield, S. B. (1999). Nursing home personnel knowledge and attitudes about hearing loss and hearing aids. *Gerontology and Geriatrics Education, 20*(2), 37–47.

Porth, C. M. (2002). *Pathophysiology: Concepts of altered health states* (6th ed.). Philadelphia: Lippincott.

Quillen, D. A. (1999). Common causes of vision loss in elderly patients. *American Family Physician, 60*(1), 99–107.

Ramponi, D. (2000). Go with the flow during an eye emergency. *Nursing 2000, 30*(8), 54–56.

Smith, S. C. (1998). Diabetic retinopathy. *Nurse Practitioner Forum, 9*(1), 13–18.

_____ . (1998). Aging, physiology, and vision. *Nurse Practitioner Forum, 9*(1), 19–22.

Stegbauer, C. C. (2000). Hallucinations in the vision-impaired elderly: The Charles Bonnet syndrome. *The Nurse Practitioner, 25*(8), 74–76.

Stone, C. M. (1999). Preventing cerumen impaction in nursing home residents. *Journal of Gerontological Nursing, 25*(5), 43–45.

Tierney, L. M., McPhee, S. J., & Papadakis, M. A. (Eds.). (2001). *Current medical diagnosis & treatment* (40th ed.). Stamford, CT: Appleton & Lange.

Tigges, B. B. (2000). Acute otitis media and pneumococcal resistance: Making judicious management decisions. *The Nurse Practitioner, 25*(1), 69–79.

Tolson, D., & McIntosh, J. (1997). Listening in the care environment—chaos or clarity for the hearing-impaired elderly person. *International Journal of Nursing Studies, 34*(3), 173–182.

Turkoski, B. B. (2000). Glaucoma and glaucoma medications. *Orthopaedic Nursing, 19*(5), 71–76.

Way, L. W., & Doherty, G. M. (2003). *Current surgical diagnosis & treatment* (11 th ed.) New York. McGraw-Hill.

Wingate, S. (1999). Treating corneal abrasions. *The Nurse Practitioner, 24*(6), 53–54, 57, 60, 65–66, 68.

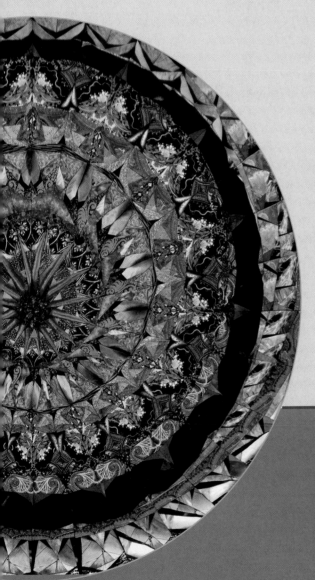

# SEXUALITY AND REPRODUCTIVE PATTERNS

Unit 14
Responses to Altered Sexual
and Reproductive Function

# Functional Health Patterns with Related Nursing Diagnosis

### HEALTH PERCEPTION HEALTH MANAGEMENT
- Perceived health status
- Perceived health management
- Health care behaviors: health promotion and illness prevention activities, medical treatments, follow-up care

### VALUE-BELIEF
- Values, goals, or beliefs (including spirituality) that guide choices or decisions
- Perceived conflicts in values, beliefs, or expectations that are health related

### COPING-STRESS-TOLERANCE
- Capacity to resist challenges to self-integrity
- Methods of handling stress
- Support systems
- Perceived ability to control and manage situations

### NUTRITIONAL-METABOLIC
- Daily consumption of food and fluids
- Favorite foods
- Use of dietary supplements
- Skin lesions and ability to heal
- Condition of the integument
- Weight, height, temperature

### Part 6
### Sexuality-Reproductive Patterns NANDA Nursing Diagnoses
- Rape-Trauma Syndrome
- Sexual Dysfunction
- Ineffective Sexuality Patterns

### SEXUALITY-REPRODUCTIVE
- Satisfaction with sexuality or sexual relationships
- Reproductive pattern
- Female menstrual and perimenopausal history

### ELIMINATION
- Patterns of bowel and urinary excretion
- Perceived regularity or irregularity of elimination
- Use of laxatives or routines
- Changes in time, modes, quality or quantity of excretions
- Use of devices for control

### ROLE-RELATIONSHIP
- Perception of major roles, relationships, and responsibilities in current life situation
- Satisfaction with or disturbances in roles and relationships

### ACTIVITY-EXERCISE
- Patterns of personally relevant exercise, activity, leisure, and recreation
- ADLs which require energy expenditure
- Factors that interfere with the desired pattern (e.g., illness or injury)

### SELF-PERCEPTION–SELF-CONCEPT
- Attitudes about self
- Perceived abilities, worth, self-image, emotions
- Body posture and movement, eye contact, voice and speech patterns

### SLEEP-REST
- Patterns of sleep and rest-/relaxation in a 24-hr period
- Perceptions of quality and quantity of sleep and rest
- Use of sleep aids and routines

### COGNITIVE-PERCEPTUAL
- Adequacy of vision, hearing, taste, touch, smell
- Pain perception and management
- Language, judgment, memory, decisions

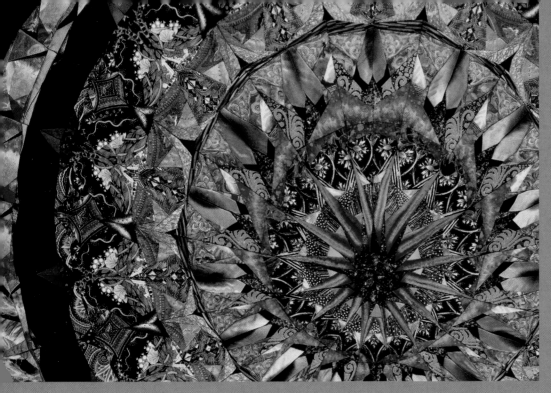

# RESPONSES TO ALTERED SEXUAL AND REPRODUCTIVE FUNCTION

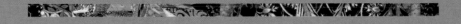

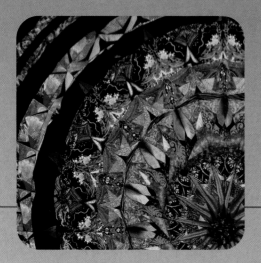

# Assessing Clients with Reproductive System Disorders

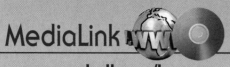

## www.prenhall.com/lemone

Additional resources for this chapter can be found on the Student CD-ROM accompanying this textbook, and on the Companion Website at www. prenhall.com/lemone. Click on Chapter 46 to select the activities for this chapter.

**CD-ROM**
• Audio Glossary
• NCLEX Review

*Animations*
• Female Reproductive System
• Male Reproductive System

**Companion Website**
• More NCLEX Review
• Functional Health Pattern Assessment
• Case Study
   Irregular Menstrual Cycle

## LEARNING OUTCOMES

After completing this chapter, you will be able to:

■ Review the anatomy and physiology of the male and female reproductive systems.

■ Explain the functions of the male and female sex hormones.

■ Identify specific topics for consideration during a health history interview of the client with health problems involving reproductive function.

■ Describe techniques for physical assessment of male and female reproductive function.

■ Identify abnormal findings that may indicate impairment in reproductive function in men and women.

Although the reproductive organs in men and women are very different, they do share common functions: enabling sexual pleasure and reproduction. The reproductive organs, in conjunction with the neuroendocrine system, produce hormones important in biologic development and sexual behavior. Parts of the reproductive organs also enclose and are integral to the function of the urinary system. The assessment of the reproductive and urinary systems is often difficult for both the beginning nurse and the client and requires skill on the part of the nurse when asking questions about sensitive topics that the client may be hesitant to talk about. Skill in conducting physical examinations of an area of the body usually considered private is also required. This chapter discusses the assessment of the reproductive system for both men and women.

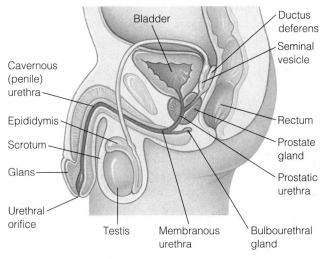

Figure 46–1 ■ The male reproductive system.

## REVIEW OF ANATOMY AND PHYSIOLOGY

### The Male Reproductive System

The male reproductive system consists of the paired testes, the scrotum, ducts, glands, and penis (Figure 46–1 ■). The location and function of the male reproductive organs are summarized in Table 46–1.

#### The Testes

The testes develop in the abdominal cavity of the fetus and then descend through the inguinal canal into the scrotum. They are homologous to the female's ovaries. These paired organs are each about 1.5 inches (4 cm) long and 1 inch (2.5 cm) in diameter. They are suspended in the scrotum by the spermatic cord. Each is surrounded by two coverings: an outer tunica vaginalis and an inner tunica albuginea. Each testis is divided into 250 to 300 lobules, with each lobule containing one to four seminiferous tubules. The testes produce sperm and testosterone.

The seminiferous tubules are responsible for sperm production. Leydig's cells (or interstitial cells) lie in the connective tissue surrounding the seminiferous tubules. They produce testosterone.

#### The Ducts and Semen

The seminiferous tubules lead into the efferent ducts and become the rete testis. From the rete testis, 10,000 to 20,000 efferent ducts join the epididymis, a long coiled tube that lies over the outer surface of each testis. The epididymis is the final area for the storage and maturation of sperm. When a man is sexually excited, the epididymis contracts to propel the sperm through the vas deferens to the ampulla, where they are stored until ejaculation.

MediaLink | MALE REPRODUCTIVE SYSTEM ANIMATION

| Male Reproductive Organ | Location | Function |
|---|---|---|
| Scrotum | Hangs from body at root of penis. | Contains testes, epididymis, and portions of the vas (ductus) deferens. |
| Testes | In the scrotal sac. | Produce sperm and testosterone. |
| Epididymis | Posterolateral to upper aspect of each testis. | Stores sperm. Promotes sperm maturation. Transports sperm to vas deferens. |
| Vas deferens (ductus deferens) | Between the epididymis and the seminal vesicle forming the ejaculatory duct. | Stores sperm. Transports sperm. |
| Penis | Attached to front and sides of the pubic arch. Proximal, ventral surface is directly continuous with the scrotum. | Excretes semen and urine. Deposits sperm in female reproductive tract. |
| Urethra | Begins at bladder and passes through prostate and penis. | Serves as passageway for urine or semen. |
| Prostate gland | Encircles the urethra at the neck of the bladder. | Contributes to ejaculatory volume. Enhances sperm motility and fertility. |
| Seminal vesicles | Lie on posterior bladder wall. | Contribute to ejaculatory volume. Contain nutrients to sustain sperm and prostaglandins to facilitate sperm motility. |
| Bulbourethral (Cowper's) glands | Inferior to the prostate. | Secrete mucus into urethra. Neutralize traces of acidic urine in the urethra. |

TABLE 46–1  Location and Function of the Male Reproductive Organs

The seminal vesicles at the base of the bladder produce about 60% of the volume of seminal fluid. Seminal fluid is also made of secretions from the accessory sex organs, the epididymis, the prostate gland, and Cowper's glands. Seminal fluid nourishes the sperm, provides bulk, and increases its alkalinity. (An alkaline pH is essential to mobilize the sperm and ensure fertilization of the ova.) Sperm mixed with this fluid is called semen. Each seminal vesicle joins its corresponding vas deferens to form an ejaculatory duct, which enters the prostatic urethra. During ejaculation, seminal fluid mixes with sperm at the ejaculatory duct and enters the urethra for expulsion.

The total amount of semen ejaculated is 2 to 4 mL, although the amount varies. The sperm count of the total ejaculate of a healthy male is from 100 to 400 million.

### The Scrotum

The scrotum is a sac or pouch made of two layers. The outer layer is continuous with the skin of the perineum and thighs. The inner layer is made of muscle and fascia. The scrotum hangs at the base of the penis, anterior to the anus, and regulates the temperature of the testes. The optimum temperature for sperm production is about 2 to 3 degrees below body temperature. When the testicular temperature is too low, the scrotum contracts to bring the testes up against the body. When the testicular temperature is too high, the scrotum relaxes to allow the testes to lie further away from the body.

### The Prostate Gland

The prostate gland is about the size of a walnut. It encircles the urethra just below the urinary bladder (see Figure 46–1). It is made of 20 to 30 tuboloalveolar glands surrounded by smooth muscle. Secretions of the prostate gland make up about one-third of the volume of the semen. These secretions enter the urethra through several ducts during ejaculation.

### The Penis

The penis is the genital organ that encloses the urethra (see Figure 46–1). It is homologous to the clitoris of the female. The penis is composed of a shaft and a tip called the glans, which is covered in the uncircumcised man by the foreskin (or prepuce). The shaft contains three columns of erectile tissue: The two lateral columns are called the corpora cavernosa, and the central mass is called the corpus spongiosum.

Erection occurs when the penile masses become filled with blood in response to a reflex that triggers the parasympathetic nervous system to stimulate arteriolar vasodilation. The erection reflex may be initiated by touch, pressure, sights, sounds, smells, or thoughts of a sexual encounter. After ejaculation, the arterioles vasoconstrict, and the penis becomes flaccid.

### Spermatogenesis

Spermatogenesis is the series of physiologic events that generate sperm in the seminiferous tubules. This process begins with puberty and continues throughout a man's life, with several hundred million sperm produced each day.

The inner layer of the seminiferous tubules consists of sustentacular cells (or Sertoli's cells), which contain the spermatocytes and sperm in different stages of development. Sertoli's cells secrete a nourishing fluid for the developing sperm, as well as enzymes that help convert spermatocytes to sperm. The events in spermatogenesis, which takes 64 to 72 days, are as follows:

1. The spermatogonia (sperm stem cells) undergo rapid mitotic division. As these cells multiply, the more mature spermatogonia divide into two daughter cells. These daughter cells grow and become the primary spermatocytes (and eventually become sperm).
2. Primary spermatocytes divide by meiosis to form two smaller secondary spermatocytes, which in turn divide to form two spermatids. This process occurs over several weeks.
3. The spermatids elongate into a mature sperm cell with a head and a tail. The head contains enzymes essential to the penetration and fertilization of the ova. The flagellar motion of the tail allows the sperm to move. The sperm cells then move to the epididymis to mature further and develop motility.

### Male Sex Hormones

The male sex hormones are called androgens. Most androgens are produced in the testes, although the adrenal cortex also produces a small amount. Testosterone, the primary androgen produced by the testes, is essential for the development and maintenance of sexual organs and secondary sex characteristics, and for spermatogenesis. It also promotes metabolism, growth of muscles and bone, and libido (sexual desire).

## The Female Reproductive System

The female reproductive system consists of the paired ovaries and fallopian tubes, uterus, vagina, mons pubis, labia majora, labia minora, and clitoris. The breasts are also a part of women's reproductive organs. In women, the urethra and urinary meatus are separated from the reproductive organs; however, they are in such close proximity that a health problem with one often affects the other. The location and function of the female reproductive organs are summarized in Table 46–2.

### The Internal Structures

The ovaries, fallopian tubes, uterus, and vagina make up the internal organs of the female reproductive system (Figure 46–2 ■). The ovaries are the primary reproductive organs in women and also produce female sex hormones. The fallopian tubes, uterus, and vagina serve as accessory ducts for the ovaries and a developing fetus.

***THE VAGINA.*** The vagina is a fibromuscular tube about 3 to 4 inches (8 to 10 cm) in length located posterior to the bladder and urethra and anterior to the rectum. The upper end contains the uterine cervix in an area called the fornix. The walls of the vagina are membranes that form folds, called rugae. These membranes are composed of mucus-secreting stratified squamous epithelial cells. The vagina serves as a route for the excretion of secretions, including menstrual fluid, and also is an organ of sexual response.

## TABLE 46–2   Location and Function of the Female Reproductive Organs

| Female Reproductive Organ | Location | Function |
| --- | --- | --- |
| Mons pubis (mons veneris) | Anterior and superior to the pubis. | Enhances sexual sensations.<br>Protects and cushions pubic symphysis during intercourse. |
| Labia majora | Extend from mons pubis to perineum. | Protect labia minora, urethral and vaginal openings.<br>Enhance sexual arousal. |
| Labia minora | Enclosed by the labia majora. | Protect clitoris.<br>Inferiorly, merge to form posterior ring of vaginal introitus (fourchette).<br>Lubricate vulva.<br>Enhance sexual arousal. |
| Vestibule | Area enclosed by labia minora. | Contains openings for urethra, vagina, Bartholin's glands, and Skene's glands. |
| Bartholin's (greater vestibular) glands | Posterior on each side of the vaginal orifice.<br>Open onto the sides of the vestibule in the groove between the labia minora and hymen. | Secrete clear, viscid mucus during intercourse. |
| Skene's (lesser vestibular, paraurethral) glands | Open onto the vestibule on each side of the urethra. | Drain urethral glands.<br>Produce lubricating mucus. |
| Clitoris | Small bud of erectile tissue just below the superior joining of the labia minora. | Stimulates and elevates levels of sexual arousal. |
| Perineum | Skin-covered muscular area between vaginal opening and anus. | Provides support for pelvic organs. |
| Mammary glands | Contained within breasts. Anterior to pectoral muscles of thorax. | Produce human milk.<br>Play a role in sexual arousal. |
| Ovaries | Lie on each side of the uterus below and behind the uterine tubes. | Produce and secrete ova.<br>Produce the hormones estrogen and progesterone. |
| Fallopian tubes (uterine tubes, oviducts) | One tube extends medially from the area of each ovary and empties into the upper portion (fundus) of the uterus. | Transport ova. |
| Uterus (adnexa of the uterus are composed of the uterine tubes and ovaries) | Anterior to the rectum and posterior/superior to the bladder. | Receives, retains, and nourishes the fertilized ovum.<br>Contracts rhythmically to expel infant. Cyclically sheds lining when ovum is not fertilized. |
| Cervix | Lower portion of uterus extending into the vagina. | Connects uterine cavity with vagina.<br>Opens to allow passage of menstrual flow and infant. |
| Vagina | Extends from the external orifice in the vestibule to the cervix. | Receives penis and semen during intercourse.<br>Passageway for menstrual flow and expulsion of infant at birth. |

The walls of the vagina are usually moist and maintain a pH ranging from 3.8 to 4.2. This pH is bacteriostatic and is maintained by the action of estrogen and normal vaginal flora. Estrogen stimulates the growth of vaginal mucosal cells so that they thicken and have increased glycogen content. The glycogen is fermented to lactic acid by Döderlein's bacilli (lactobacilli that normally inhabit the vagina), slightly acidifying the vaginal fluid.

***THE UTERUS.***   The uterus is a hollow pear-shaped muscular organ with thick walls located between the bladder and the rectum. It has three parts: the fundus, the body, and the cervix. It is supported in the abdominal cavity by the broad ligaments, the round ligaments, the uterosacral ligaments, and the transverse cervical ligaments. The uterus receives the fertilized ovum and provides a site for growth and development of the fetus.

The uterine wall has three layers. The *perimetrium* is the outer serous layer that merges with the peritoneum. The *myometrium* is the middle layer and makes up most of the uterine wall. This layer has muscle fibers that run in various directions, allowing contractions during **menstruation** (the periodic shedding of the uterine lining in a woman of childbearing age who is not pregnant) or childbirth and expansion as the fetus grows. The *endometrium* lines the uterus. Its outermost layer is shed during menstruation.

The cervix projects into the vagina and forms a pathway between the uterus and the vagina. The uterine opening of the cervix is called the internal os; the vaginal opening is called the

MediaLink | FEMALE REPRODUCTIVE SYSTEM ANIMATION

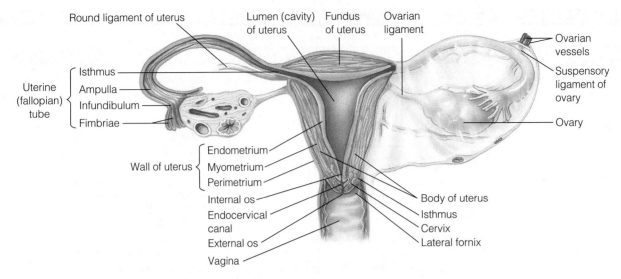

**Figure 46–2** ■ The internal organs of the female reproductive system.

external os. The space between these openings, the endocervical canal, serves as a route for the discharge of menstrual fluid and the entrance for sperm. The cervix is a firm structure that softens in response to hormones during pregnancy. It is protected by mucus that changes consistency and quantity during the menstrual cycle and during pregnancy.

*THE FALLOPIAN TUBES.*   The fallopian tubes are thin cylindrical structures about 4 inches (10 cm) long and 2.5 inches (1 cm) in diameter. They are attached to the uterus on one end and are supported by the broad ligaments. The lateral ends of the uterine tubes are open and made of projections called *fimbriae* that drape over the ovary. The fimbriae pick up the ovum after it is discharged from the ovary.

The fallopian tubes, made of smooth muscle, are lined with ciliated, mucus-producing epithelial cells. The movement of the cilia and contractions of the smooth muscle move the ovum through the tubes toward the uterus. Fertilization of the ovum by the sperm usually occurs in the outer portion of a fallopian tube.

*THE OVARIES.*   The ovaries in the adult woman are flat, almond-shaped structures located on either side of the uterus below the ends of the fallopian tubes. They are homologous to the male's testes. They are attached to the uterus by a ligament and are also attached to the broad ligament. The ovaries store the female germ cells and produce the female hormones *estrogen* and *progesterone*. A woman's total number of ova is present at birth.

Each ovary is divided into a medulla and a cortex. It contains many small structures called ovarian follicles. Each follicle contains an immature ovum, called an oocyte. Each month, several follicles are stimulated by follicle-stimulating hormone (FSH) and luteinizing hormone (LH) to mature. The developing follicles are surrounded by layers of follicle cells, with the mature follicles called graafian follicles. The graafian follicles produce estrogen, which stimulates the development of endometrium. Each month in the menstruating

woman, one or two of the mature follicles ejects an oocyte in a process called ovulation. The ruptured follicle then becomes a structure called the corpus luteum. The corpus luteum produces both estrogen and progesterone to support the endometrium until conception occurs or the cycle begins again. The corpus luteum slowly degenerates, leaving a scar on the surface of the ovary.

## The External Structures

The external genitalia collectively are called the vulva. They include the mons pubis, the labia, the clitoris, the vaginal and urethral openings, and glands (Figure 46–3 ■).

The mons pubis is a pad of adipose (fat) tissue covered with skin. It lies anterior to the symphysis pubis. After puberty, the mons is covered with hair with a diamond-shaped distribution.

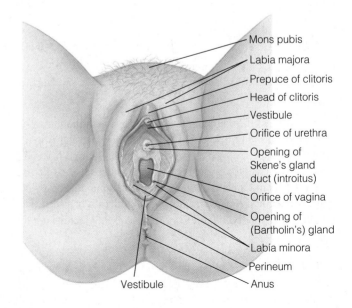

**Figure 46–3** ■ The external organs of the female reproductive system.

The labia are divided into two structures. The *labia majora,* folds of skin and adipose tissue covered with hair, are outermost; they begin at the base of the mons pubis and end at the anus. The *labia minora,* located between the clitoris and the base of the vagina, are enclosed by the labia majora. They are made of skin, adipose tissue, and some erectile tissues. They are usually light pink and hairless.

The area between the labia is called the vestibule, and contains the openings for the vagina and the urethra as well as the Bartholin's glands. Skene's glands open onto the vestibule on each side of the urethra. Bartholin's and Skene's glands secrete lubricating fluid during the sexual response cycle.

The clitoris is an erectile organ analogous to the penis in the male. It is formed by the joining of the labia minora. Like the penis, it is highly sensitive and distends during sexual arousal.

The vaginal opening, called the introitus, is the opening between the internal and the external genitals. The introitus is surrounded by a connective tissue membrane called the hymen, which determines the size and shape of the opening.

### The Breasts

The breasts (or mammary glands) are located between the third and seventh ribs on the anterior chest wall. They are supported by the pectoral muscles and are richly supplied with nerves, blood, and lymph (Figure 46–4 ■). A pigmented area called the areola is located slightly below the center of each breast and contains sebaceous glands and a nipple. The nipple is usually protrusive and becomes erect in response to cold and stimulation. The primary purpose of the breasts is to supply nourishment for the infant.

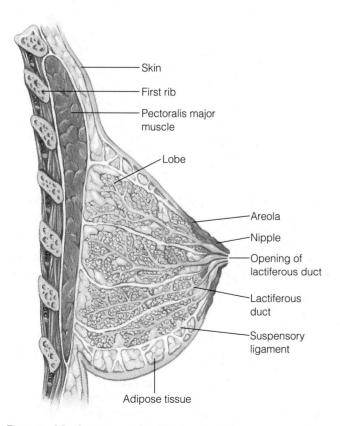

Skin

First rib

Pectoralis major muscle

Lobe

Areola

Nipple

Opening of lactiferous duct

Lactiferous duct

Suspensory ligament

Adipose tissue

**Figure 46–4 ■** Structure of the female breast.

The breasts are made of adipose tissue, fibrous connective tissue, and glandular tissue. Cooper's ligaments support the breast and extend from the outer breast tissue to the nipple, dividing the breast into 15 to 25 lobes. Each lobe is made of alveolar glands connected by ducts which open to the nipple.

### Female Sex Hormones

The ovaries produce estrogens, progesterone, and androgens in a cyclic pattern. Estrogens are steroid hormones that occur naturally in three forms: estrone ($E_1$), estradiol ($E_2$), and estriol ($E_3$). Estradiol is the most potent and is the form secreted in greatest amount by the ovaries. Although estrogens are secreted throughout the menstrual cycle, they are at a higher level during certain phases of the cycle, discussed shortly.

Estrogens are essential for the development and maintenance of secondary sex characteristics; and in conjunction with other hormones, they stimulate the female reproductive organs to prepare for growth of a fetus. Estrogens are responsible for the normal structure of skin and blood vessels. They also decrease the rate of bone resorption, promote increased high-density lipoproteins, reduce cholesterol levels, and enhance the clotting of blood. Estrogens also promote the retention of sodium and water.

Progesterone primarily affects the development of breast glandular tissue and the endometrium. During pregnancy, progesterone relaxes smooth muscle to decrease uterine contractions. It also increases body temperature. Androgens are responsible for normal hair growth patterns at puberty and may also have metabolic effects.

### Oogenesis and the Ovarian Cycle

All of a woman's ova are present as primary oocytes in primordial ovarian follicles at her birth. Each month from puberty until menopause, the remaining events of oogenesis, the production of ova, occur. Collectively, these events are known as the ovarian cycle.

The ovarian cycle has three consecutive phases that occur cyclically each 28 days (although the cycle normally may be longer or shorter). The *follicular phase* lasts from the 1st to the 10th day of the cycle; the *ovulatory phase* lasts from the 11th to the 14th day of the cycle and ends with ovulation; and the *luteal phase* lasts from the 14th to the 28th days.

During the follicular phase, the follicle develops and the oocyte matures. These processes are controlled by the interaction of FSH and LH. On day 1 of the cycle, gonadotropin-releasing hormone (GnRH) from the hypothalamus increases and stimulates increased production of FSH and LH by the anterior pituitary. FSH and LH stimulate follicular growth, and the oocyte increases in size. The structure, now called the primary follicle, becomes a multicellular mass surrounded by a fibrous capsule, the theca folliculi. As the follicle continues to increase in size, estrogen is produced and a fluid-filled space (the *antrum*) forms within the follicle. The oocyte is enclosed by a membrane, the zona pellucida. By about day 10, the follicle is a mature graafian follicle and bulges out from the surface of the ovary. There are always follicles at different stages of development in each ovary, but usually only one follicle becomes dominant and matures to ovulation, while the others degenerate.

The ovulatory phase begins when estrogen levels reach a level high enough to stimulate the anterior pituitary, and a surge of LH is produced. The LH stimulates meiosis in the developing oocyte, and its first meiotic division occurs. The LH also stimulates enzymes that act on the bulging ovarian wall, causing it to rupture and discharge the antrum fluid and the oocyte. The oocyte is expelled from the mature ovarian follicle in the process called ovulation.

During the luteal phase, the surge in LH also stimulates the ruptured follicle to change into a corpus luteum and then stimulates the corpus luteum to begin immediately to produce progesterone and estrogen. The increase of progesterone and estrogen in the blood has a negative feedback effect on the production of LH, inhibiting the further growth and development of other follicles.

If pregnancy does not occur, the corpus luteum begins to degenerate, and its hormone production ceases. The declining production of progesterone and estrogen at the end of the cycle allows the secretion of LH and FSH to increase, and a new cycle begins. The ovarian cycle is compared to the menstrual cycle in Figure 46–5 ■.

### The Menstrual Cycle

The endometrium of the uterus responds to changes in estrogen and progesterone during the ovarian cycle to prepare for implantation of the fertilized embryo. The endometrium is receptive to implantation of the embryo for only a brief period each month, coinciding with the time when the embryo would normally reach the uterus from the uterine tube (usually 7 days).

The cycle begins with the *menstrual phase,* lasting from days 1 to 5. The inner endometrial (functionalis) layer detaches and is expelled as menstrual fluid (fluid and blood) for 3 to 5 days. As the maturing follicle begins to produce estrogen (days 6 to 14), the proliferative phase begins. In response, the functionalis layer is repaired and thickens, while spiral arteries increase in number and tubular glands form. Cervical mucus changes to a thin, crystalline substance, forming channels to help the sperm move up into the uterus.

The final phase, lasting from days 14 to 28, is the secretory phase. As the corpus luteum produces progesterone, the rising levels act on the endometrium, causing increased vascularity, changing the inner layer to secretory mucosa, stimulating the secretion of glycogen into the uterine cavity, and causing the cervical mucus again to become thick and block the internal os. If fertilization does not occur, hormone levels fall. Spasm of the spiral arteries causes hypoxia of the endometrial cells, which begin to degenerate and slough off. As with the ovarian cycle, the process begins again with the sloughing of the functionalis layer.

## ASSESSING REPRODUCTIVE FUNCTION

The function of the reproductive systems in men and women is assessed both by a health assessment interview to collect subjective data and a physical assessment to collect objective data. When assessing the male or female reproductive systems, consider the psychologic, social, and cultural factors that affect

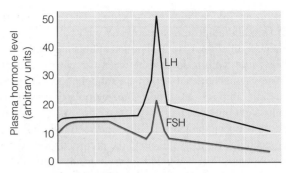

**A** Fluctuation of gonadotropin levels

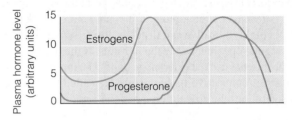

**B** Fluctuation of ovarian hormone levels

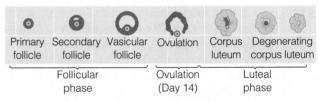

**C** Ovarian cycle

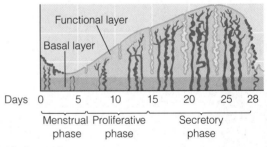

**D** Uterine cycle

**Figure 46–5** ■ Comparison of the ovarian and uterine cycles. *A,* Fluctuating levels of follicle-stimulating hormone (FSH) and luteinizing hormone (LH), the pituitary gonadotropins regulating the ovarian cycle. *B,* Fluctuating levels of ovarian hormones that cause endometrial changes during the uterine cycle. *C,* Changes in the ovarian follicles during the 28-day ovarian cycle. *D,* Corresponding changes in the endometrium during the uterine cycle.

sexual activity and sexuality. Use words that the client understands, and do not be embarrassed by the client's terminology. The client may perceive the interview as less threatening if the discussion begins with more general questions and then progresses to questions specific to the reproductive system. For example, first ask a female client about menstrual and childbirth histories before asking questions about sexually transmitted diseases. Interview questions are also less threatening if they are asked in a way that gives the client permission to report behaviors and manifestations. For example, rather than asking a man if he has difficulty achieving or maintaining an erection, ask him to describe any changes he has noticed in having an erection.

## Health Assessment Interview for Men

The health assessment for the male reproductive system is often a part of the assessment of the urinary system (see Chapter 25). ⊖⊃ Before asking questions about sexual history, explain that this information is part of a general health assessment. If a health problem is identified, collect information specific to its onset, characteristics, duration, frequency, precipitating or relieving factors, treatment and/or self-care, and outcome. For example, ask the client:

- When did you first notice that you were having difficulty urinating?
- Did you use a different brand of condoms before you noticed the rash on your penis?
- Describe the changes that occurred in your ability to have an erection after you started taking medicine for high blood pressure.

In questioning the client about past medical history, ask about chronic illnesses such as diabetes, chronic renal failure, cardiovascular disease, multiple sclerosis, spinal cord tumors or trauma, or thyroid disease. The effects of these illnesses as well as the treatment of the illnesses may cause **impotence** (inability to achieve or maintain an erection). The following drugs may cause sexual function problems: antihypertensives, antidepressants, antispasmodics, tranquilizers, sedatives, and histamine$_2$-receptor antagonists. Psychosocial stressors also may contribute to impotence.

If the man was born to a woman treated during pregnancy with diethylstilbestrol (DES), a drug used in the 1940s and 1950s to prevent miscarriage, he may have congenital deformities of the urinary tract as well as decreased semen levels. If the man had mumps as a child, sterility is possible. The risk for testicular cancer is greatest in men who have a history of an undescended testicle, an inguinal hernia, testicular swelling with mumps, a history of maternal use of DES or oral contraceptives, and a family history of testicular cancer.

Explore the lifestyle and social history of the man; the use of alcohol, cigarettes, or street drugs may affect sexual function. Frequent sexual intercourse, especially if unprotected, increases the potential for sexually transmitted diseases including HIV infection. Sexual intercourse with same-sex partners further increases the risk for HIV infection. Other questions about sexuality may include number of sexual partners; history of premature ejaculation, impotence, or other sexual problems; any history of sexual trauma; use of condoms or other contraceptives; and current level of sexual satisfaction.

Specific questions and leading statements, categorized by functional health patterns, can be found on the Companion Website.

## Health Assessment Interview for Women

The focused interview for the female reproductive system is usually extensive. However, the questions may in many instances be tailored to the specific health problem of the client. As with the assessment of other body systems, analyze and document the onset of the problem, its duration, frequency, precipitating and relieving factors, any associated symptoms, treatment, self-care, and outcome. For example, ask the client:

- Did you notice that you had increased vaginal bleeding after intercourse?
- Does the over-the-counter medication relieve the vaginal itching and discharge?
- Have you had any fever or abdominal pain with this vaginal infection?

Ask about menstrual history, obstetric history, use of contraceptives, sexual history, use of medications, and reproductive system examinations. Also assess the use of condoms during intercourse; unprotected sexual intercourse increases the risk of sexually transmitted diseases, including HIV infection. Also ask about smoking; a history of smoking increases the risk of circulatory problems in the woman taking oral contraceptives. Smoking also increases the risk for cancer of the cervix.

Chronic illnesses may affect the function of the female reproductive system. Diabetes increases the risk of vaginal infections and vaginal dryness, both of which interfere with sexual pleasure. Chronic heavy menstrual flow may result in anemia. Thyroid and adrenal disorders may affect secondary sex characteristics, the menstrual cycle, and the ability to become pregnant.

Obtaining any family history of cancer is important. The risk for endometrial cancer is higher in women with a family history of endometrial, breast, or colon cancer; the risk for ovarian cancer is higher in women with a family history of ovarian or breast cancer; and the risk for breast cancer is higher in women with a family history of breast cancer. Exposure to diethylstilbestrol (DES) in utero increases the risk of cancer of the cervix and vagina. Exposure to asbestos poses a risk of cancer of the ovary. The risk for breast cancer is also greater if the client has a history of fibrocystic disease.

Carefully explore any history of vaginal bleeding and vaginal discharge. Ask about the onset of vaginal bleeding, any related factors, the color (pink, red, dark red, brown), the character (thin, watery, presence of mucus, size and number of clots), the amount (spotting, how many pads or tampons in a specific amount of time) and relationship to menstrual cycle. Regarding vaginal discharge, ask about the onset, color (white, green, gray), character (thin, curdlike, infected), odor, itching, and rash.

Questions about sexuality may include number of sexual partners; history of **anorgasmia** (absence of orgasm), **dyspareunia** (painful intercourse), or other problems; history of sexual trauma; use of condoms or other contraceptives, and current level of sexual satisfaction.

Specific questions and leading statements, categorized by functional health patterns, can be found on the Companion Website.

MediaLink | FUNCTIONAL HEALTH PATTERN ASSESSMENT

## Physical Assessment

Physical assessment of the reproductive system usually is conducted as part of a scheduled screening (e.g., for an annual Papanicolaou smear) or for a specific reproductive health problem. If conducted as part of a total physical assessment, this is usually the final system to be assessed. The nurse must feel comfortable with the examination of clients of the opposite gender; if either the nurse or the client is not comfortable, a nurse of the same gender should be asked to conduct this part of the assessment.

The reproductive system is assessed by inspection and palpation. Ask the client to void before having the examination. Prior to the examination, collect all necessary equipment and explain the techniques to the client to decrease anxiety. Put on disposable gloves before beginning the examination and wear them throughout the examination.

### The Male Reproductive System

The equipment necessary for assessing the male reproductive system includes disposable gloves, lubricant, and a flashlight. If a culture is to be taken of any drainage or discharge, sterile cotton swabs and culture media should be available. Explain the procedures for the examination thoroughly; if the man is unfamiliar with his internal genitalia, charts may be used to demonstrate the parts that will be examined.

Ask the client to remove his clothing and put on a gown. The assessment may be done with the client sitting or standing. Ensure that the examining room is warm and private.

### Breast and Lymph Node Assessment with Abnormal Findings (✓)

(Note: Assessment of male breasts is less complicated than assessment of female breasts but should not be overlooked.)

- Inspect and palpate both breasts, including areola and nipple.
  - ✓ A smooth, firm, mobile, tender disc of breast tissue behind the areola indicates *gynecomastia,* abnormal enlargement of the breast(s) in men. Gynecomastia requires additional investigation to determine cause.
  - ✓ A hard, irregular nodule in the nipple area suggests carcinoma.
- Palpate the axillary lymph nodes.
  - ✓ Enlarged axillary nodes are common with infections of the hand or arm but may be caused by cancer.
  - ✓ Enlarged supraclavicular nodes may indicate metastasis.

### External Assessment with Abnormal Findings (✓)

- Inspect and palpate the inguinal and femoral area for bulges. Ask the client to bear down or cough as you palpate (Figure 46–6 ■).
  - ✓ A bulge that increases with straining suggests a hernia.
- Inspect the penis. If the client is uncircumcised, retract the foreskin or ask the client to do so.
  - ✓ **Phimosis** (tightness of prepuce that prevents retraction of foreskin) may be congenital or due to recurrent *balanoposthitis* (generalized infection of glans penis and prepuce).

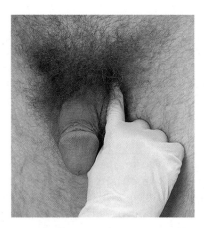

**Figure 46–6** ■ Palpating the male inguinal area for bulges.

  - ✓ Narrow or inflamed foreskin can cause paraphimosis, retraction of the foreskin that causes painful swelling of the glans.
  - ✓ **Balanitis** (inflammation of the glands) is associated with bacterial or fungal infections.
  - ✓ Ulcers, vesicles, or warts suggest sexually transmitted infection.
  - ✓ Nodules or sores seen in uncircumcised men may be cancer.
- Inspect the external urinary meatus. Press the glans between the thumb and forefinger (Figure 46–7 ■). Replace the foreskin if appropriate.
  - ✓ Erythema or discharge indicates inflammatory disease. Further assessment is required.
- Inspect the skin around the base of the penis.
  - ✓ Excoriation or inflammation suggests lice or scabies.
- Palpate the shaft of the penis.
  - ✓ Induration with tenderness along with ventral surface suggests urethral stricture with inflammation.
- Inspect the scrotum. Further assess any swelling in the scrotum using transillumination: Darken the room and place a lighted flashlight against the skin of the scrotum. The normal scrotum and epididymis appear as dark masses with regular borders.

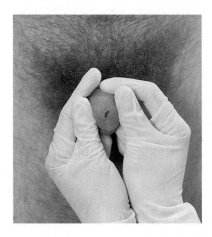

**Figure 46–7** ■ Inspecting the external urinary meatus of the male.

✓ A unilateral or bilateral poorly developed scrotum suggests **cryptorchidism** (failure of one or both testes to descend into the scrotum).

✓ Swelling of the scrotum may indicate indirect inguinal hernia, **hydrocele** (accumulation of fluid in the scrotum), or scrotal edema. Swellings containing serous fluid will transilluminate. Swellings containing blood or tissue will not transilluminate.

• Palpate each testis and epididymis.

✓ Tender, painful scrotal swelling occurs in acute epididymitis, acute orchitis, torsion of the spermatic cord, and strangulated hernia.

✓ A painless nodule in the testis is associated with testicular cancer.

### Prostate Assessment with Abnormal Findings (✓)

(Note: The prostate gland is assessed by digital rectal examination. See Chapter 23 🔗 for technique for palpation of the rectal wall.)

• Palpate the posterior surface of the prostate gland. With a gloved index finger, palpate the anterior rectal wall for the rounded, two-lobed structure of the posterior prostate.

✓ Enlargement (1-cm protrusion into the rectum) with obliteration of the median sulcus suggests benign prostatic hypertrophy.

✓ Enlargement with asymmetry and tenderness suggests prostatitis.

✓ A hard irregular nodule is seen in carcinoma.

## The Female Reproductive System

The equipment necessary for assessing the female reproductive system includes disposable latex gloves, a good light source, sterile cotton swabs, a spatula, water-soluble lubricant, slides, cytologic fixative, and specula of various sizes. If cultures are to be taken, culture media is necessary. Carefully explain the procedure for the examination, and show the speculum to the woman. If the woman is unfamiliar with her genitalia, charts may be used to demonstrate the parts that will be examined.

Ask the client to remove her clothing and put on a gown. Ensure that the examining room is private and warm.

The examination usually begins with examination of the breasts with the client in the sitting and supine positions. The nurse then helps the client move to the lithotomy position on the examining table, with the feet in the stirrups and the buttocks even with the foot of the table. Older or frail clients may not be able to tolerate this position. In this case, the client is examined in the supine position. Use draping throughout the examination so that only the part of the body being examined is exposed. Although the entire examination is described here, the internal examination is conducted only by a nurse with advanced practice in the procedure.

### Breast Assessment with Abnormal Findings (✓)

• Inspect both breasts simultaneously with the client seated in the following positions: arms at sides, arms overhead, hands pressed on hips, leaning forward. Inspect breast size, symmetry, contour, skin color, texture, venous patterns, and lesions. Lift the breasts, and inspect the lower and lateral aspects.

✓ Retractions, dimpling, and abnormal contours suggest benign lesions, but may also suggest malignancy.

✓ Thickened, dimpled skin with enlarged pores (called peau d'orange, orange peel, or pig skin) and unilateral venous patterns are also associated with malignancy.

✓ Redness may be seen with infection or carcinoma.

• Inspect the areolae and nipples.

✓ Peau d'orange may be noted first in the areola.

✓ Recent unilateral inversion of the nipple or asymmetry in the directions in which the nipples point suggests cancer.

• Palpate both breasts, axillae, and supraclavicular areas. Figure 46–8 ■ illustrates a possible pattern for breast palpation. Various palpation patterns may be used as long as every part of each breast is palpated, including the axillary tail (also called tail of Spence), which is the breast tissue that extends from the upper outer quadrant toward and into the axillae. Ask the client to assume a supine position with a small pillow under the shoulder and the arm over the head, and repeat the systematic palpation sequence. Findings of nonpathologic breast enlargement, nodularity, and tenderness are more common the week preceding and during menstrual flow. Describe identified masses by location, size, shape, consistency, tenderness, mobility, and delineation of borders.

✓ Tenderness may be related to premenstrual fullness, fibrocystic disease, or inflammation. Tenderness may also indicate cancer.

✓ Nodules in the tail of the breast may be enlarged lymph nodes.

✓ Hard, irregular, fixed unilateral masses that are poorly delineated suggest carcinoma.

✓ Bilateral, single or multiple, round, mobile, well-delineated masses are consistent with fibrocystic breast disease or fibroadenoma.

✓ Swelling, tenderness, erythema, and heat may be seen with mastitis.

• Palpate the nipple then compress it between the thumb and index finger. Note the color of any discharge.

✓ Loss of nipple elasticity is seen in cancer.

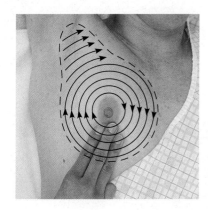

**Figure 46–8** ■ Possible pattern for palpation of the breast.

✓ Bloody or serous discharge is associated with intraductal papilloma.

✓ Milky discharge not due to prior pregnancy and found on both sides suggests **galactorrhea** (lactation not associated with pregnancy or nursing), which is sometimes associated with a pituitary tumor.

✓ Unilateral discharge from one or two ducts can be seen in fibrocystic breast disease, intraductal papilloma, or carcinoma.

### Axillary Assessment with Abnormal Findings (✓)

• Inspect the skin of the axillae.

✓ Rash may be due to allergy or other causes.

✓ Signs of inflammation and infection may be due to infection of the sweat glands.

✓ Palpate all sections of both axillae for palpable nodes (Figure 46–9 ■).

✓ Enlarged axillary nodes are most often due to infection of the hand or arm but can be caused by malignancy.

✓ Enlarged supraclavicular nodes are associated with lymphatic metastases from abdominal or thoracic carcinoma.

### External Assessment with Abnormal Findings (✓)

Help the client to the lithotomy position with the knees flexed and separated.

• Inspect and palpate the labia majora.

✓ Excoriation, rashes, or lesions suggest inflammatory or infective processes.

✓ Bulging of the labia that increases with straining suggests a hernia.

✓ Varicosities may be present on the labia.

• Inspect the labia minora. Use a gloved hand to separate the labia majora for better visualization.

✓ Inflammation, irritation, excoriation, or caking of discharge in tissue folds suggests vaginal infection or poor hygiene.

✓ Ulcers or vesicles may be symptoms of sexually transmitted infection.

• Palpate the inside of the labia minora between gloved thumb and forefinger.

✓ Small, firm, round cystic nodules in labia suggest sebaceous cysts.

✓ Wartlike lesions suggest condylomata acuminata (genital warts).

✓ Firm, painless ulcers suggest chancre of primary syphilis.

✓ Shallow, painful ulcers suggest herpes infection.

✓ Ulcerated or red raised lesions in older women suggest vulvar carcinoma.

• Inspect the clitoris.

✓ Enlargement may be a symptom of a masculinizing condition.

• Inspect the vaginal opening.

✓ Swelling or discoloration may be caused by trauma.

✓ Discharge or lesions may be symptoms of infection.

✓ Fissures or fistulas may be related to injury, infection, spreading of a malignancy, or trauma.

• Palpate Skene's glands. Using the index finger, "milk" Skene's glands on both sides and over the urethra and inspect for possible discharge (Figure 46–10 ■).

✓ Discharge from Skene's glands and/or tenderness suggests infection.

• Palpate Bartholin's glands. Palpate Bartholin's glands at the posterior labia majora (Figure 46–11 ■).

✓ A nontender mass in the posterolateral portion of the labia majora is indicative of a Bartholin's cyst.

✓ Swelling, redness, or tenderness, especially if unilateral, may indicate abscess of Bartholin's glands.

• Inspect the vaginal orifice for bulging and urinary incontinence. Ask the client to strain or "bear down."

✓ Bulging of the anterior vaginal wall and urinary incontinence suggest a cystocele.

✓ Bulging of the posterior wall suggests a rectocele.

✓ Protrusion of the cervix or uterus into the vagina indicates uterine prolapse.

• Inspect and palpate the perineum.

✓ Episiotomy scarring may be apparent.

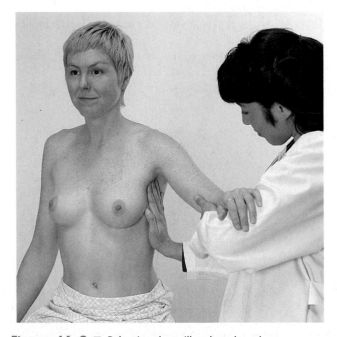

**Figure 46–9** ■ Palpating the axillary lymph nodes.

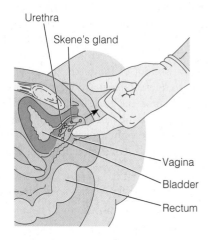

**Figure 46–10** ■ Palpating Skene's glands.

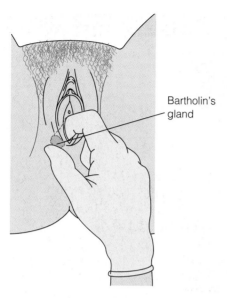

Figure 46–11 ■ Palpating Bartholin's glands.

✓ Inflammation, lesions, and growths may be seen in infections or cancer.

✓ Fistulas may be the result of injury, trauma, infection, or spreading of a malignancy.

## Vaginal and Cervical Assessment with Abnormal Findings (✓)

- Use a vaginal speculum to inspect the vaginal walls and cervix. See the guidelines in Box 46–1.

   ✓ Bluish color of the cervix and vaginal mucosa may be a sign of pregnancy.

   ✓ A pale cervix is associated with anemia.

   ✓ A cervix to the right or left of the midline may indicate a pelvic mass, uterine adhesions, or pregnancy.

   ✓ Projection of the cervix more than 3 cm into the vaginal canal may indicate a pelvic or uterine mass.

   ✓ Transverse or star-shaped cervical lacerations reflect trauma causing tearing of the cervix.

   ✓ An enlarged cervix is associated with infection.

---

**BOX 46–1** ■ **Guidelines for Intravaginal Assessment and Use of the Vaginal Speculum**

The size of the speculum that is used for an internal examination of the female reproductive system depends on the age of the woman and size of the vagina. Two types of specula are available. The Graves speculum, used most often for examinations of adult women, is available in lengths of 3½ to 5 inches and widths of ¾ to 1½ inches. The Pederson speculum, which is narrower, may be used to examine adolescents or adult women who are virgins, who have never had a baby, or who are postmenopausal with vaginal atrophy. The speculum should be warm: A heating pad is used in many institutions. If cultures or smears are to be obtained, neither water nor gel should be used either to warm or to lubricate the speculum.

If cells are to be taken for cytologic studies, the client should not douche, use vaginal medications, or take a tub bath for 24 hours before the examination. Finally, the examination is usually deferred if the client is menstruating or has a vaginal infection.

The general procedure is as follows:

1. Place the index and middle finger of one hand into the vagina, just inside the introitus, and press the fingers toward the rectum. Hold the speculum in the other hand.
2. Ask the client to bear down, and insert the closed blades of the speculum into the vagina at an oblique angle until the ends of the blades reach the fingertips (see the accompanying figure). Withdraw the fingers and rotate the speculum to a transverse position.
3. Continue to insert the speculum until it reaches the end of the vagina. Depress the lever of the speculum to open the blades. If the cervix is not in full view, try closing the blades, withdrawing the speculum about halfway, and inserting it again at a more downward angle. When the cervix is in full view, fix the depressed lever to an open position.
4. Inspect the cervix. The normal cervix is pink and midline. Assess color, position, size, projection into the vagina, surface and shape, and any discharge.

If a Papanicolaou (Pap) smear to collect cervical cells for cytologic studies is done, the following procedure may be used:

1. To collect cells from the vaginal pool, roll a sterile cotton-tipped applicator on the vaginal wall below the cervix. Paint the smear on the slide, and spray the slide with fixative.
2. To collect endocervical cells, place the groove of the spatula snugly against the cervical os, and rotate it 360 degrees. In a single stroke, spread the material from both sides of the spatula on a slide, and immediately spray with fixative.

If cultures are to be done, take a specimen from the vagina and/or cervix with a sterile, cotton-tipped applicator, and then either spread the specimen on a culture plate or place it in a culture container. Follow institutional protocols for preparing specimens for vaginal infections from suspected organisms.

At the end of the examination, loosen the lever control and slowly withdraw the speculum, closing the blades slowly and rotating the speculum while observing all areas of the vaginal wall. Assess the color of the mucosa and the color and appearance of any discharge.

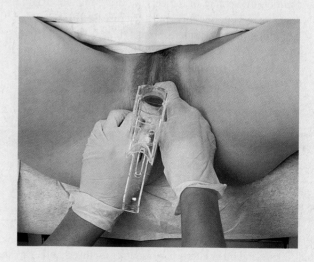

Inserting the vaginal speculum.

## BOX 46–2 ■ Guidelines for Bimanual Pelvic Examination

The bimanual pelvic examination is done to palpate the cervix, uterus, and ovaries. The examiner's hand that will be used intravaginally is held with the index and middle fingers extended, the thumb abducted, and the fourth and fifth fingers folded on the palm of the hand. The extended fingers are lubricated.

The general procedure is as follows:

1. Spread the labia with the thumb and finger of the opposite hand and insert the lubricated fingers into the vagina with the palm upward.
2. Place the opposite hand on the abdomen; it is used to press on the abdomen and gently move the internal genitals toward the intravaginal fingers (see the accompanying figure).
3. Ask the client to take deep breaths to relax the abdominal wall.
4. Palpate the cervix, assessing size, contour, position, surface, consistency, tenderness, and mobility. The cervix should be freely movable and non-tender.
5. Palpate the uterus by pressing downward on the abdomen while placing the intravaginal fingers in the anterior fornix and gently lifting against the abdominal hand. Assess the size, shape, surface; consistency, position, mobility, and tenderness of the uterus. The normal uterus is freely movable and nontender.
6. Palpate the adnexal areas, which surround the uterus and contain the fallopian tubes and ovaries. Because these struc-

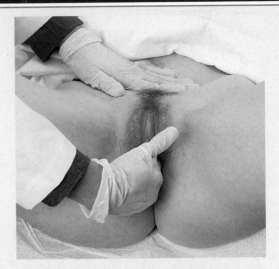

Bimanual pelvic examination.

tures are small, palpation may not be possible. If the ovaries are palpable, they should be smooth and firm. The normal ovary is sensitive to touch, firm, and highly movable.
7. Withdraw the fingers. Provide tissues for the client's use in wiping the genital area.

---

✓ An ectropion (eversion of columnar epithelium lining the cervical canal) appears plush red around the central cervical os and may bleed easily.
✓ Nabothian cysts (small, white, or yellow raised, round areas on the cervix) are considered normal but may become infected.
✓ Cervical polyps may be cervical or endometrial in origin.
• Palpate the cervix, uterus, and ovaries. See the guidelines in Box 46–2.
  ✓ The uterus may be retroverted (tilted backward) or retroflexed (angled backward).
  ✓ Pain on movement of the cervix during manual examination suggests pelvic inflammatory disease (PID).
  ✓ Softening of the uterine isthmus (Hegar's sign), softening of the cervix (Goodell's sign), and uterine enlargement may be objective signs of pregnancy.

✓ Firm, irregular nodules that vary greatly with size and are continuous with the uterine surface are likely to be myomas (fibroids).
✓ Unilateral or bilateral smooth, compressible adnexal masses are found in ovarian tumors.
✓ Profuse menstrual bleeding is seen with endometrial polyps, dysfunctional uterine bleeding (DUB), and use of an intrauterine device.
✓ Irregular bleeding may be associated with endometrial polyps, DUB, uterine or cervical carcinoma, or oral contraceptives.
✓ Postmenopausal bleeding is seen with endometrial hyperplasia, estrogen therapy, and endometrial cancer.

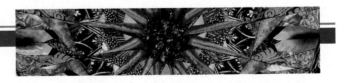

## EXPLORE MediaLink

NCLEX review questions, case studies, care plan activities, MediaLink applications, and other interactive resources for this chapter can be found on the Companion Website at www.prenhall.com/lemone.

Click on Chapter 46 to select the activities for this chapter. For animations, video clips, more NCLEX review questions, and an audio glossary, access the Student CD-ROM accompanying this textbook.

# TEST YOURSELF

1. In the male, sperm and testosterone are produced by the:
   a. Epididymis
   b. Seminal vesicles
   c. Testes
   d. Cowper's glands

2. In the female, what structure is analogous to the penis in the male?
   a. Ovaries
   b. Labia majora
   c. Labia minora
   d. Clitoris

3. Suspected abnormalities of the scrotum may be further assessed through:
   a. Transillumination
   b. Auscultation
   c. Palpation
   d. Percussion

4. What assessment technique is **primarily** used to determine abnormalities of the breast?
   a. Inspection
   b. Auscultation
   c. Palpation
   d. Percussion

5. At what anatomic location would you palpate Bartholin's glands?
   a. Above the clitoris
   b. Posterior labia majora
   c. Inferior to the urinary meatus
   d. Internal vaginal wall

See Test Yourself answers in Appendix C.

# BIBLIOGRAPHY

Andresen, G. (1998). Assessing the older patient. *RN, 61*(3), 46–56.

Billington, A. (1997). Running a nurse-led prostate assessment clinic. *Community Nurse, 3*(7), 26.

Blackwell, J., & Blackwell, D. (1997). Menopause: Life event or medical disease? *Clinical Nurse Specialist, 11*(1), 7–11.

Dumesic, D. (1996). Pelvic examinations: What to focus on in menopausal women. *Consultant, 36*(1), 39–46.

Frizzell, J. (1998). The PSA test. *American Journal of Nursing, 98*(4), 14–15.

Heath, H., & White, I. (2001). Sexuality and older people: An introduction to nursing assessment. *Nursing Older People, 13*(4), 29–31.

Klingman, L. (1999). Assessing the female reproductive system: A guide through the gynecologic exam. *American Journal of Nursing, 99*(8), 37–43.

Padbury, V. (1997). Women's health check. *Practice Nurse, 13*(9), 547–549.

Parker, S. (1997). Well-women clinics: Breast and pelvic examinations. *Practice Nurse, 14*(9), 582.

Weber, J., & Kelley, J. (2002). *Health assessment in nursing* (2nd ed.). Philadelphia: Lippincott-Raven.

Wilson, S., & Giddens, J. (2001). *Health assessment for nursing practice.* St. Louis: Mosby.

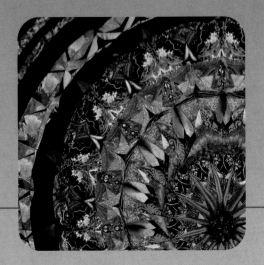

### CHAPTER 47

# Nursing Care of Men with Reproductive System Disorders

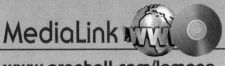

## MediaLink

### www.prenhall.com/lemone

Additional resources for this chapter can be found on the Student CD-ROM accompanying this textbook, and on the Companion Website at www. prenhall.com/lemone. Click on Chapter 47 to select the activities for this chapter.

**CD-ROM**
- Audio Glossary
- NCLEX Review

**Companion Website**
- More NCLEX Review
- Case Study
  Benign Prostatic Hyperplasia (BPH)
- Care Plan Activity
  Radical Prostatectomy
- MediaLink Application
  Prostate Cancer Prevention

## LEARNING OUTCOMES

After completing this chapter, you will be able to:

- Apply knowledge of normal male anatomy, physiology, and assessments when providing care for men with reproductive system disorders (see Chapter 46).

- Explain the pathophysiology of disorders of the male reproductive system.

- Discuss risk factors for cancers of the male reproductive system.

- Discuss the collaborative care, with related nursing implications, for men with disorders of the reproductive system.

- Provide appropriate nursing care for the man having prostate surgery.

- Use the nursing process as a framework for providing individualized care to men with disorders of the reproductive system.

Men are subject to disorders of the penis, scrotum and testes, prostate gland, and breast. These disorders may be inflammatory, structural, benign, or malignant. Young men are at increased risk for testicular cancer. As men age, both benign and malignant problems with the prostate gland become common. Many of the disorders pose significant risk to the man's fertility and sexual and urinary function, and some are life threatening. This chapter discusses disorders of the male reproductive system, including disorders of sexual expression and the male breast. As many of the treatments and disorders of the male reproductive system have the potential to affect erection and ejaculation, these problems are discussed first.

# DISORDERS OF SEXUAL EXPRESSION

## THE MAN WITH ERECTILE DYSFUNCTION

**Erectile dysfunction** is the inability of the male to attain and maintain an erection sufficient to permit satisfactory sexual intercourse. **Impotence,** a term often used synonymously with erectile dysfunction, may involve a total inability to achieve erection, an inconsistent ability to achieve erection, or the ability to sustain only brief erections. Erectile dysfunction has many possible causes (Table 47–1). Erectile dysfunction may or may not be associated with a loss of **libido** (sexual desire).

The incidence of erectile dysfunction is difficult to estimate because many affected men may not report the disorder. An estimated 10 million men in the United States have erectile dysfunction, and most are older than 65. A prevalence of 5% is noted at age 40, increasing to approximately 25% at age 65 or older (Tierney et al., 2001). Most problems with erection have an organic cause. Because this is a problem primarily of aging men, the discussion of pathophysiology focuses on this age group.

## PATHOPHYSIOLOGY

Age-related changes in sexual function involve cellular and tissue changes in the penis, decreased sensory activity, hypogonadism, and the effects of chronic illness. In the penis, a change from elastic collagen to a more rigid collagen results in decreased distensibility (a less rigid erection). This, in turn, interferes with the veno-occlusive mechanism, which prevents blood from "leaking" out of the penis into the general vasculature

## TABLE 47–1  Causes of Erectile Dysfunction

| Major Pathologic Causes | | Major Iatrogenic Causes | |
|---|---|---|---|
| | | Medications | Procedures and Infections |
| *Neurogenic*<br>Spinal cord injury<br>Cerebrovascular accident<br>Parkinson's disease<br>Multiple sclerosis | *Arterial*<br>Atherosclerosis<br>Hypertension<br>Aortic aneurysm<br>Sickle cell anemia | *Antihypertensives*<br>Hydrochlorothiazide<br>Spironolactone<br>Methyldopa<br>Clonidine | *Surgery*<br>Coronary artery bypass<br>Pelvic lymphadenectomy<br>Radical prostatectomy<br>Radical cystectomy |
| *Endocrinologic*<br>Diabetes mellitus<br>Hypogonadism<br>Hypothyroidism | *Mechanical*<br>Decreased penile<br>distensibility<br>Congenital disorders<br>Morbid obesity<br>Hydrocele<br>Hip or pelvic fractures | Prazosin<br>Propranolol<br>Reserpine<br>*Psychotropic Agents*<br>Phenothiazines<br>Butyrophenones | Abdominal perineal resection<br>Sympathectomy<br>Aortic aneurysm repair<br>Transplant surgeries<br>*Other*<br>Severe nosocomial infection |
| *Inflammatory*<br>Prostatitis<br>Cystitis | | Tricyclic antidepressants<br>MAO inhibitors | Radiation therapy to pelvis |
| *Activity Intolerance*<br>Pulmonary problems<br>Anemias<br>Myocardial infarction<br>Congestive heart failure<br>Hepatic diseases<br>Renal failure | *Psychogenic*<br>Depression<br>Stress<br>Fatigue<br>Fear of failure | Diazepam<br>Chlorodiazepoxide<br>*Endocrinologic Agents*<br>LHRH agonists<br>Estrogen compounds<br>Progesterone | |
| *Substance Dependency*<br>Alcohol<br>Marijuana<br>Narcotics<br>Sedatives<br>Tobacco | *Compulsive Food Disorders*<br>Compulsive overeating<br>Anorexia nervosa<br>Bulimia | *Other*<br>Antiparkinsonian agents<br>Anticholinergic agents<br>Immunosuppressive agents<br>Antihistamines | |

prematurely. Problems with this mechanism result in incomplete erections. Vibrotactile sensation over the skin of the penis declines with age. This decline may explain why some older men require longer stimulation to achieve an erection. Hypogonadism, common in aging men, results in decreased testosterone levels. There may be a relationship between lower androgen levels and erectile function.

Many illnesses affect erectile function. Damage to arteries, smooth muscles, and fibrous tissues are the most common causes of impotence. Diseases such as diabetes, kidney disease, chronic alcoholism, atherosclerosis, and vascular disease are responsible for about 70% of erectile dysfunction. Innervation and blood flow to the penis may be damaged during surgery, prostate surgery in particular. Given the effects of aging on erectile function, the increased incidence of chronic illness, and the multiple treatments required to manage those illnesses, it is not surprising that many older men have difficulty with erectile function.

## COLLABORATIVE CARE

The management of men with erectile dysfunction is growing in importance and scale, because the population as a whole is aging, so the incidence is increasing proportionately. Another factor is the gradual change in the willingness of men and their partners to be forthcoming about sexual concerns. Although sexuality is still a very sensitive and private area for most people, the knowledge that help is available is causing men to seek answers. Many older men are coming to believe that loss of erectile function is not an inevitable part of aging.

## Diagnostic Tests

The following diagnostic tests may be ordered.

- *Blood profiles,* including chemistry and testosterone, prolactin, thyroxin, and PSA levels, are performed to identify metabolic and endocrine problems that may be causing the dysfunction.
- *Nocturnal penile tumescence and rigidity (NPTR) monitoring* helps differentiate between psychogenic and organic causes. These tests can be performed in a sleep laboratory, although home testing with portable devices is an alternative. The number and quality of erections occurring during REM sleep can be determined.
- *Cavernosometry* and *cavernosography* of the corpora are used to evaluate arterial inflow and venous outflow of the penis.

## Medications

Erectile dysfunction can be treated with oral medications, self-administered intracavernous injections, or by topical agents.

- *Oral medications:* Sildenafil citrate (Viagra) interferes with the breakdown of a biochemical involved in the smooth muscle relaxation of the corpus cavernosum necessary to produce an erection. While sildenafil citrate has no direct effect on the corpus cavernosum, it enhances the effect of nitric oxide (NO) released during sexual stimulation. At recommended doses, no effect occurs in the absence of sexual stimulation. See the box below for nursing implications of this drug.

## Medications Administration

### Sildenafil (Viagra)

#### Sildenafil citrate (Viagra)

Sildenafil citrate is an oral medication used to treat erectile dysfunction in men. In the presence of nitric oxide released during sexual stimulation, sildenafil citrate increases smooth muscle relaxation in the corpus cavernosum, increasing the ability to achieve and maintain an erection. It may be taken once per day, approximately 1 hour before sexual activity.

#### Nursing Responsibilities

- Assess the client's health and medication history for use of nitrates. Sildenafil citrate is contraindicated for men who are currently taking nitrates such as nitroglycerine in short- or long-acting forms (including oral, sublingual transdermal, and other forms such as nitrolingual spray). Combining these drugs may cause significant hypotension.
- Inquire about the use of recreational nitrates such as amyl nitrate or nitrite ("poppers") or butyl nitrate. Use of these substances also contraindicates the use of sildenafil citrate.
- Clients who are at risk for priapism, including men with sickle cell disease, multiple myeloma, or leukemia, or who have an

anatomic abnormality of the penis should not take sildenafil citrate.
- Drugs such as ketoconazole, erythromycin, and cimetidine reduce the clearance of sildenafil citrate; concurrent administration may necessitate a reduced dosage.
- This drug is approved only for use in adult males; it is not approved for children or women.

#### Client and Family Teaching

- Take this drug as needed, approximately 1 hour before sexual activity. It can be taken within 30 minutes to 4 hours of sexual activity, although the response may be diminished after 2 hours.
- Do not take this drug more than once a day.
- Taking the drug after a high-fat meal may delay the onset of effects.
- Do not combine with other treatments for erectile dysfunction.
- If you experience chest pain or shortness of breath while using this drug, contact your physician.

• *Injectable medications:* Papaverine and prostaglandin E injections may be used. When injected directly into the penis, papaverine relaxes the arterioles and smooth muscles of the cavernosum, thus inducing tumescence (swelling). An erection usually develops that lasts from 30 minutes to 4 hours. Prostaglandin E functions much as papaverine does, but has fewer side effects. One problem with this treatment is its mode of delivery. There is a high attrition rate, and clients report dissatisfaction with lack of spontaneity, loss of interest in sex, physical limitations, cost, and occasionally, pain. Alprostadil (Caverject) is another injectable medication that may be used to treat erectile dysfunction. It may be injected into the penis or placed in the urethra as a minisuppository.

• *Hormone replacement therapy:* Testosterone injections (200 mg IM every 3 weeks) or topical patches may be used for men with documented androgen deficiency and who do not have prostate cancer.

• *Transdermal medications:* Transdermal nitroglycerin paste has restored erectile function to a few men when applied directly to the penis. The mechanism of action is probably arteriolar dilation.

## Mechanical Devices

The most frequently prescribed mechanical device for erectile dysfunction is the vacuum constriction device (VCD). The VCD draws blood into the penis with a vacuum, trapping it there with a constricting band at the base of the penis. After the device is removed for intercourse, a single small band, often called an O-ring, is left at the base of the penis to maintain the erection. If the man can attain an erection but cannot maintain it, then an O-ring alone can be used.

## Surgery

Surgical treatment for erectile dysfunction involves either revascularization procedures or implantation of prosthetic devices. Venous or arterial procedures are generally not successful. The result is often temporary, because the underlying cause of the vascular insufficiency is usually not corrected. Implantation of penile prostheses is now common (Figure 47–1 ■). Men are generally satisfied with their prostheses, and they rank the inflatable type highest. Partners are also more likely to report satisfaction with the penile implant, although not to the same degree as clients. Some partners report that the implanted penis is harder than a normal erect penis and therefore causes pain. Also, the man can have intercourse for a prolonged period of time, and some partners do not find prolonged penetration enjoyable. Client and partner teaching is mandatory. Counseling by a sex therapist may be needed to facilitate adaptation to the implant.

## NURSING CARE

Nurses in almost any health care setting may encounter men with erectile dysfunction, either through routine examinations or through careful assessment of clients' conditions and treatments that may incidentally cause erectile dysfunction. Nurses employed in clinics, operating rooms, and surgical units with urological services commonly encounter men being treated for erectile dysfunction. Nurses in a variety of settings, including long-term care, encounter men who have had surgical interventions, such as penile implants.

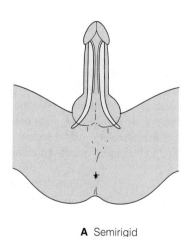 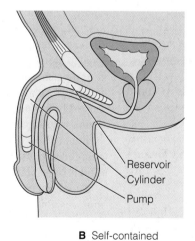 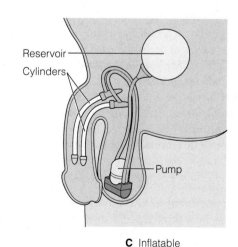

**A** Semirigid      **B** Self-contained      **C** Inflatable

**Figure 47–1** ■ Types of penile implants. *A,* With semirigid rods implanted in the corpora cavernosa, the penis is always in a state of semi-erection, which may not be acceptable to the man. *B,* With a self-contained penile implant, the penis remains flaccid until the man compresses a pump at the head of the penis, which transfers fluid from a reservoir to a cylinder within the penis to achieve an erection. The man presses a release valve to return the fluid to the reservoir. *C,* With an inflatable penile implant, the penis remains flaccid until the man compresses a pump in the scrotum, which transfers fluid from an abdominal reservoir to cylinders in the corpora cavernosa to achieve an erection. Pressing a release valve returns the fluid to the reservoir.

## Nursing Diagnoses and Interventions

Because nurses are usually accessible, they are most likely to discover problems of erectile dysfunction. Once a problem is known, nurses are involved in giving information, providing emotional support, and referring clients to physicians or counselors. Although there are many possible nursing diagnoses, this section focuses on nursing care related to sexual dysfunction and self-esteem.

### Sexual Dysfunction

Many men who lose erectile function are not aware of the cause. Often the man blames the loss on unrelated factors, such as age, a medication for an illness, a dangerous illness, or his sexual partner. Not knowing causes anxiety, which may disrupt the relationship with his partner or lead him to discontinue an important medication.

- Assess for risk factors for erectile dysfunction. Be especially alert to men who have recently begun medications or had recent surgeries that could cause erectile dysfunction. *Awareness of risk factors helps the nurse to prioritize care, although nurses must remember that almost all aging clients have at least one risk factor.*
- Assess for sexual dysfunction. Men have shown increasing willingness to discuss sexual concerns and expect nurses to be aware of the physiologic effects of their disease and side effects of treatment on all aspects of their health. *If a problem exists, information obtained in a sexual assessment guides the nurse in deciding if the next step should be client teaching, referral, or both.*

> **PRACTICE ALERT** *Many men will not volunteer information about sexual function unless asked, but then are open about concerns and appreciate being asked.* ■

- Perform a detailed assessment of current sexual practices. *It is essential for health care providers to understand the client and partner's sexual pattern in order to provide appropriate, individualized care.*
- Discuss previous methods of coping with erectile dysfunction. *Awareness of coping strategies can provide insight for the nurse and guide teaching.*
- Provide information about treatment options. *The man needs to know the details of the intervention, the chances for success, and the possible complications.*

### Situational Low Self-Esteem

The man with erectile dysfunction often believes himself to be "less than a man." In addition, the insertion of a penile implant with a semirigid prosthesis may result in disturbances in body image related to changes in sexual activity as well as the appearance and embarrassment of a permanent semierection.

- Collect data during the health history, in a nonjudgmental manner, about physiologic function, other chronic illnesses, and feelings about sexual inadequacy. *This information is necessary to establish the database for individualized interventions.*
- If the man has had a penile implant, teach him and his partner how to use the pump, including how to inflate and deflate the device. Suggest he practice inflation and deflation during the postoperative period. Suggest wearing snug-fitting underwear with the penis placed in an upright position on the abdomen and loose trousers. Provide information about length of healing, and that sexual activity may resume within 6 to 8 weeks following surgery. *Practice using the pump will maintain the pump position and promote tissue growth around the implant. The type of clothing worn can improve the ability to conceal the semi-rigid prosthesis and decrease embarrassment. Recovery from surgery is necessary before resuming sexual activity.*

### Home Care

Many nurses find that men with erectile dysfunction and their partners have lived in isolation with the problem for many years. The partner may even be unaware of the problem. The partner may believe that the man is seeing someone else or that the man has lost his attraction to the partner. The man may have kept his problem a secret because an intense feeling of shame makes him unable to admit that he cannot perform sexually. Many men greet the information about the high incidence of erectile dysfunction with a sense of relief that they are not alone in having this problem. All men and their partners also need to be aware of support services available to them.

## THE MAN WITH EJACULATORY DYSFUNCTION

There are many types of ejaculatory dysfunction. *Premature ejaculation* is usually psychogenic in origin, although diabetes can cause the problem as well. *Delayed ejaculation* can be related to aging changes, such as decreased vibrotactile sensation over the penis or decreased libido secondary to hypogonadism. Delayed ejaculation and inability to ejaculate at all may be caused by certain medications, such as antihypertensives, antidepressants, anxiolytics, and narcotics. *Retrograde ejaculation* (seminal fluid discharged into the bladder) may develop in aging men but is usually related to treatment of prostatic conditions or testicular cancer.

Among these problems, premature ejaculation has proved most responsive to medical management. The man can experiment with ways (such as wearing condoms) to decrease sensitivity. Using relaxation and guided imagery can delay sexual excitement. Mechanical devices, such as constrictive rings around the base of the penis, can help the man delay ejaculation and sustain an erection.

Nursing care focuses on assessment of the problem and teaching. The man's partner can be taught how to avoid excessive stimulation until ejaculation. If the problem persists, the man should be referred to a specialist.

# DISORDERS OF THE PENIS

## THE MAN WITH PHIMOSIS OR PRIAPISM

Two less common disorders of the penis are phimosis and priapism. Although uncommon, these disorders can cause problems with urination and sexual activity. In some cases, they are considered a medical emergency, as decreased blood flow to the penis may result in tissue ischemia and necrosis.

**Phimosis** is constriction of the foreskin so that it cannot be retracted over the glans penis. Phimosis may be congenital, or it may be related to chronic infections under the foreskin, which lead to adhesions. The major problem with this condition is that it prevents adequate hygiene, which may lead to malignant changes of the penis. It also may interfere with urinary elimination and intercourse. In a related disorder, called *paraphimosis,* the foreskin is tight and constricted, and is not able to cover the glans penis. The glans becomes engorged and edematous, and is painful. Paraphimosis may result from long-term retraction of the foreskin, such as occurs in placement of an indwelling catheter in the uncircumcised male (Porth, 2002). The tight foreskin can result in ischemia of the glans.

**Priapism** is an involuntary, sustained, painful erection that is not associated with sexual arousal. The prolonged erection may result in ischemia and fibrosis of the erectile tissue with high risk of subsequent impotence (Porth, 2002). The disorder, classified as either primary or secondary, is caused by impaired blood flow in the corpora cavernosa. Primary priapism results from conditions such as tumors, infection, or trauma. Secondary priapism is caused by blood disorders (e.g., leukemia, sickle cell anemia, and thrombocytopenia), neurologic disorders (e.g., spinal cord injury or stroke), renal failure, and some medications (see Box 47-1). Men who use intracavernous injection therapy for erectile dysfunction are at risk for priapism.

## COLLABORATIVE CARE

Severe phimosis or paraphimosis may require surgical circumcision. If infection is present, the appropriate antibiotic is administered.

| BOX 47–1 | ■ Factors Implicated in the Etiology of Priapism |
|---|---|

**Illnesses/Conditions**
- Sickle cell disease
- Leukemia
- Metastatic cancer
- Spinal cord trauma

**Drugs**
- Papaverine
- Psychotropic drugs
- Alcohol
- Marijuana

Conservative treatment of priapism includes iced saline enemas, intravenous ketamine (Ketalar) administration to induce anesthesia, and spinal anesthesia. Blood may be aspirated from the corpus through the dorsal glans, followed by catheterization and pressure dressings to maintain decompression. If necessary, more aggressive surgery to create vascular shunts to maintain blood flow is performed. When priapism is prolonged, up to 50% of men have subsequent erectile dysfunction.

## NURSING CARE

Nursing care for priapism focuses on assessing the penis, monitoring urinary output, and providing pain control. Assessment of the penis includes inspection for degree of erection and changes in color due to ischemia, and palpation of the penis for firmness and degree of rigidity. Monitor urine output, assessing for oliguria or signs of acute urinary retention. Pain is treated with analgesics.

The man usually has moderate to severe anxiety related to pain, the treatment, and the threat to his sexual function. The treatment may sound bizarre and painful, especially since the area is already extremely sensitive. The man may be acutely embarrassed by the erection and needs reassurance that the nurse understands that the erection is not within his control.

## THE MAN WITH CANCER OF THE PENIS

Cancer of the penis is a rare cancer in North America, occurring in approximately 1200 men per year (American Cancer Society [ACS], 2002). It most commonly affects men between the ages of 45 and 60. The cause is unknown. Penile cancer is rare in Jewish and Muslim men, populations in which routine circumcision is practiced, although the correlation between circumcision and this cancer is unclear. Phimosis is a risk factor, as are viral HPV and HIV infections. Ultraviolet light exposure (such as that used to treat psoriasis) also may play a role (Porth, 2002).

### PATHOPHYSIOLOGY AND MANIFESTATIONS

Squamous cell carcinoma accounts for 95% of all penile cancers. The tumor usually develops as a nodular or wartlike growth or a red velvety lesion on the glans or foreskin. The tumors tend to grow slowly. Penile cancer spreads to the superficial or deep inguinal nodes, and very late in the disease may spread to the bone, liver, or lungs. If the lesion is treated before inguinal node involvement, chances for a cure are good. Most of these lesions are painless but there may be significant ulceration and bleeding. Purulent, foul-smelling discharge may be evident under the foreskin. Occasionally, men with penile cancer may present with enlarged inguinal lymph nodes.

## COLLABORATIVE CARE

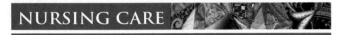

Cancer of the penis is diagnosed by a biopsy of the lesion, including any suspicious inguinal lymph nodes. The cancer is staged according to the size of the tumor, extent of invasion, status of inguinal lymph nodes, and presence or absence of distant metastasis. Small, localized lesions may be treated with fluorouracil cream, external-beam radiation, laser therapy, or surgical excision. Larger lesions with superficial or deep infiltration of penile structures require partial or total amputation of the penis. Chemotherapy may be administered to men with distant metastasis.

## NURSING CARE

Education can help prevent this disease or provide early detection. Teach men about the risks of unprotected sex and encourage condom use. Also encourage men to shield their genitals when having ultraviolet light therapy or using tanning salons. Discuss the importance of seeking prompt treatment for any lesion or abnormal drainage noted on the penis.

If the man has a penile amputation, nurses help cope with the problems of a shortened or absent penis, including the potentially devastating effect on body image and self-concept. If a total penectomy is performed, the surgeon creates a perineal urethrostomy, preserving urinary continence. However, the man must void in the sitting position, reinforcing the feeling of loss. Dribbling of urine after voiding may be a problem for a few weeks. The man should be taught to perform careful perineal hygiene following surgery, using mild soap and water. Sitz baths may be helpful to relieve pain and to promote healing. If an inguinal lymph node dissection is performed, the man may experience persistent lymphedema of the lower extremities.

# DISORDERS OF THE TESTIS AND SCROTUM

## THE MAN WITH A BENIGN SCROTAL MASS

Most scrotal masses are benign and can be managed in a manner that is satisfactory to the client. The most common are hydroceles, spermatoceles, and varicoceles (Figure 47–2 ■).

- A **hydrocele,** the most common cause of scrotal swelling, is a collection of fluid within the tunica vaginalis. The swelling ranges from slightly larger than the testicle to larger than a grapefruit. The cause of chronic hydrocele in men over the age of 40 years is an imbalance between production and reabsorption of fluid within the layers of the scrotum. Hydroceles also may occur secondary to trauma, infection, or a tumor. A hydrocele may be differentiated from a solid mass by transillumination or ultrasound of the scrotum. If the hydrocele becomes large enough to cause embarrassment or sig-

nificant pain, the fluid is aspirated and an agent is injected into the scrotal sac to sclerose the tunica vaginalis. Hydroceles are not associated with infertility.

- A **spermatocele** is a mobile, usually painless mass that forms when efferent ducts in the epididymis dilate and form a cyst. It is thought to result from leakage of sperm due to trauma or infection. Treatment is usually not necessary. Spermatoceles are not associated with infertility.

- A **varicocele** is an abnormal dilation of a vein within the spermatic cord. It is caused by incompetent or congenitally missing valves that allow blood to pool in the spermatic cord veins. The dilated vein forms a soft mass that may be painful. Most varicoceles occur after puberty on the left side. A major concern with this condition is that it can decrease blood flow through the testis, interfere with spermatogenesis, and cause infertility. Varicoceles can be felt by scrotal palpation. Sonography is also frequently used for diagnosis. If infertil-

**Figure 47–2** ■ Common disorders of the scrotum. Hydroceles and spermatoceles do not usually require treatment unless they become large and cause pain. Varicoceles are usually treated to prevent infertility.

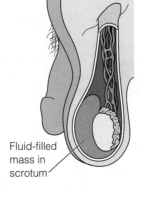
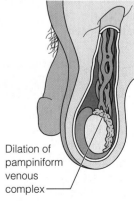

Fluid-filled mass in scrotum

Cystic mass on epididymis

Dilation of pampiniform venous complex

**Hydrocele**          **Spermatocele**          **Varicocele**

ity is a concern, the spermatic vein may be ligated or occluded with a sclerosing agent or balloon catheter. If the varicocele is small and infertility is not a concern, a scrotal support is recommended.

## NURSING CARE

Nursing care focuses on reducing anxiety and teaching about comfort measures. Almost all men are aware of the possible pain associated with scrotal manipulation. They need information and reassurance about pain management if surgical treatment is necessary. External bleeding is minimal after surgery; however, some men do develop scrotal hematomas, manifested by scrotal edema and a purple discoloration.

## THE MAN WITH EPIDIDYMITIS

**Epididymitis** is an infection or inflammation of the epididymis, the structure that lies along the posterior border of the testis. This disorder is more often seen in sexually active men who are less than 35 years of age.

Sexually transmitted urethritis caused by *C. trachomatis* or *N. gonorrhoeae* is the usual precipitating factor for epididymitis in younger men. Men who practice unprotected anal intercourse may acquire sexually transmitted epididymitis from *E. coli, H. influenzae, Cryptococcus,* or tuberculosis (McCance & Huether, 2002). In men older than 35, epididymitis usually is associated with a urinary tract infection or prostatitis. Chemical epididymitis is associated with an inflammatory response to the reflux of urine into the ejaculatory ducts from urethral strictures, congenital structural anomalies, or increased abdominal pressure from excessive heavy lifting. This type is usually self-limiting and does not require treatment.

## PATHOPHYSIOLOGY AND MANIFESTATIONS

Infectious epididymis spreads by ascending the vas deferens from an already infected urethra or bladder. Early manifestations include pain and local edema, which can progress to erythema and edema of the entire scrotum, especially on the side of the involved epididymis. Complications of the disorder include abscess formation, infarction of the testis, and infertility.

## COLLABORATIVE CARE

The infection is diagnosed with a specimen culture from a urethral swab or epididymial aspiration. Severe epididymitis may be treated with intravenous antibiotics and hospitalization. Less acute forms of the disease are treated with outpatient antibiotic therapy. The man's sexual partner should be treated with antibiotics if the causative organism is sexually transmitted.

## NURSING CARE

Nursing care involves symptomatic relief. Ice packs and a scrotal support may be applied to the scrotum to relieve pain. Ensure the man knows that complete resolution of the infection may take weeks to months, and that treatment should continue until the infection is gone. Provide information about the possibility of infertility, as the man may wish to seek evaluation for this problem at a later date.

## THE MAN WITH ORCHITIS

**Orchitis** is an acute inflammation or infection of the testes. It most commonly occurs as a complication of a systemic illness or as an extension of epididymitis. Infection may reach the testes through the vas deferens and the lymphatic and vascular channels. Trauma, including vasectomy and other scrotal surgeries, may cause inflammation of the testes.

## PATHOPHYSIOLOGY AND MANIFESTATIONS

The most common infectious cause of orchitis in postpubertal men is mumps. The manifestations have a sudden onset, usually within 3 to 4 days after the swelling of the parotid glands. Manifestations include a high fever, increased WBCs, and unilateral or bilateral scrotal redness, swelling, and pain. In about 30% of cases, atrophy of the testes with irreversible damage to spermatogenesis occurs (McCance & Huether, 2002). Although androgen production is not affected, permanent sterility may result.

## COLLABORATIVE CARE

Treatment is supportive and symptomatic, including antibiotic therapy if urine cultures are positive. Bed rest, scrotal support and elevation, hot or cold compresses, and analgesics for pain are prescribed. If a hydrocele occurs, it is aspirated. Nursing care is similar to that of the client with epididymitis and other scrotal disorders.

## THE MAN WITH TESTICULAR TORSION

**Testicular torsion,** twisting of the spermatic cord with scrotal swelling and pain, is a potential medical emergency. The condition occurs most often between birth and age 20, but can occur at any age. Testicular torsion may occur spontaneously, or it may follow trauma or physical exertion. The torsion of the arteries and veins decreases or stops testicular circulation with resultant vascular engorgement and ischemia.

Testicular torsion is usually diagnosed by history and physical examination. Testicular scanning may be used to determine if blood flow to the testicle is reduced. Treatment, which involves detorsion of the testicle and fixation to the scrotum, must begin as quickly as possible. If the testicle is necrotic or has sustained significant damage, an *orchiectomy* (surgical removal of a testes) is performed.

## THE MAN WITH TESTICULAR CANCER

Testicular cancer accounts for only 1% of all cancers in men; however, it is the most common cancer in men between the ages of 15 and 35. Annually, an estimated 7500 young men in the United States are diagnosed with this cancer (ACS, 2002). Survival from testicular cancer has improved dramatically as a result of treatment with effective combination chemotherapy.

The cause of testicular cancer is unknown, but both congenital and acquired factors have been associated with tumor development. About 5% develop in a man with a history of undescended testicle (**cryptorchidism**). Testicular cancer is more common on the right side, which parallels the incidence of cryptorchidism (Tierney et al., 2001).

## PATHOPHYSIOLOGY AND MANIFESTATIONS

Approximately 95% of testicular malignancies are germ cell tumors (Porth, 2002). Germ cell tumors are classified, depending on their origin and ability to differentiate, as seminomas and nonseminomas. Seminomas are the most common type, and are believed to arise from the seminiferous epithelium of the testes. Nonseminomas contain more than one cell type; they include embryonal carcinoma, teratoma, choriocarcinoma, and yolk cell carcinoma. The most common type in men age 20 to 30 is embryonal carcinomas. Testicular cancer may also arise from specialized cells of the gonadal stroma. These tumors are named for the cells from which they originate: Leydig cell, Sertoli cell, granulosa cell, and theca cell tumors.

Local spread of the cancer to the epididymis or spermatic cord is inhibited by the outer covering of the testicles, the tunica albuginea. Therefore, spread by lymphatic and vascular channels to other organs often causes distant disease before large masses develop in the scrotum. Lymphatic dissemination usually leads to disease in retroperitoneal lymph nodes, whereas vascular dissemination can lead to metastasis in the lungs, bone, or liver. Bilateral presentation of testicular cancer is unusual. The classic presenting manifestation of testicular cancer is a painless hard nodule. Other manifestations are summarized in the box on this page. Manifestations of metastasis include lower extremity edema, back pain, cough, hemoptysis, or dizziness. HCG-producing tumors may cause breast enlargement (*gynecomastia*).

### Risk Factors

Risk factors for testicular cancer include the following:

- Cryptorchidism
- Genetic predisposition, especially in identical twins and brothers
- Disorders of testicular development (such as Klinefelter's syndrome)
- Maternal estrogen administration during pregnancy

## Manifestations of Testicular Cancer

**Common**
- Painless swelling on one testicle
- Painless nodule on one testicle

**Occasional**
- Dull ache in pelvis or scrotum

**Uncommon (10%)**
- Acute pain in scrotum

**Metastatic symptoms**
- Neck mass
- Respiratory symptoms
- Gastrointestinal disturbance
- Lumbar back pain

**Rare (5%)**
- Infertility
- Gynecomastia

## COLLABORATIVE CARE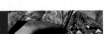

Care focuses on diagnosis, elimination of the cancer, and prevention or treatment of metastasis. Once testicular cancer is suspected, the man undergoes a number of screening tests to help determine the likelihood of the disease and its stage. If the disease is confined to the testicle, it is classified as stage I. Stage II disease is limited to the testicle and regional lymph nodes. Stage III disease involves metastasis above the diaphragm or extensive visceral involvement. Often, the man does not undergo biopsy before the beginning of treatment, but instead receives a definitive diagnosis after orchiectomy. Most men treated for testicular cancer will live a normal life span.

### Diagnostic Tests

The following diagnostic tests may be ordered.

- *Serum studies* for tumor markers. Germ cell tumors, which account for 95% of testicular cancers, produce biochemical markers such as human chorionic gonadotropin (hCG) and alpha-fetoprotein (AFP) that can be measured using radioimmunoassay techniques. Elevated levels provide strong evidence of testicular cancer. These markers are also measured after surgery to help determine the presence of residual disease that remains undetected by other means. Persistent elevation may indicate the need for further therapy.
- *Serum lactic acid dehydrogenase (LDH) levels* are elevated in testicular cancer, and may be significantly elevated when metastatic disease is present. The LDH is a less specific indicator of testicular cancer than the hCG and AFP.
- *Liver function tests, X-ray,* and *CT scans* of the chest and abdomen may be performed to evaluate the possibility of metastasis.

### Medications

Progress in chemotherapy to treat testicular cancer is one of the chief reasons why most men survive the disease. The client with advanced disease receives platinum-based combination chemotherapy. Two frequently used combinations are (1) cisplatin, bleomycin, and etoposide (BEP), and (2) etoposide plus cisplatin (EP). Toxicity from the BEP regimen can be significant, with nausea, vomiting, hair loss, bone marrow suppression, nephrotoxicity, ototoxicity, and peripheral neuropathy. Decreasing BEP cycles to 3 (rather than 4) or using the EP regimen reduces both the mortality and morbidity associated with chemotherapy. Chemotherapy is discussed in Chapter 10. ∞

## Surgery

*Radical orchiectomy* is the treatment used in all forms and stages of testicular cancer. A modified retroperitoneal lymph node dissection that preserves the nerves necessary for ejaculation often is performed at the same time.

## Radiation Therapy

Radiation therapy is used for stage I seminoma to treat cancer in the retroperitoneal lymph nodes, the most frequent site for distant metastasis. The man may experience temporary diarrhea, nausea, or a decline in bone marrow function, such as thrombocytopenia or leukopenia. These problems are usually mild and respond well to symptomatic treatment or time. Damage to the contralateral testicle is minimized by careful shielding. Pretreatment and posttreatment analysis of sperm number and function is necessary. The most common long-term complication is dyspepsia or ulcer disease. Radiation therapy is discussed in Chapter 10. ∞

## NURSING CARE

## Health Promotion

Unfortunately, even when risk factors are considered, most men who develop testicular cancer have none. Therefore, beginning at the age of 15, all men should perform monthly testicular self-examination, as described in Box 47–2.

## Nursing Diagnoses and Interventions

Nursing care of the man with testicular cancer is complex. The nurse must consider the reactions to the diagnosis, the change in body image accompanying treatment, and sexual and reproductive issues. Although chances of a cure are excellent, the long-term effect on quality of life may be extensive, requiring a change in life goals.

### Deficient Knowledge

The nurse often initiates and reinforces teaching about what to expect after radical orchiectomy. The man's knowledge about surgery is assessed, and postoperative routines such as early ambulation are explained (see Chapter 7). ∞

- Explain pain control methods. In addition to the usual analgesics used to control postoperative incisional pain, ice bags may be applied to the scrotum. A scrotal support provides relief, especially when the client ambulates. *Surgery results in incisional pain, and the scrotum is tender and slightly swollen.*
- Teach the signs and symptoms of complications. The incision is closed with Steri-Strips or staples, and, although rare, wound dehiscence is possible. If the incision gapes open, or

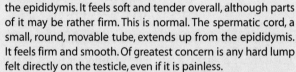

**BOX 47–2 ■ Testicular Self-Examination**

- Examine your testicles when you are taking a warm shower or bath, or just after if you prefer to use a mirror to compare size.
- The scrotum, testicles, and hands should be soapy to allow easy manipulation of the tissue.
- Gently roll each testicle between the thumb and fingers of each hand. If one testicle is substantially larger than the other, or if you feel any hard lumps, consult your physician immediately.
- Normal scrotal contents may be confusing. Just above and behind the testicle is the epididymis. It feels soft and tender overall, although parts of it may be rather firm. This is normal. The spermatic cord, a small, round, movable tube, extends up from the epididymis. It feels firm and smooth. Of greatest concern is any hard lump felt directly on the testicle, even if it is painless.
- Choose a day out of each month on which to examine yourself. Most men choose an easy day to remember, such as the first or last day of the month. Star this day on your calendar to help you remember.

if there is bleeding beyond slight oozing after 24 hours, the man should call the surgeon. Another rare complication is a hematoma in the scrotum caused by bleeding from the spermatic cord stump. Rapid onset of scrotal edema is a sign of this problem. *Because the man is usually discharged early, complications may not become apparent until he is at home.*
- Reinforce knowledge concerning the effect of surgery on sexuality. *If treatment involves only a unilateral orchiectomy, there should be no lasting effects on the client's sexual or reproductive function.*

### Ineffective Sexuality Patterns

The effect of testicular cancer and its treatment on sexual and reproductive function is varied. If the man has a retroperitoneal lymph node dissection, severing of the sympathetic plexus may result in retrograde ejaculation or failure to ejaculate. Infertility may be caused by ejaculation disorders, surgery, chemotherapy, or radiation therapy.

- Assess the man's prediagnosis sexual function. To assess this area, the nurse must establish an atmosphere of openness and permission to discuss sexual concerns. After the initial shock of the diagnosis, men report intense concern about sexual and reproductive issues, which can be relieved only by information. *Knowledge of the man's usual sexual function can guide teaching.*
- Discuss the possibility of preserving sperm in a bank prior to treatment. *This option may help relieve the man's fears about his ability to father children in the future, but must be completed prior to initiating treatment with surgery, chemotherapy, or radiation therapy.*

• Help coping with feelings about altered sexual function and appearance. Explain that testicular implants can be inserted to preserve appearance. *Many clients, regardless if they are in a significant relationship, deeply grieve the loss of the ability to father children. It is important to maintain body image despite disfiguring surgery.*

## Home Care

Families need to be included in teaching for a variety of reasons. If the man is of reproductive age, his partner will have significant anxiety and will require information. For the teenager, parents need information about the effect on sexual function and are often very involved in postoperative care. The man needs the support of the people he loves, and knowledgeable loved ones can give more effective support.

Provide teaching and reinforcement of the need for follow-up, especially if the retroperitoneal lymph nodes were not surgically explored. For men with a risk for recurrence, surveillance with periodic physical examinations, chest X-ray films, tumor markers, and CT scans of the retroperitoneal nodes could continue for a minimum of 5 years and possibly 10 years after orchiectomy.

# DISORDERS OF THE PROSTATE GLAND

## THE MAN WITH PROSTATITIS

**Prostatitis** is a term used to refer to different types of inflammatory disorders of the prostate gland. **Prostatodynia** is a condition in which the client experiences the symptoms of prostatitis but shows no evidence of inflammation or infection. Manifestations of prostatitis and prostatodynia are summarized in the box below.

## PATHOPHYSIOLOGY AND MANIFESTATIONS

The National Institutes of Health have defined four types of prostatitis: acute bacterial prostatitis, chronic bacterial prostatitis, chronic prostatitis/pelvic pain syndrome, and asymptomatic inflammatory prostatitis. Men with asymptomatic inflammatory prostatitis have no subjective symptoms, but are diagnosed when a biopsy or prostatic fluid examination is conducted.

### Acute Bacterial Prostatitis

Acute bacterial prostatitis is most often caused by an ascending infection from the urethra or reflux of infected urine into the ducts of the prostate gland. The organism most often responsible for the infection is *E. coli;* other causative organisms include *Pseudomonas, Klebsiella,* and *Chlamydia.*

Manifestations of acute bacterial prostatitis include increased temperature, malaise, muscle and joint pain, urinary frequency and urgency, dysuria, and urethral discharge. The man often experiences dull, aching pain in the perineum, rectum, or lower back. On rectal examination, the prostate is enlarged and painful.

### Chronic Bacterial Prostatitis

Men with chronic bacterial prostatitis often present with a history of recurrent urinary tract infections. The causative organisms are most often *E. coli, Proteus,* or *Klebsiella.* Calculi may form in the prostate and contribute to the chronicity of the problem.

The manifestations of chronic bacterial prostatitis include urinary frequency and urgency, dysuria, low back pain, and perineal discomfort. Epididymitis may be associated with the prostatitis.

### Chronic Prostatitis/Chronic Pelvic Pain Syndrome

This type of prostatitis is both the most common and the least understood of the syndromes (Porth, 2002). The two types (inflammatory and noninflammatory) are based on the presence of white blood cells in the prostatic fluid.

• *Inflammatory prostatitis* is believed to be an autoimmune disorder, but the actual cause is unknown. Men with this type of prostatitis have low back pain; urinary manifestations; pain in the penis, testicles, scrotum, lower back, and rectum; decreased libido, and painful ejaculations. They do not have bacteria in their urine, but do have abnormal inflammatory cells in prostatic secretions.

---

## Manifestations of Prostatitis and Prostatodynia

**Acute Bacterial Prostatitis**
• Onset (may be abrupt): obstruction, irritation, or pain upon voiding; frequency; and urgency
• Positive cultures of infectious organism
• Nonurinary symptoms: chills, fever, low back and pelvic floor pain

**Chronic Bacterial Prostatitis**
• Urinary symptoms sometimes similar to those of the acute form, except less sudden, less dramatic, or even absent
• Positive cultures of causative organism not always obtainable

**Chronic Prostatitis**
• Perineal, suprapubic, low back, or genital pain
• Irritation upon voiding
• Postejaculatory pain
• Negative cultures of organisms

**Prostatodynia**
• Pelvic, low back, or perineal pain
• Irritation or obstruction upon voiding
• No evidence of inflammation in the prostate
• No urinary tract infections
• Normal prostatic secretions

- *Noninflammatory prostatitis* (prostatodynia) has manifestations similar to those of inflammatory prostatitis, but no evidence of urinary or prostatic infection or inflammation can be found. The cause is not known, but is believed to be the result of a problem outside the prostate gland, such as obstruction of the bladder neck.

## COLLABORATIVE CARE

### Diagnostic Tests

It is often difficult to diagnose prostatitis. Urine and prostatic secretion examination and cultures are obtained to determine the presence and type of blood cells and bacteria. X-ray studies and ultrasound to visualize pelvic structures also may be useful.

### Medications

Bacterial prostatitis is treated with appropriate antibiotics. Men with the chronic form must take antibiotics for a much longer period, often up to 4 months, and may still relapse as soon as the antibiotic is discontinued. Nonbacterial prostatitis does not usually respond satisfactorily to drug therapy, although relief from symptoms is possible. Nonsteroidal anti-inflammatory drugs are useful for pain, and anticholinergics may reduce voiding symptoms. Prostatodynia is treated symptomatically to relieve muscle tension, usually with alpha-adrenergic blocking agents or muscle relaxants.

## NURSING CARE

Teaching for the man with prostatitis focuses on symptom management. Men with acute and chronic bacterial prostatitis should be taught to increase fluid intake to around 3 L daily and to void often. These measures help decrease irritation when voiding. Regular bowel movements helps ease pain associated with defecation. Local heat, such as sitz baths, may be helpful to relieve pain and irritation. It is important to teach the man to finish the course of antibiotic therapy. Men with chronic prostatitis/chronic pelvic pain syndrome need to know that the condition is not contagious and does not cause cancer (Porth, 2002).

## THE MAN WITH BENIGN PROSTATIC HYPERPLASIA (BPH)

**Benign prostatic hyperplasia (BPH),** an age-related, nonmalignant enlargement of the prostate gland, is a common disorder of the aging male. The prostate, very small at birth, grows at puberty, and reaches adult size around age 20. Benign hyperplasia (increased number of cells) begins at 40 to 45 years of age, and continues slowly through the rest of life. It is estimated that one-fourth of men over age 55 and one-half of men over 75 have manifestations of BPH (Porth, 2002). The problem that brings men to a health care provider is the associated urinary dysfunction.

## PATHOPHYSIOLOGY AND MANIFESTATIONS

The cause of BPH is unknown, but risk factors include age, family history, race, ethnicity, and hormonal factors. The incidence, which increases with age, is highest in African Americans and lowest in native Japanese. Higher rates have been associated with a family history of BPH.

The two necessary preconditions for BPH are age of 50 or greater and the presence of testes. Men who are castrated before puberty do not develop BPH. The androgen that mediates prostatic growth at all ages is dihydrotestosterone (DHT), which is formed in the prostate from testosterone. Although androgen levels decrease in aging men, the aging prostate appears to become more sensitive to available DHT. Estrogen, produced in small amounts in men, appears to sensitize the prostate gland to the effects of DHT. Increasing estrogen levels associated with aging or a relative increase in estrogen related to testosterone levels may contribute to prostatic hyperplasia.

BPH begins as small nodules in the periurethral glands, which are the inner layers of the prostate. The prostate enlarges through formation and growth of nodules (hyperplasia) and enlargement of glandular cells (hypertrophy). These changes occur over a long period of time. The pathophysiologic effects result from a combination of factors, including urethral resistance to the effects of BPH, intravesical pressure during voiding, detrusor muscle strength, neurologic functioning, and general physical health (McCance & Huether, 2002).

The expanding prostatic tissue compresses the urethra (Figure 47–3 ■) and causes partial or complete obstruction of the outflow of urine from the urinary bladder. The detrusor muscles hypertrophy to compensate for increased resistance to urinary flow; however, eventually decreased bladder compliance and bladder instability result. As a result, the man with BPH has manifestations from obstruction (weak urinary stream, increased time to void, hesitancy, incomplete bladder emptying, and postvoid dribbling) and irritation (frequency, urgency, incontinence, nocturia, dysuria, and bladder pain). Urinary retention may become chronic, resulting in overflow incontinence with any increase in intraabdominal pressure. There is little correlation between the size of the prostate gland and the urinary manifestations.

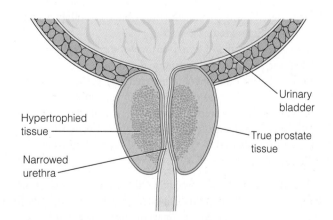

**Figure 47–3 ■** Benign prostatic hyperplasia.

Urinary bladder

Hypertrophied tissue

True prostate tissue

Narrowed urethra

## Manifestations of Benign Prostatic Hyperplasia

- Diminished force of urinary stream
- Hesitancy in initiating voiding
- Postvoid dribbling
- Sensation of incomplete emptying
- Urinary retention

- Nocturia
- Frequency
- Urgency
- Urge incontinence
- Dysuria
- Hematuria

Manifestations of BPH are summarized in the box above.

Unless the enlarging mass is reduced, multiple complications may occur. As urine is retained in the bladder, increasing bladder distention occurs. Diverticula (outpouchings) on the bladder wall result from the distention. The distention may also obstruct the ureters. Infection, more common in retained urine and in diverticula, may ascend from the bladder to the kidneys. Hydroureter, hydronephrosis, and renal insufficiency are possible complications.

## COLLABORATIVE CARE

Care of men with BPH focuses on diagnosing the disorder, correcting or minimizing the urinary obstruction, and preventing or treating complications. There is no way to reverse BPH. Treatment is often determined by the severity of the manifestations and the presence of complications. Mild cases are often monitored over time, and may remain stable or improve.

### Diagnostic Tests

The following diagnostic tests may be ordered, and include those outlined in the clinical guidelines published by the Agency for Health Care Policy and Research (1994).

- *Urinalysis* detects bacteria, WBCs, or microscopic RBCs.
- *Serum creatinine levels* are determined to estimate renal function.
- *Prostate-specific antigen (PSA) levels* are obtained to rule out prostate cancer. PSA is a glycoprotein produced only in the cytoplasm of benign and malignant prostate cells; the serum level corresponds with the volume of both benign and malignant prostate tissue.
- *DRE* examines the external surface of the prostate gland. In BPH, the prostate is asymmetrical and enlarged.
- *Residual urine* (amount of urine remaining in the bladder after voiding) may be measured with ultrasonography or postvoiding catheterization (more than 100 mL is considered high).
- *Uroflowmetry* measures urine flow rate; normal is greater than 14 mL/second. A finding of less than 10 mL/second indicates obstruction.

In addition, the man's own subjective experiences with BPH are included in the diagnosis and treatment. For example, the International Prostate Symptom Score uses a scale of 0 (not at all) to 5 (almost always) to collect data about areas such as feel-

ing as though the bladder did not empty with urinating, need to urinate within 2 hours after urinating, starting and stopping the stream several times while urinating, and straining to urinate. This questionnaire also asks how many times during the night the man gets up to urinate and how the man feels about having the disorder (Lepor, 2000).

### Medications

Treatment with medications is based on two considerations: The hyperplastic tissue is androgen dependent, and smooth muscle contraction within the prostate can exacerbate urinary obstruction. The first consideration is usually addressed by treatment for mild prostate enlargement with finasteride (Proscar), an antiandrogen agent that inhibits the conversion of testosterone to DHT and causes the enlarged prostate to shrink in size. Finasteride does cause impotence, decreased libido, and decreased volume of ejaculate. Client and family education includes the information that crushed tablets should not be handled by pregnant women, as the drug may be absorbed through the skin and be harmful to a male fetus.

Excessive smooth muscle contraction in BPH may be blocked with the alpha-adrenergic antagonists such as terazosin (Hytrin), doxazosin (Cardura), and tamsulosin (Flomax). These medications relieve obstruction and increase the flow of urine. They may cause orthostatic hypotension. Client and family teaching includes advice about making position changes slowly to avoid dizziness and accidental falls, how to take and record blood pressure, and to check with the health care provider before taking any medication for coughs, colds, or allergies (as these OTC medications may contain an adrenergic agent).

### Surgery

Men who have urinary retention, recurrent urinary tract infection, hematuria, bladder stones, or renal insufficiency secondary to BPH are candidates for surgical intervention. *Transurethral resection of the prostate (TURP), transurethral incision of the prostate (TUIP),* and open *prostatectomy* are the most common procedures.

A TURP is the surgical procedure used most often. Obstructing prostate tissue is removed using the wire loop of a resectoscope and electrocautery, inserted through the urethra (Figure 47–4 ). This surgery has potential risks, however, including postoperative hemorrhage or clot retention, inability to void, and urinary tract infection. Other possible complications are incontinence, impotence, and retrograde ejaculation.

In the TUIP procedure, a YAG laser is used to make small incisions in the smooth muscle where the prostate is attached to the bladder. The gland is split to reduce pressure on the urethra. No tissue is removed, so this procedure is most appropriate for men with smaller prostate glands. TUIP can be done on an outpatient basis, and has the additional advantage of less risk of postoperative retrograde ejaculation than is associated with TURP or other prostatectomy procedures.

When the prostate gland is very large, an open prostatectomy may be used. These procedures are discussed in the section on prostate cancer that follows. Nursing care for the client having prostate surgery is outlined on pages 1539–1540.

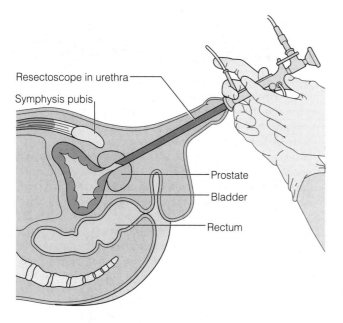

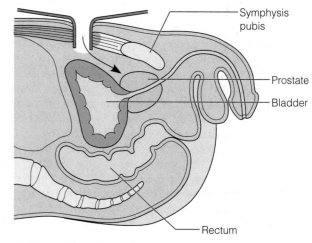

**A** Transurethral resection of the prostate

**B** Retropubic prostatectomy

**Figure 47–4** ■ *A,* In a transurethral resection of the prostate (TURP), a resectoscope inserted through the urethra is used to remove excess prostate tissue. *B,* In a retropubic prostatectomy, prostate tissue is removed through an abdominal incision.

# NURSING CARE OF THE MAN UNDERGOING PROSTATECTOMY

## PREOPERATIVE NURSING CARE

- Assess the man's and family's knowledge about the surgery. *Some men are confused about the surgical approach, because there are several, quite different, methods.*
- Inform the man that he will have a urinary catheter when he returns from surgery, and he may have a drain(s) in his incision. He also will be wearing sequential pneumatic compression stockings. *This knowledge can reduce anxiety postoperatively and increase cooperation with postoperative care.*
- Ensure that a signed consent form is in the chart and that all other preoperative tasks outlined in Chapter 7 are done. ⊖⊙
- Bowel preparation with a 2% neomycin enema may be ordered. *This cleanses the bowel if a perineal approach will be used.*
- Communicate willingness to address any concerns or anxiety. *Men may be anxious about the outcome of their surgery and potential long-term effects of the surgery on their sexuality. When a prostatectomy is performed for prostate cancer, additional fears include the extent of the cancer and surgery, chances for cure, and possible end-of-life issues.*

## POSTOPERATIVE CARE

- Maintain the usual postoperative assessments (see Chapter 7) and follow aseptic techniques in urinary drainage and irrigation care. Monitor vital signs closely for the first 24 hours and regularly thereafter. *The man who has had prostate surgery is at risk*

for hemorrhage and other postoperative complications. Vital sign changes may be early manifestations.
- Maintain accurate intake and output records, including amounts of irrigating solution used. Frequently assess patency of any catheters and drains. Monitor color and character of urine. *Catheters may become occluded by blood clots or kinks, interfering with urinary drainage and increasing the risk of hemorrhage.*
- Assess and manage the man's pain. *The man may have at least three types of pain: incisional pain, bladder spasm, and abdominal cramps due to intestinal gas. Analgesics and nonsteroidal anti-inflammatory drugs (NSAIDs) are administered on a routine and prn basis to control incisional pain. Bladder spasms may be accompanied by strong urges to void and urine leakage around the catheter. Belladona and opium (B & O) suppositories may be used to relieve bladder spasms.*
- Maintain antiembolic stockings and pneumatic compression devices as ordered. Assist with leg exercises and ambulation as ordered, usually the first postoperative day. *The man who has had prostate surgery is at risk for developing thromboemboli; these are important preventive measures.*
- Encourage the man to maintain a liberal fluid intake of 2 to 3 L a day. *Increased fluids reduce burning on urination after catheter removal and the risk of urinary tract infection.*

*(continued on page 1540)*

# NURSING CARE OF THE MAN UNDERGOING PROSTATECTOMY (continued)

## The Man with a Transurethral Resection of the Prostate (TURP)

- For the first 24 to 48 hours, monitor for hemorrhage, evidenced by frankly bloody urinary output, presence of large blood clots, decreased urinary output, increasing bladder spasms, decreased hemoglobin and hematocrit, tachycardia, and hypotension. Notify the physician if any of these manifestations occur. *Postoperative hemorrhage may be either arterial or venous, and may be precipitated by movement, bladder spasms, or an obstructed urinary drainage system.*
- Instruct the man with a three-way indwelling catheter with traction to keep the leg straight while the traction is applied. *A No. 18 to 22 Fr three-way catheter with a 30 to 45 mL balloon usually is inserted following a TURP. The inflated balloon is pulled down into the prostatic fossa and the catheter tubing is pulled down and taped to the man's leg to apply pressure against the operative site, preventing bleeding.*
- Explain that the presence of a urinary catheter will cause the sensation of needing to void, but it is important not to strain to try to void around the catheter or when having a bowel movement. Explain that bladder spasms, experienced as lower abdominal pressure or pain and a desire to urinate, may occur. Ensure that the man understands that this is an expected sensation, and that medications can help alleviate this discomfort. *Pressure on the urethra by the large catheter and on the internal sphincter by the catheter's balloon stimulate the micturition reflex. Straining to void or to have a bowel movement may stimulate bladder spasms and increase pain; it also may increase the risk for bleeding. Administer pain medications at regular intervals.*
- If the man has a continuous bladder irrigation (CBI), assess the catheter and the drainage tubing at regular intervals. Maintain the rate of flow of irrigating fluid to keep the output light pink or colorless. Assess the urinary output every 1 to 2 hours for color, consistency, amount, and presence of blood clots; assess for bladder spasms. *CBI is used to prevent the formation of blood clots, which could obstruct urinary output. Bladder distention resulting from output obstruction increases the risk of bleeding. Irrigating fluids are continuously infused and drained at a rate to keep urine light pink or colorless. Urine that is frankly bloody, contains many blood clots, or is decreased in amount, as well as bladder spasms, are indicators of obstruction and bleeding.*
- Assess for fluid volume excess and hyponatremia, called TURP syndrome, which is manifested by hyponatremia, decreased hematocrit, hypertension, bradycardia, nausea, and confusion. If these manifestations occur, notify the physician. *TURP syndrome results from the absorption of irrigating fluids during and after surgery. Untreated, it may result in dysrhythmias, seizures, or both.*
- If the man does not have CBI, follow agency procedure and physician orders for irrigating the indwelling catheter (usually when the urine is frankly bloody or has numerous larger blood clots, or when bladder spasms increase). In most in-

stances, using sterile technique, the catheter is gently irrigated with 50 mL of irrigating solution at a time, until the obstruction is relieved or the urine is clear. Ensure equal input and output of irrigating fluid. *Intermittent irrigation may be used to prevent obstruction of urinary drainage.*
- Following catheter removal, assess the amount, color, and consistency of urine. Explain that the man may experience burning on urination, that dribbling after urination is a common experience, and that the urine may contain small blood clots after catheter removal. *The CBI and catheter usually are removed in the 24 to 48 hours following surgery. Urinary control may be improved by teaching the man to start and stop the urine stream several times during each voiding and by practicing Kegel exercises. Regaining full control may take up to 1 year.*

## The Man with a Retropubic Prostatectomy

- Assess the abdominal incision for the presence of urine. *As the bladder is not entered during a retropubic prostatectomy, no urine should be found on the dressing.*
- Assess the abdominal incision for increased or purulent drainage, and the man for an increased temperature and pain. *These manifestations indicate the presence of infection.*

## The Man with a Suprapubic Prostatectomy

- Assess urinary output from both the suprapubic and the urethral catheters. *The man with a suprapubic prostatectomy often has two separate closed drainage systems: one from the suprapubic incision and one from a urethral catheter.*
- Assess the abdominal dressing for urinary drainage, and change saturated dressings frequently. Consult with a skin care specialist if necessary. *Urine is highly irritating to the skin.*
- Following removal of the urethral catheter (usually 2 to 4 days after surgery) and based on physician orders, clamp the suprapubic catheter and encourage the man to void. Assess residual urine by unclamping the suprapubic catheter and measuring urinary output after voiding. *If residual urine is 75 mL or less with several voidings, the suprapubic catheter is removed.*

## The Man with a Perineal Prostatectomy

- Assess perineal incision for drainage and manifestations of infection. *Location of the incision in the perineum increases the risk of infection.*
- Do not take rectal temperatures or administer enemas. *Insertion of a thermometer or enema tubing into the rectum may precipitate bleeding.*
- Use a T-binder or padded scrotal support to hold the dressing in place. Following removal of the dressing and perineal sutures, heat lamps or sitz baths may be used. *The location of the dressing makes application difficult: Heat lamps or sitz baths provide heat and promote healing.*
- Teach the man to perform perineal irrigations with sterile normal saline as ordered and after each bowel movement. *Because of the proximity of the incision to the anus, special wound care is necessary to prevent infection.*

Newer treatments for BPH include minimally invasive procedures such as balloon urethroplasty, destruction of excess prostate tissue using laser energy, microwave hyperthermia, and placement of intraurethral stents to maintain patency of the urethra. Balloon urethroplasty is a simple procedure in which a balloon-tipped catheter is inserted into the narrowed portion of the urethra. Inflation of the balloon widens the urethra, relieving obstruction. Obstructing prostate tissue can be destroyed using laser energy or desiccated by microwave hyperthermia. These procedures can be done as outpatient surgery.

## Phytotherapy

Phytotherapy is the use of plants or plant extracts for medical treatment. Several plant extracts have been used for years in Europe to treat BPH and are being used more often in the United States. The phytotherapy used include saw palmetto berry, the bark of *Pygeum africanum,* the roots of *Echinacea, purpurea,* and *Hypoxis rooperi,* and the leaves of the trembling poplar. The mechanisms of action of these extracts is unknown, but men report they are effective in relieving manifestations (Tierney, et al., 2001).

## NURSING CARE

Most men are unsure of the function of the prostate gland and even the prostate's exact location, though its relationship to sexual and urinary function is at least generally known. This lack of knowledge, coupled with the growing number of treatment options, is confusing to many men. There are many similarities between the nursing care of men with BPH and that of men with prostate cancer (see the section that follows). Nursing approaches to problems of urinary incontinence, sexual dysfunction, and pain are discussed there. This section provides interventions related to deficient knowledge, urinary retention, and risk of infection.

## Nursing Diagnoses and Interventions

### Deficient Knowledge

- Explain the anatomy and physiology of the prostate gland, as well as normal changes that occur with aging. *Men must know about their bodies in order to make accurate decisions about treatment.*
- Discuss treatment options, including information about effects on erectile function, ejaculation, and fertility. Counsel the man to discuss specific concerns with his urologist. *There are many different treatment options available; the choice should be a mutual decision between the man, his partner, and the urologist.*
- Discuss effects of TURP, including urinary retention and urinary incontinence. *These common transient postoperative effects are related to the surgical procedure and the postoperative indwelling catheter.*

- Explain to the man having a TURP that a catheter will be placed into the bladder, with the tubing taped to his inner thigh, and that irrigation fluid will be infusing into and out of the catheter for the first 36 to 72 hours following surgery. *The catheter and irrigation are necessary to remove blood clots from the bladder and allow drainage of urine. Gentle traction is applied to the catheter to apply pressure to the operative site (prostatic fossa) and prevent excessive bleeding.*
- Explain that, following removal of the catheter, he will most likely have urinary frequency and urgency. He may also experience dribbling of urine after voiding. Stress the importance of increasing oral fluid intake and regular Kegel exercises. *Urinary manifestations are related to the surgical procedure and the indwelling catheter. Increased fluid intake helps decrease dysuria. Kegel exercises strengthen periurethral muscles and decrease postvoiding urine leakage.*

### Urinary Retention

- Teach the manifestations of acute urinary retention: dysuria, overflow incontinence, bladder pain and distention, no urine output. *Acute urinary retention is a potential complication of BPH, requiring immediate medical attention.*
- Teach that the risk of developing urinary retention increases when the man with BPH takes over-the-counter diet or decongestant medications, or prescription medications such as antidepressants, anticholinergics, calcium channel blockers, antipsychotics, and medications to treat Parkinson's disease. Over-the-counter *decongestants and diet pills may contain alpha-adrenergic agonists that increase smooth muscle tone of the prostate, bladder neck, and proximal urethra. The prescribed medications may relax detrusor muscle contractions. Both actions may increase the risk of urinary retention (Gray & Brown, 2002).*
- Suggest avoiding intake of large volumes of liquid at any one time. *A single intake of a large volume of liquid results in rapid bladder filling and increases the risk of urinary retention.*

**PRACTICE ALERT** *In addition to avoiding a large amount of fluids at one time, it is also important to teach the man to limit liquids that stimulate voiding, such as coffee and alcoholic beverages.* ■

- Teach how to use double-voiding technique: Urinate, then sit on the toilet for 3 to 5 minutes, then urinate again. *This technique may relieve mild to moderate urinary retention.*

### Risk for Infection

- Monitor WBC and vital signs. *Infection is indicated by an increase in WBCs, body temperature, and pulse rate.*
- Maintain sterile procedures when changing irrigation fluids and emptying Foley catheter draining bag. *Sterile procedures are necessary to prevent infection.*

## Risk for Imbalanced Fluid Volume

A prostatectomy brings increased risk of imbalanced fluid volume as a result of excessive bleeding from the operative site (prostatic fossa) as well as absorption of irrigating fluid.

- Monitor pulse and blood pressure. *Manifestations of hypovolemic shock include an increasing pulse and a decreasing blood pressure.*
- Monitor color of drainage in urinary drainage bag (Table 47–2). *The appearance of urine and irrigation fluid in the urinary drainage bag is an excellent indicator of bleeding after a prostatectomy.*

### TABLE 47–2  Significance of Character of Urine After Prostatectomy and Related Nursing Care

| Urine Color | Nursing Implications |
| --- | --- |
| Light red to red | Normal day of surgery and first postoperative day |
| Very dark red | May indicate increased venous bleeding or inadequate dilution. Catheter at risk for occlusion. Increase flow rate of irrigant. If urine does not clear, notify physician. |
| Bright red | May indicate arterial bleeding. Increase flow rate of irrigant, monitor vital signs, and notify physician. |
| Contains blood clots | Occasional blood clot normal. If clots are frequent, catheter may become obstructed. Increase flow rate of irrigant. |
| Clear to light pink | Normal throughout hospitalization. |

- Monitor for manifestations of transurethral resection (TURP) syndrome: nausea and vomiting, confusion, hypertension, bradycardia, and visual disturbances. *The absorption of isotonic bladder irrigating fluids during and after surgery may cause this hypervolemic, hyponatremic state. Treatment includes diuresis and, in severe cases, hypertonic saline administration (Tierney et al., 2001).*

## Home Care

Depending on the man's choice of treatment, the procedure may be performed on an outpatient basis. If there are no complications, the man having a TURP may be discharged within 2 days after surgery. Discharge instructions after prostate surgery are given in the box below. Home care often involves care of an indwelling urinary catheter. Teaching includes the following information.

- Change from the daytime leg drainage bag to a larger night drainage bag. A larger bag suspended from the bed frame at night permits gravity drainage of urine and prevents reflux of urine back into the bladder.
- Avoid strapping the leg bag on too tightly, which can decrease venous return and increase risk for thrombophlebitis and embolic complications such as pulmonary emboli.
- Place a soft cloth between the leg bag and thigh to decrease friction and absorb dampness under the bag, reducing the risk of skin irritation.
- Empty the leg bag every 3 to 4 hours to prevent overfilling.
- Promptly report any unexpected changes in urine color, consistency, or odor; hematuria, evidence of frank bleeding, or large blood clots, as well as a lack of or significant decrease in urine output to the urologist.

## Meeting Individualized Needs

### DISCHARGE INSTRUCTIONS FOR MEN AFTER PROSTATE SURGERY

#### ACTIVITY
The healing period lasts from 4 to 8 weeks. Avoid strenuous activity and heavy lifting. Do not drive for 2 weeks, except for short rides. Do take long walks, but take stairs slowly and carefully. Continue dorsiflexion exercises that you did in the hospital to prevent blood clots in the legs. You can take showers, but avoid tub baths while the catheter is in place.

#### BLEEDING
Bleeding can occur any time after surgery. It is fairly common after a bowel movement, coughing, or increased exercise. If you notice blood in the urine, increase fluids and rest until the urine is clear. If heavy bleeding plugs the channel, call the care provider immediately. Avoid aspirin and NSAIDS for at least 2 weeks.

#### BOWEL MOVEMENTS
Keep bowel movements regular and soft to avoid pressure on the prostate area. Drink fruit juices and take mild laxatives or stool softeners as ordered.

#### DIET
Resume your normal diet. Increase fluids to ten glasses (8 oz) daily. Avoid alcohol unless otherwise advised by your physician.

#### SEXUAL INTERCOURSE
Do not have sex for 6 weeks after surgery to avoid bleeding. You may still have erections even with the catheter in place. When you resume sex, ejaculate flows back into the bladder, so you will express little or no semen.

#### URINATION
After your catheter is removed, you may experience some burning, stinging, or leakage for several weeks, and you may pass small blood clots occasionally. These symptoms will disappear as the area heals. It is best to use pads to control leakage.

#### WORK
If work is not strenuous, you may return in 4 weeks; otherwise, wait 6 to 8 weeks.

#### PLEASE CALL IMMEDIATELY IF:
- You are unable to urinate.
- Bleeding is not controlled by fluids and rest, or is excessive.
- You have chills and fever or severe abdominal pain.
- Your scrotum becomes swollen and tender.
- You have pain in one calf, chest pain, or difficulty breathing.

# THE MAN WITH PROSTATIC CANCER

Cancer of the prostate is the most common type of cancer and the second leading cause of death in North America (ACS, 2002). It is primarily a disease of older men, increasing in incidence with age, with the majority of cases diagnosed in men older than 65 years. It is estimated that each year, approximately 189,000 men will be diagnosed with prostate cancer, and 30,000 will die of it. Prostate cancer is a major health problem for older men, but the death rate is decreasing due to advances in diagnosis and treatment.

When diagnosed early, prostate cancer is curable. When the cancer is confined to the prostate at diagnosis, the 5-year survival rate is 100%. Even when the cancer has spread regionally, approximately 95% of clients are alive after 5 years. More than 75% of prostate cancer diagnoses are made at one of these stages (ACS, 2002). Many men are found to have prostate cancer on autopsy; usually the cancer has produced no manifestations or complications.

## PATHOPHYSIOLOGY AND MANIFESTATIONS

The prostate gland consists primarily of glandular epithelial cells. The exact etiology of prostate cancer is unknown, although androgens are believed to have a role in its development. Almost all primary prostate cancers are adenoncarcinomas, and develop in the peripheral zones of the prostate gland. This location increases the risk of local spread to the prostatic capsule. Despite its proximity to the rectum, metastasis to the bowel is uncommon because a tough sheet of tissue, Denonvilliers' fascia, acts as an effective physical barrier.

As the tumor enlarges, it may compress the urethra, obstructing urinary flow. The tumor may metastasize and involve the seminal vesicles or bladder by direct extension. Metastasis by lymph and venous channels is common.

Men with early-state prostate cancer are often asymptomatic. Pain from metastasis to bones is often the initial manifestation noted. Urinary manifestations depend on the size and location of the tumor and the stage of the malignancy. They are often much like manifestations of BPH: urgency, frequency, hesitancy, dysuria, and nocturia. The man may also notice hematuria or blood in the ejaculate (Porth, 2002). Manifestations are summarized in the box on this page.

Death usually occurs secondary to debility caused by multiple sites of skeletal metastasis, especially to the vertebrae. Compression fractures of the spine are common, resulting in the possible loss of mobility and bowel and bladder function. Tumors may eventually involve bone marrow, resulting in severe anemias and impaired immune function.

### Risk Factors

In addition to age, race is a significant risk factor for prostate cancer (see the Focus on Diversity box on this page). Other risk factors are as follows:

- Genetic and hereditary factors, with risk increased in men who have a family history of the disease

## Manifestations of Prostate Cancer

**Genitourinary**
- Dysuria
- Frequency of urination
- Reduction in urinary stream
- Nocturia

- Nocturia
- Hematuria
- Abnormal prostate on digital rectal examination

**Musculoskeletal**
- Bone or joint pain
- Migratory bone pain

- Back pain

**Neurologic**
- Nerve pain
- Bilateral lower extremity weakness

- Bowel or bladder dysfunction
- Muscle spasms

**Systemic**
- Weight loss

- Fatigue

## Focus on Diversity

### RISK AND INCIDENCE OF PROSTATE CANCER
- African Americans have the highest incidence of prostate cancer in the United States and the world, with rates more than twice as high as whites.
- African Americans also are more likely to be diagnosed later and to die of prostate cancer, with a mortality rate more than double that of other racial and ethnic groups.
- Asians and Native Americans have the lowest incidence of prostate cancer.

- Having a vasectomy, believed to increase the levels of circulating free testosterone
- Dietary factors, including a diet high in fat and red meats, low in vitamin A, vitamin D, lycopene, and selenium (McCance & Huether, 2002)
- Low exposure to sunlight

## COLLABORATIVE CARE

Care of the man with prostate cancer focuses on diagnosis, elimination or containment of the cancer, and prevention or treatment of complications. There are currently no proven clinical strategies to prevent the development of prostate cancer. Therefore, strategies for early detection remain the major emphasis for control of this disease.

### Diagnostic Tests

Although an increasing number of clients are now diagnosed with asymptomatic prostate cancer, many clients with prostate cancer have either locally advanced cancer or distant metastasis at the time of diagnosis. The definitive diagnosis can be made only by biopsy; however, other tests may suggest the presence of prostate cancer.

- *DRE*, with the prostate gland being nodular and fixed in prostate cancer.

- *Prostate-specific antigen (PSA) levels* are used to diagnose and stage prostate cancer, and to monitor response to treatment (normal levels are <4 ng/mL). Although men with BPH also have elevated PSA levels, almost two-thirds of those with a PSA greater than 10 ng/mL have prostate cancer (Tierney et al., 2001).
- *Transrectal ultrasonography (TRUS)* is used when the DRE is abnormal or if the PSA is elevated.
- *Prostatic biopsy* must be performed and interpreted before the diagnosis of prostate cancer can be established.

Either needle biopsy or a TRUS-guided biopsy is performed. Implications for nursing care are presented in the box below.
- *Grade* and *stage* help to determine prognosis and guide treatment decisions. Grade (cancer cell differentiation) is determined by the pathologist. Prostate cancer is staged with a variety of tests. Table 47–3 outlines treatment options according to the stage of the cancer.
- *Bone scan, MRI,* or *CT scans* may be performed to determine the presence of tumor metastasis.

## Nursing Implications for Diagnostic Tests

### Prostate Biopsy

#### Preparation
- Assess the man's understanding of the procedure. The procedure is becoming common, and many men will have heard about it from friends or family and may have significant anxiety. Especially if the man has experienced uncomfortable or perhaps painful rectal examinations in the past, the prospect of a needle advanced through the rectum into the gland can be frightening. Be sure to describe the procedure fully, and explain what the man will feel. Inform the man that he will be awake and lying on his side. (The examination can also be performed in the sitting, supine, or lithotomy position.) A local anesthetic (2% lidocaine jelly) will be applied to the rectum to minimize pain caused by stretching of the rectal wall. Because the pain receptors in the rectum respond only to stretch, the man will feel no pain as the needle penetrates the rectal wall. The ultrasound probe is inserted in the rectum approximately 10 cm, and then a balloon covering the probe is inflated with water to visualize the prostate. The man will feel a sensation of rectal fullness and possibly pain. Many men describe it as very uncomfortable. The biopsy instrument is inserted next to the probe. Men may feel a sharp pain (a "pinch") as the biopsy is obtained. Reassure the man that the nurse will be with him throughout the procedure to provide support.

- A signed consent should be in the man's chart, as this procedure is invasive.
- Some urologists require a preoperative bleeding profile and complete blood count. The man is often advised to avoid aspirin products and nonsteroidal anti-inflammatory agents for a week before the biopsy.
- An enema is usually administered prior to the examination to ensure a clean rectum.

#### Teaching
- You will be monitored for approximately 1 hour after the examination to ensure that your vital signs are stable and that you can urinate without difficulty.
- Avoid any strenuous activity for the rest of the day.
- Hematuria (blood in the urine) and some bloody streaks in the stool are expected for 24 to 48 hours after the procedure. You can also expect hematospermia (blood in the ejaculate) for a few days to 2 weeks afterward, depending on how often you ejaculate.
- Report any signs of unusual bleeding, such as blood clots in your urine or bloody stools, or infection, such as rectal pain, dysuria, and urgency.

### TABLE 47–3    Prostate Cancer Staging and Treatment

| Stage | Description | Treatment |
| --- | --- | --- |
| I | Confined to prostate, nonpalpable, focal involvement; well differentiated | Observation and follow-up<br>Interstitial or external-beam radiation therapy<br>Radical prostatectomy |
| II | Confined to prostate, palpable, involves one or both lobes; poorly differentiated | Careful observation in selected clients<br>Radical prostatectomy<br>Interstitial or external-beam radiation therapy<br>Ultrasound-guided percutaneous cryosurgery |
| III | Extension of the tumor outside the prostate capsule, possible seminal vesicle involvement | External-beam radiation therapy<br>Interstitial radiation<br>Radical prostatectomy<br>Adjunctive hormone therapy<br>Palliative surgery (TURP) |
| IV | Extension of the tumor into surrounding tissues; lymph node involvement or distant metastasis | Hormone therapy<br>External-beam radiation therapy<br>Palliative treatment with radiation therapy and/or TURP<br>Radical prostatectomy with orchiectomy<br>Chemotherapy |

## Treatments

The treatment of prostate cancer is complex and depends on the grade and stage of the cancer as well as the age, general health, and preference of the client. In some cases, for example, when the client with a slow-growing tumor is elderly or has a limited life expectancy, watchful waiting is the treatment of choice. Treatments for prostate cancer include surgery, radiation therapy, and hormone manipulation.

### Surgery

Surgery for prostate cancer includes several types of prostatectomies. For very early disease in older men, cure may be achieved with a simple prostatectomy (TURP).

- *Radical prostatectomy* involves removal of the prostate, prostatic capsule, seminal vesicles, and a portion of the bladder neck. Many clients experience varying degrees of urinary incontinence and erectile dysfunction. Refer to the box on pages 1539–1540 for nursing care of men having a prostatectomy.
- *Retropubic prostatectomy* is most often performed because it allows adequate control of bleeding, visualization of the prostate bed and bladder neck, and access to pelvic lymph nodes.
- *Perineal prostatectomy* is often preferred for older men or those who are poor surgical risks. This approach requires less time, and involves less bleeding.
- *Suprapubic prostatectomy* is rarely used, usually when problems with the bladder are expected. Control of bleeding is more difficult because the surgical approach is through the bladder.

For clients with stage III, locally advanced (beyond the prostatic capsule) cancer, surgery is controversial because of the likelihood of hidden lymph node metastasis and relapse. TURP is not performed as curative therapy but may be used to relieve urinary obstruction for men with advanced disease (stage III or IV).

Surgical intervention is now available for men with urinary sphincter insufficiency, which is the major cause of incontinence after prostatectomy. An artificial urinary sphincter is surgically implanted (Figure 47–5 ■). To be eligible, the man must be able to manipulate the pump placed in the scrotum and have adequate cognitive function to know when a problem with the appliance occurs.

### Radiation Therapy

Radiation therapy may be used as a primary treatment for prostate cancer. Long-term problems of impotence and urinary incontinence may be avoided, and survival rates often are comparable. Radiation may be delivered either by external beam or interstitial implants of radioactive seeds of iodine, gold, palladium, or iridium (*brachytherapy*). Interstitial radiation has a lower risk of impotence and rectal damage than external-beam radiation. See Chapter 10 ○ for nursing care of the client receiving radiation therapy. Table 47–4 compares the possible complications of radiation therapy with those of surgery.

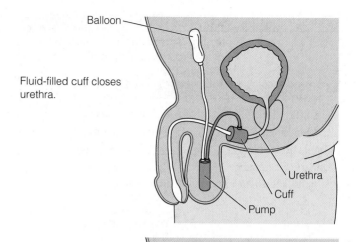

Fluid-filled cuff closes urethra.

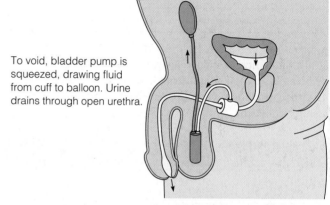

To void, bladder pump is squeezed, drawing fluid from cuff to balloon. Urine drains through open urethra.

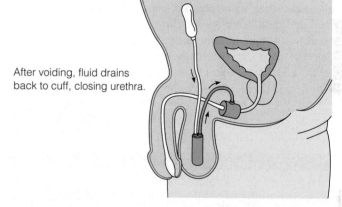

After voiding, fluid drains back to cuff, closing urethra.

**Figure 47–5 ■** Method of operation of an artificial urinary sphincter.

Radiation therapy has a palliative role for clients with metastatic prostate cancer, reducing the size of bone metastasis, controlling pain, and restoring function, such as continence or the ability to ambulate for clients with spinal cord compression.

### Hormonal Manipulation

Androgen deprivation therapy is used to treat advanced prostate cancer. Many cells in the growing tumor are androgen dependent and either cease to grow or die if deprived of androgens. Unfortunately, other cancer cells thrive without androgen and are unaffected by therapy to reduce circulating androgens. Therefore, the effects of hormone manipulations vary from complete but temporary regression of the tumor to no response

| TABLE 47-4 | Potential Complications Related to Radical Prostatectomy and Radiation Therapy | |
| --- | --- | --- |
| **Radical Prostatectomy** | **Radiation Therapy** | |
| Erectile dysfunction | Erectile dysfunction* | |
| Urethral stricture | Urethral stricture | |
| Fistula/rectal injury | Rectal/anal stricture* | |
| Urinary incontinence | Cystitis | |
| Surgical/anesthetic risk | Diarrhea | |
| | Proctitis | |
| | Rectal ulcer | |
| | Bowel obstruction* | |
| | Urinary incontinence | |

*Delayed complications; may appear months or years after completion of therapy.*

at all. Strategies to induce androgen deprivation vary from orchiectomy to oral administration of hormonal agents. Table 47–5 lists hormone therapies and the advantages and disadvantages of each.

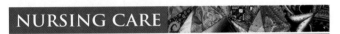

## NURSING CARE

### Health Promotion

Nurses are in a unique position to increase public awareness about detecting early prostate cancer. Every encounter with men and their families—in clinics, hospital units, or in the home—is an opportunity to provide information about early detection and identify needs. Several studies have shown a positive correlation between increased awareness of and participation in prostate cancer screening procedures. The American Cancer Society has free pamphlets about early detection of prostate cancer, which are useful in educating the public.

All men should be given information about the limitations and benefits of testing for early detection and treatment so they can make an informed decision. The American Cancer Society (2002) recommends that the PSA and DRE should be offered each year, beginning at age 50, to all men with a life expectancy of at least 10 years. Men at high risk (men of African descent and those with a first-degree relative diagnosed at a younger age) should begin testing at age 45. In addition, men with an even higher risk, due to multiple first-degree relatives diagnosed at an early age, could begin testing at age 40, with the following criteria:

PSA <1.0 ng/mL, no additional testing needed until age 45
PSA >1.0 ng/mL but <2.5 ng/mL, have annual testing
PSA >2.5 ng/mL, further evaluation with a biopsy

### Assessment

Collect the following data through the health history and physical examination (see Chapter 46). ⊙⊙ Note that a rectal examination is an advanced nursing assessment.

- Health history: risk factors, urinary elimination patterns and manifestations, hematuria, pain
- Physical assessment: DRE to assess prostate size, symmetry, firmness, and nodules

### Nursing Diagnoses and Interventions

The nursing care of men with prostate cancer must be holistic, sensitive, and individualized. The nursing diagnoses discussed for the man with BPH may also be appropriate. This section focuses on problems with urinary incontinence, sexual function, and pain.

#### Urinary Incontinence (Reflex, Stress, Total)

Urinary incontinence is a disturbing complication following treatment for prostate cancer. Both radical prostatectomy and external-beam radiation therapy can cause incontinence, rang-

| TABLE 47-5 | Surgical and Hormone* Therapy in the Management of Advanced Prostate Cancer | |
| --- | --- | --- |
| **Treatment** | **Advantages** | **Disadvantages** |
| Orchiectomy | Inexpensive Immediate effect; i.e., men report diminished pain from metastasis in the recovery room | Body image problems due to loss of testicles |
| Estrogen compounds (diethylstilbestrol) | Inexpensive Effects reversible | Increased risk of cardiovascular problems More likely to cause gynecomastia, hypertrophy of breast tissue |
| Luteinizing hormone-releasing hormone agonist (LHRH) (leuprolide) | Effects reversible No cardiovascular risk Monthly administration | Very expensive Subcutaneous injection route Slow onset: up to 4 weeks |
| Steroidal antiandrogens (megestrol [Megace]) | Effects reversible No cardiovascular risk Inexpensive | May not drop testosterone levels sufficiently Weight gain |
| Nonsteroidal antiandrogens (flutamide; often used in conjunction with LHRH) | Does not alter circulating androgens Blocks some side effects of LHRH May be effective if other methods fail | Very expensive |

*All hormonal manipulations have the potential disadvantage of loss of libido, erectile dysfunction, hot flashes, and gynecomastia.*

ing from a drop or two when the client lifts a heavy object (**stress incontinence**) to no control at all. Older men may experience **urge incontinence,** the involuntary passage of urine soon after a strong sense of urgency to void. Total and unpredictable loss of urine is classified as total incontinence. The man's reaction to incontinence may be severe even if the incontinence is not great. Many men have significant anxiety at the prospect of an incontinent episode in public, because they feel shame and often guilt about the loss of control.

- Assess the degree of incontinence and its effects on lifestyle. *The nurse needs to determine the client's previous urinary patterns and the type of incontinence currently being experienced to plan appropriate interventions.*
- Teach Kegel exercises to help restore continence. *Pelvic muscle or Kegel exercises can often either eliminate or improve stress incontinence.*
- Teach methods to control dampness and odor from stress incontinence.
  - Do not attempt to prevent accidental voiding by restricting fluids. *Not only will the client continue to have incontinent episodes, but also his urine will become concentrated, exacerbating the problem with odor.*
  - Manage occasional episodes (one to three small volume accidents per day) with absorbent pads worn inside the underwear and changed as needed. Most pads are made with a polymer gel that controls odor. *Appropriate measures help promote good hygiene, decrease anxiety, and increase comfort.*
- Refer to physical therapy or a continence specialist for additional measures to promote continence. *Special exercises, restricting some types of fluids, and other measures such as bladder training can help the client deal with incontinence.*

- Explore options such as an external collection device (external catheter or Texas catheter) for the man with total incontinence. *This device may improve the client's self-esteem and allow resumption of social activities.*
- Encourage verbalizing feelings about the impact of incontinence on his quality of life. *The degree of incontinence does not necessarily correlate to the client's perceived level of suffering. Listening to these concerns with sensitivity can help the client work through these feelings and may allow him to move toward a healthy adaptation to his disability.*

## Sexual Dysfunction

Surgical treatment for prostate cancer may cause erectile dysfunction and changes in ejaculatory function. Hormone therapy for advanced prostate cancer lowers libido and may also cause erectile dysfunction. The diagnosis of cancer and body image changes caused by hormone therapy may lower self-esteem, which in turn can diminish sexual desire and willingness to interact sexually with a partner. Most older men are active sexually and fully capable of sustaining an erection. They are likely to fear the effect of treatment on their sexual health. They may allow this concern to guide their decision about the treatment course, or they may refuse all therapy because of this fear. Client reactions vary greatly, and the nurse must maintain a nonjudgmental approach to education and support.

- Assess the man's pretreatment sexual function. *Knowledge of previous sexual function is necessary to plan appropriate interventions.*
- Teach the man about the actual or potential effects of therapy on sexual function (see the box below). *The incidence of erectile dysfunction varies with different therapies for prostate cancer.*

## Nursing Research

### Evidence-Based Practice to Identify Sexual Needs in Men with BPH and Prostate Cancer

The consequences of treatment for prostatic hyperplasia and prostate cancer often include postoperative physical effects such as erectile dysfunction, retrograde ejaculation, and loss of sexual desire. This study (Jakobsson, 2001) compared sexual problems in men with prostate cancer in comparison to men with prostatic hyperplasia and men in the general population. The men with hyperplasia and cancer, in comparison to men in the general population, reported more problems with sexual pleasure and attraction, erectile function and sexual satisfaction, and sexual performance (including a lower intercourse frequency). Despite these problems, neither the men nor their partners used medications, masturbation, or artificial aids to achieve erection. The disease and the treatment of prostatic hyperplasia and prostate cancer were found to interfere with sexual intimacy between men and their partners.

### IMPLICATIONS FOR NURSING

Men with prostate disease need information about the effects of treatment on their sexual functioning. It is important to assess the man's knowledge about his body, a past history of sexual function and satisfaction, and current dysfunction and concerns. When used as part of the total assessment, questions about sexual function

legitimize sexual concerns, establish an understanding of terminology, determine understanding of the disease and treatment options, and determine understanding of the side effects of treatments and medications and their effects on body image and sexuality.

If time is limited for assessment or if the nurse is not comfortable discussing this area of human functioning, a questionnaire may be used. In addition to information about the potential effects of treatment, men and their partners also need education about options available to achieve erection and sexual intimacy.

### Critical Thinking in Client Care

1. You are caring for a 75-year-old man who has a TURP for BPH. His wife tells you that they have always had an active sex life and she hopes this will not ruin that. What would you say to her?
2. Consider the implications for sexual dysfunction in the man diagnosed with prostate cancer. Do you believe the diagnosis of cancer, when combined with the effects of treatment, might affect sexual function even more? Why or why not?
3. Health care providers sometimes view the older adult as asexual. How does this view affect assessments and teaching? What can be done to change this situation?

- Provide an opportunity for the man and his partner to discuss implications of and concerns about the diagnosis and treatment on sexual function. *The treatments for prostate cancer often affect the physiology of erection. The man and his partner need support and counseling during the period of adjustment.*
- Discuss medical and surgical treatments for erectile dysfunction (see first section of this chapter). *Many men are as devastated by the loss of erectile function as they are by the diagnosis of cancer. Information about achieving erection and maintaining sexual intimacy is essential to quality of life.*

**PRACTICE ALERT** *A therapeutic approach to assessing how the man feels is to use an opening statement such as, "Some men are very concerned about effects of (type of treatment) on their ability to have an erection. Tell me how you feel about it."* ■

- Refer for sexual counseling as appropriate. *The man and his partner may require therapy beyond that provided by nurses.*

### Acute/Chronic Pain

The causes of pain in clients with advanced prostate cancer are many. It is not unusual for a client to have three or four distinct pains simultaneously, all from different sources. The most common cause of pain is metastasis to the spinal column, usually the thoracic spine. Other sources of pain include fractures, lymphedema of the lower extremities, gynecomastia, and mus-

cle spasms. Because most clients are over the age of 65, many also have pain associated with preexisting conditions, such as osteoarthritis, unrelated to the cancer.

- Assess the intensity, location, and quality of the client's pain. *A cardinal rule of successful pain management is the importance of reducing or eliminating the cause of pain. Appropriate interventions are based on a careful assessment of the client's pain.*
- Provide optimal pain relief with prescribed analgesics. *It is important that the man and his family understand that pain medications should be used on a regular basis to maintain comfort and should not be delayed until pain is severe.*
- Teach the client and family noninvasive methods of pain control. *Various modalities can be successful in alleviating pain or reducing its perception, thus enhancing the comfort of the client (see Chapter 4).* ⌘

### Using NANDA, NIC, and NOC

Chart 47–1 shows links between NANDA nursing diagnoses, NIC, and NOC when caring for the man with surgical treatment for prostate cancer.

### Home Care

Depending on the type of treatment, the following topics should be addressed in preparing the man and his family for home care.

---

### CHART 47–1 NANDA, NIC, AND NOC LINKAGES

#### The Client with Surgical Treatment of Prostate Cancer

| NURSING DIAGNOSES | NURSING INTERVENTIONS | NURSING OUTCOMES |
|---|---|---|
| • Acute Pain | • Analgesia Administration<br>• Anxiety Reduction<br>• Pain Management | • Pain Level<br>• Symptom Severity |
| • Risk for Infection | • Infection Control<br>• Nutrition Management<br>• Skin Surveillance<br>• Wound Care | • Risk Control<br>• Nutritional Status<br>• Tissue Integrity: Skin |
| • Impaired Urinary Elimination | • Urinary Elimination Management<br>• Bladder Irrigation<br>• Fluid Management<br>• Tube Care: Urinary<br>• Pain Management | • Urinary Elimination |
| • Disturbed Body Image | • Active Listening<br>• Coping Enhancement<br>• Teaching: Sexuality<br>• Support Group | • Acceptance: Health Status<br>• Grief Resolution |

*Note. Data from Nursing Outcomes Classification (NOC) by M. Johnson & M. Maas (Eds.), 1997, St. Louis: Mosby; Nursing Diagnoses: Definitions & Classification 2001–2002 by North American Nursing Diagnosis Association, 2001, Philadelphia: NANDA; Nursing Interventions Classification (NIC) by J.C. McCloskey & G. M. Bulechek (Eds.), 2000, St. Louis: Mosby. Reprinted by permission.*

- For the man having a surgical procedure: manifestations of infection and excessive bleeding, catheter care, wound care pain management
- For the man having radiation therapy (Greifzu, 2000):
  - Danger of radiation damage to others (sleep in a room alone for a week, avoid close contact with pregnant women, infants, and children)
  - Condom use during sexual contact (ejaculate may be discolored, distressing sexual partner)

- The importance of keeping appointments with health care providers and having yearly PSA and rectal examinations
- If appropriate, community services, such as support groups, home health nurses, and hospice
- Helpful resources:
  - American Cancer Society
  - American Urological Association
  - National Cancer Institute

## Nursing Care Plan
## A Man with Prostate Cancer

William Turner, a 71-year-old African American, lives with his wife in a small retirement community in Florida. His wife had a stroke 2 years ago, and Mr. Turner does all the cooking and housework. He has been in good health for most of his life, having only "a small touch" of osteoarthritis in his knees and hands. He has noticed a gradual onset of urinary urgency and frequency over the past 2 years, but has never had incontinence. During a routine checkup, the nurse practitioner at the local health clinic performs a digital rectal examination and palpates a hard nodule on the surface of Mr. Turner's prostate. After his PSA is found to be elevated, he is referred to a urologist, who diagnoses prostate cancer. Mr. Turner chooses to have surgery, and a radical retropubic prostatectomy and lymph node dissection are performed. The lymph nodes are negative for metastasis. Following surgery, his recovery is uncomplicated. However, the nurse caring for Mr. Turner is concerned about his ability to care for his indwelling catheter because of his arthritis and his wife's physical disabilities from the stroke. The nurse makes a referral to a home health agency to ensure Mr. Turner can manage his care at home. An initial home health assessment is scheduled for the day after Mr. Turner is discharged from the hospital.

### ASSESSMENT

The home health nurse notes that the house is clean and neat. Mr. Turner is dressing, but still wearing his night urinary drainage bag, even though it is 1300. Mr. Turner tells the nurse that his main problem is going to get groceries, because he is embarrassed to be seen with the drainage bag. He says he has not been able to remove the drainage bag and attach the leg bag because of his arthritis. Physical assessment findings include the pelvic incision to be healing without signs of infection. There is no tenderness in his calves, chest pain, or shortness of breath. The urine is yellow, without odor. Mr. Turner does state that he sees no need for the pelvic exercises since he is no longer in the hospital. He also expresses the belief that he is cured of cancer and questions the need for follow-up care.

### DIAGNOSES

- *Risk for stress urinary incontinence* related to surgical procedure
- *Ineffective health maintenance* related to inability to care for the urinary drainage system, not understanding need for postoperative exercises, and questions about follow-up care

### EXPECTED OUTCOMES
- Regain urinary continence after catheter removal.
- Change the urinary drainage bag with the appropriate assistance.
- Verbalize the rationale for performing postoperative exercise.
- Verbalize the need for continued follow-up care.

### PLANNING AND IMPLEMENTATION
- Discuss the possibility of stress incontinence after the catheter is removed.
- Reinforce the need for Kegel exercises while the catheter is still in place.
- Explore Mr. Turner's support system to identify people who could assist him with catheter care and arrange a teaching session with them.
- Teach Mr. Turner the importance of follow-up care, relating the care to the history of the disease.

### EVALUATION

Good friends from Mr. Turner's church have assisted him with care of his drainage bag, and have reminded him to do his Kegel exercises several times a day while the catheter is in place. When the catheter is removed, Mr. Turner has only a small amount of leaking of urine after voiding. He understands that it may take several weeks for this to resolve. Efforts to help him understand the need for continued medical care are less successful. Mr. Turner continues to state that he is cured, his wife needs him, and he sees no need to go back to the doctor.

### Critical Thinking in the Nursing Process

1. Outline a teaching plan for Mr. Turner for the risk for altered skin integrity related to urinary incontinence.
2. As a result of Mr. Turner's refusal to have ongoing medical care, he might be labeled as noncompliant. Would you make this nursing diagnosis? Why or why not?
3. If you were the home health nurse making a home visit and found that Mr. Turner had no urinary drainage for 16 hours, what assessments would you make? How would you handle this problem?

See Evaluating Your Response in Appendix C.

# MALE BREAST DISORDERS

## THE MAN WITH GYNECOMASTIA

**Gynecomastia,** the abnormal enlargement of the male breast, is thought to result from a high ratio of estradiol to testosterone. It is common during puberty, affecting as many as 50% of adolescent males, but usually resolves within 1 to 2 years. Any condition that increases estrogen activity or decreases testosterone production can contribute to gynecomastia. Conditions that increase estrogen activity include obesity, testicular tumors, liver disease, and adrenal carcinoma; conditions that decrease testosterone production include chronic illness such as tuberculosis or Hodgkin's disease, injury, and orchitis. Drugs such as digitalis, opiates, and chemotherapeutic agents are also associated with gynecomastia. Gynecomastia is usually bilateral. If it is unilateral, biopsy may be necessary to rule out breast cancer.

No treatment is necessary for the transient gynecomastia of puberty. If the condition becomes chronic, however, creating psychologic discomfort, surgery may be necessary to remove the subcutaneous breast tissue. When related to an underlying disorder such as tuberculosis, treatment of that disorder is required. In severe cases, tamoxifen is given to decrease estrogen activity.

Nursing care for the client with gynecomastia includes education about the cause and treatment of the condition, and emotional support for the psychosocial implications of this feminizing condition.

## THE MAN WITH BREAST CANCER

Although male breast cancer is rare, accounting for about 1% of all breast cancer cases, it is as serious to the men who have it as it is to the women. About 1500 men in the United States are estimated to be diagnosed with breast cancer each year, accounting for 400 deaths (ACS, 2002). The etiology of male breast cancer is unclear; hormonal, genetic, and perhaps environmental factors appear to be important.

Male breast cancer is clinically and histologically similar to female breast cancer, although lobular cancer is rare in males. Most tumors are estrogen-receptor positive. Because many men believe that breast cancer is only a woman's disease, they often delay seeking medical attention for symptoms and thus may present with advanced disease.

Treatment of male breast cancer is much like the treatment of female breast cancer, beginning with modified radical mastectomy, node dissection, and staging to determine the therapeutic options. Radiation, chemotherapy, or hormonal therapy (usually tamoxifen), are the conventional adjuncts to surgery. Castration is the most successful palliative measure in men with advanced breast cancer, resulting in tumor regression and prolonging life.

Nursing care for the man with breast cancer is essentially the same as for the woman with breast cancer (see Chapter 48). The nurse has an opportunity to help the man and his family cope with the psychosocial effects of having breast cancer. He may feel embarrassment or shame about his condition as well as fear about the life-threatening nature of the disease. His family may share those feelings. By listening with understanding and empathy, the nurse can help the client and family resolve their feelings and move toward healing.

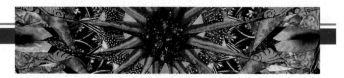

 EXPLORE MediaLink

# TEST YOURSELF

1. When conducting a health assessment, which of the following statements would most likely elicit information about sexual concerns?

   a. "Following your prostate surgery, did you first notice you had problems with sexual intercourse?"

   b. "Why do you think you should be sexually active at your age?"

   c. "Do you miss having sex?"

   d. "Tell me about your experience with sexual function since you developed prostate enlargement."

2. You are conducting a health teaching session for young men. What topic would be appropriate to reduce the risk of cancer of the penis?

   a. Wearing a condom during sexual intercourse

   b. Retracting the foreskin of the penis when showering

   c. Avoiding tight pants and very hot showers

   d. Maintaining a regular testicular self-examination schedule

3. Which of the following interventions would be appropriate for the man with prostatitis?

   a. Wear a scrotal support during the day

   b. Increase fluid intake and void often

   c. Know the manifestations of testicular torsion

   d. Surgical intervention may be necessary

4. The enlarging prostate in BPH typically is manifested by assessment of problems with:

   a. Bowel elimination

   b. Urinary elimination

   c. Peripheral vascular function

   d. Skin integrity

5. You are caring for a man who has returned to the unit following recovery from a TURP. His urinary drainage bag is filled with dark red fluid with obvious clots. He is having painful bladder spasms. What would you do first?

   a. Assess his intake and output since surgery

   b. Administer pain medication in the form of a B & O suppository

   c. Report your assessments to his urologist

   d. Nothing, as these manifestations are expected following a TURP

See Test Yourself answers in Appendix C.

# BIBLIOGRAPHY

Agency of Health Care Policy and Research. (1994). *Clinical practice guidelines for benign prostatic hyperplasia.* AHCPR Pub. no. a94-0582. Rockville, MD: U.S. Department of Health and Human Services.

American Cancer Society. (2002). *Cancer facts and figures 2002.* Atlanta: Author.

Angelucci, P. A. (1997). Caring for patients with benign prostatic hyperplasia. *Nursing, 27*(11), 54–55.

Center for Disease Control. (2001). Prostate cancer. Available www.cdc.gov/cancer/prostate/prostate.htm

Chan, E. (2001). Promoting informed decision-making about prostate cancer screening. *Comprehensive Therapy, 27*(3), 195–201, 265–266.

Germino, B. B., Mohler, J., Ware, A., Harris, L., Belyea, M., & Mishel, M. H. (1998). Uncertainty in prostate cancer. Ethnic and family patterns. *Cancer Practitioner, 6*(2), 107–113.

Gray, M., & Brown, K. (2002). Genitourinary system. In J. Thompson, G. McFarland, J. Hirsch, & S. Tucker, *Mosby's clinical nursing* (5th ed.) (pp. 917–999). St. Louis: Mosby.

Greifzu, S. (2000). Prostate cancer. *RN, 63*(6), 27–32.

Hellerstedt, B., & Pienta, K. (2002). The current state of hormonal therapy for prostate cancer. *CA: A Cancer Journal for Clinicans, 52*(3), 154–179.

Jakobsson, L. (2001). Sexual problems in men with prostate cancer in comparison with men with benign prostatic hyperplasia and men from the general population. *Journal of Clinical Nursing, 10*(4), 573–582.

Jakobsson, L., Hallberg, I., & Loven, L. (2000). Experiences of micturition problems, indwelling catheter treatment and sexual life consequences in men with prostate cancer. *Journal of Advanced Nursing, 31*(1), 59–67.

Johnson, M., Maas, M., & Moorhead, S. (Eds.). (2000). *Nursing outcomes classification (NOC)* (2nd ed.). St. Louis: Mosby.

Kee, J. (1998). *Handbook of laboratory and diagnostic tests with nursing implications* (4th ed.). Upper Saddle River, NJ: Prentice Hall.

Lepor, H. (Ed.). (2000). *Prostatic diseases.* Philadelphia: Saunders.

McCance, K., & Huether, S. (2002). *Pathophysiology: The biologic basis for disease in adults & children.* St. Louis: Mosby.

McCloskey, J. C. & Bulecheck, G. M. (Eds.). (2000). *Nursing interventions classification (NIC)* (3rd ed.). St. Louis: Mosby.

North American Nursing Diagnosis Association. (2001). *Nursing diagnoses: Definitions and classification, 2001–2002.* Philadelphia: NANDA.

Ord-Lawson, S., & Fitch, M. (1997). The relationship between perceived social support and mood of testicular cancer patients. *Canadian Oncology Nursing Journal, 7*(2), 90–95.

Porth, C. M. (2002). *Pathophysiology: Concepts of altered health states* (6th ed.). Philadelphia: Lippincott.

Shannon, M., Wilson, B., & Stang, C. (2002). *Health professional's drug guide 2002.* Upper Saddle River, NJ: Prentice Hall.

Shuster, J. (1998). Megestrol and impotence—teaching patients about this dose-related adverse effect. *Nursing, 28*(3), 25.

Therapies for the treatment of benign prostatic hyperplasia (BPH). Available http://cpmcnet.columbia.edu/dept/urology/bphtherapy.html

Tierney, L. M., McPhee, S. J., & Papadakis, M. A. (Eds.). (2001). *Current medical diagnosis & treatment* (40th ed.). Stamford, CT: Appleton & Lange.

Weinrich, S. P., Atkinson, C., Boyd, M. D., & Weinrich, M. C. (1998). The impact of prostate cancer knowledge on cancer screening. *Oncology Nursing Forum, 25*(3), 527–534.

Weinrich, S. P., Weinrich, M., Frank-Stromborg, M., Johnson, A., Cover, K., Creanga, D., Boyde, M., & Holdford, D. (1998). Prostate cancer education in African American churches. *Public Health Nursing, 15*(3), 188–195.

Yarbro, C., & Ferrans, C. (1998). Quality of life of patients with prostate cancer treated with surgery or radiation therapy. *Oncology Nursing Forum, 25*(4), 685–693.

Yarbo, C., Frogge, M., Goodman, M., & Groenwald, S. (Eds.). (2001). *Cancer nursing: Principles and practice* (5th ed.). Sudbury, MA: Jones & Bartlett.

Zaccagnini, M. (1999). Clinical snapshot: Prostate cancer. *American Journal of Nursing, 99*(4), 34–35.

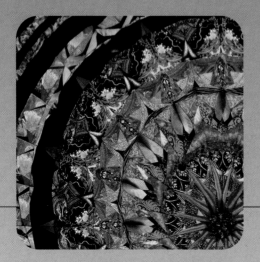

### CHAPTER 48

# Nursing Care of Women with Reproductive System Disorders

## MediaLink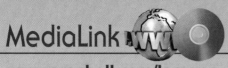

**www.prenhall.com/lemone**

Additional resources for this chapter can be found on the Student CD-ROM accompanying this textbook, and on the Companion Website at www. prenhall.com/lemone. Click on Chapter 48 to select the activities for this chapter.

**CD-ROM**
- Audio Glossary
- NCLEX Review

**Companion Website**
- More NCLEX Review
- Case Study
  Breast Cancer
- Care Plan Activity
  Postoperative Hysterectomy Care
- MediaLink Application
  Premenstrual Syndrome

## LEARNING OUTCOMES

After completing this chapter, you will be able to:

- Apply knowledge of normal female anatomy, physiology, and assessments when providing nursing care for women with reproductive system disorders (see Chapter 46).

- Explain the pathophysiology of disorders of the female reproductive system.

- Describe the physiologic process of menopause.

- Discuss risk factors for cancers of the female reproductive system.

- Discuss the collaborative care, with related nursing implications, for women with disorders of the reproductive system.

- Provide appropriate nursing care for women having diagnostic tests and gynecologic surgery.

- Provide accurate information to women about health-promoting behaviors that prevent disorders of the female reproductive system or facilitate their early diagnosis.

- Use the nursing process as a framework for providing individualized care to women with disorders of the reproductive system.

Disorders of the female reproductive system range from the minor discomfort of menstrual cramps to life-threatening diseases such as cancer. Many of these disorders can occur at any point in a woman's adult life. They may affect her ability to bear children, her sexuality, and her sense of well-being as a woman.

Women who experience reproductive system changes and disorders require a holistic approach to meet their physical, emotional, and educational needs. Because the ability to reproduce affects self-esteem, feelings of femininity, and general health, both sensitivity and understanding of caregivers are essential. Providing personal medical and family history and undergoing diagnostic tests often require women to disclose personal, intimate information, which they may find embarrassing and uncomfortable. When planning and implementing care, nurses must consider the woman within the context of her culture, socioeconomic and educational level, and lifestyle. It is also important that the nurse not make assumptions or judgments about sexual orientation.

This chapter discusses the physiologic process of menopause, menstrual disorders, structural disorders of the female reproductive system, and disorders of female reproductive tissue, including the breast. Disorders of female sexual expression are summarized. Sexually transmitted diseases, including vaginal infections and pelvic inflammatory disease, are discussed in Chapter 49. Many of the disorders result in actual or potential health problems requiring nursing care based on similar nursing diagnoses. To avoid repeating those diagnoses and interventions for each disorder, they have been divided among the nursing care discussions as appropriate. Treatment of cancer with chemotherapy and radiation is discussed in Chapter 10. ∞

## THE PERIMENOPAUSAL WOMAN

**Menopause** is the permanent cessation of menses. The *climacteric,* or *perimenopausal,* period denotes the time during which reproductive function gradually ceases. For most women, the perimenopausal period lasts several years. It begins with a decline in the production of the hormone estrogen, includes the permanent cessation of menstruation due to loss of ovarian function, and extends for 1 year after the final menstrual period, at which time a woman is said to be *postmenopausal.* The average woman will live one-third of her life after menopause.

Menopause is neither a disease nor a disorder, but a normal physiologic process. However, the hormonal changes that occur can be accompanied by unpleasant side effects. There is wide variation in how individual women experience these side effects. In the United States, most women stop menstruating between 48 and 55 years of age. A woman who had not menstruated for 1 full year or has a follicular-stimulating hormone (FSH) level of more than 30 mIU/mL is considered menopausal (Porth, 2002). Certain health risks increase after menopause, including heart disease, osteoporosis, and breast cancer.

## THE PHYSIOLOGY OF MENOPAUSE

The menopausal period marks the natural biologic end of reproductive ability. *Surgical menopause* occurs when the ovaries are removed in premenopausal women, dramatically reducing the production of estrogen and progestins. *Chemical menopause* often occurs during cancer chemotherapy, when cytotoxic drugs arrest ovarian function.

As ovarian function decreases, the production of estradiol ($E_2$), the most biologically active estrogen, decreases and is ultimately replaced by estrone as the major ovarian estrogen. Estrone is produced in small amounts and has only about one-tenth the biologic activity of estradiol. With decreased ovarian function, the second ovarian hormone, progesterone, which is produced during the luteal phase of the menstrual cycle, also is markedly reduced.

## MANIFESTATIONS

As estrogen decreases, various tissues are affected. The breast tissue, body hair, skin elasticity, and subcutaneous fat decreases. The ovaries and uterus become smaller, and the cervix and vagina also decrease in size and become pale in color. These changes may result in problems with vaginal dryness, dyspareunia, urinary stress incontinence, urinary tract infections, and vaginitis. Vasomotor instability often results in hot flashes, palpitations, dizziness, and headaches. Other problems resulting from vasomotor instability include insomnia, frequent awakening, and perspiration (night sweats). The woman may experience irritability, anxiety, and depression as a result of these events.

Long-term estrogen deprivation results in an imbalance in bone remodeling and osteoporosis, leading to fractures and kyphosis. The risk for cardiovascular diseases increases. Manifestations of the perimenopausal period are listed in the box below. These manifestations vary widely. Some women experience severe symptoms, others experience moderate symptoms, and some women experience few or no symptoms.

### Manifestations of the Perimenopausal Period

- Menstrual cycles become erratic. Menstrual flow varies widely in amount and duration and eventually ceases.
- Vaginal, vulval, and urethral tissues begin to atrophy.
- Vaginal pH rises, predisposing the woman to bacterial infections.
- Vaginal lubrication decreases, and vaginal rugae decrease in number. This may result in dyspareunia (pain during sexual intercourse), injury, and fungal infections.
- Vasomotor instability due to a decrease in estrogen may result in hot flashes and night sweats. A hot flash starts in the chest and moves upward toward the face and may last from seconds to several minutes.
- Psychologic symptoms may include moodiness, nervousness, insomnia, headaches, irritability, anxiety, inability to concentrate, and depression.

# COLLABORATIVE CARE

Care of the woman experiencing menopausal symptoms focuses on relieving symptoms and minimizing postmenopausal health risks.

## Diagnostic Tests

As estrogen secretion diminishes, levels of FSH and LH rise and remain elevated.

## Medications

Hormone replacement therapy (HRT) may be prescribed to alleviate the unpleasant manifestations of menopause. HRT may include estrogen alone for women who have had a hysterectomy, or a combination of estrogen and progestin. The addition of progestin stimulates monthly shedding of the interuterine lining, decreasing the risk of uterine cancer. HRT relieves hot flashes and night sweats and decreases problems of vaginal dryness and urogenital tissue atrophy, which can lead to painful intercourse and urinary incontinence.

Long-term benefits of HRT were once believed to be a reduced risk of coronary heart disease, osteoporosis, and Alzheimer's disease; however, research has demonstrated that estrogen plus progestin does not reduce the overall rate of coronary artery disease in postmenopausal women with established coronary disease but does increase the rate of thromboembolic events (blood clots) in the same women (Grady et al., 2000; Hulley et al., 1998). In addition, Hulley et al. (1999) and Torgerson and Bell-Syer (2001) found little evidence of the benefits of HRT in preventing fractures. In 2002, a major study of HRT was stopped, as government scientists reported that long-term use of estrogen and progestin significantly increased women's risk of breast cancer, strokes, and heart attacks. Although HRT did decrease the risk of colon cancer and hip fractures, there are other means of preventing these illnesses. Further studies are planned to evaluate using lower dose HRT, other methods of administrations (such as the patch), and estrogen alone for women who have had a hysterectomy.

Nausea, vomiting, weight gain, breast tenderness and engorgement, and vaginal bleeding are common side effects of HRT. Fluid retention may develop, worsening existing problems such as asthma, epilepsy, migraine headache, and heart and kidney diseases.

Contraindications for HRT include:

- Current diagnosis of endometrial cancer; current or past history of estrogen-dependent breast, ovarian, or cervical cancer.
- Hypertriglyceridemia.
- Active thrombotic disorders or inherited clotting disorders.
- Acute or chronic liver disease or kidney failure.
- Unexplained vaginal bleeding.
- Pregnancy.

Selective estrogen receptor modulators (SERMs) such as raloxifene (Evista) provide an alternative to HRT for preventing osteoporosis. SERMs act like estrogen in some tissues but not in others, and appear to significantly reduce the risk of breast cancer in menopausal women. Although they do not prevent manifestations of menopause, they provide an alternative for women who cannot take HRT.

## Complementary Therapies

The following complementary therapies are examples of those used by menopausal women to reduce associated discomforts (Fontaine, 2000):

- Aromatherapy: geranium, rose, fennel in bathwater or lotions
- Herbs: black cohosh, vitex, agnue castii, rehmannia, ginseng, Chinese tonic of He Shou Wu, dong quai
- Supplements: vitamin E, soy protein
- Meditation

# NURSING CARE

Nursing care during and after the menopausal period focuses on minimizing the symptoms associated with hormonal changes, reducing the risk of cardiovascular disease and osteoporosis, and educating the woman about lifestyle changes important to health and well-being.

## Health Promotion

The American Cancer Society (2002) recommends a cancer-related checkup every year after the age of 40. This checkup includes examination for cancers of the thyroid, ovaries, lymph nodes, oral cavity, and skin. Other important checkups include screening for cervical, breast, and colorectal cancer. Health counseling should also include information about alcohol and tobacco use, sun exposure, diet and nutrition, exercise, risk factors, sexual practices, and environmental and occupational exposures. It is important to discuss the benefits of rest and exercise, as well as a diet that includes fruits, vegetables, and fiber. Other health-promotion teaching is discussed later.

## Assessment

Collect the following data through the health history and physical examination (see Chapter 46). When assessing the older woman, be aware of normal changes with aging, as outlined in the box below.

## Nursing Care of the Older Adult

### VARIATIONS IN ASSESSMENT FINDING

- Menstrual irregularities during the perimenopausal period, hot flashes, night sweats
- Decreased size of vulva, loss of vaginal lubrication and flattened vaginal rugae
- Decreased size of clitoris, vagina, cervix, and ovaries
- Reduced size of breasts
- Loss of skin elasticity and turgor
- Loss of pubic and axillary hair, growth of facial hair, loss of hair pigment

- Health history: problems with urinary frequency, urgency, or incontinence; menstrual history; sexual history; dyspareunia; use of alcohol, nicotine, and drugs; medications, sleep patterns, hot flashes, night sweats, changes in emotional responses
- Physical assessment: height and weight, posture, vital signs, breast examination, pelvic examination, abdominal assessment

## Nursing Diagnoses and Interventions

Although each nursing care plan must be individualized, interventions often focus on problems with lack of information, sexuality, and self-esteem.

### Deficient Knowledge

Because menopausal manifestations vary widely, it is difficult to predict their effect on an individual woman. However, the well-informed woman is better prepared to deal with whatever symptoms she experiences.

- Discuss physiologic manifestations, such as hot flashes and night sweats. *The underlying cause of hot flashes is not known (Porth, 2002). Many physiologic effects of menopause are amenable to nonpharmacologic methods of relief, such as lifestyle changes.*

**PRACTICE ALERT** *When hot flashes occur at night and are accompanied by perspiration, they are called night sweats. Night sweats often interfere with normal sleep patterns, leading to increased fatigue and irritability.* ■

- Provide information about dietary recommendations. The recommended daily intake of calcium for women over 50 is 1200 mg. *Some women need to use calcium supplements or calcium-containing antacid tablets to meet this requirement.*
- Emphasize the importance of weight-bearing exercise. *Weight-bearing exercise reduces the rate of bone loss, helps maintain optimum weight, and reduces cardiovascular risk.*
- Provide information about the benefits and risks of HRT. Not every woman will need or want it. *Every woman needs to understand both the risks and the benefits before deciding whether to undergo HRT.*
- Encourage the woman to obtain yearly mammograms, clinical breast examinations, and Pap tests, and to perform monthly breast self-examination at the same day each month. *The increased risk for cancer of the breast and pelvic reproductive organs makes self-examination and health care provider screening during and after menopause even more important.*
- Suggest the following resources
  - National Institute on Aging
  - North American Menopause Society
  - The Hormone Foundation
  - Women's Health Initiative
  - National Women's Health Information Center

### Ineffective Sexuality Patterns

Vaginal dryness and atrophy, together with the emotional effect of menopause, can interfere with sexual expression and satisfaction. Suggesting measures to help the woman and her partner cope with these changes can enable them to continue or resume a mutually satisfying sexual relationship.

- Encourage expression of feelings and concerns about how menopause is changing her sex life. *Midlife and older women may not be comfortable in discussing their intimate sexual behavior.*
- Suggest ways to increase vaginal lubrication, such as spending more time in foreplay and/or using water-soluble gels (e.g., Replens) for vaginal lubrication. *A more leisurely approach to sexual activity can be mutually gratifying for both the woman and her partner. Use of water-soluble gels can prevent vaginal pain and irritation and improve the quality of the sexual experience.*

**PRACTICE ALERT** *Plant estrogens, found in food such as brown rice, corn, green beans, lemon and orange peels, and tofu, are mildly estrogenic and may improve vaginal dryness.* ■

- Explain that as women age, it may take longer for vaginal lubrication and orgasm to occur. *This information is important to prevent the woman from believing something is wrong with her, or her partner believing he or she is no longer interesting or sexually exciting.*

### Situational Low Self-Esteem

Each woman responds to the aging process in her own way, and most women have coping skills that adequately equip them to deal with the gradual changes associated with aging. Among the factors that may provoke a self-esteem disturbance are the loss of youth, a sense of emptiness as children leave home, and the need to redefine one's self-concept and roles as parenting becomes less important. Women who place a high value on their physical attractiveness may experience a painful psychologic response to the physical changes of menopause.

- Encourage expression of fears and concerns related to changes in interpersonal and family functions. *Many women associate aging with "uselessness" and unattractiveness.*
- Suggest volunteer activities or employment for the woman who has extra time. *This enables the woman to feel that she is still a contributing member of society. Volunteering for activities involving young people can help reduce anxiety about the loss of reproductive ability or any late regrets about not having had children.*
- Discuss the importance of a healthy lifestyle in maintaining physical attractiveness. Identify risk factors and high-risk behaviors. *Lifestyle habits and behaviors affect many body systems and physical appearance. For example, cigarette smoking and overexposure to the sun make the skin age faster, contributing to wrinkles. Active women who exercise and eat a well-balanced diet look and feel better.*

## Disturbed Body Image

As women progress through the perimenopausal period, changes in appearance and the loss of childbearing ability may combine to make the woman feel "old, ugly, and useless." Although this is far from the truth, with women living at least one-third of their lives after menopause in productive careers and activities, it nevertheless is the perception of women as well as society. The physical changes the woman often experiences include growth of facial hair, excessive perspiration and flushing of the face, and weight gain.

- Encourage the woman to describe her perceptions of her own body. *This information is necessary to obtain data to establish an individualized plan of care.*

- Encourage verbalization of feelings of concern, anger, anxiety, loss, and fear over body changes. *Expressing these emotions can facilitate the grieving process and acceptance of change.*

- Stress that certain physical characteristics of a person cannot be changed; emphasize the importance of learning to recognize and appreciate one's own special strengths. *These help the woman gain acceptance and a realistic appraisal of self.*

- Refer, as appropriate, for dietary management, exercise, stress management and cosmetic assistance (e.g., for aggravating facial hair). *These actions increase wellness and a positive sense of self.*

# MENSTRUAL DISORDERS

Monthly menstruation normally involves some minor discomfort, including breast tenderness, a feeling of heaviness and congestion in the pelvic area, uterine cramping, and lower backache. Many women, however, experience more serious effects, both physiologic and psychologic. This section discusses premenstrual syndrome, dysmenorrhea, and abnormal uterine bleeding. (The menstrual cycle is discussed in Chapter 46).

## THE WOMAN WITH PREMENSTRUAL SYNDROME

**Premenstrual syndrome (PMS)** is a complex of manifestations (e.g., mood swings, breast tenderness, fatigue, irritability, food cravings, and depression) that are limited to 3 to 14 days before menstruation and relieved by the onset of menses. It is estimated that 25% to 40% of all adult women experience mild to moderate symptoms and 1% to 8% have severe symptoms (Porth, 2002). For about 7% of women, PMS is so disabling that it is called *premenstrual dysphoric disorder (PMDD)*. The syndrome is seen less frequently during the teens and 20s, reaching a peak in women in their mid-30s. Major life stressors, age greater than 30, and depression are risk factors associated with PMS. Premenstrual syndrome can be a factor in absenteeism at school or work, decreased productivity, interpersonal relationship difficulties, and lifestyle disruption.

## PATHOPHYSIOLOGY AND MANIFESTATIONS

Although the pathophysiology of PMS is not clearly understood, it is believed that hormonal changes such as altered estrogen–progesterone ratios, increased prolactin levels, and rising aldosterone levels during the luteal phase of the menstrual cycle contribute to the problem. Increased production of aldosterone results in sodium retention and edema. Decreased

levels of monamine oxidase in the brain are associated with depression, and reduced levels of serotonin can lead to mood swings.

Manifestations of PMS occur during the luteal phase of the menstrual cycle (7 to 10 days prior to the onset of the menstrual flow), abating when the menstrual flow begins. The *Multisystem Effects of PMS* are shown on page 1557. Although PMS may produce a variety of physiologic and psychologic manifestations, the exact nature of these manifestations and their intensity are individualized for each woman with this disorder (see the Nursing Research box on page 1558). The manifestations may even differ from month to month in the same woman.

## COLLABORATIVE CARE

If no organic cause can be identified, the goals of care are to relieve manifestations and to help develop self-care patterns that will help the woman anticipate and cope more effectively with future episodes of PMS. There are no definitive diagnostic tests for PMS. The regular recurrence of manifestations preceding the onset of menses for at least 3 months leads to a diagnosis of PMS. The treatment of PMS integrates this self-monitored record of manifestations, regular exercise, avoiding caffeine, and a diet low in simple sugars and high in lean proteins (Porth, 2002).

### Medications

If the manifestations of PMS are severe or incapacitating, ovulation may be suppressed by the use of gonadotropin-releasing hormone (GnRH) agonists, oral contraceptives, or danazol. Progesterone and antiprostaglandin agents such as NSAIDs may help relieve cramping. Diuretics may be prescribed to relieve bloating. Selective serotonin reuptake inhibitors such as fluoxetine (Prozac), sertraline (Zoloft), and paroxetine (Paxil) may be used to manage mood and some physical manifestations of PMS.

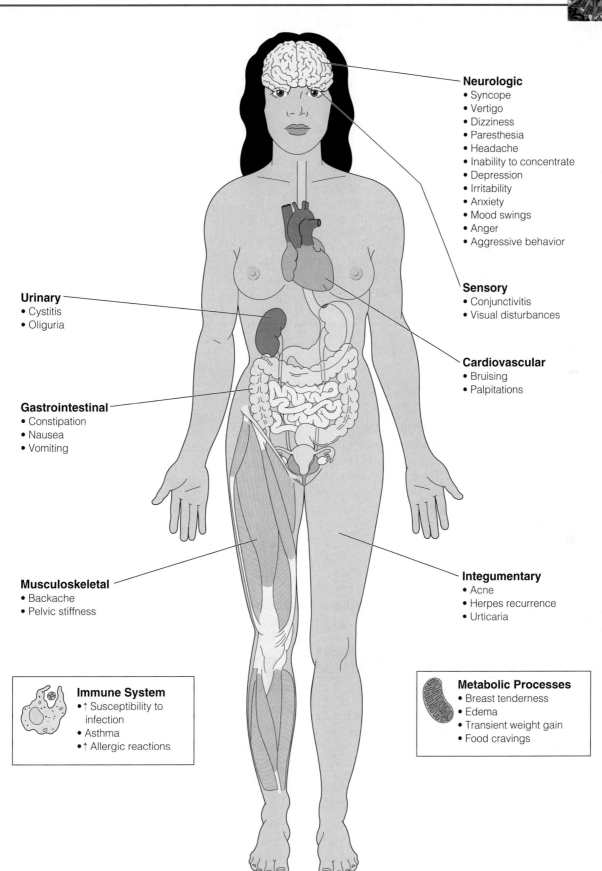

**Neurologic**
- Syncope
- Vertigo
- Dizziness
- Paresthesia
- Headache
- Inability to concentrate
- Depression
- Irritability
- Anxiety
- Mood swings
- Anger
- Aggressive behavior

**Sensory**
- Conjunctivitis
- Visual disturbances

**Cardiovascular**
- Bruising
- Palpitations

**Urinary**
- Cystitis
- Oliguria

**Gastrointestinal**
- Constipation
- Nausea
- Vomiting

**Musculoskeletal**
- Backache
- Pelvic stiffness

**Integumentary**
- Acne
- Herpes recurrence
- Urticaria

**Immune System**
- ↑ Susceptibility to infection
- Asthma
- ↑ Allergic reactions

**Metabolic Processes**
- Breast tenderness
- Edema
- Transient weight gain
- Food cravings

## Nursing Research

### Evidence-Based Practice for PMS

Many women experience varying degrees of premenstrual symptoms. Despite its prevalence, the behavioral and physiologic causes of PMS are poorly understood. This lack of understanding contributes to ineffective treatment based on symptoms rather than etiology of the disorder. Evidence suggests that stress contributes to the occurrence of premenstrual symptoms and that changes in stress hormone regulation may alter mood and affect.

In this study (Cahill, 1998), the researcher monitored symptom and cortisol secretion patterns for three menstrual cycles in three distinct groups of women: those with few premenstrual symptoms, those experiencing PMS patterns, and women with premenstrual symptoms. During the luteal phase, women in the PMS group had lower cortisol levels than did women in either of the other groups. Findings suggest that transient changes in stress hormone regulation may contribute to mood alterations associated with PMS.

### IMPLICATIONS FOR NURSING

Further study of the biochemical, physiologic, and psychologic factors that are involved in PMS is needed. With better understanding of its causes, more effective interventions for PMS can be developed. This study suggests that nursing interventions designed to limit stress effects in treating women with turmoil-type premenstrual symptoms may be appropriate.

### Critical Thinking in Client Care

1. This study looked at the effects of the menstrual cycle on mood and affect. What other manifestations of PMS do women commonly experience? What biochemical, physiologic, and psychologic factors might contribute to symptoms such as gastrointestinal, musculoskeletal, genitourinary, and other manifestations of PMS?
2. What effects might PMS have on a woman's family, social, and work interactions? What self-care measures would you suggest to the woman?

## Complementary Therapies

Complementary therapies for the woman with PMS focus on diet, exercise, relaxation, and stress management.

- A diet high in complex carbohydrates with limited simple sugars and alcohol is recommended to minimize reactive hypoglycemia, which can contribute to the manifestations of PMS.
- Reduced sodium intake helps minimize fluid retention. Increased intake of calcium (1200 mg per day), magnesium (200 mg per day), and vitamin E (400 IU per day) may be helpful (Mayo Foundation for Medical Education and Research, 2002).
- Caffeine is restricted to reduce irritability.
- Exercise is beneficial, but adequate rest also is necessary.
- Techniques for relaxation and stress management include deep abdominal breathing, meditation, muscle relaxation, and guided imagery.

## NURSING CARE

### Nursing Diagnoses and Interventions

Nursing care for the woman with PMS focuses on relieving manifestations. Most women experiencing PMS require interventions to manage pain and enhance coping.

### Acute Pain

The woman with PMS may have pain from headache (including migraine), cramps, excessive fluid retention, breast swelling, joint and muscle pain, and backache.

- Teach effective pharmacologic and nonpharmacologic self-care measures to relieve pain: application of heat, relaxation techniques (such as breathing exercises, imagery techniques, or meditation), and exercise. *Heat relieves muscle spasms and causes blood vessels to dilate, increasing blood supply to the pelvis and uterine muscles. Relaxation and exercise aid the release of naturally produced pain relievers called endorphins.*
- Review daily activities and suggest ways to balance rest periods and activity. *During rest periods, energy and oxygen requirements decrease, increasing the amount of energy and oxygen available to muscles.*
- Review manifestations and, if possible, correlate these with dietary patterns and activity levels. Encourage the woman to keep a diary of PMS manifestations. *Maintaining a diary of PMS manifestations, activity, and foods eaten can provide data to identify modifiable causes of discomfort.*
- Suggest sexual activity as a way to lessen cramps. *Orgasm may help relieve dysmenorrhea.*

### Ineffective Coping

Many women experience wide mood swings during episodes of PMS, sometimes exhibiting self-destructive or aggressive behaviors toward others. These mood swings can interfere with a woman's ability to manage her responsibilities at home or at work.

- Encourage the woman to keep a journal of her menstrual cycle and to document her mood changes in the 7 to 10 days prior to menstruation. *Recognizing the signs and timing of PMS is the first step in developing methods to cope with the problem.*
- Explore possible ways to rearrange or reschedule activities when experiencing PMS. *Planning ahead enables the woman to assume more control and promotes coping methods.*
- Explore what, if any, self-care measures have helped cope with mood alterations in the past. *Encourage healthful coping mechanisms, such as relaxation techniques and exercise. Some women may rely on alcohol or other drugs during PMS, which only exacerbate the manifestations.*

## Home Care

Teach the woman and family that PMS is not caused by a pathologic process but is a physiologic response to hormonal changes of the menstrual cycle. With an understanding of the condition, the woman is better able to manage anxiety and to become actively involved in techniques to reduce the manifestations. Teaching should also include dietary measures, relaxation techniques and exercise, stress reduction techniques, and support systems.

# THE WOMAN WITH DYSMENORRHEA

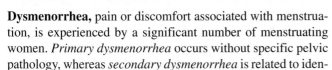

**Dysmenorrhea,** pain or discomfort associated with menstruation, is experienced by a significant number of menstruating women. *Primary dysmenorrhea* occurs without specific pelvic pathology, whereas *secondary dysmenorrhea* is related to identified pelvic disease, such as endometriosis or pelvic inflammatory disease.

## PATHOPHYSIOLOGY AND MANIFESTATIONS

In primary dysmenorrhea, excessive production of prostaglandins stimulates uterine muscle fibers to contract. As the muscles contract, uterine circulation is compromised, resulting in uterine ischemia and pain. These contractions can range from mild cramping to severe muscle spasms. Psychologic factors, such as anxiety and tension, may contribute to dysmenorrhea. Childbirth tends to decrease the incidence and severity of manifestations, possibly because of dilation of the internal cervical os. Manifestations of primary dysmenorrhea (see the box below) may be severe enough to disrupt activities of daily living, sexual function, and even fertility.

Secondary dysmenorrhea is related to underlying organic conditions that involve scarring or injury to the reproductive tract. Endometriosis, fibroid tumors, pelvic inflammatory disease, or ovarian cancer may result in painful menses.

## COLLABORATIVE CARE

Care of the woman with menstrual pain focuses on identifying the underlying cause, reestablishing functional capacity, and managing pain.

### Manifestations of Primary Dysmenorrhea

- Abdominal pain beginning with onset of menses and lasting 12 to 48 hours
- Pain radiating to lower back and thighs
- Headache
- Nausea
- Vomiting
- Diarrhea
- Fatigue
- Breast tenderness

A careful history and physical are performed to rule out any underlying organic cause of dysmenorrhea. If no organic cause can be found, the diagnosis is primary dysmenorrhea. In addition, attitudes and expectations about menstruation and lifestyle disruption are identified and explored.

### Diagnostic Tests

Various diagnostic tests are performed to identify structural abnormalities, hormonal imbalances, and pathologic conditions that could cause menstrual pain.

- *Pelvic examination,* including a Papanicolaou (PAP) smear and cervical and vaginal cultures, is performed to detect structural abnormalities, malignancy, or infections.
- *Follicle-stimulating hormone (FSH) and luteinizing hormone (LH) levels* are measured to assess the function of the pituitary gland. The results are correlated with the time of the menstrual cycle.
- *Progesterone* and *estradiol levels* are measured to assess ovarian function.
- *Thyroid function tests* ($T_3$ and $T_4$) are performed to assess thyroid function.
- *Vaginal or pelvic ultrasonography* is used to detect the presence of space-occupying lesions, including fibroid tumors, cysts, abscesses, and neoplasms (see the box below).
- *CT scan* or *MRI* can be used to detect pelvic tumors.
- *Laparoscopy* is used to diagnose structural defects and blockages caused by scarring, endometriosis, tumors, and cysts (Figure 48–1 ). See the box on page 1560 for nursing care for the woman having a laparoscopy.
- *Dilation and curettage (D&C)* of the uterus is performed to obtain tissue for evaluation or to relieve dysmenorrhea and heavy bleeding. (This procedure is presented later in this chapter in the discussion on surgery.)

### Nursing Implications for Diagnostic Tests

#### Ultrasound Examination

- If indicated, ensure that the woman's bladder is full by forcing fluids and instructing her not to void. If she is NPO, a Foley catheter may be inserted into the bladder and sterile water instilled. The catheter is then clamped to prevent the water from leaving the bladder. The full bladder lifts the pelvic organs higher into the abdomen and improves visualization.
- Explain to the woman that she will be allowed to empty her bladder as soon as possible.
- Coat the abdomen with ultrasonic transducing gel. The gel provides a better image when the scanner is applied to the abdomen. For vaginal ultrasound, a transducer is covered with a condom or vinyl glove, coated with transducing gel, and introduced into the vagina.
- Explain the procedure to the woman, indicating that she can watch the procedure and ask questions about the images on the screen. If appropriate, point out landmarks on the screen.

If it is determined that a woman has secondary dysmenorrhea due to an underlying organic cause, therapeutic measures are directed at the specific condition.

## Medications

Dysmenorrhea may be treated with analgesics, prostaglandin inhibitors such as NSAIDs, or oral contraceptives (see the Medication Administration box on this page).

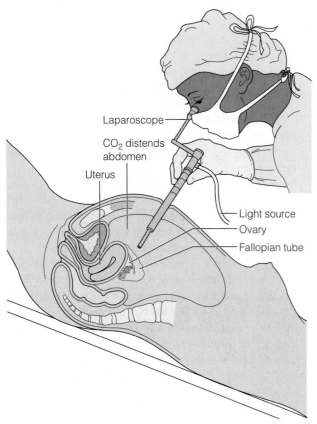

Laparoscope
CO₂ distends abdomen
Uterus
Light source
Ovary
Fallopian tube

**Figure 48–1** ■ Laparoscopy. In this surgical procedure, a flexible, lighted instrument (laparoscope) is inserted through a periumbilical incision. Laparoscopy allows visualization of the pelvic cavity.

## Complementary Therapies

The complementary therapies listed for the woman with PMS may also be useful for the woman with dysmenorrhea. Using a heating pad on the abdomen also helps reduce pain.

---

## Medication Administration

### The Woman with Dysmenorrhea

#### ORAL CONTRACEPTIVES

Norethindrone and ethinyl estradiol (Brevicon, Norinyl)
Norgestrel and ethinyl estradiol (Ovral)

Oral contraceptives inhibit ovulation and help reduce cramping and bleeding. Side effects of oral contraceptives include breast tenderness, weight gain, nausea, midcycle bleeding, mood swings, depression, chloasma (skin discoloration) on the face and chest, hypertension, vascular complications, vaginal candidiasis, migraines, and glucose intolerance. Oral contraceptives are contraindicated in women with personal or family history of breast cancer in first-degree relatives, hypertension, history of stroke or transient ischemic attack (TIA), smoking, history of estrogen-dependent cancer, pregnancy, liver disease, or thrombophlebitis.

#### Nursing Responsibilities
• Assess the client for potential contraindications to drug therapy.

#### Client and Family Teaching
• Take the drug as prescribed until the physician indicates otherwise or until side effects prevent you from continuing to take them.
• If you are taking oral contraceptives, be sure to take them at the same time every day.
• Report to the physician suspected pregnancy and any side effects such as nausea, rash, drowsiness, stomach pain, ringing in the ears, tenderness in the calf of the leg, and shortness of breath.
• Do not smoke while taking oral contraceptives.

---

## NURSING CARE OF THE WOMAN UNDERGOING LAPAROSCOPY

### PREOPERATIVE CARE
• Instruct the woman to empty the bladder prior to the surgical procedure.
• Explain to the woman that referred shoulder pain or expulsion of gas through the vagina may occur postoperatively. *During the procedure, the woman's abdomen is insufflated with carbon dioxide gas to distend the abdomen and facilitate visualization of the pelvic organs. The surgical table is then tilted so that the intestines will fall away from the pelvic organs. Some carbon dioxide gas may remain in the abdomen after the procedure.*

• Explain that pain should be minimal. Instruct the woman to report excessive pain to the nurse or physician at once. *Excessive pain signals infection or other postoperative complication.*

### POSTOPERATIVE CARE
• Apply a perineal pad. Teach the woman proper perineal hygiene, emphasizing the need to change pads at least every 4 hours. Keep a pad count. *Proper perineal hygiene reduces the risk of postoperative infection. Pad count is an indication of blood loss.*
• Assess for excessive vaginal bleeding. *Minor bleeding is normal; excessive bleeding may indicate hemorrhage.*

## NURSING CARE

Nursing care for the woman with primary dysmenorrhea focuses on controlling manifestations and providing education about the normal physiology of the menstrual cycle and self-care measures. Care of the woman with secondary dysmenorrhea varies according to the underlying cause and is discussed within sections on specific disorders. Nursing interventions for the woman with PMS are also appropriate for the woman with dysmenorrhea.

## THE WOMAN WITH DYSFUNCTIONAL UTERINE BLEEDING

**Dysfunctional uterine bleeding (DUB)** refers to vaginal bleeding that is usually painless but abnormal in amount, duration, or time of occurrence. The types of DUB include primary and secondary amenorrhea, oligomenorrhea, menorrhagia, metrorrhagia, and postmenopausal bleeding.

- **Amenorrhea** is the absence of menstruation. *Primary amenorrhea,* absence of menarche by age 16, or by age 14 if secondary sex characteristics fail to develop, may be caused by structural abnormalities, hormonal imbalances, polycystic ovary disease, or an imperforate hymen. Because a certain percentage of body fat is required for menstruation to occur, anorexia nervosa, bulimia, or excessive athletic training can also cause primary amenorrhea. *Secondary amenorrhea,* absence of menses for at least 6 months in a previously menstruating female, may also be caused by anorexia nervosa, excessive athletic activity or training, or a large weight loss. Other causes include hormonal imbalances and ovarian tumors. Normal, or physiologic, secondary amenorrhea occurs during pregnancy, breastfeeding, and menopause.
- **Oligomenorrhea,** scant menses, usually is related to hormonal imbalances.
- **Menorrhagia,** excessive or prolonged menstruation, may result from thyroid disorders, endometriosis, pelvic inflammatory disease, functional ovarian cysts, or uterine fibroids or polyps. Clotting disorders and anticoagulant medications also can cause menorrhagia. A single heavy or long cycle is not in itself a cause for concern; however, repetitive long or heavy cycles can lead to excessive blood loss, fatigue, anemia, hemorrhage, and sexual dysfunction.
- **Metrorrhagia,** bleeding between menstrual periods, may be caused by hormonal imbalances, pelvic inflammatory disease, cervical or uterine polyps, uterine fibroids, or cervical or uterine cancer. Because cancer is a possible cause of metrorrhagia, early evaluation and treatment are extremely important. *Mittleschmerz* (midcycle spotting associated with ovulation) occurs in many women and is not considered metrorrhagia.
- **Postmenopausal bleeding** may be caused by endometrial polyps, endometrial hyperplasia, or uterine cancer. The possibility of cancer makes early evaluation and treatment essential.

A number of factors may predispose a woman to DUB. These factors include stress, extreme weight changes, use of oral contraceptive agents or intrauterine devices (IUDs), and postmenopausal status. Dysfunctional uterine bleeding is usually related to hormonal imbalances or pelvic neoplasms, either benign or malignant.

## PATHOPHYSIOLOGY

Hormonal imbalances, especially progesterone deficiency with relative estrogen excess, results in endometrial hyperplasia. Estrogen stimulates endometrial proliferation. However, without the support provided by progesterone, sloughing occurs, resulting in vaginal bleeding that may be irregular, prolonged, or profuse. Defects in the follicular phase shorten the proliferative phase of the menstrual cycle, resulting in spotting and breakthrough bleeding. Defects during the luteal phase result in excessive amount or duration of flow due to persistence of the corpus luteum. This leads to a deficiency of progesterone, resulting in vaginal bleeding. *Anovulation,* absence of ovulation, is associated with both estrogen and progesterone deficiencies. Emotional upsets or stress can cause hormonal imbalances and thus affect menstruation. Pelvic neoplasms, discussed later, also cause abnormal bleeding.

## COLLABORATIVE CARE

The care of the woman with DUB focuses on identifying and treating the underlying disease. A careful history and physical examination are performed. Abdominal and pelvic examinations are performed to rule out abdominal masses. The woman may need to keep a menstrual history and basal body temperature chart for several months to determine whether ovulation is occurring.

### Diagnostic Tests

Diagnostic tests that may be ordered include the following:

- *CBC* is performed to rule out systemic disease as a contributing factor to DUB and to evaluate its effects.
- *Thyroid function studies,* including measurement of triiodothyronine ($T_3$), thyroxine ($T_4$), and thyroid-stimulating hormone (TSH) levels, are performed to rule out hyper- or hypothyroidism as a cause of DUB.
- *Endocrine studies* are done to evaluate pituitary and adrenal function. Pituitary dysfunction may first be manifested by menstrual irregularities.
- *Serum progesterone levels* are measured to determine the level of progesterone deficiency.
- *Pap smear* rules out or identifies cervical carcinoma.
- *Pelvic ultrasound* identifies luteal cysts.
- *Hysteroscopy* detects abnormalities of the uterine cavity.
- *Endometrial biopsy* is performed to obtain endometrial tissue for histologic examination.

### Medications

For many women, hormonal agents can correct menstrual irregularities. For anovulatory DUB, oral contraceptives may be prescribed for 3 to 6 months. Progesterone or medroxyprogesterone also may be prescribed to regulate uterine bleeding.

Ovulatory DUB may be treated with progestins during the luteal phase. Oral iron supplements may be prescribed to replace iron lost through menstrual bleeding.

## Surgery

Surgical intervention emphasizes the least invasive method that proves effective relief, beginning with a therapeutic dilation and curettage (D&C), then endometrial ablation, and, finally, hysterectomy.

### Therapeutic D&C

In a therapeutic D&C, the cervical canal is dilated and the uterine wall is scraped. D&C, the most frequently performed minor gynecologic surgical procedure, is used to diagnose and treat DUB and other disorders of the female reproductive system. It may be performed to correct excessive or prolonged bleeding. D&C is contraindicated in any woman who has been taking anticoagulant drugs or whose condition precludes the use of regional or general anesthesia. Nursing care of the woman having a D&C is described in the box below.

### Endometrial Ablation

In an endometrial ablation, the endometrial layer of the uterus is permanently destroyed using laser surgery or electrosurgical resection. It is performed in women who do not respond to pharmacologic management or D&C. The woman needs to understand that this procedure ends menstruation and reproduction.

### Hysterectomy

Hysterectomy, or removal of the uterus, may be performed when medical management of bleeding disorders is unsuccessful or malignancy is present, particularly if the woman no longer wishes to bear children. In premenopausal women, the ovaries are usually left in place; in postmenopausal women, a total hysterectomy, or panhysterectomy, may be performed; this procedure involves removal of the uterus, fallopian tubes, and ovaries.

Hysterectomy may involve either an abdominal or a vaginal approach. The choice depends on the underlying disorder, the need to explore the abdominal cavity, and the preference of the surgeon and woman. Nursing care of the woman undergoing a hysterectomy is described in the box on page 1563.

*Abdominal hysterectomy* is performed when a preexisting abdominal scar is present, when adhesions are thought to be present, or when a large operating field is necessary. For example, the woman with endometriosis is more likely to have an abdominal hysterectomy because endometrial tissue implants that may be present on other abdominal organs need to be removed. The surgical incision may be either longitudinal, made in the midline from umbilicus to pubis, or a *pfannenstiel incision,* also known as the bikini cut.

*Vaginal hysterectomy,* removal of the uterus through the vagina, is desirable when the uterus has descended into the vagina or if the urinary bladder or rectum have prolapsed into the vagina. Vaginal hysterectomy leaves no visible abdominal scar.

## NURSING CARE

### Nursing Diagnoses and Interventions

DUB usually causes the woman anxiety. Her self-image, sexuality, or reproductive capacity may be threatened, and she may fear the possibility of cancer. She may be embarrassed to discuss her menstrual history and hygiene practices. Interventions for the woman with DUB commonly address problems with anxiety and sexual function.

### Anxiety

The anxiety associated with abnormal uterine bleeding can be intense. Until the cause of the bleeding is identified and has been addressed, the woman may fear cancer or other life-threatening conditions.

- Discuss the results of tests and examinations with the woman. *This allows for open exchange of information.*
- Provide information about the causes, treatments, risks, long-term effects of treatments, and prognosis. *This allows the woman to assume responsibility for her own health and become involved in her own treatment plan.*

## NURSING CARE OF THE WOMAN UNDERGOING DILATION AND CURETTAGE (D&C)

### PREOPERATIVE CARE

- If ordered, ask the woman to come in 24 hours before surgery for insertion of a laminaria tent. *This device absorbs cervical secretions and slowly dilates the cervix.*
- Ensure that the woman remains NPO after midnight on the day of surgery.

### POSTOPERATIVE CARE

- Monitor circulation and sensation in the legs, and avoid compression of the popliteal area. *The lithotomy position requires the woman's legs to be elevated in stirrups, which can impair circulation.*

- Instruct the woman to use perineal pads and avoid tampons for 2 weeks. *This reduces the risk of infection and allows tissues to heal.*
- Explain that the onset of the next menstrual period may be delayed.
- Explain that intercourse should be avoided until after the postoperative checkup and after vaginal discharge has ceased. *This precaution reduces the risk of infection.*
- Instruct the woman to rest for several days after surgery, avoid heavy lifting, and report any bleeding that is bright red or exceeds that of a normal menstrual period. *Vigorous activity, lifting, or straining interferes with healing and may cause hemorrhage.*

# NURSING CARE OF THE WOMAN UNDERGOING A HYSTERECTOMY

## PREOPERATIVE CARE

- Assess the woman's understanding of the procedure. Provide explanation, clarification, and emotional support as needed. Reassure that the anesthesia will eliminate any pain during surgery and that medication will be administered postoperatively to minimize discomfort. *The woman who understands about the procedure to be performed and what to expect after surgery will be less anxious.*
- Cleanse the abdominal and perineal area, and, if ordered, shave the perineal area.
- If ordered, administer a small cleansing enema and ask the woman to empty her bladder. *This precaution helps prevent contamination from the bowel or bladder during surgery.*
- Administer preoperative medications as ordered.
- Check the chart to ensure that the consent form has been signed.

## POSTOPERATIVE CARE

- Assess for signs of hemorrhage. *Hemorrhage is more common after vaginal hysterectomy than after abdominal hysterectomy.*
- Monitor vital signs every 4 hours, auscultate lungs every shift and measure intake and output. *These data are important indicators of hemodynamic status and complications.*
- Once the catheter has been removed, measure the amount of urine voided.
- Assess for complications, including infection, ileus, shock or hemorrhage, thrombophlebitis, and pulmonary embolus.
- Assess vaginal discharge; instruct the woman in perineal care.
- Assess incision and bowel sounds every shift.
- Encourage turning, coughing, deep breathing, and early ambulation.
- Encourage fluid intake.

- Teach to splint the abdomen and cough deeply. Teach the use of the incentive spirometer.
- Instruct to restrict physical activity for 4 to 6 weeks. Heavy lifting, stair climbing, douching, tampons, and sexual intercourse should be avoided. The woman should shower, avoiding tub baths, until bleeding has ceased. *Infection and hemorrhage are the greatest postoperative risks; restricting activities and preventing the introduction of any foreign material into the vagina helps reduce these risks.*
- Explain to the woman that she may feel tired for several days after surgery and needs to rest periodically.
- Explain that appetite may be depressed and bowel elimination may be sluggish. *These are after effects of general anesthesia, handling of the bowel during surgery, and loss of muscle tone in the bowel while empty.*
- Teach the woman to recognize signs of complications that should be reported to the physician or nurse:
  a. Temperature greater than 100°F (37.7°C)
  b. Vaginal bleeding that is greater than a typical menstrual period or is bright red
  c. Urinary incontinence, urgency, burning, or frequency
  d. Severe pain
- Encourage the woman to express feelings that may signal a negative self-concept. Correct any misconceptions. *Some women believe that hysterectomy means weight gain, the end of sexual activity, and the growth of facial hair.*
- Provide information on risks and benefits of hormone replacement therapy, if indicated. *If the ovaries have also been removed, the woman is immediately thrust into menopause and may want or need hormone replacement therapy.*
- Reinforce the need to obtain gynecologic examinations regularly even after hysterectomy.

---

- Evaluate coping strategies and psychosocial support systems. Teach coping strategies if indicated. *The possibility of surgery or cancer represents a crisis for the woman and her support system. Support groups can provide assistance for the woman through crisis intervention.*

### Sexual Dysfunction

The woman with DUB may be unwilling to express herself sexually, particularly if bleeding is frequent or heavy. Additionally, fatigue may prevent her from participating in sexual activity.

- Offer information about engaging in sexual activity during menstruation. Explain that conception is possible during this time and that orgasm may help relieve symptoms. *Some women mistakenly believe that birth control measures are unnecessary during menstruation. Orgasm causes a release of tension and vascular congestion and frequently provides at least temporary relief of symptoms.*
- Provide an opportunity for the expression of concerns related to alterations in lifestyle and sexual functioning. *Some women have had a prolonged period of sexual abstinence related to DUB. Allowing women to verbalize concerns can assist them*

*in working collaboratively with the health care provider to minimize the impact of illness and optimize function.*
- Encourage frequent rest periods. *This conserves energy and may allow sexual activities to resume.*
- Provide information about alternative methods of sexual expression. *Methods of sexual expression other than vaginal intercourse may satisfy the needs of both partners.*

**PRACTICE ALERT** *If the nurse is not comfortable with frank discussions about sexual activities, referral is indicated.* ■

### Home Care

Provide support, appropriate reassurance, and information to help the woman and her family better understand her disorder and the therapeutic interventions indicated. Teaching also includes self-care measures that help minimize the effects of DUB on the daily functioning of the woman. The following topics should be included.

- Administration and side effects of prescribed medications, including iron

- The need to maintain a balanced diet, increasing iron-rich foods such as eggs, beans, liver, beef, and shrimp (Inform the woman that while orange juice may improve the absorption of iron, foods high in calcium and oxalic acid, such as spinach, may reduce its absorption.)

- Importance of maintaining a fluid intake of 2000 to 3000 mL a day
- The need to immediately report recurring episodes of DUB, particularly in postmenopausal women, to the health care provider

# STRUCTURAL DISORDERS

Structural disorders of the female reproductive system include displacement disorders and fistulas.

## THE WOMAN WITH A UTERINE DISPLACEMENT

The uterus may be displaced within the pelvic cavity or may descend into the vaginal canal. Displacement of the uterus within the pelvic cavity is classified according to the direction of the displacement (Figure 48–2 ■):

- **Retroversion** of the uterus is a backward tilting of the uterus toward the rectum.
- **Retroflexion** involves a flexing or bending of the uterine corpus in a backward manner toward the rectum.
- **Anteversion** is an exaggerated forward tilting of the uterus.
- **Anteflexion** is a flexing or folding of the uterine corpus upon itself.

**Prolapse** of the uterus into the vaginal canal can vary from mild to complete prolapse outside of the body. First-degree, or mild, prolapse involves a descent of less than half the uterine

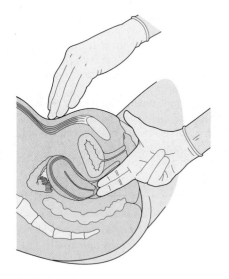

**A** Retroversion

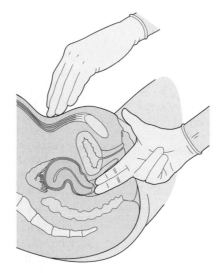

**B** Retroflexion

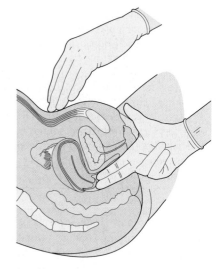

**C** Anteversion

**Figure 48–2** ■ Displacements of the uterus within the uterine cavity. *A,* Retroversion is a backward tilting. *B,* Retroflexion is a backward bending. *C,* Anteversion is a forward tilting. *D,* Anteflexion is a forward bending.

**D** Anteflexion

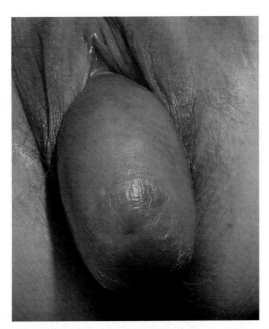

**Figure 48–3** ■ Prolapse of the uterus can vary from mild to complete. In third-degree uterine prolapse, or procidentia, the uterus prolapses completely outside the body, with inversion of the vagina.

*Source: M. English/Custom Medical Stock Photo.*

## Manifestations of Displacement Disorders

### Uterine Displacement within the Pelvic Cavity
- Dysmenorrhea
- Dyspareunia
- Backache
- Infertility

### Uterine Prolapse
- Backache
- Bearing-down sensation
- Constipation
- Urinary incontinence
- Hemorrhoids
- Dyspareunia

### Cystocele/Rectocele
- Bearing-down sensation
- Constipation
- Fecal incontinence
- Hemorrhoids
- Urinary incontinence

corpus into the vagina. Second-degree, or marked, prolapse involves the descent of the entire uterus into the vaginal canal, so that the cervix is at the introitus to the vagina. Third-degree prolapse, or *procidentia,* is complete prolapse of the uterus outside the body, with inversion of the vaginal canal (Figure 48–3 ■). Prolapse of the uterus is often accompanied by **cystocele** (herniation of the bladder into the vagina) or **rectocele** (herniation of the rectum into the vagina).

## PATHOPHYSIOLOGY AND MANIFESTATIONS

Displacement or prolapse of the uterus, bladder, or rectum can be a congenital or acquired condition. Congenital tilting or flexion of the uterus is rare. More commonly, tilting or flexion disorders in which the uterus remains within the pelvic cavity are related to scarring and inflammation of pelvic inflammatory disease, endometriosis, pregnancy, and tumors.

Downward displacement of the pelvic organs into the vagina results from weakened pelvic musculature, usually attributable to stretching of the supporting ligaments and muscles during pregnancy and childbirth. Unrepaired lacerations from childbirth, rapid deliveries, multiple pregnancies, congenital weakness, or loss of elasticity and muscle tone with aging may contribute to these disorders. The manifestations of displacement disorders are listed in the box on this page.

### COLLABORATIVE CARE

Collaborative care focuses on identifying the cause of the structural disorder, correcting or minimizing the condition, relieving pain, preventing or treating infection, and supporting and educating the woman.

A careful history and physical examination are performed. Diagnosis of uterine displacement is made after physical examination. If herniation of the rectum or bladder is suspected, the woman is asked to bear down or cough during the examination so the prolapse can be palpated and any leakage of urine or feces visualized. A history of infections, multiple pregnancies in rapid succession, and rapid labors support this diagnosis.

Treatment may include Kegel exercises to strengthen weakened pelvic muscles. Kegel exercises can be useful in the early stages of downward displacement. These exercises are discussed in Chapter 26. ⟲

### Surgery

Several surgical procedures are used to repair structural disorders. For women presenting with a cystocele, anterior *colporrhaphy* (repair of the cystocele) is the most common procedure. The anterior repair shortens the pelvic muscles, providing tighter support for the bladder. The *Marshall-Marchetti-Krantz procedure* involves resuspension of the urinary bladder in correct anatomic position. A rectocele is repaired with a posterior colporrhaphy, which shortens the pelvic muscles, providing a tighter support for the rectum.

A prolapsed uterus may be surgically repositioned and the supporting muscles shortened to provide greater support. In postmenopausal women or women with procidentia, hysterectomy is the preferred treatment.

### Pessary

When surgery is contraindicated, a *pessary* (a removable device) may be inserted into the vagina to provide temporary support for the uterus or bladder. At regular intervals, the pessary is removed, cleaned, and reinserted.

### NURSING CARE

### Nursing Diagnoses and Interventions

Nursing care focuses on education about the disorder, proposed treatments, and self-care measures for relief of symptoms.

Nursing interventions for the woman with a displacement disorder address problems with urinary incontinence and anxiety.

### Stress Incontinence

Relaxation of the pelvic floor can lead to stress incontinence. This can prove both troublesome and embarrassing and can increase the incidence of urinary tract infection.

- Teach Kegel exercises. *These exercises strengthen perineal muscle tone, minimize urinary leakage, and minimize descent of the bladder and rectum into the vagina. In postmenopausal women, estrogen supplements also can improve muscle tone in the perineal area.*
- Suggest the use of perineal pads (ranging from thin pantiliners to full-thickness incontinence pads) or special underwear (such as Depends) to absorb urine leakage. *Using pads or undergarments often allows the woman to once again take part in her usual social activities.*
- Explain perineal care and proper use of perineal pads. *Cleansing the perineum from front to back, and applying and removing perineal pads the same way minimizes cross infection from the anus to the vaginal and urethral openings. Incontinence pads need to be changed frequently to minimize surface bacterial counts.*
- Suggest reducing or eliminating caffeine intake. *Reducing caffeine intake can reduce urinary frequency and urgency.*
- Stress the importance of cleaning the perineal area. *Urine is very irritating to the skin.*

### Anxiety

Anxiety is common among women with a displacement disorder. Many women have only a cursory understanding of their reproductive anatomy. This lack of knowledge often compounds the anxiety. The nurse can use drawings and models to explain structural disorders and treatment options available.

- Encourage questions from the woman and her partner. *This helps assess the level of understanding so that teaching can be more effective.*
- Explain that the relief from discomfort and fatigue may positively influence sexual expression, and reassure the woman that the capacity for orgasm will not be affected. *Many women and their partners have major concerns about the effects of the disorder and its treatment on their sex life and capacity for sexual pleasure.*
- Explore coping mechanisms that have been previously successful. *This can help relieve anxiety and boost self-esteem.*

### Home Care

If surgery is the treatment of choice, teaching centers on what to expect in the preoperative and postoperative periods. If medical treatment is used initially, teaching focuses on measures to relieve the manifestations, such as Kegel exercises, use of incontinence pads, or the use, care, and insertion of a pessary.

Because obesity is a risk factor associated with relaxation of the pelvic and abdominal muscles, dietary counseling may be indicated. Preoperatively, a diet high in fiber may alleviate constipation, a particular concern during the postoperative period.

## THE WOMAN WITH A VAGINAL FISTULA

A **fistula** is an abnormal opening or passage between two organs or spaces that are normally separated or an abnormal passage to the outside of the body. The two types of vaginal fistulas are as follows:

- *Vesicovaginal fistula* is an abnormal opening between the urinary bladder and the vagina, leading to incontinent leakage of urine through the vagina.
- *Rectovaginal fistula* (less common) is an abnormal opening between the rectum and vagina, causing incontinent leakage of stool or flatus through the vagina.

Fistulas between the bladder and the vagina or between the rectum and the vagina may develop as a complication of childbirth, gynecologic or urologic surgery, or radiation therapy for gynecologic cancer. Cancer of the bladder is sometimes involved. The woman with a vaginal fistula often presents with a complaint of involuntary leakage of urine or flatus and symptoms of infection.

## COLLABORATIVE CARE

Fistulas are diagnosed by pelvic examination. Diagnosis of vesicovaginal fistula can be made by instilling dye into the urinary bladder through a catheter and observing the vagina for leakage. If no leakage is detected, a tampon or vaginal pack is inserted into the vagina, and the woman is asked to ambulate. If an abnormal opening is present, the tampon will absorb the dye. Dye may also be injected intravenously because it is excreted by the kidneys. Urine and vaginal cultures may be performed to rule out infections. Antibiotics are administered if infection is present.

A small vaginal fistula may resolve spontaneously. Otherwise, surgery is performed after inflammation has subsided, often a period of several months. Rarely, in the presence of a large, highly inflamed rectovaginal fistula, a temporary colostomy is performed, allowing inflammation and irritation to subside (see Chapter 24).

## NURSING CARE

Nursing care for the woman with repair of a vaginal fistula is similar to that for the woman with a displacement disorder. Teaching is an important component of nursing care. Stress the importance of careful perineal cleansing to reduce irritation and prevent further tissue breakdown. Suggest perineal irrigation or sitz baths for cleansing. Perineal pads or special underwear may be used to absorb urine or fecal drainage. For the woman with a rectovaginal fistula, provide information about avoiding gas-forming foods to minimize embarrassment from odor.

# DISORDERS OF FEMALE REPRODUCTIVE TISSUE

Both benign and malignant tissue disorders affect the female reproductive system. Benign tumors and cysts include Bartholin's gland cysts, cervical polyps, endometrial cysts and polyps, ovarian cysts, and uterine leiomyomas (fibroids). **Endometriosis** is a condition in which endometrial tissue implants outside the uterus in various locations in the pelvic cavity. Malignant tumors of reproductive tissue include cervical cancer, endometrial cancer, ovarian cancer, and vulvar cancer.

## THE WOMAN WITH CYSTS OR POLYPS

A **cyst** is a fluid-filled sac. A **polyp** is a highly vascular solid tumor attached by a pedicle, or stem. Cysts or polyps of the female reproductive system can occur in the vulva, cervix, endometrium, or ovaries.

### PATHOPHYSIOLOGY AND MANIFESTATIONS

Following are different types of female reproductive tissue cysts and polyps.

- *Bartholin's gland cysts* are the most common cystic disorder of the vulva. These cysts are caused by the infection or obstruction of Bartholin's gland.
- *Cervical polyps* are the most common benign cervical lesion in women of reproductive age. These polyps tend to occur in women over age 40 who have borne several children and have a history of using oral contraceptives. It is possible that cervical polyps develop from endocervical hyperplasia. The polyp develops at the vaginal end of the cervix, has a stem, and is highly vascular.
- *Endometrial cysts and polyps* are caused by endometrial overgrowth and are often filled with old blood (the dark color leads to the label "chocolate cysts"). Endometrial cysts are the result of endometrial implants on the ovary and are associated with endometriosis. Endometrial polyps, in contrast, are intrauterine overgrowths, similar to cervical polyps, and usually have a stalk.

- *Ovarian cysts* are classified as follicular cysts and corpus luteum cysts. Follicular cysts develop as a result of failure of the mature follicle to rupture or failure of an immature follicle to reabsorb fluid after ovulation. Corpus luteum cysts develop as a result of increased hormone secretion by the corpus luteum after ovulation. Most functional cysts regress spontaneously within two or three menstrual cycles.
- *Polycystic ovary syndrome (POS)* is an endocrine disorder characterized by numerous follicular cysts; anovulation; elevated serum estrogen, androgen, and LH levels; amenorrhea or irregular menses; hirsutism; obesity; and infertility. Women with POS often have insulin resistance and are at increased risk for early-onset type II diabetes, as well as breast and endometrial cancer.

The causes and manifestations of benign cysts and polyps of the female reproductive system are presented in Table 48–1. Complications associated with these disorders include infection, rupture, infertility, hemorrhage, and recurrence.

## COLLABORATIVE CARE

Care focuses on identifying and correcting the disorder and preventing its recurrence. A careful history and physical examination are performed, including inspection and visualization. Examination of the reproductive tract reveals the presence of most cysts and polyps. The menstrual history may reveal menstrual irregularities.

### Diagnostic Tests

The following diagnostic tests may be used to diagnose cysts and polyps of the female reproductive system.

- *Luteinizing hormone (LH) level* and *serum testosterone* are elevated and *FSH/LH ratio* is reversed in POS. *Glucose tolerance tests* also may be performed.
- *Pregnancy test* is performed to rule out early pregnancy when luteal cysts are suspected.
- *Laparoscopy* is performed to visualize ovarian cysts.
- *Ultrasonography* or *X-ray examination* is used to differentiate cysts from solid tumors.

### TABLE 48–1  Benign Cysts and Polyps of the Female Reproductive System

| Site | Type | Etiologic Origin | Manifestations |
|------|------|-----------------|----------------|
| Ovary | Functional cysts | Ovulation—include follicular cysts and corpus luteum cysts | May resolve spontaneously; can cause pain, menstrual irregularity, or amenorrhea |
| | Polycystic ovarian syndrome | Unknown; possible hypothalamic-pituitary dysfunction | Hirsutism, obesity; amenorrhea or irregular menses; hyperinsulinemia; infertility |
| Vulva | Bartholin cysts | Obstruction or infection of Bartholin's gland | Pain, redness, perineal mass, dyspareunia |
| Endometrium | Chocolate cysts | Endometrial overgrowth; filled with old blood | |
| | Endometrial polyps | Unknown | Bleeding between periods |
| Cervix | Cervical polyps | Unknown | Bleeding after intercourse or between periods |

## Medications

Pharmacologic intervention includes antibiotic treatment of any infection or abscess and, for functional ovarian cysts, regulation of ovarian hormones through administration of oral contraceptives to achieve regression of the cyst. Clomiphene (Clomid, Serophene) may be prescribed to stimulate ovulation in the woman with POS who wishes to become pregnant. Dexamethasone (Decadron) suppresses ACTH and adrenal androgens, and may be added to increase the likelihood of ovulation.

## Surgery

Cervical polyps are readily visible through a vaginal speculum and usually are removed with a clamp, using a twisting motion. To remove endometrial cysts or polyps, a transcervical approach is used. The specimen is sent to the laboratory for evaluation, and chemical or electrical cauterization is applied after cyst removal. For Bartholin's gland cysts and any abscesses, the lesion is incised and drained, and a drainage device is left in place. Follicular cysts may be punctured through laser surgery, or a wedge resection of the ovary may be performed to restore ovulation. Rarely, oophorectomy (removal of the ovary) is performed if the cysts are very large.

## NURSING CARE

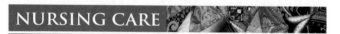

Nursing care focuses on relieving pain, implementing measures to correct the disorder, and preventing recurrence and complications. Address the following topics for self-care at home.

- The condition, its treatment, and measures to relieve pain
- The importance of keeping follow-up appointments
- Manifestations of infection (for postsurgical care) and the need to notify the physician should they occur
- If cervical polypectomy is performed, the use of external pads for 1 week (The woman must be able to state the signs of excessive bleeding and recognize that saturating more than one pad in an hour indicates the need for immediate follow-up.)
- The importance of long-term follow-up care for the woman with POS

## THE WOMAN WITH LEIOMYOMA

**Leiomyomata (fibroid tumors)** are benign tumors that originate from smooth muscle of the uterus. They are the most common form of pelvic tumor, believed to occur in 1 of every 4 or 5 women older than 35 years of age (Porth, 2002). Fibroids are seen more often and grow more rapidly in African Americans.

Fibroid tumors usually develop in the uterine corpus, and may be intramural, subserous, or submucous (Figure 48–4 ■).

- Intramural fibroid tumors (the most common type) are embedded in the myometrium. They usually present as an enlargement of the uterus.

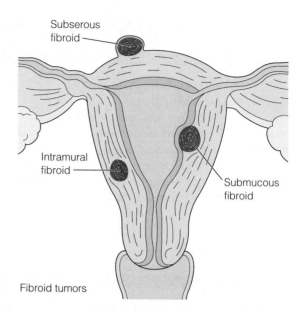

**Figure 48–4 ■** Types of uterine fibroid tumors (leiomyomata). Intramural fibroid tumors lie within the uterine wall. Subserous fibroid tumors lie beneath the serous lining of the uterus and project into the peritoneum. Submucous fibroid tumors lie beneath the endometrial lining of the uterus.

- Subserous fibroid tumors lie beneath the serous lining of the uterus and project into the peritoneal cavity. They may become pedunculated (on a stem) and displace or compress other tissues, such as the ureter or bladder.
- Submucous fibroid tumors lie beneath the endometrial lining of the uterus. They displace endometrial tissue and are more likely to cause bleeding, infection, and necrosis than the other types.

The actual cause of fibroid tumors is not clearly understood, but the association with estrogen stimulation is strong. Small tumors may be asymptomatic. The rate of growth varies, but they may increase in size during pregnancy or with use of oral contraceptives or HRT. Large fibroid tumors can crowd other organs, leading to pelvic pressure, pain, dysmenorrhea, menorrhagia, and fatigue. Depending on the location of the tumor, constipation and urinary urgency and frequency may occur. Most fibroid tumors shrink with menopause.

## COLLABORATIVE CARE

Treatment of the woman with uterine fibroids depends on the size and location of the tumors, the severity of the manifestations, and her age and childbearing status. Tests used to diagnose uterine fibroids may include an ultrasound to differentiate leiomyomata from endometriosis and a laparoscopy to visualize subserosal leiomyomata.

In asymptomatic women who wish to bear children, the fibroid tumors are monitored. Follow-up two to three times per year to monitor growth and the woman's response is recommended.

## Medications

Leuprolide acetate (Lupron) is used to decrease the size of the tumor if surgery is contraindicated or not desired. Gonadotropin-releasing hormone (GnRH) agonists are also administered.

## Surgery

*Myomectomy,* removal of the tumor without removing the entire uterus, is the surgical procedure of choice for young women who wish to retain reproductive capability. Laparoscopic laser technique is used for many women. A hysterectomy is performed if tumors are large, and if bleeding or other problems continue in perimenopausal women. A hysterectomy usually requires a hospital stay of 3 to 4 days, and a 6-week recovery time. A new method of treatment is with a *uterine fibroid embolization.* In this procedure, a catheter is guided through the femoral artery to the uterus, where tiny particles are injected into the artery supplying the fibroid to cut off the fibroid's blood supply. This procedure requires only an overnight hospital stay with a return to normal activities in 1 week.

If surgery is deferred, teaching emphasizes the importance of regular follow-up assessments to monitor tumor growth. If a hysterectomy is performed, teaching emphasizes appropriate preoperative and postoperative care. Dietary modifications to increase iron intake, prevent constipation, and promote healing are important.

## THE WOMAN WITH ENDOMETRIOSIS

**Endometriosis** is a condition in which multiple, small, usually benign implantations of endometrial tissue develop throughout the pelvic cavity. Endometriosis affects from 10% to 15% of women of childbearing age and is more common in women who postpone childbearing. Risk factors for endometriosis include early menarche, regular periods with a cycle of less than 27 days, menses lasting more than 7 days, heavier flow, increased menstrual pain, and a history of the condition in first-degree female relatives (Porth, 2002).

## PATHOPHYSIOLOGY AND MANIFESTATIONS

The cause of endometriosis is unclear, but several theories have been proposed. The metaplasia theory asserts that endometrial tissue develops from embryonic epithelial cells as a result of hormonal or inflammatory changes. The theory of retrograde menstruation suggests that menstrual tissue backs up through the fallopian tubes during menses, implants on various pelvic structures, and survives. The transplantation theory asserts that endometrial implants spread via lymphatic or vascular routes.

The abnormally located endometrial tissue responds to cyclic ovarian hormone stimulation, and bleeding occurs at the sites of implantation. Scarring, inflammation, and adhesions may develop. Endometriosis is a slowly progressive disease, responsive to ovarian hormone stimulation. Thus, the implants regress during pregnancy and atrophy at menopause unless the

---

### Manifestations of Endometriosis

- Heavy, throbbing pain of the lower abdomen and pelvis, radiating down the thighs and around the back. (The degree of pain, however, is not indicative of the severity of the disease.)
- Feeling of rectal pressure and discomfort when having a bowel movement
- Dyspareunia
- Dysfunctional uterine bleeding
- Infertility

woman is receiving HRT. Because progressive scarring may interfere with ability to conceive, women with significant endometriosis are encouraged to have children early if they wish to do so. Manifestations of endometriosis, which usually present during the luteal phase of the menstrual cycle, are summarized in the box above.

## COLLABORATIVE CARE

Endometriosis may be difficult to diagnose, but a history of dysmenorrhea, dyspareunia, and infertility strongly suggests this diagnosis. Interventions depend on the severity of symptoms, the extent of the disease, and the woman's age and desire for childbearing. Treatment goals focus on pain management and restoring fertility.

### Diagnostic Tests

Diagnostic tests are ordered to rule out other medical conditions and identify the endometrial implants.

- *Pelvic ultrasonography* may be performed to rule out other causes for pain and discomfort, including space-occupying masses
- *CBC with differential* is used to rule out pelvic abscesses and infectious processes. A low hemoglobin and hematocrit may be noted if menorrhagia accompanies endometriosis or tissue implants bleed significantly during the menses.
- *Laparoscopy* is used to visualize implants, and is the only method for definitive diagnosis.

### Medications

Medications include analgesics to control pain and prostaglandin synthesis inhibitors such as NSAIDs. Hormone therapy may include oral contraceptives or progesterone to induce pseudopregnancy, or danazol (Danocrine) to induce amenorrhea and involution of both endometrial tissue. Prolonged use of danazol, however, may result in masculinizing effects. GnRH is used to elevate levels of estrogen and progesterone and minimize bleeding.

### Surgery

Surgical interventions include laparoscopy with laser ablation (excision or removal) of endometrial implants. Refractory endometriosis may be treated with total hysterectomy.

# NURSING CARE

## Nursing Diagnoses and Interventions

Nursing care includes providing pain relief, providing education about the condition and the treatment options, and helping the woman cope with treatment outcomes. The severity of the disease and its manifestations are not necessarily related. Advanced disease may exhibit few manifestations, whereas early disease may be quite painful. Interventions for pain, discussed previously, are also appropriate for the woman with endometriosis. A priority diagnosis for the young woman with this disorder is anxiety related to loss of reproductive function.

### Anxiety

Anxiety about the unsure prognosis related to infertility is a particular problem for young women who plan to have a family in the near or distant future.

- Encourage expression of fears and anxiety about infertility, and answer questions honestly. *Knowledge helps relieve anxiety and fear.*
- Provide information on fertility awareness methods, including measurement of basal body temperature and other techniques for recognizing ovulation. *Understanding these techniques helps the woman and her partner optimize the conditions for conception.*

## Using NANDA, NIC, and NOC

Chart 48–1 shows links between NANDA nursing diagnoses, NIC, and NOC when caring for the woman with endometriosis.

## Home Care

Explain the cause of the disorder and the various treatment options, including their side effects. Discuss fertility awareness methods and the risks and benefits of long-term use of oral contraceptives. Stress the importance of exercise, smoking cessation, and weight control. If surgical treatment is chosen, provide preoperative and postoperative teaching.

# THE WOMAN WITH CERVICAL CANCER

The American Cancer Society (2002) estimates that 13,000 cases of cervical cancer will be diagnosed, with approximately 4100 deaths attributed to the disease, annually. The incidence is greater in blacks than whites. Effective screening with the Papanicolaou smear (Pap test) has reduced the death rate by 55% over the last 30 years, although the death rates for blacks continues to be more than 2 times that of whites. The age of diagnosis is between 50 and 55 years; however, it begins to appear in women in their 20s.

## PATHOPHYSIOLOGY AND MANIFESTATIONS

Most cervical cancers (90%) are squamous cell carcinomas that begin as neoplasia in the cervical epithelium. *Precancerous dysplasia (cervical intraepithelial neoplasia [CIN], cervical carcinoma in situ)* is estimated to occur in 1 of 8 women before the age of 20, often associated with human papillomavirus (HPV) infection. Studies have also found a strong association with reproductive infections with *Chlamydia trachomatis.* (These infections are discussed in Chapter 49). The precursor lesions may spontaneously regress (60%), persist (30%), or progress and undergo malignant change (10%). Only about 1% become invasive (Porth, 2002). The CIN system of grading dysplastic changes is based on the extent of involvement of the epithelial thickness of the cervix. Carcinoma in situ is localized; invasive cancer spreads to deeper layers.

Cancer in situ most often develops in the transformation zone where the columnar epithelium of the cervical lining meets the squamous epithelium of the outer cervix and vagina. Squamous cell cancers spread by direct invasion of accessory structures, including the vaginal wall, pelvic wall, bladder, and rectum. Although metastasis is most frequently confined to the pelvic area, distant metastasis may occur through the lymphatic system. Clinical staging is based on the International Federation of Gynecology and Obstetrics (FIGO) system (Table 48–2).

## CHART 48–1  NANDA, NIC, AND NOC LINKAGES

### The Client with Endometriosis

| NURSING DIAGNOSES | NURSING INTERVENTIONS | NURSING OUTCOMES |
| --- | --- | --- |
| • Fatigue<br>• Deficient Knowledge | • Energy Management<br>• Teaching: Disease Process<br>• Teaching: Sexuality<br>• Preconception Counseling | • Energy Conservation<br>• Knowledge: Disease Process |
| • Powerlessness | • Emotional Support<br>• Self-Esteem Enhancement | • Social Support<br>• Health Beliefs: Perceived Control |

*Note. Data from Nursing Outcomes Classification (NOC) by M. Johnson & M. Maas (Eds.), 1997, St. Louis: Mosby; Nursing Diagnoses: Definitions & Classification 2001–2002 by North American Nursing Diagnosis Association, 2001, Philadelphia: NANDA; Nursing Interventions Classification (NIC) by J.C. McCloskey & G. M. Bulechek (Eds.), 2000, St. Louis: Mosby. Reprinted by permission.*

## Nursing Care Plan
## A Woman with Endometriosis

Angela Hall is a 31-year-old married accountant, who relates a history of severe dysmenorrhea and menorrhagia, a feeling of pelvic heaviness and pain that radiates down her thighs. Because of her discomfort, her husband has complained about the quality of their sex life and has expressed concerns about their plans for having children. Mrs. Hall reports being so tired she doesn't care whether she has sex or not, and, in fact, would really prefer not to: "Sex hurts so much, I just can't stand it." Endometriosis is suspected, and a diagnostic laparoscopy has been scheduled.

### ASSESSMENT

Christine Brigham, RN, NP, interviews Mrs. Hall and makes the following assessments: BP 110/70, P 68, R 18, T 98.2°F (36.7°C). Mrs. Hall's weight is 130 lb (59 kg) and within normal limits for her height. Review of laboratory findings indicate a hemoglobin level of 9.8 g/dL (normal range: 12 to 16 g/dL) and a hematocrit of 33.1% (normal range: 35% to 45%). Physical examination reveals pelvic tenderness on manipulation of the cervix, and small masses that are palpable on abdominal/pelvic examination.

### DIAGNOSIS

- *Chronic pain* related to endometrial pelvic implants
- *Anxiety* related to effect of endometriosis on fertility
- *Deficient knowledge* related to diagnosis and treatment options
- *Ineffective sexuality patterns* related to the manifestations of endometriosis

### EXPECTED OUTCOMES

- Develop effective self-care measures to deal with the pain and discomfort.
- Verbalize decreased anxiety.
- Demonstrate understanding of the disease and treatment options.
- Verbalize an improvement in sexual functioning and a decrease in interpersonal stress between herself and her husband.

### PLANNING AND IMPLEMENTATION

- Identify the location, type, duration, and history of the pain.
- Recommend analgesics and heat therapy.
- Provide information on biofeedback, relaxation, and imagery to lessen pain.
- Discuss with Mr. and Mrs. Hall the causes of endometriosis and its manifestations.
- Encourage the Halls to discuss their feelings about the effect of the disease on their sex life, lifestyle, and fertility.
- Refer the couple to the local mental health center if appropriate.

### EVALUATION

Two years after the initiation of treatment, Mr. and Mrs. Hall have become parents of a baby girl. Mrs. Hall states that the discomfort and other manifestations of endometriosis have eased. Relaxation and imagery have effectively minimized her pain and brought about improvement in her function as wife, mother, and sexual partner. Counseling has improved the interpersonal and sexual relations between the Halls. Dietary management has improved her anemia, although the menorrhagia persists. The Halls are trying to have a second child, understanding the advantages of rapid succession of pregnancies. They will be followed in the nursing clinic and referred to an infertility clinic if conception does not occur within 1 year.

### Critical Thinking in the Nursing Process

1. Explain the pathophysiologic basis for Mrs. Hall's anemia.
2. How would you handle the situation if Mr. and Mrs. Hall were extremely uncomfortable and embarrassed about discussing their sexual problems?
3. Develop a plan of care for Mrs. Hall for the nursing diagnosis, *Situational low self-esteem*, related to the manifestations of endometriosis.

See Evaluating your Response in Appendix C.

---

| TABLE 48–2 | FIGO Staging Classification for Cervical Cancer |
| --- | --- |

| Stage | Description |
| --- | --- |
| 0 | Carcinoma in situ, intraepithelial carcinoma |
| I | Carcinoma that is strictly confined to the cervix |
| II | Involvement of the vagina, limited to the upper two-thirds of the vagina, or infiltration of the parametria (connective tissue surrounding the uterus) but not the side wall of the pelvis |
| III | Involvement of the lower third of the vagina or extension to the pelvic side wall |
| IV | Extension outside the reproductive tract |

Preinvasive cancer is limited to the cervix and rarely causes symptoms. Invasive cancer produces vaginal bleeding after intercourse or between menstrual periods, and vaginal discharge that increases as the cancer progresses. These changes are subtle, and may be more readily noticed by the postmenopausal woman. Manifestations of advanced disease include referred pain in the back or thighs, hematuria, bloody stools, anemia, and weight loss.

### Risk Factors

As described by the American Cancer Society (2001), risk factors for cervical cancer include infection of the external genitalia and anus with HPV, first intercourse before 16 years of age, multiple sex partners or male partners with multiple sex partners, a history of sexually transmitted infections, and infection with HIV. The most important risk factor is infection by the HPV. Other risk factors include smoking and poor nutritional status, family history of cervical cancer, and exposure to DES (diethylstilbestrol) in utero.

## COLLABORATIVE CARE

The goals of treatment are to eradicate the cancer and minimize complications and metastasis. The type of treatment depends on the degree of malignant change, the size and location of the lesion, and the extent of metastasis.

## Diagnostic Tests

Diagnostic tests used to diagnose cervical cancer include the following:

- *Pap smear* is the primary screening tool for cervical carcinoma (see the box below). If the results show atypical cells, the test is repeated. Pap test results may be reported in descriptive terms with abnormal cells described as benign, which may include infectious, inflammatory, atrophic, or other cell changes, or as epithelial cell abnormalities, including atypical squamous cells to squamous cell carcinoma, and atypical glandular cells to adenocarcinoma.

## Nursing Implications for Diagnostic Tests

### Papanicolaou (Pap) Test

The Papanicolaou smear (Pap test) is used to screen for cervical intraepithelial neoplasia (CIN) and cervical cancer. It can also be used to assess hormonal status and identify the presence of sexually transmitted diseases, such as human papilloma virus (HPV) infection.

With the woman in the lithotomy position, a speculum is inserted to visualize the cervix. A plastic or wooden spatula is used to scrape the cervical os and any suspicious-looking areas, and the material is transferred to a slide for histologic analysis. A cotton-tipped applicator or cytobrush is used to obtain a specimen from the endocervix; this specimen is then transferred to a second slide.

### Client Preparation
- Instruct the woman to empty her bladder.
- Explain that the test should be painless and quick, although slight cramping may be experienced when the endocervical specimen is obtained.

### Client and Family Teaching
- Teach the woman about recommended frequency of screening, every 3 years until age 65 after two successive negative results a year apart or more frequently if the woman has specific risk factors for cervical cancer.
- Teach the woman to schedule the Pap test for a time when she is not menstruating. Blood interferes with interpretation of the smear.
- Teach the woman to avoid intercourse, douching, or placing of any medication in the vagina for 36 hours prior to the test.

## Nursing Implications for Diagnostic Tests

### Cervical Biopsy

Cervical biopsy is performed for women whose Pap smear findings indicate possible cervical cancer or cervical intraepithelial neoplasia (CIN). The biopsy is also used to screen women at high risk for vaginal and cervical cancers due to intrauterine DES exposure. With the woman in the lithotomy position, the cervix is cleaned with 3% acetic acid, and tissue samples are taken for biopsy. Afterward, the area is cleaned and a perineal pad applied.

### Client Preparation
- Explain the procedure, indicating that the test usually involves minimal discomfort although a cramping sensation may be experienced as the cervix is dilated to obtain the specimen.
- Have the woman empty her bladder prior to the procedure.

### Client and Family Teaching
- Explain that minor bleeding and vaginal discharge are expected following this procedure. Perineal pads should be used and tampons avoided for at least one week.
- Caution to avoid sexual intercourse until discharge has stopped.
- Instruct to notify the physician if heavy bleeding or manifestations of infection (pain, foul smelling discharge, fever, malaise) occur.

- *Colposcopy* and *cervical biopsy* of the suspicious area may be performed if the second Pap test yields abnormal findings (see the box above).
- *Loop diathermy technique* (loop electrosurgical excision procedure [LEEP]) allows simultaneous diagnosis and treatment of dysplastic lesions found on colposcopy. This procedure is performed in the office, using a wire for both cutting and coagulation during excision of the dysplastic region of the cervix.
- *MRI* or *CT* of the pelvis, abdomen, or bones may be performed to detect the spread of the tumor.

## Medications

Chemotherapy is used for tumors not responsive to other therapy, tumors that cannot be removed, or as adjunct therapy if metastasis has occurred (see Chapter 10). ☍

## Treatments

The treatment for cervical cancer may include surgery and radiation therapy.

### Surgery
When combined with colposcopy, laser surgery is a viable treatment method provided that the cancer is limited to the cervical epithelium. Cryosurgery, which involves the use of a probe to freeze tissue, causing necrosis and sloughing, is also used for noninvasive lesions. Conization (Figure 48–5 ■) is performed to treat microinvasive carcinoma when colposcopy cannot define the limits of the invasion. For invasive lesions,

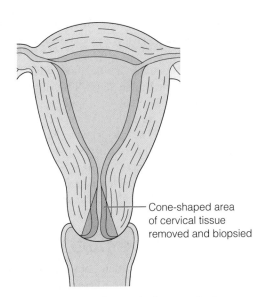

Cone-shaped area of cervical tissue removed and biopsied

**Figure 48-5** ■ Conization, the surgical removal of a cone-shaped section of the cervix, is used to treat microinvasive carcinoma of the cervix.

hysterectomy or radical hysterectomy (removal of the uterus, fallopian tubes, lymph nodes, and ovaries) is performed.

A **pelvic exenteration,** the removal of all pelvic contents, including the bowel, vagina, and bladder, is performed if the cancer recurs without involvement of the lymphatic system. An anterior exenteration is the removal of the uterus, ovaries, fallopian tubes, vagina, bladder, urethra, and lymphatic vessels and nodes. An ileal conduit is created for excretion of urine (see Chapter 26). A posterior exenteration is the removal of the uterus, ovaries, uterine tubes, bowel, and rectum. A colostomy is created for excretion of feces (see Chapter 24). ◌

### Radiation Therapy

Radiation therapy is used to treat invasive cervical cancer. External radiation beam therapy and intracavity cesium irradiation can be used.

## NURSING CARE

Nursing care involves helping the woman deal with the physical and psychologic effects of a potentially life-threatening illness, providing information needed to make informed decisions, and minimizing the adverse effects of therapy. Pain relief measures are important, as is grief work on the part of the woman and family. The woman should be encouraged to perform self-care activities and resume normal everyday activities and sexual functioning to the extent possible.

### Health Promotion

The American Cancer Society (2002) recommends that women should begin annual screening for cervical cancer with the Pap test at the age of 18, or after beginning sexual activity, whichever comes first. After three consecutive negative Pap tests, screening can be performed less frequently, at the discretion of the health care provider.

It is vital that nurses educate women of all ages about controlling risk factors for cervical cancer and about the importance of screening for this cancer throughout the life span. Teach young women about the relationship between early sexual activity, multiple partners, and risk for sexually transmitted diseases and cervical cancer. Discuss safer sex alternatives and using condoms for protection. Emphasize the importance of continued screening exams for the older woman who may not see a gynecologic specialist on a regular basis.

### Assessment

Collect the following data through a health history and physical examination (see Chapter 46).

- Health history: history of sexually transmitted infections, sexual history, family history of cervical cancer, vaginal bleeding or discharge, smoking history, maternal treatment with DES
- Physical assessment: pelvic examination, abdomen, lymph glands

### Nursing Diagnoses and Interventions

This section discusses nursing interventions for the woman who has been diagnosed with cervical cancer and requires surgical and/or radiation treatment. Other nursing diagnoses and interventions that may be appropriate for the woman with cervical cancer are discussed in the sections discussing other female reproductive system cancers.

### Fear

Many people believe that cancer equals death; however, this is no longer true in many cases, especially with early diagnosis. For cervical cancer that is diagnosed at an early stage, the 5-year survival rate is 92%. If the disease is in situ, the rate is nearly 100%.

- Explain that 70% of all women with cervical cancer survive for 5 years or more and that the earlier the cancer is detected, the better the prognosis. *This gives the woman hope, an essential ingredient in recovery.*
- Allow adequate time for the woman and her partner to express their concerns and to ask questions. *Unexpressed feelings and fears and lack of understanding may cause the woman to view the situation as worse than it is.*
- Refer to cancer counselor or support groups for additional information. *Cancer survivors who visit clients in the hospital provide proof that people can survive the diagnosis and treatment of cancer and lead normal, productive lives.*

### Impaired Tissue Integrity

Surgery interrupts the integrity of the skin surface, providing a potential portal of invasion for bacteria. Radiation therapy causes an inflammatory response in the skin and mucous membranes within the field of radiation, creating further risk of tissue reaction and breakdown.

- Teach wound and skin care, particularly if pelvic exenteration is performed. Irrigations with saline or solutions of saline and hydrogen peroxide are performed at intervals, with dry heat applied thereafter to dry the area. *Open and damaged tissue increases the risk for infection. Meticulous skin and wound care is necessary to prevent infection and further tissue destruction.*

- If appropriate, teach stoma care, and care for the skin surrounding the stoma. (These procedures are discussed in Chapters 24 and 26.) ⊙⊙ *Urine and stool are irritating to the skin. Without proper care, the skin surrounding the stoma can become excoriated.*
- Apply non-oil-based lotions to skin surface. This may minimize itching and help maintain integrity. *Oil-based lotions are not recommended for tissue undergoing radiation.*
- Instruct the woman not to remove the markings used to localize the radiation beam to the target area. *Markings are used in future radiation treatments.*
- Monitor for evidence of fistula formation, and teach the woman to do the same. *Fistula formation is a potential complication of radiation to the pelvic or abdominal cavities. Vaginal fistulas may form between the vagina and the bladder or rectum. Fistulas may also develop between the bladder and rectum, resulting in the expulsion of stool in the urine or loss of urine through the anus.*

### Using NANDA, NIC, and NOC

Chart 48–2 shows links between NANDA nursing diagnoses, NIC, and NOC when caring for the woman with cervical cancer.

### Home Care

Teaching varies according to the stage of the cancer and the treatment selected. Provide information concerning radiation, chemotherapy, or surgery, as indicated. Preoperative teaching focuses on postoperative expectations, including management of urinary or fecal diversion, if indicated (see Chapters 24 and 26). Help the woman and family recognize signs of infection and understand the importance of follow-up care. In addition, suggest the following resources:

- American Cancer Society
- National Cancer Institute
- Women's Cancer Network

## THE WOMAN WITH ENDOMETRIAL CANCER

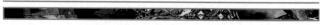

Endometrial carcinoma is the most frequently diagnosed pelvic cancer in the United States. The American Cancer Society (2002) estimates that each year approximately 39,000 women are diagnosed with endometrial cancer, and 6600 die from this disease. The incidence is higher in whites than blacks, but the mortality rate is nearly twice as high in blacks. Most endometrial cancer is diagnosed in postmenopausal women, with the peak incidence in the late 50s and early 60s. When diagnosed and treated early in the disease, the 5-year survival rate is about 90%.

### PATHOPHYSIOLOGY AND MANIFESTATIONS

Most endometrial malignancies are adenocarcinomas that are slow to grow and metastasize. These cancers develop in the glandular cells or endometrial lining of the uterus (the same tissue that is shed each month during a normal menstrual period). Endometrial hyperplasia (excessive growth) is a precursor of endometrial cancer. These tumors tend to grow slowly in the early stages.

Tumor growth usually begins in the fundus, invades the vascular myometrium, and spreads throughout the female reproductive tract. Metastasis occurs by means of the lymphatic system, through the fallopian tubes to the peritoneal cavity, and to the rest of the body via the bloodstream. Target areas for metastasis include the lungs, liver, and bone. The FIGO classification of endometrial cancer is presented in Table 48–3.

The major manifestation of endometrial hyperplasia or overt endometrial cancer is abnormal, painless vaginal bleeding. In menstruating women, this bleeding is manifested as menorrhagia or metrorrhagia. In postmenopausal women, any bleeding is abnormal. Later manifestations include pelvic cramping, bleeding after intercourse, and lower abdominal pressure. In advanced disease, lymph node enlargement, pleural effusion, abdominal masses, and ascites may be present.

### CHART 48–2 NANDA, NIC, AND NOC LINKAGES

#### The Client with Cervical Cancer

| NURSING DIAGNOSES | NURSING INTERVENTIONS | NURSING OUTCOMES |
|---|---|---|
| • Deficient Knowledge | • Teaching: Safe Sex<br><br>• Teaching: Disease Process | • Knowledge: Infection Control<br>• Risk Control: STD<br>• Knowledge: Disease Process<br>• Knowledge: Health Behaviors |
| • Anticipatory Grieving | • Active Listening<br>• Emotional Support | • Coping<br>• Grief Resolution |
| • Ineffective Protection | • Risk Identification<br>• Chemotherapy Management<br>• Surgical Precautions | • Infection Status |

*Note. Data from Nursing Outcomes Classification (NOC) by M. Johnson & M. Maas (Eds.), 1997, St. Louis: Mosby; Nursing Diagnoses: Definitions & Classification 2001–2002 by North American Nursing Diagnosis Association, 2001, Philadelphia: NANDA; Nursing Interventions Classification (NIC) by J.C. McCloskey & G. M. Bulechek (Eds.), 2000, St. Louis: Mosby. Reprinted by permission.*

## Nursing Care Plan
## A Woman with Cervical Cancer

Anna Eliza Gillam is a 45-year-old divorced mother of four children ranging in age from 16 to 23. She was married at age 18 and had several sexual partners prior to her marriage. She has had three sexual partners since her marriage ended. Last year she was treated with cryosurgery for venereal warts. The Pap smear taken 2 weeks ago showed atypical cells, and she has come in for a repeat test.

### ASSESSMENT

Judy Davis, RN, the admitting nurse, interviews Mrs. Gillam and records the following assessment findings: BP 130/80, P 72, R 18, T 99.2°F (37.3°C). Ms. Gillam weighs 142 lb (64.5 kg), approximately 15% over her ideal body weight. Examination of the cervix reveals a large necrotic lesion at the 7 o'clock position. She has reduced her smoking to less than 10 cigarettes per day, and she does not drink alcohol.

Ms. Gillam is extremely fearful and anxious and has told no one about her abnormal Pap smear. She reveals that she has had back pain radiating down her thighs for several months and a foul vaginal discharge that increases after intercourse. Until 2 weeks ago, she had not had a Pap smear for 5 years. Ms. Davis performs the repeat Pap smear, which is positive for squamous cell carcinoma of the cervix. A CT scan and lymphangiography are scheduled. Laparoscopy shows the disease to be widespread in the pelvic cavity.

### DIAGNOSES

- *Decisional conflict* related to treatment options
- *Chronic and acute pain* related to metastasis and surgery
- *Risk for impaired skin integrity* related to radiation
- *Fear* related to diagnosis of cervical cancer
- *Anticipatory grieving* related to potential loss of life

### EXPECTED OUTCOMES

- Gain knowledge to make informed decisions about treatment options.
- Develop strategies for pain control.
- Maintain skin and tissue integrity during radiation treatment.
- Express her feelings about the fear of cancer and death.

- Develop effective coping strategies for dealing with life-threatening illness and pain.

### PLANNING AND IMPLEMENTATION

- Discuss treatment alternatives, including the prognosis with each option.
- Administer pain medications as prescribed.
- Inspect skin surfaces daily before and after radiation therapy.
- Provide information on biofeedback training and relaxation techniques for control of moderate pain.
- Refer to a local cancer support group so that she can interact with cancer survivors.
- Refer Mrs. Gillam to a social worker in preparation for her altered level of functioning.

### EVALUATION

Mrs. Gillam has begun radiation therapy following pelvic extenteration. She controls her pain with relaxation and imagery techniques, requiring only occasional analgesics. She uses a water-based lotion to soothe the skin surface and is careful not to remove the skin markings. She seems optimistic and has quit smoking. She and her family have continued to attend the cancer support group meetings. Mrs. Gillam is planning for the future and has talked with her family about what it means to live with cancer.

### Critical Thinking in the Nursing Process

1. Compare and contrast your teaching plan for health promotion interventions to decrease the risks of cervical cancer for a young woman of 17 and an older woman of 70. Would they differ, and if so, how?
2. Develop a teaching plan to help Mrs. Gillam cope with the effects of radiation.
3. During a home visit, Mrs. Gillam tells the nurse that she has been so tired since beginning radiation treatments that all she can do is sit in her chair. Design a plan of care for the nursing diagnosis, *Fatigue*.

See Evaluating Your Response in Appendix C.

---

| TABLE 48–3 | FIGO Staging Classification for Endometrial Cancer |
|---|---|

| Stage | Description |
|---|---|
| I | Tumor limited to endometrium or myometrium |
| II | Endocervical glandular involvement or invasion of cervical stroma |
| III | Metastasis or invasion of serosa, adnexae, vagina, and pelvic or para-aortic lymph nodes |
| IV | Tumor invasion of bladder or bowel mucosa; distant metastases |

## Risk Factors

A significant risk factor for endometrial cancer is prolonged estrogen stimulation with hyperplasia. Other factors that increase the risk are obesity, anovulatory menstrual cycles, decreasing ovarian function (as with menopause), estrogen-secreting tumors, and unopposed estrogen (e.g., estrogen therapy without progesterone). Medical conditions that may alter estrogen metabolism and increase the risk of endometrial cancer are diabetes mellitus, hypertension, and polycystic ovary syndrome (Porth, 2002). Tamoxifen, a drug that blocks estrogen receptor sites and is used to treat breast cancer, has a weak estrogenic effect on the endometrium, and is also a risk factor.

## COLLABORATIVE CARE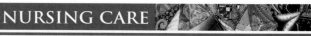

The goals of care for the woman with endometrial cancer are to eradicate the cancer and minimize complications and metastasis.

### Diagnostic Tests

Tests used to diagnose cancer of the endometrium include the following:

- *Vaginal ultrasonography* is sometimes used to determine endometrial thickening, which may indicate hypertrophy or malignant changes.
- *Endometrial biopsy* (see the box below) or dilation and curettage (D&C) provides definitive diagnosis.
- *Transvaginal ultrasound* is used to measure endometrial thickness.
- *Laparoscopy* may be performed to determine the stage of the cancer.
- Other tests to determine the extent of the disease include *chest X-ray, intravenous urography, cystoscopy, barium enema, sigmoidoscopy, MRI,* and *bone scans.*

### Medications

Although the treatment of choice for primary endometrial carcinoma is surgery, progesterone therapy may be used for recurrent disease. About one-third of women respond favorably, primarily those with well-differentiated tumors. Chemotherapy is less effective than other forms of therapy, although cisplatin or combination chemotherapy may be used for women with disseminated disease.

### Surgery

After the diagnosis is confirmed, a total abdominal hysterectomy and bilateral salpingo-oophorectomy is performed. A radical hysterectomy with node dissection is performed if the disease is stage II or beyond.

### Radiation Therapy

Treatment with external and internal radiation may be performed as a preoperative measure or as adjuvant treatment in advanced cases.

## NURSING CARE

### Health Promotion

All perimenopausal and postmenopausal women need annual pelvic examinations. Those in high-risk groups are advised to have endometrial biopsies every 2 years. Any vaginal bleeding in postmenopausal women should be reported at once to the physician. In addition, control of diseases such as diabetes mellitus and hypertension decreases the risk of endometrial hyperplasia.

### Assessment

Collect the following data through a health history and physical examination (see Chapter 46).

- Health history: abnormal vaginal bleeding, menstrual history, use of estrogen (without progesterone) to treat menopausal symptoms, breast cancer treated with tamoxifen, childbearing status, presence of chronic illnesses
- Physical assessment: height and weight, pelvic examination, abdomen, lymph glands

### Nursing Diagnoses and Interventions

Nursing care involves helping the woman deal with the physical and psychologic effects of a potentially life-threatening illness, make informed decisions, and minimize the adverse effects of therapy. Pain relief is a key component of care, as is grief work on the part of the woman and family. Encourage the woman to perform self-care and resume normal activities of daily living.

### Acute Pain

Total abdominal hysterectomy can involve severe and prolonged pain, not only from the surgical incision but also from the manipulation of internal organs during surgery. Abdominal viscera are highly vascular and easily bruised by handling.

- Administer analgesics as ordered. *Analgesics provide pain relief and promote early ambulation.*
- Encourage ambulation. *Ambulation facilitates the expulsion of flatus, which can cause distention as well as discomfort.*

## Nursing Implications for Diagnostic Tests

### Endometrial Biopsy

Endometrial biopsy is performed to detect endometrial cancer or hyperplasia. With the woman in the lithotomy position, the cervix is cleaned with iodine solution and the biopsy specimen is taken from the endometrial lining, using a transcervical approach and either curettage or vacuum aspiration.

#### Client Preparation
- Explain that this procedure is uncomfortable but that post-procedure pain medication can offer relief.
- Explain that the procedure causes vaginal bleeding, and instruct the woman to use perineal pads rather than tampons.

- When the physician has informed the woman about the results of the biopsy, encourage her to ask questions and express her feelings and concerns.

#### Client and Family Teaching
- Instruct to avoid intercourse until advised by the physician.
- Provide information about treatment options or health maintenance activities related to regular examinations and health screening.

- Apply heat to the abdomen, and recommend that the woman use a heating pad at home. *Heat dilates blood vessels, increasing blood supply to the pelvis.*

### Disturbed Body Image

For many women, the side effects of cancer treatment can be almost as difficult and painful as the disease itself. Although side effects of the different therapies vary among individuals, the woman's body image and quality of life are always affected. Such side effects as alopecia (hair loss), nausea, vomiting, fatigue, diarrhea, stomatitis, and surgical scarring disturb body image.

- Review the side effects of the treatment regimen proposed, and assist the woman to develop a plan to deal with these effects. *This promotes a sense of control.*
- Remind the woman and family that side effects are usually manageable and may be temporary. *Over-the-counter agents can be used to alleviate stomatitis. Frequent rest periods can relieve fatigue. Medications can be prescribed for nausea, vomiting, and diarrhea.*

### Ineffective Sexuality Patterns

Altered sexuality may result from a feeling of unattractiveness, fatigue, or pain and discomfort. The woman's partner may fear that sexual activity will be harmful.

- Encourage expression of feelings about the effect of cancer on their lives and sexual relationship. *Verbalizing feelings helps relieves stress and maximizes relaxation.*
- Suggest that the couple explore alternative sexual positions and coordinate sexual activity with rest periods and periods that are relatively free from pain. *This creates a more favorable environment for satisfying sexual activity.*

### Home Care

Provide information about the specific treatment and prognosis for the cancer. Explain the expected side effects of radiation implant therapy (see Chapter 10). ⊖ Pain control measures are also an essential part of the teaching plan (see Chapter 4). ⊖ The resources listed for the woman with cervical cancer are also appropriate for the woman with endometrial cancer.

## THE WOMAN WITH OVARIAN CANCER

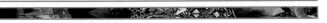

Ovarian cancer is the second most common gynecologic cancer. It is the most lethal, killing an estimated 14,000 women in the United States each year. Approximately 23,000 women in the United States were diagnosed with ovarian cancer in 2002 (ACS, 2002). The incidence increases with age, peaking in women between the ages of 40 and 80 years; half of all cases are in women over 65 years of age. Ovarian cancer is more common in whites than blacks, and mortality rate is highest in whites.

**TABLE 48–4 FIGO Staging Classification for Ovarian Cancer**

| Stage | Description |
| --- | --- |
| I | Growth limited to the ovaries |
| II | Growth involving one or both ovaries with pelvic extension |
| III | Tumor involving one or both ovaries, with peritoneal implants outside the pelvis or positive retroperitoneal or inguinal nodes |
| IV | Growth involving one or both ovaries with distant metastasis |

## PATHOPHYSIOLOGY AND MANIFESTATIONS

There are several types of ovarian cancers: epithelial tumors, germ cell tumors, and gonadal stromal tumors. Most ovarian cancers are epithelial tumors, originating from the surface epithelium of the ovary. Ovarian cancer usually spreads by local shedding of cancer cells into the peritoneal cavity and by direct invasion of the bowel and bladder. Cancer cells in peritoneal fluid can implant in the intestines, bladder, and mesentary. Tumor cells also spread through the lymph and blood to such organs as the liver, and across the diaphragm to involve the lungs. Both pelvic and para-aortic lymph nodes may be involved and tumor cells can block lymphatic drainage from the abdomen, resulting in ascites. Staging for ovarian cancer is based on surgical and histologic evaluation (Table 48–4).

In early stages, ovarian cancer generally causes no warning signs or manifestations. When manifestations do develop, they are often vague and mild, such as indigestion, urinary frequency, abdominal bloating, and constipation. Abnormal vaginal bleeding may occur if the endometrium is stimulated by a hormone-secreting tumor or if the tumor erodes the vaginal wall. Pelvic pain sometimes occurs. An enlarged abdomen with ascites signals later-stage disease.

### Risk Factors

Family history is a significant risk factor, with a 50% risk of developing the disease if two or more first- or second-degree relatives have site-specific ovarian cancer. Other types of inherited risk are *breast-ovarian cancer syndrome* (first- and second-degree relatives have both breast and ovarian cancer) and *family cancer syndrome* (Lynch syndrome II), in which male or female relatives have a history of colorectal, endometrial, ovarian, pancreatic, or other types of cancer (Porth, 2002). The breast cancer susceptibility genes BRAC1 and BRAC2 are implicated in 5% to 10% of hereditary ovarian cancers.

Risk factors also include a high-fat diet and use of powders containing talc in the genital area. Other factors associated with increased risk are prior use of fertility drugs or HRT, and a diet low in fruits and vegetables (ACS, 2001a).

## COLLABORATIVE CARE

As with other malignancies, care of the woman with ovarian cancer is focused on surgery to determine the stage of the tumor and to remove as much of the tumor as possible. Unfortunately, because there are no early manifestations, the disease is often well advanced prior to diagnosis.

### Diagnostic Tests

Tests used in the diagnosis of ovarian cancer may include the following:

- *Blood test* in which patterns of proteins in blood serum can reflect the presence of disease. This preliminary test was able to accurately identify 100% of a small sample of patients with stage I ovarian cancer (National Cancer Institute, 2002).
- *Laparoscopy* is performed to determine definitive diagnosis and organ involvement.
- *Pap smears* are abnormal in up to 30% of women with ovarian cancer.
- *CA125 antigen level* can be useful in detecting ovarian cancer. CA125 is a tumor marker that is highly specific to epithelial ovarian cancer. Transvaginal or transabdominal ultrasonography is used to measure ovarian size and detect small masses. These tests, however, are not appropriate screening measures because they cannot differentiate between cystic or benign ovarian masses and malignancy.
- *CT scans* and *X-ray films* can reveal areas of metastasis.

### Medications

While surgery is the treatment of choice for ovarian cancer, chemotherapy may be used to achieve remission of the disease. Chemotherapy is not curative for ovarian cancer. Combination chemotherapy regimens using cyclophosphamide and cisplatin or other agents may be employed. Chemotherapy with paclitaxel (Taxol) may prolong survival. Close monitoring of bone marrow and renal function is vital while the woman is on chemotherapy because these drugs have significant toxic effects.

### Surgery

In young women with stage I disease who wish to bear children, treatment may be limited to removal of one ovary. Usually, however, total hysterectomy with bilateral salpingo-oophorectomy (removal of the ovaries and fallopian tubes) and removal of the omentum are performed.

### Radiation Therapy

Radiation therapy using external-beam or intracavitary implants is performed for palliative purposes only and is directed at shrinking the tumor at selected sites.

## NURSING CARE

Nursing care for the woman with ovarian cancer is similar to the nursing care for women with other gynecologic cancers.

The side effects of treatment and generally poor prognosis diminish the woman's quality of life and involve major psychosocial implications (see Chapter 10). ⬠

### Home Care

Address the following topics in preparing the woman and her family for home care.

- If a positive family history of the disease or previous breast cancer exists, stress the importance of obtaining regular pelvic examinations. Inform women in this risk group that annual screening with transvaginal ultrasound and CA125 measurements may be recommended.
- Long-term use of oral contraceptives may reduce the risk of developing ovarian cancer.
- It is crucial not to ignore symptoms such as indigestion, nausea, or urinary frequency, as these seemingly unrelated manifestations may be early signs of ovarian tumors. Emphasize, however, that ovarian cancer usually is asymptomatic in early stages.
- Discuss treatment options and their side effects and provide information on ways to minimize or manage side effects.
- Refer to hospice services when appropriate. The resources suggested for the woman with cervical cancer are also appropriate for the woman with ovarian cancer.

# THE WOMAN WITH CANCER OF THE VULVA

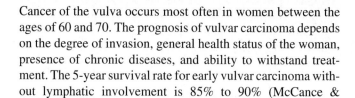

Cancer of the vulva occurs most often in women between the ages of 60 and 70. The prognosis of vulvar carcinoma depends on the degree of invasion, general health status of the woman, presence of chronic diseases, and ability to withstand treatment. The 5-year survival rate for early vulvar carcinoma without lymphatic involvement is 85% to 90% (McCance & Huether, 2002).

## PATHOPHYSIOLOGY AND MANIFESTATIONS

The cause of vulvar cancer is unknown, but there is evidence to associate it with sexually transmitted diseases, particularly human papilloma virus (HPV). Nearly 85% of malignant and premalignant cervical and vulvar lesions have been found to contain HPV DNA, HPV structural antigens, or both. Herpes simplex type 2 (HSV2) infection has also been associated with vulvar cancer. Other risk factors include advanced age, diabetes, and a history of leukoplakia.

Most vulvar cancers are epidermoid or squamous cell carcinomas. The primary site is usually the labia majora, but vulvar cancer is also found on the labia minora, clitoris, vestibule, and occasionally in multiple locations. Metastasis occurs by direct extension into the vagina, perineal skin, anus, and urethra. The cancer also spreads through the lymphatic system via the superficial and deep inguinal and femoral nodes, and to the pelvic lymph nodes.

The woman with vulvar cancer is often asymptomatic, and lesions are discovered on routine examination or self-examination. Discoloration can vary from white macular patches to red painless sores. Lesions may be *exophytic* (proliferating outwardly), *endophytic* (proliferating inwardly), ulcerative, or *verrucous* (resembling a wart).

Pruritus is the most common manifestation, and the woman often has had a history of prolonged vulvar irritation. Perineal pain and bleeding indicate large tumors and advanced disease. In very advanced disease, dysuria related to urethral involvement may be the presenting symptom.

## COLLABORATIVE CARE

The report of itching, burning, or a sore on the vulva merits careful investigation and biopsy of any lesions found. Inguinal lymph nodes may be enlarged. The goal of care is to eradicate the lesion and reduce the risk of recurrence. Surgical resection is the preferred treatment. If lymph nodes are involved, radiation therapy is used postoperatively. Chemotherapy is reserved for distant metastases.

Diagnosis is based on the results of an excisional biopsy of the lesion. Metastasis, if suspected, can be evaluated by chest X-ray examination, barium enema, intravenous pyelogram, cystoscopy, CT and MRI scans, and proctoscopy. Lymphangiography can also be used.

Surgery is the most common treatment for vulvar cancer. The specific procedure depends on the stage of the cancer. Early, noninvasive lesions may be treated with laser surgery,

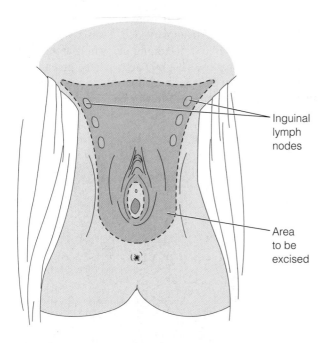

**Figure 48–6** ■ Vulvectomy for vulvar carcinoma. A radical vulvectomy involves removal of the vulva, labia majora, labia minora, clitoris, prepuce, subcutaneous tissue, and regional lymph nodes.

cryosurgery, or electrocautery. For more advanced disease, vulvectomy may be performed (Figure 48–6 ■). A simple vulvectomy involves the removal of the vulva, labia majora and minora, clitoris, and prepuce. A radical vulvectomy is performed if invasion is suspected. This procedure involves removal of all the tissue in a simple vulvectomy, as well as the subcutaneous tissue and regional lymph nodes.

## NURSING CARE

### Nursing Diagnoses and Interventions

Nursing care is similar to that for the woman with endometrial cancer. The woman fears death as the ultimate outcome as well as the possible pain and suffering that surgery and other treatments may cause. Many older women are still sexually active, and radical surgery represents a great loss to them. Disruption of perineal tissues is a priority nursing problem for these women.

### Impaired Tissue Integrity

The woman who has undergone a vulvectomy is at high risk for infection and impaired healing because of proximity of the surgical site to urinary and anal orifices. In addition, the women are often older and may have age-related changes in healing and immune function.

- Teach the woman and/or her partner or other family member the procedure for irrigation of the vulvectomy. If neither is able to perform this procedure, arrange for home health nursing. *Irrigation helps prevent skin breakdown and infection.*
- After irrigation, apply dry heat using a heat lamp positioned about 18 inches from the area; emphasize safety precautions, including use of a low-wattage bulb (40 to 60 watts). *Dry heat helps promote healing and comfort.*
- Provide information on maintaining a diet high in protein, iron, and vitamin C. *These nutrients promote collagen formation and wound healing.*

### Home Care

Explain the association between sexually transmitted diseases such as human papilloma virus (genital warts) and cancer of the vulva. Provide information about safer sex practices such as abstinence, limiting the number of sexual partners, and using condoms (male or female). Explain that early diagnosis and treatment of STIs and other irritative conditions of the external genitalia may reduce the risk of developing vulvar cancer. Teaching for the woman undergoing a vulvectomy should emphasize the potential for skin breakdown, particularly with radiation therapy. Explain that removal of lymph nodes leads to lymphedema and that recurrent cellulitis and sexual dysfunction are common complications of vulvar cancer.

# DISORDERS OF THE FEMALE BREAST

Breast disorders are common conditions that primarily affect women (disorders of the male breast are discussed in Chapter 24). ⊙⊙ When a woman discovers a breast lump, her first response is often fear: of breast cancer, of losing her breast, and perhaps of losing her life. Because American society views the breast as a significant component of feminine beauty, any problem that threatens the breast often strikes at the core of a woman's self-image.

Nurses play a critical role in the care of women experiencing breast disorders by providing education, support, and advocacy. Part of the nurse's role is educating women about normal breast tissue, common benign breast disorders, available screening techniques and risk factors for breast cancers, and breast self-examination.

## THE WOMAN WITH A BENIGN BREAST DISORDER

Benign breast disorders occur frequently in women and may be a source of anxiety. Changes in a woman's breast tissue often correspond to hormonal changes of the menstrual cycle. Most women notice increased tenderness and lumpiness prior to menses. (For this reason, it is best to perform BSE after the menstrual period.) Breast tissue changes in response to hormonal, nutritional, physical, and environmental stimuli. More than half of all women who menstruate regularly will find a lump in the breast; 80% of these lumps are benign. Benign breast disorders include fibrocystic breast changes, fibroadenomas, intraductal papillomas, duct ectasia, fat necrosis, and mastitis (Table 48–5).

## PATHOPHYSIOLOGY AND MANIFESTATIONS
### Fibrocystic Changes

**Fibrocystic changes (FCC)** (*fibrocystic breast disease*) is the physiologic nodularity and breast tenderness which increases and decreases with the menstrual cycle. An estimated 50% to 80% of all women experience some of these changes, which include fibrosis, epithelial proliferation, and cyst formation. FCC is most common in women 30 to 50 years of age, and is rare in postmenopausal women who are not taking hormone replacement (Porth, 2002).

FCC includes many different lesions and breast changes. The more common nonproliferative form does not increase the risk for breast cancer. The proliferative form, accompanied by giant cysts and proliferative epithelial lesions, does increase the risk for breast cancer.

Nonproliferative changes may be cystic or fibrous. Cystic change refers to the dilation of ducts in the subareolar, lobular, or lobe areas. Cysts often go unnoticed unless there is pain and tenderness associated with menses. Fibrous changes are infrequent but can occur during the menstrual years. A firm, palpable mass, 2 to 3 cm in size, is typically located in the upper outer breast quadrant following an inflammatory response to ductal irritation.

Women with fibrocystic changes experience bilateral or unilateral pain or tenderness in the upper, outer quadrants of their breasts, and report that their breasts feel particularly thick and lumpy the week prior to menses. Nipple discharge may be present. Pain is due to edema of the connective tissue of the breast, dilation of the ducts, and some inflammatory response; some women report an increase in breast size. Multiple, mobile cysts may form, usually in both breasts (Figure 48–7 ■). Fluid aspirated from these cysts ranges in color from milky white to yellow, brown, or green. If the fluid is tinged with blood, there is reason to suspect malignancy.

### Intraductal Disorders

An **intraductal papilloma** is a tiny, wartlike growth on the inside of the peripheral mammary duct that causes discharge from the nipple. The discharge may be clear and sticky or bloody. When more than one of these growths is present, the condition is called *intraductal papillomatosis*. This condition is most common in women in their 30s and 40s. The lesion must be investigated to rule out malignancy.

**Mammary duct ectasia** (*plasma cell mastitis*) is a palpable lumpiness found beneath the areola. Duct ectasia involves periductal inflammation, dilation of the ductal system, and accumulation of fluid and dead cells that block the involved ducts. The condition usually occurs in perimenopausal women and is difficult to differentiate from cancer.

Manifestations of mammary duct ectasia include sticky, thick nipple discharge with burning and itching around the nipple, and inflammation. The discharge may be green, greenish brown, or bloody. Nipple retraction often is associated with duct ectasia in postmenopausal women.

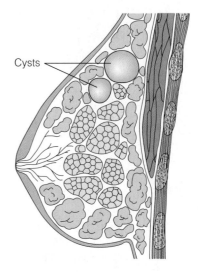

Cysts

**Figure 48–7** ■ Fibrocystic breast changes.

**TABLE 48–5  Summary of Common Breast Disorders**

| Condition | Age | Pain | Nipple Discharge | Location | Consistency and Mobility | Diagnosis and Treatment |
|---|---|---|---|---|---|---|
| Duct ectasia | 35 to 55 years; median age 40 | Burning around nipple | Sticky, multicolored; usually bilateral | No specific location | Retroareolar mass with advanced disease | Open biopsy; local excision of diseased portion of breast |
| Fibroadenoma | 15 to 39 years; median age 20 | No | No | No specific location | Mobile, firm, smooth, well delineated mass | Mammography, surgical or needle biopsy; excision of the tumor |
| Fibrocystic breast disease | 20 to 49 years; median age 30 (may subside with menopause) | Yes | No | Upper outer quadrant | Bilateral multiple lumps influenced by the menstrual cycle | Needle aspiration; observation; biopsy if there is an unresolved mass or mammographic changes |
| Intraductal papilloma | 35 to 55 years; median age 40 | Yes | Serous or sanguineous; usually unilateral from one duct | No specific location | Usually soft, poorly delineated mass | Pap smear of nipple discharge; biopsy; wedge resection |
| Mastitis, acute | Childbearing years | Tenderness, pain | No | No specific location | Generalized redness of overlying skin | Antibiotic therapy; incision and drainage if mastitis progresses to an abscess |
| Mastitis, chronic | Any age | Tenderness, pain; headache; high fever | No | No specific location | Generalized redness and swelling | Antibiotics, usually penicillin |
| Fat necrosis | Any age | Tenderness | No | No specific location | Firm, irregular, palpable | Surgical biopsy to rule out cancer |

## COLLABORATIVE CARE

Diagnosis of fibrocystic breast changes is based on complete history, physical examination, and imaging studies. A biopsy may be required for diagnosis.

Analysis of nipple discharge, mammography, and possibly ductography may be used to diagnose ductal disorders. The affected duct is excised in an open biopsy procedure. Nursing care for the woman is similar to that for any client with an open biopsy. It also is important to reassure the woman that these disorders are not breast cancer.

The treatment is usually symptomatic. Cyst aspiration may relieve pain, and also allows examination of fluid to confirm the cystic nature of the disease. A well-fitting brassiere that provides good support worn day and night helps relieve discomfort. Some women report that eliminating xanthines (found in coffee, tea, cola and chocolate) from the diet decreases symptoms. Aspirin, mild analgesics, local heat or cold, and vitamin E may help relieve breast pain. Hormone therapy is controversial because of the benign nature of the disease and potential adverse effects of therapy. Danazol, a synthetic androgen, may be prescribed for women with severe pain.

## NURSING CARE

When a woman presents with a breast mass, nursing responsibilities include taking a careful history and facilitating follow-up care. If a palpable mass is present, it is important to ask how long the lesion has been present and whether the woman has noticed any pain associated with the mass, any change in its size, and any changes in association with the menstrual cycle.

In many cases, definitive diagnosis of the breast disorder requires surgical biopsy to rule out cancer. During the diagnostic process, the nurse can provide emotional support and education about diagnostic and therapeutic procedures, self-care and comfort measures, and resources to help the woman cope with the experience.

## THE WOMAN WITH BREAST CANCER

**Breast cancer** is the unregulated growth of abnormal cells in breast tissue. Breast cancer is the most commonly occurring cancer in women and the second leading cause of death in women in the United States. The American Cancer Society (2002a) estimates that more than 200,000 women will be diagnosed with breast cancer each year, and approximately 40,000 women will die from it annually. There are racial differences in the incidence and mortality of breast cancer (see the Focus on Diversity box below).

Possible causes of breast cancer include environmental, hormonal, reproductive, and hereditary factors. Two breast cancer susceptibility genes have been identified: BRCA1 on chromosome 17 and BRCA2 on chromosome 13. These genes may be responsible for the approximately 8% of women with hereditary breast cancer. A woman with identified mutations in BRCA1 (known to be involved in tumor suppression) has a lifetime risk of 56% to 85% for breast cancer and also has an increased risk for ovarian cancer (Porth, 2002). Mutations of a tumor suppressor gene, are also linked to increased risk for breast cancer

## PATHOPHYSIOLOGY

Cancer of the breast begins as a single transformed cell and is hormone dependent. Cancers of the breast are classified as noninvasive (in situ) or invasive, depending on the penetration of the tumor into surrounding tissue. Breast cancer may remain a noninvasive disease, or an invasive disease without metastasis, for long periods of time. Two atypical types of breast cancer are inflammatory carcinoma and Paget's disease.

Breast cancer may be categorized as carcinoma of the mammary ducts, carcinoma of mammary lobules, or sarcoma of the breast. Most breast cancers are adenocarcinomas and

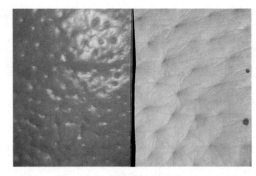

**Figure 48–8** ■ *Left,* Orange peel; *Right,* Peau d'orange sign.

*Source: CNRI/Phototake, Inc.*

appear to arise in the terminal section of the breast ductal tissue. There are many histologic types of breast cancer, and only examples are described here. The most common type is *infiltrating ductal carcinoma,* accounting for approximately 70% of cases (McCance & Huether, 2002). Inflammatory carcinoma of the breast, a systemic disease, is the most malignant form of breast cancer. Edema of the skin (*peau d'orange*) is usually present (Figure 48–8 ■). *Paget's disease* is a rare type of breast cancer involving infiltration of the nipple epithelium (Figure 48–9 ■).

Breast cancer can metastasize to other sites through the bloodstream or lymphatic system. The common sites of metastasis of breast cancer are bone, brain, lung, liver, skin, and lymph nodes. Staging is a system of classifying cancer according to the size of the tumor, involvement of lymph nodes, and metastasis to distant sites, and the presence/absence of distant metastasis (Table 48–6). The staging of the breast cancer provides important information for making decisions about treatment options and is also used as a basis for prognosis.

## MANIFESTATIONS

The manifestations of breast cancer may include a nontender lump in the breast (most often in the upper outer quadrant, the area with the most glandular tissue), abnormal nipple discharge, a rash around the nipple area, nipple retraction, dim-

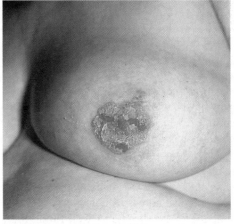

**Figure 48–9** ■ Paget's disease of the nipple.

*Source: Carroll H. Weiss/Camera M.D. Studios.*

## Focus on Diversity

### INCIDENCE AND MORTALITY FOR BREAST CANCER IN WOMEN

• Breast cancer is more prevalent in African American women up to the age of 40 years.
• Breast cancer is more prevalent in Caucasian women over the age of 40 years.
• Asian, Hispanic, and American Indian women have a lower risk of developing breast cancer.
• African American women are more likely to die from the cancer because they are often diagnosed at an advanced stage.

## TABLE 48-6   Staging of Breast Cancer

| Stage | Tumor | Node | Metastasis |
|---|---|---|---|
| 0 | Tis–Carcinoma in situ or Paget's disease of the nipple | N0–No regional lymph node metastasis | M0–No evidence of distant metastasis |
| I | T1–Tumor no larger than 2 cm | N0 | M0 |
| IIA | T0–No evidence of primary tumor<br>T1 | N1–Metastasis to movable ipsilateral axillary nodes | M0 |
| | T2–Tumor no larger than 5 cm | N0 | M0 |
| IIB | T2 | N1 | M0 |
| | T3–Tumor larger than 5 cm | N0 | M0 |
| IIIA | T0<br>T1<br>T2 | N2–Metastasis to ipsilateral fixed axillary nodes | M0 |
| | T3 | N1 | M0 |
| | | N2 | M0 |
| IIIB | T4–Tumor of any size with direct extension to chest wall or skin | Any N | M0 |
| | Any T | N3–Metastasis to ipsilateral internal mammary lymph nodes | M0 |
| IV | Any T | N0 and N1 | M1–Distant metastasis |

## Manifestations of Breast Cancer

- Breast mass or thickening
- Unusual lump in the underarm or above the collarbone
- Persistent skin rash near the nipple area
- Flaking or eruption near the nipple
- Dimpling, pulling, or retraction in an area of the breast
- Nipple discharge
- Change in nipple position
- Burning, stinging, or pricking sensation

pling of the skin, or a change in the position of the nipple (see the box above). Breast cancer is usually painless, but some women report a burning or stinging sensation. Many women with breast cancer have no symptoms, and their tumors are detected by mammography. However, most breast cancers are found by the women themselves (during breast self-examination or a shower) or by their partners during sexual activity.

### Risk Factors

Of the various kinds of risk factors for breast cancer, some can be changed and some cannot. Those that cannot be changed are:

- Being an aging woman (see the box below). Women are 100 times more likely to have breast cancer than are men, with the risk increasing with age. About 77% of women with breast cancer are over the age of 50 when diagnosed (ACS, 2001).
- Genetic risk factors (as previously described).

## Nursing Care of the Older Adult

### OLDER WOMEN WITH BREAST CANCER

- Although the incidence of breast cancer is increasing among premenopausal women, it is still primarily a disease of older women. However, the needs of older women with breast cancer have been inadequately addressed in the professional literature and in the popular media.
- Women between the ages of 50 and 65 are the group most likely to benefit from annual screening mammography, yet many women in this age group have never had a mammogram. Failure of physicians to refer older women for mammography is the reason most frequently cited for this statistic; nurse practitioners and female physicians are more likely to refer women for mammography. Promotional campaigns for mammography send a confusing message by showing images of women in their 20s and 30s for whom mammography is largely ineffective, rather than women in older age groups who are more likely to benefit from mammography.

- For too long, mastectomy was perceived as the only treatment option open to most older women with breast cancer, even those with early-stage disease. Slowly that perception is changing as breast-conservation treatment gains greater acceptance. The choice of surgical treatment, particularly for older women, is highly individual. Many older women wish to preserve their breasts.
- Although older women with breast cancer may experience coexisting chronic illnesses and impaired physical function, research suggests that they show lower levels of emotional distress than younger women. Obviously the need for services such as personal care, shopping, housekeeping, and transportation increases as the ages of the woman and the caregiver increase.

- Family history of breast cancer. Relatives from either the maternal or paternal side of the family. Having a first-degree relative (mother, sister, or daughter) with breast cancer approximately doubles the risk, and having two first-degree relatives increases it fivefold. Having a male family member with breast cancer also poses an increased risk.
- Personal history of breast cancer. A woman with cancer in one breast has a three to fivefold increase in risk for developing a new cancer in the other breast or in a different part of the same breast.
- Previous breast biopsy. If earlier breast biopsies were diagnosed as proliferative, then breast disease without atypical hyperplasia increases risk by 1.5 to 2 times. A previous biopsy of atypical hyperplasia increases risk by 4 to 5 times.
- Previous breast irradiation. Radiation of the chest as a child or young woman for other cancer (such as Hodgkin's disease) significantly increases the risk.
- Menstrual history. Women who begin menstruating before the age of 12 or who have menopause after the age of 50 are at a slightly higher risk.

Lifestyle related factors and breast cancer risk include using oral contraceptives, not having children or having them after the age of 30, using HRT for more than 5 years, not breast feeding, drinking alcohol (especially two to five drinks daily), obesity, high-fat diets, physical inactivity, and (possibly) environmental pollution. Risk factors that have been postulated, but have not been proven, include using antiperspirants, wearing underwire bras, smoking, induced abortion, and breast implants.

## COLLABORATIVE CARE

Diagnosis of breast cancer begins with detection, either detection of asymptomatic lesions discovered through screening or symptomatic lesions discovered by the woman. Any palpable mass requires evaluation. Once the diagnosis is made, a number of treatment options are available. The choice of treatment depends on several factors, such as the stage of the cancer, the age of the woman, and the woman's preferences.

### Diagnostic Tests

The following diagnostic tests may be ordered to diagnoses breast cancer.

- *Clinical breast examination (CBE)* is the inspection and palpation of the breasts and axillae performed by a trained health professional. The physical examination includes inspection, palpation, and a check for nipple discharge (see Chapter 46).
- *Mammogram* is a low-dose X-ray study of the breast used to detect breast lesions. Although mammography can detect breast tumors 2 years before they reach palpable size, most of these tumors have been present for 8 to 10 years. Although controversy exists about the ability of screening mammography to improve mortality rates for women under 50, the American Cancer Society (2002) recommends annual screening beginning at age 40.

- *Percutaneous needle biopsy* defines cystic masses or fibrocystic changes and provides specimens for cytologic examination. In aspiration biopsy or fine-needle aspiration biopsy, a fine needle is used to remove cells or fluid from the breast lesion (Figure 48–10A ■). In many facilities, fine-needle aspiration biopsies are performed using a stereotactic biopsy device; mammography and a computer are used to guide the needle.
- *Stereotactic needle biopsy* obtains cells for histologic evaluation.
- *Excisional biopsy* removes the entire lump (Figure 48–10B). See the box on page 1585 for nursing implications for a breast biopsy.
- *Ductal lavage and nipple aspiration* withdraw fluid to analyze for abnormal cells.

### Medications

Adjuvant (additional) systemic therapy following primary treatment for early-stage breast cancer refers to the administration of chemotherapy or hormonal therapy. This type of therapy has been widely studied; its use reduces the rates of recurrence and death from breast cancer.

Tamoxifen citrate (Nolvadex) is an oral medication that interferes with estrogen activity. It is used to treat advanced breast

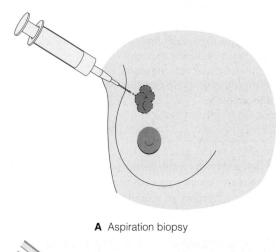

**A** Aspiration biopsy

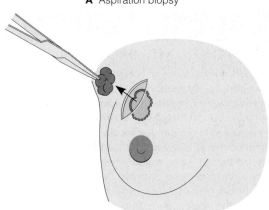

**B** Excisional biopsy

**Figure 48–10** ■ Types of breast biopsy. *A,* In an aspiration biopsy, a needle is used to aspirate fluid or tissue from the breast. *B,* In an excisional biopsy, tissue from the breast lesion is removed surgically.

## Nursing Implications for Diagnostic Tests

### Breast Biopsy

#### PREPARATION OF THE WOMAN

##### All Biopsies
- Ensure that the consent form is signed.
- Acknowledge that preoperative anxiety is normal. It is important to remember that 80% of all breast lesions are benign.

#### WOMAN AND FAMILY TEACHING

##### Aspiration Biopsy (Fine-Needle Aspiration Biopsy)
- A needle will be used to remove tissue and/or fluid from the breast lesion. This procedure may be done in the surgeon's office and takes only a few minutes.
- Aspirated tissue is sent for histologic examination to determine whether it is cancerous. Results are sent to the surgeon within a few days.
- Mild analgesics are usually sufficient to relieve postbiopsy pain.

##### Stereotactic Core Biopsy (Tru-Cut Biopsy)
- The woman lies face down on a special stereotactic biopsy table with a hole through which her breast protrudes. The breast is anesthetized, the lesion located by mammography, and a computer-guided hollow-core needle enters the breast at high speed and withdraws a core of tissue.
- The tissue is sent for histologic examination to determine whether it is cancerous. Results are available within 36 hours.
- Mild analgesics are usually sufficient to relieve postbiopsy pain.

##### Incisional or Excisional Biopsy
- The needle-wire localization procedure provides a guide for the surgeon to follow. This procedure involves a mammogram followed by insertion of a hollow needle and one or more wires into the lesion. Dye may be injected through the hollow needle; the dye may cause a stinging sensation. The woman is then taken to the operating room with the wires in place for the biopsy.
- The biopsy is generally performed in an ambulatory surgery center using local anesthesia. If the woman has large breasts or is at high risk for complications, the surgeon may prefer to use the standard operating room.
- In an incisional biopsy, a section of tissue is removed from the breast lesion and sent for histologic examination.
- In an excisional biopsy, the entire lesion is removed along with a surrounding margin of normal-looking tissue. The specimen is then sent for mammographic and histologic analysis, to be sure that the entire lesion has been removed and to determine whether it is cancerous.
- A screen shields the operative area from view. A nurse stands within view of the woman to explain what's happening, answer questions, and offer emotional support.
- If there is any painful sensation, the woman needs to ask for additional anesthesia.
- The surgeon closes the internal incision with absorbable sutures and secures the skin with sutures or tape. A gauze dressing is applied to protect the area.
- Postoperative pain, bruising, or scarring varies according to the surgeon's technique and the woman's tissue. It is helpful to wear a bra and to apply ice packs periodically. Mild analgesics are generally sufficient to control pain.
- Results of the biopsy are usually available within a few days.

## Medication Administration

### Tamoxifen

#### Tamoxifen (Nolvadex)

Tamoxifen is the most widely prescribed breast cancer drug, commonly given to prevent recurrence of estrogen-positive breast cancer in postmenopausal women. It inhibits tumor growth by blocking the estrogen receptor sites of cancer cells. Tamoxifen increases a woman's risk of developing endomerial cancer, deep vein thrombosis (DVT), and pulmonary embolism.

#### Nursing Responsibilities
- Assess for potential contraindications to therapy.
- Assess liver function tests; tamoxifen may interfere with liver function.

#### Client and Family Teaching
- If in childbearing years, use a nonhormonal, barrier form of contraception; tamoxifen has adverse effects on the developing fetus.
- Take the drug as prescribed until the physician indicates otherwise.
- Side effects such as hot flashes, vaginal dryness, irregular periods, and weight gain are commonly experienced by women taking tamoxifen.
- Do not smoke while taking tamoxifen; smoking further increases the risk of DVT.
- Promptly report any abnormal vaginal bleeding (nonmenstrual bleeding, bleeding after menopause) to your primary care provider.

cancer, as an adjuvant for early-stage breast cancer, and as a preventive treatment for women at high risk of developing breast cancer. Nursing implications for tamoxifen are presented in the Medication Administration box above.

Chemotherapy has become the standard of care for the majority of breast cancer cases with axillary node involvement. In late metastatic disease, chemotherapy becomes the primary treatment to prolong the woman's life. Chemotherapy is discussed in Chapter 10. ∞

Immunotherapy, using trastuzumab (Herceptin), is used to stop the growth of breast tumors that express the HER2/neu receptor (which binds an epidermal growth factor that contributes to cancer cell growth) on their cell surface. This drug is a recombinant DNA-derived monoclonal antibody that binds to the receptor, inhibiting tumor cell proliferation.

## Treatments

The choice of systemic treatment depends on the woman's age, stage of cancer, and other individual factors. Breast cancer tends to be more aggressive in premenopausal women, probably because of hormonal factors. Thus, treatment regimens for premenopausal women are also more aggressive.

### Surgery

Until recently, the treatment of choice for breast cancer was a radical mastectomy. The trend now is toward more conservative surgery combined with chemotherapy, hormone therapy, or radiation, depending on the stage of the tumor and the age of the woman.

**MASTECTOMY.** There are various types of mastectomy for breast cancer. *Radical mastectomy* is the removal of the entire affected breast, the underlying chest muscles, and the lymph nodes under the arms. *Simple mastectomy* is the removal of the complete breast only. *Segmental mastectomy* or *lumpectomy* (Figure 48–11A ■) is the removal of the tumor and the surrounding margin of breast tissues. *Modified radical mastectomy* is the removal of the breast tissue and lymph nodes under the arm (axillary node dissection), leaving the chest wall muscles intact (Figure 48–11B). See the box on page 1587 for the nursing care of a woman having a mastectomy.

Axillary node dissection is generally performed with all invasive breast carcinoma to stage the tumor. Because this surgery can cause **lymphedema** (accumulation of fluid in the soft tissues of the arm caused by removal of lymph channels), nerve damage, and adhesions, and because of the role of the lymph nodes in immune system function, nonsurgical methods of detecting lymph node involvement are being used. *Sentinel node biopsy* is conducted by injecting a radioactive substance or dye into the region of the tumor. The dye is carried to the first (sentinel) lymph node to receive lymph from the tumor and would therefore be the node most likely to contain cancer cells if the cancer had metastasized. If the sentinel node is positive, more nodes are removed. If it is negative, further node evaluation is usually not indicated.

Breast conservation surgery (*lumpectomy*) may be defined as excision of the primary tumor and adjacent breast tissue followed by radiation therapy. Many women are candidates for this procedure; however, women who have multicentric breast neoplasms and those who have large tumors in relation to their breast size are examples of unsuitable candidates. Selection of women for this procedure is guided by the need for local control of the lesion, cosmetic results, and personal preference.

**BREAST RECONSTRUCTION.** After a mastectomy, some women may choose to have their breast reconstructed. They report that surgical reconstruction of the breast simplifies their lives and restores a sense of body integrity. Other women choose to use a removable breast prosthesis, and some women are comfortable without reconstruction or a prosthesis.

Breast reconstruction may be performed at the time of the mastectomy or at any time thereafter, depending on the woman's preference. A number of procedures may be used for the breast reconstruction (Figure 48–12 ■). These include placement of a submuscular implant, the use of a tissue expander followed by an implant, the transposition of muscle and blood supply from the abdomen or back, or using (most often) the transverse rectus abdominis myocutaneous (TRAM) free tissue flap. Nursing implications for the care of women undergoing breast reconstruction surgery are summarized in the box on page 1588.

### Radiation Therapy

Radiation therapy is typically used following breast cancer surgery to destroy any remaining cancer cells that could cause

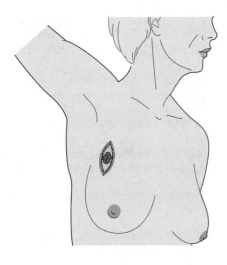

**A** Lumpectomy

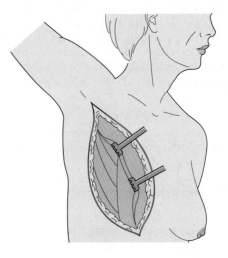

**B** Modified radical mastectomy

**Figure 48–11** ■ Types of mastectomy. *A*, In a lumpectomy, only the tumor and a small margin of surrounding tissue are removed. *B*, In a modified radical mastectomy, all breast tissue and the underarm lymph nodes are removed, but the underlying muscles remain.

## NURSING CARE OF THE WOMAN HAVING A MASTECTOMY

### NURSING RESPONSIBILITIES

- Ensure that the woman or family member signs informed consent form.
- See Chapter 7 ⊂⊃ for preoperative preparation.

### Client and Family Teaching

- Deep-breathing exercises are important because after general anesthesia, it is difficult for air to reach the lungs, particularly with the restrictive surgical dressing that decreases chest expansion.
- A suction apparatus will be placed in the wound to allow drainage of excess body fluids that accumulate when the lymph nodes are removed. This device is usually removed 3 to 5 days after surgery.
- An IV line may be in place for fluid replacement and antibiotics to reduce the risk of postoperative infection.
- Control pain by using the patient-controlled analgesia device or requesting analgesics before pain becomes severe. Take analgesics as needed before performing recommended exercises to facilitate full movement.
- Note any signs of bleeding on the dressing or on the bedding.
- Numbness or feelings of "pins and needles" in the axillary area are common.

- Lying on one's back or on the side not operated on helps fluid drain from the site.
- Moving the arm on the operated side helps regain mobility; specific exercises will be prescribed for increasing mobility after the incisions have healed.
- If fluid builds up after the drains have been removed, it can be aspirated by the surgeon.
- Use caution about lifting heavy objects with the arm on the operated side.
- Be careful about injury and infection on the affected side; wear rubber gloves when washing dishes, garden gloves when working outside. Request that caregivers not perform blood pressures or venipunctures on the operative side to reduce the risk of injury and infection.
- Feelings of anxiety, sadness, and fear of looking at the incision are normal; mastectomy means abrupt change in body image. It is normal to mourn the loss of a breast and to fear the loss of one's life after a cancer diagnosis.
- Sexual intimacy can be affected by mastectomy; it often helps to be able to discuss potential sexual problems with one's partner, with a counselor, or with a breast cancer support group.

recurrence or metastasis. If a tumor is unusually large, radiation may be used to shrink the tumor prior to surgery. Radiation therapy is most commonly used in combination with lumpectomy for early stage (I or II) breast cancer. Palliative radiation therapy is also used to treat chest wall recurrences and some bone metastases to help control pain and prevent fractures. Radiation therapy is administered by means of an external-beam or tissue implants (see Chapter 10). ⊂⊃

A new experimental radiation treatment (*intraoperative radiotherapy*) is provided by a single, concentrated dose of radiation. During surgery, a probe is inserted into the cavity created by the lumpectomy and radiation equivalent to 6 weeks of doses is emitted for about 25 minutes. If this proves successful, the treatment could make lumpectomy available to more women and prevent the woman from having 6 weeks of daily radiation treatments following surgery.

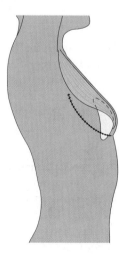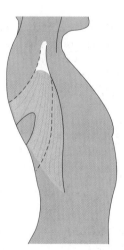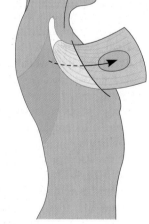

**A** Implant          **B** Latissimus dorsi musculocutaneous flap

**Figure 48–12** ■ Types of breast reconstruction surgeries. *A,* A breast implant is inserted under the pectoris muscle. *B,* Autogenous procedures transfer a flap of skin, muscle, and fat from the donor site on the woman's body to the mastectomy site. The most frequently used donor muscle sites are the latissimus dorsi and the rectus abdominis (the TRAM-flap or transrectus abdominis muscle flap).

## NURSING CARE OF THE WOMAN HAVING BREAST RECONSTRUCTION

### CLIENT AND FAMILY TEACHING

- Controversy exists about the health effects of silicone. While there is no conclusive evidence that silicone implants induce cancer or autoimmune disease, they are associated with hardening and pain due to contracture of the capsule around the implant. The implant may rupture, releasing silicone gel, or infection may occur. Saline-filled breast implants may be an alternative.
- Reconstruction can be done immediately after a mastectomy, or at any time later on. Some surgeons believe that delayed reconstruction offers better cosmetic results.
- Reconstructive surgery can create a natural looking breast that makes clothes fit better. Since it has no nerve endings, however, the reconstructed breast has no feeling or sensations.
- If a simple mastectomy is done, an implant approximately the same size as the other breast is placed under the pectoral muscle on the operative side. This creates a breast mound that closely resembles the natural breast in shape and softness. If the implant is placed over the pectoral muscle, a high degree of firmness may occur.

- With a simple mastectomy or modified radical mastectomy, a tissue expander may be used to replace the breast. The tissue expander is placed under the pectoral muscle and gradually expanded with saline injections every 2 to 3 weeks to stretch the overlying skin and create a pocket. After a period of time, usually 1 to 2 months, the tissue expander is exchanged for a saline implant.
- With more extensive surgery such as radical mastectomy, a flap of skin, fat, or muscle is transferred from a donor site to the operative area. A new nipple may be created by using tissue from the opposite nipple or from the inner thigh.
- Reconstructive surgery may require multiple surgeries, including all the risks associated with anesthesia. As the complexity of the procedures increases, so does the risk of complications such as infection.
- To decrease the risk of a fibrous capsule forming around the implant, it is important to perform breast massage as instructed.

## NURSING CARE

Breast cancer is not one disease entity, but many, depending on the affected breast tissue, the tissue's estrogen dependency, and the age of the person at onset. The psychosocial impact of breast cancer extends beyond the fear and threat of death. The diagnosis may transform the woman's sense of self and lead to reintegration or negotiation of family relationships.

### Health Promotion

The American Cancer Society (2002a) recommends that all women conduct a monthly breast self-examination (BSE) beginning at age 20, have a clinical breast examination every 3 years from ages 20 to 39 years, and have a clinical breast examination and mammogram each year starting at age 40 years.

All women should be taught to perform BSE monthly (Figure 48–13 ■). Premenopausal women should perform BSE after their menstrual period, because hormonal changes increase breast tenderness and lumpiness prior to menses.

Educational messages about breast cancer screening need to be culturally sensitive to the intended audience. Media campaigns promoting mammography often show young white women, an approach that has proved ineffective among women of color (see the Nursing Research box on page 1590). By working with women of different races and cultures, nurses can help make breast cancer education more meaningful to women in these groups.

### Assessment

Collect the following data through the health history and physical examination (see Chapter 46). Further focused assessments are described with nursing interventions following.

- Health history: family history of breast cancer, breast changes, nipple discharge, use of HRT, personal history of breast cancer, previous diagnostic tests and treatment for cancer, menstrual history, pregnancies, alcohol intake, physical activity, dietary history
- Physical assessment: height and weight, breast, lymph glands

### Nursing Diagnoses and Interventions

Although each woman has individual needs, nursing diagnoses prior to surgery are concerned with anxiety, decisional conflict, knowledge deficit, and grief over the loss of a breast. Because the typical hospital stay is short, usually 2 to 3 days, preoperative teaching is done on an outpatient basis.

### Anxiety

The woman with breast cancer is often anxious about the diagnoses, the surgery, the outcome of surgery if nodal involvement is found, and the possible changes in sexual and family relationships. Studies show that young women with breast cancer, a growing population, are particularly vulnerable for anxiety and other psychosocial effects, as are their spouses and their children.

- Provide opportunities to express thoughts and feelings. In this process, the woman can name her fears. *Once the fears are named, the nurse may simply listen, educate, or dispel fears that stem from lack of understanding.*
- Discuss with the woman her knowledge of breast cancer. *Assessing the woman's knowledge of breast cancer helps the nurse plan more effective teaching.*
- Encourage discussion relating to immediate concerns about resuming her life at home and the changes she must make. *Anticipatory guidance can help plan for and cope with changes in her life and relationships.*

**Figure 48–13** ■ Teaching Breast Self-Examination (BSE)

**Step 1** Teach the woman to observe her breasts in front of a mirror and in good lighting. Tell her to observe her breasts in four positions:

- With her arms relaxed and at her sides
- With her arms lifted over her head
- With her hands pressed against her hips
- With her hands pressed together at her waist, leaning forward

Instruct her to look at each breast individually, and then to compare them. She should observe for any visible abnormalities, such as lumps, dimpling, deviation, recent nipple retraction, irregular shape, edema, discharge, or asymmetry.

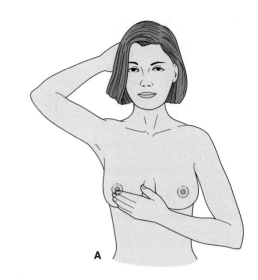

A

**Step 2** Teach the woman to palpate both breasts while standing or sitting, with one hand behind her head (Figure A). Tell her that many women palpate their breasts in the shower because water and soap make the skin slippery and easier to palpate. Show the woman how to use the pads of her fingers to palpate all areas of her breast, using the concentric circles technique (Figure B). Tell her to press the breast tissue gently against the chest wall, and to be sure to palpate the axillary tail.

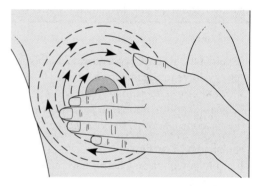

B

**Step 3** Instruct the client to palpate her breasts again while lying down, as described in step 2. Suggest that she place a folded towel under the shoulder and back on the side to be palpated. The arm on the examining side should be over the head, with the hand under the head (Figure C).

**Step 4** Teach the woman to palpate the areola and nipples next. Show her how to compress the nipple to check for discharge (Figure D).

**Step 5** Remind the woman to use a calendar to keep a record of when she performs BSE. Teach her to perform BSE at the same time each month, usually 5 days after the onset of menses, when there is less hormonal influence on tissues.

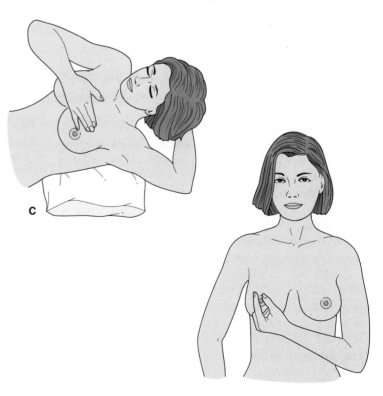

C

D

## Nursing Research

### Evidence-Based Practice for Cancer Screening for African American Women

African American women have a higher mortality from breast cancer than do European American women, despite a lower incidence. This difference may be due to the later stage of diagnosis for African American women when compared with European American women. This study (Champion & Scott, 1997) describes the development of culturally sensitive scales to measure beliefs related to mammography and breast self-examination screening. The researchers found that barriers to mammography such as understanding the procedure, scheduling, child care, and transportation are more relevant to low-income African American than to the predominantly European American, middle-class population with whom previous screening scales were developed. It is important to note that many of the identified barriers related to socioeconomic status rather than race; tools used for screening purposes may translate better among socioeconomic groups than ethnic groups.

### IMPLICATIONS FOR NURSING

Further study is needed to identify the barriers to breast cancer screening among different populations of women. Increasing breast self-examination practices and mammography can eventually help decrease the mortality from breast cancer among African American women.

### Critical Thinking in Client Care

1. What other barriers to breast cancer screening would you identify in women in lower socioeconomic groups? Why are these barriers specific to this group of women?
2. Are there barriers to breast cancer screening that are unique to African American women? To Hispanic women? To Asian American women? How could your teaching and interventions to increase breast cancer screening be tailored to women of different cultural groups?

---

- Explain the surgical procedure, including information about preoperative medications, anesthesia, and recovery. *Knowing what to expect helps to decrease anxiety.*
- Explain that it is normal to have decreased sensation in the surgical area. *Severed or damaged nerves reduce sensation.*

### Decisional Conflict

The woman with breast cancer must make life-changing decisions about treatment within a relatively brief and highly stressful time. Her age, menopausal status, and stage of cancer are only some of the factors that affect her decisions. Culture, values, lifestyle, socioeconomic status, and self-esteem also are considered.

- Provide an opportunity for the woman to ask questions; answer questions as simply and directly as possible. Make eye contact and pay attention to body language. *During this time, the woman can process information and make informed decisions.*
- Focus on immediate concerns, and provide up-to-date written material for the woman to review. *Written material provides easy reference to information not processed immediately because of anxiety and stress.*
- Listen to the woman in a nonjudgmental manner during her decision-making process. *Nonjudgmental, empathic listening helps the woman process information and make informed decisions. Only she knows the context of her life.*
- If the woman wishes, provide opportunities for her to meet with other women who have had breast cancer surgery. *Not all women are ready to meet others in their situation, but opening the door to this resource is appropriate. The woman may choose to talk with these women after the surgery.*
- Facilitate a team approach with the surgeon, anesthesiologist, oncologist, plastic surgeon, and other health professionals. *Being the woman's advocate during this time of anxiety and decision making reduces the stress of coordinating multiple health care provider schedules.*

### Anticipatory Grieving

Breast surgery, even lumpectomy, alters the appearance of the breast. This loss is expressed through grief.

- Listen attentively to expressions of grief and watch for nonverbal cues (failure to make eye contact, crying, silence). *Not all women will express grief clearly; sometimes unspoken grief is the most painful. Grief is relieved only when expressed in a nonthreatening environment.*
- Allow time to interact and do not rush interactions. *Taking time to be with the woman communicates caring.*
- Explain that it is normal to have periods of depression, anger, and denial after breast surgery. *All these feelings are appropriate expressions of grief.*
- If the woman wishes to do so, involve the partner in helping the woman cope with her grief. *Remember that the partner may also be grieving. Not all women want to share their grief, and not all partners are interested and supportive.*

### Risk for Infection

Like any surgical client, the woman who has breast surgery is at risk for infection. Removal of lymph nodes and the presence of a draining wound increase the risk.

- Assess the surgical dressings for bleeding, drainage, color, and odor every 4 hours for 24 hours and document your findings. Circle any visible bleeding and drainage on the dressing as a baseline for subsequent assessment. *Excessive bleeding or drainage signals postoperative complications that may require emergency attention.*
- Observe the incision and IV sites for pain, redness, swelling, and drainage. Assess the drainage system for patency and adequate suction; note the color and amount of drainage. *Careful observation for any signs of infection is essential because the woman's immune system is compromised. IV catheters should be placed on the uninvolved side only.*
- Change dressings and IV tubing using aseptic technique. *Moist dressings and intravenous tubing provide sites for bac-*

terial growth. Routine dressing and IV tubing changes using aseptic technique reduce the risk for infection.

- Encourage a protein-rich diet. Discuss the woman's nutritional status with the dietitian and request a consultation for the woman. Adequate nutrition promotes healing and boosts the immune system.
- Teach the woman how to care for the drainage system, if present (clean the site, empty the device, and record the amount, color, and type of drainage). The woman is often discharged prior to removal of the drainage system and dressings and needs teaching to provide self-care.
- At discharge, teach the woman to watch for and report to her health care provider the manifestations of infection: fever, redness or hardness at the surgical site, or purulent drainage. Any of these manifestations should be reported to the physician/surgeon. Knowing the signs and symptoms of infection prepares the woman to seek prompt treatment if infection occurs.
- Explain that she may experience scaling, flaking, dryness, itching, rash, or dry desquamation of the skin, particularly after radiation therapy. Impaired skin integrity increases the risk of infection.
- Tell the woman to avoid deodorants and talcum powder on the affected side until the incision is completely healed. These substances may irritate the skin and impede healing.

### Risk for Injury

Removal of the lymph nodes puts the woman at risk for injury and long-term complications such as lymphedema and infection.

- When obtaining blood pressure and starting IVs, use the nonsurgical side. Compression of the arm on the surgical side may cause lymphedema.
- Elevate the affected arm on a pillow higher than shoulder, but do not abduct it; the hand should be higher than the elbow. Elevating the arm permits drainage, prevents swelling, and promotes circulation.
- Encourage range-of-motion exercises in the affected arm. Exercise helps develop collateral drainage.
- Explain that lymphedema massage and an elastic compression bandage may help control the swelling after she has recovered from surgery. It is important that women know about the resources available after recovery.

### Body Image Disturbance

Breast surgery can change the woman's body image. The surgical changes may be compounded by weight gain and other side effects of chemotherapy or hormone therapy. Self-esteem also affects adjustment to a changed body image.

- Assess how the woman views her body. Discuss with the woman what image of herself she had prior to surgery. Self-image is related to self-esteem. Discuss whether her self-image has changed.
- Explain that redness and swelling in the scar will fade with time. The knowledge that the scar will fade may give the woman a more realistic view of the changes.

- Include the partner and family if possible when discussing the plan of care and ADLs. Request consultation with a psychologist or other professional if the woman is interested. Discussion with the partner and family can facilitate the woman's emotional healing process.
- Offer pamphlets and suggest books and videos that might increase knowledge about what lies ahead. Knowing what to expect can help the woman cope.

**PRACTICE ALERT** Offer referral to support groups with women experiencing similar problems. Some women may prefer one-on-one counseling. ■

- Encourage the woman to look at her incision when she feels ready; often the reality is not as frightening as the woman had imagined. Explain that it is normal to be afraid to look. Reassurance that her behavior is normal decreases anxiety.
- If the woman is interested in breast reconstruction, provide written material and encourage her to talk with a plastic surgeon and with women who have had reconstruction. It is important that the woman is fully informed about available options to make an informed decision.

### Using NANDA, NIC, and NOC

Chart 48–3 shows links between NANDA nursing diagnoses, NIC, and NOC when caring for the woman with breast cancer.

### Home Care

The woman with breast cancer and her family have much to learn to provide self-care at home. Address the following topics in preparation for home care.

- Manifestations of infection and the need to report any that occur to her health care provider
- The importance of ADLs, such as eating, combing her hair, and washing her face
- Postmastectomy exercises (Figure 48–14 ■) as discussed with physicians and physical therapists
- The need for adequate rest and emotional support
- Participation in a breast cancer support group and on-line information services and bulletin boards for sources of education and support
- Prosthesis management, if this option is chosen (A temporary lightweight prosthesis may be worn immediately after the drains and sutures have been removed from the surgical site. Because prostheses are expensive, a permanent one should not be purchased until the wound has completely healed. Prostheses are available at medical stores and many larger department stores. Most private and government insurance policies pay for the first prosthesis.)
- Helpful resources:
  - Reach to Recovery
  - American Cancer Society
  - National Breast Cancer Coalition
  - National Lymphedema Network

## CHART 48–3 NANDA, NIC, AND NOC LINKAGES

### The Client with Breast Cancer/Mastectomy

| NURSING DIAGNOSES | NURSING INTERVENTIONS | NURSING OUTCOMES |
|---|---|---|
| • Acute Pain | • Analgesia Administration<br>• Anxiety Reduction<br>• Pain Management | • Pain Level<br>• Symptom Severity |
| • Risk for Infection | • Infection Control<br>• Nutrition Management<br>• Skin Surveillance<br>• Wound Care | • Risk Control<br>• Nutritional Status<br>• Tissue Integrity: Skin |
| • Risk for Injury<br>• Impaired Physical Mobility | • Postanesthesia Care<br>• Exercise Promotion: Stretching<br>• Teaching: Prescribed Activity/Exercises | • Safety Status<br>• Mobility Level |
| • Fear | • Anxiety Reduction<br>• Progressive Muscle Relaxation<br>• Spiritual Support<br>• Support Group | • Fear Control |

*Note. Data from Nursing Outcomes Classification (NOC) by M. Johnson & M. Maas (Eds.), 1997, St. Louis: Mosby; Nursing Diagnoses: Definitions & Classification 2001–2002 by North American Nursing Diagnosis Association, 2001, Philadelphia: NANDA; Nursing Interventions Classification (NIC) by J.C. McCloskey & G. M. Bulechek (Eds.), 2000, St. Louis: Mosby. Reprinted by permission.*

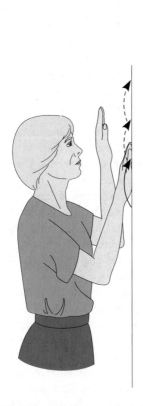

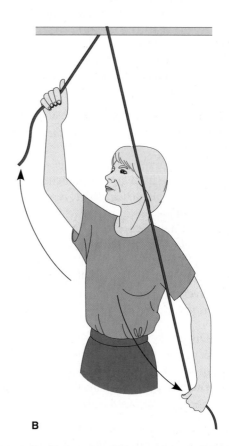

A                                                    B

**Figure 48–14** ■ Postmastectomy exercises. *A,* Wall climbing: Stand facing wall with toes 6 to 12 inches from wall. Bend elbows and place palms against wall at shoulder level. Gradually move both hands up the wall parallel to each other until incisional pulling or pain occurs. (Mark that spot on wall to measure progress.) Work hands down to shoulder level. Move closer to wall as height of reach improves. *B,* Overhead pulley: Using operated arm, toss 6-foot rope over shower curtain rod (or over top of a door that has a nail in the top to hold the rope in place for the exercise). Grasp one end of rope in each hand. Slowly raise operated arm as far as comfortable by pulling down on the rope on opposite side. Keep raised arm close to your head. Reverse to raise unoperated arm by lowering the operated arm. Repeat.

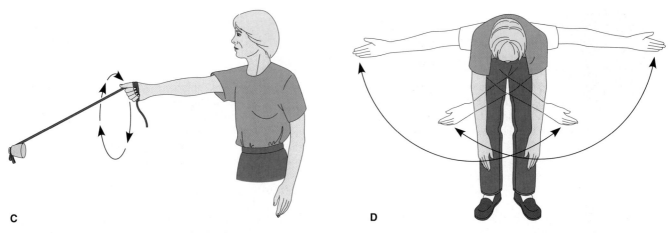

**C**      **D**

**Figure 48–14** ■ *(Continued)* *C,* Rope turning: Tie rope to door handle. Hold rope in hand of operated side. Back away from door until arm is extended away from body, parallel to floor. Swing rope in as wide a circle as possible. Increase size of circle as mobility returns. *D,* Arm swings: Stand with feet 8 inches apart. Bend forward from waist, allowing arms to hang toward floor. Swing both arms up to sides to reach shoulder level. Swing back to center, then cross arms at center. Do not bend elbows. If possible, do this and other exercises in front of mirror to ensure even posture and correct motion.

## Nursing Care Plan
## A Woman with Breast Cancer

Rachel Clemments is a 42-year-old mother of two, Sarah, age 12, and Jennifer, age 18. Because of a family history of breast cancer, she has been closely monitored (annual mammograms and clinical breast examination, monthly BSE, a needle aspiration biopsy with negative findings) for 4 years prior to her diagnosis. Mrs. Clemments discovers a lump in her left breast during her monthly BSE. An incisional biopsy reveals invasive lobular carcinoma in the left breast. Mrs. Clemments is debating whether to have reconstructive breast surgery. Her oncologist has recommended a 6-month course of adjuvant chemotherapy, and she is concerned about side effects. One of her greatest concerns is how her illness will affect her ability to support and care for her daughters. She is afraid that recovering from the mastectomy and completing the chemotherapy regimen will limit her ability to keep her part-time job, complete her academic work, and continue to meet the needs of her daughters. Also, this breast cancer diagnosis seems part of the family legacy. She wonders, "When will it happen to Jennifer? To Sarah?"

### ASSESSMENT
During the history, Laura Nelson, RN, the nurse admitting Mrs. Clemments, learns that her mother, two of her aunts, and one sister had been diagnosed with breast cancer. Her mother and one of the aunts died before age 45. Physical assessment findings include T 98.5°F (37.0°C), BP 110/62, P 65, R 14. Her weight is 120 lb (54 kg); she is 66 inches (168 cm) tall. Modified radical mastectomy is performed; histologic examination shows a 3 cm tumor; axillary node dissection shows that 4 of 16 lymph nodes are positive.

### DIAGNOSES
- *Risk for infection* related to surgical incision
- *Ineffective tissue perfusion* related to edema
- *Acute pain* related to surgery
- *Disturbed body image* related to loss of breast

- *Decisional conflict* about treatment, related to concerns about risks and benefits
- *Interrupted family processes* related to effect of surgery and therapy on family roles and relationships
- *Fear* related to disease process/prognosis

### EXPECTED OUTCOMES
- Remain free of infection.
- Maintain adequate tissue perfusion.
- Experience minimal pain or discomfort during her recovery.
- Maintain a positive body image, regardless of her decision about reconstruction.
- Evaluate the treatment options in relation to personal values and decide on a course of action.
- Together with her daughters, acknowledge the need for a change in family roles during her illness and identify new coping patterns.
- Identify the sources of her fear and demonstrate behaviors that may reduce fears.

### PLANNING AND IMPLEMENTATION
- Teach her about handwashing and wound care.
- Discuss the postoperative drainage device and its management after she goes home.
- Assess her pain tolerance and administer analgesics as prescribed.
- Teach her to use caution when moving the arm on the operated side, to avoid lifting heavy objects, and to wear gloves when gardening.
- Encourage her to discuss her thoughts and feelings about her body changes.
- Suggest that she talk with a Reach to Recovery volunteer about her thoughts and feelings.

*(continued on page 1594)*

## Nursing Care Plan
## A Woman with Breast Cancer (continued)

- Assess her interest in spiritual/religious support and refer if appropriate.
- Discuss medication and dietary changes that will minimize the effects of chemotherapy; request a consultation with the dietitian.
- Provide a list of educational resources about chemotherapy and breast reconstruction.
- Discuss the use of a temporary prosthesis and later the fitting of a permanent prosthesis (6 to 8 weeks after surgery), the need to be fitted by an experienced person, and insurance reimbursement for the prosthesis.
- Discuss the possibility of attending a breast cancer support group where she can draw on the experiences of other women who have undergone mastectomy, chemotherapy, or radiation.
- Refer her and her daughters to social services for a consultation about the changed family roles during her recovery and treatment.
- Encourage her to verbalize her fears about her own prognosis and about her daughters' future risk of breast cancer; assess the need/interest for referral to psychologic counseling.
- Teach her about dietary and lifestyle changes that can help reduce the risk of breast cancer for her daughters (low-fat, high-fiber diet; regular exercise; avoidance of obesity, alcohol, and oral contraceptives).

### EVALUATION

At discharge, Mrs. Clemments has no signs of physical complications and is looking forward to being at home with her daughters as temporary caregivers. Together they decide to try a vegetarian diet and buy a new vegetarian cookbook. Mrs. Clemments met with a Reach to Recovery volunteer, who brought her a temporary prosthesis and booklets about postmastectomy exercises, chemotherapy, and breast reconstruction. The volunteer also referred her to a local breast cancer support group. Mrs. Clemments has talked about her concerns related to breast reconstruction, which center on the possible health risks of silicone. "I want to wait and talk with women who have had reconstruction before I decide," she said. "I want to avoid anything that would increase the risk of complications. The possibility of recurrence and my fear for my daughters' future health are more than enough to worry about."

### Critical Thinking in the Nursing Process

1. What role could genetic counseling play in helping Mrs. Clemments and her daughters better understand the daughters' risk of breast cancer?
2. Describe the types of mastectomies and their implications for nursing care.
3. What medications might help minimize the side effects of chemotherapy?
4. Develop a plan of care for Mrs. Clemments for the nursing diagnosis, *Sleep pattern disturbance*.

See Evaluating Your Response in Appendix C.

# DISORDERS OF SEXUAL EXPRESSION

The normal female sexual drive can persist well into the eighth and ninth decade. The body maintains the capacity for sexual activity and orgasm long after menopause (see the Meeting Individualized Needs box on page 1595). In a typical sexual event, two physiologic sexual responses occur: vasocongestion and myotonia. Sexual stimulation results in vasocongestion of the blood vessels surrounding the vagina, causing engorgement, increased lubrication, and genital swelling and enlargement. Arousal, or myotonia, increases muscular tension, resulting in voluntary and involuntary muscle contraction.

The sexual response cycle has four phases: excitement, plateau, orgasm, and resolution. These phases always occur in the same sequence; however, the duration of each phase may vary. Sexual arousal typically ends in orgasm, or climax, but sometimes fails to do so. The refractory period, or period in which the sexual organs are incapable of responding to stimulus, does not occur in the female. Multiple orgasms are physically possible in all women.

Although nurses may not do sexual counseling, they should be able to obtain a sexual history without embarrassment, discuss sexual concerns with women, and make appropriate referrals.

## PATHOPHYSIOLOGY

Disorders of sexual expression may include dyspareunia, inhibited sexual desire, and orgasmic dysfunction.

### Dyspareunia

The woman with **dyspareunia** (pain during intercourse) may find it difficult to express her feelings to her partner. This condition is more likely to manifest itself as decreased desire or inhibited orgasm. The causes of dyspareunia range from organic to psychogenic.

Physical conditions, such as imperforate hymen, vaginal scarring, or vaginismus, may cause dyspareunia. *Vaginismus* is a rare condition in which the vaginal muscles at the introitus contract so tightly that an erect penis cannot be inserted. An

## Meeting Individualized Needs

### SEXUAL FUNCTION IN THE AGING WOMAN

Myths, taboos, and stereotypes held by society may foster the belief that older women are no longer interested in expressing their sexuality. Two commonly held myths are that menopause is the death of a woman's sexuality and that hysterectomy results in the inability to function sexually. Loss of sexual function is not an inevitable result of aging, although physical changes related to aging do affect the female sexual response. These physical changes, along with chronic conditions common in aging women, may alter a woman's sexual function. In addition, some medications used to treat the chronic conditions associated with aging can also alter the sexual response. It is the role of the nurse to educate women about the myths and misinformation about changes in sexual functioning and to provide information about ways to achieve optimal sexual health.

#### Physiologic Changes

Changes in aging women's sexual function begin in the perimenopausal period as estrogen levels decrease. Estrogen-sensitive cells are found throughout the central nervous system and the cardiovascular system. These cells are involved in the female sexual response. With menopause comes a decrease in the levels of estradiol, which affects nerve transmission and the response in the peripheral vascular system. As a result, the timing and degree of vasocongestion during the sexual response are affected.

Specific changes in the female sexual response occur in all phases. During the plateau phase, the capacity for vasocongestion decreases, as does muscle tension. In the orgasmic phase, the contractions are fewer and less intense. During the resolution phase, vasocongestion subsides more quickly.

#### Nursing Care

The nurse's role in assisting aging women to reach optimal sexual functioning centers on teaching them about the physiologic and psychologic changes associated with menopause. In addition, the nurse should instruct the woman in how the effects of chronic illness and the medications used to treat these illnesses affect sexual functioning. The woman should be taught the importance of maintaining a healthy lifestyle, which includes a balanced diet, weight-bearing and aerobic exercises, stress management, and routine health examinations.

For problems related to vaginal dryness and dyspareunia, the nurse can recommend water-soluble vaginal lubricants or vaginal gels before intercourse. Intercourse on a regular basis and estrogen replacement therapy can also be recommended for these problems. Women who experience joint pain or other musculoskeletal pain due to conditions such as arthritis can benefit from instruction in how to adapt positions for intercourse.

---

early traumatic event, such as sexual abuse, fear of men, rape, or ignorance of sexual functioning contribute to this disorder. However, it is estimated that 90% of dyspareunia is psychogenic in origin. The woman develops an anxiety-fear-guilt cycle in which negative thoughts become associated with the act of vaginal penetration, initiating a conditioned involuntary reflex. Other sexual activity may be quite pleasurable.

## Inhibited Sexual Desire

Inhibited sexual desire may be a result of pathophysiologic processes or may be psychogenic in origin. Often, inhibited sexual desire is rooted deeply in childhood teaching or experiences that may be too painful to recall. Cultural and religious values can also affect the processing of sexual stimuli. Fear of pregnancy or sexually transmitted diseases and depression also contribute to decreased libido.

## Orgasmic Dysfunction

Inhibited female orgasm (**anorgasmia**) is the most prevalent sexual problem among women. However, fewer than 20% of cases are physiologic in origin. It is estimated that from 8% to 15% of women have never experienced an orgasm in the waking state. Psychogenically induced anorgasmia may result from unresolved conflicts about sexual activity. Organic causes of anorgasmia include the presence of disease that re-

sults in general debilitation or that affects the sexual response cycle, and the use of drugs that depress the central nervous system.

Primary anorgasmia exists when a woman has never experienced an orgasm during the waking state, either through self-stimulation or intercourse. Secondary anorgasmia exists when a woman who previously experienced orgasms is no longer able to do so.

## NURSING CARE

Nursing care focuses on identifying the type of disorder of sexual expression through a thorough history, including the onset, duration, frequency, and context or situation in which the problem occurs. The woman's partner should be included in discussions when possible.

Teach the woman and her partner about varied normal and acceptable sexual responses. The goal is to increase self-awareness and understanding of communication and their relationship to sexual desire. Explain the differences in the behaviors that men and women consider sexually stimulating. Sex therapists may provide training in autostimulation techniques (masturbation) after inhibitions against this practice are discussed. Group therapy may be encouraged to help the woman discuss her problem and to decrease the sense of isolation it gives her.

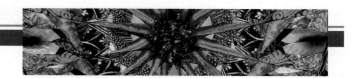

 EXPLORE MediaLink

NCLEX review questions, case studies, care plan activities, MediaLink applications, and other interactive resources for this chapter can be found on the Companion Website at www.prenhall.com/lemone.

Click on Chapter 48 to select the activities for this chapter. For animations, video clips, more NCLEX review questions, and an audio glossary, access the Student CD-ROM accompanying this textbook.

## TEST YOURSELF

1. Your aunt tells you that her health care provider has asked her to begin short-term HRT. She asks you to tell her what good it would do her. Your reply is based on the knowledge that HRT:

   a. Prevents breast cancer
   b. Relieves perimenopausal discomforts, such as hot flashes and vaginal dryness
   c. Increases the risk of bone loss
   d. Has little effect on the physiologic effects of menopause

2. An intervention for the woman with a uterine displacement disorder is to teach Kegel exercises. These exercises may help reduce:

   a. Stress incontinence
   b. Menorrhagia
   c. Vaginal discharge
   d. Retroversion

3. Which of the following topics would you include in a health-promotion seminar to reduce the risk of cervical cancer?

   a. Weight loss
   b. Safe sex methods
   c. Yearly mammograms
   d. A diet high in iron

4. Of the following women, which one would be most at risk for breast cancer?

   a. Age 23, two children
   b. Age 33, never pregnant
   c. Age 45, very thin
   d. Age 64, positive family history

5. You are caring for a woman who is scheduled to have a lumpectomy later in the day. She is crying. What would be an appropriate nursing diagnosis?

   a. *Disturbed body image*
   b. *Fatigue*
   c. *Anticipatory grieving*
   d. *Risk for injury*

See Test Yourself answers in Appendix C.

## BIBLIOGRAPHY

American Cancer Society. (2002a). *Cancer facts & figures 2002.* Atlanta: Author.

_____. (2002b). *New test may spot women at high risk for breast cancer.* Available wysiwyg://19?http://www.cancer.org/epris. . .pot_women_at_high_risk_for_breast_cancer

_____. (2001a). *What are the risk factors for breast cancer?* Available wysiwyg://13/http:/www.cancer.org/epris. . .factors_for_breast_cancer

_____. (2001b) *What are the risk factors for ovarian cancer?* Available http://www.c. . ./CRI_2_4_2X_What_are_the_risk_factors_for_ovarian_cancer

_____. (2001c) *What are the risk factors for cervical cancer?* Available http://What_are_the_risk_factors_for_cervical_cancer

Andrews, G. (2000). Alleviating the misery of premenstrual syndrome. *Community Nurse, 5*(12), 23–24.

Cadman, L. (1998). Lifelong protection from cervical cancer. *Community Nurse, 3*(12), 12–13.

Cahill, C. (1998). Differences in cortisol, a stress hormone, in women with turmoil-type premenstrual symptoms. *Nursing Research, 47*(5), 278–284.

Champion, V. L., & Scott, C. (1997). Reliability and validity of breast cancer screening belief scales in African American women. *Nursing Research, 46*(6), 331–337.

Eliopoulos, C. (2001). *Gerontological nursing* (5th ed.). Philadelphia: Lippincott.

Fentiman, I., & Hamed, H. (2001). Assessment of breast problems. *International Journal of Clinical Practice, 55*(7), 458–460.

Fontaine, K. (2000). *Healing practices: alternative therapies for nursing.* Upper Saddle River, NJ: Prentice Hall.

Foxall, M. J., Barron, C. R., & Houfek, J. (1998). Ethnic differences in breast self-examination practice and health beliefs. *Journal of Advanced Nursing, 27*(2), 419–428.

Grady, D., Wenger, N., Herrington, D., Khan, S., Furberg, C., Hunninghake, D., Vittinghoff, E., & Hulley, S. (2000). Hormone replacement

therapy and blood clots. *Annals of Internal Medicine,* May 2. Available www.coloradohealthsite.org/CHNReports/hrtandclots.html

Hoskins, C., & Haber, J. (2000). Adjusting to breast cancer. *American Journal of Nursing, 100*(4), 26–32.

Hulley, S., Grady, D., Bush, T., Furberg, C., Herrinton, D., Riggs, B., & Vittinghoff, E. (1999). Randomized trial of estrogen plus progestin for secondary prevention of coronary heart disease in postmenopausal women. *Journal of the American Medical Association,* August 19, p. 605. Available www.coloradohealthsite.org/women/women_estrogen.html

Institute of Medicine. (2002). Hormone replacement therapy: Project summary. Available www4/matopma;academies.org/IO

Irvine, D. M., Vincent, L., Graydon, J. E., & Bubela, N. (1998). Fatigue in women with breast cancer receiving radiation therapy. *Cancer Nursing, 21*(2), 127–135.

Jemal, A., Thomas, A., Murray, T., & Thun, M. (2002). Cancer statistics, 2002. *CA: A Cancer Journal for Clinicians, 52*(1), 45.

Johnson, M., & Maas, M. (Eds.). (1997). *Nursing outcomes classification.* St. Louis: Mosby.

Kee, J. (1998). *Handbook of laboratory and diagnostic tests with nursing implications* (4th ed.). Upper Saddle River, NJ: Prentice Hall.

Machia, J. (2001). Breast cancer: Risk, prevention, and tamoxifen. *American Journal of Nursing, 101*(4), 26–36.

Mayo Foundation for Medical Education and Research. (2002). Premenstrual syndrome. Available www.mayoclinic.com/diseases & conditions A-Z.>P> Premenstrual syndrome

Mazmanian, C. (1999). Hysterectomy: Holistic care is key. *RN, 62*(6), 32–35.

McCance, K., & Huether, S. (2002). *Pathophysiology: The biologic basis for disease in adults & children* (4th ed.). St. Louis: Mosby.

McCloskey, J. C., & Bulecheck, G. M. (Eds.). (2000). *Nursing interventions classification (NIC)* (3rd ed.). St. Louis: Mosby.

Murray, R., & Zentner, J. (2001). *Health promotion strategies through the life span* (7th ed.). Upper Saddle River, NJ: Prentice Hall.

National Cancer Institute. (February 7, 2002). Protein patterns may identify ovarian cancer. Available wysiwyg://23/http://newscenter. cancer.gov/pressreleases/proteomics07feb02. html

North American Nursing Diagnosis Association. (2001). *Nursing diagnoses: Definitions and classification, 2001–2001.* Philadelphia: NANDA.

Peters, S. (1997). The puzzle of premenstrual syndrome: Putting the pieces together. *Advance for Nurse Practitioners, 5*(10), 41–42, 44, 79.

Peters, S. (1998). Menopause: A new era. *Advance for Nurse Practitioners, 6*(7), 61–64.

Porth, C. M. (2002). *Pathophysiology: Concepts of altered health states* (6th ed.). Philadelphia: Lippincott.

Resnick, B., & Belcher, A. (2002). Breast reconstruction. *American Journal of Nursing, 102*(4), 26–34.

Shannon, M., Wilson, B., & Stang, C. (2002). *Health professional's drug guide 2002.* Upper Saddle River, NJ: Prentice Hall.

Smith, A., & Hughes, P. L. (1998). The estrogen dilemma. *American Journal of Nursing, 98*(4), 17–20.

Smith, R. et al. (2002). American Cancer Society guidelines for the early detection of cancer. *CA A Cancer Journal for Clinicians, 52*(1), 8–22.

Tiedemann, D. (2000). Ovarian cancer. *RN, 63*(10), 36–42.

Tierney, L. M., McPhee, S. J., & Papadakis, M. A. (Eds.). (2001). *Current medical diagnosis & treatment* (40th ed.). Stamford, CT: Appleton & Lange.

Torgerson, D., & Bell-Syer, S. (2001). Hormone replacement therapy and prevention of nonvertebral trials: A meta-analysis of randomized trials. *Journal of the American Medical Association,* June 13. Available www. coloradohealthsite.org/CHNReports/HRT_ fractures.html.

U.S. National Library of Medicine. (2002). Caution on hormone replacement therapy. Available www.nlm.nih.gov/medlilneplus/ news/fullstory_8434.html

Wolf, L. (1999). Dysmenorrhea. *Journal of the American Academy of Nurse Practitioners, 11*(3), 125–133.

Yarbo, C., Frogge, M., Goodman, M., & Groenwald, S. (Eds.). (2001). *Cancer nursing: Principles and practice* (5th ed.). Sudbury, MA: Jones & Bartlett.

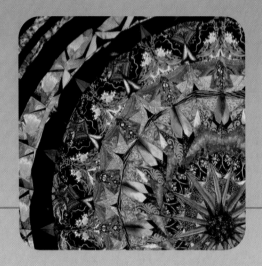

### CHAPTER 49

# Nursing Care of Clients with Sexually Transmitted Infections

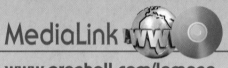

## MediaLink

**www.prenhall.com/lemone**

Additional resources for this chapter can be found on the Student CD-ROM accompanying this textbook, and on the Companion Website at www.prenhall.com/lemone. Click on Chapter 49 to select the activities for this chapter.

**CD-ROM**
- Audio Glossary
- NCLEX Review

**Companion Website**
- More NCLEX Review
- Case Study
  Syphilis
- Care Plan Activity
  Gonorrhea

## LEARNING OUTCOMES

After completing this chapter, you will be able to:

- Apply knowledge of normal anatomy, physiology, and assessments when providing nursing care for the client with a sexually transmitted infection (STI) (see Chapter 46).

- Explain the pathophysiology and manifestations of the most common STIs.

- Identify diagnostic tests and collaborative care used to diagnose and treat STIs.

- Describe teaching to prevent and control STIs.

- Use the nursing process as a framework for providing individualized care to clients with STIs.

Any infection transmitted by sexual contact, including vaginal, oral, and anal intercourse, is referred to as a **sexually transmitted infection (STI).** Infections transmitted by sexual intercourse are also labeled as **sexually transmitted diseases (STDs)** or venereal diseases. STIs are transmitted by intimate and sexual contact, and include systemic diseases (such as tuberculosis and hepatitis) that can be transmitted from an infected person to a partner. This chapter discusses STIs that involve the urogenital system and are sexually transmitted. Every sexually active person is at risk for STIs, and some of these diseases can be life threatening, particularly for women and infants.

This chapter provides an overview of the most common STIs with related collaborative and nursing care. Vaginal infections and pelvic inflammatory disease are included in this chapter as they are often transmitted by intimate contact.

## OVERVIEW OF STIs

### Incidence and Prevalence

STIs have reached epidemic proportions in the United States and continue to increase worldwide. They are the most frequent infections encountered by professionals in the field of reproductive health. According to the Centers for Disease Control and Prevention (CDC) (2000a, b), an estimated 15 million people contract an STI from an infected person each year in the United States and more than two-thirds of those infected are younger than age 25. In addition, viral STIs (considered incurable) affect more than 56 million people: 1 million with HIV, 20 million with genital warts, and 45 million with genital herpes. Some authorities believe that at least half of all Americans have been infected by an STI by age 35.

Women and infants are disproportionately affected by STIs. Many STIs are more easily transmitted from a man to a woman than from a woman to a man. Women often experience few early manifestations of the infection, delaying diagnosis and treatment. Furthermore, women are at greater risk for complications of STIs such as PID and genital cancers.

Several factors help explain the escalating incidence of STIs. The so-called sexual revolution of the 1960s and 1970s, fueled by "the pill" and the freedom from unplanned pregnancy, led to a more permissive attitude about sexuality and increases in sexual activity and the number of sexual partners. In addition, since oral contraceptives were introduced to American women in 1961, they have replaced the condom as a birth control method for many couples. However, oral contraceptives do not protect against STIs, a fact of increasing importance in the age of HIV/AIDS. Indeed, by making the vaginal environment less acidic, oral contraceptives predispose women to infection.

Finally, the emergence of HIV/AIDS has created a kind of "epidemiologic synergy" among all STIs. Other STIs, such as syphilis, HSV, and chancroid, facilitate the transmission of HIV/AIDS, and the immune suppression caused by HIV potentiates the infectious process of other STIs. In fact, individuals who are infected with STIs are 2 to 5 times more likely than uninfected individuals to acquire HIV if they are exposed to the virus. This is the result of several factors: Genital ulcers create a portal of entry for HIV, nonulcerative STIs increase the concentration of cells in genital secretions that can be targets for HIV, and infection with both an STI and HIV results in an increased likelihood of having HIV in genital secretions and semen.

The incidence of STIs is highest in populations with multiple sexual partners and among people of color in urban populations of lower socioeconomic status. People in these groups generally have little information about prevention of STIs and limited access to medical care, two factors that often delay diagnosis and treatment and sometimes limit compliance. Drug abuse, unprotected sexual activity, and sexual activity with multiple partners also are associated with increased incidence of STIs.

All states require reporting of syphilis, gonorrhea, and AIDS to state and federal agencies. Chlamydia is reportable in most states; however, requirements for reporting other STIs vary by state. This uneven reporting of cases means that the exact incidence of many STIs is unknown.

## Characteristics of STIs

Although sexually transmitted diseases are caused by various organisms, they have several common characteristics.

- Most can be prevented by the use of latex condoms.
- They can be transmitted during both heterosexual and homosexual activities.
- For treatment to be effective, sexual partners of the infected person must also be treated.
- Two or more STIs frequently coexist in the same client.

The complications of STIs include pelvic inflammatory disease (PID), ectopic pregnancy, infertility, chronic pelvic pain, neonatal illness and death, and genital cancer. Some STIs can be cured through appropriate early treatment with antibiotics. Others, such as genital herpes and genital warts, are chronic conditions that can be managed but not cured. The most serious STI is AIDS, which at this time is incurable. HIV/AIDS is discussed in Chapter 9. ⊖⊖ Treatment guidelines for STIs are updated regularly and are available from the Centers for Disease Control and Prevention. Nurses have a critical role in the prevention of STIs by teaching clients about these diseases, their prevention, treatment, and potential complications. Table 49–1 summarizes the most common STIs.

## Prevention and Control

The prevention and control of STIs is based on the principles of education, detection, effective diagnosis, and treatment of infected persons; and evaluation, treatment, and counseling of sex partners of people who are infected. The ability of the health care provider to obtain an accurate sexual history is essential to prevention and control efforts.

The most effective way to prevent sexual transmission of HIV and other STIs is to avoid sexual intercourse with an

## TABLE 49-1   Selected Sexually Transmitted Infections*

| Condition/Organism | Signs & Symptoms | Medical Treatment[†] | Complications |
|---|---|---|---|
| Syphilis[‡]<br>*Treponema pallidum* | **Primary:** Painless chancre at site of exposure; regional lymphadenopathy<br>**Secondary:** Skin rash; oral mucous patches; generalized lymphadenopathy; condyloma lata; fever; malaise; patchy alopecia<br>**Tertiary (late):** Infiltrating tumors of skin, bone, liver; *cardiovascular changes:* aortitis, aneurysms; *central nervous system degeneration:* paresthesias, shooting pains, abnormal reflexes, dementia, psychoses | Benzathine penicillin G IM in a single injection *or* doxycycline PO for 14 days<br>Syphilis of indeterminate length or more than 1 year's duration: benzathine penicillin G IM weekly for 3 weeks *or* doxycycline PO for 28 days | Disease progression and transmission<br><br>Disease progression and transmission<br><br><br>Disease progression and transmission<br>Heart failure, blindness, paralysis, skin ulcers, liver failure, mental illness |
| Gonorrhea[‡]<br>*Neisseria gonorrhoeae* | **In females:** Often asymptomatic, but can include abnormal vaginal discharge, abnormal menses, dysuria<br>**In males:** Dysuria, increased urinary frequency, purulent urethral discharge | Cefixime PO *or* ciprofloxacin PO *or* ceftriaxone IM in a single injection *plus* azithromycin PO in a single dose *or* doxycycline PO for 7 days to treat possible coexisting chlamydia | **In females:** Pelvic inflammatory disease (PID), sterility, ectopic pregnancy, abdominal adhesions<br>**In males:** Prostatitis, urethritis, nephritis, epididymitis, sterility |
| Chancroid[‡] (rare in U.S.)<br>*Haemophilus ducreyi* | **In females:** Frequently asymptomatic<br>**In males:** Painful penile ulcers and lymphadenopathy | Azithromycin PO once *or* ceftriaxone IM once *or* ciprofloxacin PO for 3 days *or* erythromycin PO for 7 days | Secondary infection of lesions, fistulas, chronic ulcers |
| Granuloma inguinale[‡] (donovanosis) (rare in U.S.)<br>*Calymmatobacterium granulomatis* | Single or multiple subcutaneous nodules that erode to form painless, bleeding, enlarging ulcers | Trimethoprim-sulfamethoxazole PO for 21 days *or* doxycycline PO for 21 days | Secondary infection of lesions, keloid formations on genitals, tissue necrosis, fever, malaise, secondary anemia, cachexia, and death |
| Lymphogranuloma venereum[‡] (LGV) (rare in U.S.)<br>*Chlamydia trachomatis* (immunotypes L1, L2, or L3) | Painless vesicle or nonindurated ulcer, followed by regional lymphadenopathy, inguinal abscess | Doxycycline PO for 21 days *or* erythromycin PO for 21 days | Ruptured inguinal or perianal abscesses producing draining sinuses or fistulas, nephropathy, hepatomegaly, or phlebitis |
| Chlamydial infections<br>*Chlamydia trachomatis* | **In females:** Asymptomatic but can include dysuria, mucopurulent vaginal or cervical discharge, vaginal bleeding or pelvic pain<br>**In males:** Sometimes asymptomatic but can include dysuria, white or clear urethral discharge, testicular pain (epididymitis) | Doxycycline PO for 7 days *or* azithromycin PO once | **In females:** Pelvic inflammatory disease (PID), infertility, pelvic abscesses, spontaneous abortion, still-birth, postpartum endometritis<br>**In neonates:** Ophthalmia neonatorum or pneumonia<br>**In males:** Nongonococcal urethritis, epididymitis, prostatitis, disease transmission |

\* This table does not include the following STIs discussed in other chapters: AIDS/HIV, viral hepatitis, sexually transmitted enteritis and proctitis, and ectoparasitic infections.

† Treatment recommendations are based on 1998 treatment guidelines by the Centers for Disease Control and Prevention.

‡ Reporting to state and federal agencies required by law.

TABLE 49-1   Selected Sexually Transmitted Infections* (continued)

| Condition/Organism | Signs & Symptoms | Medical Treatment† | Complications |
|---|---|---|---|
| Genital herpes<br>  Herpes simplex virus, usually type 2 but rarely type 1 | Single or multiple vesicles, on the genitals with associated pruritus, followed by painful ulcers | No cure; acyclovir PO *or* famcyclovir PO *or* valacyclovir PO for 7–10 days or until symptoms resolve | **In females:** Potentially fatal infection of fetus or neonate; possible cervical cancer<br>**In neonates:** Neonatal herpes affecting eye, skin, mucous membranes, and possibly central nervous system<br>**In males:** Neuralgia, meningitis, ascending myelitis, urethral strictures, lymphatic suppuration<br>**In both males and females:** Herpes keratitis, a severe eye infection, caused by autoinoculation |
| Genital warts<br>  (Condyloma acuminatum)<br>  Human papillomavirus (HPV) | Single or multiple painless warts on genitals or perianal area | No cure, recurrence in 80% of cases; cryotherapy with liquid nitrogen or cryoprobe, *or* podophyllin 10%–25% in tincture of benzoin compound applied to wart, *or* client-applied podofilox topical solution or gel *or* imiquimod cream | **In females:** Enlargement during pregnancy and obstruction of the birth canal; transmission to fetus or neonate; increased risk of cancer of the cervix, vagina, vulva, and anus<br>**In neonates:** Respiratory papillomatosis, a chronic condition requiring multiple surgeries<br>**In males and females:** Urinary obstruction and bleeding |
| Bacterial vaginosis<br>  *Gardnerella vaginalis,*<br>  *Mycoplasma hominis* | Excessive or foul-smelling vaginal discharge; erythema, edema, and pruritus of the external genitals | Metronidazole PO *or* clindamycin cream 2% *or* metronidazole gel intravaginally for 7 days | Recurrent infections; increased risk of PID |
| Mucopurulent cervicitis<br>  *Chlamydia trachomatis,*<br>  *Neisseria gonorrhoeae* | Mucopurulent cervical discharge | Depends on causative organism; *Chlamydia* involved in 50% of cases | **In females:** Pelvic inflammatory disease (PID), infertility, pelvic abscesses, spontaneous abortion, stillbirth, postpartum endometritis<br>**In neonates:** Opthalmia neonatorum or pneumonia |
| Nongonococcal urethritis (NGU)<br>  *Chlamydia trachomatis,*<br>  *Urea plasma urealyticum,*<br>  *Trichomonas vaginalis,*<br>  herpes simplex | Dysuria, urinary frequency, mucoid to purulent urethral discharge; some men asymptomatic | Depends on causative organism; azithromycin PO in a single dose *or* doxycycline PO for 7 days | Urethral strictures or epididymitis; if transmitted to female partners, may result in mucopurulent cervicitis and PID; if female is pregnant, can cause neonatal ophthalmia or pneumonia |
| Pelvic inflammatory disease (PID)<br>  *Chlamydia trachomatis,*<br>  *Neisseria gonorrhoeae,*<br>  *Mycoplasma hominis,*<br>  and others | Asymptomatic or can include pain and tenderness in lower abdomen, uterus and adnexa, possibly with fever, chills, and elevated white blood count and erythrocyte sedimentation rate | Combined drug therapy such as cefotetan IV *plus* doxycycline IV or PO *or* clindamycin IV *plus* gentamicin IV or IM; may require hospitalization | Ectopic pregnancy, pelvic abscess; infertility, recurrent or chronic PID, chronic abdominal pain, pelvic adhesions, depression |
| Trichomoniasis<br>  *Trichomonas vaginalis* | **In females:** Asymptomatic or can include frothy, excessive vaginal discharge, erythema, edema and pruritus<br>**In males:** Usually asymptomatic but can include urethritis, penile lesions, or inflammation | Metronidazole PO in a single dose *or* for 7 days | **In females:** Recurrent infections, salpingitis, low birth weight infants, prematurity |

## Meeting Individualized Needs

### HEALTH PROMOTION IN CLIENTS WITH STIs

| Barrier Protection | Teaching Topics |
|---|---|
| • Male condoms | ✓ Use a new condom with each act of sexual intercourse.<br>✓ Handle carefully to avoid damaging the condom.<br>✓ Be sure no air is trapped in the end of the condom.<br>✓ Put the condom on when the penis is erect and before genital contact with partner.<br>✓ Ensure adequate lubrication exists during intercourse, using only water-based lubricants (e.g., K-Y® Jelly, Astroglide®, AquaLube, and glycerine) and latex condoms. Oil-based lubricants, such as petroleum jelly, massage oil, mineral oil, or body lotions can weaken latex.<br>✓ Withdraw while the penis is erect and hold the condom firmly against the base of the penis during withdrawal. |
| • Female condoms | ✓ The female condom (Reality®) is a lubricated polyurethane sheath with a ring on each end that is inserted into the vagina. It is an effective mechanical barrier to viruses. |
| • Vaginal spermicides, sponges, diaphragms | ✓ Vaginal spermicides used alone without condoms reduce the risk for cervical gonorrhea and chlamydia. They do not reduce the risk of HIV infection.<br>✓ The vaginal sponge has the same benefit as spermicides.<br>✓ The diaphragm protects against cervical gonorrhea, chlamydia, and trichomoniasis, but not HIV. |

infected partner. It is recommended that both partners be tested for STIs, including HIV, before beginning to have sexual intercourse. If a person chooses to have intercourse with an infected partner or one whose infection status is unknown, a new condom should be used for each act of intercourse (CDC, 1998). See the box above for recommended STI barrier guidelines (CDC, 1998).

Prevention teaching for the person who is an injecting-drug user includes:

• Enroll or continue in a drug treatment program.
• Do not use injection equipment that has been used by another person. If equipment is shared, first clean the syringe and needle with bleach and water (to reduce the rate of HIV transmission).
• If needles can legally be obtained in the community, obtain and use clean needles.

Eliminating further transmission and reinfection of STIs is critical to control. For treatable STIs, this means that referral of sex partners for diagnosis, treatment, and counseling is essential. Gonorrhea, syphilis, and AIDS are reportable diseases in every state, and chlamydial infections are reportable in most states. When a health care professional refers infected clients to a local or state department of health, every effort is made to identify and contact sex partners. Reports of STI and HIV infections are maintained in strictest confidence, and are protected by law from subpoena. Suggested resources for people with STIs are listed in Box 49–1.

### BOX 49–1 ■ Resources for Clients with STIs

■ CDC National STD Hotline
■ CDC National Prevention Information Network
■ National Center for HIV, STD, and TB Prevention
■ National HPV and Cervical Cancer Resource Center and Hotline
■ National Herpes Hotline
■ American Social Health Association

## THE CLIENT WITH A VAGINAL INFECTION

The vagina may be infected by yeasts, protozoa, or bacteria. These infections can be sexually transmitted, but the male partner does not usually have manifestations of the infection. Risk factors include the use of oral contraceptives or broad-spectrum antibiotics, obesity, diabetes, pregnancy, unprotected sexual activity, multiple sexual partners, and poor personal hygiene. Manifestations of vaginal infections are outlined in Table 49–2.

Preventive measures include educating women about personal hygiene practices and safer sex. Women need to avoid frequent douching and wearing nylon underwear and/or tight pants. Unprotected sexual activity, particularly with multiple partners, increases the risk of vaginal infections.

TABLE 49-2   Vaginal Infections

| Infection | Type of Discharge | Typical Manifestations | Treatment | Nursing Care |
|---|---|---|---|---|
| Candidiasis (*Monilia*, yeast) | Thick white patches adhering to cervix and vaginal wall, resembling cottage cheese; little odor | Itching of vulva and vaginal area, redness, painful intercourse | Miconazole, clotrimazole, or terconazole creams or suppositories; povidone-iodine (Betadine) or vinegar douches | Teach perineal hygiene and proper use of vaginal applicators. Instruct the client to complete the entire treatment. |
| Simple vaginalis (bacterial vaginosis, *Gardnerella* vaginosis) | Thin, white, "milklike," or gray with fishy odor, especially when mixed with potassium hydroxide | None to mild itching or burning in vulvar area; clue cells on microscopic examination | Oral metronidazole for client; topical metronidazole or clindamycin for client's sexual partner | Teach proper perineal hygiene. Instruct client to complete treatment. Teach client relationship of infection to PID. |
| Trichomoniasis | Frothy, yellow or white, foul odor | Burning and itching of vulva | Oral metronidazole for client and sexual partner | Teach perineal hygiene |
| Atrophic vaginitis (Senile vaginitis) | Thin, opaque discharge, occasionally blood-tinged, odorless; pale, smooth, thin, dry vaginal walls | Painful intercourse, itching, vaginal dryness | Use of topical estrogen cream; use of water-soluble lubricant for intercourse. Evaluate need for HRT and antibiotic therapy | Counsel client on symptoms of menopause and sexual techniques to minimize trauma |

## PATHOPHYSIOLOGY

Alterations in pH, changes in the normal flora, and low estrogen levels are conducive to the development of vaginal infections. When conditions are favorable, microorganisms invade the vulva and vagina.

### Bacterial Vaginosis

**Bacterial vaginosis** (nonspecific vaginitis) is the most common cause of vaginal infection in women of reproductive age. *Gardnerella vaginalis* is one of the causative organisms, but others are also implicated. The relationship of sexual activity to this infection is not clear, and is believed to be the catalyst instead of the cause. The primary manifestation is a vaginal discharge that is thin and grayish-white, and has a foul, fishy odor. Complications include pelvic inflammatory disease, preterm labor, premature rupture of the membranes, and postpartum endometritis.

### Candidiasis

**Candidiasis** (moniliasis or yeast infection) is caused by the organism *Candida albicans,* which has several strains of different virulence. Candida organisms are part of the normal vaginal environment, causing problems only when they multiply rapidly. When increased estrogen levels, antibiotics, diabetes mellitus, fecal contamination, or other factors alter the normal vaginal flora, the organism proliferates, resulting in a yeast infection. The manifestations include an odorless, thick, cheesy vaginal discharge. This is often accompanied by itching and irritation of the vulva, dysuria, and dyspareunia.

### Trichomoniasis

**Trichomoniasis** is caused by *Trichomonas vaginalis,* a protozoan parasite. Symptoms usually appear in 5 to 28 days of exposure. It most commonly infects the vagina in women and the urethra in men. Most men are asymptomatic. Women have a frothy, green-yellow vaginal discharge with a strong odor, often accompanied by itching and irritation of the genitalia. Trichomoniasis during pregnancy may cause premature rupture of the membranes and preterm delivery. A woman with HIV who becomes infected has an increased risk of transmitting HIV to her sex partner.

## COLLABORATIVE CARE

Collaborative care focuses on identifying and eliminating the infection and preventing recurrence.

### Diagnostic Tests

Diagnostic tests vary with the suspected organism. The following tests may be ordered.

- *Culture of vaginal secretions* is performed and discharge is examined microscopically for the presence of "clue cells" if bacterial vaginitis is suspected.
- If candidiasis is suspected, the discharge is examined microscopically to detect hyphae (filaments or threads) and spores.
- *Normal saline wet prep* is used to detect the presence of protozoa if trichomoniasis is suspected
- *Glucose tolerance tests* or *HIV screening* are performed at the time of the initial assessment, if indicated.

## Medications

The pharmacologic treatment varies with the organism, as shown in Table 49–2. The sexual partner must also be treated to prevent reinfection. Some antifungal agents are available without prescription, which can lead to self-medication with the incorrect agent or allow repeated infections to go unreported.

## NURSING CARE

### Nursing Diagnoses and Interventions

Nursing care focuses on teaching the client and, if necessary, her sexual partner to comply with the treatment regimen, use safer sex practices, and prevent future transmission of the infection. Careful history taking may also reveal high-risk sexual practices that require intervention, particularly if the client has had repeated yeast infections. The initial presenting symptom for many HIV-positive women is vaginal candidiasis, which may be refractory to over-the-counter treatments. Treatment with some antibiotics destroys normal vaginal flora, resulting in superinfection with yeast. Although each nursing care plan must be individualized, nursing diagnoses that often apply to clients with vaginal infections are presented below.

### Deficient Knowledge

Many women are unaware of the causes of vaginal infections and the self-care measures to prevent and treat these infections. If possible, both the woman and her sexual partner should be taught the following information.

- Explain the transmission of the infection. Many infections are transmitted most easily during certain times of the menstrual cycle; some can also be transmitted by towels or other inanimate objects, or by certain types of sexual activity. *A frank discussion of disease transmission and prevention with the woman and her partner can reduce the risk of reinfection.*
- The need to complete the course of treatment. *Many infections are asymptomatic in one partner. Incomplete treatment allows for recurrence of the infection and reinfection of the partner.*

### BOX 49–2 ■ Self-Care Comfort Measures

- Do not wear pantyhose; wear loose fitting pants or skirts.
- Double-rinse underwear; do not use fabric softener on underwear.
- Do not use bubble bath, perfumed soaps, or feminine hygiene products.
- Use 100% cotton menstrual pads and tampons.
- Use white, unscented toilet paper.
- Use a water-soluble lubricant for intercourse.
- Apply ice or a frozen blue gel pack wrapped in a towel to the vulva after intercourse to relieve burning.
- Rinse vulva with cool water after voiding and intercourse.

### Acute Pain

The symptoms of vaginitis can lead to dysuria, painful excoriation or ulceration of tissue, and painful intercourse (**dyspareunia**). Often these symptoms can be relieved by relatively simple self-care measures. See Box 49–2 for additional comfort measures.

- Suggest the use of cool compresses and vinegar or povidone-iodine douches (if approved by the primary health care provider). *Cool compresses relieve itching. Vinegar and iodine are fungicidal and bactericidal in effect.*
- Recommend sitz baths to alleviate discomfort. *Sitz baths cleanse the perineal area and the warmth is soothing to inflamed, irritated skin and membranes.*
- Wear cotton underwear. *Cotton absorbs moisture and allows better air circulation than other types of material.*
- Avoid sexual contact until treatment is completed. *Treatment of the infected woman and her sex partner as well as sexual abstinence are necessary to prevent reinfection.*

### Home Care

Teaching focuses on eradicating the infection, preventing further disease transmission, and relieving discomfort associated with the condition. Educating the client and her partner(s) about safer sex and improved genital hygiene practices can reduce the incidence of recurrence. Unless contraindicated, encourage the client with repeated mild candidiasis infections to consume 8 oz of yogurt containing live active cultures daily to help restore normal vaginal flora.

## INFECTIONS OF THE EXTERNAL GENITALIA

### THE CLIENT WITH GENITAL HERPES

**Genital herpes** (*herpes simplex genitalis*) is the most common infectious genital ulceration in the United States, and is considered epidemic. Although not a reportable disease, it is estimated to affect 1 million individuals each year. Recurrent infections affect an estimated 45 million people annually. The incidence is highest in teens and young adults, and in nonwhite lower socioeconomic populations (McCance & Huether, 2002). Genital herpes is chronic and, in many people, largely asymptomatic. Currently, it is incurable.

While the majority of infected people are asymptomatic, others experience frequent, painful recurrences. Other than recurrences, however, men are not likely to experience serious physical complications of genital herpes. Women, however, face concerns about childbearing (and infection of the newborn during delivery, resulting in death for 6 of 10 infants) and possible cervical cancer, although the risk of malignancy is not clearly established.

## PATHOPHYSIOLOGY AND MANIFESTATIONS

Genital herpes is transmitted by vaginal, anal, or oral-genital contact. Although it may be caused by either the herpes simplex viruses HSV-type 1 (HSV-1) or HSV-type 2 (HSV-2), 80% of initial infections and 95% of recurrent infections are caused by HSV-2. The incubation period is 3 to 7 days. Within 1 week after exposure to genital herpes, painful red papules appear in the genital area. In men, the lesions generally occur on the glans or shaft of the penis. In women, the lesions commonly occur on the labia, vagina, and cervix. Anal intercourse may result in lesions in and around the anus.

Soon after the papules appear, they form small painful blisters filled with clear fluid containing virus particles (Figure 49–1 ■). The blisters break, shedding the highly infectious virus and creating patches of painful ulcers that last 6 weeks (or longer if they become infected). Touching these blisters and then rubbing or scratching in another place can spread the infection to other areas of the body (*autoinoculation*).

The first outbreak of herpes lesions is called *first episode infection,* with an average duration of 12 days. Subsequent occurrences, usually less severe, are termed *recurrent infections* (average duration of 4 to 5 days). The period between episodes is called *latency,* during which time the person remains infectious even though no symptoms are present. During latency, the virus withdraws into the nerve fibers that lead from the infected site to the lower spine, remaining dormant until recurrence, at which time it retraces its path to the genital area.

The manifestations of genital herpes are presented in the box on this page. Prodromal symptoms of recurrent outbreaks of genital herpes can include burning, itching, tingling, or throbbing at the sites where lesions commonly appear. These sensations may be accompanied by pain in the legs, groin, or buttocks. Some authorities believe that prodromal symptoms signal increased levels of infectiousness, during which sexual contact should be avoided.

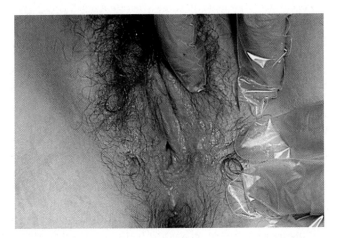

**Figure 49–1** ■ Genital herpes blisters as they appear on the labia.

*Source: Biophoto Associates/Photo Researchers, Inc.*

### Manifestations of Genital Herpes

- Herpetic lesions
- Regional lymphadenopathy
- Headache
- Fever
- General malaise
- Dysuria
- Urinary retention
- Vaginal discharge
- Urethral discharge (men)

In rare cases, the herpes virus spreads to the brain, causing herpes encephalitis, a life-threatening disorder. Prompt treatment with acyclovir (Zovirax) can cure the encephalitis, but more than 60% of survivors have permanent neurologic damage.

## COLLABORATIVE CARE

Because there is no cure for genital herpes, treatment focuses on relieving symptoms and preventing spread of the infection. Client education is essential to prevent further transmission of the disease and to help clients integrate management of a chronic disease into their lifestyles.

Presumptive diagnosis of genital herpes is based on history and physical examination of the client, including lesions and patterns of recurrence. Definitive diagnosis requires isolation of the virus in tissue culture. Ideally, tissue specimens should be obtained within 48 hours of the appearance of the blisters.

### Medications

Acyclovir (Zovirax) helps reduce the length and severity of the first episode and is the treatment of choice for genital herpes. The oral form is considered most effective for first episode as well as recurrences and is given for 7 to 10 days or until lesions heal. It may also be administered intravenously. Evidence shows that some strains of HSV are becoming resistant to acyclovir, particularly in HIV-positive people. In those cases, foscarnet (Foscavir) is used. Other antivirals used for treatment and prevention are valacyclovir (Valtrex), penciclovir (Denavir), and famcyclovir (Famvir).

## NURSING CARE

### Nursing Diagnoses and Interventions

In planning and implementing holistic nursing care for the client with genital herpes, the nurse needs to consider both short-term and long-term implications. Although the immediate priority is symptom relief and prevention of further transmission, the client needs assistance to deal with the life-changing diagnosis of a chronic disease (see the Nursing Research box on page 1606). Nursing diagnoses discussed in this section focus on pain, sexual dysfunction, and anxiety regarding childbearing and possible malignancy.

## Nursing Research

### Evidence-Based Practice for the Client with Genital Herpes

Researchers studied 70 young adults to determine the physical and psychosocial effects of living with genital herpes (Swanson et al., 1995). Stress was found to be the major cause of recurrence, headaches the major stress symptom, and acyclovir the major treatment. Findings indicated that young adults with genital herpes had lower self-concept, more psychopathology, greater frequency of daily hassles, and less intense emotional uplifts than non-patient control subjects. The researchers found no differences between the two groups in scores on depression.

### IMPLICATIONS FOR NURSING

Clients with genital herpes need psychosocial support and counseling as well as education in self-care measures to deal with physical effects of the disease. Teaching stress-management techniques and suggesting alternatives to sexual intercourse, such as masturbation, may be useful. Allowing clients to express feelings and perceptions about how genital herpes has affected their lives can be an important part of counseling. Teaching safer sex practices and communication skills to use with a partner needs to be part of the care of all clients with STIs.

### Critical Thinking in Client Care

1. Do you believe that the threat of contracting genital herpes or another chronic STI will change established sexual behavior patterns among high school and college students? Why or why not?
2. Do people with genital herpes who take appropriate precautions have the right to enter into sexual relationships without revealing that they are infected? Why or why not?
3. Why would the presence of genital herpes increase the likelihood of contracting other STIs?

## Acute Pain

Herpetic lesions are very painful and can become infected. Because the virus resides in the nerve ganglia, pain may also occur in the legs, thighs, groin, or buttocks. Although acyclovir diminishes the pain of herpes and accelerates the healing process, additional measures can relieve the discomfort further.

- Teach how to keep herpes blisters clean and dry. A solution of warm water, soap, and hydrogen peroxide can be used to cleanse the lesions two or three times daily. Burrow's solution can also be used. Lesions should be dried using a hair dryer turned to a cool setting. It is important to wear loose cotton clothing that will not trap moisture; panty hose and tight jeans are to be avoided. *Keeping the lesions clean and dry reduces the possibility of secondary infection and speeds the healing process.*
- For dysuria, suggest pouring water over the genitals while urinating. Drinking additional fluids also helps dilute the acidity of the urine; however, fluids that increase acidity, such as cranberry juice, should be avoided. *These measures dilute the acid content of urine and thereby reduce the burning sensation.*

## Sexual Dysfunction

Clients who learn that they are infected with an incurable STI may believe they can no longer have a normal sex life. Fortunately, many people have learned to live with and manage genital herpes without infecting their partners or their children.

- Provide a supportive, nonjudgmental environment for the client to discuss feelings and ask questions about what this diagnosis means to future sexual relationships. *Feelings of guilt, shame, and anger are natural responses to such a diagnosis and can lead to a total avoidance of sexual intimacy.*

- Offer information about support groups and other resources for people with herpes such as the National Herpes Information Hotline. *Information about how others cope with this disease can offset feelings of shame and hopelessness.*

## Anxiety

The woman with genital herpes faces two serious potential complications: elevated risk of cervical cancer and infection of her neonate during delivery. Some evidence suggests that the risk of cervical cancer is higher among women with genital herpes, although a direct causal link has not been identified. There is no question about the risk of neonatal infection from a mother with herpes, however, and such infection can range from asymptomatic to widely disseminated fatal disease. Transmission occurs during passage through the birth canal. The risk is highest during the first episode of infection.

- Advise the client about need for regular Papanicolaou (Pap) smears; some authorities suggest Pap smears every 6 months for women with genital herpes. *Careful monitoring will detect cervical dysplasia at a time when treatment is most likely to be effective.*
- Discuss with women of childbearing age that cesarean delivery can prevent transmission of infection to the neonate. In women without signs or symptoms of recurrence, vaginal delivery is possible. *Understanding that infection of the neonate can be prevented helps relieve anxiety.*

## Home Care

Health teaching for clients with genital herpes involves helping them manage this chronic disease with the least possible disruption in lifestyle and relationships. Understanding the disease process and factors that affect it helps the client regain a sense of control and see the potential for future sexual intimacy without transmission of infection. The following topics should be addressed.

- How to recognize prodromal symptoms of recurrence and factors that seem to trigger recurrences (such as emotional stress, acidic food, sun exposure)
- The need for abstinence from sexual contact from the time prodromal symptoms appear until 10 days after all lesions have healed
- If lesions become infected, use of topical acyclovir. (Painful lesions can be protected with sterile vaseline or aloe vera gel.)
- Use of latex condoms due to viral shedding at any time and careful hygiene practices (such as not sharing towels or other personal items) even during latency periods

## THE CLIENT WITH GENITAL WARTS

**Genital warts,** also known as *condyloma acuminatum* or *venereal warts,* are caused by human papilloma virus (HPV) and are transmitted by all types of sexual contact. The incubation period for genital warts ranges from 6 weeks to 8 months, with an average of 3 months. The four specific types of warts are as follows:

- *Condyloma acuminata:* cauliflower-shaped lesions that appear on moist skin surfaces such as the vagina or anus
- *Kerototic warts:* thick, hard lesions that develop on dry keratinized skin such as the labia major, penis, or scrotum
- *Papular warts:* smooth lesions that also develop on keratinized skin
- *Flat warts:* slightly raised lesions, often invisible to the naked eye, also develop on kertinized skin

HPV is not a reportable disease, so its exact incidence is unknown, but it is believed to be one of the most common STIs in the United States. Most HPV infections are asymptomatic or unrecognized. An estimated 20 million Americans are infected with the virus, and up to 1 million new cases are diagnosed annually. Like most STIs, genital warts are most commonly found in young, sexually active adults and are associated with early onset of sexual activity and multiple sexual partners.

Several subtypes of HPV are strongly associated with cervical dysplasia. More than 90% of cervical cancers contain DNA of oncogenic (cancer-promoting) HPV subtypes. HPV also is associated with a higher risk of vaginal, vulvar, penile, and anal cancers.

## PATHOPHYSIOLOGY AND MANIFESTATIONS

Although most people carry HPV without symptoms, others exhibit characteristic manifestations: single or multiple painless, cauliflowerlike growths on the vulvovaginal area, perineum, penis, urethra, or anus (Figure 49–2 ■). In women, the growths may appear in the vagina or on the cervix and be apparent only during a pelvic examination.

Potential complications of genital warts include obstruction of the urethra, causing bleeding, and transmission of the virus to the fetus during pregnancy or delivery. Infants infected with HPV can develop respiratory papillomatosis, a respiratory condition causing chronic distress and requiring multiple surgeries. There is also a relationship between HPV and the development of genital malignancies, with the risk believed to be increased by smoking, immunosuppression, and using oral contraceptives.

## COLLABORATIVE CARE

Treatment is directed at removal of the warts, relief of symptoms, and health teaching to reduce the risk of recurrence and future transmission. The HPV is considered chronic, however, with recurrence experienced in 80% of those infected.

### Diagnostic Tests

Genital and anal warts are diagnosed primarily by clinical appearance or by examination of Pap smear specimens. However, therapy is not determined until a VDRL test for syphilis and a gonorrheal culture have been done. Because HPV infection has been associated with various genital and anal cancers, biopsy is performed if lesions bleed.

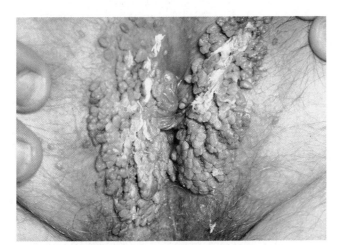 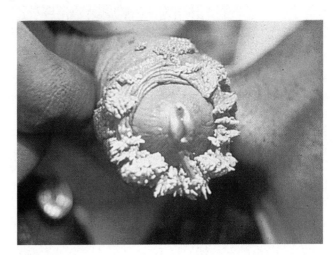

**Figure 49–2** ■ Genital warts (condyloma acuminatum) on the vulva and penis.

## Medication Administration
### The Client with Genital Warts

**TOPICAL APPLICATIONS**

Podophyllin resin (Pod-Ben-25, podofilox 0.5% solution)
Trichloroacetic acid

Although cryotherapy using liquid nitrogen or a cryoprobe is more commonly used to treat genital warts, podophyllum preparations or trichloroacetic acid are sometimes used. Podophyllin resin, 25% in compound tincture of benzoin, is applied topically to the warts by the physician once weekly for 3 to 5 weeks.

Podophyllin resin is contraindicated during pregnancy; the alternative is cryotherapy or topical treatment with trichloroacetic acid. Podophyllin resin is also contraindicated in cervical, urethral, oral, or anorectal warts. It is important to avoid contact of podophyllin resin with the eyes.

Adverse effects of podophyllin resin include local irritation, severe ulceration of surrounding tissue, nausea, diarrhea, lethargy, paralysis, and coma.

**Nursing Responsibilities**
- Establish baseline data, including mental status, vital signs, and weight.

- Document and report any existing lesions (genital, anal, or oral).
- Cover the tissue surrounding the warts with petrolatum or a paste of baking soda and water to protect the tissue from the caustic treatment solution.

**Client and Family Teaching**
- Wash off the treated area thoroughly within 1 to 4 hours after the first application; gradually increase this period to 6 to 8 hours after the second and subsequent applications.
- Return for regular treatment until warts are gone.
- Refer partners for examination and any necessary treatment.
- Report any adverse effects (nausea, diarrhea, local irritation, lethargy, numbness)
- Avoid sexual activity until you and your partners have been free of disease for 1 month.
- Use condoms to prevent future infections.
- Return for an annual Pap smear.

## Medications

Topical agents used to treat genital warts include podofilox or podophyllin. Podophyllin (Condylox, Podofin) is contraindicated during pregnancy and can have serious side effects in any client, ranging from nausea, diarrhea, and lethargy to paralysis and coma (see the box above).

## Other Treatments

Genital warts may also be removed by cryotherapy, electrocautery, or surgical excision. Carbon dioxide laser surgery is becoming increasingly common for removal of extensive warts (see Chapter 14 ⬩⬩ for a discussion of these procedures).

## NURSING CARE

### Nursing Diagnoses and Interventions

Nursing care for the client with genital warts includes pretreatment teaching, treatment of the lesions, health teaching for self-care, and health promotion.

### Deficient Knowledge

HPV is spread by contact with infectious lesions or secretions, with up to 70% of genital warts spread by people who do not know they have the infection. Although there is no known cure, it is essential to prevent secondary infections.

- Discuss the need for prompt treatment and the necessity for sexual abstinence until lesions have healed. *This reduces the risk of reinfection and further transmission of the disease.*

- Discuss the increased risk of cervical cancer and the importance of an annual Pap smear. *Understanding the risk, the client will be more motivated to seek annual screening.*
- Stress the importance of thorough handwashing. *Handwashing is essential to prevent hand-to-eye spread of HPV, which is the most frequent cause of corneal damage and subsequent blindness in the United States (Porth, 2002).*

### Fear

Surgery engenders some degree of fear in most clients: fear of the procedure itself, of pain and possible complications. Surgery or cryotherapy in the genital area involves all these fears plus fear of possible impaired sexual function.

- Allow the client to express specific fears and feelings about the procedure. Explain the procedure, approximate recovery time, possible complications and ways to avoid them, and ways to cope with complications that do occur. *Knowing what to expect reduces the client's fear and helps the client feel a greater sense of control.*
- Explain that the procedure is performed with a local anesthesia. *Being awake during surgery gives the client a greater sense of participation in the treatment process.*

### Home Care

Health teaching emphasizes the need for the client and infected partners to return for regular treatment until lesions have resolved, and to use condoms to prevent reinfection. Because of the increased risk of cervical cancer, annual Pap smears are essential for female clients.

# UROGENITAL INFECTIONS

## THE CLIENT WITH CHLAMYDIA

**Chlamydia** are a group of syndromes, all caused by *Chlamydia trachomatis,* a bacterium that behaves like a virus, reproducing only within the host cell. The bacterium is spread by any sexual contact and to the neonate by passage through the birth canal of an infected mother. The syndromes include acute urethral syndrome, nongonococcal urethritis, mucopurulent cervicitis, and pelvic inflammatory disease (PID); all are commonly called chlamydia.

Chlamydia is the most commonly reported bacterial STI in the United States, affecting an estimated 3 million people each year. Of that number, three of every four reported cases occurred in people under age 25. Chlamydia is so common in young women, that by age 30, 50% of sexually active women have evidence that they have had chlamydia at some time during their lives (CDC, 2001). Risk factors for chlamydia are listed in Box 49–3.

Because chlamydia is asymptomatic in most women until they have invaded the uterus and uterine tubes, treatment is delayed, resulting in devastating long-term complications. Nearly a third of men with urethral chlamydia are also asymptomatic. Chlamydia is a leading cause of preventable blindness, particularly in the newborn.

## PATHOPHYSIOLOGY AND MANIFESTATIONS

The incubation period is from 1 to 3 weeks; however, chlamydia may be present for months or years without producing noticeable symptoms in women. Chlamydia typically invades the same target organs as gonorrhea (cervix and male urethra) and result in similar manifestations (dysuria, urinary frequency, and discharge). Clients may be asymptomatic; however, they are still potentially infectious.

If chlamydial infections in women are not treated, they ascend into the upper reproductive tract, causing such complications as PID, which includes endometritis, salpingitis, and chronic pelvic pain. These infections are a major cause of infertility and ectopic pregnancy, a potentially life-threatening disorder in women. Complications of chlamydial infections in men include epididymitis, prostatitis, sterility, and Reiter's syndrome.

| BOX 49–3 | ■ Risk Factors for Chlamydial Infection |
|---|---|

- Personal or partner history of STD
- Pregnancy
- Adolescent sexual activity
- Oral contraceptive use
- Unprotected sexual activity
- Multiple sexual partners

## COLLABORATIVE CARE

*C. trachomatis* is treated with medications to eradicate the infection. Its prevalence, particularly in younger populations, makes widespread screening necessary if the disease is to be controlled. Because chlamydia is often asymptomatic, treatment is often begun on a presumptive basis. The CDC recommends screening asymptomatic women who are at high risk for chlamydial infection.

### Diagnostic Tests

The following diagnostic tests may be ordered.

- *Cultures of tissue* from the female endocervix and urethra, or from the male urethra
- *Tests for antibodies* to chlamydia such as direct fluorescent antibody (DFA) test and an enzyme-linked immunosorbent assay (ELISA)
- *Polymerase chain reaction (PCR)* or *ligase chain reaction (LCR) tests,* highly sensitive and specific tests, on urine and vaginal swab specimens (Porth, 2002)

### Medications

The drug of choice for chlamydial infections in men and nonpregnant women is oral azithromycin (Zithromax) or doxycycline (Vibramycin, Vivox) given as prescribed for 7 days. For pregnant women, erythromycin (E.E.S., Wyamycin E) is the alternative therapy. Ofloxacin (Floxin, Ocuflox) given twice daily for 7 days is another alternative treatment.

## NURSING CARE

Nursing care of the client with chlamydia focuses on eradication of the infection, prevention of future infections, and management of any chronic complications. Nursing diagnoses for the client with chlamydia are the same as for clients with any STI. Interventions are similar to those previously discussed for gonorrhea and genital herpes.

### Home Care

Health teaching for the client with chlamydia centers on the need to comply with the treatment regimen, refer partners for examination and necessary treatment, and the use of condoms to avoid reinfection. If the infection has progressed to pelvic inflammatory disease (discussed later), the client needs additional information on self-care and health promotion. The CDC recommends annual screening for chlamydia for clients who are young, sexually active, and do not use condoms correctly with every act of sexual intercourse. All pregnant women should be screened for chlamydia.

## THE CLIENT WITH GONORRHEA

**Gonorrhea,** also known as **GC** or **clap,** is caused by *Neisseria gonorrhoeae,* a gram-negative diplococcus. The incubation period is 2 to 8 days after exposure. Gonorrhea is transmitted by direct sexual contact and during delivery as the neonate passes through the birth canal. Gonorrhea is the most common reportable communicable disease in the United States. The CDC estimates that approximately 300,000 new cases occur annually, with the rate of reported gonorrhea increasing. Women age 15 to 19 have the highest rate, along with men age 20 to 24 (CDC, 2000).

Gonorrhea rates for African Americans are 30% higher than for non-Hispanic whites. Other risk factors include residence in large urban areas, transients, early onset of sexual activity, multiple serial or consecutive sex partners, drug use, prostitution, and previous gonorrheal or concurrent STI infection (McCance & Huether, 2002).

## PATHOPHYSIOLOGY AND MANIFESTATIONS

The organism initially targets the female cervix and the male urethra. Without treatment, the disease ultimately disseminates to other organs. In men, gonorrhea can cause acute, painful inflammation of the prostate, epididymis, and periurethral glands and can lead to sterility. In women, it can cause pelvic inflammatory disease (PID), endometritis, salpingitis, and pelvic peritonitis. In the neonate, gonorrhea can cause ophthalmia neonatorum, rhinitis, or anorectal infection.

Manifestations of gonorrhea in men include dysuria and serous, milky, or purulent discharge. Some men also experience regional lymphadenopathy. About 20% of men and 80% of women remain asymptomatic until the disease is advanced. Those women with symptoms experience dysuria, urinary frequency, abnormal menses (increased flow or dysmenorrhea), increased vaginal discharge, and dyspareunia (pain with intercourse).

Anal and rectal gonorrhea occurs in 30% to 50% of women diagnosed with gonorrhea. In women it is often asymptomatic and may not be connected with anal intercourse. Anorectal gonorrhea is seen most often in homosexual men. The manifestations include pruritus, mucopurulent rectal discharge, rectal bleeding and pain, and constipation. Gonococcal pharyngitis occurs primarily in homosexual or bisexual men or heterosexual women after oral sexual contact (fellatio) with an infected partner. The manifestations include fever, sore throat, and enlarged lymph glands.

### Complications

The complications of untreated gonorrhea in both men and women may be permanent and serious. They include:

- Pelvic inflammatory disease (PID) in women, leading to internal abscesses, chronic pain, ectopic pregnancy, and infertility.
- Blindness, infection of joints, and potentially lethal infections of the blood in the newborn, contracted during delivery.

- Epididymitis and prostatitis in men, resulting in infertility and dysuria.
- Spread of the infection to the blood and joints.
- Increased susceptibility to and transmission of HIV

## COLLABORATIVE CARE

The goals of treatment for the client with gonorrhea include eradication of the organism and any coexisting disease, and prevention of reinfection or transmission. It is important to emphasize the importance of taking all medications as prescribed and abstaining from sexual contact until the infection is cured in both client and partners. Condom use to prevent future infections is essential, particularly for pregnant women whose partners may be infected.

### Diagnostic Tests

Diagnosis of gonorrhea is based on the following diagnostic tests.

- *Fluid analysis* from the infected mucous membranes (cervix, urethra, rectum, or throat)
- *Urinalysis* from an infected person
- *Gram stain,* allowing visualization of the bacteria under the microscope

### Medications

Because of the many penicillin-resistant strains of *N. gonorrhoeae,* an alternative antibiotic, such as oral cefixime (Suprax), ciprofloxacin (Cipro), or ofloxacin (Floxin); or intramuscular ceftriaxone (Rocephin), is used to treat gonorrhea. A single dose of oral azithromycin (Zithromax) or a 7-day course of oral doxycycline (Vibramycin, Vivox) usually is added to treat any coexisting chlamydial infection. Infected sexual partners also need to be treated.

## NURSING CARE

### Nursing Diagnoses and Interventions

In planning and implementing care for the client with gonorrhea, the nurse considers the possible coexistence of other STIs such as syphilis and HIV, the impact of the disease and its treatment on the client's lifestyle, and the likelihood of noncompliance. Nursing diagnoses discussed in this section focus on noncompliance and impaired social interaction.

### Noncompliance

Although one-time treatment with the recommended antibiotic is highly effective in curing gonorrhea, noncompliance with the doxycycline regimen may leave any coexisting chlamydial infection unresolved. Noncompliance with recommendations for abstinence, follow-up, or condom use fosters a high rate of reinfection. Failure to refer partners for examination and treatment also leads to reinfection.

- Reinforce the need for taking all medications as directed and keeping follow-up appointments to be sure no reinfection has occurred. Discuss the prevalence of gonorrhea and the potential complications if it is not cured. *The client who understands the complications of incomplete or failed treatment is more likely to comply with the medication regimen.*

- Discuss the importance of sexual abstinence until the infection is cured, referral of partners, and condom use to prevent reinfection. *Understanding that cure is possible and reinfection is avoidable helps the client cope with the disease and its treatment and is likely to increase compliance.*

## Impaired Social Interaction

Diagnosis of any STI can make clients feel "dirty," ashamed, and guilty about their sexual behaviors, and unworthy to be with others.

- Provide privacy, confidentiality, and a safe, nonjudgmental environment for expression of concerns. Help the client understand that gonorrhea is a consequence of sexual behavior, not a punishment, and that it can be avoided in the future. *Being treated with respect and privacy helps the client realize that the disease does not change an individual's worth as a person. This knowledge enhances the client's ability to relate to others.*

## Home Care

Health teaching focuses on helping clients understand the importance of (1) taking any and all prescribed medication, (2) referring sexual partners for evaluation and treatment, (3) abstaining from all sexual contact until the client and partners are cured, and (4) using a condom to avoid transmitting or contracting infections in the future. Clients also need to understand the need for a follow-up visit 4 to 7 days after treatment is completed.

---

## Nursing Care Plan
## A Client with Gonorrhea

Janet Cirit, a 33-year-old legal secretary, lives in a suburban midwestern community. She is unmarried but dating a man named Jim Adkins, who lives in an adjacent suburb. Ms. Cirit visits her gynecologist because her periods have become irregular and she is experiencing pelvic pain and an abnormal amount of vaginal discharge. Recently she has developed a sore throat. The pelvic pain has begun to disrupt her sleeping pattern, and she is concerned that she might have cancer because her mother recently died of ovarian cancer.

### ASSESSMENT

When Ms. Cirit arrives for her appointment at the gynecologist's office, Marsha Davidson, the nurse practitioner, interviews her. Ms. Davidson completes a thorough medical and sexual history, including questions about her menstrual periods, pain associated with urination or sexual intercourse, urinary frequency, most recent Pap smear, birth control method, history of STI and drug use, and types of sexual activity. Ms. Cirit reports her symptoms and her concern about ovarian cancer. She also indicates that she is taking oral contraceptives and therefore sees no need for her boyfriend to use a condom because she believes their relationship is monogamous.

Physical examination reveals both pharyngeal and cervical inflammation, and lower abdominal tenderness. Her temperature is 98.5°F (37.0°C). There are no signs or symptoms of pregnancy.

The gynecologist orders a Pap smear and cultures of the cervix, urethra, and pharynx to evaluate for gonorrhea and chlamydial infection. Blood is drawn for WBC. Test results are positive for gonorrhea and negative for chlamydia. The WBC is slightly elevated, indicating possible salpingitis. Because Mr. Adkins has been Ms. Cirit's only sexual partner, it is clear that he is the source of infection and needs to be treated as well.

### DIAGNOSIS

- *Pain* related to the infectious process
- *Anxiety* related to fear about possible cancer
- *Situational low self-esteem* related to shame and guilt because of having an STI

- *Ineffective sexuality patterns* related to the impaired relationship and fear of reinfection

### EXPECTED OUTCOMES

- Experience relief of pain, indicating that the infection had been eradicated.
- Express relief that the Pap smear showed no abnormal cells.
- Verbalize that she has nothing to be ashamed of and that she has been wise to seek treatment as soon as symptoms occurred.
- Verbalize that she will insist her partner use condoms during future sexual activity.

### PLANNING AND IMPLEMENTATION

- Administer ceftriaxone IM as ordered.
- Emphasize the need for regular Pap smears and pelvic examinations because of the family history of ovarian cancer.
- Discuss feelings and concerns about the diagnosis of gonorrhea. Stress that such a diagnosis does not reflect on one's self-worth as a person.
- Teach how to talk with a future sexual partner about condom use.

### EVALUATION

A week later during her follow-up visit, Ms. Cirit states that she is feeling much better and sleeping well at night since the pain has ended. She has terminated her relationship with Mr. Adkins and is considering joining a health club in the hope of increasing her level of fitness and perhaps meeting someone new.

### Critical Thinking in the Nursing Process

1. How are Ms. Cirit's manifestations related to the infectious process of gonorrhea?
2. Should the nurse have suggested that Ms. Cirit also be tested for HIV? Why or why not?
3. Develop a care plan for Ms. Cirit for the nursing diagnosis, *Impaired social interaction.*

See Evaluating Your Response in Appendix C.

## THE CLIENT WITH SYPHILIS

**Syphilis** is a complex systemic STI caused by a spirochete, *Treponema pallidum,* which may infect almost any body tissue or organ. It is transmitted from open lesions during any sexual contact (genital, oral-genital, or anal-genital). The organism is highly susceptible to heat and drying, but can survive for days in fluids; thus, it may also be transmitted by infected blood or other body fluid such as saliva. The incubation period ranges from 10 to 90 days, averaging 21 days. If not treated appropriately, syphilis can lead to blindness, paralysis, mental illness, cardiovascular damage, and death. Syphilis often occurs with one or more other STIs, such as HIV/AIDS or chlamydial infection. Pregnant women with syphilis can also infect the fetus, causing eye damage, dental and bone deformities, blindness, brain damage, and death.

With the advent of penicillin in the 1940s and 1950s, the incidence of syphilis plummeted. While in 1996 the rate of syphilis infection reached its lowest level in many years, it remains a significant problem in certain geographic regions, and among specific populations such as African Americans. Rates also remain high in many urban centers, with higher infection rates found in drug users, transients, and the homeless. The rate of syphilis infection is declining among most racial and ethnic groups, with the exception of American Indians and Alaska Natives (CDC, 2001).

## PATHOPHYSIOLOGY AND MANIFESTATIONS

Any break in the skin or mucous membrane is vulnerable to invasion by the spirochete. Once it has entered the system, the spirochete is spread through the blood and lymphatic system. Congenital syphilis is transferred to the fetus through the placental circulation. Syphilis is generally characterized by three clinical stages: primary, secondary, and tertiary. Each stage has characteristic manifestations (see the box below). The client with syphilis also may experience a latency period when no signs of the disease are evident.

### Primary Syphilis

The primary stage of syphilis is characterized by the appearance of a **chancre** (Figure 49–3 ■) and by regional enlargement of lymph nodes; little or no pain accompanies these warning signs. The chancre appears at the site of inoculation (genitals, anus, mouth, breast, finger) 3 to 4 weeks after the infectious contact. In women, a genital chancre may go unnoticed, disappearing within 4 to 6 weeks. In both primary and secondary stages, syphilis remains highly infectious, even if no symptoms are evident.

### Secondary Syphilis

Manifestations of secondary syphilis may appear any time from 2 weeks to 6 months after the initial chancre disappears. These symptoms can include a skin rash, especially on the

## Manifestations of Syphilis

**REPRODUCTIVE**

Primary
- Genital chancre (may be internal in female)

Secondary
- Condyloma lata

**INTEGUMENTARY SYSTEM**

Secondary
- Rash on palms and soles

Tertiary
- Granulomatous lesions involving mucous membranes and skin

**GASTROINTESTINAL SYSTEM**

Secondary
- Anorexia
- Oral mucous patches

**NEUROLOGIC SYSTEM**

Secondary
- Asymptomatic
- Headache
- Meningitis
- Cranial neuropathies

Tertiary
- Asymptomatic
- Neurosyphilis
- Tabes dorsalis
- Seizures, hemiparesis, hemiplegia
- Personality changes, hyperactive reflexes, Argyll Robertson pupil, decreased memory, slurred speech, optic atrophy

**MUSCULOSKELETAL SYSTEM**

Secondary
- Arthralgia
- Bone and joint arthritis
- Myalgia
- Periostitis

Tertiary
- Gummas

**CARDIOVASCULAR SYSTEM**

Tertiary
- Aortic insufficiency
- Aortic aneurysm
- Stenosis of openings to coronary arteries

**RENAL SYSTEM**

Secondary
- Glomerulonephritis
- Nephrotic syndrome

**OTHER**

Primary
- Regional lymphadenopathy

Secondary
- Generalized lymphadenopathy
- Fever
- Malaise
- Hepatitis
- Alopecia

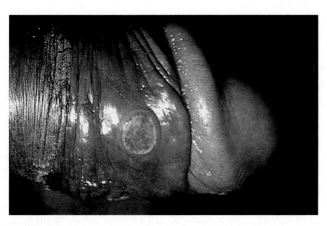

**Figure 49–3** ■ Chancre of primary syphilis on the penis.

*Source: Biophoto Associates/Photo Researchers, Inc.*

palms of the hands (Figure 49–4 ■) or soles of the feet, mucous patches in the oral cavity; sore throat; generalized lymphadenopathy; condyloma lata (flat, broad-based papules, unlike the pedunculated structure of genital warts) on the labia, anus or corner of the mouth; flulike symptoms; and alopecia. These manifestations generally disappear within 2 to 6 weeks, and an asymptomatic latency period begins.

## Latent and Tertiary Syphilis

The latent stage of syphilis begins 2 or more years after the initial infection and can last up to 50 years. During this stage, no symptoms of syphilis are apparent, and the disease is not transmissible by sexual contact. It can be transmitted by infected blood, however; thus, all prospective blood donors must be screened for syphilis. In two-thirds of all cases, the latent stage persists without further complications. Unless treated, the remaining one-third of infected people progress to late-stage or tertiary syphilis. In the presence of HIV infection, disease progression seems to be more rapid.

Two types of late-stage syphilis occur. Benign late syphilis, of rapid onset, is characterized by localized devel-

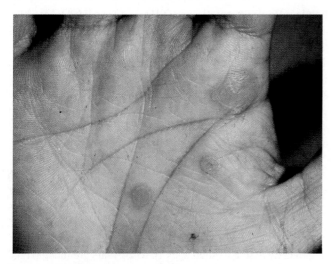

**Figure 49–4** ■ Palmar rash of secondary syphilis.

*Source: Dr. Carroll Weiss, Camera MD Studios.*

opment of infiltrating tumors (*gummas*) in skin, bones, and liver, generally responding promptly to treatment. Of more insidious onset is a diffuse inflammatory response that involves the central nervous system and the cardiovascular system. Though the disease can still be treated at this stage, much of the cardiovascular and central nervous system damage is irreversible.

## COLLABORATIVE CARE

The goals of treatment are to inactivate the spirochete and educate the client about how to prevent reinfection or further transmission. Treatment includes antibiotic therapy and identification and referral of partners for testing and treatment if necessary, follow-up testing, and education about condom use to prevent reinfection of self and transmission of disease to partners. In addition, clients should be screened for chlamydial infection and advised to have an HIV test.

## Diagnostic Tests

Diagnosis of syphilis is complex because it mimics many other diseases. A careful history and physical examination are obtained, as well as laboratory evaluations of lesions and blood. The following tests are widely used.

- The *VDRL (Venereal Disease Research Laboratory)* and *RPR (rapid plasma reagin) blood tests* measure antibody production. People with syphilis become positive about 4 to 6 weeks after infection. However, these tests are not specific for syphilis, and other diseases may also cause positive results. Additional tests are required for definitive diagnosis.
- *FTA-ABS (fluorescent treponemal antibody absorption) test* is specific for *T. pallidum* and can be used to confirm VDRL and RPR findings. It may be used for clients whose clinical picture indicates syphilis but who have negative VDRL results.
- *Immunofluorescent staining* during which a specimen obtained from early lesions or aspiration of lymph nodes is specially treated and examined microscopically for the presence of *T. pallidum*.
- *Darkfield microscopy* involves examining a specimen from the chancre for the presence of *T. pallidum* using a darkfield microscope.

## Medications

The treatment of choice for primary and secondary syphilis is benzathine penicillin G, given intramuscularly (IM) in a single dose. For syphilis of indeterminate length or more than 1 year's duration, the total dosage is increased and given in three weekly injections. Clients allergic to penicillin are given oral doxycycline. The length of therapy depends on the estimated duration of infection. If the client cannot tolerate doxycycline, oral erythromycin is substituted.

Treatment of syphilis in pregnant women may result in a severe reaction called the *Jarisch-Herxheimer reaction*, involving fever, musculoskeletal pain, tachycardia, and sometimes hypotension. This is not a reaction to the penicillin itself, but to the sudden and massive destruction of spirochetes by the penicillin and the resulting release of toxins into the bloodstream. The Jarisch-Herxheimer reaction generally begins within 24 hours of treatment and subsides in another 24 hours. Treatment should not be discontinued unless symptoms become life threatening.

## NURSING CARE

### Nursing Diagnoses and Interventions

In planning and implementing nursing care for the client with syphilis, the nurse needs to consider the client's age, lifestyle, access to health care, and educational level. Although each client has individualized needs, nursing diagnoses for the client with syphilis would be the same as for any client with an STI. Nursing diagnoses discussed in this section focus on high risk for injury, anxiety, and self-esteem.

#### Risk for Injury

If syphilis is not diagnosed and treated promptly and effectively, it can have devastating effects on all body systems, particularly the neurologic and cardiovascular systems, eventually leading to a painful death.

- Teach the importance of taking any prescribed oral medication. *Completion of the prescribed course of antibiotic is important to ensure eradication of the infecting organism.*
- Encourage referral of any sexual partners for evaluation and any necessary treatment. *Without treatment of both partners, reinfection can occur or the disease may be transmitted to other people through sexual activity.*
- Teach abstinence from sexual contact until client and partners are cured and to use condoms to prevent future infections. *Abstinence until the organism is eradicated prevents reinfection. Condoms provide barrier protection, reducing the risk of infection during sexual activity.*
- Emphasize the importance of returning for follow-up testing at 3- and 6-month intervals for early syphilis, and 6- and 12-month intervals for late latent syphilis. *Follow-up testing is performed to assure eradication of the disease.*
- Provide information about signs and symptoms of reinfection. *Successful treatment of the disease does not prevent possible subsequent infections.*

#### Anxiety

The diagnosis of syphilis understandably causes the client anxiety, not only about personal well-being but about the well-being of partners and, in the expectant woman, her fetus.

- Emphasize that syphilis can be effectively treated, preventing the serious complications of late-stage disease. *This information provides a sense of control and helps decrease anxiety.*
- Teach the pregnant client that taking medications as directed and returning each month for follow-up testing will help ensure the well-being of her baby. *Knowing that treatment can reduce the risk to her baby relieves anxiety and possibly increases compliance.*

#### Low Self-Esteem

Living with any chronic disease can be damaging to a person's self-esteem. However, the client with syphilis or any STI needs additional support to cope with the stigma of this kind of infection. Unfortunately, the populations most affected by STIs often lack family and other social support networks.

- Create an environment where the client feels respected and safe to discuss questions and concerns about the disease and its effect on the client's life. *Being treated with respect helps enhance self-esteem.*
- Provide privacy and confidentiality. *Clients are often embarrassed to discuss the intimate details of their sex lives.*
- Let clients know that the nurse and other health care providers care about them and the successful treatment of their disease. *Feeling valued enhances self-esteem.*

### Home Care

Education is an essential part of nursing care for the client with any STI, and syphilis is no exception. The nurse emphasizes that syphilis is a chronic disease that can be spread to others even though no symptoms are evident. Address the following topics.

- Taking any and all prescribed medication
- Referring sexual partners for evaluation and treatment
- Abstaining from all sexual contact for a minimum of 1 month after treatment
- Using a condom to avoid transmitting or contracting infections in the future
- The need for follow-up testing (at 3 and 6 months for clients with primary or secondary syphilis, and at 6 and 12 months for those with late-stage disease). If clients are HIV-positive, follow-up visits are recommended 1, 2, 3, 6, 9, and 12 months after treatment

## THE CLIENT WITH PELVIC INFLAMMATORY DISEASE

**Pelvic inflammatory disease (PID)** is a term used to describe infection of the pelvic organs, including the fallopian tubes (**salpingitis**), ovaries (**oophoritis**), cervix (**cervicitis**), endometrium (**endometritis**), pelvic peritoneum, and the pelvic vascular system. PID can be caused by one or more infectious agents, including *Neisseria gonorrhoeae, Chlamydia trachomatis, Escherichia coli,* and *Mycoplasma hominis. N. gonorrhoeae* and *C. trachomatis* are responsible for as much as 80% of PID; dual infection with both agents is common.

PID is not a reportable disease in the United States; however, it is estimated that about 1 million women experience PID each year. As a result of the infection, more than 100,000 women become infertile and a large proportion of the ectopic pregnancies occurring each year are the result of PID. The disease may also cause pelvic abscesses and chronic abdominal pain.

Sexually active women ages 16 to 24 years are most at risk. Risk factors include a history of sexually transmitted disease (especially gonorrhea and chlamydia), bacterial vaginosis,

## Nursing Care Plan
## A Client with Syphilis

Eddie Kratz, age 22, works as a bellman at a large hotel. For the past year, he has shared a small apartment with Marla Jones, who is 5 months pregnant with his child. Although he intends to marry Ms. Jones before the baby is born, he has continued a previous relationship with a woman named Justine Simpson. His sexual activities with Ms. Simpson have increased in frequency as Ms. Jones's pregnancy has advanced. Recently Mr. Kratz has noticed a swelling in his groin and a sore on his penis.

### ASSESSMENT

When Mr. Kratz comes to the community clinic, he is interviewed by the nurse practitioner, Sally Morovitz. She takes a thorough medical and sexual history, including questions about drug use, allergies, difficulty with urination, urinary frequency, itching or discharge from the penis, recent sexual activities, precautions taken against infection, history of STIs, and sexual function. She determines that Mr. Kratz has been having unprotected sex with both Ms. Jones and Ms. Simpson. He believes that Ms. Jones is not having sex with anyone except him, but he is not sure.

Physical assessment reveals a classic syphilitic chancre on the shaft of the penis and regional lymphadenopathy. A specimen of exudate from the chancre is sent for darkfield examination. Ms. Morovitz discusses with Mr. Kratz the likelihood that he has syphilis and the need to tell both Ms. Jones and Ms. Simpson so that they can be tested and, if necessary, treated. Ms. Morovitz also suggests that Mr. Kratz be tested for HIV since he has been having unprotected sex with two women, at least one of whom may be sexually active with other partners. He agrees, and blood is drawn for an ELISA test. Darkfield analysis of the chancre exudate confirms the diagnosis of syphilis; the ELISA results are negative for HIV.

### DIAGNOSES

- *Risk for injury* to the client, his partners, and the infant, related to the disease process
- *Ineffective health maintenance* related to a lack of knowledge about the disease process, its transmission, and the need for treatment
- *Interrupted family processes* related to the effects of the diagnosis of syphilis on the couple's relationship
- *Anxiety* related to the effects of the infection on the unborn child

### EXPECTED OUTCOMES

- Prompt treatment will cure the syphilis.

- Will verbalize understanding for the need to abstain from sexual contact during treatment, complete all medications, return for follow-up visits, and use condoms to prevent reinfection.
- Will verbalize ability to cope with the effect of diagnosis and treatment on the relationship.
- Will verbalize decreased anxiety following education and treatment.

### PLANNING AND IMPLEMENTATION

- Administer IM injection of benzathine penicillin G as ordered, and document.
- Discuss the importance of abstaining from sexual activity until he and his partners are cured, and of using condoms to prevent reinfection.
- Explain the need to return for follow-up testing in 3 months and again at 6 months. Provide a copy of the STI prevention checklist, and document that reminders need to be sent at 3- and 6-month intervals.
- Notify sexual partners that they need to come to the clinic for testing.
- Refer to a social worker for counseling about the impact of the disease on their relationship.
- Teach the couple about the importance of treatment to the health of their infant.

### EVALUATION

At the 3-month follow-up visit, the chancre on Mr. Kratz's penis has healed, and he reports that he is using a condom any time he has sex. Ms. Jones has also tested positive for syphilis and negative for HIV, so she, too, is given benzathine penicillin G, and verbal and written follow-up instructions, including follow-up until the infant is born. The couple is meeting every other week with the social worker and say that their relationship is improving. Ms. Simpson has received similar test results and is given a prescription for doxycycline because she is allergic to penicillin.

### Critical Thinking in the Nursing Process

1. What signs and symptoms might a client with early syphilis experience?
2. List some appropriate questions for taking a sexual history when you suspect the presence of one or more STIs.
3. How might you counsel Mr. Kratz to help him break the news of the diagnosis to Ms. Jones?

See Evaluating Your Response in Appendix C.

---

multiple sexual partners, douching, and previous PID. Oral contraceptives and barrier contraceptive devices such as condoms reduce the risk of PID.

The prognosis depends on the number of episodes, promptness of treatment, and modification of risk-taking behaviors. Prevention includes educating women, especially young women, regarding the causes and transmission of infection and methods of self-protection, such as appropriate personal hygiene and avoiding unprotected sexual activity.

## PATHOPHYSIOLOGY AND MANIFESTATIONS

Pelvic inflammatory disease is usually polymicrobial (caused by more than one microbe) in origin. Pathogenic microorganisms enter the vagina and travel to the uterus during intercourse or other sexual activity. They can also gain direct access to the uterus during childbirth, abortion, or surgery of the reproductive tract. The organisms ascend to the endocervical canal to the fallopian tubes and ovaries. Abscess formation is common.

Manifestations of PID include fever, purulent vaginal discharge, severe lower abdominal pain, and a painful cervical movement. However, the manifestations may be so mild that the infection is not recognized. Complications include pelvic abscess, infertility, ectopic pregnancy, chronic pelvic pain, pelvic adhesions, dyspareunia, and chronic pelvic pain.

## COLLABORATIVE CARE

The goals of treatment are to eliminate the infection and prevent complications and recurrence. The physical examination may reveal abdominal, adnexal, and cervical pain.

### Diagnostic Tests

Tests used in the diagnosis of PID may include the following:

- *CBC* with differential reveals a markedly elevated WBC.
- *Sedimentation rate* increases with infection.
- *Laparoscopy* or *laparotomy* may reveal inflammation, edema, or hyperemia of the fallopian tubes, or tubal discharge and, possibly, generalized pelvic involvement, abscesses, and scarring.

### Medications

Combination antibiotic therapy with at least two broad-spectrum antibiotics administered IV or orally is the typical treatment for PID. If PID is not acute, outpatient antibiotic therapy is prescribed. In acute cases, however, the client may be hospitalized. Analgesics are given, and antibiotics and fluids are administered intravenously. Commonly prescribed antibiotics include doxycycline (Vibramycin), cefoxitin (Mefoxin), clindamycin (Cleocin), gentamicin (Garamycin), ofloxacin (Floxin), and ceftriaxone (Rocephin). The antiprotozoal agent, metronidazole (Flagyl) may also be administered. Nursing implications for these drugs are discussed in Chapter 8. ⟳

### Surgery

The surgeon may insert a drain into an abscess, if present, and remove any adhesions. If the client does not respond to conservative therapy, surgical removal of the uterus, uterine tubes, and ovaries may be necessary.

## NURSING CARE

### Nursing Diagnoses and Interventions

The goals of nursing care are to treat the infection and to prevent complications, such as scarring and infertility. The client who is hospitalized maintains bed rest in the semi-Fowler's position to promote drainage and to localize the infectious process in the pelvic cavity. Nursing diagnoses that often apply to the client with PID are described below.

### Risk for Injury

PID can have severe, even life-threatening, complications. Scarring of fallopian tubes can lead to ectopic pregnancy or pelvic abscess. Infertility is a common complication, as are re-current or chronic PID, chronic abdominal pain, pelvic adhesions, premature hysterectomy, and depression.

- Administer antibiotic therapy as ordered, and monitor closely for adverse effects. *Antibiotics used in acute PID are potent agents; some can have life-threatening side effects.*
- Practice thorough handwashing and strict adherence to universal precautions when handling perineal pads and linens. Appropriate disinfection of bedpans, toilet seats, linens, and utensils is also important. *These practices help avoid disseminating the infection to others.*

### Deficient Knowledge

PID is most common in young women, many of whom have limited understanding of their own anatomy and physiology, and of sexually transmitted disease. Diagnosis and treatment of PID offer an opportunity to increase that understanding, thereby preventing complications and recurrent infection.

- Explain how infection is spread and what measures to take to prevent future infection. *Understanding can improve compliance with treatment regimens and perhaps change high-risk behavior.*
- Explain the need to complete the treatment regimen and the importance of follow-up visits. If the client or partner fails to take all of the medication as prescribed, the infection may not be completely cured. *Noncompliance and recurrence are common, particularly if follow-up appointments are not kept.*
- Teach proper perineal care, especially wiping from front to back. *This reduces transmission of fecal organisms to reproductive tissues and reduces the incidence of urinary tract infections.*
- Caution the client about using tampons, particularly if they previously have caused problems. Instruct the client to change tampons or pads at least every 4 hours. *Menstrual flow and other discharges provide a favorable environment for microorganisms to multiply.*
- Provide information about safer sex practices and family planning. Instruct the client to remove diaphragms within 6 hours after use. IUDs are contraindicated. Latex condoms offer the most effective protection against infection. *These measures help prevent recurrence of infection.*
- Teach the client to report any unusual vaginal discharge or odor to the health care provider. *Treatment is most effective early in the disease process.*

### Home Care

Teach measures to eradicate the infection and prevent recurrence, and help the client deal with the physical and psychosocial implications of treatment, including possible infertility. Provide general information related to sexually transmitted diseases. Inform the client that the patency of the fallopian tubes can be evaluated after several menstrual cycles; this delay allows for complete resolution of the inflammatory process.

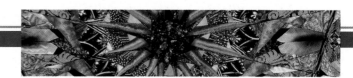

 **EXPLORE MediaLink**

NCLEX review questions, case studies, care plan activities, MediaLink applications, and other interactive resources for this chapter can be found on the Companion Website at www.prenhall.com/lemone.

Click on Chapter 49 to select the activities for this chapter. For animations, video clips, more NCLEX review questions, and an audio glossary, access the Student CD-ROM accompanying this textbook.

## TEST YOURSELF

1. Which population is most often affected by STIs?
   a. Men
   b. Women and infants
   c. Adolescent males
   d. Older adults

2. Which of the following statements would indicate a client understands teaching to treat an STI?
   a. "My sex partner and I must both take medications."
   b. "I know I can never have sex again."
   c. "I will douche after every sexual encounter with my partner."
   d. "My sex partner does not have an infection, so won't need medications."

3. You are assessing a young male. He has both blisters and ulcerations on the shaft of his penis. What is his most likely medical diagnosis?
   a. Chlamydia
   b. Gonorrhea

   c. Genital warts
   d. Genital herpes

4. The infective organism responsible for gonorrhea *initially* targets what body parts?
   a. Male urethra and female cervix
   b. Female vulva and vagina
   c. Male prostate
   d. Male and female external genitalia

5. Which of the following is true about syphilis?
   a. Syphilis is caused by a virus
   b. Syphilis is transmitted only through intimate genital contact
   c. Syphilis is spread through the blood and lymphatic system
   d. Syphilis has no effect on the developing fetus

See Test Yourself answers in Appendix C.

## BIBLIOGRAPHY

Centers for Disease Control and Prevention. (1998). Guidelines for treatment of sexually transmitted diseases. *MMWR, 47* (No. RR-1).

Centers for Disease Control and Prevention. (2001a). *Division of sexually transmitted diseases; facts.* Available www.cdc.gov/nchstp/dstd/Fact_Sheets

_____ . (2001b). National Center for Health Statistics. *Fastats A to Z: Sexually transmitted disease* Available www.cdc.gov/nchswww/fastats/stds.htm

_____ . (2000). *STD surveillance 2000.* Available www.cdc.gov/std/stats/2000NatOverview.htm

Champion, J., Piper, J., Shain, R., Perdue, S., & Newton, E. (2001). Minority women with sexually transmitted diseases: Sexual abuse and risk for pelvic inflammatory disease. *Research in Nursing & Health, 24*(1), 38–43.

Currie, S. (2001). Sexually transmitted infections and older people. *Elderly Care, 12*(1), 15–19.

Hutchinson, M., Sosa, D., & Thompson, A. (2001). Sexual protective strategies of late adolescent females: More than just condoms. *JOGHN-*

*Journal of Obstetric, Gynecologic, & Neonatal Nursing, 30*(4), 429–438.

McCance, K., & Huether, S. (2002). *Pathophysiology: The biologic basis for disease in adults & children* (4th ed.). St. Louis: Mosby.

McEwan, A., & Pittam, D. (2001). Clinical update: Sexually transmissible infections. *Australian Nursing Journal, 9*(2) (insert 1-4), 23–26.

Miller, K., & Graves, J. (2000). Update on the prevention and treatment of sexually transmitted diseases. *American Family Physician, 61*(2), 379–386.

Nicholas, H. (1998). Sexually transmitted diseases. Gonorrhoea: Symptoms and treatment. *Nursing Times, 94*(8), 52–54.

North American Nursing Diagnosis Association. (2001). *Nursing diagnoses: Definitions and classification 2001–2002.* Philadelphia: NANDA.

Porth, C. M. (2002). *Pathophysiology: Concepts of altered health states* (6th ed.). Philadelphia: Lippincott.

Ricchini, W. (1997). Break the silence: Talking to your patients about STDs. *Advance for Nurse Practitioners, 5*(6), 55–56, 83.

Shannon, M., Wilson, B., & Stang, C. (2002). *Health professional's drug guide 2002.* Upper Saddle River, NJ: Prentice Hall.

Slade, C. S. (1998). HPV and cervical cancer: Breaking the deadly link. *Advance for Nurse Practitioners, 6*(3), 39–40, 42, 54.

Swanson, J., Dibble, S., & Chenitz, W. (1995). Clinical features and psychosocial factors in young adults with genital herpes. *Image: Journal of Nursing Scholarship, 27*(1), 16–22.

Thomas, D. (2001). Sexually transmitted viral infections: Epidemiology and treatment. *Journal of Obstetric, Gynecologic, & Neonatal Nursing, 30*(3), 316–323.

Tierney, L. M., McPhee, S. J., & Papadakis, M. A. (Eds.). (2001). *Current medical diagnosis & treatment* (40th ed.). Stamford, CT: Appleton & Lange.

Weston, A. (1998). Striking back at syphilis. *Nursing Times, 94*(3), 30–32.

_____ .(1998). Warts and all. *Nursing Times, 94*(3), 26–28.

Wright, T. (1998). Genital warts: Their etiology and treatment. *Nursing Times, 94*(7), 52–54.

## Standard Precautions

Standard precautions are designed to reduce the risk of transmission of microorganisms from both recognized and unrecognized sources of infection. They are the primary strategies for preventing nosocomial infections within institutions, and are important to protect health care workers as well. Standard precautions apply to (1) blood; (2) all body fluids, secretions, and excretions except sweat, regardless of whether or not they contain visible blood; (3) nonintact skin; and (4) mucous membranes. Standard precautions are applied to all clients receiving care in hospitals, regardless of their diagnosis or presumed infection status. These precautions are specifically designed for hospitals; however, they also may be implemented in extended and long-term care facilities, and to a more limited extent in providing home care or in other community-based care settings.

### HANDWASHING

- Wash your hands (a) after touching blood, body fluids, secretions, excretions, and contaminated items, whether or not gloves are worn; (b) immediately after removing gloves, even if gloves appear to be intact; (c) between contacts with clients; and (d) when otherwise indicated to prevent transfer of organisms to other clients. You may need to wash your hands between tasks and procedures on the same client to prevent cross-contaminating different body sites.

- Use soap and warm water for handwashing when hands are visibly dirty or contaminated with blood or other body fluids.

- If hands are not visibly soiled, use an alcohol-based hand rub for routinely decontaminating hands in all other situations.

### GLOVES

- Wear clean, nonsterile gloves when touching blood, body fluids, secretions, excretions, and contaminated items.

- Put on clean gloves just before touching mucous membranes and nonintact skin.

- Change your gloves between tasks and procedures on the same client after contacting material that may contain a high concentration of microorganisms.

- Wear gloves for all invasive procedures such as performing venipuncture or other vascular or surgical procedures.

- Wear gloves if you have cuts, scratches, or other breaks in the skin.

- Remove gloves promptly after use, before touching noncontaminated items and surfaces, and before going to another client; wash hands immediately after removing gloves.

### MASK, EYE PROTECTION, FACE SHIELD

Wear a mask and eye protection or a face shield to protect mucous membranes of your eyes, nose, and mouth during procedures and client care activities that are likely to generate splashes or sprays of blood, body fluids, secretions, or excretions.

### GOWN

Wear a gown (clean, disposable) to protect your skin and prevent soiling of clothing during procedures and client care activities that are likely to generate splashes or sprays of blood, body fluids, secretions, or excretions. Remove soiled gowns promptly, washing your hands immediately after gown removal.

### EQUIPMENT

Handle used client care equipment that is soiled with blood, body fluids, secretions, and excretions in a way that prevents exposing your skin and mucous membranes, contaminating your clothing, and transferring microorganisms to other clients or environments. Ensure that reusable equipment is cleaned and appropriately reprocessed before using for the care of another client.

### ENVIRONMENTAL CONTROL

Follow hospital procedures for routine care, cleaning, and disinfecting environmental surfaces, beds, bed rails, bedside equipment, and other frequently touched surfaces.

### LINEN

Handle and transport linens soiled with blood, body fluids, secretions, and excretions in a manner that prevents exposing your skin and mucous membranes, contaminating your clothing, and transferring microorganisms to other clients and environments. Place soiled linen in leakage-resistant bags at the location where it is used.

### OCCUPATIONAL HEALTH AND BLOODBORNE PATHOGENS

- Take care to prevent injuries when using needles, scalpels, and other sharps; when handling sharp instruments after

*Sources.* Centers for Disease Control and Prevention (2002). Guidelines for hand hygiene in health-care settings: Recommendations of the Healthcare Infection Control Practices Advisory Committee and the HICPAC/SHEA/APIC/IDSA Hand Hygiene Taskforce. *MMWR, 51*(RR-16), 1–56; Hospital Infection Control Practices Advisory Committee (1997). Part II. Recommendations for isolation precautions in hospitals. Atlanta: Public Health Service, U.S. Department of Health and Human Services, Centers for Disease Control and Prevention.

procedures; when cleaning used instruments; and when disposing of used needles.

- Never recap used needles, manipulate them using both hands, or handle them in a manner that directs the point of a needle toward any part of your body. If it is necessary to protect the needle prior to disposal, use a one-handed "scoop" technique or mechanical device to hold the needle sheath.

- Do not remove used needles from disposable syringes by hand; do not bend, break, or otherwise manipulate used needles by hand.

- Place used disposable syringes and needles, scalpel blades, and other sharp items in appropriate puncture-resistant containers located as close as practical to the area in which the items were used.

- Place reusable syringes and needles in a puncture-resistant container for transport to the reprocessing area.

- Use mouthpieces, resuscitation bags, or other ventilation devices as an alternative to mouth-to-mouth resuscitation methods whenever possible.

## CLIENT PLACEMENT

Place clients who contaminate the environment or who do not (or are not expected to) assist in maintaining appropriate hygiene or environmental control (e.g., an ambulatory, confused client with fecal incontinence) in a private room.

## 2003–2004 NANDA-Approved Nursing Diagnoses

Activity Intolerance
Activity Intolerance, Risk for
Adaptive Capacity: Intracranial, Decreased
Adjustment, Impaired
Airway Clearance, Ineffective
Anxiety
Anxiety, Death
Aspiration, Risk for
Attachment, Parent/Infant/Child, Risk for Impaired
Body Image, Disturbed
Body Temperature: Imbalanced, Risk for
Bowel Incontinence
Breastfeeding, Effective
Breastfeeding, Ineffective
Breastfeeding, Interrupted
Breathing Pattern, Ineffective
Cardiac Output, Decreased
Caregiver Role Strain
Caregiver Role Strain, Risk for
Communication, Readiness for Enhanced
Communication: Verbal, Impaired
Confusion, Acute
Confusion, Chronic
Constipation
Constipation, Perceived
Constipation, Risk for
Coping: Community, Ineffective
Coping: Community, Readiness for Enhanced
Coping, Defensive
Coping: Family, Compromised
Coping: Family, Disabled
Coping: Family, Readiness for Enhanced
Coping (Individual), Readiness for Enhanced
Coping, Ineffective
Decisional Conflict (Specify)
Denial, Ineffective
Dentition, Impaired
Development: Delayed, Risk for
Diarrhea
Disuse Syndrome, Risk for
Diversional Activity, Deficient
Dysreflexia, Autonomic
Dysreflexia, Autonomic, Risk for
Energy Field, Disturbed
Environmental Interpretation Syndrome, Impaired
Failure to Thrive, Adult
Falls, Risk for
Family Processes, Dysfunctional: Alcoholism
Family Processes, Interrupted
Family Processes, Readiness for Enhanced
Fatigue
Fear
Fluid Balance, Readiness for Enhanced
Fluid Volume, Deficient
Fluid Volume, Deficient, Risk for
Fluid Volume, Excess
Fluid Volume, Imbalanced, Risk for
Gas Exchange, Impaired
Grieving, Anticipatory
Grieving, Dysfunctional
Growth, Disproportionate, Risk for
Growth and Development, Delayed

Health Maintenance, Ineffective
Health-Seeking Behaviors (Specify)
Home Maintenance, Impaired
Hopelessness
Hyperthermia
Hypothermia
Identity: Personal, Disturbed
Infant Behavior, Disorganized
Infant Behavior: Disorganized, Risk for
Infant Behavior: Organized, Readiness for Enhanced
Infant Feeding Pattern, Ineffective
Infection, Risk for
Injury, Risk for
Knowledge, Deficient (Specify)
Knowledge (Specify), Readiness for Enhanced
Latex Allergy Response
Latex Allergy Response, Risk for
Loneliness, Risk for
Memory, Impaired
Mobility: Bed, Impaired
Mobility: Physical, Impaired
Mobility: Wheelchair, Impaired
Nausea
Neurovascular Dysfunction: Peripheral, Risk for
Noncompliance (Specify)
Nutrition, Imbalanced: Less than Body Requirements
Nutrition, Imbalanced: More than Body Requirements
Nutrition, Imbalanced: More than Body Requirements, Risk for
Nutrition, Readiness for Enhanced
Oral Mucous Membrane, Impaired
Pain, Acute
Pain, Chronic
Parenting, Impaired
Parenting, Readiness for Enhanced
Parenting, Risk for Impaired
Perioperative Positioning Injury, Risk for
Poisoning, Risk for
Posttrauma Syndrome
Posttrauma Syndrome, Risk for
Powerlessness
Powerlessness, Risk for
Protection, Ineffective
Rape-Trauma Syndrome
Rape-Trauma Syndrome: Compound Reaction
Rape-Trauma Syndrome: Silent Reaction
Relocation Stress Syndrome
Relocation Stress Syndrome, Risk for
Role Conflict, Parental
Role Performance, Ineffective
Self-Care Deficit: Bathing/Hygiene
Self-Care Deficit: Dressing/Grooming
Self-Care Deficit: Feeding
Self-Care Deficit: Toileting
Self-Concept, Readiness for Enhanced
Self-Esteem, Chronic Low
Self-Esteem, Situational Low
Self-Esteem, Risk for Situational Low
Self-Mutilation

Self-Mutilation, Risk for
Sensory Perception, Disturbed (Specify: Visual, Auditory, Kinesthetic, Gustatory, Tactile, Olfactory)
Sexual Dysfunction
Sexuality Patterns, Ineffective
Skin Integrity, Impaired
Skin Integrity, Risk for Impaired
Sleep Deprivation
Sleep Pattern Disturbed
Sleep, Readiness for Enhanced
Social Interaction, Impaired
Social Isolation
Sorrow, Chronic
Spiritual Distress
Spiritual Distress, Risk for
Spiritual Well-Being, Readiness for Enhanced
Spontaneous Ventilation, Impaired
Sudden Infant Death Syndrome, Risk for
Suffocation, Risk for
Suicide, Risk for
Surgical Recovery, Delayed
Swallowing, Impaired
Therapeutic Regimen Management: Community, Ineffective
Therapeutic Regimen Management, Effective
Therapeutic Regimen Management: Family, Ineffective
Therapeutic Regimen Management, Ineffective
Therapeutic Regimen Management, Readiness for Enhanced
Thermoregulation, Ineffective
Thought Processes, Disturbed
Tissue Integrity, Impaired
Tissue Perfusion, Ineffective (Specify: Renal, Cerebral, Cardiopulmonary, Gastrointestinal, Peripheral)
Transfer Ability, Impaired
Trauma, Risk for
Unilateral Neglect
Urinary Elimination, Impaired
Urinary Elimination, Readiness for Enhanced
Urinary Incontinence, Functional
Urinary Incontinence, Reflex
Urinary Incontinence, Stress
Urinary Incontinence, Total
Urinary Incontinence, Urge
Urinary Incontinence, Risk for Urge
Urinary Retention
Ventilatory Weaning Response, Dysfunctional
Violence: Other-Directed, Risk for
Violence: Self-Directed, Risk for
Walking, Impaired
Wandering

*Source. NANDA Nursing Diagnoses: Definitions and Classification, 2003–2004.* Philadelphia: North American Nursing Diagnosis Association. Used with permission.

# APPENDIX C

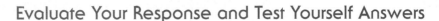

## Evaluate Your Response and Test Yourself Answers

Answers to Test Yourself

**Chapter 1: The Medical-Surgical Nurse**
1. D 2. A 3. B 4. C 5. C

**Chapter 2: The Adult Client in Health and Illness** 1. D 2. A 3. B 4. B 5. B

**Chapter 3: Community-Based and Home Care of the Adult Client** 1. B 2. D 3. C 4. A 5. B

**Chapter 4: Nursing Care of Clients in Pain** 1. B 2. A 3. B 4. D 5. C

**Chapter 5: Nursing Care of Clients with Altered Fluid, Electrolyte, or Acid-Base Balance** 1. A 2. D 3. B 4. D 5. A

**Chapter 6: Nursing Care of Clients Experiencing Trauma and Shock** 1. D 2. A 3. B 4. C 5. B

**Chapter 7: Nursing Care of Clients Having Surgery** 1. B 2. D 3. C 4. B 5. D

**Chapter 8: Nursing Care of Clients with Infection** 1. C 2. B 3. D 4. A 5. B

**Chapter 9: Nursing Care of Clients with Altered Immunity** 1. D 2. A 3. C 4. D 5. B

**Chapter 10: Nursing Care of Clients with Cancer** 1. C 2. A 3. C 4. B 5. C

**Chapter 11: Nursing Care of Clients Experiencing Loss, Grief, and Death** 1. C 2. D 3. B 4. A 5. C

**Chapter 12: Nursing Care of Clients with Problems of Substance Abuse** 1. B 2. A 3. D 4. C 5. B

**Chapter 13: Assessing Clients with Integumentary Disorders** 1. B 2. C 3. A 4. D 5. D

**Chapter 14: Nursing Care of Clients with Integumentary Disorders** 1. C 2. B 3. D 4. A 5. B

**Chapter 15: Nursing Care of Clients with Burns** 1. A 2. C 3. D 4. B 5. C

**Chapter 16: Assessing Clients with Endocrine Disorders** 1. D 2. A 3. C 4. B 5. B

**Chapter 17: Nursing Care of Clients with Endocrine Disorders** 1. A 2. C 3. C 4. D 5. B

**Chapter 18: Nursing Care of Clients with Diabetes Mellitus** 1. A 2. C 3. D 4. C 5. C

**Chapter 19: Assessing Clients with Nutritional and Gastrointestinal Disorders** 1. A 2. C 3. D 4. A 5. D

**Chapter 20: Nursing Care of Clients with Nutritional Disorders** 1. C 2. B 3. A 4. C 5. D

**Chapter 21: Nursing Care of Clients with Upper Gastrointestinal Disorders** 1. D 2. B 3. A 4. D 5. C

**Chapter 22: Nursing Care of Clients with Gallbladder, Liver, and Pancreatic Disorders** 1. A 2. C 3. D 4. B 5. C

**Chapter 23: Assessing Clients with Bowel Elimination Disorders** 1. D 2. A 3. D 4. D 5. C

**Chapter 24: Nursing Care of Clients with Bowel Disorders** 1. B 2. C 3. A 4. D 5. B

**Chapter 25: Assessing Clients with Urinary System Disorders** 1. D 2. C 3. B 4. C 5. A

**Chapter 26: Nursing Care of Clients with Urinary Tract Disorders** 1. B 2. D 3. A 4. C 5. C

**Chapter 27: Nursing Care of Clients with Kidney Disorders** 1. B 2. D 3. A 4. C 5. B

**Chapter 28: Assessing Clients with Cardiac Disorders** 1. C 2. D 3. C 4. A 5. B

**Chapter 29: Nursing Care of Clients with Coronary Heart Disease** 1. C 2. B 3. D 4. A 5. B

**Chapter 30: Nursing Care of Clients with Cardiac Disorders** 1. A 2. C 3. B 4. D 5. C

**Chapter 31: Assessing Clients with Hematologic, Peripheral Vascular, and Lymphatic Disorders** 1. D 2. A 3. B 4. C 5. A

**Chapter 32: Nursing Care of Clients with Hematologic Disorders** 1. C 2. D 3. A 4. B 5. A

**Chapter 33: Nursing Care of Clients with Peripheral Vascular and Lymphatic Disorders** 1. C 2. A 3. D 4. B 5. A

**Chapter 34: Assessing Clients with Respiratory Disorders** 1. D 2. C 3. B 4. D 5. C

**Chapter 35: Nursing Care of Clients with Upper Respiratory Disorders** 1. B 2. D 3. C 4. A 5. C

**Chapter 36: Nursing Care of Clients with Lower Respiratory Disorders** 1. D 2. B 3. A 4. C 5. D

**Chapter 37: Assessing Clients with Musculoskeletal Disorders** 1. C 2. A 3. B 4. D 5. A

**Chapter 38: Nursing Care of Clients with Musculoskeletal Trauma** 1. B 2. C 3. C 4. A 5. D

**Chapter 39: Nursing Care of Clients with Musculoskeletal Disorders** 1. B 2. D 3. D 4. A 5. C

**Chapter 40: Assessing Clients with Neurologic Disorders** 1. D 2. C 3. B 4. A 5. B

**Chapter 41: Nursing Care of Clients with Cerebrovascular and Spinal Cord Disorders** 1. B 2. D 3. C 4. A 5. B

**Chapter 42: Nursing Care of Clients with Intracranial Disorders** 1. D 2. B 3. B 4. A 5. C

**Chapter 43: Nursing Care of Clients with Neurologic Disorders** 1. C 2. A 3. B 4. D 5. B

**Chapter 44: Assessing Clients with Eye or Ear Disorders** 1. B 2. C 3. A 4. D 5. C

**Chapter 45: Nursing Care of Clients with Eye and Ear Disorders** 1. B 2. D 3. C 4. A 5. D

**Chapter 46: Assessing Clients with Reproductive System Disorders** 1. C 2. D 3. A 4. C 5. B

**Chapter 47: Nursing Care of Men with Reproductive System Disorders** 1. D 2. A 3. B 4. B 5. C

**Chapter 48: Nursing Care of Women with Reproductive System Disorders** 1. B 2. A 3. B 4. D 5. C

**Chapter 49: Nursing Care of Clients with Sexually Transmitted Infections** 1. B 2. A 3. D 4. A 5. C

Evaluate Your Response: Cues for Critical Thinking Questions

Chapter 4: Nursing Care of Clients in Pain

**A Client with Chronic Pain**

1. Review the factors that affect an individual's response to pain. What have you observed in your own family and friends, as well as clients for whom you have cared?

2. Reflect on the benefits and disadvantages of each alternative. Make your decision based on knowledge about pain and about medications for pain.

3. What factors in Ms. Akers's illness and treatment increase her risk for constipation? What would you include in the plan specific to fluid intake and diet?

## Chapter 5: Nursing Care of Clients with Altered Fluid, Electrolyte, or Acid-Base Balance

### A Client with Fluid Volume Excess

1. Review the homeostatic mechanisms that control fluid balance and cardiac output. Which mechanisms are employed in this situation?

2. Review the anatomy and physiology of the respiratory system, including cardiopulmonary blood flow. Think about the effects of the upper abdominal organs on respiratory function as well.

3. Use therapeutic communication techniques: What is behind the client's statement? How can you facilitate Mrs. Rainwater's involvement in care decisions?

4. Review the actions and precautions for diuretic therapy. Think about what the client needs to know in terms of timing, possible adverse effects, and other information about diuretic therapy.

### A Client with Hypokalemia

1. Review the physiologic effects of potassium, especially its intracellular and neuromuscular effects.

2. Review the potential sites and causes of excess potassium loss.

3. Think about the effects of diuretics on potassium balance and the effects of hypokalemia on digitalis therapy. What is the primary indication for digitalis therapy and how does this contribute to the interaction of these three factors?

4. Review the section in Chapter 24 on constipation and its management. ⊖⊃

### A Client with Hyperkalemia

1. Review the causes and manifestations of hyperkalemia.

2. What are the potential effects of hyperkalemia on cardiac conduction? At what level of hyperkalemia are these likely to be seen?

3. Review collaborative treatment measures to rapidly reduce potassium levels. Why would these be used with a K+ of 8.5?

4. Think about the effects of anxiety on learning as you develop a plan to provide teaching to avoid future episodes of hyperkalemia. As you develop your plan, remember the potential long-term effects of chronic renal failure.

### A Client with Acute Respiratory Acidosis

1. Review normal gas exchange across the alveolar-capillary membrane and the processes that drive this exchange. Then review the role that carbon dioxide plays as a potential acid.

2. Describe the effect of acidosis on mental function.

3. Consider risk factors for choking: alcohol consumption, taking large bites of food, inadequate chewing, and so forth.

## Chapter 6: Nursing Care of Clients Experiencing Trauma and Shock

### A Client with Multiple Injuries

1. The definition of *Deficient fluid volume* is decreased intravascular, interstitial, and/or intracellular fluid. Which of Mrs. Souza's vital signs would support this definition? What other assessments could you make that would further support this diagnosis?

2. Consider the physiology of cellular metabolism. How long do brain cells live without oxygen? What happens if circulation is improved but the airway is blocked?

3. What can cause restlessness? Consider comfort, elimination, oxygenation, emotional status, and immobility.

4. List the multiple possibilities for entry of pathogens into the human body. Would age and physical condition increase the risk? What about transmission from health care personnel?

### A Client with Septic Shock

1. Review the pharmacologic effects of vasopressors. Consider the pathologic basis for septic shock and how these medications may be effective.

2. Review the content on respiratory acidosis in Chapter 5. ⊖⊃ What do these findings tell you? What is present in Ms. Huang's physical status that would cause these manifestations?

3. Review the content about colloidal intravenous solutions in the chapter. What would you expect them to do when they are administered? How does this correlate to cardiac output? How do you assess increased circulatory volume?

## Chapter 7: Nursing Care of Clients Having Surgery

### A Client Having Surgery

1. Safety concerns include ambulating and not tripping over scatter rugs or clutter. See information in Chapter 3 on safety in the home. ⊖⊃

2. Medications used to prevent an occurrence such as infection are called prophylactic medications. Her risks for infection are from the surgical wound and microvascular circulation in bone. Teach her to take the complete course of antibiotics prescribed and the possible side effects of the antibiotic. Encourage her to notify the physician if side effects or adverse events occur.

3. When blood stops flowing, it clots. Her immobility is a concern and puts her at risk for thrombosis and emboli. She has a risk for bleeding secondary to the anticoagulant and should inform any health care providers such as dentists that she is taking the anticoagulant.

4. Consider the risk for osteoporosis in addition to the degenerative changes Mrs. Overbeck experienced. She will need calcium sources and vitamin D.

## Chapter 8: Nursing Care of Clients with Infection

### A Client with Acquired Immunity

1. Review the adult immunizations listed in Table 8–8. ⊖⊃ Consider the geographical area in which the client lives. For example, clients living in areas at risk for Lyme disease should check with their physician about the new Lyme disease vaccine.

2. Review the concept of acquired immunity and the discussion of immunization in this chapter. What affect could nonimmunized persons have on their family and community?

3. Identify possible systemic and local reactions associated with immunizations. List manifestations that the client should report to the primary caregiver.

### Chapter 9: Nursing Care of Clients with Altered Immunity

#### A Client with HIV Infection

1. Considering Ms. Lu's age, how effective is her immune system? How could lifestyle factors affect immune status?

2. At this stage of Ms. Lu's diagnosis, would you expect the physician to order a viral load test? Why or why not?

3. You have been asked to discuss AIDS and safe sex practices to a group of high school freshmen. What information would you present to them?

4. What resources could you provide to Ms. Lu and her fiancé regarding their desire to have a child?

### Chapter 10: Nursing Care of Clients with Cancer

1. Review content on altered nutrition in Chapter 20 and the content in this chapter on the nursing diagnosis Altered Nutrition: Less than Body Requirements. Make a list of diagnostic tests for malnutrition with normal values.

2. Consider the type of cancers Mr. Casey has been diagnosed as having. Where in the body do these malignancies commonly metastasize? What would cause the pain?

3. Review a pharmacology book for medications that increase appetite and make a list of those appropriate to Mr. Casey.

4. Sepsis is discussed in Chapter 6. ⊕ Review the content in that chapter on septic shock and outline manifestations. Develop a plan of care for Mr. Casey that is structured by priority of nursing diagnoses.

### Chapter 11: Nursing Care of Clients Experiencing Loss, Grief, and Death

#### A Client Experiencing Loss and Grief

1. Review the physical manifestations of grief described in the chapter and compare and contrast those with the ones verbalized by Mrs. Rogers.

2. Consider the benefits of including Mrs. Rogers's daughter in a meeting of the staff. What type of questions would be most useful in making the daughter feel a part of the plan of care? Why would a statement such as, "Why don't you do more for your mother," be inappropriate?

3. Consider the losses Mrs. Rogers has experienced. Review the material in the chapter on responses to loss. Think about the reasons you would not say, "Oh, you have a lot to live for." Think of two or three questions or statements that would help you assess the reason why Mrs. Rogers said this to you.

### Chapter 12: Nursing Care of Clients with Problems of Substance Abuse

1. Consider the interactions of prescribed or over-the-counter medications with alcohol. What if the client has not taken prescribed medications because of chronic alcoholism?

2. Review the effects of Anatbuse. Make a list of possible interactions and side effects.

3. *Imbalanced nutrition: Less than body requirements* is an appropriate nursing diagnosis when a client does not have sufficient nutritional intake to meet metabolic needs. What in Mr. Russell's history and physical assessment supports this diagnosis? What nutritional information should you provide?

### Chapter 14: Nursing Care of Clients with Integumentary Disorders

#### A Client with Herpes Zoster

1. Consider environmental, economic, and language barriers. What agencies in your own city or state exist to provide help? What can you do other than make referrals? If you do make a referral, to whom would it be?

2. Review skin assessment guidelines in Chapter 13. ⊕ How would you determine that the lesions had not improved? What manifestations would indicate secondary infection of the lesions? What would you do next if the lesions are still very painful and have not improved?

3. *Ineffective role performance* is defined as patterns of behavior and self-expression that do not match the environmental context, norms, and expectations. Related factors include inadequate or inappropriate linkage with the health care system and poverty. Based on this information, what interventions would you use? How would you evaluate the effectiveness of your interventions?

#### A Client with Malignant Melanoma

1. List reasons why people do not seek health care. Do you believe nurses can effect change? If so, what community activities would be most effective?

2. Consider attitudes toward the possibility of future illnesses. How would this affect your plan? What do you believe would be most effective in teaching this age group?

3. Think about what you know about taking prescribed antibiotics as well as the side effects of antibiotic therapy. What would you suggest that Mr. Sanders do?

4. *Powerlessness* is the perception that one's own actions will not significantly affect an outcome. Is this a common response to the diagnosis of cancer? Consider types of communications and interventions that would allow greater decision making for Mr. Sanders.

### Chapter 15: Nursing Care of Clients with Burns

#### A Client with a Major Burn

1. Review the effects of the major burn wound on the renal and gastrointestinal systems. What assessments would indicate effective fluid resuscitation?

2. What type of burns did Mr. Howard have on his arms? Consider the effect of compression on the peripheral vascular system. What assessments would you make to identify this complication?

3. Consider the type of pain the client has. What do you think might happen if the narcotics were given by other routes, such as oral or intramuscularly?

4. Review the effects of a major burn. Consider the damage to cell wall integrity and capillary beds. What effect does the shift of proteins and sodium have on intravascular volume?

## Chapter 17: Nursing Care of Clients with Endocrine Disorders

### A Client with Graves' Disease

1. What effect does increased TH have on metabolism and cardiac rate and stroke volume? How does this effect compare to that of sympathetic stimulation?

2. Consider the effect of elevating any body part, such as elevating your leg above heart level for a sprained ankle. How does this affect venous return?

3. You will need to consider Mrs. Manuel from both a medical and a surgical perspective. How would you teach her to care for her incision? With removal of most of the thyroid gland, what symptoms would you be sure she knew about? What should she do if these occur?

### A Client with Hypothyroidism

1. Make a list of changes in body systems with aging and with decreased TH levels. How would you determine what assessment findings were abnormal?

2. Consider the effects of the following factors: weakness, fatigue, problems with memory. What would you recommend she do in her home to increase her safety?

3. Prepare a list of manifestations of hyperthyroidism. Be sure they are in terms a client would understand.

### A Client with Cushing's Syndrome

1. Review Ms. Domico's lab results and compare them to normal results. What altered the findings in her case?

2. How many ways can you think of to assess fluid balance? Consider weight, I&O, and skin. What other assessments provide information?

3. Review Box 17–3. ⊙⊙ How does fatigue differ from "just being tired"? Would increasing hours of sleep be an intervention you would include? Why or why not?

### A Client with Addison's Disease

1. Review the functions of the hormones of the adrenal cortex in Chapter 16. ⊙⊙ Consider the effects of stress, and formulate your response with rationale.

2. Review content on fluid imbalance in Chapter 5. ⊙⊙ Make a list of assessments you might make that would indicate severe dehydration. What is the pathophysiology of fluid loss in the client with Addison's disease?

3. Review content on sodium and potassium in Chapter 5 ⊙⊙ and make a list of foods you would suggest Mr. Sardoff eat.

## Chapter 18: Nursing Care of Clients with Diabetes Mellitus

### A Client with Type 1 Diabetes

1. How do the increased urinary output and increased osmolarity of the blood plasma affect the fluid status of the body? What is the response of the body to decreased intravascular volume?

2. Consider the effects of nicotine on blood vessels. How would these effects, when combined with the pathologic effects of long-standing hyperglycemia, affect blood vessel walls?

3. Review the information about chronic illness in Chapter 2. ⊙⊙ *Powerlessness* is a perceived lack of control over a situation and/or one's ability to significantly affect an outcome. What types of statements by a client would help you make this nursing diagnosis?

4. Compare and contrast the developmental needs and tasks of the young adult and the older adult (see Chapter 2 ⊙⊙ ). Consider the teaching materials that might have to be adapted to physical changes in the older adult.

## Chapter 20: Nursing Care of Clients with Nutritional Disorders

### A Client with Obesity

1. Review the physiology of cholesterol formation in the body and the factors that affect this process.

2. Consider developmental stages and teaching strategies for adult learners.

3. Think about individual factors, family and support group influences, and cultural factors that may affect recommended weight loss and exercise strategies.

### A Client with Malnutrition

1. Review the physiology of albumin and cholesterol formation in the body.

2. Review Mrs. Chow's diet and compare it to the food pyramid or recommendations for food intake to formulate your response.

3. Consider cultural influences and the client's preferred foods as you plan a diet that is high in calories and protein.

## Chapter 21: Nursing Care of Clients with Upper Gastrointestinal Disorders

### A Client with Oral Cancer

1. Review the major risk factors for oral cancer and identify the populations most likely to have these risk factors.

2. Work with your classmates to plan (and implement) an education program, considering the developmental/teaching needs of this group of young people.

3. Think about the possible causes for Mr. Chavez's refusal to talk (remember that assessment is the first step of the nursing process). How will you identify factors contributing to his behavior?

### A Client with Peptic Ulcer Disease

1. Review the physiology of the gastric mucosal barrier and the pathogenesis of peptic ulcer disease, and the effect of *H. pylori* infection on these processes.

2. Review physiologic responses to stress in your physiology or nursing fundamentals text; compare and apply this information with the physiology of the gastric mucosal barrier and the pathophysiology of ulcer development.

3. Consider Mr. O'Donnell's occupation and schedule, as well as the prescribed medications and when each should be taken.

4. Using journal and text resources as well as your classmates, identify as many stress reduction techniques as possible. Then sort your list into those which could be used while working, and identify ways to effectively teach each technique.

### A Client with Gastric Cancer

1. Review the healing process and the normal physiology of the stomach as you formulate your answer to this question.

2. Consider the surgery, immediate postoperative care, and what the client and family should expect in developing your teaching plan.

3. Review Chapter 10 ⊝ and nursing care related to chemotherapy.

4. Again, review Chapter 10 ⊝ for nursing care measures for clients with cancer; also review Chapter 20 ⊝ for strategies to prevent and manage malnutrition.

### Chapter 22: Nursing Care of Clients with Gallbladder, Liver, and Pancreatic Disorders

### A Client with Cholelithiasis

1. Review the composition of gallstones, as well as the physiology of gallbladder function and bile. Research and discuss dietary practices of the Chickasaw tribe (or of Native Americans).

2. Review Chapter 7 ⊝ for care related to a laparotomy (incision into the abdomen).

3. As you develop your plan, consider Mrs. Red Wing's culture, job, and family obligations.

### A Client with Hepatitis A

1. In your plan, consider the transmission and pathophysiology of hepatitis A. Review developmental considerations when teaching clients to adapt your teaching to Mr. Johns's level.

2. Review Table 22–2, ⊝ as well as the pathophysiology of hepatitis.

3. Review Tables 22–2 and 22–3, ⊝ as well as standard precautions.

4. In your plan, consider the living situation (group home), the developmental level of the residents, and the resident care managers (largely unskilled). Work with your study or clinical group to develop this plan.

### A Client with Alcoholic Cirrhosis

1. Review the anatomy and physiology of the liver and its circulation, as well as the pathophysiology of cirrhosis and its complications.

2. Consult your nutrition textbook as needed for foods that are high in calories but low in protein and sodium. When planning for limited protein intake, be sure to include high-quality proteins and limit intake of lower-quality proteins such as legumes.

3. Review the pathophysiology of hepatic encephalopathy and the medication box on page 591 ⊝ to develop your responses to this question.

4. Review therapeutic communication skills; consult your nursing diagnosis and care planning text book as you develop this care plan.

### A Client with Acute Pancreatitis

1. Review Chapter 12 ⊝ for assessment data indicative of alcohol withdrawal.

2. Review both the pathophysiology of acute pancreatitis and the acute inflammatory process.

3. Consult your nutrition textbook or the American Dietetic Association web site: www.eatright.org

4. Consult your nursing care planning textbook to develop this care plan.

### Chapter 24: Nursing Care of Clients with Bowel Disorders

### A Client with Acute Appendicitis

1. Review the acute inflammatory response to an infectious process and the role WBCs play in the immune response.

2. Review Chapter 7. ⊝ Consider factors such as incision size, abdominal muscle disruption, and manipulation of the bowel in developing your response.

3. Consider points such as pain management, resumption of activities, incision care, and potential complications in developing your teaching plan. Consider the client's education and developmental stage as well.

4. Review the effects of anxiety on recovery and learning. Identify nursing measures to reduce situational anxiety.

### A Client with Ulcerative Colitis

1. Review normal functions of the small and large intestine. Review the usual location of an ileostomy. Review fluid volume deficit in Chapter 5 ⊝ for manifestations and assessment data.

2. Think about the effect of chronic blood loss and review the effect of malnutrition on the hemoglobin and hematocrit.

3. Review the home care section of inflammatory bowel disease for teaching points to include.

4. Review nursing care for the client with diarrhea, as well as the procedure for ileostomy care.

### A Client with Colorectal Cancer

1. Review peripheral innervation and impulse transmission in your anatomy and physiology textbook; think about how nerves in the rectal region are disrupted in an abdominoperineal resection. Also review the phantom pain phenomenon in Chapter 4. ⊝

2. Compare elimination through a colostomy with "normal" bowel elimination through the anus. How do they differ in terms of the passage of flatus?

3. Review Procedure 24–1 ⊝ and the nursing care box on page 672. ⊝ Also review the procedure for administering an enema in your fundamentals or skills textbook.

4. Review this nursing diagnosis in your nursing diagnosis or nursing care planning handbook; be sure to individualize your plan to Mr. Cunningham's situation and needs.

### A Client with Diverticulitis

1. Review Mrs. Ukoha's presenting symptoms and laboratory data. Then review the collaborative care section related to diverticulitis.

2. Consider how long Mrs. Ukoha may have been on bowel rest (NPO) prior to having a bowel movement, and the manifestations of diverticular disease.

3. Review the risk factors for and pathophysiology of diverticular disease and diverticulitis.

4. Consult your nutrition textbook and see Table 24–13 ⬯ to develop your teaching plan.

## Chapter 26: Nursing Care of Clients with Urinary Tract Disorders

### A Client with Cystitis

1. Consider risk factors for UTI as well as factors affecting Mrs. Waisanen's immune function.

2. Consider the indications for short-course antibiotic therapy and the indications for conventional therapy. Think about factors such as cost, compliance, and the risk for adverse effects, as well as how antibiotics work to eradicate bacteria.

3. Identify why *Ineffective health maintenance* may be an appropriate nursing diagnosis for Mrs. Waisanen and the individual factors contributing to this diagnosis as you plan care.

### A Client with Urinary Calculi

1. Review the risk factors for urinary lithiasis.

2/3. Using the medications section of collaborative care for the client with urinary calculi in Chapter 26 ⬯ as well as Chapter 4, ⬯ and your pharmacology textbook or drug handbook, review analgesia for the client with renal colic and the intended and adverse effects of the drugs given to Mr. Leton.

### A Client with a Bladder Tumor

1. Review the physiology of the bladder and the risk factors for urinary tract tumors.

2. Review Mr. Hussain's health history for possible contributing factors.

3. See Chapter 12 ⬯ for nursing care of clients with problems of substance abuse.

4. Use your nursing care planning and nursing diagnoses textbooks to identify possible outcomes and interventions for *Sexual dysfunction*.

### A Client with Urinary Incontinence

1. Review the desired and adverse effects of the prescribed medications.

2. Review the effects of menopause and estrogen deficiency on perineal tissues.

3. Review Mrs. Giovanni's physical examination findings and risk factors for UTI.

4. Identify factors that may contribute to *Situational low self-esteem* in Mrs. Giovanni and nursing measures to address this diagnosis.

## Chapter 27: Nursing Care of Clients with Kidney Disorders

### A Client with Acute Glomerulonephritis

1. Review Chapter 8 ⬯ and the use of antibiotics to treat infection.

2. Review Mr. Chang's history and the risk factors for acute glomerulonephritis.

3. Review the diagnostic tests used to differentiate different forms of glomerulonephritis on page 750. ⬯

### A Client with Acute Renal Failure

1. Review common causes and the pathophysiology of acute renal failure.

2. Review the sections on peptic ulcer disease and stress gastritis in Chapter 21. ⬯

3. Consider the position requirements to maintain body and bone alignment in skeletal traction (Chapter 38). ⬯

### A Client with End-Stage Renal Disease

1. Review the usual onset, pathophysiology, and long-term effects of type 1 and type 2 diabetes (Chapter 18). ⬯

2. Consider the effects of urea and ammonia (both neurologic toxins) on brain function.

3. Review the manifestations of uremia.

4. Consider the composition of the dialysate and its possible effect on blood glucose control.

## Chapter 29: Nursing Care of Clients with Coronary Heart Disease

### A Client with Coronary Artery Bypass Surgery

1. Identify Mr. Clements's modifiable risk factors as you develop your plan. What barriers might need to be overcome to implement strategies to reduce his risk factors?

2. What strategies can you use to overcome denial without creating hostility or impairing the client-nurse relationship?

3. Consider traditional family roles as well as those roles that are unique to these individuals. Identify measures you can use to enlist the spouse's support.

4. Think about therapeutic communications as you formulate your response. Will your age or gender potentially affect your ability to respond effectively to these concerns? Would referral to another health care provider be appropriate?

### A Client with Acute Myocardial Infarction

1. Review immediate treatment measures for MI. Are other means available for reestablishing coronary artery perfusion? If you are in a rural area without immediate access to a cardiac catheterization lab, how will this affect your response?

2. Review the section of this chapter on dysrhythmias and their treatment. Research protocols for treating frequent PVCs in the post-MI client at your clinical facility.

3. Review the goals of cardiac rehabilitation and Mrs. Williams's individual risk factors as you develop your teaching plan.

4. Consider the value of using a therapeutic response to Mrs. Williams's statement concerning smoking. Also consider the risks associated with cigarette smoke. How can you respond without supporting Mrs. Williams's desire to smoke and without precipitating anger or resistance? Review Chapter 12. ⬯

### A Client with Supraventricular Tachycardia

1. Review the effects of sympathetic and parasympathetic nervous system stimulation on cardiac function.

2. Review the section on supraventricular tachycardias, as well as the antidysrhythmic medications for other treatment options.

3. Use your pharmacology textbook as you develop your teaching plan.

## Chapter 30: Nursing Care of Clients with Cardiac Disorders

### A Client with Heart Failure

1. Review the prescribed medications and their interactions. Do not forget to consider Mr. Jackson's age in assessing his risk for toxicity and interactions.

2. Review therapeutic communications skills and the use of open-ended statements to evaluate the underlying message of Mr. Jackson's statement.

3. Review exercise recommendations for the client with heart failure (page 885) ⊂⊃ as well as cardiac rehabilitation principles (Chapter 29). ⊂⊃

4. Review the rationale for aspirin therapy in the client with CHD and its effects on platelets and clotting as you formulate your response.

5. Review Chapter 41 ⊂⊃ for causes of CVA and the section of Chapter 29 ⊂⊃ on atrial fibrillation.

### A Client with Mitral Valve Prolapse

1. Review the pathophysiology and manifestations of MVP, as well as the general treatment measures for valve disorders.

2. Think about the effects of progressive conditioning on cardiac function.

3. Consider the anxiety associated with heart conditions and with a potentially progressive disorder that could affect childbearing and other life activities, as well as ultimately necessitate surgery.

4. Review the manifestations of MVP and of mitral regurgitation.

## Chapter 32: Nursing Care of Clients with Hematologic Disorders

### A Client with Anemia

1. Consider the effects of Mrs. Matthews's rapid weight loss on fluid balance, as well as the effects of tissue hypoxia on cardiac output.

2. Refer to Box 32–6 ⊂⊃ and your nutrition text. Be sure to consider Mrs. Matthews's age in designing your menu.

3. Consider factors such as Mrs. Matthews's recent dietary history, the folic acid content of foods, and

other pertinent factors in the history and physical assessment

4. In addition to general factors to consider for the older adult (don't forget transportation among other factors), also consider the possible effect of Mrs. Matthews's recent loss and the grieving process.

### A Client with Hemophilia

1. Review the pathophysiology of hemophilia and its effect on the clotting process.

2. Consider both the ABCs and Maslow's hierarchy of needs as you respond to this question.

3. Think about the genetic transmission of hemophilia. How might Mr. Cruise's hemophila affect any children that he has? Grandchildren?

4. Review your nursing fundamentals book, nursing skills book, and intravenous therapy text to develop your teaching plan. Also consider previous learning and developmental levels.

5. Consult your nursing care planning text. Consider why this might be an appropriate nursing diagnosis for Mr. Cruise.

### A Client with Leukemia

1. Review the physiology of white blood cells, and the immune and inflammatory responses.

2. Think about the risks created by hospitalization in terms of exposure to infection and invasive procedures.

3. Think about the effect of inability to perform self care on self-esteem, self-confidence, and perception of power and control.

4. Use information provided in the nursing care and home care sections of this chapter as well as in Chapter 8. ⊂⊃

5. Use your nursing care planning and fundamentals texts to develop your care plan.

### A Client with Hodgkin's disease

1. Review Chapter 10 ⊂⊃ and the effects of chemotherapy and radiation on cancerous cells. Think about the advantages of combining these two therapies in terms of short and long-term desired and adverse effects.

2. Consider the primary and potential risks for infection in community settings as you design your teaching plan. What teaching strategies will you use for a young adult with Mr. Quito's education and experience?

3. Review theories of development and the developmental tasks for the young adult.

4. Use your nursing fundamentals and nursing care planning texts for reference in developing your care plan.

## Chapter 33: Nursing Care of Clients with Peripheral Vascular and Lymphatic Disorders

### A Client with Hypertension

1. Review Mrs. Spezia's assessment data and the risk factors for primary hypertension.

2. Review the pathophysiology of primary hypertension and of obesity (Chapter 20), ⊂⊃ as well as the relationship between hypertension and coronary heart disease.

3. Think about resources that are available in your community for homeless people. Talk to community health and social service agencies to identify additional resources.

4. Again, review Mrs. Spezia's assessment data, the pathophysiology of hypertension, and the long-term effects of stress.

5. Use your nursing care planning and nursing diagnosis textbooks to help develop your care plan.

### A Client with Peripheral Atherosclerosis

1. Review treatments for peripheral atherosclerosis, as well as lifestyle measures for preventing and treating atherosclerosis and coronary heart disease (Chapter 29). ⊂⊃

2. Compare the pathophysiology of peripheral atherosclerosis, intermittent claudication, and coronary heart disease (Chapter 29 ⊂⊃ ) to identify similarities and differences.

3. Review the actions of beta blockers and their role in angina prophylaxis.

4. Use your nursing care planning and nutrition textbooks to help develop your care plan.

### A Client with Deep Vein Thrombosis

1. Review the pathophysiologic processes of venous thrombosis and inflammation as you develop your answer.

2. Think about questions you could ask for further information as well as potential resources for Mrs. Hipps.

3. Consider assessment data to evaluate Mrs. Hipps's limitations and resources, as well as community resources to help meet her needs.

4. Use your nursing diagnosis and care planning textbooks to develop your plan of care.

### Chapter 35: Nursing Care of Clients with Upper Respiratory Disorders

### A Client with Peritonsillar Abscess

1/2. Review the manifestations of upper respiratory infections and management of these disorders.

3. Think about the primary uses of the nose, mouth, and pharynx as you consider nursing diagnoses related to upper respiratory disorders.

### A Client with Nasal Fracture

1. Consider other measures to restore the client's sense of control over the situation. Consider the potentially traumatic effects of suction on the mucous membranes as well as possible infection control risks.

2. Review the implications and potential dangers of CSF leakage to help you develop your care plan.

3. Think about the benefits and drawbacks of immediate and delayed rhinoplasty.

### A Client with Total Laryngectomy

1. Review the options for speech rehabilitation. If available, practice using a speech generator. Practice esophageal speech.

2. Use your nursing care planning and nursing diagnoses handbook to develop your care plan. Consider Mr. Tom's age, occupation, and marital status in your plan of care.

3. Review Chapter 7 ⊙⊙ for surgical nursing care interventions, as well as your nursing fundamentals textbook for wound care strategies.

4. Consider measures to promote airway clearance and ventilation of all lung fields.

### Chapter 36: Nursing Care of Clients with Lower Respiratory Disorders

### A Client with Pneumonia

1. Review Mrs. O'Neal's assessment data and compare her history with identified risk factors for pneumonia.

2. Review normal immune and inflammatory responses and the role of white blood cells in these processes.

3. Review Chapter 9 ⊙⊙ and altered immune responses for the physiology and effects of anaphylactic shock.

4. Use your nursing care planning and nursing diagnosis textbooks to help develop your care plan.

### A Client with Tuberculosis

1. Consider available resources for mentally ill clients, as well as community and public health resources. Consider measures to ensure compliance with the prescribed treatment.

2. Contact your local public health department, the discharge planner for your unit, or the social services department in your clinical facility to help identify available resources.

3. Use your nursing fundamentals text, the nursing care section under Pneumonia, and your nursing diagnosis or care planning handbook as you develop your care plan.

### A Client with COPD

1. Review the processes by which cigarette smoke inflicts damage on lung tissue. Use your pediatric and pathophysiology texts for additional information.

2. Review the physiology of the respiratory drive, as well as the effects of chronic elevated carbon dioxide levels in the blood.

3. Review the manifestations of COPD and its complications as well as the section of this chapter on respiratory failure.

4. Use your nursing diagnosis handbook to help identify appropriate goals and interventions for this nursing diagnosis.

### A Client with Lung Cancer

1. Review Chapter 10 ⊙⊙ and use your pharmacology text to research the effects of these drugs and the rationale for combination chemotherapy.

2. Use Chapter 10 ⊙⊙ and your pharmacology text to identify probable side effects of this treatment regimen. Then use your nursing care planning book to identify appropriate nursing diagnoses and interventions.

3. Review the pathophysiology and collaborative care sections for lung cancer to develop your response to this question.

### A Client with ARDS

1. As you respond to this question, consider additional treatment measures for ARDS and respiratory failure. Also consider the potential long-term consequences and complications of intubation and mechanical ventilation. Discuss strategies for communicating with Ms. Adamson's family and supporting coping and decision-making by Ms. Adamson and her family in an instance such as this.

2. Think about the precipitating factors for ARDS and the factors that may precipitate respiratory failure in a client with COPD. Consider the probable overall respiratory and general health status of the individual affected by each of these conditions.

3. Review the precipitating factors for ARDS and discuss strategies to prevent them.

4. Use your nursing care planning book to identify appropriate goals and nursing interventions for this nursing diagnosis.

### Chapter 38: Nursing Care of Clients with Musculoskeletal Trauma

### A Client with a Hip Fracture

1. Consider Mrs. Carbolito's age and the fact that she is postmenopausal. What effect does estrogen have on bone health? What might have increased her risk for falls?

2. Review the principles of traction application. What purpose does it

serve prior to surgery? What words could you use that she would understand? Think about the effects of trauma, pain, and suddenly finding oneself in a strange environment on listening and understanding verbal communications.

3. List how each of these manifestations would affect skin integrity, food intake, and bone healing.

### A Client with a Below-the-Knee Amputation

1. Design a sequential plan for Mr. Rocke's self-care of the stump. Consider his readiness to learn and the complexity of the care. Is there a risk in letting him assume total responsibility from the beginning? Why or why not?

2. List the factors used to describe Mr. Rocke. How do these affect his ability or willingness to follow up with medical care? What community agencies are available where you live or go to school that would be good sources of assistance and support for Mr. Rocke?

3. Review the information about exercise. How would Mr. Rocke's choice not to do exercises affect his ability to use a prosthesis to walk?

### Chapter 39: Nursing Care of Clients with Musculoskeletal Disorders

### A Client with Osteoporosis

1. Review the effects of nicotine and caffeine on blood circulation to bones. What effect does alcohol play in bone loss?

2. Review foods that increase blood cholesterol levels. What is considered a normal cholesterol level? You may need to read content in Chapter 29. ⊕ Knowing the client needs calcium, what type of dairy products would you recommend?

3. List activities for the client who is not able to be ambulatory. How many of the activities on your list would help prevent osteoporosis?

4. *Risk for trauma* is defined as an increased risk for accidental tissue injury, such as a fracture. What

interventions would you teach Mrs. Bauer to reduce this risk?

### A Client with Osteoarthritis

1. Review information about serum creatinine and BUN in a laboratory studies textbook or on the web. What medications is Mr. Cerulli taking that may be affecting these findings? Consider what teaching is necessary related to these findings.

2. What assessments are significant for confusion? If necessary, review content related to confusion. Review Mr. Cerulli's history in the case study and determine factors that may have contributed to his risk for confusion before, during, and after surgery.

3. *Acute confusion* is defined as an abrupt onset of a cluster of global, transient changes and disturbances in attention, cognition, psychomotor activity, level of consciousness, and/or sleep/wake cycle. What assessments could you make to support this diagnosis for Mr. Cerulli? What interventions might you design for this diagnosis?

### A Client with Rheumatoid Arthritis

1. Think about the role differences in a 42-year-old woman and a 72-year-old woman. On the other hand, consider the effects of a chronic illness that may have been present for 30 years. Would your plan differ? Why or why not?

2. List the possible disabilities that may be caused by rheumatoid arthritis. How do you believe these would affect Mrs. James? What agencies in your community are available for support of people with this type of illness? Where would you go for literature to give Mrs. James?

3. *Ineffective role performance* is defined as behaviors and expressions that do not match norms or expectations. Do you believe this is an appropriate nursing diagnosis for Mrs. James? Why or why not? What interventions could be implemented for this diagnosis?

### Chapter 41: Nursing Care of Clients with Cerebrovascular and Spinal Cord Disorders

### A Client with a Stroke

1. What subjective manifestations does the client with hypertension have? (Review content in Chapter 33.) ⊕

2. How does increased blood pressure affect the walls of blood vessels in the cerebral circulation?

3. Consider referral to community resources as a volunteer tutor for adult literacy, gardening, and/or woodworking. Tutoring college students is another option.

4. Use statements that will encourage Mr. Boren to talk about his arm and how he feels about being unable to use it.

### A Client with a SCI

1. What are the developmental tasks of a 19-year-old? How does the inability to meet these tasks affect emotional responses?

2. Think about questions that explore Mr. Valdez's fears in relation to sexuality. Practice questions and statements with friends until you are not embarrassed to ask them.

3. Consider how your own values and beliefs may differ from those of a client.

4. What baseline assessments and information are necessary before developing a plan for urinary elimination needs? Why would self-catheterization be an option? What are the risks of long-term Foley catheterization?

### A Client with an Intervertebral Disk

1. What emergency management of any possible spinal cord injury is necessary, and why?

2. Consider social and economic needs. What types of community and health care resources are available for a young single mother?

3. What type of clothing would be most useful for Mrs. Ivans? In what sequence should she dress? What about shoes?

## Chapter 42: Nursing Care of Clients with Intracranial Disorders

### A Client with a Migraine Headache

1. Review the content in the chapter on migraine headaches. List questions that you would ask specific to onset, length, manifestations, stages, pain, diet, and factors associated with the headache onset.

2. Consider foods that are high in sodium. What would you suggest if Ms. Friedman eats fast foods at least five times a week? Review the food pyramid in Chapter 2 ⊙⊙ and outline a weekly meal plan for Ms. Friedman.

3. Discuss with members of your class those factors that interfere with their normal sleep patterns. What suggestions might you give Ms. Friedman to help her improve her sleep? Why is this important?

### A Client with a Seizure Disorder

1. List the teaching topics you would include for Ms. Carlson. Consider how her needs (e.g., for safety) would differ if she lived alone.

2. Describe statements you could use to help Ms. Carlson understand not only the dangers but also the legal issues involved. What if Ms. Carlson does not recognize these concerns?

3. What type of questions could you ask Ms. Carlson to determine why she feels this way? Would you personally find it embarrassing? How can you facilitate Ms. Carlson's understanding for this recommendation?

### A Client with Subdural Hematoma

1. Review the manifestations of the types of intracranial hematomas. What assessments are specific to a subdural hematoma? Why is it important to know this?

2. What are some other interventions that might be used? How could family help? What if no family members are available?

3. Acute confusion is a sudden onset of changes in attention, cognition, psychomotor activity, level of consciousness, and/or sleep/wake cycle. What would you determine as priority nursing diagnoses and interventions for Mr. Lee?

### A Client with Bacterial Meningitis

1. List the environmental stimuli in the hospital setting. How could these be decreased? What effect do these stimuli have on cognition and behavior that is altered by an intracranial infection?

2. Think about how you would feel if Mr. Cook tried to hit you. How would you respond to him? To whom would you report this?

3. Why would Mr. Cook have pain? How would pain be manifested during the initial treatment period for Mr. Cook? Is it important to consider the respiratory effects of narcotics for him? Defend your answer.

### A Client with a Brain Tumor

1. Review content in the chapter on increased intracranial pressure and intracranial surgery. List collaborative and nursing interventions to decrease increased intracranial pressure.

2. What do these manifestations indicate? What would be your priority assessment? Who would you notify?

3. Practice the use of therapeutic communications and what response you would make.

4. Consider the reasons Ms. Lange feels powerless. What nursing interventions might decrease this feeling?

## Chapter 43: Nursing Care of Clients with Neurologic Disorders

### A Client with AD

1. Think about what information you would need and how you would collect it. Consider such factors as the age of family members, educational level of family members, and stage of the client's AD. What else would you need to know?

2. Review the suggested activities in this section of the chapter. What others can you think of or have you seen used successfully? Osteoarthritis often results in joint stiffness and pain as well as problems with mobility. Would this affect your interventions? If so, how could they be adapted?

3. Consider the type of foods that might be prepared, the timing of meals, and interventions that might be used to decrease agitation before or during meals.

### A Client with MS

1. Outline a typical day's activities for Mr. McMurphy that would provide a balance between activity and rest. What assessments would you make to evaluate the effectiveness of this plan?

2. Consider how respiratory infections are spread. Why is Mr. McMurphy at increased risk?

3. The definition of *Risk for injury* is that one is at risk as a result of environmental conditions interacting with the person's adaptive and defensive resources. What factors in this client's history and physical status would support this diagnosis? What interventions would you include in the care plan and why?

### A Client with Parkinson's Disease

1. Consider the adaptations that might be made to clothing and shoes. What adaptive devices might be useful?

2. What information would you need to know before you develop your interventions? Include that from Mr. Avneil and what might be available in the community and the long-term care facility.

3. *Chronic sorrow* is a recurring pattern of sadness in response to continual loss. Consider the type of communications you would need to use with Mr. Avneil to identify his degree of sorrow. What other assessment might provide cues to support this diagnosis (think about eating and sleeping)? How might an activity such as reminiscence help?

### A Client with Myasthenia Gravis

1. Review the pathophysiology of myasthenia gravis. What is the action of Tensilon?

2. Consider teaching topics for Mrs. Avis that would assist her in conserving energy while preparing meals. List suggestions to conserve energy while eating.

3. *Ineffective role performance* is the state in which behaviors and self-expression do not match such factors as norms and expectations. What changes occur as a result of this illness? What do you think Mrs. Avis expects of herself? What are some interventions you could implement to facilitate acceptance of the change she is experiencing?

## Chapter 45: Nursing Care of Clients with Eye and Ear Disorders

### A Client with Glaucoma and Cataracts

1. What is the pathophysiology of glaucoma? How does a cataract affect glaucoma?

2. Consider the effects of corticosteroids on glaucoma. If Mrs. Rainey is to administer several medications at home, identify specific teaching guidelines for her.

3. Consider referral for home health visits. Think about the effect of transferring her for a brief admission to an assisted-living facility.

## Chapter 47: Nursing Care of Men with Reproductive System Disorders

### A Man with Prostate Cancer

1. Why would Mr. Turner be at risk for altered skin integrity? Outline the interventions you would include on his teaching plan that would promote skin integrity as he cares for himself at home.

2. *Noncompliance* is defined as behaviors that do not coincide with the therapeutic plan agreed upon by the person and the health care professional. Do you think Mr. Turner fully understood his treatment and agreed with his follow-up care? What could be done in the preoperative phase of Mr. Turner's care to better ensure his understanding and desire to have continued medical care?

3. What assessments indicate that Mr. Turner does or does not have bladder distention? Would you report this? If so, to whom?

## Chapter 48: Nursing Care of Women with Reproductive System Disorders

### A Woman with Endometriosis

1. What is the relationship between Mrs. Hall's manifestations and a decreased RBC count? Review the information in Chapter 32 ⊝ and list assessments you would make to identify anemia.

2. List nonthreatening questions you would use to begin the discussion. How might it help to ask these questions at the beginning of the interview? Then list questions that you might use to collect data about the couple's sexual history. Would you be embarrassed to ask them? If so, how might this in turn affect their responses?

3. *Situational low self-esteem* is the state in which a person develops a negative perception of self-worth in response to a current situation. What information in Mrs. Hall's history might provide data to support this nursing diagnosis?

### A Woman with Cervical Cancer

1. Review the risk factors for cervical cancer. Consider what might differ for a young woman and an older woman.

2. Review the information in Chapter 10 ⊝ on radiation as a treatment for cancer. What interventions would be appropriate for Ms. Gillam?

3. Based on your review of the information on radiation, explain how radiation might cause fatigue. How does fatigue differ from being tired? What interventions would you include in a plan of care for this nursing diagnosis?

### A Woman with Breast Cancer

1. Review the information in the chapter on the genetic factors that pose a risk for developing breast cancer. How could you explain this in terms understandable by Mrs. Clemments and her daughters?

2. List the different types of mastectomies. Consider the implications of the differences, and how this would affect your nursing care.

3. Review the information on chemotherapy in Chapter 10. ⊝ List the types of chemotherapy and its common side effects. Consider the classifications of medications that are used to treat these side effects.

4. What factors in the treatment of Mrs. Clemments treatment might disrupt the amount and quality of her sleep? What interventions might be used to improve her sleep pattern?

## Chapter 49: Nursing Care of Clients with Sexually Transmitted Infections

### A Client with Gonorrhea

1. What manifestations does Ms. Cirit have that are typical of the disease? Would you make other assessments? If so, what are they?

2. Review the discussion of HIV in Chapter 9. ⊝ Do you believe it is true that infection with gonorrhea may increase the risk of HIV? If so, how would you explain this to Ms. Cirit?

3. *Impaired social interaction* is a state of aloneness or rejection experienced by an individual that is perceived as negative. What assessments of Ms. Cirit might support this diagnosis? What interventions and expected outcomes would you develop?

### A Client with Syphilis

1. Describe the assessments you would expect to find in a man with early syphilis.

2. Consider topics such as number of sex partners, patterns of sexual activity, and use of safe sex practices. What other topics should be explored? How can you ask these questions without being embarrassed or embarrassing the client?

3. List possible statements you might make. Do you believe this is a nursing responsibility? If you do not feel comfortable with this topic, what could you do?

# CREDITS

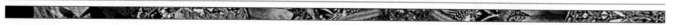

All photographs/illustrations not credited on page, under or adjacent to the piece, or not credited below, were photographed/rendered on assignment and are property of Pearson Education/Prentice Hall Health.

**Illustrations:**

Figure 28–3     Todd A. Buck
Figure 28–7     Todd A. Buck
Figure 34–1     Todd A. Buck
Figure 19–1     Todd A. Buck
Figure 12–2     Todd A. Buck
Figure 44–1     Todd A. Buck
Figure 37–1     Todd A. Buck
Figure 37–4     Todd A. Buck
Figure 44–11    Todd A. Buck

# INDEX

## A

Abacavir, 261
Abciximab, 833
Abdomen
  nutrition and, 303
    quadrants of, 516, 519
    peritonitis and, 636
    radiologic examination of, 222
Abdominal aorta, 920, 929, 995
Abdominal aortic aneurysms, 995, 997
Abdominal arteries, 519
Abdominal assessment, 518–21, 615, 702, 929
Abdominal CT scan, 974
Abdominal hysterectomy, 1562
Abdominal injuries, 140
Abdominal muscles, 1183
Abdominal perineal resection, 1527
Abdominal pulse generator, 857
Abdominal reflexes, 1304
Abdominal surgery, shaving for, 176
Abdominal thrusts, 1061
Abdominal ultrasound/ultrasonography, 589,
    632, 996
Abdominal X-rays, 575, 632, 636, 681, 684, 749
Abducens nerves, 1297, 1298, 1300
Abduction, 1181
A-beta fibers, 55
ABGs. See Arterial blood gases
Ablative surgical procedures, 166
Above-elbow amputation, 1213
Above-knee amputation, 1213, 1214
Abrasions, 139, 140
Abscesses
  anorectal, 690
  brain, 1384–86
  liver, 598–99
  lung, 1091–92
  peritonsillar, 1050, 1052, 1628
Absence seizures, 1367
Absolute refractory period, 841
Absorbants, 619
Absorption, impaired, 661. See also
    Malabsorption syndrome
Abstinence, 334
Abstinence medications, 338
Acanthamoeba protozoa, 1384
Acantholysis, 384
Acarbose, 492
Acceleration, 1324
Acceleration-deceleration injury, 1373
Acceleration injuries, 138, 1373
Acceptance, 318
Accessory digestive organs, 508, 510–11
Accessory nerves, 1297, 1298, 1301
Accessory pancreatic duct, 509
Accidents, young adults and, 21. See also Motor
    vehicle accidents
Accolate, 1109, 1111
Accupril, 879, 987

Accutane, 383–384
Acebutolol, 854, 987
ACE inhibitors. See Angiotensin-converting
    enzyme inhibitors
Acetaminophen, 207, 897, 1321, 1357, 1362
Acetazolamide, 879, 1369, 1479, 1481
Acetic acids, 62, 208, 363
Acetaminophen, 1046
Acetylated, 62
Acetylcholine (ACh), 1291, 1366, 1480, 1481
Acetylcholine receptors, 1431
Acetylcholine release site, 1431
Acetylcholinesterase inhibitor, 1432
Acetylsalicylic acid. See Aspirin
Achalasia, 552
Achilles reflex, 1303
Achilles tendon, 1184
Acid-base balance, regulation of, 119–21
Acid-base imbalances, 121–22, 123, 1622
  compensation, 122, 124
  metabolic acidosis, 121, 122, 124–27
  metabolic alkalosis, 121, 122, 127–29
  respiratory acidosis, 121, 123, 129–32
  respiratory alkalosis, 121, 123, 132–34
Acid excretion, 123
Acid-fast bacilli, 1097
Acidifying foods, 718
Acidosis, 108, 120, 123, 1237. See also
    Metabolic acidosis; Respiratory acidosis
Acid phosphatase (ACP), 288
Acid production, 123
Acids, 119
Aciphex, 548, 549
Acne, 381–384
Acne conglobata, 382
Acne-Dome, 383
Acne rosacea, 382, 383
Acne vulgaris, 382
Aceon, 987
Acoustic nerves. See Vestibulocochlear nerves
Acoustic neuroma, 1389, 1501
Acquired hemolytic anemia, 939, 941
Acquired immunity, 210–14, 215, 1622–23
Acquired immunodeficiency syndrome. See
    AIDS
Acral lentiginous melanoma, 392
Acromegaly, 469
ACS. See American Cancer Society
Acthar, 1411
Actidil, 1043
Actifed, 1043
Actigall, 576
Actinic keratosis, 386–387
Action potential, 840–41, 1291
Actiq, 61, 73
Activase rt-pa, 1312
Activated partial thromboplastin time (aPTT),
    1013, 1131
Active chronic hepatitis, 244
Active immunity, 210, 211

Active transport, 81, 699
Activity
  heart failure and, 881
  prostate surgery and, 1542
Activity-exercise pattern, 12
Activity intolerance
  cardiac disorders, 883–84, 890, 895, 899, 909
  coronary heart disease, 860
  endocrine disorders, 456
  erectile dysfunction, 1527
  fluid volume excess and, 93
  hematologic disorders, 944
  hyperkalemia, 106
  hypokalemia, 102
  lung cancer, 1141
  nutritional disorders, 527, 528
  peripheral atherosclerosis, 1006
  pneumonia, 1086–87
Actonel, 1226
Actos, 492
Actylcholinesterase, 1291
Acupuncture, 68, 1109
Acute abdomen, 555, 635
Acute bronchitis, 1077
Acute care
  burns, 423
  home health care and, 44
Acute coronary syndromes, 827
Acute illnesses, 32–33
Acute renal failure (ARF), 124
  collaborative care, 764–70
  course and manifestations, 762–64
  nursing care, 770–73, 1626
  nursing care plan, 774
  pathophysiology, 761–62, 763
  physiology, 761
Acute respiratory distress syndrome (ARDS),
    1169–75, 1628
Acute tubular necrosis (ATN), 761–62, 763
Acutrim, 526
Acyclovir, 226, 247, 377, 542, 1385, 1601, 1605
Adalat, 818
Addiction, 61, 334
Addictive substances, 333–36
Addisonian crisis, 465
Addison's disease, 244, 463–67, 468, 1624
Additives, food, 91
Adduction, 1181
Adductor longus, 1183
Adductor magnus, 1184
A-delta fibers, 55, 56
Adenocarcinoma, 1136
Adenocard, 854
Adenohypophysis, 439
Adenoids, 1031
Adenomas
  pituitary, 1389
  tubular, 667
  tubulovillous, 668
  villous, 668